Advanced Pharmacology for Prescribers

Brent Luu, PharmD, BCPS, BCACP, is an associate clinical professor for the Master of Science–Nurse Practitioner, Master of Health Sciences–Physician Assistant Studies, and Master Entry Program in Nursing degree programs at the Betty Irene Moore School of Nursing, University of California, Davis, where he teaches the Pharmacology series courses across the UC Davis programs. Dr. Luu earned his Doctor of Pharmacy degree from the University of the Pacific School of Pharmacy in 2000. With two decades of experiences in pharmacy practice, Dr. Luu brings a broad perspective of various pharmacy practice settings, including inpatient, outpatient, acute care, ambulatory care, and home infusion. Dr. Luu has authored and coauthored multiple manuscripts and book chapters in various publications. In addition, he has been a reviewer for *Journal of the American Academy of Physician Assistants*, *Journal for Nurse Practitioners*, and the *Annals of Internal Medicine*. Prior to teaching, Dr. Luu was a clinical pharmacist practitioner at Kaiser Permanente, a Wal-Mart Pharmacy manager, and a co-owner of an independent pharmacy. Dr. Luu's focus is on patient care and medication safety. As an educator, he hopes to train students to optimize therapeutic outcomes while minimizing adverse drug events, as well as improve patient and medication safety. His clinical interests include pain management, neurology, and chronic disease management.

Gerald Kayingo, PhD, MMSc, PA-C, is the executive director of the Physician Assistant Leadership and Learning Academy and an assistant dean and professor at the graduate school of the University of Maryland Baltimore. He previously worked at the University of California, Davis, where he served in various capacities including director of the Master of Health Services–Physician Assistant program. Prior to joining University of California, Davis, Dr. Kayingo was a faculty member at the Yale School of Medicine Physician Associate Program and practiced at the Yale New Haven Hospital Primary Care Center in Connecticut. He has extensive experience in health professions education and clinical practice.

Dr. Kayingo is an alumnus of the Harvard Management Development Program following a Master of Medical Science–Physician Assistant Degree at Yale University School of Medicine in Connecticut and a Doctor of Philosophy in Microbiology from Orange Free State University in South Africa. He completed his postdoctoral education in infectious diseases at Yale University School of Medicine, where he studied microbial pathogenesis, membrane transport, and signal transduction. He is in the process of completing his Master of Business Administration at the University of Illinois Urbana–Champaign, specializing in strategic leadership and management.

Nationally, Dr. Kayingo has served as a director at large on the Physician Assistant Education Association Board of Directors, member of the editorial board for the *Journal of Physician Assistant Education*, and associate editor of *BMC Health Services Research*. He was a pioneering member of the Commission on the Health of the Public and served on the national health disparities working group for the American Academy of Physician Assistants. He was recently inducted into the prestigious Uganda National Academy of Sciences. Dr. Kayingo has coauthored three books on health professions education and published extensively on health systems science and infectious diseases in peer-reviewed journals. He is a recipient of several awards, including a university book prize, the 2016 PA Student Academy mentor award, the 2015 American Academy of Physician Assistant Research Publishing Award, and the 2014 Jack Cole Society Award at Yale.

Virginia McCoy Hass, DNP, MSN, RN, FNP-C, PA-C, has more than 20 years of experience in graduate nursing and medical education, teaching advanced pharmacology, applied clinical pharmacology, and primary care medicine to family nurse practitioner and physician assistant students. She is a graduate of the Rush University Doctor of Nursing Practice Program, following a Master of Science in nursing from California State University, Sacramento, and family nurse practitioner and physician assistant certification from the University of California, Davis. Dr. McCoy Hass has extensive experience in the development and implementation of active learning strategies, simulation pedagogy, distance education using innovative technology, and instructional design strategies. She has led a variety of initiatives to create new interdisciplinary models for the delivery of primary care and student training opportunities. Dr. McCoy Hass coedited *The Health Professions Educator: A Practical Guide for New and Established Faculty*, authored book chapters on chronic illness management and interprofessional education, and published in a variety of peer-reviewed journals. Dr. McCoy Hass has presented extensively at regional, state, and national meetings on a wide variety of topics, including pharmacology, primary care, interprofessional education, and educational innovation. She has served on the editorial board of the *Journal of the American Academy of Physician Assistants* and the board of directors of the California Association for Nurse Practitioners. While retired from clinical practice and teaching, she continues to serve as a medicolegal expert witness and expert witness for the California Board of Registered Nursing.

Advanced Pharmacology for Prescribers

BRENT LUU, PHARMD, BCPS, BCACP

GERALD KAYINGO, PHD, MMSc, PA-C

VIRGINIA MCCOY HASS, DNP, MSN, RN, FNP-C, PA-C

Section Editors:

Elaine D. Kauschinger, PhD, MSN, APRN, FNP-C

Sandhya Venugopal, MD, MS-HPEd

Xiaodong Feng, PhD, PharmD

SPRINGER PUBLISHING

Springer Publishing Company, LLC
11 West 42nd Street, New York, NY 10036
www.springerpub.com
connect.springerpub.com/

Acquisitions Editor: Adrianne Brigido
Developmental Editor: Taylor Ball
Compositor: S4Carlisle Publishing Services

ISBN: 978-0-8261-9546-3
ebook ISBN: 978-0-8261-9547-0
DOI: 10.1891/9780826195470

Qualified instructors may request supplements by emailing textbook@springerpub.com

Instructor Manual ISBN: 978-0-8261-9548-7
Chapter PowerPoints ISBN: 978-0-8261-9549-4
Test Bank ISBN: 978-0-8261-9616-3
Image Bank ISBN: 978-0-8261-9616-0

21 22 23 24 / 5 4 3 2

Medicine is an ever-changing science. Research and clinical experience are continually expanding our knowledge, in particular our understanding of proper treatment and drug therapy. The authors, editors, and publisher have made every effort to ensure that all information in this book is in accordance with the state of knowledge at the time of production of the book. Nevertheless, the authors, editors, and publisher are not responsible for any errors or omissions or for any consequence from application of the information in this book and make no warranty, expressed or implied, with respect to the content of this publication. Every reader should examine carefully the package inserts accompanying each drug and should carefully check whether the dosage schedules therein or the contraindications stated by the manufacturer differ from the statements made in this book. Such examination is particularly important with drugs that are either rarely used or have been newly released on the market.

Library of Congress Cataloging-in-Publication Data

Names: Luu, Brent, editor. | Kayingo, Gerald, editor. | Hass, Virginia
  McCoy, editor.
Title: Advanced pharmacology for prescribers / editors, Brent Luu, Gerald
  Kayingo, Virginia McCoy Hass ; section editors, Elaine Kauschinger,
  Sandhya Venugopal, Xiaodong Feng.
Description: First Springer Publishing edition. | New York : Springer
  Publishing Company, [2022] | Includes bibliographical references and
  index.
Identifiers: LCCN 2020055324 (print) | LCCN 2020055325 (ebook) | ISBN
  9780826195463 (cloth) | ISBN 9780826195470 (ebook) | ISBN 9780826195487
  (instructor manual) | ISBN 9780826195494 (chapter powerpoints) | ISBN
  9780826196163 (test bank) | ISBN 9780826196160 (image bank)
Subjects: MESH: Drug Therapy | Pharmacology—methods
Classification: LCC RM300 (print) | LCC RM300 (ebook) | NLM WB 330 | DDC
  615.5/8—dc23
LC record available at https://lccn.loc.gov/2020055324
LC ebook record available at https://lccn.loc.gov/2020055325

Contact sales@springerpub.com to receive discount rates on bulk purchases.

Publisher's Note: **New and used products purchased from third-party sellers are not guaranteed for quality, authenticity, or access to any included digital components.**

Printed in the United States of America.

Contents

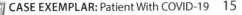
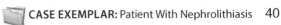

Integrative Behavioral Treatments   527
Conclusion   527
CASE EXEMPLAR: Patient With Depression
and Generalized Anxiety Disorder   529
CASE EXEMPLAR: Patient With Bipolar Disorder   529

33. PHARMACOTHERAPY FOR PAIN MANAGEMENT   533

Theresa Mallick-Searle, Joy Vongspanich, Aliyah Ali,
Paramjit Kaur, Erielle Anne P. Espina, Phil Emond, and Brent Luu

Introduction   533
Characterizing Pain   534
Acute Versus Chronic Pain   534
Types of Pain Based on Pathophysiology   534
The Pain Pathway   535
Assessment of Pain   535
Standardized Tools for Measuring Pain Intensity   535
Standardized Tools to Assess Neuropathic Pain   536
Other Standardized Tools   536
Managing Pain   536
Acute Pain   536
Chronic Pain   537
Pharmacology of Analgesic Agents   538
Nonopioid Agents   538
Opioid Analgesia and Safe Opioid Prescribing   542
Opioid Agents   543
Conclusion   548
CASE EXEMPLAR: Patient With Chronic Pain   548
CASE EXEMPLAR: Patient With Shingles   548

34. SUBSTANCE USE DISORDER   553

James Anderson and Kathleen Nowak

Introduction   553
Background   553
Diagnosis of Substance Use Disorder   554
Treatment of Substance Use Disorder   554
Alcohol Use Disorder   554
Tobacco Use Disorder   559
Opioid Use Disorder   563
CASE EXEMPLAR: Patient With Opioid
Dependence   566
CASE EXEMPLAR: Patient With Tobacco Use
Disorder   567

PART III: HEALTH PROMOTION AND MAINTENANCE

35. OVER-THE-COUNTER MEDICATIONS   573

Ashley Taylor, Janel Bailey Wheeler, and Kristi Isaac Rapp

Introduction   573
Over-the-Counter Medications for Cough and Cold   573
Antitussives   573

Expectorants   575
Herbals and the Common Cold   575
Over-the-Counter Medications for Allergic Rhinitis   575
Intranasal Corticosteroids   575
Antihistamines   575
Decongestants   576
Over-the-Counter Medications for Pain   576
Nonsteroidal Anti-Inflammatory Drugs   578
Acetaminophen   578
Topical Agents   578
Herbals and Natural Products   578
Nutrition and Supplementation   578
Vitamins and Minerals   578
Enteral Supplements   579
Cosmetics   580
Over-the-Counter Medications for Treatment
of Acne   580
Over-the-Counter Medications for Treatment of Dry Skin,
Psoriasis, and Dandruff   582
Over-the-Counter Medications for Treatment
of Warts   582
Over-the-Counter Medications for the Treatment
of Alopecia   582
First-Aid Products   583
Conclusion   583
CASE EXEMPLAR: Patient With Knee Pain Secondary
to Osteoarthritis   584
CASE EXEMPLAR: Pediatric Patient With Nonproductive
Cough   585

36. PHARMACOTHERAPY FOR OBESITY   589

Seleda Williams and Dennis M. Styne

Introduction   589
Part I: Adult Obesity   589
Definition and Prevalence of Adult Obesity   589
Comorbidities Associated With Overweight and
Obesity   589
Etiology of Obesity   590
Physiologic Pathways Related to Obesity   590
Satiety (Anorectic) Hormones   590
Hunger (Orexigenic Hormone)   591
History of Pharmacotherapy for Obesity   592
Current Treatment of Adult Obesity   593
Medications That Contribute to Weight Gain   600
Conclusion   600
CASE EXEMPLAR: Patient With Obesity and Unsuccessful
Weight Loss   601
Part II: Pediatric Obesity   602
Definition of Pediatric Overweight and Obesity   602
General Considerations of Treatment for Pediatric
Obesity   602
Conclusion   605
CASE EXEMPLAR: Patient With Obesity and Fatigue   605

Index   611

Contributors

Aliyah Ali, BSc
Medical Student (MS4)
International University of the Health Sciences
University of Western Ontario
Ontario, Canada

Ezra A. Amsterdam, MD
Distinguished Professor of Cardiology
Division of Cardiovascular Medicine
Department of Internal Medicine
University of California–Davis Medical Center
Sacramento, California

James Anderson, PA-C, MPAS, DFAAPA
Physician Assistant
Evergreen Treatment Services
Seattle, Washington

Veronica T. Bandy, PharmD, MS, FCPhA, FCSHP, BCACP
Clinical Professor and Regional Coordinator
Thomas J. Long School of Pharmacy
University of the Pacific
Sacramento, California

Erica Barr, PharmD
Assistant Clinical Professor
Thomas J. Long School of Pharmacy
University of the Pacific
Stockton, California

Tedi Begaj, MD
Ophthalmology Resident
Massachusetts Eye and Ear
Harvard Medical School
Boston, Massachusetts

Sara Boullt
Research Assistant
Department of Medical Microbiology
University of California–Davis
Sacramento, California

Diane M. Bruessow, MPAS, PA-C, DFAAPA
Instructor in the Physician Assistant Online Program
Department of Internal Medicine
Yale School of Medicine
President-Elect, American Academy of PAs
New Haven, Connecticut

Reamer Bushardt, PharmD, PA-C, DFAAPA
Senior Associate Dean for Health Sciences
Professor of PA Studies
The George Washington University School of Medicine
    and Health Sciences
Washington, District of Columbia

Martin Cadeiras, MD
Associate Professor of Cardiology
Division of Cardiovascular Medicine
Department of Internal Medicine
University of California–Davis Medical Center
Sacramento, California

Michael Casner, PhD
Interdisciplinary Scientist
The Office of Regulatory Affairs
U.S. Food and Drug Administration
Rockville, Maryland

Patrick Chan, PharmD, PhD
Associate Professor
Department of Pharmacy Practice and Administration
Western University of Health Sciences
Pomona, California

Doris Chen, MD
Clinical Fellow, Memory and Aging Center
University of California–San Francisco
San Francisco, California

Nipavan Chiamvimonvat, PhD
Roger Tatarian Endowed Professor of Cardiovascular
    Medicine
Division of Cardiovascular Medicine
Department of Internal Medicine
University of California–Davis Medical Center
Sacramento, California

Ricketta Clark, DNP, FNP-BC
Assistant Professor
College of Nursing
University of Tennessee Health Science Center
Memphis, Tennessee

Jeremy M. DeMartini, MD
Internist/Psychiatrist
Assistant Clinical Professor
Director of Internal Medicine/Psychiatry Training Program
University of California–Davis
Sacramento, California

Alexandra (Sasha) Duffy, DO
Assistant Professor
Program Director Neurology Residency
Department of Neurology
University of California–Davis Medical Center
Sacramento, California

Felix D. Emond, Jr., MS, PA-C, DFAAPA
Assistant Clinical Professor
Betty Irene Moore School of Nursing
University of California—Davis
Sacramento, California

Ahmed El-Shamy, PhD
Assistant Professor of Virology
Colleges of Pharmacy and Medicine
California Northstate University
Elk Grove, California

Melanie A. Felmlee, PhD
Assistant Professor
Department of Pharmaceutics and Medicinal Chemistry
Thomas J. Long School of Pharmacy
University of the Pacific
Stockton, California

Xiaodong Feng, PhD, PharmD
University Vice President of Admissions and Student
    Services
Associate Dean of Student Affairs, Admissions, and
    Outreach
California Northstate University College of Medicine
Elk Grove, California

Jaclyn K. Gaulden, DNP, NP-C
Assistant Professor of Nursing
DNP Program Coordinator
Anderson University
Anderson, South Carolina

David S. Grega, PA-C, MPAS, DFAAPA
Assistant Clinical Professor
Betty Irene Moore School of Nursing
University of California—Davis
Sacramento, California

Tegest Hailu, MD
Assistant Clinical Professor
UCSF Fresno Family Community
Fresno, California
Palliative Care and Hospice Physician
Providence Sound Home Care and Hospice
Lacey, Washington

Virginia McCoy Hass, DNP, MSN, RN, FNP-C, PA-C
Associate Clinical Professor (Retired)
Betty Irene Moore School of Nursing
University of California—Davis
Sacramento, California

Matthew Horton, PharmD, BCPS
Assistant Professor
Clinical and Administrative Sciences
California Northstate University College of Pharmacy
Elk Grove, California

Stanley Hsia, MD
Health Science Associate Clinical Professor
General Endocrinology, Diabetes, Lipid Metabolism
UCLA Medical Center
Southern California Endocrine Medical Group
Orange, California

Ragan Johnson, DNP, FNP-BC, CNE
Assistant Professor
School of Nursing
Duke University School of Nursing
Durham, North Carolina

Paramjit Kaur, MSN, FNP-C
Past Family Practice Nurse Practitioner
Adventist Medical Clinic
Sanger, California

Gerald Kayingo, PhD, MMSc, PA-C
Associate Clinical Professor
Physician Assistant Studies
Betty Irene Moore School of Nursing
University of California–Davis
Davis, California

Manoj Kesarwani, MD
Clinical Assistant Professor
Department of Cardiology
Division of Cardiovascular Medicine
Department of Internal Medicine
University of California–Davis Medical Center
Sacramento, California

Thamer Khasawneh, PharmD, BCPS
Clinical Inpatient Pharmacist and Pharmacy
  Informatics
Automated Data Processing Application Coordinator
Department of Inpatient Pharmacy
Sacramento VA Medical Center
VA Northern California Health Care System
Mather, California

Lucy W. Kibe, DrPH, MS, MHS, PA-C
Chief Medical Quality Officer
Community Access Network
Lynchburg, Virginia

Vasco Deon Kidd, DHSc, MPH, MS, PA-C
Director of Advanced Practice Providers
University of California–Irvine
Irvine, California

Simeon O. Kotchoni, PhD
Associate Professor of Molecular Physiology
  and Biochemistry
Department of Pharmaceutical and Biomedical
  Sciences
Colleges of Pharmacy and Medicine
California Northstate University
Elk Grove, California

Jennifer Kuretski, DNP, APRN, FNP-C, AAHIVS
Degree Track Chair, Nurse Practitioner Program
Palm Beach Atlantic University
Family Nurse Practitioner
Midway Specialty Care Center
West Palm Beach, Florida

Simone T. Lew, MD, MS
Resident Physician
Internal Medicine/Psychiatry Resident
University of California–Davis
Sacramento, California

Tianhong Li, MD, PhD
Associate Professor
Division of Hematology/Oncology
Department of Internal Medicine
University of California–Davis School of Medicine
University of California–Davis Comprehensive Cancer
  Center
Sacramento, California

Andrew G. Lowe, PharmD, APh
Clinical Director of Pharmacy
Arrowhead Regional Medical Center
Vice-President for Clinical Services
Comprehensive Pharmacy Services
Colton, California

Brent Luu, PharmD, BCPS, BCACP
Associate Clinical Professor
Betty Irene Moore School of Nursing
University of California–Davis
Sacramento, California

Erin Lyden, MSN, BSN, BS, FNP-C
Nurse Practitioner
Baptist Health
Miami, Florida

Weijie Ma, MD
Division of Hematology/Oncology
Department of Internal Medicine
University of California–Davis School of Medicine
University of California–Davis Comprehensive Cancer
  Center
Sacramento, California

Niti Madan, MD
Associate Professor
Division of Nephrology
Department of Internal Medicine
University of California–Davis
Sacramento, California

Theresa Mallick-Searle, MS, PMGT-BC, ANP-BC
Adult Nurse Practitioner
Stanford Health Care
Division of Pain Medicine
Stanford, California

Steadman McPeters, DNP, CRNP, CPNP-AC, RNFA
Assistant Professor of Nursing
University of Alabama at Birmingham
Birmingham, Alabama

Eric C. Nemec, II, PharmD, MEHP, BCPS
Director of Research and Assessment
Clinical Associate Professor
Master of Physician Assistant Program
Sacred Heart University
Stamford, Connecticut

Andrew Nevins, MD
Clinical Associate Professor
Stanford University School of Medicine
Stanford, California

Kwan L. Ng, MD, PhD
Associate Professor
Director of Comprehensive Stroke Center
Department of Neurology
University of California–Davis Medical Center
Sacramento, California

Kathleen Nowak, PharmD, BCACP, AAHIVP
Clinical Pharmacist
Medical Group of the Carolinas
Spartanburg, South Carolina

Kevin C. O'Connor, DO, FAAFP
Associate Professor of Medicine
Senior Medical Advisor, Health Sciences Programs
The George Washington University School
    of Medicine & Health Sciences
Washington, District of Columbia

Kevin Michael O'Hara, MMSc, MS, PA-C
Assistant Professor
School of Medicine
Yale University
New Haven, Connecticut

Lisa M. O'Neal, NP-C
Nurse Practitioner
Surgical Intensive Care Unit
Charlotte, North Carolina

Adebola Olarewaju, PhD (Candidate), MS, CPNP, BSN
Nurse Practitioner
Betty Irene Moore School of Nursing
University of California–Davis
Sacramento, California

Katherine Park, MD
Assistant Professor
Associate Program Director–Neurology Residency
Department of Neurology
University of California–Davis Medical Center
Sacramento, California

Simon Paul, MD, AAHIVS
Internal Medicine Physician/HIV Specialist
Health Officer
Department of Public Health
Madera County, California

Courtney J. Perry, PharmD
Assistant Professor
Department of PA Studies
Wake Forest School of Medicine
Pediatric Pharmacist
Department of Pharmacy
Wake Forest Baptist Medical Center
Winston-Salem, North Carolina

Amir Ramezani, PhD
Psychologist, Associate Clinical Professor
Director of Neuropsychology and Health Psychology
    Training Program
University of California–Davis
Sacramento, California

Carly A. Ranson, PharmD, MS, BCGP
Assistant Professor and Director of Pharmacy
    Co-Curricular Programming
Department of Pharmacy Practice
Thomas J. Long School of Pharmacy
University of the Pacific
Stockton, California

Kristi Isaac Rapp, PharmD, BCACP
Clinical Professor and Associate Dean
College of Pharmacy
Xavier University of Louisiana
New Orleans, Louisiana

Angela Richard-Eaglin, DNP, MSN, FNP-BC, CNE, FAANP
Assistant Clinical Professor
Duke University School of Nursing
Co-Director of the VA Nursing Academic Partnership
    in Graduate Education (VANAP-GE)
Adult Gerontology Primary Care Residency Program
Durham, North Carolina

Joanne Rolls, MPAS, PA-C, MEHP
Clinical Assistant Professor
University of Utah School of Medicine
Division of Physician Assistant
University of Utah Hospitals and Clinics
Salt Lake City, UT

Prem Sahasranam, MD
Assistant Clinical Professor
Loma Linda University School of Medicine
American Board Certified in Internal Medicine
American Board Certified in Endocrinology, Diabetes
 & Metabolism
CEO & Medical Director Central Valley Endocrinology,
 APC
CEO & Medical Director, My Diabetes Tutor, Inc
Central Valley Endocrinology
Hanford, California

Sumathi Sankaran-Walters, MBBS, PhD
Associate Adjunct Professor
Department of Medical Microbiology
University of California–Davis
Davis, California

Shlomit Schaal, MD, PhD
Professor and Chair
Department of Ophthalmology and Visual Sciences
University of Massachusetts Medical School
Worcester, Massachusetts

Vishwa C. Sheth, MD
Nephrology Fellow
Division of Nephrology
Department of Internal Medicine
University of California–Davis
Sacramento, California

Jon E. Siiteri, PhD, PA-C
Urology and Urologic Oncology (retired)
Dignity Health Medical Foundation
Woodland Memorial Hospital
Woodland, California

Tyrell Simkins, DO, PhD
Neurology Fellow
Department of Neurology
Oregon Health and Science University
Portland, Oregon

Elizabeth F. Snyder, DNP, APRN, FNP-BC
Assistant Professor of Nursing
Graduate Chair, School of Nursing
Anderson University
Anderson, South Carolina

Dennis M. Styne, MD
Professor of Pediatrics
Yocha Dehe Endowed Chair in Pediatric
 Endocrinology
School of Medicine
University of California–Davis
Sacramento, California

Rahnea Sunseri, MD
Medical Director
Assistant Professor at University of the Pacific
Department of Physician Assistant Education
University of the Pacific
Stockton, California

Ashley Taylor, PharmD, BCGP, BCACP
Clinical Assistant Professor
College of Pharmacy
Xavier University of Louisiana
New Orleans, Louisiana
Clinical Pharmacy Specialist at U.S. Department of
 Veterans Affairs-Endocrine Clinic
Frances Place, Los Angeles

Peter Tenerelli, PHARMBSC
Assistant Professor of Pharmacology
College of Pharmacy
California Northstate University
Elk Grove, California

Michael Tran, MD, FACP, FACE
Clinical Instructor of Medicine
Endocrinology, Diabetes, and Metabolism
David Geffen UCLA School of Medicine
Los Angeles, California;
Medical Director
Southern CA Endocrine Medical Group
Orange, California

James Uchizono, PharmD, PhD
Professor and Associate Provost for Research
Thomas J. Long School of Pharmacy
University of the Pacific
Stockton, California

**Cynthia S. Valle-Oseguera, PharmD, APh,
BCACP, BCGP**
Assistant Clinical Professor
Department of Clinical Pharmacy
UCSF School of Pharmacy
San Francisco, California

Sandhya Venugopal, MD, MS-HPEd
Professor of Cardiology
Division of Cardiovascular Medicine
Department of Internal Medicine
University of California–Davis Medical Center
Sacramento, California

Joy Vongspanich, PharmD
Residency Program Director PGY-1
Ambulatory Care-HIV
Senior Pharmacist
University of California–Davis
Sacramento, California

Hongbing Wang, PharmBS, MS, PHD
Assistant Professor of Pharmacology
Colleges of Pharmacy and Medicine
California Northstate University
Elk Grove, California

Elyse Watkins, DHSc, PA-C, DFAAPA
Associate Professor
Doctor of Medical Science Program
School of PA Medicine
University of Lynchburg
Lynchburg, Virginia

Janel Bailey Wheeler, PharmD, BCACP
Clinical Assistant Professor
College of Pharmacy
Xavier University of Louisiana
New Orleans, Louisiana

Sampath Wijesinghe, DHSc, MS, MPAS, PA-C, AAHIVS
Principal Faculty
MSPA Program
Stanford School of Medicine
Primary Care PA-C/HIV Specialist
Adventist Health Central Valley Network
Stanford, California

Seleda Williams, MD, MPH
Clinical Professor
Department of Internal Medicine
School of Medicine
University of California–Davis
Sacramento, California

Catherine C. Wilson, DNP, APRN, NNP-BC, FNP-BC, FNP
Assistant Professor of Nursing
Anderson University
Anderson, South Carolina

Catherine F. Yang, PhD
Vice President of Academic Affairs and Associate
    Dean of Medical Education
Professor of Molecular Pharmacology/Medicinal
    Chemistry/Biomedical Sciences
Department of Basic Sciences
College of Medicine
California Northstate University
Elk Grove, California

Alan H. Yee, DO
Assistant Professor
Associate Director Neurology Residency
Department of Neurology
University of California–Davis Medical Center
Sacramento, California

Brian Y. Young, MD
Health Sciences Clinical Professor
School of Medicine
University of California–Davis
Sacramento, California

Erika Young, PharmD
Pharmacy Intern
Anticoagulation Clinics
Brigham and Women's Hospital
Harvard Medical School
Cambridge, Massachusetts

Emmanuel A. Zamora, PsyD
Psychologist
Physical Medicine and Rehabilitation
University of California–Davis
Sacramento, California

Reviewers

Nicole B. Burwell, PhD, MSHS, PA-C
Director of Pre-Clerkship Education
Clinical Associate Professor of Medicine
Stanford School of Medicine
Stanford, California

Brigitte Chiu, PharmD (retired)
Inpatient Pharmacist
Sutter Health
Roseville, California

Ashook Joshua Dayanathan, MD
Health Sciences Assistant Clinical Professor
Neurology—Movement Disorders
University of California—Davis Health System
Sacramento, California

Charles De Mesa, DO, MPH
Director of Pain Medicine Fellowship
Director of Musculoskeletal Pain Medicine
Assistant Professor
Department of Anesthesiology and Pain Medicine
University of California–Davis
Sacramento, California

Dale Cai Dong, PharmD
Pain Management and Palliative Care Resident
    Pharmacist
Department of Pharmacy Services
University of California–Davis
Sacramento, California

Susan M. Fernandes, LPD, PA-C
Associate Dean for PA Education and Clinical
    Professor of Pediatrics and Medicine
Stanford University School of Medicine
Stanford, California

David Grega, PA-C, MPAS, DFAAPA
Assistant Clinical Professor
Betty Irene Moore School of Nursing
University of California–Davis
Sacramento, California

Charity Hale, PharmD
Pain Management and Palliative Care Pharmacist
Pain Management and Palliative Care Residency
    Program Director
Inpatient Clinical Services
Assistant Clinical Professor
Department of Pharmacy
University of California–San Francisco School
    of Pharmacy
San Francisco, California

Kimberly A. Hoffmann, PharmD, APh, BCPP, BCGP
Clinical Professor, Regional Coordinator—Bakersfield
University of the Pacific School of Pharmacy
Stockton, California

Susan LeLacheur, DrPH, PA-C
Associate Professor of Physician Assistant Studies
School of Medicine and Health Scences
The George Washington University
Washington, DC

Han Duong Lund, PharmD, BCPS, BCIDP
Inpatient Clinical Pharmacist
San Diego County, California

Ricky Norwood, DNP, MSN, RN, FNP-BC
Assistant Clinical Professor
Betty Irene Moore School of Nursing, UC Davis
Sacramento, California

Onyema Ogbuagu, MBBCh, FACP
Associate Professor of Medicine
Section of Infectious Disease
Yale University School of Medicine
New Haven, Connecticut

Michael T. Sim, MD
Associate Physician
General Nephrology
UC Davis Medical Center
Sacramento, California

Johnson Thomas, MD, FACE
Section Chair
Department of Endocrinology
Mercy, St. Louis
St. Louis, Missouri

Randall Udouj, PharmD
Clinical Pharmacy Specialist
Portland Veterans Affairs Medical Center
Portland, Oregon

Laura Van Auker, DNP, RN, FNP-BC, SNC
Assistant Clinical Professor
Betty Irene Moore School of Nursing
University of California–Davis
Sacramento, California

Joy Vongspanich, PharmD
Senior Pharmacist
Residency Program Director PGY-1
Ambulatory Care—HIV
UC Davis Health
Sacramento, California

Sampath Wijesinghe, DHSc, MS, MPAS, PA-C, AAHIVS
Principal Faculty
MSPA Program
Stanford School of Medicine
Primary Care PA-C/HIV Specialist
Adventist Health Central Valley Network
Stanford, California

Jane Yeun, MD
Clinical Professor of Medicine
University of California—Davis Health System
Sacramento, California

Section Editor Biographies

Elaine D. Kauschinger, PhD, MSN, APRN, FNP-C, is an assistant professor of clinical nursing at the Duke University School of Nursing (DUSON). She is a board-certified family nurse practitioner (FNP) and DUSON course coordinator for the primary care adolescent and adult courses. Previously, she was the program director for the FNP program at the University of Miami. Her area of research is in virtual simulation in nurse practitioner education. Dr. Kauschinger has presented on a variety of primary care topics and nursing education at national and international conferences. She has authored several book chapters on primary care, nursing education, and board review preparation for nurse practitioners. Her diverse experience in teaching includes clinical and nonclinical courses in Master's and Doctorate of Nursing Practice (DNP) programs and serving as chairperson of numerous DNP scholarly projects. Her clinical experience includes family practice, HIV/AIDS, substance abuse, retail health, and occupational health. Additionally, she has international experience working in Mexico in association with various embassies and multinational companies. Dr. Kauschinger is a member of the National Organization of Nurse Practitioner Faculties (NONPF) Simulation in Nurse Practitioner Committee and is the chair of the Simulation Special Interest Group. Dr. Kauschinger has been appointed as a National League for Nursing (NLN) onsite evaluator and has served as a Sigma Theta Tau International Honor Society in Nursing (STTI) and NONPF conference abstract reviewer.

Sandhya Venugopal, MD, MS-HPEd, is a clinical professor in the Division of Cardiovascular Medicine, School of Medicine at the University of California Davis Health, and associate dean for Continuing Medical Education. She is a noninvasive cardiologist and specialist in the use of frontline assessments to determine cardiac health. She received her medical degree from the University of Kentucky and completed her Internal Medicine residency training at Oregon Health and Science University Medical Center and fellowship training in Cardiovascular Diseases at Rush Medical Center in Chicago. She received her master's degree in Health Professions Education through Massachusetts General Hospital Institute of Health Professions. Since joining the faculty of UC Davis Health in 2006, Dr. Venugopal has held major roles at all levels of educational programs, from MS1 to 4, NP/PA training program and with residents, fellows, and CME functions. In her role as associate dean, Dr. Venugopal oversees the design, development, delivery, evaluation, and certification of continuing medical education curriculum. She has a proven track record of being an innovative educator, having served as a Master Clinical Educator in the School of Medicine from 2012 to 2016, and as the codirector of the Health Professions Education program at Massachusetts General Hospital Institute of Health Professions from 2016 to 2017. She is a successful team leader and is advancing continuing education to address pressing health issues for changes in clinical care outcomes. Dr. Venugopal has authored numerous publications in the field of cardiology and on topics in medical education. Her passion lies in imparting optimal medical education to the adult learner and reshaping the role of clinical educator. Dr. Venugopal's scholarly interests are focused on health professions, educational program evaluation, and curriculum development.

Xiaodong Feng, PhD, PharmD, is a professor of both oncology and pharmacology at the College of Medicine and College of Pharmacy at Northstate University, Elk Grove, California. He also serves as dean of the College of Pharmacy and university vice president for Admissions and Student Services. Previously, he served as the associate dean of Admissions and Student Affairs and Outreach for 5 years. Dr. Feng received his Doctor of Philosophy degree in cellular and molecular physiology from the Chinese Academy of Medical Sciences and Doctor of Pharmacy degree from Albany College of Pharmacy and Health Sciences. He completed his fellowship at the Department of Dermatology, State University of New York at Stony Brook. Dr. Feng has more than 20 years of clinical and biomedical research experience in cancer, wound healing, and cardiovascular disease. He also has extensive experience in cancer education, clinical practice, community service activities, and cancer research to effectively deliver high-quality patient care and medical education. He previously practiced as a clinical pharmacist at Sutter Davis Hospital and an Oncology Pharmacy Specialist at Dignity Health Medical Foundation. Dr. Feng has recently been issued two U.S. patents on strategies for antiangiogenesis and cancer treatments and has edited a textbook on pharmacogenomics, *Applying Pharmacogenomics in Therapeutics*. This textbook was selected as a reference for the pharmacy board exam by the American Association of Colleges of Pharmacy.

Preface

Pharmacotherapy is a significant piece of a puzzle in medicine that can impact the outcomes of virtually all health-related conditions. While it may bring relief of symptoms, improve quality of life, and cure diseases, it may also cause unwanted adverse reactions. Pharmacology is an area of "rich, fertile soil" filled with a variety of unexpected outcomes. Many drug responses or mechanisms of action related to pharmacotherapy are not fully understood or well characterized. The current understanding of pharmacology can be likened to a drop of water within an ocean because the human body is a hidden universe. The interactions of therapeutic agents and pharmacologic responses within the body could be compared to the billions of stars and galaxies that have been discovered, or are yet to be discovered, within deep space.

To utilize pharmacotherapy to create impactful results and benefits for patients, prescribers must not only understand the principles of pharmacology, but also be able to effectively apply these principles to individual therapeutic agents. There are many textbooks on the market, created by experts in various medical specialties, that provide necessary foundational knowledge—often with a tremendous level of detail and exhaustive coverage of the core principles of pharmacology—but lack guidance on how to apply these principles in clinical practice. Alternatively, there are references that provide too little coverage of pharmacology principles, condensing key information into "pocket guides" that require prerequisite background knowledge.

As educators and clinicians, we recognized that what is needed is a textbook that falls between those two ends of the spectrum, a "bridge" between the standard, lengthy pharmacology texts and quick pocket references. *Advanced Pharmacology for Prescribers* is designed to be that bridge. The major themes for this textbook include:

1. general principles of pharmacotherapeutics, including guideline analysis, pharmacokinetics, pharmacodynamics, pharmacogenomics, and promoting adherence to therapy

2. evidence-based prescribing across the life span, including patient populations such as pediatrics, geriatrics, and pregnancy and lactation
3. alterations in prescribing based upon comorbid disease

CONTENT AND ORGANIZATION

Advanced Pharmacology for Prescribers provides an applied therapeutic approach to major disorders and their pharmacologic treatment. With a focus on how medications act on the body and vice versa, readers will learn the rationale for utilizing specific therapeutic agents or drug classes. Chapters include learning objectives, relevant diagnostic studies, applicable guidelines, genomics, and important life span considerations, as well as case studies that apply the concepts discussed with questions to promote critical thinking, clinical pearls, and key takeaways. Chapters focus on the most evidence-based and effective pharmacologic treatments and, therefore, may not necessarily be inclusive of all drug treatments.

It is a multidisciplinary textbook, featuring contributions from authors in a wide range of disciplines, including nurse practitioners, pharmacists, physician assistants, and physicians. Each chapter is a product of true collaboration between authors of various disciplines because we believe that in clinical practice, a collaborative model is required to achieve optimal patient outcomes and medication safety.

Our goal is to provide students and prescribers a concise, well-balanced perspective of various principles of pharmacology and therapeutics while managing diseases. The information presented in each chapter is evidence-based and relevant to daily clinical practice. We designed the textbook with a patient-centered approach, organizing the chapters in a manner designed to enhance patient outcomes and benefits. The textbook is divided into three parts: Part I, "Foundations of Pharmacology and Prescribing"; Part II, "System-Specific and Patient-Focused Prescribing"; and Part III, "Health Promotion and Maintenance."

PART I: FOUNDATIONS OF PHARMACOLOGY AND PRESCRIBING

Part I focuses on the foundations of pharmacology, providing the fundamental information required for evidence-based prescribing. It begins with an introduction to evidence-based clinical practice guidelines. This essential chapter offers background rationale on why drug treatments are recommended and how to interpret data from various treatment guidelines to make sound clinical decisions. In addition to chapters on pharmacokinetics and pharmacodynamics, a chapter on pharmacogenomics and pharmacogenetics provides the basic principles underlying our current understanding of genetic variations in response to pharmacotherapy and adverse drug reactions. It also examines precision medicine, which has advanced significantly and gained much momentum during the last two decades. An effective clinician should be familiar with these concepts, as well as knowing how and when to implement them to improve patient outcomes. Pharmacology is then examined under various lenses of patient characteristics across the life span, from pediatric and pregnant and lactating patients to geriatric patients.

Part I includes chapters on the process of drug development and approval, as well as the fundamentals of prescription writing—vital knowledge for all prescribers, but a topic often ignored in textbooks. It also sets the stage for new prescribers to practice safe and responsible prescribing. As opioid overdose continues to be a crisis within the United States, responsible controlled-substance prescribing must be relentlessly emphasized and reminded about. Part I concludes with chapters on antimicrobial stewardship, promoting adherence, and a unique chapter on applied calculations. Calculations that are typically spread amongst various chapters in other textbook have been combined into one convenient chapter for easy reference.

PART II: SYSTEM-SPECIFIC AND PATIENT-FOCUSED PRESCRIBING

In Part II, the pharmacotherapies of the most common conditions of each organ system are discussed. In addition to chapters on organ systems, this part includes chapters on renal, acid–base, and fluid and electrolyte disorders; men's and women's health conditions; and transgender care. Immunology and vaccines and antimicrobial and antiviral pharmacotherapy are examined, as well as psychopharmacology, integrative health, and pain management. The treatment guidelines from various organizations are included for prescribers to apply and implement drug treatments accordingly.

PART III: HEALTH PROMOTION AND MAINTENANCE

The textbook concludes with a focus on health promotion and maintenance, helping clinicians to treat patients and educate them on how to lead healthier lives. Topics such as treatment of substance use disorders, over-the-counter medications, and treatment of obesity are discussed.

INSTRUCTOR RESOURCES

Advanced Pharmacology for Prescribers is accompanied by comprehensive instructor resources, including an Instructor's Manual with learning objectives, chapter summaries, case studies, and discussion questions; summary PowerPoint slides for each chapter; a test bank; and an image bank. **Qualified instructors can access these resources by emailing textbook@ springerpub.com.**

We hope you enjoy using the book as much as we enjoyed creating it.

—Brent Luu, Gerald Kayingo,
and Virginia McCoy Hass

Acknowledgements

On behalf of the Editorial Team, I would like to express our sincere appreciation to the authors and reviewers from across the country and disciplines for your contributions. Your willingness to share your expertise and the spirit of professionalism as well as collaboration have touched us deeply. Your insights of evidence-based clinical practice will serve new practitioners in a very meaningful way. We are humbly grateful to work with all of you on various levels during the project. We hope you have enjoyed the project as much as we have.

On a personal note, I would like to thank each member of the Editorial Team—Virginia, Gerald, Sandhya, Elaine, and Xiaodong—for your commitment. Thank you for your valuable ideas and suggestions to move the project along. Thanks to my colleagues who provided words of encouragement and checked on me regularly to make sure I was on track. I also would like to thank the team at Springer Publishing Company, particularly Adrianne Brigido, Jaclyn Koshofer, Kris Parrish, and Margaret Zuccarini (retired), for sharing our vision and providing feedback and invaluable suggestions throughout the project. I am grateful for your efforts in bringing the text to production and publication. I would like to thank my deceased parents and my eight dear siblings for instilling a strong perseverance personality within me to complete the project. In addition, I would like to thank my parents-in-law for their many years of relentless support in caring for our two children and cooking for us many delicious meals. I would also like to thank my brother-in-law for reminding me of what a high level of professionalism and a strong work ethic are. Finally, many thanks to my immediate family, my wife, SangSang, and my two teenagers, Leianna and Jess, for their love and laughter. They are the primary source of my motivation and energy to thrive because:

"Being deeply loved by someone gives you strength, while loving someone deeply gives you courage." —Lao Tzu

—*Brent Luu*

I

Foundations of Pharmacology and Prescribing

An Introduction to Evidence-Based Clinical Practice Guidelines

Adebola Olarewaju and George W. Rodway

LEARNING OBJECTIVES

- Understand the purpose and importance of evidence-based medicine guidelines.
- Describe the source of published evidence-based guidelines and clinical practice guidelines.
- Analyze the process required to develop useful rigorous practice guidelines.
- List the potential pitfalls inherent in creating clinical practice guidelines.

INTRODUCTION

The concept of evidence-based medicine can be aggregated into what has popularly been termed in the clinical world of healthcare as "evidence-based practice." A central component to evidence-based practice is clinical practice guidelines.[1] Evidence-based practice and clinical practice guidelines are often used interchangeably in the literature. The goal of the guidelines is to set some standards in practice using the best evidence, but not to dictate practice. The purpose of this chapter is to introduce the brief history of guidelines, their use in clinical practice, their benefits and limitations, and the rigorous process in their development.

BACKGROUND

Some of the earliest published clinical guidelines were from professional organizations and government agencies such as the American Academy of Pediatrics (AAP), the Canadian Task Force on the Periodic Health Examinations, the U.S. Preventive Services Task Force,

and the American College of Physicians in the 1970s and 1980s.[1] The Institute of Medicine (IOM)[2] report on quality and the health system for the 21st century focused on closing the gap between the concept of quality healthcare delivery on one hand and the actual clinical care on the other hand. The IOM had six aims for the improvement of healthcare delivery: (a) safety, (b) effectiveness, (c) patient-centeredness, (d) timeliness, (e) efficiency, and (f) equity. These aims should also be at the core of clinical practice guidelines. The inclusion or exclusion of these aims potentially differentiates high- from low-quality guidelines. An increasingly significant degree of importance has been placed on the use of clinical guidelines, but insufficient time is spent in training clinicians on their interpretation and application. Furthermore, the commitment made to training students in the evaluation and grading of peer-reviewed literature in clinician education has wide variation across academic institutions.[3] For example, a cross-sectional survey exploring how physician assistant programs teach evidence-based practice found that across 186 programs, training ranged from 4 to 550 hours. Of those who reported barriers to evidence-based practice training, 27% reported time constraints as the most common barrier. Observably, time (or lack thereof) is also a barrier in guideline implementation in clinical practice.

CLINICAL GUIDELINES

UTILIZATION OF CLINICAL GUIDELINES

In general, guidelines improve health outcomes by promoting clinical practice based on the best evidence.[4–6] Guidelines should be used in the first instance to reduce unnecessary practice variation. Variations in practice occur at the clinician and institution level. This may be due to insufficient knowledge, historical preferences, or inherent biases that propagate health disparities. Second, guidelines should be used to reduce the use of low-quality or minimum-value interventions. Intervention strategies should be based on the most up-to-date information. Use of low-quality interventions does not improve patient outcomes and is not cost-effective. Third, guidelines should increase the use of valuable interventions that are under-utilized. This is demonstrated in all areas of healthcare from diagnostic testing to medication recommendations. Lastly, guidelines should target interventions to populations that would receive the most benefit.[1] However, one important caveat is that clinicians must be aware of underrepresented populations, whom may not be well represented during clinical trials, potentially requiring personalization of guideline recommendations.

BENEFITS AND LIMITATIONS OF CLINICAL GUIDELINES

The use of guidelines provides multiple benefits. The primary advantage is the best current evidence being implemented in patient care and subsequently improves outcomes. There is also the potential to reduce unjustified variations in healthcare delivery and possibly health disparities. Additionally, for patients who seek health information online, clinical guidelines generated by professional organizations may be a source of more credible information. Guidelines can also assist in the identification of knowledge gaps and facilitate discussions about the future direction of the research topic.[7]

Despite the stated benefits, guidelines also have limitations that need to be recognized. Some limitations affect guideline development—as well as guideline application.[1,5] In the search for evidence, the authors may find it lacking, misleading, or misinterpreted, affecting the strength of the recommendations. Guidelines that are rigid or limited in their scope leave little room for clinicians to adapt recommendations to the patient's specific circumstances. It is most helpful when guidelines allow clinicians to adapt them to specific patient needs.[8] Adoption of guidelines in public policies may cause insurers to be less flexible in covering those interventions if they are not a part of a guideline or best practice recommendation, hindering the clinician's decision-making and patient access to effective treatment. Critical thinking and clinical judgment should always be at the forefront of applying guidelines to practice. Time and resources are needed for both guideline implementation and, perhaps more importantly, to overcome the resistance to change.[5] Another important limitation is that proper adherence to guidelines requires the ability to competently interpret the evidence, as well as the clinical skills to effectively apply them.

CLINICAL GUIDELINE DEVELOPMENT

Guidelines are ideally intended to summarize the available literature and be formatted in a way that increases the accessibility of peer-reviewed information to clinicians. Guidelines are meant to be practical for everyday use.[1] Although guidelines are not a recipe for practice, clinicians do not typically use recommendations that are not easily understood. In addition, due to the decentralized nature of guideline development, guidelines created by independent professional groups or agencies can be duplicating or contradicting each other. Contradicting information, based on the grading of evidence and recommendations, hinders the potentially beneficial effects of guidelines.[1]

According to Ardern and Winters,[9] there are three things to consider when creating a guideline. The authors must first decide which evidence to include. They also need to grade the quality of the evidence. The evidence should then be synthesized in a meaningful way that is practical for the user. However, grading the strength of the recommendation is as important as grading the quality of the evidence. The Grades of Recommendation, Assessment, Development, and Evaluation (GRADE) Working Group[8] took it a step further and recommended implementation and evaluation of guidelines to address barriers to change, evaluation of the implementation, and to continue updating the materials. It is recommended that guidelines are reassessed and updated every 3 years.[1]

Per the IOM, the standards of guideline development include the involvement of a multidisciplinary panel and a comprehensive systematic review of the evidence. Biases can be found in research as well as guideline recommendations.[1,6] It is important to recognize that professional groups may have internal and external pressures to make certain recommendations.[1] Members of the panel may have financial or contractual obligations that influence decision-making. Professional organizations and panel members should disclose conflicts of interest prior to reviewing the evidence. The best evidence should move forward to support clinical practice recommendations.[7]

A good guideline is one that is based on consistent and systematic judgment of the evidence, clear in its recommendations and translatable into practice. There are sequential steps that should be utilized in evaluating the strengths of the evidence and recommendations.[8] The quality of the evidence across studies is examined at the beginning. The evidence is evaluated for rigor, quality, and the risks and benefits of the clinical practice to the patient.[7] Next, outcomes critical to decision-making are identified and the quality of the evidence across outcomes is then evaluated by weighing the degree of harm and benefit to the patient. Lastly, the strength of the recommendation is assessed.[8,10]

Grading the Quality of the Evidence

When judging the quality of the evidence, it is important to consider the study design, quality, consistency, and directness.[8] Study design is categorized into randomized controlled trials (RCTs), observational studies, and all others. The level of evidence is graded accordingly to the following: RCTs = high; observational studies = low; and all other studies = very low.[8]

RCTs are awarded the highest rank of evidence, but they do have limitations.[11] Inadequate sample size and research findings may be limited to the study population with limited generalizability to actual practice. Due to well-defined inclusion and exclusion criteria, certain characteristics of trial subjects in terms of age, therapy, and comorbidity may not be represented.[6] Outcome measures may not correlate with actual outcomes of interest. RCTs are impractical for urgent situations or rare diseases.[11,12] RCTs are also costly to conduct in regard to time and resources. New treatment methods may be introduced prior to trial completion; therefore, RCTs may not be readily available in clinical practice. When the availability of high-quality studies is limited or absent, low-quality studies should be judiciously considered.[9] Sometimes the authors have to rely on reviews and expert opinions. Good reviews lead to appropriate clinical decisions, but weak reviews are misleading and undermine clinical guidelines and practice.[4] Position statements from a group of experts on a specific topic may provide valuable information on a clinically relevant topic regardless of whether robust or limited research exists.[9] Research often lags behind clinical practice.[9] It has been suggested that it takes approximately 17 years to fully translate research evidence to clinical practice.[13] Expert opinion based on clinical practice can fill these gaps in the literature.[9]

The overall grade of the quality of the evidence is impacted by the remaining three elements of study quality, consistency, and directness. Study quality refers to the study methods. If the methods used by the researchers have serious limitations, the grade for the quality of evidence decreases. Consistency examines whether the effects reported across studies are similar.[8] Directness assesses the extent to which the study population, interventions, and outcome measures match the target population for the guideline.[8] After all elements are taken into consideration, a categorical grade for the quality of evidence is generated. The grade ranges from high (further research is unlikely to change outcomes) to very low (outcome effects are very uncertain). The quality of the evidence is a major contributor to the strength of the recommendation.

Grading the Strength of the Recommendation

Recommendations should be based on the effective size of the main outcomes, the quality of the evidence, the application of the evidence into specific practice settings, and the baseline risk to population. Additional attention should be given to the cost of the intervention relative to the added benefit to the patient.[8] The American College of Chest Physicians (ACCP) created a grading system for evidence and recommendations based on the GRADE Working Group platform in order to simplify the evaluation process (**Table 1.1**). This systematic approach attempts to minimize biases and improve interpretation.[14]

TABLE 1.1 The Grading of Recommendations

Grade	Benefit Versus Risk/Burdens	Supporting Evidence
1A: Strong recommendation, high-quality evidence	Benefits clearly outweigh risks/burdens or vice versa	RCTs without significant limitations or tremendous evidence from observational studies
1B: Strong recommendation, moderate-quality evidence	Benefits clearly outweigh risks/burdens or vice versa	RCTs with significant limitations or extremely strong evidence from observational studies
1C: Strong recommendation, low- or very low-quality evidence	Benefits clearly outweigh risks/burdens or vice versa	Observational studies or case series
2A: Weak recommendation, high-quality evidence	Benefits balanced with risks/burdens	RCTs without significant limitations or tremendous evidence from observational studies
2B: Weak recommendation, moderate-quality evidence	Benefits balanced with risks/burdens	RCTs with significant limitations or extremely strong evidence from observational studies
2C: Weak recommendation, low- or very low-quality evidence	Estimates of benefits and risks/burdens closely balanced or unknown	Observational studies or case series

RCT, randomized controlled trial.

Source: Reproduced with permission from Guyatt G, Gutterman D, Baumann MH, et al. Grading strength of recommendations and quality of evidence in clinical guidelines: a report from an American College of Chest Physicians task force. *Chest.* 2006;129(1):174–181. doi:10.1378/chest.129.1.174

The strength of a recommendation is influenced by the balance of the risks, burdens, and benefits of an intervention to a specific population and the quality of the evidence supporting the treatment outcomes.[14] The ACCP grades recommendations as strong or weak. Although this strategy is simplified into two categories, the ACCP recommends considering patients' values and preferences when making recommendations.

CONCLUSION

Judgments about clinical evidence and recommendations in healthcare are complex. Since available resources are always limited and money that is allocated for a certain treatment must be weighed against other worthwhile pharmacological interventions, clinicians may also need to decide whether any incremental health benefits are worth the additional costs.

Systematic reviews may provide essential, but not sufficient, information for making well-informed decisions. Reviewers and people who use reviews draw conclusions about the quality of the evidence, either implicitly or explicitly. Similarly, people who use practice guidelines draw conclusions about the strength of recommendations. Such judgments and conclusions will guide subsequent decisions. As a result, a systematic and explicit approach to making judgments can help to prevent errors, facilitate critical appraisal of these judgments, and improve communication of the information.

Clinical guidelines provide a problem-solving approach to healthcare delivery using the best evidence.[4] Randomized clinical trials and systematic reviews are important to the evidence base but they have their own inherent limitations. Expert opinion can be valid and clinical-based evidence can fill important research gaps. Tailoring guidelines to the individual patient supports patient-centered care and shared decision-making may be applicable and appropriate in a specific setting.[5,8] The best guidelines integrate clinical experience and research evidence.[15] Clinicians should consider guidelines as tools to identify gaps in knowledge. They should not be considered as the holy grail nor a substitute for clinical judgment.

CLINICAL PEARLS

- Clinical practice guidelines and their application to evidence-based medicine were initially developed as a means of reducing variability in clinical practice.
- Guidelines are not meant to mandate a particular practice pattern or therapeutic choice, but to help clinicians understand and apply the current state-of-the-art care based on rigorous scientific studies.
- The quality of clinical practice guidelines depends heavily on the selected data sources, preferably based on large randomized controlled trials rather than smaller case studies with limited applicability.
- It is incumbent upon the reader and user of clinical practice guidelines to assess the quality of the source, often relying on the integrity and rigor of the publisher and reviewers.
- Well-designed clinical practice guidelines can improve patient care outcomes and guide future research directions.

KEY TAKEAWAYS

- Well-designed and presented clinical guidelines can improve the efficiency and reduce the variability of clinical practice in select patients.
- The most reliable clinical practice guidelines are derived through rigorous statistical analysis of high-quality studies with low risk of bias.
- Guidelines are not mandates and may not apply to every patient scenario, and the treating clinician should exercise care in the application of published clinical practice guidelines.
- The strength of a recommendation is influenced by the balance of the risks, burdens, and benefits of an intervention in a specific population and the quality of the evidence supporting the treatment outcomes.
- Not all published clinical practice guidelines are reliable and immune from bias.

REFERENCES

1. Eden J, Wheatley B, McNeil B, Sox H, eds. *Knowing What Works in Health Care: A Roadmap for the Nation.* National Academies Press; 2008. https://www.nap.edu/read/12038/chapter/1
2. Institute of Medicine. *Crossing the Quality Chasm: A New Health System for the 21st Century.* National Academies Press; 2001.
3. White DM, Stephens P. State of evidence-based practice in physician assistant education. *J Physician Assist Educ.* 2018;29(1):12–18. doi:10.1097/JPA.0000000000000183
4. Beitz JM, Bolton LL. Systematic reviews and meta--analyses—literature-based recommendations for evaluating strengths, weaknesses, and clinical value. *Ostomy Wound Manage.* 2015;61(11):26–42. https://www.o-wm

.com/article/systematic-reviews-and-meta-analyses-literature-based-recommendations-evaluating-strengths

5. Hollon SD, Areán PA, Craske MG, et al. Development of clinical practice guidelines. *Ann Rev Clin Psychol*. 2014;10:213–241. doi:10.1146/annurev-clinpsy-050212-185529

6. Sheridan DJ, Julian DG. Achievements and limitations of evidence-based medicine. *J Am Coll Cardiol*. 2016;68(2):201–213. doi:10.1016/j.jacc.2016.03.600

7. Kredo T, Bernhardsson S, Machingaidze S, et al. Guide to clinical practice guidelines: the current state of play. *Int J Qual Health Care*. 2016;28(1):122–128. doi:10.1093/intqhc/mzv115

8. Grades of Recommendation, Assessment, Development, and Evaluation (GRADE) Working Group. Grading quality of evidence and strength of recommendations. *BMJ*. 2004;328:1490–1494. doi:10.1136/bmj.328.7454.1490

9. Ardern CL, Winters M. Synthesizing 'best evidence' in systematic reviews when randomized controlled trials are absent: three tips for authors to add value for clinician readers. *Br J Sports Med*. 2018;52(15):948–949. doi:10.1136/bjsports-2017-097881

10. Guyatt G, Vist G, Falck-Ytter Y, et al. An emerging consensus on grading recommendations? *Evid Based Med*. 2006;11(1):2–4. doi:10.1136/ebm.11.1.2-a

11. Hohmann E, Brand JC, Rossi MJ, et al. Expert opinion is necessary: Delphi panel methodology facilitates a scientific approach to consensus. *Arthroscopy*. 2018;34(2):349–351. doi:10.1016/j.arthro.2017.11.022

12. Frieden TR. Evidence for health decision making—beyond randomized, controlled trials. *N Engl J Med*. 2017;377:465–475. doi:10.1056/NEJMra1614394

13. Morris ZS, Wooding S, Grant J. The answer is 17 years, what is the question: understanding time lags in translational research. *J R Soc Med*. 2011;104:510–520. doi:10.1258/jrsm.2011.110180

14. Guyatt G, Gutterman D, Baumann MH, et al. Grading strength of recommendations and quality of evidence in clinical guidelines: a report from an American College of Chest Physicians Task Force. *Chest*. 2006;129(1):174–181. doi:10.1378/chest.129.1.174

15. Sackett DL, Rosenberg WMC, Gray JAM, et al. Evidence based medicine: what it is and what it isn't. It's about integrating individual clinical expertise and the best external evidence. *Br Med J*. 1996;312(7023):71–72. doi:10.1136/bmj.312.7023.71

Pharmacokinetics

Patrick Chan and James Uchizono

INTRODUCTION

An understanding of pharmacokinetics (PK) allows healthcare providers to optimize doses and dosing regimens to maximize efficacy and minimize toxicities. Physiological processes affect drug kinetic and dynamic behavior of clinical response(s). As research continues to provide more information, it is apparent that these processes are extremely complex. Colloquially, PK is described as "what the body does to the drug," or the study of the physiological processes that affect drug concentration in the body. Pharmacodynamics (PD) is described as "what the drug does to the body," or the study of the pharmacological response and subsequent clinical outcome resulting from the drug concentration. Furthermore, physiological processes that convert drug concentrations into responses serve as the link between PK and PD processes. PK encompasses all of the kinetic processes from the drug released from its dosage form (e.g., oral, intravenous, subcutaneous) to the delivery of drug to its site or tissue responsible for initiating the translation of drug concentration/exposure into a response (shown as the solid arrows in **Figure 2.1**). Where PK ends, PD begins by explaining the time-course translation/transduction of drug concentration into a "biological signal" or "messenger" (e.g., intracellular Ca^{2+} concentration) that ultimately leads to the end desired response or effect (e.g., increased pain relief) (shown as the broken line arrow in Figure 2.1).

Upon closer examination, PK includes even the kinetics of a drug released from the dosage form prior to absorption—such as a drug being transferred from syringe to systemic circulation (i.e., IV bolus) or the complex disintegration, solvation, and dissolution of a drug released by an advanced drug delivery system (ADDS) into the gastrointestinal (GI) tract milieu for permeation (passive diffusion and active or facilitated transport) across the GI endothelial barrier to the systemic circulation. Additional terms associated with the PK of a drug include *absorption, distribution, excretion,* and *metabolism* (see Figure 2.1). A general term describing the sum of drug excretion and metabolism is *elimination*. An even more general PK term, *disposition*, describes the kinetic time-course of drug distribution, excretion, and metabolism. The input function of a drug (e.g., IV bolus, oral administration) combined with the disposition is the drug PK. *Most importantly, clinicians can generally only control the input function of drugs, while the "body" or physiology controls the disposition.*

An essential hypothesis of PK is that there is a quantitative relationship between drug concentration and pharmacological effect.[1] Clinical PK incorporates the fundamentals of PK to dose calculations, infusion rates, predictions of drug concentrations, dosing intervals, and time to eliminate the drug from the body. The primary objective of clinical PK is to maximize efficacy while minimizing toxicities, through a process

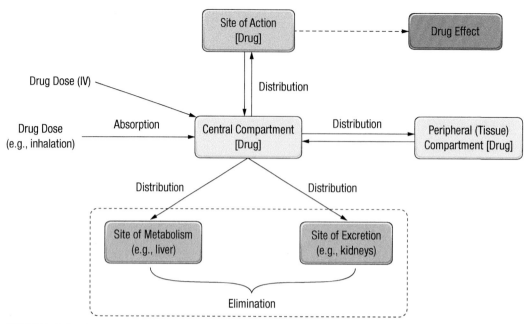

FIGURE 2.1 Absorption, distribution, excretion, and metabolism. The relationship among the pharmacokinetic processes of absorption, distribution, metabolism, and excretion with the central, peripheral, and site-of-action compartments.

IV, intravenous.

called therapeutic drug monitoring (TDM). A complete TDM protocol entails monitoring defined therapeutic endpoints (which includes plasma drug concentration if appropriate) and adverse reactions. Adjustments of doses can be guided by TDM to provide individualized regimens. Clinical PK can be affected by numerous covariates, such as age, genetics, gender, race, comorbid disease states, and concomitant medications resulting in drug interactions. These factors should be considered into the dosing regimen for each patient.

There is a trend to incorporate newly acquired pharmacogenomic knowledge into pharmacokinetics. *Pharmacogenomics* is the study of how a patient's genetics may influence drug response. Genetic information may provide insight to a patient's metabolism, distribution, and excretion or perhaps pharmacological response or toxicities which will further maximize patient outcomes. Pharmacogenomic information may have a role in providing empiric therapy for patients along with more personalized TDM.

BACKGROUND

In the mid-19th century, Dr. Andrew Buchanan of Great Britain studied the effects of ether, an inhaled anesthetic. Through his studies, he correlated blood concentrations of ether with the dose of inhaled ether. Furthermore, brain concentrations of ether determined the level of anesthesia. Although the term "pharmacokinetics" was not yet conceived, Dr. Buchanan's mathematical

calculations of ether in the body was one of the first known studies in the area of pharmacokinetics. "Pharmakon" is the Greek word for drugs and poisons while "kinetics" is the study of the changes to a variable(s) with respect to time.

In 1937, Swedish physiologist Torsten Teorell published two seminal papers utilizing a physiological-based model to describe the kinetics of drugs after administration.[2] These papers have been recognized as providing the foundations of pharmacokinetics.[3,4] Forty years later, Gibaldi and Levy described the study of pharmacokinetics as characterizing the time course of drug absorption, distribution, metabolism, and excretion in relationship with the time course and magnitude of drug effect and toxicity.[5] As studies of pharmacokinetics along with pharmacodynamics developed over the next several decades, this paved the way for the emergence of TDM. TDM focuses on individualization of drug dosing within the framework of a patient and their concurrent disease-states.

PHARMACOKINETIC PROCESSES

ABSORPTION

The absorption of a drug is largely dependent on the route of delivery. Drugs can be administered by different routes, including oral, inhaled, subcutaneous, intramuscular, sublingual, rectal, intraocular, intranasal, vaginal, and transdermal (**Table 2.1**). Although intravenous and intra-arterial technically do have an as-

TABLE 2.1 Routes of Drug Administration

Route	Drug Administration
Inhalation or nebulization	Breathed into the lungs through the mouth; absorbed by lungs
Intramuscular	Inserted into muscle of upper arm, thigh, or buttock
Intranasal	Breathed into nose; absorbed through thin mucous membrane that lines the nasal passages
Intraocular	Applied to or inserted onto affected eye
Intrathecal	Injected into the spinal canal
Intravenous	Inserted into a vein
Oral	Taken by mouth; absorbed by mouth, stomach, or small intestine
Otic	Applied to affected ear
Rectal	Inserted into rectum; absorbed through rectal wall
Subcutaneous	Injected into fatty tissue just beneath the skin
Sublingual or buccal	Placed under the tongue (sublingual) or between the gums and teeth (buccal); absorbed into small blood vessels that lie beneath the tongue
Transdermal	Delivered through a patch on the skin
Vaginal	Inserted into vagina; absorbed through vaginal wall

pect of absorption (i.e., release of drug from a syringe or IV or IA bag), these routes deliver drug directly into the systemic circulation and are a special subset of PK input (i.e., instantaneous absorption processes having a bioavailability of 1.0). The physicochemical properties (solubility, pKa, ionization, polarity, molecular weight, partition coefficient) play a critical role in the absorption of drugs. The route of delivery impacts the rate of absorption as well as the extent of absorption. The absorption rate constant, frequently denoted as k_a or K_a, can be found in drug package inserts or most drug information references.

DISTRIBUTION

Once in systemic circulation, drugs distribute into the tissue. Drugs must cross lipid membranes to reach the site of action. Passive diffusions, presence of transport proteins, hemodynamics, and the physicochemical properties of the drug influence the extent of distribution of the drug.

Protein Binding

Protein- and tissue-binding influence drug distribution. The free, unbound drug in the plasma is frequently denoted as f_u (fraction unbound). It is the unbound fraction of drugs that may distribute into the tissue, undergo metabolism and excretion, and exert its pharmacological and toxicological effects. Important factors influencing drug binding to plasma proteins are described in **Table 2.2**.

Acidic drugs in the plasma frequently bind to albumin while basic drugs frequently bind to α_1-acid glycoprotein (AAG).[6] Hypoalbuminemia resulting from disease complications (e.g., liver disease, kidney disease, poor nutrition) may result in reduced protein binding. Elevated urea levels in patients with end-stage renal disease (ESRD) have been shown to have reduced phenytoin binding to albumin, therefore increasing the free fraction.[7] AAG is an acute-phase reactant which is elevated in inflammatory states and therefore reduces the free fraction of basic drugs.[8]

DRUG METABOLISM

It is estimated that more than 75% of drugs are metabolized.[9] Drug metabolism occurs primarily in the liver, though metabolism can also occur at other sites such as the gastrointestinal wall, kidneys, and blood–brain barrier. Metabolism can be characterized as phase 1 or 2 reactions. Phase 1 reactions include oxidation, epoxidation, dealkylation, and hydroxylation reactions catalyzed by the cytochrome P450 enzyme system. A majority of the cytochrome P450 enzymes reside in the microsomes of hepatocytes where it metabolizes the highest number of substrates (chemical, drugs, and pollutants) in the body. Phase 2 reactions are glucuronidation and sulfation processes.

Many drug interactions involve the cytochrome P450 enzyme system. Certain drugs, termed *inducers*, may increase the activity of specific cytochrome P450 isozymes, leading to increased metabolism of drugs that are substrates of that particular isozyme. The reduction in plasma concentration of the drug substrates may lead to decreased therapeutic effects. Other drugs are inhibitors of cytochrome P450 enzymes and therefore decrease the metabolism of drugs that are substrates. The increase in substrate plasma concentration may

TABLE 2.2 Factors That Influence Drug Binding

Factor	Influence on Drug Binding
Drug	Physicochemical properties Total drug concentration
Plasma protein	Total concentration of available plasma protein
Binding affinity	Binding affinity of a drug to a plasma protein is determined by both the physicochemical properties of the drug and protein[10]
Comorbid conditions	Diseases may alter plasma protein levels or binding affinity[11]
Drug interactions	Competitive binding by two drugs for same plasma protein[12] Alterations in binding affinity by one drug affecting another drug

result in not only enhanced pharmacological effects, but enhanced toxicological effects. Clinicians are encouraged to consider dosing adjustments based on known drug interactions to achieve therapeutic effects while minimizing adverse reactions.

EXCRETION

Excretion refers to the irreversible loss of an intact drug. Excretion of a drug typically occurs through the kidneys and ultimately through urine. Other routes of excretion of an intact drug include bile, breast milk, saliva, and sweat. The three major physiological processes occurring in the kidneys governing renal excretion are glomerular filtration, active secretion, and reabsorption. Drugs that are filtered through the glomerulus are typically small molecules (MW <500 Da) and not protein-bound. Glomerular filtration rate (GFR) is a measurement that indicates how much of the plasma volume has been filtered by the glomerulus per unit of time (e.g., minute); it also correlates well with body surface area (BSA). Normal GFR is approximately 125 to 130 mL/minute. Active secretion through the kidneys is an active transport process requiring energy. Drugs may compete for the same transport process, resulting in a drug interaction. Reabsorption occurs following glomerular filtration. Reabsorption may be an active or passive process that places drugs back into the plasma. The pH of the renal tubules largely influences the amount of drug that is reabsorbed.

PHARMACOKINETIC PARAMETERS

BIOAVAILABILITY

Bioavailability is defined as the rate and extent of drug absorption, or the percentage or fraction of the parent compound that reaches systemic (plasma) circulation. The bioavailability of the same drug in the same patient may be different depending on the route of administration. Drug references frequently provide the bioavailabilities of drugs and are typically denoted as F. The extent of absorption, but not the rate, can be described by the parameter Area Under the Curve (AUC). In an acute setting, the rate of absorption, generally k_a, tends to be more important whereas the extent of absorption tends to be more important in chronic use medications. The salt factor (S) is the fraction of a dose that is the active base form of the drug, and pragmatically can be viewed as an attenuation of F (e.g., "effective dose" = $F \times S \times$ dose). The most frequently used routes of administration of drugs are oral and intravenous.

The absolute bioavailability, F, is determined by comparing the availability for any given extravascular (e.v.) route of administration measured against an i.v. point of reference of availability of the drug administered intravenously (Equation 2.1).

$$F = \frac{\text{AUC}_{e.v.}/\text{Dose}_{e.v.}}{\text{AUC}_{i.v.}/\text{Dose}_{i.v.}}$$

(Equation 2.1)

The value of F is important in determining the "effective dose" for these e.v. drugs. The physicochemical properties of the drug affect the drug's ability to partition from lipid to aqueous phases, and therefore, F. Food, drug interactions, and gastrointestinal (GI) motility can all affect drug solubility and absorption. First-pass metabolism, which is presystemic metabolism of the drug, can occur in the GI tract and the liver prior to reaching systemic circulation. All of these factors can affect F and the route will sometimes dictate the countersalt needed, thus affecting S, as well.

It is important to note that F does not account for the rate of absorption. The rate of absorption influences the onset of action for drugs. For most medications taken chronically, the rate of absorption may not be an issue.

CLEARANCE

Clearance is an independent PK parameter quantifying the rate the body is able to eliminate a drug. More specifically, clearance is the volume of blood that is completely cleared of the drug per unit time. The units are in volume/time, usually liters per hour or milliliters per minute. While the liver is primarily responsible for drug metabolism and the kidneys are primarily responsible for parent drug and metabolite excretion (filtration and secretion), other routes of elimination include the chemical decomposition, feces, skin, and lungs. Hepatic metabolism and elimination are components of drug clearance. Total clearance is characterized by Equation 2.2:

$$Cl_{Total} = Cl_{Hepatic} + Cl_{Renal} + Cl_{Other} \qquad \text{(Equation 2.2)}$$

Total clearance Cl_{Total} is used in most dose calculations without taking into account the specific route of elimination. Clearance is an important parameter because it controls the steady-state concentration Cp_{ss} as shown in Equation 2.3:

$$Cp_{ss} = \frac{(S)(F)(\text{Dose}/\tau)}{Cl} \qquad \text{(Equation 2.3)}$$

S is the salt factor, F is the bioavailability, and tau (τ) is the dosing interval. Rearranging the equation, the clearance of a drug can be calculated from steady-state concentrations of a drug (Equation 2.4):

$$Cl = \frac{(S)(F)(\text{Dose}/\tau)}{Cp_{ss}} \qquad \text{(Equation 2.4)}$$

The glomerular filtration of an adult patient may be estimated by the Cockcroft-Gault equation[13] (Equation 2.5):

$$Cl_{Cr} (\text{mL / minute}) = \frac{(140 - \text{age}) \times \text{IBW}}{72 \times \text{SCr}} \text{ for males}$$

$$Cl_{Cr} (\text{mL/minute}) = \frac{(140 - \text{age}) \times \text{IBW}}{72 \times \text{SCr}}$$
$$\times 0.85 \text{ for females} \qquad \text{(Equation 2.5)}$$

Cl_{Cr} is the creatinine clearance in milliliters per minute, the age of the patient is in years, SCr is the serum creatinine, and IBW is the ideal body weight of the patient in kilograms (kg). For female patients, the resultant Cl_{Cr} is multiplied by 85% to account for lower muscle mass. The Cockcroft-Gault equation utilizes serum creatinine, which is a by-product of muscle metabolism and is freely filtered by the glomerulus. Creatinine is not actively secreted nor is it reabsorbed.[14] The equation is limited to use in adult patients and cannot be applied for pediatric or dialysis patients. For drugs that are primarily eliminated via the renal route, dose adjustments may be made on the basis of creatinine clearance (Cl_{Cr}) and are provided by drug package inserts or drug information references.

VOLUME OF DISTRIBUTION

The volume of distribution V_d is a PK parameter characterizing the extent of drug distribution into the tissue from the blood. The physicochemical properties of a drug, plasma protein binding, and tissue binding influence V_d. It has also been termed *apparent* volume of distribution because it does not correlate with an actual physiological volume compartment in the human body, but rather, it is the inferred volume in which the drug appears to dissolve in. It is inferred because the clinician knows the dose given and Cp (drug plasma concentration) is measured; the V_d is inferred or calculated from the two values of dose and Cp. The lower limit for nearly all drugs is 3 L or the actual average volume of human plasma. As the apparent or inferred volume of distribution increases in size, the interpretation begins to focus on the distribution of drug into extravascular tissues. The apparent or inferred V_d can be calculated using Equation 2.6.[15]

$$V_d = \frac{\text{Dose}_{i.v.}}{Cp} \qquad \text{(Equation 2.6)}$$

If the plasma concentration Cp of a drug is small immediately following a single bolus dose, this generally indicates substantial drug permeation into the tissue(s) and the resultant V_d is >40 to 80 L, indicating extensive distribution into the tissue. In contrast, if V_d is small (close to 3 L), a large fraction of the drug is assumed to reside in the blood plasma, thus suggesting a little amount of drug has permeated into the extravascular tissue(s). While V_d provides insight as to whether the drug is residing in the blood or tissue, its value does not determine which specific tissue compartment the drug permeates into.

V_d is useful in determining the loading dose necessary to achieve a targeted Cp. Equation 2.7 illustrates the usual loading dose equation:

$$\text{Loading Dose} = V_d \times Cp_{target} \qquad \text{(Equation 2.7)}$$

For drugs that have a large V_d, a greater loading dose is necessary to achieve the targeted Cp. Drugs with a small V_d require a reduced loading dose to obtain the targeted Cp.

ELIMINATION RATE CONSTANT

The dependent parameter K is a first-order rate constant. It is a function of V_d and Cl. K can be described as the percentage or fraction of the amount of drug that is cleared from the body per unit time. The units are typically expressed as 1/hour (h^{-1}) or 1/minute (min^{-1}). As shown in Equation 2.8, K can be viewed as a proportionality constant between V_d and Cl:

$$K = \frac{Cl}{V_d} \qquad \text{(Equation 2.8)}$$

A large K value indicates rapid elimination of the drug. If two drug concentrations are drawn within the same dosing interval, K can be determined using Equation 2.8.[16] Another way of expressing Equation 2.8 is as follows (Equation 2.9):

$$K = \frac{Ln\left(\frac{Cp_1}{Cp_2}\right)}{\Delta t} \qquad \text{(Equation 2.9)}$$

Ln is natural log and Δt is the time elapsed between Cp_1 and Cp_2. In other words, the value of K may be determined if two drug levels are measured within a known time lapse between the levels.

HALF-LIFE

The determination of K is integral to calculating half-life, $t_{1/2}$, as shown in Equation 2.10:

$$t_{1/2} = \frac{Ln(2)}{K} = \frac{(V_d) \times Ln(2)}{Cl} \qquad \text{(Equation 2.10)}$$

Equation 2.10 also shows the relationship among $t_{1/2}$, V_d, and Cl. The $t_{1/2}$ is the amount of time it takes for the drug currently in the body to reduce by 50%. The $t_{1/2}$ can also predict the amount of time it takes for a patient to achieve steady-state drug concentrations (assuming no loading dose and the same dose was administered at the same interval). For example, after one $t_{1/2}$, Cp is 50% of the final steady-state Cp_{ss}. Under these conditions, a patient is considered to be clinically at steady state

TABLE 2.3 Number of Half-Lives and Expected Percent of True Steady-State Concentration Cp_{ss} or Percent of Drug Eliminated

Number of $t_{1/2}$	Percent of Cp_{ss} or Percent Eliminated
1	50
2	75
3	87.5
4	93.8
5	96.9
6	98.5
7	99.2

if the drug concentration is >90% of the true steady-state level. As shown in **Table 2.3**, it would take approximately 3.3 half-lives for a patient to achieve 90% of the true steady state. Conversely, it would take 3.3 half-lives for a patient to eliminate 90% of the drug once the administration of the drug has ceased. To note, $t_{1/2}$ determines the dosing interval, but V_d and Cl determine the size of the dose.

CONCLUSION

An understanding of pharmacokinetics and the physiological processes affecting absorption, distribution, metabolism, and excretion aids in optimizing therapeutic effects while minimizing adverse reactions of medications. Drug doses and expected concentrations can be calculated utilizing pharmacokinetic models. New doses can be calculated from plasma drug levels. For drugs with narrow therapeutic windows, monitoring of plasma drug concentrations, clinical outcomes, and adverse reactions are often required.

CASE EXEMPLAR: Patient With New-Onset Seizures

CP, a 32-year-old woman, visits the clinic for her annual well-woman examination. She has been taking oral contraceptive pills consistently for the past 3 years and is in a consistent monogamous relationship. She and her partner are not ready to have children.

Past Medical History
- Recent closed-head injury that occurred as a result of a motor vehicle accident. Since the accident, she has experienced two grand mal seizures, which have been controlled by medication.
- Otherwise healthy

Medication
- Phenobarbital, 15 mg once daily

Physical Examination
- Unremarkable

Labs
- Therapeutic blood levels of phenobarbital
- Pregnancy test: negative

Discussion Questions
1. How do oral contraceptives and phenobarbital interact?
2. What other medications interact with birth control pills?
3. How might patients of child-bearing age who are on birth control pills be counseled?

CASE EXEMPLAR: Patient With COVID-19

MS, a 56-year-old Black male with multiple comorbidities, presents with coronavirus 2019 (COVID-19). He has known stage 4 renal insufficiency and takes multiple medications for his various medical conditions.

Past Medical History
- Obesity
- Type 2 diabetes mellitus
- Hypertension

Physical Examination
- Height: 5'11"; weight: 232 lbs; blood pressure: 152/102; pulse: 102; respiration rate: 24; temperature: 103.6°F

Labs
- Consistent with dehydration and marked systemic inflammation
- Liver function: consistent with low-grade nonviral hepatitis
- Glomerular filtration rate: 20 mL/min/1.73 m^2 (estimated)
- Blood sugar (random): 181 mg/dL
- Serum creatinine: 5.2 mg/dL

Next Step
MS is admitted to the hospital for treatment with systemic corticosteroids, antiviral agents, and hydroxychloroquine.

Discussion Questions
1. What baseline medical problems are impacting this patient's pharmacokinetic and pharmacodynamic profile?
2. What acute medical problems will impact on the dosage requirements for treating COVID-19?
3. What problems will MS's proposed treatment cause for his underlying and acute medical conditions?

CLINICAL PEARLS

- Approximately 75% of medications are eliminated through metabolism while the other 25% are directly excreted through the liver, kidneys, sweat, saliva, and breast milk.
- Medications administered through depot delivery systems (intramuscular injections, pills, ointments, and sprays) are absorbed more slowly and require more time to achieve steady-state blood levels.
- Changes in a patient's physiologic status (age, lean body mass, inflammation, fever, dehydration, malnutrition) may profoundly affect the pharmacokinetics and pharmacodynamics of a drug.
- Drugs that are highly protein-bound or fat soluble require a longer time to achieve steady state or to be eliminated from the body.
- Drug-drug interactions can significantly affect the bioavailability of an agent through changes in hepatic metabolism and renal excretion.

KEY TAKEAWAYS

- Every chemical compound that is introduced into the body has its own unique pharmacodynamic profile.
- A given pharmacologic agent's levels and distribution in the body vary in different physiologic situations.
- Protein-bound drugs tend to have a longer half-life in the body than nonprotein-bound drugs.
- Polypharmacy can impact efficacy and toxicity of a drug by affecting its absorption, volume of distribution, enzymatic degradation, or renal excretion.
- Knowledge of a medication's specific pharmacokinetic profile can help clinicians make informed choices on dosing and monitoring of that drug.

REFERENCES

1. Buxton ILO, Benet LZ. Pharmacokinetics: the dynamics of drug absorption, distribution, metabolism, and elimination. In: Brunton LL, Chabner BA, Knollmann BC, eds. *Goodman & Gilman's The Pharmacological Basis of Therapeutics*. 12th ed. McGraw-Hill; 2011:17–40.
2. Teorell T. Studies on the diffusion effect upon ionic distribution: II. Experiments on ionic accumulation. *J Gen Physiol*. 1937;21(1):107–122. doi:10.1085/jgp.21.1.107.
3. Wagner, J. G. History of pharmacokinetics. *Pharmacol Ther*. 1981;12(3):537–562. doi:10.1016/0163-7258(81)90097-8.
4. Paalzow, L. K. Torsten Teorell, the father of pharmacokinetics. *Ups J Med Sci*. 1995;100(1):41–46. doi:10.3109/030097395091788955.
5. Gibaldi M, Levy G. Pharmacokinetics in clinical practice. I. Concepts. *JAMA*. 1976;235:1864–1867. doi:10.1001/jama.1976.03260430034020
6. Pike E, Skuterud B, Kierulf P, et al. Binding and displacement of basic, acidic and neutral drugs in normal and orosomucoid-deficient plasma. *Clin Pharmacokinet*. 1981;6:367–374. doi:10.2165/00003088-198106050-00003
7. Odar-Cederlof I, Borga O. Kinetics of diphenylhydantoin in uraemic patients: consequences of decreased plasma protein binding. *Eur J Clin Pharmacol*. 1974;7:31–37. doi:10.1007/BF00614387
8. Piafsky KM. Disease-induced changes in the plasma binding of basic drugs. *Clin Pharmacokinet*. 1980;5:246–262. doi:10.2165/00003088-198005030-00004
9. Benet LZ. The role of BCS (biopharmaceutics classification system) and BDDCS (biopharmaceutics drug disposition classification system) in drug development. *J Pharm Sci*. 2013;102:34–42. doi:10.1002/jps.23359
10. Du X, Li Y, Xia YL, et al. Insights into protein-ligand interactions: mechanisms, models, and methods. *Int J Mol Sci*. 2016;17(2):144. doi:10.3390/ijms17020144
11. Reidenberg MM, Affrime M. Influence of disease on binding of drugs to plasma proteins. *Ann N Y Acad Sci*. 1973;226:115–126. doi:10.1111/j.1749-6632.1973.tb20474.x
12. Dahlqvist R, Borga O, Rane A, et al. Decreased plasma protein binding of phenytoin in patients on valproic acid. *Br J Clin Pharmacol*. 1979;8:547–552. doi:10.1111/j.1365-2125.1979.tb01042.x
13. Cockcroft DW, Gault MH. Prediction of creatinine clearance from serum creatinine. *Nephron*. 1976;16:31–41. doi:10.1159/000180580
14. Traynor J, Mactier R, Geddes CC, et al. How to measure renal function in clinical practice. *Br Med J*. 2006;333(7577). doi:10.1136/bmj.39035.465174.68
15. Wagner JG, Northam JI. Estimation of volume of distribution and half-life of a compound after rapid intravenous injection. *J Pharm Sci*. 1967;56:529–531. doi:10.1002/jps.2600560424
16. Gibaldi M, Perrier D. *Pharmacokinetics*. 2nd ed. M. Dekker; 1982.

Pharmacodynamics

James Uchizono and Patrick Chan

INTRODUCTION

Chapter 2 focused on the pharmacokinetics (PK) of drugs within the body (absorption, distribution, metabolism, and elimination). In 2003, the Food and Drug Administration (FDA) elevated its standards and guidance[1] for new drugs that can be introduced into the marketplace. One such guidance requires both PK and pharmacodynamic (PD) analyses (prior to 2003, only PK analysis was required) to better ensure patient safety of these new drugs. Combining PK and PD (i.e., PK/PD) together provides the clinician with a more complete pharmacological understanding from dose to the observed response or effect. **Figure 3.1** illustrates the PK/PD general schematic.

In Figure 3.1B, the shorthand schematic shows how closely PK and PD are linked together with overlap in the compartment labeled "Ce." The time course of increased/decreased drug concentration [drug] in Ce is driven by the PK of the drug. Ultimately, changes in [drug] in Ce initiates the downstream pharmacological

pathways (PD pathways) that are responsible for the resulting drug effect or response. In Figure 3.1, clinicians provide the input (dose and frequency = regimen), while the body converts the regimen into the clinical response or effect.

In pharmacokinetics, the plot of drug concentration versus time (i.e., C vs. t) contains most of the relevant information to determine the PK parameters (e.g., Cl, F, V_d, k). In PD, the familiar plot, commonly called the "dose-response curve" in **Figure 3.2**, provides an easily accessible view of the relationship between dose and response.

In Figure 3.2, two commonly used curves for dose–response data are shown. Curve A shows a linear relationship and Curve B is a nonlinear relationship between dose and responses. Both curves are useful for clinicians because one or the other tends to reflect real-life experiences; however, there are underlying assumptions and governing principles that guide the choice of an appropriate-shaped curve. Further, when these assumptions are not true, the resulting dose versus response curves take on unusual characteristics and shapes. This chapter will only briefly discuss the more complex curves and their underlying assumptions. The variable E (for "effect"; substituted for "response" in the remainder of the chapter) represents the response, similarly to how "effect" is used in the common term *side effect*. The variable C is the concentration of drug, which is analogous to dose/volume in PK. When volume is constant, C is analogous to dose.

LINKING DOSE TO RESPONSE

The therapeutic goal is to understand how changes in dose alter the patient's response to that dosing change (see Figure 3.1). Clinically, two models

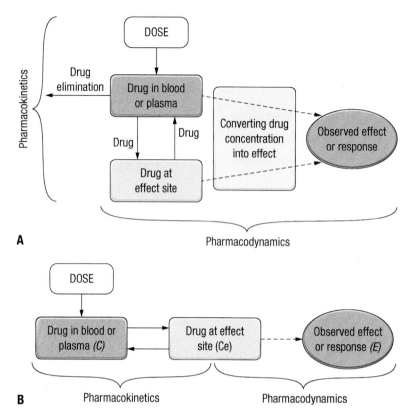

A

B

FIGURE 3.1 Relationship between dose and response in the pharmacokinetics and pharmacodynamics framework in longform (A) and shorthand (B).

Source: Sheiner LB, Stanski DR, Vozeh S, et al. Simultaneous modeling of pharmacokinetics and pharmacodynamics: application to *d*-tubocurarine. *Clin Pharmacol Ther.* 1979;25(3):358–371. doi:10.1002/cpt1979253358

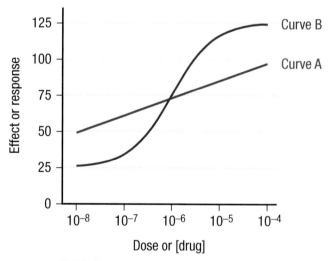

FIGURE 3.2 Response versus log_{10}[drug].

(linear effect or nonlinear E_{max} effect models) usually work well provided their underlying assumptions are upheld.[2] Many small molecules (molecular mass <~400 Da) can be described by these simple models because many small-molecule drugs work via a receptor system that produces the familiar sigmoidal curve (Curve B; Figure 3.2). Drugs that work by affecting pharmacological pathways (e.g., blocking the production of a critical protein necessary to produce the response) tend to have complex PD that usually do not produce the simple sigmoidal curve seen in Figure 3.2.

LINEAR MODEL

The linear model with baseline (Equation 3.1) relates the dose to the response with two parameters (E_0 and m) that describe a straight line and baseline.

$$E = E_0 + mC \qquad \text{(Equation 3.1)}$$

E is the measured or observed effect, E_0 is the baseline or effect in the absence of drug y-intercept of the E versus C line, and m is the slope of the line relating C (drug concentration) and E. This model works well over a smaller range of drug concentrations near the mid-range of clinical dose-responses. When C falls outside of this small range, it will fail to accurately predict E. For example, a dose cannot be increased infinitely to achieve higher and higher values of E; *at some point, the body will limit its response to the increased drug doses because the body has limited receptors, co-factors, energy stores, and other resources.*

E_{MAX} MODEL

The limitations of the linear model shown in Equation 3.1 led to the most popular PD nonlinear model, the E_{max} model[2,3] (Equation 3.2 and Figure 3.2 [Curve B]).

$$E = E_0 + \frac{E_{max}C^{\gamma}}{EC_{50}^{\gamma} + C^{\gamma}} \qquad \text{(Equation 3.2)}$$

E_0 is the baseline when no drug is present, E_{max} is the maximal effect that can be achieved, EC_{50}^{γ} describes the potency of the drug, and γ indicates if the drug exhibits positive, negative, or no cooperativity. **Figures 3.3 and 3.4** show the impact of different values of each of these parameters. When $C = 0$ (corresponding to no dose), the numerator is zero, leaving $E = E_0$. When C^{γ} (i.e., dose) is much larger than EC_{50}^{γ} (i.e., $C \gg EC_{50}^{\gamma}$), EC_{50}^{γ} is insignificant in the denominator and the fraction in Equation 3.2 becomes

$$E \approx E_0 + \frac{E_{max}C^{\gamma}}{EC_{50}^{\gamma} + C^{\gamma}} = E_0 + \frac{E_{max}C^{\gamma}}{C^{\gamma}}$$

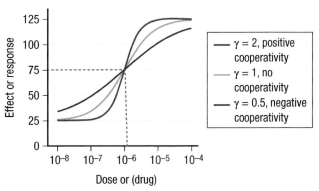

FIGURE 3.3 Influence of γ on the E_{max} model.

and the numerator and denominator C^{γ} terms cancel, leaving $E = E_0 + E_{max}$. In other words, when the dose is large, the observed E is the baseline plus the maximum effect achievable by the drug.

Noncompetitive and Competitive Antagonists

One benefit of the E_{max} model is its utility to describe clinical observations. The framework of the E_{max} model can help clinicians make therapeutic decisions. In the E_{max} model, there are four parameters (E_0, E_{max}, EC_{50}, γ) that describe or control the pharmacological effect. In pure noncompetitive antagonism, the antagonist drug reduces E_{max} and does not affect E_0, EC_{50}, or γ (see Figure 3.4B). The blue curve has no antagonist present, the green curve has some noncompetitive antagonism present, and the purple curve has the most noncompetitive antagonism. Note: The baseline (E_0), EC_{50}, and γ remain unchanged; only the maximum response, Emax, has been reduced by the antagonist. Conversely, when pure competitive antagonism is present, EC_{50}, increases (see Figure 3.4A, green = no antagonism). Note, as dose continues to increase, the effects of competitive antagonism can be overcome (i.e., E_{max} can still be reached). However, the antagonism of noncompetitive inhibitors

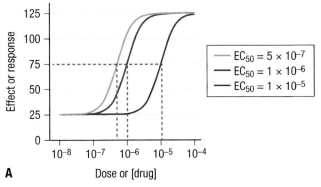

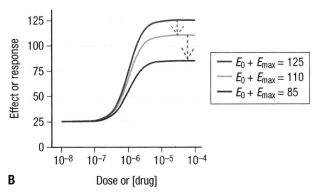

FIGURE 3.4 Competitive inhibition (A) and noncompetitive inhibition (B).
Source: Data adapted from Holford NH, Sheiner LB. Understanding the dose-effect relationship: Clinical application of pharmacokinetic-pharmacodynamic models. *Clin Pharmacokinet.* 1981;6(6):429–453. doi:10.2165/00003088-198106060-00002

cannot be overcome by increasing the dose. A more convoluted form of antagonism, uncompetitive inhibition, alters both E_{max} and EC_{50} is beyond the scope of this chapter, which will not be discussed here.

Clinical Observations Related to the E_{max} Model

The E_{max} model captures four major PD behaviors that clinicians observe in their patients, which usually manifest as clinical intuition. E_0 is the baseline or the measured effect without drug present. For example, if one is measuring a patient's pulse before administering epinephrine, E_0 would be the pulse prior to giving epinephrine. The E_{max} parameter is the maximum limit of the effect in response to the drug. In other words, as the patient is given larger and larger doses, at some point the increase in the dose does not improve or increase the effect. Hydrochlorothiazide (HCTZ) is a classic example of this. Diuresis does increase with increasing doses of HCTZ, but at some point, the amount of diuresis changes very little despite larger changes in dose (e.g., from 100 mg to 200 mg). In this example, HCTZ has reached its E_{max} at approximately 80 to 100 mg; no further diuresis is gained by increasing the dose.

Another parameter in this equation that is clinically useful is the EC_{50}, which is associated with the potency of the drug. The smaller the value of EC_{50}, the greater its potency. The EC_{50} is defined as the concentration of the drug (or "dose") that is needed to produce 50% of E_{max}. Comparing the EC_{50} of opioid analogs (e.g., morphine, fentanyl, and codeine) is clinically relevant. Fentanyl (most potent in this example) has the smallest EC_{50} value while codeine (least potent) has the largest. The last parameter in the E_{max} model is γ (also known as the Hill coefficient) and it accounts for effect or response behavior of the drug known as *cooperativity*. Drugs can exhibit positive cooperativity ($\gamma > 1$), negative cooperativity ($\gamma < 1$), or no cooperativity ($\gamma = 1$). Although cooperativity and sensitivity are pharmacologically different, clinically they are similar and changes in sensitivity are easier to clinically understand, so cooperativity will be loosely described as "sensitivity." Positive cooperativity (i.e., $\gamma > 1$) occurs when the "sensitivity" increases as drug exposure increases; negative cooperativity occurs when the "sensitivity" decreases as drug exposure increases. Many drugs behave with no cooperativity (i.e., $\gamma = 1$), meaning the amount of drug exposure does not increase or decrease future response(s). Figure 3.3 shows how each of these parameters affect the shape of the concentration versus effect curves.

COMPLEX PHARMACODYNAMIC BEHAVIORS AND LIMITATIONS

In the clinical setting, while the E_{max} model does work reasonably well for small-molecule drugs (molecular weight 400–800 Da) where the blood or effect compartment rapidly equilibrate to produce the desired effect or response, there are other more complex PD behaviors that cannot be well described by an E_{max} model. For example, many patients develop drug tolerance to morphine (or other opioids). A similar phenomenon occurs in many patients in the Intensive Care Unit (ICU) with the medications ("drips") used to optimize heart function. In both cases, the clinician considers whether to increase the medication dose to achieve the similar outcome previously achieved with a lower dose prior to the patient's body developing drug tolerance. The E_{max} model as written in Equation 3.2 cannot describe this PD behavior.

Other complex behaviors or limitations poorly described by the E_{max} model are patient responses to macromolecule therapies (e.g., antibody therapy, DNA/RNA therapies, most therapies where the drug is a protein). The complexity of these macromolecule therapies frequently requires models known as "indirect models" or models with mathematical sophistication to describe the significant complexity. Other examples of clinically relevant clinically PD behaviors[4,5] include: circadian rhythms, all-or-none responses, tachyphylaxis, and hypersensitivity reactions. In therapeutic regimens involving complex PD behavior, indirect models or other models known as "differential equation models"[6] may be needed to appropriately model the PD.

CASE EXEMPLAR: Patient With Syncope

OH is a 76-year-old White male with a history of osteoarthritis who presents for a follow-up of his urinary symptoms. He has a history of benign prostatic hypertrophy with frequent nocturia, approximately three to four times per night. OH was started on a medicine to help with his symptoms, but he has not been tolerating it well. Even though his clinician told him it was a "small dose," he keeps fainting when he stands up too fast. Even after his first dose he fainted and fell.

Past Medical History
- Osteoarthritis
- Benign prostatic hypertrophy (BPH)
- Osteoporosis

Medications
- Terazosin, 2 mg at bedtime
- Acetaminophen, 500 mg, two tablets two to four times per day as needed for pain

Physical Examination
- Height: 73 inches; weight: 152 lbs.; blood pressure: 92/60 mmHg; pulse: 82; respiration rate: 16; temperature: 97.2 °F
- BP drops to 80/48 when standing, and pulse rises to 108
- Lungs: Clear
- Heart: Regular rate and rhythm

Labs
- Prostate-specific antigen (PSA): Normal
- Complete blood count (CBC): Normal

Discussion Questions
1. Terazosin is known to cause orthostatic hypotension. What risk factors does OH have for this reaction?
2. Terazosin is among a group of several medications that are known for the "first-dose effect." What does this mean?
3. Given the pharmacodynamics of terazosin demonstrated by OH, what alternatives exist for his treatment?

CASE EXEMPLAR: Patient With Pulmonary Embolism

BC is a 48-year-old female patient following up after a pulmonary embolism. She had been in her usual state of health until 2 months ago when, after a long transoceanic flight, she experienced sudden onset of right-sided severe chest pain, shortness of breath, and cough. She was transported to a local emergency department where she was diagnosed with a deep vein thrombosis and a right-sided pulmonary embolus. BC was treated initially with heparin, and warfarin was initiated shortly thereafter. She was ultimately discharged on warfarin therapy. She has had some difficulties maintaining a therapeutic level with her anticoagulation and is in today for advice.

Past Medical History
- Gravida 2 para 2, last menstrual period 3 weeks ago
- Deep vein thrombosis with pulmonary embolus

Medications
- Warfarin, 5 mg daily

Physical Examination
- Well-developed, well-nourished female in no distress
- No significant findings

Labs
- International normalized ratio (INR): 2.5

Discussion Questions
1. Most patients require anywhere between 3 and 10 days to achieve a therapeutic INR after initiation of warfarin therapy. Why is there such a wide range?
2. What factors negatively impact the clinical response to warfarin?
3. What factors heighten the clinical response to warfarin?

CLINICAL PEARLS

- Combining PK and PD (i.e., PK/PD) together provides the clinician with a more complete pharmacological understanding, from dose to the observed response or effect.
- The therapeutic goal is to understand how changes in dose alter the patient's response to that dosing change.
- Many small molecules can be described by simple models of pharmacodynamics because they work via a receptor system that produces the familiar sigmoidal dose–response curve.
- Drugs that work by affecting pharmacological pathways (e.g., blocking the production of a critical protein necessary to produce the response) tend to have more complex pharmacodynamics.
- The clinical significance of antagonism is that the effects of noncompetitive inhibitors cannot be overcome by increasing the dose, whereas increasing the dose can overcome competitive inhibition.

KEY TAKEAWAYS

- FDA guidelines require both PK and PD analyses for new drugs to better ensure patient safety.
- The time course of increased or decreased drug concentration is driven by the PK of the drug, while the resulting drug effect is driven by PD pathways.
- The E_{max} model captures four major PD behaviors that clinicians observe in their patients, which usually manifest as clinical intuition.
- Complex behaviors or limitations poorly described by the E_{max} model are patient responses to macromolecule therapies (e.g., antibody therapy, DNA/RNA therapies, most therapies where the drug is a protein).

REFERENCES

1. Exposure-Response Working Group. *Guidance for Industry: Exposure-Response Relationships—Study Design, Data Analysis, and Regulatory Applications*. U.S. Department of Health and Human Services; 2003. https://www.fda.gov/media/71277/download
2. Holford NH, Sheiner LB. Understanding the dose-effect relationship: clinical application of pharmacokinetic-pharmacodynamic models. *Clin Pharmacokinet*. 1981;6(6):429–453. doi:10.2165/00003088-198106060-00002
3. Williams PJ, Uchizono JA, Ette EI. Pharmacometric knowledge-based oncology drug development. In: Figg WD, McLeod HL, eds. *Handbook of Anticancer Pharmacokinetics and Pharmacodynamics*. Humana Press/Springer; 2004:149–167. doi:10.1007/978-1-59259-734-5_11
4. Uchizono JA, Lane J. Empirical pharmacokinetic/pharmacodynamic models. In: Ette EI, Williams PJ, eds. *Pharmacometrics: The Science of Quantitative Pharmacology*. John Wiley & Sons; 2007:529-545.
5. Mager D, Jusko W. Mechanistic pharmacokinetic/pharmacodynamic models II. In: Ette EI, Williams PJ, eds. *Pharmacometrics: The Science of Quantitative Pharmacology*. John Wiley & Sons; 2007:607–631. doi:10.1002/9780470087978.ch23
6. Gabrielsson J, Weiner D. *Series: Pharmacokinetic & Pharmacodynamic Data Analysis: Concepts and Applications*. 5th ed. Swedish Pharmaceutical Press; 2017.

Pharmacogenetics and Pharmacogenomics

Kevin C. O'Connor, Xiaodong Feng, and Brent Luu

LEARNING OBJECTIVES

- Formulate a rational diagnostic workup for a patient requiring pharmacological intervention related to their genomic makeup.
- Select a drug from a class of drugs likely to be effective for a patient based on their pharmacogenomic profile.
- Classify a patient based on their predicted rate of metabolism of a drug based on their pharmacogenomic profile.
- Predict which patients from a cohort of patients are more likely to develop adverse events from a drug based on their pharmacogenomic profile.
- Describe the various ways in which the patient's genetic makeup might influence drug reactions.
- Recall the ways that a patient's genome might affect drug metabolism.

INTRODUCTION: PHARMACOGENETICS VERSUS PHARMACOGENOMICS

Since the publication of the full mapping of the human genome in April 2003 from the international collaborative Human Genome Project (HGP),[1] literature related to the human genome has grown drastically. Research interest of this field within the scientific community has elevated to a new height. In addition, the previously used terminologies have also evolved. Historically, *pharmacogenetics* is a term that was introduced in the late 1950s by an American geneticist, Arno Motulsky, which has been used to define the variability of drug responses due to a person's heredity.[2] It refers to the study

of gene(s) that determine the drug metabolism. As the whole human genome was unfolded, the term *pharmacogenomics (PGx)* emerged, which covers a broader meaning that includes all genes in the genome that may influence drug responses.[3] In other words, *pharmacogenetics* is the study of genetic variation in drug response at the individual gene level, whereas *pharmacogenomics* involves all genes in the genome.[4] *Pharmacogenomics* is now an important aspect of precision medicine, in which it studies how the genetic makeup of a patient may determine their drug responses.[5] Clinicians are now able to use PGx information to decide which drug treatment will be most appropriate for a specific patient; which medication to avoid to prevent serious adverse drug reactions; or which drug needs to have a dose adjustment and close monitoring for a specific population. Not only has PGx assisted clinicians in decision-making during a drug therapy, but it has opened new windows in drug development processes and opportunities for new targeted drug discovery.[5]

BACKGROUND

As early as 510 BCE, Pythagoras, an ancient Greek philosopher, noticed the inter-individual differences in responding to a certain food. He observed that some patients developed hemolytic anemia after ingesting fava beans.[3,6,7] Therefore, he may be thought of as one of the earliest pioneers in the field of PGx. In retrospect, we now can postulate that it was likely a result of a glucose-6-dehyrogenase (G6PD) deficiency.[3]

By the late 1950s, Werner Kalow at the University of Toronto discovered abnormal butyrylcholinesterase enzyme in psychiatric patients who experienced prolonged paralysis after the neuromuscular blocking agent succinylcholine was administered before electroconvulsive therapy.[8] During the same period, Beutler served that African American males who were treated with primaquine for malaria developed hemolytic anemia with alarming frequency. Subsequently, the relationship between this adverse drug reaction and G6PD deficiency was established.[7,9,]

By the 1960s, important work was being done by David Pryce Evans and his team at Johns Hopkins. They pursued a genetic linkage to previous reports of genetic variation in the N-acetylation of isoniazid, which was used to treat tuberculosis.[10] In the mid-1970s, important discoveries noted that certain ethnic groups were "slow acetylators" who demonstrated variations in their abilities to metabolize the anti-tuberculosis drug isoniazid.[7,11,] Research on this phenomenon continued, and by 1999 this slow acetylation, and a resultant peripheral neuropathy seen in some patients, was clearly associated with diversity of the enzyme N-acetyltransferase.[7,12,]

Because of this *genotype–phenotype* relationship observed in drug metabolism, scientists continued to explore the *polymorphism* of a trait and distinguish between common and rare phenotypes, which occur by spontaneous mutations. *Phenotype* is the corresponding observations or character trait(s) that are expressed by the presence of the specific genotype within the organism. Meanwhile, *genotype* is the set of genes of an organism or group of organisms that determines and influences a specific characteristic or trait. These are hereditary genetic materials transmitted from gametes, which are mature haploid germ cells from both male and female in sexual reproduction.[13] Nevertheless, the phenotypical expression of an organism may also involve other factors beyond the genotype of the organism including cellular environment, mechanical forces, symbionts, temperature, and many others.[13] In other words, the genotype of an organism is only one of the many factors that leads to the expression of its phenotype. In the mid-1980s, scientists arbitrarily defined that if the frequency of a trait is greater than 1%, it is considered as a common trait in the spectrum of polymorphism. When the frequency of a trait is expressed less than 1% within a population, it would be considered as a rare phenotype that occurs by spontaneous mutations. However, this grouping of phenotypes did not specify if the genotypes are heterozygous or homozygous.[14]

Researchers once thought the human genome shared 99.9% of the same DNA sequences. It is this 0.1% of the differences that contribute to the human's phenotypic diversity.[15] However, as new technologies and techniques become available, many more variations were identified; for example, the Copy Number Variations (CNVs), relatively newly identified genetic variations, revealed as deletions and/or duplications of 1 kb or larger of DNA fragments that are found throughout the entire genome.[15] Moreover, these variants are thought to play important roles in disease susceptibility and the ability for human individuals to adapt to the surrounding environment.[15] Other forms of polymorphisms may involve smaller insertions or deletions of DNA sequence, variable numbers of repetitive sequences, or structural alterations.[16]

The discovery of the even more precise element of single-nucleotide polymorphisms (SNPs) has also been described. This is the most common type of variation among individuals. SNP occurs on an average of once per every 1,000 nucleotides within a person's genome, which translates to approximately 4 to 5 million of SNP in the whole human DNA.[17] These variations in a single nucleotide may be unique or occur in many individuals. Thus far, scientists have identified more than 100 million SNPs worldwide from various human populations.[18] Most of these SNPs have no effect on the person's health or development; however, many SNPs have been found to associate with drug responses or susceptibility to developing certain diseases or reactions. As a result, these SNPs can be used as a tracking tool to trace hereditary diseases within families or measure risk of an individual developing certain diseases.[18]

GENOMIC DATABASES

There are two robust, nationally accessible reference databases that classify and annotate genomic variation: the Clinical Pharmacogenetics Implementation Consortium (CPIC) and the Pharmacogenomics Knowledgebase, PharmGKB.[19]

CPIC was established in 2009 (https://cpicpgx.org). It is a shared project between the PharmGKB (www.pharmgkb.org) and the Pharmacogenomics Research Network (PGRN). It is unique in that it provides evidence-based genotype-based drug guidelines and clinical recommendations to the end-user, thus linking the genetic laboratory test results to clinically relevant and actionable prescribing guidance. CPIC guidelines help clinicians understand how the results of genetic tests can be used in optimizing drug treatment. The levels of recommendations are shown in **Figure 4.1**.

The key underlying assumption for all CPIC guidelines is that clinical high-throughput and preemptive genotyping will eventually become common practice and clinicians will increasingly have patients' genotypes available before a prescription is written.[20] These guidelines closely follow the National Academy of Medicine's Standards. Their recommendations are free and readily accessible at https://cpicpgx.org/guidelines and www.guidelines.gov.

Another national effort that has drawn much attention is the National Institutes of Health (NIH) National Human Genome Research Institute (NHGRI)–funded Clinical Genome Resource, ClinGen. ClinGen is a collaborative effort from over 29 countries with more than 970 contributors.[21] The effort's goal is to enhance patient care through genomic medicine and build a

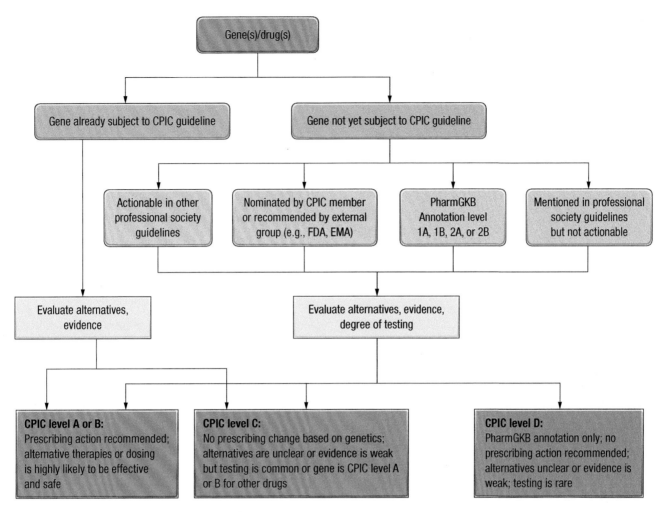

FIGURE 4.1 Considerations for assignment of CPIC level for genes/drugs.
CPIC, Clinical Pharmacogenetics Implementation Consortium; EMA, European Medicines Agency; FDA, Food and Drug Administration; PharmGKB, Pharmacogenomics Knowledgebase.
Source: PharmGKB. https://cpicpgx.org/prioritization

knowledge base that is clinically relevant by sharing information among the stakeholders, patients, clinicians, laboratories, and researchers.

All of these initiatives are noncommercial, national efforts with the central goal of integrating pharmacogenomic test results in clinical information systems with clinical decision support (CDS) tools to facilitate the application of patient genomic data at the point of care.[19]

VARIATIONS OF ENZYMES IN DRUG METABOLISM

Drug metabolism generally involves conversion of substances into more easily excreted water-soluble forms. It takes place mostly in the hepatocytes and is divided into two primary categories: *Phase I reactions* (oxidation, reduction, and hydrolysis reactions) and *Phase II conjugation reactions* (e.g., addition of a glucuronyl or methyl group to the metabolite). Once drugs are metabolized

and ready for excretion, metabolism primarily occurs via the kidneys, hepatobiliary system, or lungs.

Phase I: Enzymes Metabolisms

Phase I, enzymes metabolisms, are implicated in 55% to 60% of all adverse drug reactions (ADRs). The most widely considered Phase I enzymes belong to the Cytochrome P450 superfamily. The prefix "Cyto" means "cell" and "chrome" means color. These enzymes contain an iron-porphyrin ring center. During the oxidation reaction, the oxidative state of iron in the porphyrin ring changes, resulting in a spectrophotometric absorption maximum observed at 450 nm, hence the name Cytochrome P450 (CYP450).

There are approximately 60 P450 proteins, which are categorized into 18 families and 43 subfamilies. CYP1, CYP2, and CYP3 are the main families involved in human drug metabolism.[22,23] In particular, CYP2D6, CYP2C9, and CYP2C19 are highly polymorphic and account for

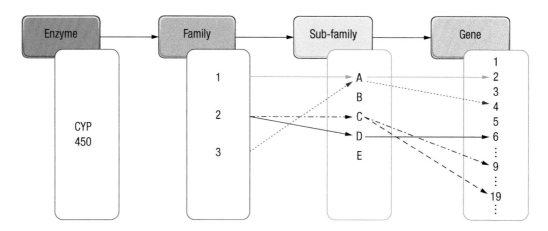

FIGURE 4.2 Summary of main families of cytochrome P450 involved in drug metabolism.

more than 40% of hepatic Phase I metabolism. How-ever, there are five specific CYP isoenzymes that me-tabolize 90% of all drugs, namely CYP1A2, CYP3A4, CYP2C9, CYP2C19, and CYP2D6 **(Figure 4.2)**.[24]

The "star system" is the most commonly used no-menclature in the CYP450 when referring to genes and variant (mutant) copies of genes. It was developed and implemented in the 1990s to describe variations of alleles and haplotypes of genes that are involved in absorption, distribution, metabolism, and elimination (ADME).[25] The gene is expressed in italics, which is then followed by a "star" and a number to indicate the sequence of the identified variant of the gene, which is then followed with a dot and a string of subvariant num-bers.[26] For example, the wild-type enzyme is expressed as *CYP1A2*1*, which indicates the first identified vari-ant of the gene. Any identified variant found after the *1 will be assigned a number following. In many cases, the *1 allele indicates the reference gene that was initially studied but does not necessarily imply the most com-mon allele in all populations.[4,25,26]

With respect to drug metabolism, there are four dif-ferent phenotypes observed, which categorize the ef-fects genetic polymorphisms have on individuals:

1. Poor Metabolizers (PM) have markedly reduced or lack of enzyme activity to metabolize the drug.
2. Intermediate Metabolizers (IM) have reduced enzyme activity.
3. Extensive Metabolizers (EM) have high enzyme activity.
4. Ultra-rapid Metabolizers (UM) have very high enzyme activity.

CYP1A2

The enzyme *CYP1A2* gene was sequenced and published in 1989.[27] It is one of the four enzymes that are responsi-ble for approximately 40% of all the drugs' metabolism[28];

however, individually, it metabolizes approximately 20% of clinically available drugs.[29] According to the Phar-macogene Variation Consortium report, 21 alleles have been reported.[26] There are at least nine variants with re-duced enzyme activity both in vivo and in vitro, namely *CYP1A2*1C, *1K, *3, *4, *7, *8, *11, *15, *16*.[26] Never-theless, the reported highly inducible variant was **1F*, which carries a C>A substitution at position –163 rela-tive to the "A" in the initiation codon (i.e., AUG).[30]

Typical substrates of *CYP1A2* include propranolol, clozapine, imatinib, thalidomide, leflunomide, lido-caine, theophylline, tizanidine, and zolpidem. Further-more, it is also a major enzyme activating many of the procarcinogens, such as polycyclic aromatic hydro-carbons or heterocyclic aromatic amines or amides.[29] As a result, the polymorphism of *CYP1A2* may play an important role in drug toxicities and malignancy asso-ciated with its many substrates; however, there is no CPIC guideline for *CYP1A2* at this point in time.

CYP3A4

The *CYP3A4* enzyme metabolizes approximately 40% to 50% of all medications used in clinical practice.[24] Currently, 34 variants of *CYP3A4* have been reported; however, eight variants (*CYP3A4*8, *11, *12, *13, *16A, *16B, *17,* and **22*) have shown reduced en-zyme activity mostly in vitro.[26] Extrapolating from the in vitro data, drug concentration of substrates that are metabolized by CYP3A4, such as calcium channel blockers, macrolide antibiotics, statins (simvastatin, lovastatin, atorvastatin), fentanyl, sufentanil, alfentanil, rivaroxaban, and apixaban, might be elevated in these patients. In addition, drug levels of neurokinin-1 (NK-1) receptor antagonists used in chemotherapy-induced nausea and vomiting, such as rolapitant, aprepitant and netupitant, might also be affected. Although the U.S. Food and Drug Administration (FDA) has not approved any biomarker screening test for the 3A4 enzyme, it is likely that screening tools will be recommended in the future as more data become available. Since 3A4 is one of the most abundant enzymes that plays a critical role in drug metabolism, enzyme inducers such as carbamazepine, phenobarbital, phenytoin, rifampin, and St. John's wort extract, or the inhibitors of 3A4, namely the "azole" antifungal agents such as ketoconazole or itraconazole, protease inhibitors (indinavir, nelfinavir, ritonavir) and macrolides (erythromycin or clarithromycin), may add more complications in patients who carry various variants of the defective enzyme.[24]

CYP2C9

The CYP2C9 is another important enzyme involved in drug metabolism. It is the second highest isoform of the CYP450 subfamilies in the liver and responsible for up to 20% of all drugs that undergo Phase I metabolism.[31] The substrates that are metabolized by 2C9 involve many drug classes such as anticoagulants, antihypertensives, nonsteroidal anti-inflammatory drugs, oral antihyperglycemics, or antiepileptics.[31,32]

CYP2C9 is a highly polymorphic enzyme. As of 2018, there have been 61 variants reported.[33] Studies have shown that many polymorphisms of CYP2C9 play significant roles in drug–drug interactions as well as drug metabolism in vivo. Some variants are found at higher frequency in a certain population relative to the others.[32] For example, the CYP2C9*2 variant is more common in White Europeans; however, the *3 variant has higher frequencies in the South Asian population. Meanwhile, CYP2C9*5, *8, *9, and *11 are more common in the African population.[32] Recently, the CYP2C9*61 variant has also been identified in Puerto Ricans who require low doses of warfarin (i.e., 3 mg/day).[33] Since these variants of CYP2C9 are associated with reduction of enzymatic activities, metabolic clearance of their substrates may be significantly affected; therefore, therapeutic dose reduction might be warranted in vivo, especially for agents that have narrow therapeutic index, such as warfarin and phenytoin.[32,33] In fact, studies have shown that CYP2C9*2 and *3 impair the metabolism of S-warfarin up to 40% and 90%, respectively.[34] Patients who carry one or two alleles of these variants will have higher risk of bleeding while taking warfarin and require a lower dose to achieve a therapeutic international normalized ratio (INR). Most FDA-approved CYP2C9 panels include *2 and *3 variants, which may not be applicable for patients with African ancestry; thus, an expanded panel should be ordered to capture the other variants (i.e., *5, *6, *8, and *11). The current CPIC guidelines recommended dose reduction by as much as 30% of the calculated dose of warfarin when these variants are detected.[34]

CYP2C19

Proton pump inhibitors (PPIs) are widely used to treat a variety of acid-related disorders such as peptic ulcer disease, gastro-esophageal reflux disease (GERD), and Helicobacter pylori infections. PPIs are cleared in the liver, primarily by CYP2C19, and to a lesser extent by CYP3A4. At traditional standard doses, there is compelling evidence that poor metabolizers (PM) have the highest drug concentrations and the greatest response rates. Meanwhile, IM, RM (rapid metabolizers), and UM have progressively lower drug concentrations and poorer response rates. This is particularly true for omeprazole, lansoprazole, and pantoprazole, which are highly dependent on CYP2C19 for their metabolism.[35] Clearly, a genotype-guided dosing of PPIs would be likely to optimize both the efficacy and safety of patients.[35] As of the writing of this chapter, 35 variants of CYP2C19 have been reported, of which there are five variants that resulted in nonfunctional enzyme with definitive level of evidence, namely CYP2C19*2.002, *2.003, *3.002, *4.001, and *35.001.[26] The current CPIC guidelines have not recommended screening for CYP2C19 polymorphism in patients who are taking PPI; however, they are recommended for patients taking SSRI, TCA, voriconazole, and clopidogrel.[36] Decreased doses of citalopram, escitalopram, and sertraline are recommended in patients who are known to be CYP2C19 poor metabolizers. In these cases, paroxetine and fluvoxamine could possibly be alternative options, as they are metabolized by another enzyme, CYP2D6.[37]

Furthermore, clopidogrel is a thienopyridine antiplatelet prodrug used for prevention of atherothrombotic events. Its active metabolites selectively and irreversibly inhibit adenosine diphosphate-induced platelet aggregation. This oxidation reaction is processed chiefly by CYP2C19, which converts the parent compound to its active thiol metabolite. Patients who have CYP2C19 polymorphisms experience variations in drug response. For instance, patients with CYP2C19*2 alleles are at increased risk for cardiovascular events, since the antiplatelet activity is greatly reduced, as the oxidation reaction was compromised. This is particularly significant with acute coronary syndrome managed by percutaneous coronary intervention (PCI). The CPIC recommends using alternative agents (such as prasugrel or ticagrelor) for the PM or IM undergoing PCI. Fortunately, for other indications, such as atrial fibrillation and stroke, the effect of CYP2C19*2 is less significant.[38]

CYP2D6

Perhaps the most appropriate polymorphic gene to illustrate how pharmacogenomics can have a profound impact on patient care is CYP2D6. This enzyme was estimated to be involved in approximately 25% of all drug metabolism; 119 different variants have been identified.[4,26] The variants that expressed as poor metabolizers are CYP2D6*3, *4, *5, and *6 in Caucasians but CYP2D6*17 in Black people.[4] Since codeine is a pro-drug that metabolized by CYP2D6 to morphine, patients with variants expressed as poor metabolizers have poor analgesic response.[4,39] On the contrary, patients who have high or very high enzyme activity (i.e., EM or UM) would quickly convert codeine to morphine; therefore, they have enhanced analgesic effects and risk for toxicities or overdose.

Other opioid analgesics such as tramadol, oxycodone, and hydrocodone can also be affected by this enzyme. Although the parent compounds of these agents have some biological activities, their enzymatic metabolism by *CYP2D6* provide even more potent metabolites. Tramadol is converted into *O*-desmethyltramadol, oxycodone to the active metabolite oxymorphone, and hydrocodone into hydromorphone.[40]

Clinicians must always guard against any assumption that a patient is "dishonest" when the anticipated effects of these agents are not realized. It may be simply that science has not caught up with them. Landmark case-reports include a 13-day infant who died from morphine toxicity via breastfeeding from the mother with *CYP2D6* ultra-rapid metabolizing activity, who was prescribed "appropriate" doses of codeine.[41] In addition, tramadol-related respiratory depression was reported in both a child with obstructive sleep apnea[42] and in an adult with kidney failure[43]—both patients had ultra-rapid metabolic phenotype due to *CYP2D6* gene duplications.

CYP2D6 polymorphisms also significantly impact the efficacy and safety of selective serotonin reuptake inhibitors (SSRIs). For example, paroxetine is not recommended in UM or PM because significant drug exposure may be reduced for the UM while elevated for the PM. Fluvoxamine is another example that requires a 25% to 50% reduction of dosage in PM of *CYP2D6*. In such cases, citalopram, escitalopram, or sertraline may be good alternatives, as they are metabolized by *CYP2C19*.[37] Of course, that is assuming the patient does not also have other variants of *CYP2C19*.

In addition to the catabolism of SSRIs and opioids, *CYP2D6* also activates tamoxifen, a chemotherapeutic drug, to its active form endoxifen, inside the cell. This active metabolite is known to display nearly 100-fold antiestrogenic potency compared to the parent compound.[44] As a result, genetic variations of *CYP2D6* can also provide varying therapeutic outcomes.[45] The current CPIC guidelines recommended alternative therapies such as aromatase inhibitor or using higher dose of tamoxifen (e.g., 40 mg/day) for patients who are PM, IM, or NM (normal metabolizers).[44]

DPYD

Dihydropyrimidine dehydrogenase (DPD), encoded by the *DPYD* gene, is the first and rate-limiting step in pyrimidine catabolism. It is also paramount to the elimination of fluoropyrimidine chemotherapy drugs. Three fluoropyrimidine drugs are commonly used to treat solid tumors such as breast and colorectal cancers. 5-Fluorouracil (5-FU), capecitabine, and tegafur (not available in the United States) all have 5-FU as their active component. Capecitabine and tegafur are oral prodrugs, which metabolized to 5-FU after administration. Typically, only 1% to 3% of the 5-FU is converted to the active cytotoxic metabolites, while 80% are degraded and the remaining are eliminated renally.[46]

The most commonly observed polymorphism of the *DPYD* gene is *DPYD*2A*, which can lead to significantly reduced clearances of 5-FU. This results in risk of severe dose-dependent fluoropyrimidine toxicity, such as myelosuppression, neurotoxicity, hand and foot syndrome, mucositis, and diarrhea. The current CPIC guidelines recommended to reduce dose of fluoropyrimidine by 25% to 50% for patients who are IM, while avoiding use for those who are PM or have an enzyme activity score of 0.5 or 0.[46] Although the 5-FU related toxicities have been consistently found to associate with various *DPYD* variants, not all patients with decreased or non-functional enzyme variants developed toxicity. Meanwhile, patients without decreased or nonfunctional enzyme variants may still develop severe toxicity due to other genetic or environmental factors.[46] Therefore, the current genetic testing only detects selected variants with decreased or nonfunctional enzymatic activity but does not fully explain whom will develop severe toxicities.

Phase-II ("Conjugating") Enzymes

In Phase II metabolism, the elimination of drugs is primarily affected by the nonfunctional enzymes; therefore, the issues with drug toxicities are commonly observed. However, during Phase I reactions, both activation and elimination are affected.

Uridine 5′-Diphosphoglucuronosyl Transferase 1

The uridine 5′-diphosphoglucuronosyl transferase 1 gene (*UGT1A1*) conjugates glucuronic acid onto lipophilic molecules such as bilirubin, and onto many drug substrates, so they can be more readily excreted into bile. While polymorphisms of *UGT1A1* are relatively rare, one particular allele stands out—the *28* allele. The homozygous *UGT1A1*28* carriers are recognized to have Gilbert's syndrome.[47] This condition is generally benign, but many such patients will have increased levels of unconjugated bilirubin. Patients with this variant could be at an increased risk for adverse drug reactions with *UGT1A1* drug substrates.[38] One such drug is irinotecan, a chemo-agent, which metabolizes into a cytotoxic metabolite, SN-38. It is used commonly for metastatic carcinoma of the colon or rectum. Since the inactivation of the SN-38 is carried out via *UGT1A1*, patients with *UGT1A1*28* variant are thus at increased risk for life-threatening toxicities such as neutropenia and diarrhea.[38]

Uridine 5′-Diphosphoglucuronosyl Transferase 2B7

Uridine 5′-diphosphoglucuronosyl transferase 2B7 (*UGT2B7*) is involved in the conversion of morphine into morphine-3-glucuronide (M3G) and the active metabolite morphine-6-glucuronide (M6G). It has been suggested that *UGT2B7* polymorphisms may be implicated in morphine-associated nausea, but thus far studies were still inconclusive.[40]

Thiopurine S-Methyltransferase

Thiopurine *S*-methyltransferase (*TPMT*) is responsible for the deactivation of thiopurine drugs, which include mercaptopurine, thioguanine, and azathioprine (a prodrug for mercaptopurine). These are antineoplastic and immunosuppressive agents used to treat a variety of cancers, as well as inflammatory bowel diseases. Because of its clinical importance, *TPMT* was the first gene selected by the FDA for public hearings if it should be included in drug labeling. Subsequently, the clinical testing for the gene is now widely available and applied.[48]

Genetic variation in the *TPMT* gene leading to enzymatic deficiency is associated with a potentially life-threatening myelosuppression because this enzyme catalyzes *S*-methylation reaction that inactivates the thiopurine drugs. The most common variants involve *TPMT*2, *3A*, and *3C*; furthermore, the homozygous *3A* is found in 1 of 300 people of European descent.[2] This mutation results in misfolding, which in turn leads to rapid degradation of the enzyme. When patients have *TPMT* deficiency, they cannot inactivate mercaptopurine and thioguanine; instead, these drugs are converted into thioguanine nucleotides (TGNs). The buildup of TGNs may lead to potentially fatal myelosuppression in 100% of cases.[48] Consequently, patients would have a lack of enzyme and the ability to metabolize thiopurines. They may develop up to 10-fold increase of drug level of these cytotoxic agents when a "standard" dose is administered.[2] Patients who carry only one allele of the inactive variants may have reduced enzyme activity; therefore, they are still at increased risk of serious myelosuppression.[48]

Glucose-6-Phosphate Dehydrogenase

Glucose-6-phosphate dehydrogenase (G6PD) is an important enzyme involved in the pentose phosphate pathway (PPP), which converts glucose to pentose for nucleic acid synthesis.[49] Within the PPP, nicotinamide adenine dinucleotide phosphate (NADP+) undergoes reduction to form NADPH, which is a "protectant" that prevents cells from oxidative damages, especially on red blood cells (RBCs). Individuals who have G6PD deficiency are at high risk for hemolytic anemia when RBCs are exposed to stressors such as infection, ingestion of fava beans, or taking drugs such as primaquine, dapsone, or rasburicase.[49] The *G6PD* gene is located on the X-chromosome; more than 200 variants have been identified. Therefore, males who carry a single mutated allele will express G6PD deficiency. However, females must have a homozygous genotype to develop G6PD deficiency. Females with heterozygous genotype may develop a 50:50 ratio of deficient to normal RBCs.[49,50]

Polygenic Effects

Polygenic effects refer to traits that are determined by multiple genes, usually at different loci on different chromosomes. Perhaps the best example of such effect is seen with *CYP2C9* and *VKORC1*. It had been long established that a narrow therapeutic medication, warfarin, was subject to variable responses. Interpatient differences in dosing requirements can be as much as 20-fold![38] This was partly associated with variable *CYP2C9* metabolism. However, variants in *VKORC1* which encode a subunit of the vitamin K epoxide reductase complex (the target of warfarin) may cause different levels of sensitivity toward warfarin.[51] These variants have been found to account for 21% of drug variability, versus 6% in *CYP2C9*.[52] Patients with decreased *VKORC1* expression are at increased risk for excessive anticoagulation with standard warfarin dosing. This is also seen with reduced function of *CYP2C9* genotypes. When both polymorphisms exist in the same patient, the risk of serious bleeding is tremendously increased.

In 2008, the FDA recommended that manufacturers update the package insert for warfarin to include the application of pharmacogenomics to warfarin dosing. They "recommended" testing for CYP2C9, VKORC1, as well as Protein C deficiency. There are three broad categories of FDA packaging requirements: "Test Required," "Test Recommended," and "Information Only." Detailed FDA recommendations can be found at: www.fda.gov/Drugs/ScienceResearch/ucm572698.htm.

VARIATIONS IN TRANSPORTERS

In addition to mutations of enzymes involved in the elimination of drugs, other variations seen in humans are mutations in transport proteins. These transport proteins are often seen at the apical membranes of cells which interact most specifically with xenobiotic compounds such as intestinal enterocytes, hepatocytes, and renal epithelium—even endothelial cells forming the blood–brain barrier. They mediate selective permeability.

Transporters are generally categorized into ATP-binding cassette (ABC) and solute carrier (SLC) transporters. ABC and SLC are super-families of membrane-bound transport proteins that are involved in the absorption, distribution, and elimination of drugs. ABC proteins are exclusively involved in efflux, or waste elimination, whereas SLC proteins can be involved in both efflux and influx activities.[37]

ATP-Binding Cassette Transporters

The ATP-binding cassette superfamily transports drugs and other substances against the concentration gradient, using ATP as an energy source. They include over 50 genes, divided into seven subfamilies, from *ABCA* to *ABCG*.

ABCB1 (a.k.a. Multi-Drug Resistance 1 or P-Glycoprotein)

ABCB1 (also known as P-glycoprotein, or "Pgp") is a membrane-bound, ATP-dependent transport system which is responsible for the efflux of many xenobiotics, including numerous chemotherapeutic agents, metabolites, and carcinogens, from cells out to the extracellular fluids. If this transporter is over-expressed in cancer cells, a profound chemo-resistance is seen; therefore, it is also named "multi-drug resistance 1 (MDR1)."[7] Other names of this transporter include: ABC20, CD243, CLCS, GP170, and PGY1.[53]

An interesting example of *ABCB1* variation playing an important and clinically relevant role can be seen in patients who experience nausea with chemotherapy. Two variants, the CG haplotype (*C3435T* and *G2677T*), have been identified in patients who were more likely to experience chemotherapy-induced nausea and vomiting despite appropriate treatment with ondansetron. Researchers suggested that the CG haplotype was associated with greater *ABCB1* expression. Patients with these variants might have a decrease in levels of CNS accumulation of ondansetron (i.e., not efficiently crossing the blood–brain barrier), thus demonstrating variation in the genotype of transport proteins.[54] The *ABCB1* variants have also been implicated with a large variety of morphine-associated adverse events, including nausea and vomiting, as well as sweating and sedation.[40]

ABCB1 rs1045642 (GG) has been shown to be associated with a higher incidence of drug-resistant epilepsy, which suggests that some anti-epileptic drugs' ability to cross the blood–brain barrier may be impacted by *ABCB1* function. It is believed that this association goes beyond the single implication for phenytoin.[37]

ABCC1/C2

The *ABCC1/C2* are involved in transport and excretion of several chemotherapeutic agents and organic anion molecules. Both require glutathione cotransporter to transport certain substances, such as estrone sulfate. Allelic variants have been associated with differences in response to doxorubicin in non-Hodgkin's lymphoma patients.[55] The role of *ABCC2* variants is also highly studied in drug resistance development in cancer and HIV-infected patients.[56]

ABCG2

ABCG2 was first discovered in multidrug-resistant cell lines. *ABCG2* is also known as breast cancer resistance protein (BCRP), mitoxantrone resistance protein (MXR), or placenta-specific ABC protein.[57] The substrates of *ABCG2* are the inhibitors of epidermal growth factor receptor (EGFR) tyrosine kinase; that is, gefitinib. When there is a presence of the SNP *C421A* variant in the *ABCG2* gene, cancer patients treated with gefitinib developed drug accumulation, with a resultant significant increase in diarrhea as compared to patients with wild-type allele.[58]

Similarly, plasma levels of diflomotecan (chemotherapeutic agent) were tripled when heterozygous *C421A* was present.[59] However, this same variant can be beneficial in LDL-lowering efficacy of rosuvastatin in Chinese patients with hypercholesterolemia. The variant was found to be at a significantly lowered LDL level in a gene-dose-dependent manner. In other words, patients with *C421A* variant were able to suppress LDL level 6.9% more than the wildtype, which is approximately equivalent to doubling the dose of rosuvastatin.[60]

Solute-Carrier Transporters

SLC is a superfamily of transporters which contains over 360 genes, divided into 46 subfamilies. Of those 46, organic anion transporter (OAT), organic anion transporting polypeptides (OATP), and organic cation transporter (OCT) subfamilies are particularly relevant to the disposition of medications.[57]

SLC22A1

The *SLC22A1* gene has several well-established "loss-of-function" polymorphisms (*2, *3, *4, *5, *6). Any of these variants results in prolonged effects and increased toxicity at usual doses for both morphine and tramadol. When two or more loss-of-function polymorphisms are present, clearance is particularly impaired and toxicity is more frequent. *SLC22A1* deficient alleles may be especially relevant for patients who also carry the *CYP2D6* UM status, as both genetic variants lead to an increase in opioid toxicity and potentially severe effects.[40]

Organic Anion Transporting Polypeptides

OATPs are membrane-bound influx transporters, regulating cellular uptake of many substances, including bile salts, hormones, and drugs such as antibiotics, cardiac glycosides, and anti-cancer. There are 11 human OATP; for example, OATP1A2, OATP1B1, OATP1B3, OATP2B1, and OATPC all affect drug pharmacokinetics.[58] In particular, *OATPC*5* and *OATPC*9* variants are associated with reduced uptake of estrogens. Furthermore, the *AOTPC*5* allele is also associated with very high plasma levels of pravastatin.[61]

SLCO1B1

OATP1B1 is encoded by *SLCO1B1*, which is required for the hepatic uptake of the simvastatin acid, an active metabolite of simvastatin.[62] Simvastatin is a popular drug used to treat hyperlipidemia, which inhibits 3-hydroxy-3-methylglutaryl coenzyme A (HMG-CoA) reductase, the rate-limiting enzyme of cholesterol biosynthesis. A *SLCO1B1*5* variant (rs4149056) is associated with reduced OATP1B1 activity, which impaired the transportation of simvastatin into hepatic cells, thus leading to higher drug concentrations in blood.[63] Studies have shown patients who carry this variant have approximately 2.5- to-4.6-fold increase in risk of developing myopathy when a dose of simvastatin was given at 40 or 80 mg, respectively.[64]

Cough is the most common side effect of angiotensin-converting enzyme inhibitor (ACEI). The *SLCO1B1* gene variant *T521C* (Val174Ala, rs4149056) is well established to have a strong association with increased risk for enalapril-induced cough. *SLCO1B1* encodes the OATB1B1, which is involved with the hepatic drug clearance of enalapril. Since enalapril and other ACEIs are cleared less efficiently in patients carrying this variant, the plasma levels of the drug remain high, leading to a reduction of bradykinin breakdown (or accumulation of bradykinin) within the lungs and inducing cough.[65]

Organic Cation Transporters

OCTs are proteins encoded by the *SLC22A* family. Three isoforms are found in humans—OCT1, OCT2, and OCT3. OCT2 is highly expressed in the kidneys, which regulate the cellular uptake of drugs such as metformin, which is used in the treatment of type 2 diabetes mellitus. Since metformin is excreted principally by the kidneys, its drug level will be significantly affected by the variants of *OCT2*.[66,67,] The *rs316019 (c.808G>T)* is the most common variant of *SLC22A2*, which significantly reduces the clearance of metformin. The variant leads to a protein (p.270A>S) that is present in 15% or more of many populations. The 270S variant can clear metformin from the circulation much slower than the 270A form.[67] A patient who is homozygous for the *270A* variant will see a higher renal clearance and lower plasma concentration of metformin than a patient homozygous for the *270S* variant.[68] In other words, the change of 270A>S may further increase risk of metformin-associated lactic acidosis in patients carrying a homozygous genotype of this variant.[67]

VARIATIONS IN IMMUNE SYSTEM FUNCTION

HLA-B*57:01

Perhaps one of the well-known pharmacogenomic associations is between abacavir and *HLA-B*57:01*. Abacavir is a medication that is metabolized intracellularly into its active form, carbovir 5′-triphosphate (CBV-TP), by various enzymes and used to treat HIV infection.[69] CBV-TP inhibits HIV reverse transcriptase, which is critical to HIV replication. For most individuals, aba-

cavir is well-tolerated; however, 5% to 8% of patients experience a hypersensitivity reaction within the first month or two of treatment. Symptoms are initially mild (e.g., fever, rash, nausea), and they respond well to discontinuation of the abacavir. However, re-challenge with the drug can lead to potentially life-threatening hypersensitivity reactions. This phenomenon is strongly linked to an *HLA-B*57:01* variant.[48]

Multiple guidelines on CPIC and DPWG (Dutch Pharmacogenetics Working Group) have been published, which recommend the use of an alternate drug when patients with *HLA-B*57:01* variants are identified. In fact, the FDA-approved drug labeling for abacavir specifically states that genetic testing for this variant is required prior to initiating or reinitiating abacavir, and that the drug is contraindicated for patients with known *HLA-B*57:01*-positive serologic status.[48]

HLA-B*15:02

The *HLA-B*15:02* haplotype is associated with a four-fold increased risk for severe cutaneous adverse reactions with the use of phenytoin, a very common anti-epileptic drug.[70]

Another anti-seizure drug, carbamazepine, also induces high risk of developing Stevens–Johnson syndrome (SJS) or toxic epidermal necrolysis (TEN) in patients carrying *HLA-B*15:02* allele. In 2007, the FDA issued a Black-Box Warning that recommended testing for the *HLA-B*15:02* allele in patients with Asian Han ancestry before initiating the therapy.[7]

Interferon Lambda-3 (Interleukin-28B)

Interferon lambda-3 (IFNL3), also known as interleukin-28B (IL-28B), belongs to the family of type III interferon lambda cytokines. These cytokines help to mount antiviral responses in cells. The *IFNL3* gene has been found to have a very strong association with hepatitis C treatment responses to pegylated interferon with ribavirin. The *rs12979860* variant near *IFNL3* is thought to be the strongest predictor of a cure for patients with HCV-1 receiving this therapy. This favorable allele is inherited most frequently in Asians (90%).[38]

Mu-Opioid Receptor Gene

Opiates and opioids such as morphine and fentanyl exert their analgesic effect primarily via the mu-opioid-receptor (MOR), which is encoded by the mu-opioid receptor (*OPRM1*) gene. The most prominent variant of this gene is *118A>G*. Carriers of the *OPRM1 118A>G* variant have a higher opioid requirement and a lower risk for adverse events. Interestingly, this seems to be the case with morphine, alfentanil, and oxycodone. However, the effect of the genetic variant seems inconclusive for codeine, tramadol, and sufentanil. This genetic variant of *OPRM1* may serve as a potential biomarker for use in clinical practice. Although the current evidence of mu-opioid receptor gene is less conclusive than in other genetic variants (e.g., *CYP2D6* and *SLC22A1*), the polymorphism of *OPRM1* may factor in significantly for opioid selection and dosing guidelines.[40]

Catechol-*O*-Methyltransferase

With respect to pain management research, the *COMT* gene is one of the most frequently analyzed candidates, after *OPRM1* and *CYP2D6*. It codes for the enzyme catechol-*O*-methyltransferase (*COMT*), which has shown to regulate the expression of MOR and the perception of pain.[40,71,] Nevertheless, the studies on COMT genetic variability and opioid therapy have been controversial and non-conclusive. More research is necessary to better understand the importance of the polymorphism of this enzyme in pain management.

DRUG–DRUG INTERACTIONS AND GENETIC POLYMORPHISM

Evidence demonstrates that an individuals' pharmacogenomic signatures can have a profound effect on how drugs are metabolized by enzymes or transported into or out of cells by various transporters. The polymorphisms of enzymes in drug metabolism and protein transporter genes are important risk factors of drug–drug interactions and interindividual drug responses.[72] Furthermore, a given drug level may elevate even more following the co-administration of an enzyme inhibitor, while the patient is carrying a genotype that significantly impacts drug metabolism. For example, voriconazole (an antifungal) is metabolized by *CYP3A4* and *CYP2C19*. Ritonavir (an antiviral) strongly inhibits *CYP3A4* and induces *CYP2C19* activity. If a *CYP2C19* poor metabolizer (PM) is treated with voriconazole and ritonavir at the same time, up to 461% area under the curve (AUC) for voriconazole was observed as reduced *CYP2C19* and *CYP3A4* caused the patient to be incapable of metabolizing the voriconazole.[57,73]

There is significant anticipation of how pharmacogenomics may help guide clinicians to the optimal treatment for Parkinson's disease (PD). PD is known to be exceptionally multifactorial, with the net effect being a mishandling of dopamine pathways. There is wide interindividual variation in both efficacy and toxicity of dopaminergic drugs. L-dopa and dopamine agonists can lead to psychosis, and almost half of patients develop dyskinesia within the first 5 years of starting L-dopa. Several frequently studied polymorphisms in Parkinson's disease drug metabolism include dopamine receptors (*DRD1*, *DRD2*, *DRD3*, *DRD4*, *DRD5*), dopamine transporters (*DAT1* or *LSC6A3*), monoamine oxidase (*MAO-B*),

and catechol-*O*-methyltransferase (*COMT*), which degrades dopamine. Multiple polymorphisms can make interindividual responses very complex.[74]

Drug–gene interactions (DGIs) and drug–drug–gene interactions (DDGIs) account for approximately 34% (i.e., 14.7% DGIs and 19.2% DDGIs)[75] of significant interaction warnings that can potentially lead to toxic effects or decreased effectiveness. A study noted that 20% of drug interactions were in fact DDGIs, which are often missed without a clinical decision support tool (CDST),[75] which are now routinely incorporated into existing electronic health records (EHRs). Furthermore, a drug may induce a change of phenotype, creating a mismatch between the genotype-derived phenotype and the "real" phenotype, a phenomenon referred to as *phenoconversion*.[76] Another study also noted that 54.6% of patients taking medications that interacted with genes were also taking medications that modulate the same enzyme activity. Drug–drug–gene interactions are not uncommon and must be built in CDSTs when possible.[76]

COST-EFFECTIVENESS OF PHARMACOGENOMICS

PGx has the potential to personalize pharmaceutical treatments. Many relevant gene–drug associations have been discovered, but PGx-guided treatment must be cost-effective as well as clinically beneficial to be incorporated into standard healthcare. A 2017 review from *The Pharmacogenomics Journal* found PGx-guided treatment to be cost-effective and/or cost-saving over alternative strategies. According to this report, 57% of the 44 economic evaluations of 10 different drugs favored PGx testing. In other words, 30% of the studies showed cost-effectiveness, whereas 27% showed cost-savings. Thus, PGx-guided treatment could be both cost-effective and -saving strategies.[77]

Arguments against pharmacogenomics testing include a review by Relling and Evans,[78] in which they concluded that only approximately 7% of FDA-approved medications are affected by "actionable" inherited genes. They also showed that these medications constitute 18% of all prescriptions written in the United States. With a steady and logarithmic increase in the publishing of genetic information, that percentage will likely grow.[78]

A recent comparative study demonstrated that genetic profiles of cytochrome enzymes in elderly patients 65 or older may reduce the hospitalization and emergency department (ED) visit rate within 4 months, showing potential for total healthcare dollars savings. In fact, the relative risk of hospitalization and ED visits in patients with pharmacogenetic testing versus untested patients is reported at 0.61 ($p = .027$)

and 0.29 (p = .0002), respectively.[79] This translates to an estimated average potential cost savings of $218 per patient in the tested group, including the cost of the test.[79]

In a year-long prospective study involving outpatient mental health patients, researchers compared 1-year pharmacy claims between a pharmacogenomic test (PGx)–guided cohort and a propensity-matched control group. The claims were followed for 1 year following testing, comparing eligible patients (n = 2,168) to a 5-to-1 propensity-matched treatment-as-usual (TAU; n = 10,880) standard-of-care control group. Patients who received PGx testing saved $1,035 in total medication costs over 1 year compared to the non-tested standard-of-care cohort. In addition, PGx testing improved adherence compared to the standard-of-care cohort, and the pharmacy cost savings averaged $2,774 for patients who were changed to a medication regimen that is congruent with pharmacogenomics results compared to those who were not.[80]

A 2018 publication studying major depressive disorder built a Markov state-transition probability model that predicted very similar results as the previously mentioned prospective study. The model estimated a cumulative effect over 3 years of 2.07 quality-adjusted life years (QALYs) for the PGx-guided treatment group and 1.97 QALYs for the standard-of-care (SOC) group, including a lower probability of death by suicide. Total costs over 3 years were $44,697 (PGx guided) and $47,295 (SOC). The difference includes a savings of $2,918 in direct medical costs and $1,680 in indirect costs. Results were even more pronounced when only severely depressed patients were evaluated.[81]

Some have pondered whether or not disparities in benefits of pharmacogenomics will be an unintended consequence of this emerging capability. A study from the United Kingdom that reviewed 4,978 abstracts showed that only five met their rigorous inclusion criteria. While three studies of genotype-guided dosing of warfarin reported that ethnic disparities in healthcare may widen, two other studies (one reporting on warfarin, the other reporting on clopidogrel) suggested that disparities in healthcare may be reduced. There is a paucity of studies that evaluate the impact of pharmacogenomics on health disparities. Further work is required to evaluate health disparities not only between ethnic groups and differing countries, but also within ethnic groups in the same country, and solutions must be identified to overcome these disparities.[82]

FUTURE OF PHARMACOGENOMICS

Preemptive Pharmacogenetic Testing

Recent surveys have found that 80% of clinicians surveyed believe pharmacogenetic testing will become standard in psychiatry,[83] and that patients who received CDST-guided treatment reported more positive perceptions of care.[84] Another recent survey found that up to 98% of physicians surveyed agreed that drug response may be influenced by genetic variation, yet only 13% indicated they had ordered a CDST-guided treatment within the last 6 months.[85] Another survey of 300 psychiatrists found that about 7% had ordered a CDST-guided treatment.[86]

See **Tables 4.1 to 4.5** for a summary of genetic tests recommended by clinical guidelines.

TABLE 4.1 Clinical Recommendations for Drug-Metabolizing Enzymes Related to Biomarkers in Cancer Therapy			
PGx Biomarkers and Affected Cancer Drugs	**Significant Polymorphisms**	**Genetic Testing**	**Clinical Recommendations**
UGT1A1 (UDP-glucuronyltransferase) Irinotecan (Camptosar) Nilotinib (Tasigna)	*UGT1A1*28* (insertion of an additional seventh TA sequence in the promoter region of *UGT1A1* gene)[21]	*UGT1A1* gene polymorphism (TA repeat) testing by PCR	Reduction in starting dose of irinotecan in patients with homozygous *UGT1A1*28* genotype[20] Routine use of genotyping may be useful for high dose of irinotecan (>200 mg/m²)[22] The FDA recommends, but does not require, genetic testing for *UGT1A1* variants prior to initiating or reinitiating treatment with nilotinib.[23]
DPD (dihydropyrimidine) Fluorouracil (5-FU) (Adrucil) Capecitabine (Xeloda)	*DPYD*2A*	AmpliChip	Genetic screening recommended before starting 5-FU therapy[24,25]
TPMT (thiopurine methyltransferase) 6-Mercaptopurine (6-MP)	*TPMT*2* *TPMT*3A* *TPMT*3C*[26]	*TPMT* Activity Assay	Substantial dose reductions are generally required for patients with homozygous *TPMT* deficiency[27]

(continued)

TABLE 4.1 Clinical Recommendations for Drug-Metabolizing Enzymes Related to Biomarkers in Cancer Therapy (*continued*)

PGx Biomarkers and Affected Cancer Drugs	Significant Polymorphisms	Genetic Testing	Clinical Recommendations
CYP2D6 Tamoxifen (Nolvadex)	*CYP2D6*3* *CYP2D6*4* *CYP2D6*5* *CYP2D6*6*[28]	AmpliChip CYP450 test[29]	No current clinical recommendations regarding *CYP2D6* polymorphisms and tamoxifen therapy from National Comprehensive Cancer Network (NCCN) 2016 Breast Cancer Guidelines, nor the American Society of Clinical Oncology (ASCO) Breast Cancer Guidelines[30]
CYP2B6 Cyclophosphamide (Cytoxan) Ifosfamide (Ifex)	*CYP2B6*5* *CYP2B6*6*	Pyrosequencing assays for *CYP2B6* polymorphisms[31]	*CYP2B6* is highly inducible. The interindividual difference of *CYP2B6* enzyme activity can be 20- to 250 -fold, which can affect drug efficacy and toxicity.[32]
MTHFR (methylenetetrahydrofolate reductase) Methotrexate (Rheumatrex)	*C677T*	Methotrexate sensitivity 2 mutations assay (ARIP lab)	*C677T* homozygous variant with 35% of normal enzyme activity occurs in up to 10% of Caucasians. Oral mucositis occurrence rate was 36% higher for chronic myelogenous leukemia patients with *C677T* polymorphism.[33,34]
G6PD (glucose-6-phosphate dehydrogenase) Rasburicase (Elitek)	G6PD deficiency	G6PD activity assay	FDA recommends not to administer rasburicase to patient with G6PD deficiency, which may trigger acute hemolysis.

PGx, pharmacogenomics

Source: Data from References 20–34, FDA drug package inserts, and Lexi-Comp drug.

TABLE 4.2 Pharmacogenomic Biomarkers That Influence Efficacy and Toxicities in Cancer Therapy

PGx Biomarkers	Therapeutic Agents	PK/PD Impact	Frequency of Variant	Clinical Impact
UGT1A1 (UDP-glucuronyltransferase)[5,6]	Irinotecan (Camptosar) Nilotinib (Tasigna)	Poor metabolism Increased systemic exposure to SN-38 with *UGT1A1*28* Increased bilirubin level	Deficiency of the enzyme may occur in 35% of Caucasians and African Americans.	Homozygous *UGT1A1*28* genotype is a risk factor for severe diarrhea, neutropenia at doses >200 mg/m². Largest increase of bilirubin with homozygous *UGT1A1*28*
DPD (dihydropyrimidine dehydrogenase)[7,8]	Fluorouracil (5-FU), (Adrucil) Capecitabine (Xeloda)	Deficiency of this enzyme due to mutation Causes systemic increase in 5-FU	3% of Caucasians may have deficiency.	Deficiency can lead to fatal neurological and hematological toxicities. Grade 3 diarrhea and hand-foot syndrome linked with 5-FU plasma levels more than 3 mg/L in males.
TPMT (thiopurine methyltransferase)[2,4,9]	6-Mercaptopurine (6-MP, Purinethol)	*TPMT* inactivates 6-MP, low or absent *TPMT* activity increases systemic drug exposure	10% of Caucasians are PMs of this enzyme; 0.3% have complete deficiency.	Patients with low or absent *TPMT* activity are at an increased risk of developing severe, life-threatening myelotoxicity. Dose adjustment required.
CYP3A4/3A5[4,10–12]	Cyclophosphamide (Cytoxan)	Activate the prodrug to its active form	A variant allele occurs in 45% of African Americans and 9% of Caucasians.	Deficiency of this enzyme causes interindividual variability in efficacy and enhanced toxicity.

(*continued*)

TABLE 4.2 Pharmacogenomic Biomarkers That Influence Efficacy and Toxicities in Cancer Therapy (*continued*)

PGx Biomarkers	Therapeutic Agents	PK/PD Impact	Frequency of Variant	Clinical Impact
CYP2B6[10–12]	Cyclophosphamide (Cytoxan) Ifosfamide (Ifex)	CYP2B6 is a major metabolizing enzyme for cyclophosphamide and ifosfamide.	Polymorphisms of CYP2B6 are prevalent in more than 45% of individuals.	Standard dosing for patients with dysfunctional CYP2B6 may increase risk of nephrotoxicity (data variable).
CYP2D6[11–13]	Tamoxifen (Nolvadex)	Tamoxifen is converted to the potent active metabolite endoxifen.	Polymorphisms that cause absence of CYP2D6 activities found in 7% of Caucasians, 3% of African Americans, and 1% of Asians.	Deficiency of CYP2D6 causes reduction of endoxifen and may vary levels of toxicity. Routine genotyping is not recommended due to variability.
GST1 (glutathione-**S**-transferase alpha 1)[14]	Cyclophosphamide (Cytoxan) Busulfan (Myleran)	A family of enzyme detoxifying electrophilic group of some chemotherapeutic agents	57% of Caucasians and 13% of African Americans have deficiency.	Deficiency of this enzyme may result in enhanced drug toxicity.
Excision repair cross-complementing rodent repair deficiency group 1 (ERCC1) and group 2 (ERCC2)[15]	Cisplatin (Platinol) Carboplatin Oxaliplatin (Eloxatin)	ERCC1 is an endonuclease, repairing damaged DNA segments.	No data	Not conclusive; high gene expression associated with inferior outcomes for bladder cancer
ABCB1 (aka MDR1), ABCB2 (MRP2)[16]	Paclitaxel (Taxol and Onxol)	Encodes for P-glycoprotein responsible for efflux of drugs from the cell	More than 50 SNPs and three insertion/deletion polymorphisms have been reported.	Overexpression of ABCB1 leads to drug resistance. Patients with wild type demonstrated reduced neuropathy.

PD, pharmacodynamics; PK, pharmacokinetics; PM, poor metabolizer; SNP, single-nucleotide polymorphism.

TABLE 4.3 Pharmacogenomic Biomarkers for Selection of Cancer Therapy

PGx Biomarker	Therapeutic Agents	Mutations Detected	Potential Clinical Impact	ASCO or NCCN Guidelines
EGFR (HER1) in nonsmall-cell lung cancer (NSCLC)	Erlotinib (Tarceva) Gefitinib (Iressa)	Activating tumor EGFR mutations: mainly deletions in exon 19 and L858R Resistance tumor mutation: T790M	Presence of EGFR-activating mutations predicts response to gefitinib and erlotinib. Presence of EGFR T790M mutation predicts resistance to gefitinib.	Recommends testing for EGFR mutation before gefitinib or erlotinib treatment.
HER2/neu (ErbB2) in breast cancer and gastric tumor	Trastuzumab (Herceptin) Lapatinib (Tykerb)	Use immunohistochemistry (IHC) or fluorescence *in situ* hybridization (FISH) to detect HER2 gene overexpression	Overexpression of HER2 (+3 by IHC or FISH) predicts response to trastuzumab and lapatinib.	Recommends to test HER2 expression for all breast cancer tumors; overexpression of HER2 qualifies patient for trastuzumab. Allow lapatinib to be used in combination with capecitabine as an option for trastuzumab-refractory breast cancer patients.

(continued)

TABLE 4.3 Pharmacogenomic Biomarkers for Selection of Cancer Therapy *(continued)*

PGx Biomarker	Therapeutic Agents	Mutations Detected	Potential Clinical Impact	ASCO or NCCN Guidelines
KRAS in metastatic colon cancer and squamous cell carcinoma of head and neck	Cetuximab (Erbitux) Panitumumab (Vectibix)	Activating tumor *KRAS* mutations: mainly exon 2 codon 12 and 13	Presence of *KRAS* mutations predicts nonresponse to cetuximab and panitumumab. Absence of *KRAS* mutations predicts response to cetuximab and panitumumab.	Recommends genotyping tumor tissue for *KRAS* mutation in all patients with metastatic colorectal cancer. Patients with known codon 12 and 13 *KRAS* gene mutation are unlikely to respond to EGFR inhibitors and shouldn't receive cetuximab.
BCR-ABL or Philadelphia chromosome in chronic myelogenous leukemia (CML)	Imatinib (Gleevec) Nilotinib (Tasigna) Dasatinib (Sprycel)	Detecting Philadelphia chromosome by fluorescence in situ hybridization (FISH) Detecting *BCR-ABL* mutations	Presence of *BCR-ABL* or Philadelphia chromosome predicts response to imatinib and nilotinib. Presence of *BCR-ABL* mutation predicts resistance to imatinib. Dasatinib overcome most *BCR-ABL* mutation (except T315I)	Recommends cytogenetics and mutation analysis for patients receiving imatinib therapy and an 18-month follow-up evaluation with treatment recommendations based upon cytogenetic response. Recommends Dasatinib for the treatment of adults with chronic, accelerated, or myeloid or lymphoid blast-phase chronic myeloid leukemia with resistance or intolerance to prior therapy, including imatinib.
c-Kit in gastrointestinal stromal tumors (GIST)	Imatinib (Gleevec)	Oncogenic c-Kit mutation in exon 9 and 11 D816V mutation of c-Kit	Presence of a c-Kit mutation in exon 11 is associated with a more favorable prognosis and greater likelihood of response to imatinib therapy in patients with advanced GIST. Presence of D816V mutation of c-Kit predicts resistance to imatinib.	Mutational analysis of c-Kit is strongly recommended in the diagnostic work-up of GIST patients. In locally advanced, inoperable, and metastatic GIST, imatinib 400 mg daily is the standard of care. In patients whose GIST harbors KIT exon 9 mutations, imatinib 800 mg daily is the recommended dose.
PML-RAR-α translocation in patients with acute promyelocytic leukemia (APL)	Arsenic trioxide (Trisenox)	t(15:17) translocation determined by FISH or *PML-RAR-α* gene expression	Presence of *PML-RAR-α* fusion gene predicts clinical outcome following arsenic trioxide treatment.	Arsenic trioxide induces *PML-RAR-α* degradation. Diagnostic testing of *PML-RAR-α* is required for the treatment of arsenic trioxide. Used for remission induction and consolidation in patients with relapsed or refractory AP characterized by *PML-RAR-α* expression.

ASCO, American Society of Clinical Oncology; NCCN, National Comprehensive Cancer Network.

TABLE 4.4 U.S. Food and Drug Administration-Approved Pharmacogenomic Testing Recommendations in Cardiology

Drug	Pharmacogenomic Marker	Example of Pharmacogenomic Testing	FDA Recommendation	Pharmacology
Carvedilol	CYP2D6	AmpliChip CYP450 test (Roche Diagnostics)	Increase blood levels of the R(+) enantiomer of carvedilol in poor 2D6 metabolizers and potentially associated with higher rate of dizziness during up-titration. Potent inhibitors of CYP2D6 isoenzyme (such as quinidine, fluoxetine, paroxetine, and propafenone) may add to complication.	Carvedilol is subject to the effects of genetic polymorphism with poor metabolizers of debrisoquine (a marker for CYP450 2D6) exhibiting two-to-three-fold higher plasma concentrations of the R(+)-carvedilol.
Quinidine	CYP2D6	AmpliChip CYP450 test (Roche Diagnostics)	Precaution with prodrugs, such as codeine, that are activated by CYP2D6	Quinidine is not metabolized by CYP2D6 but it is a potent competitive inhibitor of CYP2D6. At therapeutic level of quinidine, it can effectively convert extensive metabolizers into poor metabolizers.
Clopidogrel	CYP2C19	AmpliChip CYP450 test (Roche Diagnostics)	Boxed Warning: Diminished antiplatelet effect in CYP2C19 PMs who have two loss-of-function alleles of the CYP2C19 gene	CYP2C19 converts the prodrug clopidogrel to its active metabolite. PMs of CYP2C19 (with two inactive copies of CYP2C19) will have inadequate antiplatelet activity.
Warfarin	CYP2C9; VKORC1	Infiniti 2C9-VKORC1 multiplex assay (AutoGenomic) Verigene warfarin metabolism nucleic acid test (Nanosphere)	Dosing recommendations of warfarin varies in patients who have CYP2C9 and/or VKORC1 polymorphism. Patients who carry CYP2C9 *1/*3, *2/*2, *2/*3, and *3/*3 may need longer time (>2 to 4 weeks) to achieve maximum INR effect. The variant CYP2C9*2 and *3 result in reduction of CYP2C9 enzymatic activity in vitro. The frequencies in Caucasians are approximately 11% and 7% for CYP2C9*2 and CYP2C9*3, respectively. Other CYP2C9 alleles occur at lower frequencies, such as *5, *6, and *11; observed in African ancestry and *5, *9, and *11 alleles in Caucasians, and are also associated with reduced enzymatic activity.	Warfarin inhibits vitamin K-dependent coagulation factor synthesis (II, VII, IX, X, Protein C and S) by reducing the regeneration of vitamin K through inhibition of VKOR. The S-enantiomer of warfarin is mainly metabolized by CYP2C9. PM of CYP2C9 increases risk of bleeding associated with warfarin. Poor metabolizer of VKORC1 increases risk of bleeding associated with warfarin.

FDA, Food and Drug Administration; INR, international normalized ratio; PM, poor metabolizer.

TABLE 4.5 U.S. Food and Drug Administration-Approved Pharmacogenomic Testing Recommendations for Anesthesiology

Drug	Pharmacogenomic Marker	Example of Pharmacogenomic Testing	FDA Warnings	Pharmacology
Codeine	CYP2D6	XTAG CYP2D6 Kit V3 (Luminex Molecular Diagnostics)	Black-Box Warning: Death related to ultra-rapid metabolism of codeine to morphine. Respiratory depression and death have occurred in children who received codeine following tonsillectomy and/or adenoidectomy and had evidence of being ultra-rapid metabolizers of codeine due to a CYP2D6 polymorphism.	CYP2D6 converts the prodrug codeine to its active metabolite, morphine. PMs of CYP2D6 (with two inactive copies of CYP2D6) will have reduced levels of morphine and inadequate pain relief. Ultra-rapid metabolizers (with more than two copies of CYP2D6) have increased levels of morphine following codeine administration, leading to higher risk of toxicity.
Tramadol	CYP2D6	XTAG CYP2D6 Kit V3 (Luminex Molecular Diagnostics)	Black-Box Warning: Patients who have risk factors for life-threatening respiratory depression in children and those who have ultra-rapid metabolism	Tramadol is subjected to variability in metabolism based upon CYP2D6 genotype, which can lead to increased exposure to an active metabolite (same polymorphic metabolism as codeine).
Lofexidine	CYP2D6	XTAG CYP2D6 Kit V3 (Luminex Molecular Diagnostics)	Caution if poor CYP2D6 metabolizer	It is primarily metabolized by CYP2D6.
Lidocaine and Prilocaine	G6PD (glucose-6-phosphate dehydrogenase)	CareStart G6PD (AccessBio)	Warning: Patients with G6PD deficiency or congenital or idiopathic methemoglobinemia are more susceptible to drug-induced methemoglobinemia.	Patients with G6PD deficiencies and patients taking oxidizing drugs such as antimalarials and sulfonamides are more susceptible to drug-induced methemoglobinemia.
Succinylcholine	BCHE (butyrylcholinesterase)		Precaution: The likelihood of prolonged neuromuscular blockade following administration of succinylcholine must be considered in patients who carry BUCHE genotypes that express reduced plasma butyrylcholinesterase activity.	Succinylcholine is rapidly hydrolyzed by plasma butyrylcholinesterase to succinylmonocholine and choline. Patients with heterozygous or homozygous for atypical plasma cholinesterase gene may have diminished enzymatic activity (i.e., PM) and extreme sensitivity to the effects of succinylcholine. A 5- to 10-mg test dose of succinylcholine may be administered to evaluate sensitivity to succinylcholine.

PM, poor metabolizer.

Research and Education in Pharmacogenomics

Collaboration between the basic and the clinical sciences must continue to thrive. Translational medicine has finally moved into the forefront of the best institutions. Many medical schools have taken deliberate and proactive measures to enhance collaboration at every level, including the physical location of the basic science researchers and the clinicians. To keep this in perspective, the *TPMT* and *CYP2D6* genetic polymorphisms that are now being implemented into clinical practice were discovered more than 35 years ago, whereas researchers realized that they may have clinical utility at least 25 years ago. The discovery that statin-induced myopathy was associated with a SNP in the *SLCO1B1* gene was achieved more than a decade ago, yet very few clinicians have the knowledge or the means to consider this before prescribing statins. Moreover, the cost-effectiveness of these tests is an inarguable consideration. At the current stage of healthcare development, only very generous insurance policies will consider paying for preemptive testing. As poignantly stated by Weinshilboum and Wang, "The processes of 'discovery,' 'translation,' and 'implementation' are not separate and distinct activities, but rather they are tightly intertwined, and they inform each other...."[2]

In order for the clinical utility of this growing capability to flourish, educational institutions must continually invest in genetics and genomics research, facilitating a healthy ecosystem that provides widespread support for ongoing programs in translational pharmacogenomics. Academic leadership must invest wisely, which may involve focusing efforts on discovery, education, clinical implementation, and testing, which are collaboratively accomplished by multiple departments, institutes, laboratories, companies, and colleagues. Focus areas have included drug-response association studies and allele discovery, multiethnic pharmacogenomics, personalized genotyping and survey-based education programs, preemptive clinical testing implementation, and novel assay development.[87]

Unraveling the human genome has unlocked a limitless list of possibilities for researchers and clinicians to collaborate with the goal of delivering medicine with individual precision, while promoting health, preventing disease, and treating illness both effectively and safely. Each patient's unique biologic, environmental, and lifestyle condition must be acknowledged. It will require complex, habitual, inter-professional interactions, as well as the harnessing of artificial intelligence and optimization of clinical decision support tools within electronic health records. Clinicians must champion necessary restructuring at their home institutions.

CASE EXEMPLAR: Patient With Post-Concussive Syndrome

AC is a 45-year-old Asian American female presenting for primary care. She is new to the clinic. She is experiencing postconcussive syndrome after a closed head injury, which she sustained several months prior. She was prescribed amitriptyline by a neurologist. She states that her headaches worsened for a couple weeks after taking prescribed medication. She also complains of a vague difficulty with her vision, as well as constipation. She is interested in "precision medicine," and would like to proceed with pharmacogenomic testing.

Medication
- Amitriptyline, 25 mg nightly

Physical Examination
- Height: 5'0"; weight: 134 lb; blood pressure: 118/78; pulse: 72; respiration rate: 14; temperature: 98.7 °F

Next Step
- A comprehensive PGx panel was ordered; see **Exhibit 4.1** for the results.

Discussion Questions

1. What is a "poor metabolizer?"
2. Amitriptyline is cited on the PGx results as a potential interaction with CYP2C19 poor metabolizers. What is the most appropriate next step in this patient?

CASE EXEMPLAR: Patient With Nephrolithiasis

LR presents to a primary care office 24 hours after being discharged from the emergency department (ED) with a diagnosis of nephrolithiasis. He appears to be uncomfortable. He is diaphoretic, and his voice has a tone of despair. LR was discharged home from the ED with a prescription for acetaminophen with codeine (Tylenol #3). He states that he experiences excellent pain relief for about an hour, but then it seems to wear off, and he is in agony until his next dose in 6 hours. LR is aware of and concerned with the potential for acetaminophen toxicity; therefore, he has not taken extra doses.

Medications
- Codeine (Tylenol #3), 300 mg/30 mg; 1 tablet orally every 6 hours as needed

Physical Examination
- Height: 5′6″; weight: 220 lb; blood pressure: 44/90; pulse: 88, respiration rate: 16; temperature: 98.8 °F

Discussion Questions
1. What could be a potential explanation for what LR is describing?
2. What is the most significant potential risk with LR?

EXHIBIT 4.1 GENETIC ANALYSIS REPORT

Pgx Comprehensive Genetic Analysis Report

PATIENT	ORDERING CLINICIAN		LABORATORY INFORMATION
			Lab ID:
DOB:			Collection Date:
			Test Date:
			Report Date:

ASSAY	RESULT	PHENOTYPE	CLINICAL CONSEQUENCES
ANKK1_DRD2	T/C	Heterozygous	Consistent with a reduced dopamine receptor D2 function.
APOE	E3/E3	Normal APOE function	Not associated with type III hyperlipoproteinemia—No increased risk of cardiovascular disease
COMT	G/G	Normal	Consistent with a normal catechol O-methyltransferase (COMT) function.
CYP2C19	*2/*2	Poor metabolizer	Consistent with a significant deficiency in CYP2C19 activity. Increased risk for side effects or loss of efficacy with drug substrates.
CYP2C9	*1/*1	Normal metabolizer	Consistent with a typical CYP2C9 activity. This test did not identify risks for side effects or loss of efficacy with drug substrates.
CYP2D6	*2/*10	Normal metabolizer	Consistent with a typical CYP2D6 activity. This test did not identify risks for side effects or loss of efficacy with drug substrates.
CYP23A4	*1/*1	Normal metabolizer	Consistent with a typical CYP3A4 activity. Caution is advised when prescribing narrow therapeutic index drugs. Alternative drugs or dose adjustment may be required if CYP3A inhibitors or inducers are co-prescribed.
CYP23A5	*1/*1	Normal metabolizer	Consistent with a normal CYP3A5 activity. Caution is advised when prescribing narrow therapeutic index drugs. Alternative drugs or dose adjustment may be required if CYP3A inhibitors or inducers are co-prescribed.

(continued)

EXHIBIT 4.1: GENETIC ANALYSIS REPORT *(continued)*

FACTOR 2	G/G	Normal	Unless other genetic or circumstantial risk factors are present, the patient is not expected to have an increased risk for thrombosis.
FACTOR5	C/C	Normal	Unless other genetic or circumstantial risk factors are present, the patient is not expected to have an increased risk for thrombosis.
MTHFR C677T	C/C	Normal—Patient does not carry the c677T mutation.	The patient does not carry the *MTHFR C677T* mutation (wild-type) and the patient's *MTHFR* activity is normal. This is not associated with an increased risk of hyperhomocysteinemia.

Psychotropic

Drug Class	Standard Precautions	Use With Caution	Consider Alternatives
Anti-ADHD agents	Dexmethylphenidate (Focalin®) Dextroamphetamine (Dexedrine®) Guanfacine (Intuniv®)		
Antidepressants	Amoxapine (Amoxapine®) Desipramine (Norpramin®) Desvenlafaxine (Pristiq®) Duloxetine (Cymbalta®) Fluoxetine (Prozac®, Sarafem®) Fluvoxamine (Luvox®) Levomilnacipran (Fetzima®) Maprotiline (Ludiomil®) Mirtazapine (Remeron®) Nefazodone (Serzone®) Nortriptyline (Pamelor®) Paroxetine (Paxil®, Brisdelle®) Protriptyline (Vivactil®) Trazodone (Oleptro®) Venlafaxine (Effexor®) Vilazodone (Viibryd®) Vortioxetine (Trintellix®)	Citalopram (Celexa®) Escitalopram (Lexapro®) Sertraline (Zoloft®)	Amitriptyline (Elavil®) Clomipramine (Anafranil®) Doxepin (Silenor®) Imipramine (Tofranil®) Trimipramine (Surmontil®)

CLINICAL PEARLS

- If a patient does not respond to treatment by a certain medication, or quickly develops adverse reactions to a certain medication, there may be a genetic explanation for their unexpected results rather than an issue of compliance.
- It is particularly important to perform pharmacogenomic profiling of a patient prior to the use of a drug with a narrow therapeutic window and extensive side effect profile.
- Several drugs are metabolized by enzyme systems that can be up- or down-regulated by other medications, requiring careful monitoring.
- Bioactive metabolites or unchanged active forms of some drugs may be passed in higher-than-expected concentrations to nursing babies depending on a breastfeeding mother's pharmacogenomic profile.
- Excellent databases exist to help analyze the results of a pharmacogenomic profile panel in relation to the use of a certain medication.
- The FDA has introduced Black-Box Warnings on several medications suggesting pharmacogenomic analysis prior to use or adjustment of the drug.

KEY TAKEAWAYS

- *Phenotype* is the set of character traits that are expressed by the presence of the specific genotype, and *genotype* is the set of genes that determine a specific characteristic or trait.
- *Pharmacogenetics* is the study of genetic variation in drug response at the individual gene level, and *pharmacogenomics* involves all genes in the genome.
- Clinicians are now able to use PGx information to decide which drug treatment will be most appropriate for a specific patient, which medication to avoid to prevent serious adverse drug reactions, or which drug needs to have a dose adjustment and close monitoring for a specific population.
- Single-nucleotide polymorphisms (SNPs) are the most common type of variation among individuals.
- CPIC guidelines help clinicians understand how the results of genetic testing can be used in optimizing drug treatment.
- Differences in drug handling by a patient may result from differences in metabolic enzymes, differences in drug transporter systems, variations in immune system functions, and variations in drug–drug interactions and the genetic background of a patient.

REFERENCES

1. National Human Genome Research Institute. An overview of the human genome project. Published November 5, 2016. https://www.genome.gov/sites/default/files/media/files/2020-09/HGP_Timeline.pdf
2. Weinshilboum RM, Wang L. Pharmacogenomics: precision medicine and drug response. *Mayo Clin Proc.* 2017;92(11):1711–1722. doi:10.1016/j.mayocp.2017.09.001
3. Pirmohamed M. Pharmacogenetics and pharmacogenomics. *Br J Clin Pharmacol.* 2001;52:345–347. doi:10.1046/j.0306-5251.2001.01498.x
4. Belle DJ, Singh H. Genetic factors in drug metabolism. *Am Fam Physician.* 2008;77(11):1553–1560. https://www.aafp.org/afp/2008/0601/p1553.html
5. U.S. Food and Drug Administration. Pharmacogenomics: overview of the genomics and targeted therapy group. Published March 30, 2018. https://www.fda.gov/drugs/scienceresearch/ucm572617.htm
6. Nebert DW, Zhang G, Vesell ES. From human genetics and genomics to pharmacogenetics and pharmacogenomics: past lessons, future directions. *Drug Metab Rev.* 2008;40(2):187–224. doi:10.1080/03602530801952864
7. Malhotra A. An introduction to pharmacogenomics. In: Robinson MV, Woo TM, eds. *Pharmacotherapeutics for Advanced Practice Nurse Prescribers.* F.A. Davis; 2015:103–114.
8. Kalow W. Familial incidence of low pseudocholinesterase level. *Lancet.* 1956;26871(6942):576–577. doi:10.1016/S0140-6736(56)92065-7
9. Beutler E. The hemolytic effect of primaquine and related compounds: a review. *Blood.* 1959;14(2):103–139. doi:10.1182/blood.V14.2.103.103
10. Price Evans DA, Manley KA, McKusick VA. Genetic control of isoniazid metabolism in man. *Br Med J.* 1960;2(5197):485–491. doi:10.1136/bmj.2.5197.485
11. Ellard GA. Variations between individuals and populations in the acetylation of isoniazid and its significance for the treatment of pulmonary tuberculosis. *Clin Pharmacol Ther.* 1976;19(5 pt 2):610–625. doi:10.1002/cpt1976195part2610
12. Yamamoto M, Sobuea G, Mukoyama M, et al. Demonstration of slow acetylator genotype of N-acetyltransferase in isoniazid neuropathy using an archival hematoxylin and eosin section of a sural nerve biopsy specimen. *J Neurol Sci.* 1996;135(1):51–54. doi:10.1016/0022-510X(95)00254-Y
13. Orgogozo V, Morizot B, Martin A. The differential view of genotype-phenotype relationships. *Front Genet.* 2015;6:179. doi:10.3389/fgene.2015.00179
14. Meyer UA. Genotype or phenotype: the definition of a pharmacogenetic polymorphism. *Pharmacogenetics.* 1991;1(2):66–67. doi:10.1097/00008571-199111000-00002
15. Tchinda J, Lee C. Detecting copy number variation in the human genome using comparative genomic hybridization. *Biotechniques.* 2006;41(4):385–392. doi:10.2144/000112275
16. Iafrate AJ, Feuk L, Rivera MN, et al. Detection of large-scale variation in the human genome. *Nat Genet.* 2004;36(9):949–951. doi:10.1038/ng1416
17. U.S. Department of Health & Human Services, National Institutes of Health. *Help Me Understand Genetics—Genomic Research.* Lister Hill National Center for Biomedical Communications; 2019:1–15.
18. Genetics Home Reference. *What are single nucleotide polymorphisms (SNPs)?* https://ghr.nlm.nih.gov/primer/genomicresearch/snp
19. Hoffman JM, Dunnenberger HM, Hicks JK, et al. Developing knowledge resources to support precision medicine: principles from the Clinical Pharmacogenetics Implementation Consortium (CPIC). *J Am Med Inform Assoc.* 2016;23(4):796–801. doi:10.1093/jamia/ocw027
20. Caudle KE, Klein TE, Hoffman JM, et al. Incorporation of pharmacogenomics into routine clinical practice: the Clinical Pharmacogenetics Implementation Consortium (CPIC) guideline development process. *Curr Drug Metab.* 2014;15(2):209–217. doi:10.2174/1389200215666140130124910
21. ClinGen. *Get started with ClinGen.* 2019. https://clinicalgenome.org/start/#loc_1550536143-7476-1
22. Behrooz A. Pharmacogenetics and anaesthetic drugs: implications for perioperative practice. *Ann Med Surg (Lond).* 2015;4(4):470–474. doi:10.1016/j.amsu.2015.11.001

23. Genetics Home Reference. *Cytochrome P450*. Published April 30, 2019. https://ghr.nlm.nih.gov/primer/genefamily/cytochromep450

24. Sychev DA, Ashraf GM, Svistunov AA, et al. The cytochrome P450 isoenzyme and some new opportunities for the prediction of negative drug interaction in vivo. *Drug Des Devel Ther.* 2018;12:1147–1156. doi:10.2147/DDDT.S149069

25. Kalman LV, Agúndez J, Appell ML, et al. Pharmacogenetic allele nomenclature: international workgroup recommendations for test result reporting. *Clin Pharmacol Ther.* 2016;99(2):172–185. doi:10.1002/cpt.280

26. Pharmacogene Variation Consortium. *Genes*. Published February 6, 2019. https://www.pharmvar.org/genes

27. Ikeya K, Jaiswal AK, Owens RA, et al. Human CYP1A2: sequence, gene structure, comparison with the mouse and rat orthologous gene, and differences in liver 1A2 mRNA expression. *Mol Endocrinol.* 1989;3(9):1399–1408. doi:10.1210/mend-3-9-1399

28. Preissner SC, Hoffmann MF, Preissner R, et al. Polymorphic cytochrome P450 enzymes (CYPs) and their role in personalized therapy. *PLoS One.* 2013;8(12):e82562. doi:10.1371/journal.pone.0082562

29. Wang B, Zhou SF. Synthetic and natural compounds that interact with human cytochrome P450 1A2 and implications in drug development. *Curr Med Chem.* 2009;16(31):4066–4218. doi:10.2174/092986709789378198

30. Sim SC. CYP1A2*1E [corrected] contains the −163C>A substitution and is highly inducible. *Pharmacoge net Genomics.* 2013;23(2):104–105. doi:10.1097/FPC.0b013e32835ccc76

31. Van Booven D, Marsh S, McLeod H, et al. Cytochrome P450 2C9-CYP2C9. *Pharmacogenet Genomics.* 2010;20(4):277–281. doi:10.1097/FPC.0b013e3283349e84

32. Daly AK, Rettie AE, Fowler DM, et al. Pharmacogenomics of CYP2C9: functional and clinical considerations. *J Pers Med.* 2017;8(1):1. doi:10.3390/jpm8010001

33. Claudio-Campos KI, González-Santiago P, Renta JY, et al. CYP2C9*61, a rare missense variant identified in a Puerto Rican patient with low warfarin dose requirements. *Pharmacogenomics.* 2019;20(1):3–8. doi:10.2217/pgs-2018-0143

34. Johnson JA, Caudle KE, Gong L, et al. Clinical Pharmacogenetics Implementation Consortium (CPIC) guideline for pharmacogenetics-guided warfarin dosing: 2017 update. *Clin Pharmacol Ther.* 2017;102(3):397–404. doi:10.1002/cpt.668

35. El Rouby N, Lima JJ, Johnson JA. Proton pump inhibitors: from CYP2C19 pharmacogenetics to precision medicine. *Expert Opin Drug Metab Toxicol.* 2018;14(4):447–460. doi:10.1080/17425255.2018.1461835

36. CPIC. *Guidelines*. Published March 5, 2019. https://cpicpgx.org/guidelines

37. Adams SM, Conley YP, Wagner AK, et al. The pharmacogenomics of severe traumatic brain injury. *Pharmacogenomics.* 2017;18(15):1413–1425. doi:10.2217/pgs-2017-0073

38. Hibma JE, Giacomini KM. Pharmacogenomics. In: Katzung BG, Masters SB, Trevor AJ, eds. *Basic & Clinical Pharmacology.* 13th ed. McGraw-Hill Education; 2015:74–86.

39. de Leon J, Dinsmore L, Wedlund P. Adverse drug reactions to oxycodone and hydrocodone in CYP2D6 ultrarapid metabolizers. *J Clin Psychopharmacol.* 2003;23(4):420–421. doi:10.1097/01.jcp.0000085421.74359.60

40. Matic M, de Wildt SN, Tibboel D, et al. Analgesia and opioids: a pharmacogenetics shortlist for implementation in clinical practice. *Clin Chem.* 2017;63(7):1204–1213. doi:10.1373/clinchem.2016.264986

41. Koren G, Cairns J, Chitayat D, et al. Pharmacogenetics of morphine poisoning in a breastfed neonate of a codeine-prescribed mother. *Lancet.* 2006;368(9536):704. doi:10.1016/S0140-6736(06)69255-6

42. Orliaguet G, Hamza J, Couloigner V, et al. A case of respiratory depression in a child with ultrarapid CYP2D6 metabolism after tramadol. *Pediatrics.* 2015;135(3):e753–e755. doi:10.1542/peds.2014-2673

43. Stamer UM, Stüber F, Muders T, et al. Respiratory depression with tramadol in a patient with renal impairment and CYP2D6 gene duplication. *Anesth Analg.* 2008;107(3):926–929. doi:10.1213/ane.0b013e31817b796e

44. Goetz MP, Sangkuhl K, Guchelaar H-J, et al. Clinical Pharmacogenetics Implementation Consortium (CPIC) guideline for CYP2D6 and tamoxifen therapy. *Clin Pharmacol Ther.* 2018;103(5):770–777. doi:10.1002/cpt.1007

45. Schroth W, Hamann U, Fasching PA, et al. CYP2D6 polymorphisms as predictors of outcome in breast cancer patients treated with tamoxifen: expanded polymorphism coverage improves risk stratification. *Clin Cancer Res.* 2010;16(17):4468–4477. doi:10.1158/1078-0432.CCR-10-0478

46. Amstutz U, Henricks LM, Offer SM, et al. Clinical Pharmacogenetics Implementation Consortium (CPIC) guideline for dihydropyrimidine dehydrogenase genotype and fluoropyrimidine dosing: 2017 update. *Clin Pharmacol Ther.* 2018;103(2):210–216. doi:10.1002/cpt.911

47. Thoguluva Chandrasekar V, John S. Gilbert syndrome. [Updated August 16, 2020]. In: *StatPearls* [Internet]. StatPearls Publishing; 2020. https://www.ncbi.nlm.nih.gov/books/NBK470200.

48. Barbarino JM, Whirl-Carrillo M, Altman RB, Klein TE. PharmGKB: a worldwide resource for pharmacogenomic information. *Wiley Interdiscip Rev Syst Biol Med.* 2018;10(4):e1417. doi:10.1002/wsbm.1417

49. Belfield KD, Tichy EM. Review and drug therapy implications of glucose-6-phosphate dehydrogenase deficiency. *Am J Health Syst Pharm.* 2018;75(3):97–104. doi:10.2146/ajhp160961

50. U.S. National Library of Medicine. *G6PD gene glucose-6-phosphate dehydrogenase.* 2019. https://ghr.nlm.nih.gov/gene/G6PD#conditions

51. Rost S, Fregin A, Ivaskevicius V, et al. Mutations in VKORC1 cause warfarin resistance and multiple coagulation factor deficiency type 2. *Nature.* 2004;427:537–541. doi:10.1038/nature02214

52. Gulseth MP, Grice GR, Dager WE. Pharmacogenomics of warfarin: uncovering a piece of the warfarin mystery. *Am J Health Syst Pharm.* 2009;66(2):123–133. doi:10.2146/ajhp080127

53. National Institutes of Health. *ABCB1 gene.* 2019. https://ghr.nlm.nih.gov/gene/ABCB1#location

54. He H, Yin J-Y, Xu Y-J, et al. Association of ABCB1 polymorphisms with the efficacy of ondansetron in chemotherapy-induced nausea and vomiting. *Clin Ther*. 2014;36(8):1242–1252.e2. doi:10.1016/j.clinthera.2014.06.016

55. Wojnowski L, Kulle B, Schirmer M, et al. NAD(P)H oxidase and multidrug resistance protein genetic polymorphisms are associated with doxorubicin-induced cardiotoxicity. *Circulation*. 2005;112(24):3754–3762. doi:10.1161/CIRCULATIONAHA.105.576850

56. Izzedine H, Hulot J-S, Villard E, et al. Association between *ABCC2* gene haplotypes and tenofovir-induced proximal tubulopathy. *J Infect Dis*. 2006;194(11):1481–1491. doi:10.1086/508546

57. Ahmed S, Zhou Z, Zhou J, et al. Pharmacogenomics of drug metabolizing enzymes and transporters: relevance to precision medicine. *Genomics Proteomics Bioinformatics*. 2016;14(5):298–313. doi:10.1016/j.gpb.2016.03.008

58. Niemi M. Role of OATP transporters in the disposition of drugs. *Pharmacogenomics*. 2007;8(7):787–802. doi:10.2217/14622416.8.7.787

59. Sparreboom A, Gelderblom H, Marsh S, et al. Diflomotecan pharmacokinetics in relation to ABCG2 421C>A genotype. *Clin Pharmacol Ther*. 2004;76(1):38–44. doi:10.1016/j.clpt.2004.03.003

60. Tomlinson B, Hu M, Lee VWY, et al. ABCG2 polymorphism is associated with the low-density lipoprotein cholesterol response to rosuvastatin. *Clin Pharmacol Ther*. 2010;87(5):558–562. doi:10.1038/clpt.2009.232

61. Tirona RG, Leake BF, Merino G, et al. Polymorphisms in OATP-C: identification of multiple allelic variants associated with altered transport activity among European- and African-Americans. *J Biol Chem*. 2001;276(38):35669–35675. doi:10.1074/jbc.M103792200

62. Kalliokoski A, Niemi M. Impact of OATP transporters on pharmacokinetics. *Br J Pharmacol*. 2009;158(3):693–705. doi:10.1111/j.1476-5381.2009.00430.x

63. Lauschke VM, Milani L, Ingelman-Sundberg M. Pharmacogenomic biomarkers for improved drug therapy-recent progress and future developments. *AAPS J*. 2017;20(1):4. doi:10.1208/s12248-017-0161-x

64. SEARCH Collaborative Group; Link E, Parish S, Armitage J, et al. SLCO1B1 variants and statin-induced myopathy—a genomewide study. *N Engl J Med*. 2008;359(8):789–799. doi:10.1056/NEJMoa0801936

65. Flaten HK, Monte AA. The pharmacogenomic and metabolomic predictors of ACE inhibitor and angiotensin II receptor blocker effectiveness and safety. *Cardiovasc Drugs Ther*. 2017;31(4):471–482. doi:10.1007/s10557-017-6733-2

66. Dresser MJ, Leabman MK, Giacomini KM. Transporters involved in the elimination of drugs in the kidney: organic anion transporters and organic cation transporters. *J Pharm Sci*. 2001;90(4):397–421. doi:10.1002/1520-6017(200104)90:4<397::AID-JPS1000>3.0.CO;2-D

67. Sajib AA, Islam T, Paul N, et al. Interaction of rs316019 variants of SLC22A2 with metformin and other drugs-an in silico analysis. *J Genet Eng Biotechnol*. 2018;16(2):769–775. doi:10.1016/j.jgeb.2018.01.003

68. Wang ZJ, Yin OQP, Tomlinson B, et al. OCT2 polymorphisms and in-vivo renal functional consequence: studies with metformin and cimetidine. *Pharmacogenet Genomics*. 2008;18(7):637–645. doi:10.1097/FPC.0b013e328302cd41

69. Yuen GJ, Weller S, Pakes GE. A review of the pharmacokinetics of abacavir. *Clin Pharmacokinet*. 2008;47(6):351–371. doi:10.2165/00003088-200847060-00001

70. Dean L. Phenytoin therapy and *HLA-B*15:02* and *CYP2C9* genotypes. In: Pratt V, McLeod HL, Rubinstein WS, et al, eds. *Medical Genetics Summaries*. National Center for Biotechnology Information; 2016. https://www.ncbi.nlm.nih.gov/books/NBK385287.

71. Hu B, Zhang X, Xu G, et al. Association between COMT polymorphism Val158Met and opioid consumption in patients with postoperative pain: a meta-analysis. *Neurosignals*. 2018;26(1):11–21. doi:10.1159/000487038

72. Magro L, Moretti U, Leone R. Epidemiology and characteristics of adverse drug reactions caused by drug-drug interactions. *Expert Opin Drug Saf*. 2012;11(1):83–94. doi:10.1517/14740338.2012.631910

73. Tannenbaum C, Sheehan NL. Understanding and preventing drug–drug and drug–gene interactions. *Expert Rev Clin Pharmacol*. 2014;7(4):533–544. doi:10.1586/17512433.2014.910111

74. Payami H. The emerging science of precision medicine and pharmacogenomics for Parkinson's disease. *Mov Disord*. 2017;32(8):1139–1146. doi:10.1002/mds.27099

75. Verbeurgt P, Mamiya T, Oesterheld J. How common are drug and gene interactions? Prevalence in a sample of 1143 patients with CYP2C9, CYP2C19 and CYP2D6 genotyping. *Pharmacogenomics*. 2014;15(5):655–665. doi:10.2217/pgs.14.6

76. Blagec K, Kuch W, Samwald M. The importance of gene-drug-drug-interactions in pharmacogenomics decision support: an analysis based on Austrian claims data. *Stud Health Technol Inform*. 2017;236:121–127. doi:10.3233/978-1-61499-759-7-121

77. Verbelen M, Weale ME, Lewis CM. Cost-effectiveness of pharmacogenetic-guided treatment: are we there yet? *Pharmacogenomics J*. 2017;17(5):395–402. doi:10.1038/tpj.2017.21

78. Relling MV, Evans WE. Pharmacogenomics in the clinic. *Nature*. 2015;526(7573):343–350. doi:10.1038/nature15817

79. Brixner D, Biltaji E, Bress A, et al. The effect of pharmacogenetic profiling with a clinical decision support tool on healthcare resource utilization and estimated costs in the elderly exposed to polypharmacy. *J Med Econ*. 2016;19(3):213–228. doi:10.3111/13696998.2015.1110160

80. Winner JG, Carhart JM, Altar CA, et al. Combinatorial pharmacogenomic guidance for psychiatric medications reduces overall pharmacy costs in a 1 year prospective evaluation. *Curr Med Res Opin*. 2015;31(9):1633–1643. doi:10.1185/03007995.2015.1063483

81. Groessl EJ, Tally SR, Hillery N, et al. Cost-effectiveness of a pharmacogenetic test to guide treatment for major depressive disorder. *J Manag Care Spec Pharm*. 2018;24(8):726–734. doi:10.18553/jmcp.2018.24.8.726

82. Martin A, Downing J, Maden M, et al. An assessment of the impact of pharmacogenomics on health disparities: a systematic literature review. *Pharmacogenomics.* 2017;18(16):1541–1550. doi:10.2217/pgs-2017-0076

83. Walden LM, Brandl EJ, Changasi A, et al. Physicians' opinions following pharmacogenetic testing for psychotropic medication. *Psychiatry Res.* 2015;229(3):913–918. doi:10.1016/j.psychres.2015.07.032

84. McKillip RP, Borden BA, Galecki P, et al. Patient perceptions of care as influenced by a large institutional pharmacogenomic implementation program. *Clin Pharmacol Ther.* 2017;102(1):106–114. doi:10.1002/cpt.586

85. Stanek EJ, Sanders CL, Johansen Taber KA, et al. Adoption of pharmacogenomic testing by US physicians: results of a nationwide survey. *Clin Pharmacol Ther.* 2012;91(3):450–458. doi:10.1038/clpt.2011.306

86. Salm M, Abbate K, Appelbaum P, et al. Use of genetic tests among neurologists and psychiatrists: knowledge, attitudes, behaviors, and needs for training. *J Genet Couns.* 2014;23(2):156–163. doi:10.1007/s10897-013-9624-0

87. Scott SA, Obeng AO, Botton MR, et al. Institutional profile: translational pharmacogenomics at the Icahn School of Medicine at Mount Sinai. *Pharmacogenomics.* 2017;18(15):1381–1386. doi:10.2217/pgs-2017-0137

5

Pharmacology Across the Life Span

Cynthia S. Valle-Oseguera, Melanie A. Felmlee, and Carly A. Ranson

LEARNING OBJECTIVES

- Recall how the primary pharmacokinetic parameters, clearance and volume of distribution, change over the lifespan for a given drug.
- Explain how the clearance of a drug and its volume of distribution in a pediatric, geriatric, or gravid patient is different from that of an average adult.
- Apply the physiologic principles associated with each phase of life in treatment planning.
- Categorize the effects of aging and pregnancy on a class of drugs.
- Design an intelligent treatment plan using a particular drug for patients as they enter each life phase (childhood, pregnancy, elderly).
- Assess the risks (if any) of using the same dosage of a selected drug across all phases of life.

INTRODUCTION

There are three distinct stages of life with unique pharmacokinetic (PK) and pharmacodynamic (PD) characteristics that dictate particular considerations when it comes to the therapeutics of disease management: pediatrics, pregnancy and lactation, and geriatrics. For each stage, unique elements must be factored into the decision-making process when determining appropriate pharmacologic therapy. The primary PK parameters, clearance (CL) and volume of distribution (V_D), may change over the lifespan for a given drug. However, the fundamental equations used for calculating

these parameters from patient-specific data are not age dependent. When evaluating PK/PD changes over the lifespan, it is critical to understand the underlying physiological changes that contribute to alterations in clearance and volume. Currently, there are significant gaps in our knowledge of physiological changes in pediatric, pregnant and lactating women, and the geriatric populations; therefore, clinical judgment based on individual patient characteristics is crucial for therapy optimization. While there is wide variability in response to treatment, understanding concepts of PK, PD, and therapeutic specific considerations will help to guide therapy. In this chapter, PK and PD changes seen in pediatric patients, pregnant and lactating women, and the geriatric population, as well as therapeutic approaches and caveats to treating each stage, will be discussed.

PEDIATRIC POPULATION

OVERVIEW

While the medical treatment of pediatric patients is extremely variable, there are some overall concepts that assist clinicians to better anticipate therapeutic response. Pediatric populations are more likely to experience adverse drug reactions, with those younger than 12 months of age being at highest risk. Additionally, these reactions, when experienced, often lead to more serious complications than what is seen in adults.[1,2] Successful predictions of response and risks can maximize positive therapeutic outcomes and assist in early identification of adverse reactions to minimize the risk of patient harm. However, most drug trials prohibit pediatric patients from participation due to perceived ethical concerns. This results in limited data regarding the risks of drugs in pediatric patients. Despite these concerns and lack of evidence, there continues to be many off-label uses for medications in pediatric patients, which results in an increased risk for unknown reactions.[2-4]

Pharmacokinetics and Pharmacodynamics in the Pediatric Population

Drug therapy in pediatric patients requires an understanding of the developmental changes in PK and PD to determine a safe and effective drug dose. Typically, pediatric doses are based on empiric recommendations for specific age groups based on body weight. The values should not be scaled directly from adult dosing values as drug disposition varies in pediatric patients, and it is crucial to account for the maturation of drug absorption, metabolism, elimination, and distribution. The following paragraphs describe developmental maturation of PK and PD processes in full-term infants; development may differ in preterm infants.

Drug absorption in pediatric patients is influenced by developmental changes in gastrointestinal physiology (gastric pH, gastric emptying, intestinal motility, and expression of drug transporters). These changes may impact the rate and extent of drug absorption leading to changes in maximum plasma concentration (Cmax), bioavailability (F), and area under the plasma concentration time curve (AUC). Gastric pH is neutral at birth[5] and decreases over weeks to years to reach adult values.[6] Variations in gastric pH influence drug ionization, with any increases in ionization leading to a decrease in drug absorption. Currently, there is very limited information on gastric emptying and intestinal motility[5]; therefore, a prediction of their impact on drug absorption in pediatric patients cannot be made. Further, drug transporter expression in enterocytes influences drug absorption; however, there is a large informational gap in our understanding of developmental maturation of intestinal transporters.[7]

Protein binding, body composition, blood flow, and permeability at organ barriers govern V_D. Pediatric patients have a higher percentage of body water, which leads to an increased V_D for hydrophilic drugs, including aminoglycosides and beta-lactams.[8] As children age the percentage of body water decreases as does the V_D. As a result, younger children will require a higher dose (per kilogram body weight) to achieve the same plasma concentrations as an older child. These distribution changes are not observed with lipophilic drugs.[8] In addition, infants and children have decreased albumin and alpha1-acid glycoprotein concentrations, which can contribute to alterations in protein binding.[5,8] Lower protein concentrations lead to a higher free fraction of drug (higher unbound drug concentration), which translates into a higher V_D as only free drugs can diffuse across cell membranes. The impact of these changes is limited to drugs that exhibit a high degree of protein binding, including phenytoin and etoposide.[5]

Developmental changes in systemic clearance will reflect changes in hepatic and renal clearance pathways, with each pathway maturing at its own rate. As an infant matures, there may be a shift in the major clearance pathway due to maturation of elimination mechanisms. Renal drug elimination is dependent on filtration, tubular secretion, and reabsorption. Drug filtration is governed by glomerular filtration rate (GFR), which is low at birth and reaches adult values by 6 months of age.[5] For drugs primarily eliminated by renal filtration, GFR estimates are required to inform dose adjustments.[5] In adults, GFR is estimated using the Cockcroft-Gault equation; however, in children under 12 years old this equation does not accurately estimate GFR, and the Schwartz equation should be utilized.[9] Drug transporters are involved in renal tubular secretion; however, there is limited information on their maturation, and therefore the impact on renal clearance in pediatric patients is largely unknown.[7]

Developmental changes in hepatic clearance are generally mediated by maturation of drug metabolizing enzymes (DMEs); neonates have decreased or nonexistent expression of DMEs, and they demonstrate isoform-specific maturation patterns. A discussion of developmental changes in DME expression is beyond the scope of this chapter; however, a number of recent reviews described the DME maturation in pediatric patients.[5,8] In general, lower DME expression results in decreased hepatic clearance and increased systemic drug concentrations; therefore, a lower dose would be required to obtain the same plasma concentration observed in adults.

For pediatric PD, the common assumption is that the plasma concentrations associated with efficacy and toxicity are similar to those seen in adults. However, the concentration-effect relationship may differ between adults and children and age-dependent differences in PD are seen for valproic acid, diphenhydramine, atypical antipsychotic agents, and warfarin.[5] There are limited studies assessing developmental PD, and a lack of translational juvenile animal models to study maturation of PD pathways.[10]

Therapeutics in the Pediatric Population

Therapeutic options in pediatric populations require specific considerations into the physiology of the patient as well as the pharmacologic recommendations available for the condition. Clinicians must balance predicted adverse drug reactions with age-appropriate drug delivery models to compare the risks of potential treatments with their perceived benefits. Historically, many of the reported adverse reactions involve the skin and gastrointestinal tract of pediatric patients due to the continual growth and developmental changes that occur in this population.[4] Therefore, therapies requiring patches, topical creams, gels, and sprays may result in wide absorption variability leading to difficulties in predicting response.

Respiratory conditions in pediatric patients, while common, are extremely difficult to treat. The younger the patient, the greater the difficulty in administering treatment; therapeutic considerations such as drug delivery methods become even more important. While there has been an increase in the inclusion of pediatric patients in both disease identification and drug delivery trials, there are still very few that capture the appropriateness and effectiveness in pediatric age groups.[3,11] Clinicians must be cognizant that younger patients frequently have difficulty managing inhalers, particularly multidose inhalers. Therefore, it is often recommended that pediatric patients use a pressurized valve spacer to ensure appropriate medication delivery. Dry powder inhalers may offer a more simplified and appropriate delivery mechanism for pediatrics due to a decreased reliance on hand-eye coordination and fewer administration steps. However, these devices require a more forceful breathing technique for proper use, which may be difficult for younger patients to achieve.[12,13] Some therapies offer a form of drug delivery that is more conducive to pediatric patient care, such as liquid oral formulations. However, the lack of pediatric specific options poses a challenge, which requires careful coordination between clinicians, patients, and caregivers. **Figure 5.1** illustrates some of the preferred and nonpreferred drug delivery methods for pediatric patients.

Resources for Clinicians

Many drug database systems offer a pediatric section with age-specific recommendations for subscribers. **Box 5.1** contains a few of the available resources to aid clinicians in the prescribing of pharmacologic therapy in a pediatric patient population.

BOX 5.1
ELECTRONIC PEDIATRIC PRESCRIBING RESOURCES

American Academy of Pediatrics
- https://www.aap.org

healthychildren.org
- https://www.healthychildren.org

Micromedex Neofax and Pediatric Drug Database
- https://www.micromedexsolutions.com/

Clinical Pharmacology—Pediatrics monographs
- https://www.clinicalkey.com/pharmacology

Lexicomp—Pediatric sections and monographs
- http://online.lexi.com

Note: Not all-inclusive.

Preferred   Nonpreferred

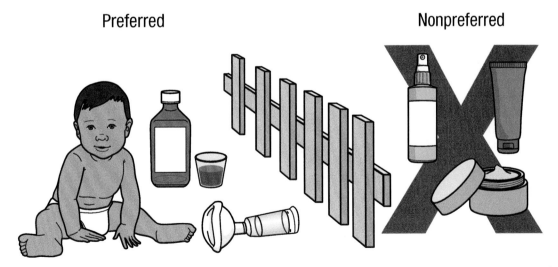

FIGURE 5.1 Drug delivery methods in pediatrics. Preferred and nonpreferred agents which, as outlined in the chapter, are dictated largely by predictability in the patient population. Pressurized valve spacers and liquid medication formulations tend to provide better results while creams, sprays, and lotions often result in variable absorption. Image is not all-inclusive.

CASE EXEMPLAR: Patient With Newly Diagnosed Asthma

CJ is a 5-year-old male who comes into the clinic with newly diagnosed asthma. He was recently prescribed a low-dose fluticasone propionate hydrofluoroalkane (HFA) inhaler for control of the condition. His mother believes the medication is not working and has seen no change in his condition since starting the medications.

Past Medical History

- Up-to-date on all vaccines
- Asthma × 1 month
- No other conditions reported

Medications

- Fluticasone propionate HFA, 88 mcg twice daily

- Cetirizine oral solution, 2.5 mg daily as needed for seasonal allergies

Labs

- Normal

Discussion Questions

1. What is the first step to identify the appropriateness of CJ's therapy?
2. After asking CJ and his mom to show you their inhaler technique, you identify that improper inhaler technique is being used, both when CJ administers it himself, as well as when his mother assists. What options can you provide to ensure proper administration occurs?
3. What other asthma-related considerations must be addressed in CJ?

PREGNANT AND LACTATING POPULATION

OVERVIEW

Since the mid-1970s there has been more than a 65% increase in the average number of medications used during pregnancy with over 90% of pregnant patients taking one or more medications, and close to 50% taking at least four.[14] Recent literature revealed that even after omitting vaccines, supplements, and vitamins, 73% of pregnant females take one or more medications.[15] When looking at the first trimester, a crucial development period, about 55% of expectant mothers report taking medications.[15] During this trimester, there are a variety of recognized types of pharmacologic agents used by pregnant patients, including cough and cold therapies, asthma agents, analgesics, antibiotics, antacids, antihistamines, laxatives, and oral contraceptives.[16] Nonprescription medications tend to be more frequently used during pregnancy and the use of some of those agents in the months prior to pregnancy is lower than in the first, second, or third trimester of pregnancy. Interestingly, at least 15% of expectant mothers report taking ibuprofen, while over 65% report taking acetaminophen while pregnant.[17]

Concerns regarding the safety of medications follow the baby during gestation and throughout the breast-feeding period. According to the latest data provided by the Centers for Disease Control and Prevention (CDC) over 80% of mothers breastfeed their babies at birth, which decreases to less than 60% at 6 months, and fur-

ther declines to about 35% at 1 year.[18] While medication use during pregnancy and lactation is not to be discouraged, the appropriateness of the therapy should be considered to ensure the safety of both mother and child.

Pharmacokinetics and Pharmacodynamics in the Pregnant and the Lactating Population

Pregnancy-induced changes in the gastrointestinal system (stomach pH, intestinal transit time, intestinal drug metabolism, and drug transport) may influence drug absorption and bioavailability.[19] Decreased gastric acid production (increased stomach pH) leads to increased ionization of weak acids, such as aspirin, decreasing their absorption, while increasing the absorption of weak bases such as caffeine.[19] Delayed gastric emptying and decreased intestinal transit time may decrease the maximum concentration (C_{max}) and delay the time to reach C_{max} following oral drug administration[20]; however, no PK studies have demonstrated these changes.[21] Current literature suggests that gastrointestinal changes in pregnancy have minimal effects on drug absorption and bioavailability.

Volume of distribution governs the calculation of a drug's loading dose and is influenced by body composition and drug protein binding. During pregnancy, total body water and fat increase, leading to an increase in V_D for both hydrophilic and lipophilic drugs, and a corresponding decrease in plasma drug concentrations. As a result, a higher-loading dose may be required to achieve the same plasma concentrations. In addition, pregnancy decreases systemic concentrations of albumin and alpha1-acid glycoprotein, leading to an increase in the fraction of free drug in plasma and an increase in V_D. This will have the greatest impact for highly bound drugs. Due to the changes in plasma protein binding, total plasma drug concentrations may not be a good therapeutic predictor due to the increase in free drug concentration, which is the case for phenytoin.[19]

In pregnancy, changes in total clearance result from changes in both hepatic clearance, due to changes in hepatic metabolism, and renal clearance. Changes in both phase 1 and 2 metabolic enzymes are observed during pregnancy, with enzyme-specific variations in direction and magnitude. Increased expression of metabolic enzymes can lead to increased drug clearance, and decreased plasma concentrations, with the potential for therapeutic failure. Additionally, metabolic activity is governed by genetic variation in metabolizing enzymes. The reviews by Anderson[22] and Feghali et al.[19] provide a thorough discussion of enzyme-specific changes during pregnancy and the impact of pharmacogenomics variants, which is beyond the scope of this chapter. Renal clearance is determined by GFR, tubular secretion, and reabsorption. GFR increases by 50% within the first trimester and continues to increase uniformly throughout pregnancy.[20,22] However, pregnancy-induced changes in GFR do not result in consistent changes in renal clearance, due to differences in drug transporters involved in tubular secretion.[19,22] Renal clearance has been demonstrated to double (lithium), increase 30% (digoxin), or increase 12% (atenolol) during the third trimester.[23–25] Therapeutic adjustments should be made on a case-specific basis. Currently, there is a lack of information on renal transporter expression in pregnancy, which precludes a generalized approach to adjusting therapy.

There is very limited data on PD changes in pregnancy. Most PK studies did not evaluate outcome measures[21]; however, the assumption that the concentration-effect relationship is not altered in pregnancy does not hold for all drugs. In some cases, the clinical outcome corresponds to the pregnancy-induced changes in PK (lamotrigine and indinavir).[26] In contrast, significant PK changes have been observed with no correlation to clinical outcome (emtricitabine, levetiracetam, topiramate)[27–29] suggesting a change in the underlying concentration-effect relationship. For other drugs, there are conflicting studies on the correlation of PK and clinical outcome data in pregnancy.

Therapeutics in the Pregnant and the Lactating Population

Pregnancy Categories in Medications
The widespread use of medication therapy for management of health conditions, coupled with the need for safety assessment of such therapy in pregnant patients, led to the U.S. Food and Drug Administration

(FDA) releasing regulations for drug labeling in 1979. Under FDA regulations, drugs were categorized into five different pregnancy classes (A, B, C, D, X). Categories A to C included medications largely based on their potential for fetal harm, whereas the latter categories also took into consideration pregnant females' benefits from therapy.[30,31] In 2015, the FDA provided updated regulations for prescription and biologic medications that discontinued the use of pregnancy drug categories. Under the new regulations, both the data on the risks associated with drug use during pregnancy and lactation, as well as a discussion of pertinent material to aid clinicians in the prescribing and consultation of these drugs in a pregnant or breastfeeding patient, are provided. This new style of narrative drug labeling summarizes the risks and corresponding evidence for medication use and was implemented to address a lack of clarity and the concerns regarding misinterpretation with prior pregnancy categorization.[32,33]

Prescribing in Pregnancy
Complete elimination of drug therapy use during pregnancy is often not feasible. Management of chronic conditions, such as human immunodeficiency virus infection, epilepsy, cardiovascular disorders, and addiction management, must continue and acute conditions requiring therapeutic intervention may arise. However, practicing evidence-based medicine when it comes to a pregnant patient has its challenges. Usually, pregnancy is a condition for exclusion in trials, thus limiting available literature to animal, cohort, and case control studies.[34] Regardless of evidence limitations, the utmost care must be provided to ensure that medications used are safe and effective for the mother and fetus, with consideration for the stage of fetal development. Physiological changes happen progressively throughout the pregnancy and it can be challenging to identify fetal changes by trimester. Therefore, therapeutic modification may be necessary to ensure adequate drug exposure in the mother, while avoiding unwanted exposure to the fetus. Clinicians face the conundrum of whether to initiate, continue, or discontinue treatment for conditions depending on the potential implications of the decision.[34] Close monitoring of patients on chronic therapy, especially narrow therapeutic index drugs, is the optimal approach to maintaining therapeutic benefit during pregnancy. **Table 5.1** offers a brief overview of recommended therapies for common conditions encountered in pregnancy.

Generally, at around 3 weeks post-conception, pregnant females will have their first missed menstruation.[34] Often, by the time a pregnancy is confirmed, the fetus may have already been exposed to a potentially harmful agent. Therefore, potential for pregnancy should be considered when initiating a medication in any woman of childbearing age. For example, a patient trying to conceive who is also indicated for anticoagulation therapy

TABLE 5.1 Common Conditions and Their Pharmacologic Management in Pregnancy

Medical Condition/ Disease State	Pharmacologic Management
Allergic rhinitis	Intranasal steroids (preferred: budesonide), cetirizine, loratadine
Asthma	Inhaled corticosteroids (preferred: budesonide), beta2-agonists
Pain	Acetaminophen
Chronic hypertension	Methyldopa, labetalol, nifedipine
Thrombosis	Low molecular weight heparin, unfractionated heparin
Infection	Cephalosporins, penicillins, azithromycin
Diabetes	Insulin
Gastroesophageal reflux disease	Antacids

Note: Not all-inclusive.

Sources: Gonzalez-Estrada A, Geraci SA. Allergy medications during pregnancy. *Am J Med Sci*. 2016;352(3):326–331. doi:10.1016/j.amjms.2016.05.030; Mehta N, Chen K, Powrie RO. Prescribing for the pregnant patient. *Cleve Clin J Med*. 2014;81(6):367–372. doi:10.3949/ccjm.81a.13124; National Heart, Lung, and Blood Institute; National Asthma Education, and Prevention Program Asthma and Pregnancy Working Group. NAEPP expert panel report. Managing asthma during pregnancy: recommendations for pharmacologic treatment—2004 update. *J Allergy Clin Immunol*. 2005;115(1):34–46. doi:10.1016/j.jaci.2004.10.023; Rayburn WF, Amanze AC. Prescribing medications safely during pregnancy. *Med Clin North Am*. 2008;92(5):1227–1237, xii. doi:10.1016/j.mcna.2008.04.006; Whelton PK, Carey RM, Aronow WS, et al. 2017 ACC/AHA/AAPA/ABC/ACPM/AGS/APhA/ASH/ASPC/NMA/PCNA guideline for the prevention, detection, evaluation, and management of high blood pressure in adults: a report of the American College of Cardiology/American Heart Association Task Force on clinical practice guidelines. *J Am Coll Cardiol*. 2018;71(19):e127–e248. doi:10.1161/HYP.0000000000000075

may not be the ideal candidate for warfarin therapy given its teratogenic effects. Thus, the clinician should consider initiation of a more appropriate alternative such as a low molecular weight heparin. **Figure 5.2** contains a depiction of agents with teratogenic potential.

Prescribing During Lactation

The American Academy of Pediatrics (AAP) recommends the review of several elements when deciding the course of treatment for a breastfeeding mother as it relates to continuation or discontinuation of either pharmacologic therapy or nursing. These elements involve therapeutic necessitation for an agent, quantity excreted into the milk, its impact on milk production, degree of infant absorption, and subsequent adverse effects.[34] Per limited case reports, it appears that almost 80% of cases involving adverse effects from maternal medications in nursing infants occurred in the first 2 months of age, with over half occurring in the first month postpartum.[35]

An enormous responsibility is placed upon all members of the healthcare team to ensure that neither a mother nor a breastfeeding infant is adversely affected by a medication used by the mother. To facilitate the process of prescribing and dispensing to this group, the AAP recommends the use of the LactMed® database when researching the safety of individual agents, excluding radioactive compounds that entail permanent or temporary termination of breastfeeding.[34] The database is updated monthly providing evidence-based data regarding the levels of drugs found in breast milk and infant blood, potential effects on the infant, and, if applicable, possible therapeutic substitutes for consideration. As with all patients, clinicians must assess the risk versus the benefit of therapies recommended to a nursing mother. While many agents are not explicitly deemed to be a risk to the infant, caution should still be employed to monitor medications that may lead to clinically significant infant exposure. Medications that potentially pose the most risk include those that exhibit increased serum concentration or relative infant dose, agents that concentrate in the milk, those lacking evidence of benefit, drugs with known toxicity to baby or mother, and agents with long half-lives and thus potential for accumulation.[34]

Resources for Clinicians

There are various resources to assist in the safe prescribing of drug therapy during pregnancy and lactation. **Box 5.2** contains a select number of them to aid when reviewing the safety and evidence for the use of medications in this stage of life.

BOX 5.2
ELECTRONIC PREGNANCY AND LACTATION RESOURCES

Drugs and Lactation Database (LactMed®), U.S. National Library of Medicine
• https://toxnet.nlm.nih.gov/newtoxnet/lactmed.htm

Developmental and Reproductive Toxicology Database (DART), U.S. National Library of Medicine
• https://toxnet.nlm.nih.gov/newtoxnet/dart.htm

Treating for Two: Medicine and Pregnancy (CDC)
• https://www.cdc.gov/pregnancy/meds/treatingfortwo/

Mother To Baby, Organization of Teratology Information Specialist (OTIS)
• https://mothertobaby.org/

REPROTOX, Reproductive Toxicology Center
• https://reprotox.org/

Natural Medicines, Therapeutic Research Center
• https://naturalmedicines.therapeuticresearch.com/

Note: Not all-inclusive.

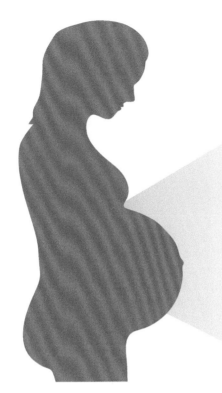

Angiotensin-converting-enzyme (ACE) inhibitors

Angiotensin II receptor blockers (ARBs)

Carbamazepine

Lithium

Methotrexate

Misoprostol

Phenytoin

Retinoids

Statins

Topiramate

Valproic acid

Warfarin

FIGURE 5.2 Teratogenic agents. Agents with teratogenic effects likely to result in fetal harm if taken by a pregnant patient. Figure is not all-inclusive.

Sources: AstraZeneca Pharmaceuticals. Crestor (rosuvastatin calcium) tablets. Updated 2010. https://www.accessdata.fda.gov/drugsatfda_docs/label/2010/021366s016lbl.pdf; Brent RL. How does a physician avoid prescribing drugs and medical procedures that have reproductive and developmental risks? *Clin Perinatol.* 2007;34(2):233–262. doi:10.1016/j.clp.2007.03.003; Janssen Pharmaceuticals. Topamax (topiramate) tablets label. Updated October 2012. https://www.accessdata.fda.gov/drugsatfda_docs/label/2012/020844s041lbl.pdf; Merck Sharp & Dohme. Cozaar (losartan potassium) tablets label. Revised March 2013. https://www.accessdata.fda.gov/drugsatfda_docs/label/2013/020386s058lbl.pdf; Parke-Davis. Dilantin (phenytoin sodium) capsule. Updated January 2009. https://www.accessdata.fda.gov/drugsatfda_docs/label/2009/084349s060lbl.pdf

CASE EXEMPLAR: Patient With Suspected Pregnancy

PK is a 32-year-old female who presents to her primary care appointment to determine if she is pregnant. She admits to missing "a couple pills" of her birth control. She used a home pregnancy test after becoming suspicious of her missing period.

Past Medical History

- Migraines (well controlled)
- Hypertension (well controlled)
- Allergic rhinitis (well controlled)

Medications

- Topiramate IR, 50 mg twice daily for migraine prophylaxis
- Naratriptan, 1 mg as needed for migraine

- Lisinopril, 20 mg daily for blood pressure
- Loratadine, 10 mg daily for allergies
- Ethinyl estradiol and drospirenone, one tablet daily

Labs

- hCG: positive

Diagnosis

- Pregnancy

Discussion Questions

1. PK, while surprised, is happy to learn the unexpected news and asks the clinician if

(continued)

CASE EXEMPLAR: Patient With Suspected Pregnancy (*continued*)

her current medications are safe to take in pregnancy. What is the most appropriate way to correctly address this question?

2. What alternative therapies can be recommended by PK's primary care clinician?

3. After delivery, should her clinician consider the potential for baby harm when making treatment recommendations?

GERIATRIC POPULATION

OVERVIEW

A substantial growth in prescription use in the geriatric population has occurred in recent years with 40% taking five or more medications.[36] This increase in medication use brings along additional considerations for this population, such as polypharmacy, potentially inappropriate medications (PIMs), prescribing cascades, and an increased risk for adverse effects. While the exact number of medications that constitutes polypharmacy has been debated, it is generally defined as the concomitant use of five or more medications by the same patient.[37] This is often the case given the higher incidence of chronic conditions generally seen in this population. However, it is further exacerbated by the addition of unnecessary therapies. A Veterans Affairs study found that almost 50% of older adults were taking at least one medication deemed unnecessary at discharge.[38] PIMs are defined by the American Geriatrics Society (AGS) Beers Criteria as medications that should generally be avoided due to an unnecessarily higher risk for adverse reactions in the geriatric population where an alternate option is available.[39] Their use is often encountered in practice; Patel et al.[40] reported that 29% of their study's elderly population were found to be taking at least one PIM.[40] The term "prescribing cascade" (**Figure 5.3**) describes the common pattern that occurs when clinicians prescribe new medications to address adverse drug reactions and side effects of an existing drug, instead of adjusting the offending agent.[41] While each issue provides its own set of complications, they typically occur together. This creates a challenge when attempting to identify the root cause, resulting in less optimal treatment strategies.

These phenomena, while not unique to the geriatric population, contribute strongly to the complicated nature of treating this population. While the PK and PD properties associated with aging affect the appropriateness of therapy, this is also further complicated by the additional medications and chronic conditions clinicians must navigate in order to treat a geriatric patient.

Pharmacokinetics and Pharmacodynamics in the Geriatric Population

The process of aging involves a decline in the physiological function of organs involved in drug absorption, distribution, and elimination. Drug-specific PK and PD studies are confounded due to polypharmacy and multiple comorbidities in this population. The consequences of age-related physiological changes should be considered in combination with any patient-specific confounding factors when optimizing therapeutic regimens and dose selection.

Increased gastric pH, delayed gastric emptying, and decreased intestinal motility are observed in the elderly; however, changes in drug absorption and bioavailability with age are not seen clinically. Data on intestinal transporter expression and activity changes with age are not available in the literature.

Body composition changes with age, with elderly individuals having decreased total body water and plasma volume, and increased body fat.[42] These changes can result in an increased V_D for lipophilic drugs, such as diazepam, and decreased V_D for polar drugs, such as lithium and digoxin.[42] Albumin concentrations decline with age, while alpha1-acid glycoprotein concentrations increase[43]; however, changes in plasma protein binding have not shown clinical significance in the elderly.[44]

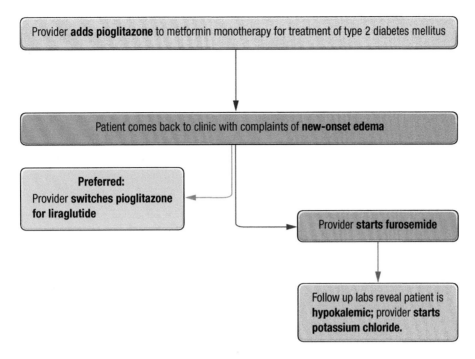

FIGURE 5.3 Example of a prescribing cascade. In this example, furosemide was added to treat new-onset edema, a result of pioglitazone therapy. This also led to hypokalemia and addition of an agent for its treatment. It would have been more appropriate to switch pioglitazone for a different agent, avoiding this cascade altogether.

Liver mass and hepatic blood flow decrease with age, leading to decreased hepatic clearance for drugs with flow-limited metabolism (propranolol and amitriptyline).[42] Phase 1 and 2 enzyme expression and activity are not altered by aging; however, metabolic drug interactions are more common in the elderly due to polypharmacy, and this may mask underlying changes in enzyme activity. GFR declines moderately with age[42] and can be estimated using the Cockcroft-Gault or the Modification of Diet in Renal Disease (MDRD) Study equations. In an attempt to better fit the Cockcroft-Gault equation, many settings may use an adjusted serum creatinine in geriatric patients, but this approach has been shown to be less accurate than the MDRD equation and results in a less accurate depiction of renal function; therefore, the MDRD equation remains preferred. Currently, there is no information in the literature on renal transporter activity in the elderly.

As with studies in pregnancy, there is limited PD data in aging populations due to the complexity of the analyses. Therapeutic outcome differences in the elderly may be related to PD changes (reduced receptor density), a decline in baseline function, or altered concentrations at the drug's site of action.[45] There are currently no general rules for predicting PD changes in the elderly, and therapeutic decisions should be based on an individual's PK and response.

Therapeutics in the Geriatric Population

Medication prescribing in the geriatric population utilizes many of the same methodologies as the adult population despite some of the differences observed in the former. However, additional guidance is available to assist clinicians in avoiding unwanted side effects and unnecessary therapies in geriatric patients. The following are some of the most utilized resources and concepts for appropriate prescribing in this population.

Beers Criteria

Since its inception in 1991, the Beers Criteria have focused on decreasing inappropriate medication use in the elderly.[46] While originally dedicated to the nursing home setting, through its many updates, it provides clinician guidance on all patient care settings excluding hospice and palliative care.[46–48] The 2015 AGS Beers Criteria was categorized into tables comprising of PIMs given older age, PIMs in specific conditions, medications to be used with caution, drug–drug interactions to be avoided, and drugs that require dose adjustment or avoidance based on renal function.[47] The 2019 AGS Beers Criteria further refines the content within these tables by removing agents no longer available in the United States (e.g., ticlopidine), medication use in specific conditions that is potentially inappropriate but not limited to the geriatric population (e.g., oral decongestants in those with insomnia), and recommendations with weak supporting evidence (e.g., avoidance of histamine-2 receptor antagonists in those with cognitive impairment or dementia), among others. Alternatively, it contains new PIM additions (e.g., glimepiride given increased risk of prolonged hypoglycemia), modifications to existing recommendations based on new evidence (e.g., age for caution regarding aspirin use in primary prevention was decreased from 80 to 70 years given increased risk for bleeding), and drug–drug interactions (e.g., concurrent opioid and benzodiazepine use given increased risk for overdose), among others.[48]

It is important to note that inclusion of a medication into these criteria does not mean that said therapy is categorically inappropriate, but rather that it has an increased risk of unwanted effects and thus warrants further review.[49] These criteria are meant to educate both clinicians and patients to improve pharmacological therapy utilization and decrease patient harm.[47] Of note, a publication was released alongside the 2015 AGS Beers Criteria containing guidance on alternative therapies to use in place of medications included in the Potentially Harmful Drug–Disease Interactions in the Elderly and Use of High-Risk Medications in the Elderly quality measures.[50] The 2019 AGS Beers Criteria endorse the review of this 2015 publication while recognizing that updates are needed to reflect new recommendations and available therapies.[37]

STOPP/START

In 2008, the Screening Tool of Older People's Prescriptions (STOPP) and Screening Tool to Alert to Right Treatment (START) criteria were published, undergoing updates in 2015.[51,52] The first component, STOPP, is similar to the Beers Criteria in that it provides guidance on potentially inappropriate medications in older adults. START is comprised of potential prescribing omissions or medications that should be recommended for elderly patients in the absence of legitimate rationale for omission.[51]

Deprescribing

Deprescribing comprises of removing pharmacologic therapy when it is harmful, no longer beneficial, or no longer indicated.[53] While not readily attributed to the prescribing continuum, deprescribing is a crucial component in chronic condition management that decreases pill burden and adverse effects.[54–56] Overlooking the deprescribing end of the prescribing continuum may potentially lead to an increase in polypharmacy, PIM usage, and prescribing cascades. When oppor-

---

BOX 5.3
ELECTRONIC GERIATRIC PRESCRIBING RESOURCES

2019 AGS Beers Criteria Pocketcard
- https://geriatricscareonline.org/ProductAbstract/2019-ags-beers-criteria-pocketcard/PC007

AGS Deprescribing Toolkit
- https://geriatricscareonline.org/ProductAbstract/ags-deprescribing-toolkit/TK013

Canadian Deprescribing Network
- https://www.deprescribingnetwork.ca

Deprescribing
- https://deprescribing.org

MedStopper
- http://medstopper.com

Note: Not all-inclusive.

---

tunities are identified for decreasing or discontinuing medications, open discussion and collaboration should take place to identify the safest mode of deprescribing based on the disease state being treated, drug(s) in question, and patient-specific factors.

Resources for Clinicians

Box 5.3 contains several available resources to aid clinicians in the prescribing and deprescribing of pharmacologic therapy in a geriatric patient.

CONCLUSION

These three separate stages of human development are unique in the challenges they pose when it comes to selecting the most appropriate pharmacologic therapy. These patients are encountered every day in primary care practice, but their management can also extend to specialists as dictated by the specific clinical case. Therefore, the safe and effective treatment of pediatric and geriatric patients as well as pregnant and nursing mothers is pertinent to all clinicians and members of the healthcare team. It is imperative that prescribing clinicians and nurses work together with pharmacists in the assessment of therapy appropriateness via comprehensive medication reviews. These collaborations will allow for the optimal therapy initiation or modification, monitoring, and, when pertinent, deprescribing of harmful or unnecessary medications.

CASE EXEMPLAR: Patient With Recent Fall and Dizziness

RG is a 76-year-old female who presents to the clinic for a follow up after a recent fall from getting "dizzy" while getting out of bed one morning. RG is very concerned this will happen again as she is afraid of "ending up in a nursing home."

Past Medical History

- Barrett's esophagus
- Hypertension (controlled)
- Neuropathic pain
- Osteoarthritis
- Osteoporosis

Medications

- Esomeprazole, 40 mg daily
- Doxazosin, 4 mg daily
- Amitriptyline, 100 mg at bedtime
- Naproxen, 250 mg twice daily
- Denosumab, 60 mg subcutaneous every 6 months
- Vitamin D, 800 IU daily

- Calcium citrate (elemental calciʉ one tablet three times per day
- Aspirin, 81 mg for primary prevention of cardiovascular events

Labs

- Normal

Discussion Questions

1. According to the 2019 AGS Beers Criteria, which of RG's medications is/are potentially inappropriate given her age, and what is the rationale for its/their inclusion?
2. According to the 2019 AGS Beers Criteria, which of RG's medications is/are potentially inappropriate given her falls history, and what is the rationale for its/their inclusion?
3. Based on the medication(s) identified in the previous question, what are potential therapeutic recommendations or medication alternatives for this patient?

CLINICAL PEARLS

- Dosing recommendations that are based on data derived from an average, nonpregnant adult population may not apply to pediatric patients, pregnant or lactating patients, or geriatric patients.
- Children have a higher proportion of lean body mass than do elderly patients, affecting their volumes of distribution for water- or fat-soluble medications.
- Administration of medication to pregnant or breastfeeding women must also consider the welfare of the baby.
- The physiologic responsiveness and clearance of drugs is often slower in geriatric patients than in children, and correcting the adverse effects of a medication in seniors may require more time.

- The LactMed® database can provide helpful information regarding the use of medications during lactation.
- Deprescribing of redundant or nonessential medications in elderly patients reduces the risk of drug–drug interactions.

KEY TAKEAWAYS

- When evaluating PK/PD changes over the life span, it is critical to understand the underlying physiological changes that contribute to alterations in clearance and volume.
- Pediatric doses should not be scaled directly from adult dosing values as drug disposition varies in pediatric patients, and it is crucial to

(continued)

- account for the maturation of drug absorption, metabolism, elimination, and distribution.
- Drug absorption in pediatric patients is influenced by developmental changes in gastrointestinal physiology (gastric pH, gastric emptying, intestinal motility, and expression of drug transporters), which may impact the rate and extent of drug absorption.
- While medication use during pregnancy and lactation is not to be discouraged, the appropriateness of the therapy should be considered to ensure safety of both mother and child.
- During pregnancy, the utmost care must be provided to ensure that medications used are safe and effective for the mother and fetus, with consideration for the stage of fetal development.
- While the exact number of medications that constitutes polypharmacy has been debated, it is generally defined as the concomitant use of five or more medications by the same patient.
- Body composition changes with age, with elderly individuals having decreased total body water and plasma volume, and increased body fat.
- The Beers Criteria have focused on decreasing inappropriate medication use in the elderly.
- Deprescribing comprises of removing pharmacologic therapy when it is harmful, no longer beneficial, or no longer indicated, and is a crucial component in chronic condition management that decreases pill burden and adverse effects.

REFERENCES

1. Priyadharsini R, Surendiran A, Adithan C, et al. A study of adverse drug reactions in pediatric patients. *J Pharmacol Pharmacother.* 2011;2(4):277–280. doi:10.4103/0976 -500X.85957
2. Smyth RM, Gargon E, Kirkham J, et al. Adverse drug reactions in children—A systematic review. *PLoS One.* 2012;7(3):e24061. doi:10.1371/journal.pone.0024061
3. Chien JY, Ho RJ. Drug delivery trends in clinical trials and translational medicine: evaluation of pharmacokinetic properties in special populations. *J Pharm Sci.* 2011;100(1):53–58. doi:10.1002/jps.22253
4. Napoleone E. Children and ADRs (adverse drug reactions). *Ital J Pediatr.* 2010;36:4. doi:10.1186/1824-7288-36-4
5. van den Anker J, Reed MD, Allegaert K, et al. Developmental changes in pharmacokinetics and pharmacodynamics. *J Clin Pharmacol.* 2018;58(suppl 10):S10–S25. doi:10.1002/jcph.1284
6. Yu G, Zheng QS, Li GF. Similarities and differences in gastrointestinal physiology between neonates and adults: a physiologically based pharmacokinetic modeling

perspective. *AAPS J.* 2014;16(6):1162–1166. doi:10.1208/s12248-014-9652-1
7. Mooij MG, Nies AT, Knibbe CA, et al. Development of human membrane transporters: drug disposition and pharmacogenetics. *Clin Pharmacokinet.* 2016;55(5):507–524. doi:10.1007/s40262-015-0328-5
8. Eidelman C, Abdel-Rahman SM. Pharmacokinetic considerations when prescribing in children. *Int J Pharmacokinet.* 2016;1(1):69–80. doi:10.4155/ipk-2016-0001
9. Schwartz GJ, Brion LP, Spitzer A. The use of plasma creatinine concentration for estimating glomerular filtration rate in infants, children, and adolescents. *Pediatr Clin North Am.* 1987;34(3):571–590. doi:10.1016/S0031-3955(16)36251-4
10. Mulla H. Understanding developmental pharmacodynamics: importance for drug development and clinical practice. *Paediatr Drugs.* 2010;12(4):223–233. doi:10.2165/11319220-000000000-00000
11. Dunne J, Margaryants L, Murphy MD, et al. Globalization facilitates pediatric drug development in the 21st century. *Drug Inf J.* 2010;44(6):757–765. doi:10.1177/009286151004400612
12. Das P, Nof E, Amirav I, et al. Targeting inhaled aerosol delivery to upper airways in children: insight from computational fluid dynamics (CFD). *PLoS One.* 2018;13(11):e0207711. doi:10.1371/journal.pone.0207711
13. Dolovich M. Aerosol delivery to children: what to use, how to choose. *Pediatr Pulmonol Suppl.* 1999;18:79–82. doi:10.1002/(SICI)1099-0496(1999)27:18+<79::AID -PPUL27>3.0.CO;2-9
14. Mitchell AA, Gilboa SM, Werler MM, et al. Medication use during pregnancy, with particular focus on prescription drugs: 1976-2008. *Am J Obstet Gynecol.* 2011;205(1):51.e1–51.e8. doi:10.1016/j.ajog.2011.02.029
15. Haas DM, Marsh DJ, Dang DT, et al. Prescription and other medication use in pregnancy. *Obstet Gynecol.* 2018;131(5):789–798. doi:10.1097/AOG.0000000000002579
16. Thorpe PG, Gilboa SM, Hernandez-Diaz S, et al. Medications in the first trimester of pregnancy: most common exposures and critical gaps in understanding fetal risk. *Pharmacoepidemiol Drug Saf.* 2013;22(9):1013–1018. doi:10.1002/pds.3495
17. Werler MM, Mitchell AA, Hernandez-Diaz S, et al. Use of over-the-counter medications during pregnancy. *Am J Obstet Gynecol.* 2005;193(3, pt 1):771–777. doi:10.1016/j.ajog.2005.02.100
18. Centers for Disease Control and Prevention. *Health, United States.* National Center for Health Statistics; 2018.
19. Feghali M, Venkataramanan R, Caritis S. Pharmacokinetics of drugs in pregnancy. *Semin Perinatol.* 2015;39(7):512–519. doi:10.1053/j.semperi.2015.08.003
20. Costantine MM. Physiologic and pharmacokinetic changes in pregnancy. *Front Pharmacol.* 2014;5:65. doi:10.3389/fphar.2014.00065
21. Pariente G, Leibson T, Carls A, et al. Pregnancy-associated changes in pharmacokinetics: a systematic review. *PLoS Med.* 2016;13(11):e1002160. doi:10.1371/journal.pmed.1002160
22. Anderson GD. Pregnancy-induced changes in pharmacokinetics: a mechanistic-based approach. *Clin Pharmacokinet.* 2005;44(10):989–1008. doi:10.2165/00003088-200544100-00001

23. Hebert MF, Carr DB, Anderson GD, et al. Pharmacokinetics and pharmacodynamics of atenolol during pregnancy and postpartum. *J Clin Pharmacol.* 2005;45(1):25–33. doi:10.1177/0091270004269704

24. Luxford AM, Kellaway GS. Pharmacokinetics of digoxin in pregnancy. *Eur J Clin Pharmacol.* 1983;25(1):117–121. doi:10.1007/BF00544027

25. Schou M, Amdisen A, Steenstrup OR. Lithium and pregnancy. II. Hazards to women given lithium during pregnancy and delivery. *Br Med J.* 1973;2(5859):137–138. doi:10.1136/bmj.2.5859.137

26. Pennell PB, Newport DJ, Stowe ZN, et al. The impact of pregnancy and childbirth on the metabolism of lamotrigine. *Neurology.* 2004;62(2):292–295. doi:10.1212/01.WNL.0000103286.47129.F8

27. Colbers AP, Hawkins DA, Gingelmaier A, et al. The pharmacokinetics, safety and efficacy of tenofovir and emtricitabine in HIV-1-infected pregnant women. *AIDS.* 2013;27(5):739–748. doi:10.1097/QAD.0b013e32835c208b

28. Tomson T, Palm R, Kallen K, et al. Pharmacokinetics of levetiracetam during pregnancy, delivery, in the neonatal period, and lactation. *Epilepsia.* 2007;48(6):1111–1116. doi:10.1111/j.1528-1167.2007.01032.x

29. Westin AA, Nakken KO, Johannessen SI, et al. Serum concentration/dose ratio of topiramate during pregnancy. *Epilepsia.* 2009;50(3):480–485. doi:10.1111/j.1528-1167.2008.01776.x

30. Ramoz LL, Patel-Shori NM. Recent changes in pregnancy and lactation labeling: retirement of risk categories. *Pharmacotherapy.* 2014;34(4):389–395. doi:10.1002/phar.1385

31. Food and Drug Administration. Content and format of labeling for human prescription drug and biological products; requirements for pregnancy and lactation labeling. In: Department of Health and Human Services, ed. *Federal Register.* Office of the Federal Register; 2008 https://www.federalregister.gov/documents/2008/05/29/E8-11806/content-and-format-of-labeling-for-human-prescription-drug-and-biological-products-requirements-for.

32. Pernia S, DeMaagd G. The new pregnancy and lactation labeling rule. *P T.* 2016;41(11):713–715. https://www.ncbi.nlm.nih.gov/pmc/articles/PMC5083079

33. Food and Drug Administration. Content and format of labeling for human prescription drug and biological products; requirements for pregnancy and lactation. In: Department of Health and Human Services. *Federal Register.* Office of the Federal Register; 2014 https://www.federalregister.gov/documents/2014/12/04/2014-28241/content-and-format-of-labeling-for-human-prescription-drug-and-biological-products-requirements-for4.

34. Sachs HC, Committee on Drugs. The transfer of drugs and therapeutics into human breast milk: an update on selected topics. *Pediatrics.* 2013;132(3):e796–e809. doi:10.1542/peds.2013-1985

35. Anderson PO, Manoguerra AS, Valdes V. A review of adverse reactions in infants from medications in breastmilk. *Clin Pediatr (Phila).* 2016;55(3):236–244. doi:10.1177/0009922815594586

36. Charlesworth CJ, Smit E, Lee DS, et al. Polypharmacy among adults aged 65 years and older in the United States: 1988–2010. *J Gerontol A Biol Sci Med Sci.* 2015;70(8):989–995. doi:10.1093/gerona/glv013

37. Golchin N, Frank SH, Vince A, et al. Polypharmacy in the elderly. *J Res Pharm Pract.* 2015;4(2):85–88. doi:10.4103/2279-042X.155755

38. Hajjar ER, Hanlon JT, Sloane RJ, et al. Unnecessary drug use in frail older people at hospital discharge. *J Am Geriatr Soc.* 2005;53(9):1518–1523. doi:10.1111/j.1532-5415.2005.53523.x

39. American Geriatrics Society Beers Criteria Update Expert Panel. American Geriatrics Society updated Beers Criteria for potentially inappropriate medication use in older adults. *J Am Geriatr Soc.* 2012;60(4):616–631. doi:10.1111/j.1532-5415.2012.03923.x

40. Patel R, Zhu L, Sohal D, et al. Use of 2015 Beers Criteria medications by older medicare beneficiaries. *Consult Pharm.* 2018;33(1):48–54. doi:10.4140/TCP.n.2018.48

41. Rochon PA, Gurwitz JH. The prescribing cascade revisited. *Lancet.* 2017;389(10081):1778–1780. doi:10.1016/S0140-6736(17)31188-1

42. Klotz U. Pharmacokinetics and drug metabolism in the elderly. *Drug Metab Rev.* 2009;41(2):67–76. doi:10.1080/03602530902722679

43. Butler JM, Begg EJ. Free drug metabolic clearance in elderly people. *Clin Pharmacokinet.* 2008;47(5):297–321. doi:10.2165/00003088-200847050-00002

44. Benet LZ, Hoener BA. Changes in plasma protein binding have little clinical relevance. *Clin Pharmacol Ther.* 2002;71(3):115–121. doi:10.1067/mcp.2002.121829

45. Corsonello A, Pedone C, Incalzi RA. Age-related pharmacokinetic and pharmacodynamic changes and related risk of adverse drug reactions. *Curr Med Chem.* 2010;17(6):571–584. doi:10.2174/092986710790416326

46. Beers MH, Ouslander JG, Rollingher I, et al. Explicit criteria for determining inappropriate medication use in nursing home residents. *Arch Intern Med.* 1991;151(9):1825–1832. doi:10.1001/archinte.1991.00400090107019

47. American Geriatrics Society Beers Criteria Update Expert Panel. American Geriatrics Society 2015 updated Beers Criteria for potentially inappropriate medication use in older adults. *J Am Geriatr Soc.* 2015;63(11):2227–2246. doi:10.1111/jgs.13702

48. American Geriatrics Society Beers Criteria Update Expert Panel. American Geriatrics Society 2019 updated ags Beers Criteria® for potentially inappropriate medication use in older adults. *J Am Geriatr Soc.* 2019. 67(4):674–694. doi:10.1111/jgs.15767

49. Steinman MA, Beizer JL, DuBeau CE, et al. How to use the American Geriatrics Society 2015 Beers Criteria—A guide for patients, clinicians, health systems, and payors. *J Am Geriatr Soc.* 2015;63(12):e1–e7. doi:10.1111/jgs.13701

50. Hanlon JT, Semla TP, Schmader KE. Alternative medications for medications in the use of high-risk medications in the elderly and potentially harmful drug–disease interactions in the elderly quality measures. *J Am Geriatr Soc.* 2015;63(12):e8–e18. doi:10.1111/jgs.13807

51. O'Mahony D, O'Sullivan D, Byrne S, et al. STOPP/START criteria for potentially inappropriate prescribing in older people: version 2. *Age Ageing.* 2015;44(2):213–218. doi:10.1093/ageing/afu145

52. Gallagher P, Ryan C, Byrne S, et al. STOPP (Screening Tool of Older Person's Prescriptions) and START

(Screening Tool to Alert doctors to Right Treatment). Consensus validation. *Int J Clin Pharmacol Ther.* 2008;46(2):72–83. doi:10.5414/CPP46072

53. Farrell B, Conklin J, Dolovich L, et al. Deprescribing guidelines: an international symposium on development, implementation, research and health professional education. *Res Social Adm Pharm.* 2019;15(6):780–789. doi:10.1016/j.sapharm.2018.08.010

54. American Geriatrics Society Expert Panel on the Care of Older Adults with Multimorbidity. Patient-centered care for older adults with multiple chronic conditions: a stepwise approach from the American Geriatrics Society *J Am Geriatr Soc.* 2012;60(10): 1957–1968. doi:10.1111/j.1532-5415.2012.04187.x

55. Scott IA, Hilmer SN, Reeve E, et al. Reducing inappropriate polypharmacy: the process of deprescribing. *JAMA Intern Med.* 2015;175(5):827–834. doi:10.1001/jamaint ernmed.2015.0324

56. deprescribing.org. What is deprescribing? Accessed January 10, 2019. https://deprescribing.org/what-is -deprescribing

Drug-Therapy Prescribing in Special Populations

Reamer Bushardt and Courtney J. Perry

LEARNING OBJECTIVES

- Identify populations at higher risk for medication-induced adverse events based on their individual risk factors.
- Discuss the impact of renal and hepatic dysfunction on drug metabolism.
- Interpret the results of laboratory tests that may identify those in need of adjustments to their medication regimens.
- Analyze which combinations of medications may pose a significant health risk for certain populations.
- Compose a list of safe alternative treatments for patients with certain risk factors.
- Evaluate a medication list for a patient with medical risk factors.

INTRODUCTION

The United States spends between $323 and $477 billion annually on pharmaceuticals, making drug prescribing and consumption of over-the-counter medications a major part of healthcare expenditures.[1] Effective medications, immunizations, and novel pharmaceutical devices have ushered in numerous benefits for Americans and transformed how we support health and treat and prevent illness. At the same time, no medication is without risks, and those risks can increase when prescribing is not optimized for individual patients. An adverse drug event (ADE) is "an injury resulting from medical intervention related to a drug" and a large majority of them are preventable; ADEs encompass issues like medication errors, adverse drug reactions,

allergic reactions, and overdoses.[2] In hospital settings, ADEs comprise a third of hospital adverse events, impact around 2 million hospitalizations each year, and increase costs and length of stays.[3,4] In outpatient settings, ADEs account for more than 3.5 million clinic visits, a million emergency room visits, and nearly 125,000 hospitalizations.[5-7] As prescribers, it is critical that we apply evidence-based decision-making to identify and prescribe drug therapy and engage patients and families. Issues like safety, tolerability, efficacy, price, ease of administration, drug cost, genetic factors, medical comorbidities, and concurrent medications are examples of those to consider prior to prescribing. Select patient populations and physiologic factors are known to influence the risk of drug injury, thus compelling prescribers to be particularly cautious when selecting, dosing, and monitoring medications. Commonly recognized special populations include those related to these factors: age, pregnancy or breastfeeding, race/ethnicity, hepatic and renal function, weight, and genetic factors.

The pharmacokinetics (see Chapter 2) of a drug depend on drug-related and patient-related factors. Commonly recognized patient-related factors (e.g., age, weight, renal or liver function) are often used to estimate pharmacokinetic parameters for specific populations. Alterations in renal or liver function can cause wide variability in these parameters, which has implications for drug selection, dosing, and monitoring. This chapter presents principles, practical guidance, and tools to support appropriate prescribing for commonly encountered special populations.

OPTIMIZING DRUG THERAPY FOR RENAL FUNCTION

Medications that require clearance of active metabolites through the kidneys will have reduced elimination in patients with significant renal dysfunction or kidney disease. Kidney disease can impact glomerular filtration, tubular secretion, and reabsorption. Inadequate adjustment in dosage of medications in this population is known to lead to increased risk of adverse effects and toxicities. Efforts to evaluate renal function are key for prescribers to appropriately dose medications in this population.

Appropriate dosage of renally cleared medications depends on an accurate estimate of glomerular filtration rate (GFR) or creatinine clearance (CrCl). It is important to note that estimated GFR is expressed as mL/min/1.73 m^2 while CrCl is expressed as mL/min and should be considered while analyzing values and their implications. Many equations exist to provide prescribers with an estimation of GFR and CrCl in adult patients. Guidelines, including the Kidney Disease Improving Global Outcomes (KDIGO), recommend use of the following three: Cockcroft-Gault,[8] Modification of Diet in Renal Disease (MDRD),[9] or Chronic Kidney Disease Epidemiology Collaboration (CKD-EPI)[10] (**Exhibit 6.1**).[11] Another option for calculation of CrCl is a 24-hour urine collection; however, this is rarely used due to complexity and overestimation of GFR.[12]

While Cockcroft-Gault is used commonly, the MDRD and CKD-EPI equations have been found to be more accurate. The Cockcroft-Gault equation, expressed in mL/min, often overestimates renal function in obese patients.[13] Additionally, it is not normalized to body surface area (BSA) and must be adjusted in order to compare to normal values. Lastly, prescribers should note that the equation was created before the availability of standardized creatinine assays, often resulting in overestimation of CrCl.[14] MDRD, expressed in mL/

min/1.73 m^2, also overestimates renal function in obese patients and is less accurate in patients with normal renal function or patients of Asian descent.[13,15–17] However, the MDRD and CKD-EPI equations appear to be most accurate in patients with known chronic kidney disease (i.e., GFR <60 mL/min/1.73 m^2).[15,17] CKD-EPI, expressed in mL/min/1.73 m^2, appears to be the most accurate equation for use in patients with normal or near normal function and those with higher body mass indices.[10,18] Modifications to the CKD-EPI and MDRD equation, to account for difference in race and ethnicity, can provide increased accuracy and help account for their preference over other equations.[11,18]

All three of the discussed equations are limited in their use of creatinine, which is affected by numerous variables aside from renal function (e.g., obesity and increased muscle mass). Additionally, they do not provide accurate estimates of GFR in patients with rapidly changing glomerular filtration, as in acute kidney injury. Prescribers must be cautious when using estimated GFR or CrCl calculations to make dose adjustments in patients affected by these variables.

The U.S. Food and Drug Administration (FDA) has recommended that pharmaceutical industries use Cockcroft-Gault to measure estimated CrCl in pharmacokinetic studies of patients with impaired renal function to characterize the impact on pharmacokinetics.[19] Because of this recommendation, drug monographs most often recommend dosing adjustments based on estimated CrCl in mL/min, which has been calculated by the Cockcroft-Gault equation. It is important to remember that this recommendation came from the FDA prior to the availability of the MDRD or CKD-EPI equations. Recent studies have

---

EXHIBIT 6-1 EQUATIONS FOR ESTIMATION OF GLOMERULAR FILTRATION RATE

Cockcroft-Gault

$$\text{CrCl (mL/min)} = \left(\frac{(140 - \text{age}) \times \text{Weight(kg)}}{\text{serum creatine(mg/dL)} \times 72} \right) \times 0.85 \text{ for women}$$

MDRw

Estimated GFR (mL/min/1.73 m^2) = $175 \times S_{cr}$ (mg/dL)$^{-1.154} \times$ age$^{-0.203} \times 0.742$ [if female] $\times 1.212$ [if Black]

CKD-EPI

GFR (mL/min/1.73 m^2) = $141 \times \min (S_{cr}/k, 1)^{a} \times \max (S_{cr}/k, 1)^{-1.209} \times 0.993^{Age} \times 1.018$ [if female]
$\times 1.159$ [if Black]
min = indicates the minimum of S_{cr}/k or 1
max = indicates the maximum of S_{cr}/k or 1
S_{cr} = serum creatinine (mg/dL)
k = 0.7 [females] or 0.9 [males]
a = −0.329 [females] or −0.411 [males]

CKD-EPI, Chronic Kidney Disease Epidemiology Collaboration; CrCl, creatinine clearance; GFR, glomerular filtration rate; K, potassium; MDRD, Modification of Diet in Renal Disease; S$_{cr}$, serum creatinine.
Source: Adapted from Cockcroft DW, Gault MH. Prediction of creatinine clearance from serum creatinine. *Nephron.* 1976;16(1):31–41. doi:10.1159/000180580; Levey AS, Bosch JP, Lewis JB, et al. A more accurate method to estimate glomerular filtration rate fcrom serum creatinine: a new prediction equation. *Ann Intern Med.* 1999;130(6):461–470. doi:10.7326/0003-4819-130-6-199903160-00002 Levey AS, Stevens LA, Schmid CH, et al. A new equation to estimate glomerular filtration rate. *Ann Intern Med.* 2009;150(9):604–612. doi:10.7326/0003-4819-150-9-200905050-00006

shown reasonable concordance of the MDRD equation with the Cockccroft-Gault equation, and the CKD-EPI with the MDRD equation.[15] This suggests they can be appropriate to use for drug dosing, accompanied by mindfulness of the units expressed.[20] In patients whose body size is significantly different than average (BSA 1.73 m²) the MDRD and CKD-EPI equations may be discordant with Cockcroft-Gault and may require conversion of units (**Figure 6.1**) or utilization of measured versus estimated GFR or CrCl.[21] Measured values may also be more appropriate when prescribing medications with a narrow therapeutic index or any time there is discordance between estimated GFR or CrCl.[21]

Because of the increased accuracy of the MDRD and CKD-EPI equations, the KDIGO clinical update suggests selection of an equation for estimation of GFR or CrCl that is most appropriate for the patient as opposed to consistent use of the Cockcroft-Gault equation.[22] Commonly pre-scribed medications whose clearance is impacted by renal function are presented in **Table 6.1**, along with suggested dose adjustments for the given severity of renal dysfunction. Prescribers should seek official dosing recommendations from the drug monograph or an approved drug reference. Adjustments discussed in the table are not inclusive of recommendations for patients receiving dialysis.

OPTIMIZING DRUG THERAPY FOR LIVER FUNCTION

Metabolism of drugs by the liver is a critical pharmacokinetic pathway for many medications used in the United States, including prescription and over-the-counter drugs. Hepatic impairment and other alterations in metabolic capacity, such as those observed in drug interactions or due to genetic variations, are important considerations in optimizing a drug therapy plan to support both safety

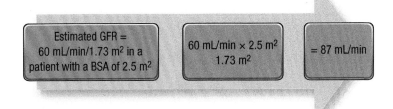

FIGURE 6.1 Conversion of units from mL/min/1.73 m² to mL/min.

TABLE 6.1 Common Medications That Require Dose Adjustments in Kidney Dysfunction

Medication	CrCl 50 to 10 mL/min	CrCl <10 mL/min
Antimicrobials		
Cephalosporins		
Cefazolin	50%–100% of dose every 8–12 hours	50% of dose every 18–24 hours
Ceftazidime	25%–100% of dose every 12–24 hours	25%–50% of dose every 24–48 hours
Cefdinir	100% of dose every 12–24 hours	100% of dose every 24 hours
Penicillins		
Amoxicillin (immediate-release form)	25%–100% of dose every 8–12 hours	25%–100% of dose every 24 hours
Piperacillin/tazobactam	50%–75% of dose every 6–8 hours	50%–75% of dose every 6–8 hours
Carbapenems		
Meropenem	50%–100% of dose every 12 hours	50% of dose every 24 hours
Aminoglycosides		
Gentamicin	100% of dose every 12–48 hours	100% of dose every 48–72 hours
Amikacin	100% of dose every 24–72 hours based on levels	100% of dose every 48–72 hours based on levels
Pain Medications		
Opioids		
Hydromorphone	25%–50% of starting dose	50% of starting dose
Oxycodone	33%–50% of starting dose	33%–50% of starting dose
NSAIDs		
Ibuprofen	Avoid or use with caution	Avoid use
Naproxen	Avoid or use with caution	Avoid use

(continued)

TABLE 6.1 Common Medications That Require Dose Adjustments in Kidney Dysfunction *(continued)*

Medication	CrCl 50 to 10 mL/min	CrCl <10 mL/min
Cardiovascular Medications		
Antihypertensives		
Lisinopril	25%–100% of starting dose	25%–100% of starting dose
Bisoprolol	25%–100% of starting dose	25%–100% of starting dose
Diuretics		
Spironolactone	Avoid or use with caution	Avoid use
Thiazides	Less effective <30 mL/min	Avoid use

BSA, body surface area; CrCl, creatinine clearance; GFR, glomerular filtration rate.

Source: Data from Lexicomp Online. Pediatric and Neonatal Lexi-Drugs Online. Lexicomp, Inc.; 2019. https://online.lexi.com

and effectiveness. Drugs with small margins of safety, or a narrow therapeutic index, that require hepatic metabolism must be carefully managed given a heightened risk of accumulation and toxicity. While the effects of a dysfunctional liver on drug metabolism are easy to appreciate, the liver plays an important role in the absorption, distribution, and elimination of many drugs. Liver problems can affect metabolic enzyme activity, liver blood flow, plasma protein binding, and biliary excretion.[23] Another consideration is the role of the liver for medications known as prodrugs, which are biologically inactive until metabolized in the body to produce an active drug. **Box 6.1** provides examples of prodrugs by therapeutic class. Liver dysfunction that impairs activation of a prodrug has significant ramifications for the utility of that treatment which should be assessed prior to prescribing. Drug developers have increasingly targeted cytochrome P450 enzymes in recent years for prodrug activation, making this issue relevant for prescribers.[24]

Clinicians will encounter adult patients more frequently than children or adolescents that require drug therapy adjustments based on liver dysfunction. Consider adults with liver disease, those on complex medication regimens or using biologics, and patients with medical comorbidities that may impact liver health. The metabolism of drugs is, however, the most complicated pharmacokinetic difference between adult and pediatric patients. The cytochrome P450 enzyme system becomes active in the fetus. Increases in enzyme activity occur during the later stages of pregnancy with considerable variability in enzyme development among preterm infants. Typically, pediatric liver enzyme activity has reached or exceeded adult levels by age 2 years, but the pattern can change significantly during the first few months of life. Among cytochrome P450 enzymes, there are those that continue to increase in activity and others that are replaced by new enzymes. A developmental difference to consider in infants is their relatively high liver blood flow, which can impact first-pass metabolism and significantly alter the effects of high extraction drugs.[25]

Unfortunately, there is not a single, reliable biochemical marker to predict liver function related to drug

BOX 6.1
EXAMPLES OF PRODRUGS ACTIVATED BY CYTOCHROME P450 ENZYME

Therapeutic Class and Prodrug(s)

Antiplatelet
- Clopidogrel
- Prasugrel

Nonsteroidal Anti-Inflammatory
- Nabumetone

Antihistamine
- Loratadine

Antihypertensive
- Losartan

Antiviral
- Pradefovir

elimination. The Child-Pugh score is often used to evaluate the severity of hepatic impairment, but the results offer prescribers limited guidance for subsequent drug therapy adjustment.[23] The Child-Pugh classification combines five variables to estimate the severity of hepatic disease: serum bilirubin, serum albumin, prothrombin time, and the presence of encephalopathy and/or ascites.[26] A point system then classifies the severity of liver disease as mild, moderate, or severe (refer to www.hepatitisc .uw.edu/page/clinical-calculators/ctp for an online calculator). The Model for End-Stage Liver Disease (MELD) is another classification system used in patients with advanced disease.[27,28] If a drug requires liver elimination, there are several important factors to consider before prescribing it to a patient with hepatic impairment or disease (**Box 6.2**). Clinicians should try to avoid prescribing a drug (or consider significant dose reductions) with a narrow margin of safety to a patient with liver disease

BOX 6.2
PRESCRIBING CONSIDERATIONS FOR PATIENTS WITH HEPATIC DISEASE OR IMPAIRMENT

Before prescribing drugs that require liver metabolism:
* Consider the extent of total drug elimination that is liver-dependent.
* Estimate the severity of liver impairment (e.g., Child-Pugh classification).
* Identify potential drug-drug interactions with current drug therapies.
* Evaluate for concurrent comorbidities that may impact drug safety (e.g., malnutrition, proteinemia, alcoholism, heart failure, renal disease).

Source: Data from Sloss A, Kubler P. Prescribing in liver disease. *Austr Prescr.* 2009;32(2):32–35. doi:10.18773/austprescr.2009.018

if it requires significant liver metabolism (e.g., greater than 20% of overall elimination is liver-dependent).[29]

While there is considerable work to be done to better understand the connection between liver function and drug safety, improvements are being seen. Cases of severe liver injury caused by prescription drugs, over-the-counter medications, and alternative products (e.g., herbal products, dietary supplements) are regularly collected and analyzed by the National Institute of Diabetes and Digestive and Kidney Diseases' Drug-Induced Liver Injury Network (DILIN). The DILIN is growing our understanding of clinical, immunological, and environmental risk factors for drug injury, facilitating research, and disseminating the results.[30] The FDA has also enhanced guidance, regulations, and reporting requirements related to liver safety, resulting in a major reduction in the number of approved drugs that have been removed from market because of liver injury.[31]

DRUG THERAPY IN PEDIATRICS

Almost three-fourths of medications lack and FDA-approved indication for use in pediatric patients. Furthermore, the availability of pharmacokinetic and pharmacodynamic data on pediatric patients is limited. This often results in prescribers extrapolating pediatric doses from adult doses. The need for adjustment in dosing of medications in pediatrics arises predominantly from significant differences in pharmacodynamic and pharmacokinetic properties of medications in this population, compared to adults. Differences in all major pharmacokinetic principles (i.e., absorption, distribution, metabolism, and excretion) exist across the life span of pediatric patients. Dosage adjustments in pediatric

patients result predominantly from differences that relate to changes in metabolism, excretion, and distribution of medications. Just as pediatric patients cannot be dosed similarly to adult patients; there is variation in pharmacokinetic properties of neonates, infants, children, and adolescents that also require prescribers to make dosage adjustments across the pediatric age-span.[32]

Phase 1 (e.g., the cytochrome P450 system) and phase 2 (e.g., sulfation and glucuronidation) enzyme systems responsible for hepatic metabolism of medications are immature at birth and can be responsible for significant toxicities and therapeutic failures in neonates and young infants.[32–34] Inability of neonates and young infants to convert a medication to an inactive form can result in drug accumulation and therefore toxicities, as seen with many antibiotics and pain medications. This can lead to a longer half-life and the need for extended dosing intervals.[35,36] Conversely, the inability to activate a prodrug can lead to diminished therapeutic effect as seen with codeine and tramadol.

As the enzyme systems mature throughout the first years of life, they approach and then exceed adult levels through childhood and often into adolescence.[32] Rapid metabolism of medications in children and adolescents can result in reduced concentrations of active drugs and the need for shortened dosing intervals or higher doses, as seen with opioids such as morphine and oxycodone.[35,36] In contrast, rapid conversion of prodrugs in children and adolescents can lead to accumulation of active metabolites and is responsible for respiratory depression and sedation seen with the use of tramadol and codeine in this population. Because of this outcome, the FDA has recommended against the use of these agents in children under 18 for most indications and they are contraindicated for patients less than 12 years of age.[37]

Similar to the hepatic enzyme system, renal excretion of medications is immature at birth and into infancy due to reduced glomerular filtration. Reduced GFR can lead to significant toxicities as a result of accumulation of medications that are cleared predominantly through the kidneys. Similar to metabolism, as GFR increases through the first year of life, it will also approach and then exceed adult levels in early childhood and often into adolescence.[32,38] Rapid clearance of medications in children and adolescents can result in rapid clearance of medications and often requires a shortened dosing interval or higher doses, as seen with opioids and antibiotics.

As with adults, we can estimate glomerular filtration using serum creatinine (SCr). In children, most commonly the Schwartz, Updated "Bedside" Schwartz, and "1B" equations are used by prescribers as validated methods to estimate GFR and therefore renal function (**Exhibit 6.2**).[38,39] Many medications require a dosage adjustment when GFR or CrCl fall below 50 mL/min/1.73 m² or 50 mL/min, respectively.[11] In neonates, prescribers must be cautious when using these equations as SCr is not reflective of renal function for the first week of life.

It is important for prescribers to consider the impact of medications eliminated through breast milk in children and infants that are breastfed and that of medications that cross the placenta in pregnant patients. Classification of the safety of medications to be used in pregnancy and lactation were updated in 2015 with the goal of removing the labeling of medications as A, B, C, D, X for prescription products. The new labeling system is designed to better allow the clinician to understand risks and benefits of use of medications in pregnancy and lactation. It is crucial that clinicians reference the appropriate resources to safely dose and administer medications in pregnant and lactating patients such as: the drug monograph, the FDA pregnancy registry, and books such as *Drugs in Pregnancy and Lactation* by Briggs and colleagues.[40,41]

Alteration in distribution of medications in pediatric patients compared to adults stems largely from differences in total body water composition. Neonates and young infants have significantly higher total body water content, necessitating higher doses of hydrophilic medications, such as gentamicin. Conversely,

lower doses of hydrophilic medications are required as children grow and their total body water content declines. Additionally, neonates have a decrease in the plasma binding protein, albumin. Medications that are highly bound to albumin can displace bilirubin and increase risk of jaundice and kernicterus, as seen with ceftriaxone and sulfamethoxazole.[13,32,37]

Differences in pharmacokinetics contribute to the necessity of age-appropriate dose adjustments for many medications. **Table 6.2** reviews common medications that require dose adjustments due to developmental differences in metabolism, excretion, and distribution of medications for pediatric patients across the age-span. Dosing considerations may also be important when considering the route of administration as pediatric patients have varied absorption of medications across the age-span (see Chapter 5) and as compared to adults (**Box 6.3**).

Drug dosing in pediatric patients is often discussed as a product of the patient's weight or BSA. While this approach is practical, it does not account for differences in maturation of absorption, distribution, and metabolism of medications between patients. Major differences in pharmacokinetic properties of medications

EXHIBIT 6.2 PEDIATRIC EQUATIONS TO ESTIMATE GLOMERULAR FILTRATION RATE

Schwartz Equation

$$\text{GFR (mL / min/ 1.73 m}^2) = \frac{k \times \text{height (cm)}}{\text{Serum Creatinine (mg / dL)}}$$

k = constant
k = 0.45 for infants 1–52 weeks old
k = 0.55 for children 1–13 years old
k = 0.55 for adolescent females 13–18 years old
k = 0.7 for adolescent males 13–18 years old

Updated Schwartz Equatihn

$$\text{GFR (mL / min/ 1.73 m}^2) = \frac{0.413 \times \text{height (cm)}}{\text{Serum Creatinine (mg / dL)}}$$

1B equation
$$\text{GFR (mL/min/1.73 m}^2) = 40.7 \times (\text{height/SCr [mg/dL]})^{0.64} \times (30/\text{BUN [mg/dL]})^{0.202}$$

BUN, blood urea nitrogen; GFR, glomerular filtration rate; SCr, serum creatinine.

Source: Adapted from Food and Drug Administration. Pregnancy registry information for health professionals. Published 2018. https://www.fda.gov/ScienceResearch/SpecialTopics/WomensHealthResearch/ucm256789.htm; Schwartz GJ, Muñoz A, Schneider MF, et al. New equations to estimate GFR in children with CKD. *J Am Soc Nephrol.* 2009;20(3):629–637. doi:10.1681/ASN.2008030287

TABLE 6.2 Medications That Commonly Require Dose Adjustments in Pediatric Patients

Medication	Major Principles	Dosing Adjustments*
Antibiotics		
Cephalosporins Ceftazidime Ceftriaxone	↓ Excretion Distribution (protein bound)	Neonates: Longer dosing interval at lower PMA
		Neonates: Avoid due to decreased albumin and displacement of bilirubin
Penicillins Ampicillin Nafcillin	↓ Excretion	Neonates: Longer dosing interval at lower PMA

(continued)

TABLE 6.2 Medications That Commonly Require Dose Adjustments in Pediatric Patients (*continued*)

Medication	Major Principles	Dosing Adjustments*
Aminoglycosides Gentamicin	↓ Excretion and ↑ distribution (hydrophilic)	Neonates: Longer dosing interval and higher dose at lower PMA
Sulfamethoxazole	Distribution (protein bound)	Neonates: Avoid use due to decreased albumin and displacement of bilirubin
Clindamycin	↓ Metabolism	Neonates: Longer dosing interval and lower doses at lower PMA
Pain Medications		
Morphine	↓ Metabolism and excretion ↑ Metabolism and excretion	Neonates: Lower doses needed Children and adolescents: Higher (mg/kg) doses
Ibuprofen	↓ Metabolism	Infants and children <6 months: Avoid in this population
Codeine	↑ Metabolism	Children <12 years: Contraindicated due to rapid metabolism to morphine Children <18 years: Avoid use due to rapid metabolism to morphine
Antiepileptic Drugs		
Carbamazepine	↑ Metabolism	Children and adolescents: Higher (mg/kg) doses needed
Phenytoin	↓ Metabolism Distribution (protein bound) ↑ Metabolism	Neonates: Lower doses needed Infants and young children: Higher maintenance doses may be needed
Phenobarbital	↓ Metabolism Distribution (protein bound)	Neonates: Longer dosing interval at lower PMA

*Dosing intervals suggested in absence of renal or hepatic dysfunction unrelated to age. PMA, post-menstrual age.

Source: Data from Arant BS Jr. Developmental patterns of renal functional maturation compared in the human neonate. *J Pediatr.* 1978;92:705–712. doi:10.1016/S0022-3476(78)80133-4; IBM Micromedex® (electronic version). IBM Watson Health. 2019; O'Hara K. Paediatric pharmacokinetics and drug doses. *Aust Prescr.* 2016;36(6): 208–210. doi:10.18773/austprescr.2016.071; Ortiz de Montellano PR. Cytochrome P450-activated prodrugs. *Future Med Chem.* 2013;5(2):213–228. doi:10.4155/fmc.12.197

BOX 6-3
ABSORPTION-RELATED CONCERNS IN PEDIATRIC PATIENTS

Skin
- Thinner stratum corneum
- Increased BSA:weight ratio
- Increased absorption
- Caution using topical medications in neonates and young children

Muscle
- Reduced mass and perfusion
- Reduce absorption of drug
- Pain on administration
- Caution in pediatric patients <6 years
- Caution administering volumes >0.5 mL per injection site

BSA, body surface area.
Source: Data from Ortiz de Montellano PR. Cytochrome P450-activated prodrugs. *Future Med Chem.* 2013;5(2):213–228. doi:10.4155/fmc.12.197; Porter RS, Kaplan JL, Beers MH, eds. *The MERCK Manual of Diagnosis and Therapy.* Merck Sharp & Dohm; 2006

in pediatric patients highlight the need for continued research and the risk of extrapolating pediatric dosing strictly from adult literature.

DRUG THERAPY IN THE ELDERLY

More than 49.2 million people in the United States are age 65 years or older, representing 15.2% of the population or about one in every seven Americans.[42] These individuals consume around 30% of all prescription medications and half of over-the-counter medications.[43] Higher rates of drug-related problems, such as polypharmacy, are observed among elderly versus younger adults, and these problems are associated with high rates of medical comorbidities, overprescribing, and inadequate monitoring. Polypharmacy, or concomitant use of multiple medications, is common in the United States, with 30% to 40% of elderly adults consuming five or more daily drugs simultaneously.[44–46] Using four billion patient-months of outpatient prescription drug claims data in the United States from 2007 to 2014, Quinn and Shah determined that among patients taking any prescription medication, half are exposed to two or more drugs and 5% are exposed to eight or more.[47] Given these facts, prescribers must understand the benefits and risks associated with medication use in older adults.

The physiologic process of aging makes elderly patients more vulnerable to the therapeutic or toxic effects of many medications, increasing the risk of ADE. Age-related physiologic decline and changes in body composition result in pharmacokinetic and pharmacodynamic mechanisms of altered drug responses.[48] Common observations of such effects with implications for drug safety include decreased total body water, decreased lean body mass, increased body fat, decreased serum albumin and altered protein binding, decreased liver blood flow and hepatic metabolism, reduced renal plasma flow and GFR decreased tubular secretion function, and various changes in determinants of tissue sensitivity.[49] Table 6.3 cites examples of common physiologic changes in aging that have implications for prescribing. There are some examples of pharmacodynamic changes in aging, such as increased sensitivity among elderly patients to opioid analgesics or warfarin as well as decreased sensitivity to beta-agonist medications.[49,50] Beyond physiologic changes, elderly patients may experience acute or chronic illness, poor nutrition, cognitive impairment, or drug interactions (e.g. drug–drug, drug–food, drug–disease, or drug–dietary supplement interactions) that complicate medication therapy safety and effectiveness.

The physiologic effects of aging may vary considerably from elderly patient to patient, making some more vulnerable than others to medication effects. Likewise, this variability makes it problematic for clinicians to generalize prescribing practices for older patients. Table 6.4 presents age-related changes that relate to drug pharmacokinetics, which practically relates to the movement of drugs through the body. To describe the disposition of a drug within the body, discussion of pharmacokinetics is organized around four processes: absorption (e.g., gastrointestinal), distribution, metabolism (e.g., hepatic), and elimination (e.g., renal excretion), or "ADME." Clinicians should also remember that the number of elderly patients evaluated in clinical trials, which are similar to the target population for treatment, may be quite small, limiting the empiric evidence on safety and efficacy of a drug. However, the advice of "start low and go slow" when dosing a drug for an older patient is worth considering. Box 6.4 also provides common characteristics and selected risk factors for drug injury in elderly patients.

Assessing and managing polypharmacy in older patients can be overwhelming and time intensive. Various tools and resources exist to help prescribers overcome this challenge and improve the efficiency of screening for and addressing polypharmacy. We recommend adoption of a systematic approach, whether it be a digital tool integrated with an electronic health record,[4] a polypharmacy assessment instrument,[52] or an informal approach.[53] Bushardt and Jones proposed a structured, informal assessment system based on various definitions of polypharmacy, which consists of nine questions (see Box 6.5). Incorporating this system into a primary care visit, together with educating the patient regarding

TABLE 6.3 Examples of Physiologic Changes in Aging That Impact Medication Effects by Body System

Body System	Potential Effect in Aging
Body composition	Decreased total body water, decreased lean body mass, increased body fat, altered serum albumin or α_1-acid glycoprotein concentrations
Cardiovascular	Decreased baroreceptor activity resulting in orthostatic hypotension, decreased cardiac output, decreased heart rate (e.g., resting, maximal)
Central nervous system	Decreased receptor number and increased receptor sensitivity, decreased short-term memory, altered sleep patterns
Endocrine	Altered insulin signaling
Gastrointestinal	Decreased large intestine motility, decreased vitamin absorption, decreased bowel surface area
Genitourinary	Detrusor hyperactivity
Hepatic	Decreased liver size, decreased liver blood flow, decreased phase I metabolism
Oropharyngeal	Altered dentition, dry mouth
Pulmonary	Decreased respiratory muscle strength, decreased arterial oxygenation and carbon dioxide elimination, decreased vital capacity
Renal	Decreased glomerular filtration rate, decreased renal blood flow, decreased tubular secretion
Musculoskeletal	Decreased skeletal bone mass
Dermatologic	Thinning of stratum corneum, decreased depth of subcutaneous fat

Source: Adapted from Wells BG, Schwinghammer TL, DiPiro JT, DiPiro CV. *Pharmacotherapy Handbook.* 10th ed. McGraw-Hill; 2017:902–903.

TABLE 6.4 Pharmacokinetic Changes Related to Aging

ADME Phase	Pharmacokinetic Parameters
Gastrointestinal absorption	Unchanged passive diffusion, no change in bioavailability for most drugs Decreased active transport, decreased bioavailability for some drugs Decreased first-pass metabolism, increased bioavailability for some drugs, decreased bioavailability for some prodrugs
Distribution	Decreased volume of distribution, increased plasma concentration for water-soluble drugs Increased volume of distribution, increased accumulation of lipid-soluble drugs
Liver metabolism	Decreased clearance of drugs with high hepatic extraction
Renal elimination	Decreased clearance of renally eliminated drugs and active metabolites

ADME, absorption, distribution, metabolism, and excretion.

Source: Adapted from Sera LC, McPherson ML. Pharmacokinetics and pharmacodynamic changes associated with aging and implications for drug therapy. *Clin Geriatr Med.* 2012;*28*(2):273–286. doi:10.1016/j.cger.2012.01.007; Wells BG, Schwinghammer TL, DiPiro JT, DiPiro CV. *Pharmacotherapy Handbook.* 10th ed. McGraw-Hill; 2017:903

BOX 6.4
COMMON CHARACTERISTICS AND SELECTED RISK FACTORS FOR DRUG INJURY IN ELDERLY PATIENTS

Patient and Physiologic Factors
- Advanced age (>85 years)
- Female sex
- Low body weight or body mass index (<22 kg/m²)
- Hepatic impairment or liver disease
- Renal impairment (estimated CrCl <50 mL/min) or kidney disease
- History of falls

Disease-Related Factors
- Comorbidities (e.g., more than six chronic illnesses, cognitive impairment or limited ADLs)
- Concurrent cardiovascular disease, cancer, diabetes, or depression

Drug-Therapy Factors
- Prior significant adverse drug effect
- Taking nine or more daily medications, or taking more than 12 doses of medications daily
- Drug–drug interactions
- Use of certain high-risk medications (e.g., antihypertensive, anticoagulant/antithrombotic, antibacterial, diabetes medication, nonsteroidal anti-inflammatory drug, psychotropic agent)

ADLs, activities of daily living.

Source: Adapted from Alhawassi TM, Krass I, Bajorek BV, Pont LG. A systematic review of the prevalence and risk factors for adverse drug reactions in the elderly in the acute care setting. *Clin Interv Aging.* 2014;9:2079–2086. doi:10.2147/CIA.S71178; Bushardt RL, Jones KW. Nine key questions to address polypharmacy in the elderly. *JAAPA.* 2005;18(5): 32–37. doi:10.1097/01720610-200505000-00005

BOX 6.5
KEY QUESTIONS TO ASSESS POLYPHARMACY IN OLDER PATIENTS

1. Is the drug necessary (e.g., active diagnosis, drug is indicated)?
2. Is the drug contraindicated in the elderly?
3. Are there duplicate drugs?
4. Is the patient taking the lowest effective dosage?
5. Is the drug intended to treat an adverse effect of another prescribed drug?
6. Can the drug regimen be simplified?
7. Are there potential drug interactions?
8. Is the patient adherent to the drug therapy?
9. Is the patient taking an over-the-counter medication, dietary supplement, or another person's medication?

Source: From Bushardt RL, Jones KW. Nine key questions to address polypharmacy in the elderly. *JAAPA.* 2005;*18*(5):32–37. doi:10.1097/01720610-200505000-00005

medication use, can provide opportunities to address polypharmacy and help patients' drug therapy-related problems. Prescribers may also find value in numerous other tools that are suitable for use at the point of care that support appropriate prescribing for older patients. The American Geriatrics Society Updated Beers Criteria offer evidence-based guidance on potentially inappropriate medications for older adults and can aid prescribers in considering the safest alternatives within a therapeutic area.[54] To readily identify medications with anticholinergic effects and quantify the effects by severity and body system, prescribers can use various anticholinergic drug indices or scales.[55,56] The screening tool of older people's prescriptions (STOPP) and the screening tool to alert to right treatment (START) criteria offer practical tools for clinicians and help ensure that current drug therapy regimens reflect evidence-based options for a wide array of therapeutic areas.[57]

The optimal drug therapy regimen for any patient, including older adults, considers the patient's current health, medical conditions, and long-term goals from treatment. Elderly patients are more likely to be harmed by medications, even when used at normal doses, so weighing the risks and benefits, and considering the individual patient's prognosis and personal wishes, are key. In addition to routine, ongoing surveillance for appropriate drug therapy in older adults, clinicians should keep in mind common opportunities that may arise to reconcile medications or revisit therapy in the context of a care transition. Such opportunities may include whenever a new drug is prescribed, at an annual or semi-annual outpatient appointment to evaluate overall medication management, and during care transitions (e.g., hospital admission or discharge, long-term care facility admission or discharge, after an injury or surgery).[50] Finally, clinicians can embrace the principle of "start low, go slow" and take time to introduce new medications and taper medications that require discontinuation as slowly as the clinical circumstance allows.

CONCLUSION

Alterations in pharmacodynamics and pharmacokinetic properties in the previously noted special populations are related to normal developmental changes and anticipated and disease-related modifications in organ function. These changes have a significant impact in efficacy and toxicity of medications. Alterations in kidney and liver function can be objectively assessed to allow for dose-adjustments. Prescribers must take care to appropriately adjust medications in accordance with current recommendations to ensure optimal outcomes. Knowledge of resources available for adjustment of medications in renal or hepatic dysfunction is key to providing appropriate care for patients across their life span.

CASE EXEMPLAR: Patient With Altered Mental Status

AD is a 79-year-old woman brought from a nursing home to the emergency department for evaluation of altered mental status. The staff has noticed changes evolving over the past few weeks, but now she is unable to eat or take fluids without assistance. About 1 month ago she was able to feed herself. The clinician covering the long-term care facility is worried about the need for enteral or parenteral feedings.

Past Medical History
- Hypertension
- Hyperlipidemia
- Hypothyroidism
- Allergic rhinitis
- Urinary tract infection
- Osteoarthritis
- Presbycusis
- Constipation/diarrhea intermittently

Medications
- Lisinopril, 20 mg orally once daily
- Atenolol, 50 mg orally once daily
- Lovastatin, 20 mg orally once daily
- Hydrochlorothiazide, 25 mg orally once daily
- Cetirizine, 10 mg orally once daily
- Levothyroxine, 100 mcg orally once daily
- Diphenoxylate/atropine, 2.5 mg orally every 12 hours as needed for diarrhea
- Melatonin, 5 mg orally before bed
- Acetaminophen, 500 mg 2 tablets orally every 6 hours as needed for pain

- Diphenhydramine, 25 mg orally every 6 hours as needed for agitation
- Amoxicillin/clavulanate, 500 mg/125 mg orally three times a day for a recent bladder infection
- Lorazepam, 1 mg orally before bed as needed for sleep
- Multivitamin

Physical Examination
- Blood pressure: 82/50; pulse: 108; respiration rate: 16; temperature 97.2°F
- Cachectic female without contractures
- Awake but nonresponsive
- Lungs: Bilateral scattered rhonchi
- Heart regular rate and rhythm, grade I systolic murmur
- Stage I decubitus ulcer over the coccyx

Labs and Imaging
- Complete blood count (CBC): Normal
- Albumin: 2.8 mg/dL

Discussion Questions

1. What is the clinician's first step in caring for this patient?
2. What laboratory tests should the clinician order?
3. The patient's renal and hepatic functions are relatively normal, but her albumin is low. How will this affect her medication regimen?

CASE EXEMPLAR: Patient With Acute Renal Failure

HG is a 52-year-old man with a long history of type 2 diabetes mellitus who presents to the emergency department with acute shortness of breath. He is being seen by another clinician for management of his conditions. He takes insulin along with metformin for control of his blood sugar. Recently his blood pressure has been increasing even though he tries to exercise. Understanding the impact of diabetes on kidneys, 2 weeks ago his clinician decided to start him on lisinopril for hypertension.

Past Medical History
- Hypertension
- Type 2 diabetes mellitus
- Chronic renal insufficiency

Medications
- Humulin 70/30 (insulin isophane and insulin regular), 25 U, subcutaneously once a daily
- Metformin, 850 mg orally twice a day
- Aspirin, 81 mg orally once daily

Physical Examination
- Body mass index: 21 kg/m^2; blood pressure: 154/98; pulse: 104; respiration rate: 24; temperature: 98.2°F
- Moderate respiratory distress
- Lungs: Bilateral wheezes and rhonchi with poor air exchange
- Heart tachycardic, regular rate and rhythm
- 3+ peripheral edema

Labs and Imaging
- Hemoglobin A1C: Normal
- Creatinine: 8.2 mg/dL
- Potassium: 5.9 mEq/L
- Chest x-ray: Pulmonary edema

Discussion Questions
1. Why did the patient develop acute respiratory distress?
2. What other diagnostic tests should the clinician order?
3. What should be the clinician's next steps in caring for this patient?

CLINICAL PEARLS

- Clinicians are advised to review a patient's complete medication list, including over-the-counter drugs and supplements, before prescribing a new medicine. Avoidance of drug–drug interactions is imperative. This may include the decision to not prescribe a particular agent or to adjust its starting dose.
- Medications such as antibiotics, opioids, and antihypertensives may need adjustment in patients with chronic renal failure. Creatinine clearance can guide therapy.
- Liver activity of cytochrome P450 can significantly affect the metabolism of certain medications. Assessment of liver function prior to prescribing may help avoid adverse drug effects. The Child-Pugh classification or the Model for End-Stage Liver Disease (MELD) are useful tools for assessment of liver function.
- Dosing of medicines in children must consider age, weight, and stage of bony development. Some medications are contraindicated in children, while others may be given after appropriate dosing adjustments.
- Older patients accumulate medicines and supplements on their medication lists over time. They cannot tolerate some medicines used in younger patients, and some drugs can impair cognition or the function of unrelated body systems like the bone marrow. Clinicians should weigh the risks and benefits of new medications, and work to de-prescribe certain medicines on their medication list that are no longer relevant.
- Electronic medical records systems maintained by the clinician and/or the pharmacy may help avoid drug–drug interactions.

KEY TAKEAWAYS

- Polypharmacy in all patients, particularly in vulnerable populations, poses a significant health risk for patients. Prescribers should review medication lists on every patient at every visit to look for potential drug–drug interactions and to eliminate unneeded, redundant medications.
- Certain drugs are renally excreted while others are nephrotoxic. Patients with underlying kidney disease are at higher risk of adverse drug effects from these medications. The doses or dosing regimen of many of the medicines can be adjusted to allow for their safe use even in the face of renal disease.
- Certain other medications are excreted or metabolized by the liver, and some are hepatotoxic. Liver disease is common in adults, and dosing considerations must be made before prescribing these pharmaceutical agents.
- Pediatric patients have both a rapid metabolism and a smaller volume of distribution for drugs. Some medicines can adversely affect the growing structures in a child. Clinicians must be aware of indications and contraindications based on age and weight.
- Elderly people have a higher fat-to-muscle ratio with alterations in volume of distribution of drugs. Medications are eliminated more slowly in these patients, particularly lipophilic agents. Many older patients are on multiple over-the-counter medications and supplements that may interact with prescribed pharmaceuticals. Clinicians must adjust the dose or schedule of many medications in this vulnerable population.

REFERENCES

1. Yu NL, Atteberry P, Bach PB. *Spending on prescription drugs in the US: Where does all the money go?* Published July 31, 2018. https://www.healthaffairs.org/do/10.1377/hblog20180726.670593/full
2. Kohn LT, Corrigan JM, Donaldson MS, eds. *To Err Is Human: Building a Safer Health System*. National Academies Press; 2000.
3. Levinson DR. *Adverse events in hospitals: national incidence among Medicare beneficiaries*. U.S. Department of Health and Human Services Office of Inspector General. Report No.: OEI-06-09-00090. Published November, 2010. https://www.oig.hhs.gov/oei/reports/oei-06-09-00090.pdf
4. Lucado J, Paez K, Elixhauser A. Medication-related adverse outcomes in U.S. hospitals and emergency departments, 2008. *HCUP Statistical Brief #109*. Published April, 2011. https://www.ncbi.nlm.nih.gov/books/NBK54566/..
5. U.S. Department of Health and Human Services, Office of Disease Prevention and Health Promotion. *National Action Plan for Adverse Drug Event Prevention*. U.S Department of Health and Human Services; 2014. https://health.gov/sites/default/files/2019-09/ADE-Action-Plan-508c.pdf.
6. Weiss AD, Freeman WJ, Heslin KC, et al. Adverse drug events in U.S. hospitals, 2010 versus 2014.*HCUP Statistical Brief #234*. Published January 2018. https://www.hcup-us.ahrq.gov/reports/statbriefs/sb234-Adverse-Drug-Events.pd.
7. Bourgeois FT, Shannon MW, Valim C, et al. Adverse drug events in the outpatient setting: an 11-year national analysis. *Pharmacoepidemiol Drug Saf*. 2010;19(9):901–910. doi:10.1002/pds.198.
8. Cockcroft DW, Gault MH. Prediction of creatinine clearance from serum creatinine. *Nephron*. 1976;16(1):31–41. doi:10.1159/00018058.
9. Levey AS, Bosch JP, Lewis JB, et al. A more accurate method to estimate glomerular filtration rate from serum creatinine: a new prediction equation. *Ann Intern Med*. 1999;130(6):461–470. doi:10.7326/0003-4819-130-6-199903160-0000.
10. Levey AS, Stevens LA, Schmid CH, et al. A new equation to estimate glomerular filtration rate. *Ann Intern Med*. 2009;150(9):604–612. doi:10.7326/0003-4819-150-9-200905050-0000.
11. Kidney Disease: Improving Global Outcomes (KDIGO) CKD Work Group. KDIGO 2012 clinical practice guideline for the evaluation and management of chronic kidney disease. *Kidney Int Suppl*. 2013;3(1):1–150. doi:10.1038/kisup.2012.73.
12. Proulx NL, Akbari A, Garg AX, et al. Measured creatinine clearance from timed urine collections substantially overestimates glomerular filtration rate in patients with liver cirrhosis: a systematic review and individual patient meta-analysis. *Nephrol Dial Transplant*. 2005;20:1617–1622. doi:10.1093/ndt/gfh839
13. Porter RS, Kaplan JL, Beers MH, eds. *The MERCK Manual of Diagnosis and Therapy*. Merck Sharp & Dohme; 2006.
14. Shoker A, Hossain MA, Koru-Sengul T, et al. Performance of creatinine clearance equations on the original Cockcroft-Gault population. *Clin Nephrol*. 2006;66(2):89–97. doi:10.5414/CNP6608.
15. Froissart M, Rossert J, Jacquot C, et al. Predictive performance of the modification of diet in renal disease and Cockcroft-Gault equations for estimating renal function. *J Am Soc Nephrol*. 2005;16(3):763–773. doi:10.1681/ASN.200407054.
16. Zuo L, Ma Y-C, Zhou Y-H, et al. Application of GFR-estimating equations in Chinese patients with chronic kidney disease. *Am J Kidney Dis*. 2005;45(3):463–472. doi:10.1053/j.ajkd.2004.11.01.
17. Poggio ED, Wang X, Greene T, et al. Performance of the modification of diet in renal disease and Cockcroft-Gault equations in the estimation of GFR in health and in chronic kidney disease. *J Am Soc Nephrol*. 2005;16(2):459–466. doi:10.1681/ASN.2004060447

18. Stevens LA, Schmid CH, Greene T, et al. Comparative performance of the CKD Epidemiology Collaboration (CKD-EPI) and the Modification of Diet in Renal Disease (MDRD) study equations for estimating GFR levels above 60 mL/min/1.73 m². *Am J Kidney Dis*. 2010;56(3):486–495. doi:10.1053/j.ajkd.2010.03.02.

19. Food and Drug Administration. Guidance for industry: pharmacokinetics in patients with impaired renal function—Study design, data analysis, and impact on dosing and labeling. U.S. Department of Health and Human Services; 1998. https://www.fda.gov/media/71334/download

20. National Institute of Diabetes and Digestive and Kidney Diseases. *CKD and drug dosing: information for providers*. Published 2005.

21. Mosteller RD. Simplified calculation of body-surface area. *N Engl J Med*. 1987;317:1098. doi:10.1056/NEJM198710223171717.

22. Matzke GR, Aronoff GR, Atkinson AJ Jr, et al. Drug dosing consideration in patients with acute and chronic kidney disease—a clinical update from Kidney Disease: Improving Global Outcomes (KDIGO). *Kidney Int*. 2011;80(11):1122–1137. doi:10.1038/ki.2011.323.

23. Verbeek RK. Pharmacokinetics and dosage adjustment in patients with hepatic dysfunction. *Eur J Clin Pharmacol*. 2008;64:1147–1161. doi:10.1007/s00228-008-0553-z

24. Ortiz de Montellano PR. Cytochrome P450-activated prodrugs. *Future Med Chem*. 2013;5(2):213–228. doi:10.4155/fmc.12.197

25. O'Hara K. Paediatric pharmacokinetics and drug doses. *Aust Prescr*. 2016;*36*(6):208–210. doi:10.18773/austprescr.2016.071

26. Pugh RN, Murray-Lyon IM, Dawson JL, et al. Transection of the oesophagus for bleeding oesophageal varices. *Br J Surg*. 1973;*60*:646–649. doi:10.1002/bjs.180060081

27. Kamath PS, Kim WR. The Model for End-Stage Liver Disease (MELD). *Hepatology*. 2007;*45*:797–805. doi:10.1002/hep.21563

28. Peng Y, Qi X, Guo X. Child-Pugh versus MELD score for the assessment of prognosis in liver cirrhosis: a systematic review and meta-analysis of observational studies. *Medicine*. 2016;*95*(8):e2877. doi:10.1097/MD.0000000000002877

29. Sloss A, Kubler P. Prescribing in liver disease. *Austr Prescr*. 2009;*32*(2):32–35. doi:10.18773/austprescr.2009.018

30. Drug-Induced Liver Injury Network. *DILIN overview*. Updated September 16, 2011. http://www.dilin.org/for-researchers/dilin-overview

31. U.S. Food and Drug Administration. *Drug induced liver toxicity*. Published September 2017.

32. Kearns GL, Abdel-Rahman SM, Alander SW, et al. Developmental pharmacology—Drug disposition, action, and therapy in infants and children. *N Engl J Med*. 2003;349:1157–1167. doi:10.1056/NEJMra035092

33. Koren G. Special aspects of perinatal and pediatric pharmacology. In: Katzung BG, Trevor AJ, eds. *Basic and Clinical Pharmacology*. 13th ed. McGraw-Hill; 2015:1013–1024.

34. Hines RN, McCarver DG. The ontogeny of human drug-metabolizing enzymes: phase I oxidative enzymes. *J Pharmacol Exp Ther*. 2002;300:355–360. doi:10.1124/jpet.300.2.355

35. IBM Micromedex® (electronic version). *IBM Watson Health*. 2019. https://www.micromedexsolutions.com/home/dispatch/ssl/true

36. Food and Drug Administration. *FDA Drug Safety Communication: FDA restricts use of prescription codeine pain and cough medicines and tramadol pain medicines in children; recommends against use in breastfeeding women*. Published 2017. https://www.fda.gov/drugs/drug-safety-and-availability/fda-drug-safety-communication-fda-restricts-use-prescription-codeine-pain-and-cough-medicines-and

37. Arant BS Jr. Developmental patterns of renal functional maturation compared in the human neonate. *J Pediatr*. 1978;92:705–712. doi:10.1016/S0022-3476(78)80133-4

38. Schwartz GJ, Gauthier BJ. A simple estimate of glomerular filtration rate in adolescent boys. *J Pediatr*. 1985;106(3):522–526. doi:10.1016/S0022-3476(85)80697-1

39. Schwartz GJ, Muñoz A, Schneider MF, et al. New equations to estimate GFR in children with CKD. *J Am Soc Nephrol*. 2009;20(3):629–637. doi:10.1681/ASN.2008030287

40. Food and Drug Administration. *Pregnancy registry information for health professionals*. Published 2018. https://www.fda.gov/ScienceResearch/SpecialTopics/WomensHealthResearch/ucm256789.htm

41. Briggs GG, Freeman RK, Yaffe SJ. *Drugs in Pregnancy and Lactation*. 9th ed. Lippincott Williams & Wilkins; 20142.

42. Roberts AW, Ogunwole SU, Blakeslee L, Rabe MA. *The Population 65 years and Older in the United States: 2016*. U.S. Department of Commerce, Economics and Statistics Administration, U.S. Census Bureau; 2018. https://www.census.gov/content/dam/Census/library/publications/2018/acs/ACS-38.pdf

43. Qato DM, Alexander GC, Conti RM, et al. Use of prescription and over-the-counter medications and dietary supplements among older adults in the United States. *JAMA*. 2008;300(24):2867–2878. doi:10.1001/jama.2008.892

44. Gu Q, Dillon CF, Burt VL. Prescription drug use continues to increase: U.S. prescription drug data for 2007–2008. *NCHS data brief, no 42*. National Center for Health Statistics; 2010. https://www.cdc.gov/nchs/products/databriefs/db42.htm

45. Sutherland JJ, Daly TM, Liu X, et al. Co-prescription trends in a large cohort of subjects predict substantial drug-drug interactions. *PLoS ONE*. 2015;10(3):e0118991. doi:10.1371/journal.pone.0118991

46. Bushardt RL, Massey EB, Simpson TW, et al. Polypharmacy: misleading, but manageable. *Clin Interv Aging*. 2008;*3*(2):383–389. doi:10.2147/CIA.S2468

47. Quinn KJ, Shah NH. A dataset quantifying polypharmacy in the United States. *Sci. Data*. 2017;4:170167. doi:10.1038/sdata.2017.167

48. Turnheim K. Drug therapy in the elderly. *Exp Gerontol*. 2004;39:1731–1738. doi:10.1016/j.exger.2004.05.011

49. Lavan AH, Gallagher P. *Predicting risk of adverse drug reactions in older adults*. Published 2016. https://www.ncbi.nlm.nih.gov/pmc/articles/PMC4716390/pdf/10.1177_2042098615615472.pdf

50. Wallace J, Paauw DS. Appropriate prescribing and important drug interactions in older adults. *Med Clin N Am*. 2015;99:295–310. doi:10.1016/j.mcna.2014.11.005

74 I · Foundations of Pharmacology and Prescribing

51. Wells BG, Schwinghammer TL, Dipiro JT, DiPiro CV. *Pharmacotherapy Handbook*, 10th ed. McGraw-Hill; 2017

52. Young A, Tordoff J, Dovey S, et al. Using an electronic decision support tool to reduce inappropriate polypharmacy and optimize medicines: rationale and methods. *JMIR Res Protoc*. 2016;5(2):e105. doi:10.2196/resprot.5543

53. Bushardt RL, Jones KW. Nine key questions to address polypharmacy in the elderly. *JAAPA*. 2005;18(5):32–37. doi:10.1097/01720610-200505000-00005

54. American Geriatrics Society 2015 Beers Criteria Update Expert Panel. *American Geriatrics Society 2015 updated Beers Criteria for potentially inappropriate medication use in older adults*. Published 2015. https://www.sigot.org/allegato_docs/1057_Beers-Criteria.pdf

55. Salahudeen MS, Duffull SB, Nishtala PS. *Anticholinergic burden quantified by anticholinergic risk scales and adverse outcomes in older people: a systematic review*. Published 2015. https://www.ncbi.nlm.nih.gov/pmc/articles/PMC4377853/pdf/12877_2015_Article_29.pdf

56. Regenstrief Institute. *Aging brain care*. Published 2012. http://www.miltonkeynesccg.nhs.uk/resources/uploads/ACB_scale_-_legal_size.pdf

57. O'Mahony D, O'Sullivan D, Byrne S. *STOPP/START criteria for potentially inappropriate prescribing in older people: version 2*. Published 2018. https://www.ncbi.nlm.nih.gov/pmc/articles/PMC4339726

Drug Development and Approval

Hongbin Wang, Peter Tenerelli, Simeon O. Kotchoni, Ahmed El-Shamy,
Erika Young, Michael Casner, and Catherine F. Yang

LEARNING OBJECTIVES

- Define and contrast the phases of drug trials.
- Illustrate the purpose of each phase of a drug trial in the development of a novel drug.
- Explain the role of microorganisms and plants in the genesis of new drugs.
- Compare a drug that has been approved for generic prescribing versus a brand-name drug.
- Analyze the advantages and disadvantages of releasing a prescription drug as a nonprescription medication.

INTRODUCTION

Drug development involves lengthy procedures such as the identification of new chemical entities, clinical trials, regulatory approval, and the final postmarketing or phase 4 clinical trials. In the past decade, these processes have been substantially shortened due to cutting-edge innovations and novel technologies. It is prudent for clinicians to understand this process to make well-informed decisions and plan for the best course of action during patient care.

Drug discovery usually stems from developing an intervention to fill the gaps of a specific disease or a clinical condition. A drug may be broadly defined as a substance that interferes with biological processes that are "intended for use in the diagnosis, cure, mitigation, treatment, or prevention of disease."[1] Prior to the 20th century, clinicians commonly used a wide range of natural products obtained from plant, animal, vegetable, and mineral sources for medicinal purposes with empirical benefit.[2] To minimize the toxicities, scientists began to purify substances from natural products to seek better pharmacologic reagents. In the early 1900s, Paul Ehrlich developed the concept of the chemotherapeutic index, the ratio of maximum-tolerated dose to the minimum curative dose, which has spurred the rational drug development. Meanwhile, new insights of a disease process allow researchers to design a therapeutic agent to stop or reverse the effects of the disease.[2,3] Once the initial therapeutic agents have been developed and approved for marketing, they are available as *brand* name drugs. Other formulations of the same drugs may be available at a later time in the form of *generic* medications.

Since the passage of the Drug Price Competition and Patent Term Restoration Act in 1984 (Hatch-Waxman Amendment), the U.S. Food and Drug Administration (FDA) has approved thousands of generic drug products. The availability of these generic products has become a cost-containment measure for many patients by switching from a branded to a generic medication. The approved generic drugs are expected to have the same performance and quality as their branded counterparts. They are marketed after the patent of the innovator drugs or other exclusive authority has expired. They must meet the rigorous standards established by the FDA, which include identity, purity, strength, quality, and efficacy. Their bioequivalence must be tested to ensure quality. According to the World Health Organization (WHO), two drugs are bioequivalent when they have similar bioavailability profiles (i.e., T_{max}, C_{max}, and area under the curve [AUC]) after the administration of the same molar dose and conditions that are expected to provide the same therapeutic effects.[4] This chapter will summarize the drug development and approval process. It will also discuss the clinical decision-making process during drug selection in the context of generic versus brand. The process of conversion of *legend* drugs (or prescription-only) to over-the-counter (OTC) will also be reviewed.

THE PROCESS OF NEW DRUG DEVELOPMENT AND U.S. FOOD AND DRUG ADMINISTRATION APPROVAL

The process of drug discovery and development involves the identification of a target that causes the disease, followed by modeling of that target (e.g., a protein, an antigen, or a receptor type) to design a drug candidate.[3] To develop a new therapeutic agent, a pharmaceutical company must bring together appropriate cross sections of scientists, clinicians, statisticians, regulatory agencies, marketing, and even economists as well as attorneys. Furthermore, preclinical investigations involve toxicology, pharmacodynamics (PD), and pharmacokinetics (PK) studies, as well as optimization of the drug delivery system.[3] Once a selection of a candidate molecule for clinical development has been identified, an FDA Investigational New Drug (IND) application will be filed. **Figure 7.1** shows the de novo drug discovery process and the approximate timeline during each of the steps.

TARGET IDENTIFICATION

Typically, researchers begin the drug discovery process by thoroughly examining the critical pathways within a cell, which may directly regulate a phase of the disease. It is crucial to identify a potential drug target in a pathway since there may be multiple metabolic sites of action that can impact the metabolic flow.[5] These potential targets may include enzymes, receptors, or oligonucleotides. A promising drug target may have the following properties:

1. A defined role in the pathophysiology of a disease and/or one that is disease-modifying
2. Not evenly distributed throughout the body
3. Easily "assayable" enabling high-throughput screening
4. Possesses potential adverse effects that can be predicted using phenotypic data

TARGET VALIDATION

Drug-target validation is a critical step before moving onto the developmental stage.[6] A new drug often takes more than 10 years to develop with a cost close to $1 billion.[3,6] Furthermore, more than 50% of failures in clinical phase 2 and 3 trials are due to insufficient efficacy. Consequently, an in-depth understanding of a molecular target is required, since later success or failure of the potential drug candidate is dependent on this early step. While the validation of a drug's efficacy and toxicity in numerous disease-relevant cell and animal models is highly valuable, the ultimate test is whether the drug works in a clinical setting. The *target-validation* process may be summarized in three key steps:

1. Once a drug candidate is identified via a specific technique, procedure, or review of literature, a confirmatory experiment is repeated to confirm if the data are successfully reproducible.
2. Modulation of the activities of the drug candidate or the binding sites are performed. By varying different parameters, such as introducing mutations into the binding domain or using a different cell or tissue type, researchers are able to further determine the characteristics of the potential drug target. In other words, the introduction of manipulations of either the environment, the ligand, or the binding sites helps to further characterize the potential drug target.
3. Establishment of the druggable toxicities and pharmacological profile is achieved.

ASSAY DEVELOPMENT

One of the first steps in drug development and toxicity testing is creating assays, which evaluate the effects of chemical compounds on cellular, molecular, or biochemical processes of interest. An assay is defined as a method by which the activity of a compound is measured. When active compounds are identified, they may become potential therapeutic candidates in the drug development pipeline.

LEAD GENERATION

A chemical lead is defined as a synthetically feasible, stable, and druglike molecule active in primary and secondary assays with acceptable *specificity* and *selectivity* for the target. The characteristics of a chemical lead include:

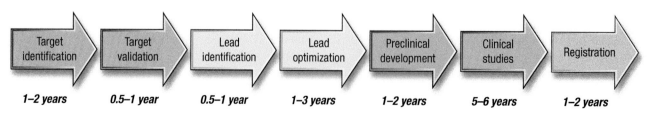

Target identification	Target validation	Lead identification	Lead optimization	Preclinical development	Clinical studies	Registration
1–2 years	0.5–1 year	0.5–1 year	1–3 years	1–2 years	5–6 years	1–2 years

FIGURE 7.1 De novo drug discovery process and timeline.

1. A defined structure-activity relationship (SAR)
2. Druggability
3. Synthetic feasibility
4. Selective mechanistic assays
5. In vitro assessment of drug resistance and efflux potential
6. Evidence of in vivo efficacy of chemical class
7. Pharmacokinetics/toxicity of the chemical class that are known based on preliminary toxicity or in silico studies

To increase the success rate from the compound candidates during the drug development process, a druggability assessment is conducted. This assessment is crucial in transforming a compound from a lead molecule to a drug. For a compound to be considered druggable, it should have the potential to bind to a specific target at high affinity. Other assay screenings such as the Ames test and cytotoxicity assay may be applied to evaluate the potential toxicity of the new compound. Of note, when compounds are being developed, a positive result in the cytotoxicity assays may not necessarily limit the development of the compound. In fact, the other more relevant druggability factors (such as the PK profile) would be the potential determining factors for a drug development.

LEAD OPTIMIZATION

Once a lead structure is identified, a detailed SAR can be carefully constructed to increase the activity of the *lead compound*. Subsequently, an optimized *lead molecule* will enter IND-enabling studies in compliance with good laboratory practices (GLP) and good manufacturing practices (GMP).[7] The criteria for selecting optimized candidates are as follows:

1. Acceptable in vivo PK and toxicity
2. Feasible formulation
3. In vivo preclinical efficacy (properly powered)
4. Dose range finding (DRF) pilot toxicology
5. Scale up feasibility of chemistry assessment
6. Regulatory and marketing assessments[3,8]

When a promising compound for development is identified, various experiments are conducted to determine how it is absorbed, distributed, metabolized, and excreted. Its potential benefits, best dosage, and mechanisms of action are determined. The best route of administration (e.g., by mouth or injection) is described. Side effects, adverse events, or toxicities are also recorded. Furthermore, the effects of how the optimized compound has influenced different populations by gender, race, or ethnicity and how it interacts with other drugs and treatments are observed. Additionally, its effectiveness as compared with similar drugs is also noted.

NEW CHEMICAL ENTITY SOURCES

New chemical entity (NCE) is a new molecule with a physiological or pharmacological bioactive response that has not been used before as a medicinal product. NCEs can be obtained from various sources, which may be natural, semi-synthetic, or synthetic. The NCEs are the major contributors to the new drug discovery process that may take up to 10 years depending on the advance of technology employed.[9,10]

Natural products are biologically active chemical compounds found in nature of biological organisms or systems regardless of modes of preparation (e.g., by extraction or total synthesis). These compounds are generally secondary metabolites that are not crucial for the growth, development, or reproduction of the organism.[11] They are often a product of defense mechanisms against predators or adaptation of the organism to its environment.[12,13] The NCEs from natural products are highly potent and selective because they result from an "optimized" biological process to help the organism cope with its environment. They are generally an important source of NCEs throughout history and continue to deliver a great variety for drug discovery.[13–15]

Plants as a Source of a New Chemical Entity

Many drugs are derived from plants. For example, *artemisinin* was isolated from *wormwood, Artemisia annua*, in 1972. It has been used for centuries in traditional Chinese medicine to treat malaria and fevers. *Artemisinin* and its derivative, *artemether*, have been used until today to effectively treat chloroquine-resistant malaria.[16,17] In 2006, the FDA-approved *sinecatechins*, which was extracted from green tea leaves, *Camellia sinensis*, containing more than 95% catechins, which is used for the treatment of external genital or perianal warts. In 2012, another botanical drug, *crofelemer*, extracted from "dragon's blood," *Croton lechleri*, was approved for the treatment of non-infectious diarrhea.[18]

Microorganisms as a Source of a New Chemical Entity

Screening of microorganisms for NCEs has resulted in many important pharmaceutical products.[19–21] In 1928, Alexander Fleming discovered penicillin from the filamentous fungus *Penicillium notatum*, and in 1943 Selman Waksman and colleagues discovered streptomycin from the soil bacteria Actinomycete, *Streptomyces griseus*.[22] These discoveries have transformed the drug discovery industry and the search for NCEs in biological systems. Up to 2013, 69% of all antibacterial agents approved by the FDA originated from natural products, of which 97% were isolated from microorganisms.[18] Furthermore, during the 2000 to 2013 time period, 77%

of antibiotics approved by the FDA were natural products, and all were derived from microorganisms.[18] To date, less than 1% of microorganisms available in nature have been screened thus far for NCEs.[20] This suggests there is much potential for further discoveries of microbe-derived therapeutic agents.

Other Sources of a New Chemical Entity

Other sources of NCEs may include the synthesis or purification of bioactive peptides acting against a disease process. Exenatide and lepirudin are examples of bioactive peptide-derived drugs that may be classified under this category. Exenatide, a peptide extracted from the saliva of the Gila monster lizard, *Heloderma suspectum*, is a well-known glucagon-like peptide-1 analog approved for the treatment of type 2 diabetes mellitus.[20,23] In addition, the hirudin was produced from the salivary gland of the medical leech, *Hirudo medicinalis*. Hirudin is a potent thrombin inhibitor, which acts as a potent anticoagulant. The gene encoding for this protein was later identified and cloned. In 1998, a recombinant product of this protein (i.e., hirudin) known as lepirudin was approved by the FDA as an alternative anticoagulant for patients who developed heparin-induced thrombocytopenia (HIT) with heparin.[24]

Over the past decades, the drug discovery paradigm has shifted toward rational design. This target-based approach involves specific proteins or "targets," which are often chosen according to the current understandings of the pathophysiology of the disease process. Although the application of rational design has systematically outlined and identified new drugs, serendipity still plays a significant role in the new entity discoveries.[25]

CLINICAL TRIALS

Once a promising NCE has been identified, clinical trials are the ultimate step to translate laboratory-research findings to patient-oriented applications. Simply, new treatments that work in laboratory animal studies (i.e., preclinical trials) need to be tested in humans to determine if the treatment would provide benefits or harms. Generally, clinical trials are controlled by ethical principles of respect for the persons, beneficence of the patient, and justice. These principles are presented in the form of *informed consent*, which has to be explained and signed by every participant in the study. Additionally, all clinical trials are overseen by the Institutional Review Boards (IRBs) ensuring that human research conforms to local and national standards of safety and ethics.[25–27] Study populations are properly selected based on two major characteristics: (a) a sound "internal validity" with predefined characteristics; and (b) a high degree of "external validity" to represent a general patient population.[27]

Before initiating a clinical trial on humans, all data from preclinical studies must be first submitted to the FDA in the form of *IND application*. If the IND is approved, the new drug may be studied in human in phases 1 to 3. If a drug showed high safety and efficacy, a second application referred to as *New Drug Application (NDA)* may be also submitted to the FDA to determine if it can be prescribed and marketed for the intended population. Subsequently, the drug continues to be studied and monitored post marketing as a phase 4 trial.[28]

PHASE 1 CLINICAL TRIALS

Phase 1 clinical trials are the first stage during drug testing on human subjects. The purpose of this phase is to test the safety and dosage ranges, as well as potential toxicity of the new drug. Phase 1 trials are usually designed as "open-labeled" studies where the clinician and the participant are aware of the given drug. This phase is often conducted on a small number of healthy volunteers for a few months.

PHASE 2 CLINICAL TRIALS

Phase 2 clinical trials evaluate the efficacy and side effects of the new drug. In this phase, the safety and dosage specifications are conducted on patients affected with the condition for which the drug is intended to treat, rather than on healthy volunteers. These trials are designed as "controlled" studies that involve one group of patients who receive the new drug and a control group who receives a placebo or gold-standard treatment. They are usually carried out in "double-blinded" fashion in which neither the clinicians nor the patients know if the given therapy is the new drug or a placebo.

PHASE 3 CLINICAL TRIALS

Phase 3 clinical trials are studies of the new drug prior to getting the final FDA approval for marketing. The purposes of this phase are to determine the efficacy and to monitor adverse reactions. In this stage, the safety, efficacy, and dosage modification of the new drug compared to the current gold-standard treatment or placebo are intensively evaluated in thousands of participants. Although only one-third of new drugs successfully progress to phase 3 clinical trials, approximately 80% of those that enter phase 3 receive an NDA approval and move on to phase 4 clinical trials.[29]

PHASE 4 CLINICAL TRIALS

Phase 4 clinical trials are conducted after getting the FDA approval for NDA and post marketing to identify and evaluate the long-term effect of new drugs over a lengthy period on a massive number of "real-world" patients. Through phase 4 clinical studies, new drugs can be tested continuously post marketing approval to uncover more information about efficacy, safety, and side effects. Approximately 20% of new drugs in the market acquire new Black-Box Warnings post marketing, and approximately 4% of drugs are ultimately withdrawn from the market for safety reasons.

GENERIC VERSUS BRAND-NAME DRUGS

The initial therapeutic agents developed and approved for marketing are referred to as brand name drugs. Once the current patents of the brand-name products have expired, their generic counterparts may become available. The FDA requires that the generic drugs have the same performance and quality as their brand-name counterparts. Approved generic drugs must meet rigorous standards established by the FDA in terms of their identity, purity, strength, quality, and efficacy. Since they carry the same active ingredients as the brand, they are expected to provide the same therapeutic effects. In clinical practice, prescribers often use generic drugs interchangeably with the innovator brand products. As reported by the Intercontinental Marketing Statistics (IMS) Institute for Healthcare Informatics, generic drugs now account for approximately 88% of prescriptions dispensed in the United States. From 2005 to 2014, generic medications saved Americans $1.68 trillion—a rate of more than $1 billion in savings every other day.

THE U.S. FOOD AND DRUG ADMINISTRATION APPROVAL OF GENERIC DRUGS

Over the last several decades, the numbers of abbreviated new drug applications (ANDAs) have grown substantially. In the United States, drug companies can submit an ANDA for approval to market a generic drug that is bioequivalent to the brand-name version. Manufacturers seeking an approval of a generic drug product must submit data to demonstrate that it has the same active ingredient(s), strength, type of product, route of administration, use of indication(s), strict manufacture standard, and the same rate and extent of absorption (i.e., bioequivalence) as the innovator drug product. In other words, the generic drug has to show that it is the same type of product and uses the same time-release technology, such as immediate-release or extended-release. Nevertheless, the inactive ingredients from the generic version, which do not affect the active drug function, can be different from the copied brand drug.[30]

Generic manufacturers must provide evidence that the ingredients used in their product are safe.

Drug label information for generic should also be the same as for the brand-name drug. In addition, the FDA must evaluate the container information to make sure it is appropriate for storage.[30] However, the ANDA process does not require the drug applicant to repeat the costly animal and pre- or clinical research on ingredients or dosage forms already proven safe and effective. Consequently, the generic formulations are brought to the market more quickly and at much lower cost, which allows increased medication accessibility to the public.[30]

BIOEQUIVALENCE STUDY OF GENERIC MEDICATIONS

As part of developing and approving generic drugs, manufacturers must provide proof of bioequivalence. This involves submitting data demonstrating that the generic drug has the same rate and extent of absorption as the innovator drug product. Bioequivalence measures drug peak plasma concentration (C_{max}) and area under the plasma drug concentration versus time curve (AUC). These measurements are expressed as geometric mean ratios (GMRs) of generic to innovator C_{max} and AUC.

Both C_{max} and AUC (average bioequivalence) must be within the limits of 80% to 125%.[31] In 2000, the FDA guidance for ANDA applicants recommended that age, sex, and race be considered while selecting patients to represent the general population. To support the validity of the FDA bioequivalence approach, post marketing safety and efficacy data of approved generic drug products also need to be followed and analyzed.[30]

THE IMPACT OF SWITCHING TO GENERIC DRUGS

In clinical settings, prescribers usually switch between branded drugs to generic formulations. This practice has become a common cost-containment measure in the United States. However, generic substitution continues to be a topic of debate among government officials, consumers, pharmaceutical companies, and healthcare professionals; particularly, the controversy is over the methods of evaluation of bioequivalence in vivo between the generic and innovator products.[32–34] In other words, the current FDA standards for generic bioequivalence may not be sufficient for patients treated with drugs that have a narrow therapeutic index. Drugs with variable absorption patterns or with nonlinear pharmacokinetics may also be significantly impacted with generic substitution.[35–37] In general, the potential impacts of switching from brand to generic drugs may be classified into three categories: (a) Clinical and safety outcomes, (b) general attitudes toward generic drugs and adherence, and (c) cost and resource utilization.[38]

Clinical and Safety Outcomes

The clinical outcomes of a patient may be affected by the substitution of generic for brand products. There are case reports of breakthrough seizures or increased seizure frequency in patients who were switched from brand to generic or vice versa.[39] Consequently, the American Academy of Neurology (AAN) opposes generic substitution of anticonvulsants for the treatment of epilepsy without the approval of the attending physician.[36] Additionally, a retrospective study demonstrated that a higher dose of the generic warfarin was needed to maintain a previously stabilized international normalized ratio (INR) value when patients were switched from the brand Coumadin.[40] Furthermore, the American Society of Transplantation (AST) has recommended that generic immunosuppressive medications should be clearly labeled and distinguished from innovator drugs. Patients who are taking these medications should inform their physician of any switch to or among generic formulations to prevent disturbances of therapeutic drug levels[41]; as a result, generic substitution may not be applicable for all patients and conditions. It should be evaluated on an individual basis in certain therapeutic areas, such as antiepileptic, immunosuppressive, and narrow therapeutic index drugs.

General Attitudes Toward Generic Drugs and Adherence

Perception and knowledge of generic medications can be influenced by a consumer's inherent beliefs. Generally, one of the common perceptions that most patients have is the notion that lower drug price equates to lower quality.[42] They usually face generic medication with skepticism due to changes in size and shape of the tablet. Even the taste of the medicine and packaging of the generic formulation may look very different from the brand, which leads to confusion and stress. Although no such tangible proof exists, generic drugs are usually considered inferior medications. Therefore, switching from branded drugs could negatively impact adherence.[38] A study revealed that the generic substitution of risperidone in patients with schizophrenia in Germany was not cost-effective due to a reduction in adherence rates. Patients with generic substitution had poor adherence, poor symptom control, and increased probability of more intensive and expensive hospitalization.[43] Ideally, clinicians should prescribe using the international nonproprietary name (INN), leaving it up to the pharmacist to choose the generic best-suited formulation for the patient.

Cost and Resource Utilization

Switching a generic to a branded drug or vice versa may significantly impact the cost and resource use. A large study by Helmers et al. reported that treating patients with generic antiepileptic drugs was associated with higher medical service costs and total costs than the branded drugs.[44] In another study, the use of generic topiramate was correlated with a higher utilization of other prescription drugs, higher hospitalization rates, and longer hospital stays compared to branded drugs.[45] As a result, the evaluation of economic benefits of switching to and from generic medications may be very complex. Each case, condition, or therapeutic entity may represent a unique situation requiring careful study before identifying its true impacts. Nevertheless, it seems that the current system in place does not offer all the necessary securities regarding pharmacovigilance, notably for the products with narrow therapeutic margin, antiepileptic, and immunosuppressive medications.

CONVERSION OF DRUGS FROM LEGEND TO OVER-THE-COUNTER

Millions of Americans rely on over-the-counter (OTC) medications as the first line of therapy for common diseases or conditions. Most of these OTC products entered the market first as prescription-only medications. Once they demonstrate a proven track record of safety and effectiveness, the drug manufacturer can petition to have them reclassified as OTC and made available to consumers without a prescription. This process is known as an Rx-to-OTC switch.

The migration of some prescription medications to the status of OTC takes place on an almost yearly basis. In fact, since 1976 more than 100 formerly prescription ingredients, indications, or dosage strengths have made the switch to OTC, adding up to over 700 OTC products available to the public.[46]

HISTORY OF PRESCRIPTION VERSUS NONPRESCRIPTION MEDICATIONS

The Durham-Humphrey Amendment of 1951 to the Federal Food, Drug, and Cosmetic Act of 1938 classified the existence of two specific categories of medications: Legend prescription (Rx) and OTC.[47] Prescription medications are drugs deemed as not safe in self-administration; therefore, they require a physician's supervision. The amendment went on to stipulate that these drugs bear a label stating "Caution: Federal law prohibits dispensing without prescription."[47] Meanwhile, OTC became a classification representative of all other drugs that "did not meet the definition of a prescription drug."[48] In 1962, the Kefauver-Harris Amendment required manufacturers of prescription medications to also show evidence of drug effectiveness for its intended use.[49] As such, any application submitted for a drug conversion from Rx status to OTC must show evidence that the drug is safe and effective.

THE CONVERSION PROCESS OF PRESCRIPTION TO OVER-THE-COUNTER

After consumers have used the prescription medication for a period of time and the evidence sufficiently affirms the drug's safety and efficacy, the manufacturer may make application to the FDA requesting the prescription medication to be moved to the OTC status. There are two main pathways of converting a drug from prescription (Rx) to OTC, namely the *NDA* and the *OTC Monograph Process*. For further details of these processes, please visit the FDA website at: www.accessdata.fda.gov/scripts/cder/training/OTC/topic3/topic3/da_01_03_0190.htm

Primarily, most of the Rx-to-OTC switches follow the same NDA process as prescription drug applications.[50] The process may be further complicated if the drug manufacturer requests a change in the indications or a change in drug strength.

Nevertheless, changes of indications and/or strength are common in the OTC environment. For example, in the case of several antihistamines, they may be prescribed to alleviate allergic reactions or rashes, though they may possess the unwanted side effects of drowsiness. These medications are subsequently marketed as OTC drugs for sleep enhancement.

As part of the Rx-to-OTC switch application, the FDA examines the safety and effectiveness of the medication and determines if the instructions for the products are written in a way to provide reasonable assurance that the products will be used correctly and safely by the consumers. This information is determined through Label Comprehension Studies. These studies provide insight into the consumer's ability to understand and properly administer the OTC medication.[47] Ultimately the manufacturer must demonstrate that the drug's benefits to the general public will outweigh any potential risks from the Rx-to-OTC switch.

LABELING OF OVER-THE-COUNTER PRODUCTS

The labeling of OTC products must adhere to a standard format regarding minimum type size, bullet lists, and warnings to present the "Drug Facts."[51]

BENEFITS OF THE PRESCRIPTION-TO-OVER-THE-COUNTER SWITCH

Once a former Rx is evaluated and approved for OTC classification, the foremost benefit to consumers is immediate access in various pharmacies without waiting for appointments.[47] Furthermore, the medications may become more affordable after the Rx-to-OTC switch. Although these switched medications may no longer be eligible to be paid by health insurance, the cost of many OTC preparations may be roughly the same amount as many insurance copayments. In general, OTC medications allow millions of patients to access affordable treatments in a timely manner.[52] Studies have estimated a combined cost savings of approximately $146 billion annually.[53,54] In other words, for each dollar used to purchase an OTC medication, the U.S. Healthcare system realizes $6 to $7 of savings.[53]

RISKS ASSOCIATED WITH OVER-THE-COUNTER MEDICATIONS

While most OTC medications have proven themselves to be safe and effective for the treatment of many health-related issues, there have been instances of misuse or abuse of these drugs. For example, high doses of the common OTC cough suppressant dextromethorphan (DM) can affect memory cognition and motor function.[55] DM packaging gives explicit directions for use with a warning not to exceed 120 mg in a 24-hour period[55]; however, patients with substance use disorder may exceed this maximum in hoping to attain euphoria, leading to dangerous side effects. A dose of 200 to 400 mg may lead to hallucinations; 300 to 600 mg may cause loss of motor coordination and visual distortions; and 500 to 1,500 mg may lead to out-of-body sensations. Additionally, doses exceeding those listed previously may induce breathing problems, heart palpitations, and brain damage.[55]

CONCLUSION

To offer patients the ideal therapies and promote evidence-based clinical practice, it is important for clinicians to understand the key concepts involved in drug development and approval, as well as the involved clinical trials. Well-designed and executed clinical trials can contribute significantly to improve the effectiveness and efficiency of healthcare. Constant improvement of the practices applied to new drug candidates will provide a significant boost of patients' confidence in the treatment prescribed. Widespread access to nonprescription medications has enabled consumers to experience greater convenience and cost savings with treatments, while minimizing associated risks. Although switching branded medications to generic formulations has become a common cost-containment measure, it may potentially impact clinical and safety outcomes, as well as general attitudes of patients and prescribers toward generic drugs. The financial impact of OTC drugs on the healthcare system alone is saving billions of dollars per year, and the trend is not expected to slow down.

CASE EXEMPLAR: Patient With Urinary Retention

BP is a 72-year-old man who presents with the inability to urinate. This is a new symptom for him and started about 1 week ago. It has gotten progressively worse, and now he has a fever. He is very uncomfortable. He recently started over-the-counter diphenhydramine, 25 mg every 6 hours as needed for allergies.

Past Medical History
- Hypertension
- Hyperlipidemia
- Allergic rhinitis
- Benign prostatic hypertrophy (BPH)

Medications
- Hydrochlorothiazide, 25 mg once daily
- Atorvastatin, 20 mg once daily

Physical Examination
- Well-developed white male in mild distress
- Blood pressure: 152/102; pulse: 84; respiration rate: 16; temperature: 100.2 °F
- Lungs clear
- Heart regular rate and rhythm
- Abdomen obese but with palpable bladder to the umbilicus
- Prostate 3+ enlarged on digital rectal exam

Labs
- Complete blood count: White blood cell (WBC) 12.5k
- Urine analysis (catheterized specimen): Innumerable WBC/HPF, 5–10 RBC/HPF

Discussion Questions
1. What caused the patient's acute urinary retention?
2. What is the best approach, after acute management, to managing BP's urinary outflow obstruction?
3. Is there a better way to treat BP's allergies?

CASE EXEMPLAR: Patient With Skin Rash

AD is a 42-year-old Asian female complaining that her eczema is becoming severe. She describes a chronic, itchy rash on the hands and arms. She has had this rash for about two months and has tried numerous over-the-counter creams and lotions to no avail. She says she is "going crazy" from the rash. She wants a more powerful steroid cream than the nonprescription treatments she has been using.

Past Medical History
- Gravida 3 para 3; very active with her kids in school
- In good health

Medications
- OTC hydrocortisone, 1% ("Kind of a lot" she says)
- Ibuprofen, 200 mg two to three tabs every 4–6 hours as needed

Physical Examination
- Well-developed, well-nourished female in mild distress—scratching at her arms
- Heart and lungs normal
- Skin of arms with numerous excoriations in various stages of healing; some thickening; some areas of epithelial atrophy; some burrow patterns noted between the webs of the fingers, creases of the wrists, and antecubital fossae

Labs
- Skin scrapings: *Sarcoptes scabiei*

Discussion Questions
- Why isn't AD's eczema getting better?
- How can some of the findings on AD's skin exam be explained?
- What treatment is likely to be more helpful for AD?

84

CLINICAL PEARLS

- Development of a new drug often takes more than 10 years with a cost close to $1 billion.
- Switching from branded to generic medications may significantly impact cost and resource use, sometimes lowering costs but on occasion resulting in more frequent medical system utilization and higher costs than the branded drugs.
- Millions of Americans rely on over-the-counter (OTC) medications as the first line of therapy for common diseases or conditions, most of which entered the market first as prescription-only medications.
- Dextromethorphan, like several other drugs, was initially controlled by prescription laws but now contributes to overdoses and toxicities in abuse-prone individuals.

KEY TAKEAWAYS

- Approved generic drugs are expected to have the same performance and quality as their branded counterparts.
- While the validation of a drug's efficacy and toxicity in numerous disease-relevant cell and animal models is highly valuable, the ultimate test is whether the drug works in a clinical setting.
- Before initiating a clinical trial on humans, all data from preclinical studies must be first submitted to the FDA in the form of an IND application.
- Phase 1 clinical trials are undertaken to test the safety and dosage ranges as well as the potential toxicity of the new drug in healthy volunteers.
- In phase 2 trials, the safety and dosage specifications are conducted on a small number of patients affected with the condition that the drug is intended to treat, rather than on healthy volunteers.
- Phase 3 trials are conducted on thousands of participants to evaluate the safety, efficacy, and dosage modification of the new drug compared to the current gold-standard treatment or placebo.

- Phase 4 clinical trials are condu ting the FDA approval for NDA keting to identify and evaluate effect of new drugs over a lengthy perio massive number of "real-world" patients.
- Once the current patents of the brand-name products have expired, their generic counterparts may become available.
- Once a drug has demonstrated a proven track record of safety and effectiveness, the drug manufacturer can petition to have it reclassified as over-the-counter (OTC) and made available to consumers without a prescription.

REFERENCES

1. Food and Drug Administration. *Human drugs.* Published September 14, 2018. https://www.fda.gov/industry/regulated-products/human-drugs#drug
2. Cummings JL, Morstorf T, Zhong K. Alzheimer's disease drug-development pipeline: few candidates, frequent failures. *Alzheimers Res Ther.* 2014;6(4):37. doi:10.1186/alzrt269
3. Mohs RC, Greig NH. Drug discovery and development: role of basic biological research. *Alzheimers Dement (NY).* 2017;3(4):651–657. doi:10.1016/j.trci.2017.10.005
4. World Health Organization. *Guidance for organizations performing in vivo bioequivalence studies* (Technical Report Series No. 996, 2016, Annex 9). Published 2016. https://www.who.int/medicines/publications/pharmprep/WHO_TRS_996_annex09.pdf?ua=15.
5. DiMasi JA, Feldman L, Seckler A, et al. Trends in risks associated with new drug development: success rates for investigational drugs. *Clin Pharmacol Ther.* 2010;87(3):272–277. doi:10.1038/clpt.2009.295
6. Sams-Dodd F. Target-based drug discovery: is something wrong? *Drug Discov Today.* 2005;10(2):139–147. doi:10.1016/S1359-6446(04)03316-1
7. DeRoo D. *GLPs and GMPs: when are they necessary?* (NAMSA Whitepaper No. 13). December 2014.
8. Becker RE, Greig NH. Lost in translation: neuropsychiatric drug development. *Sci Transl Med.* 2010;2(61):61rv66. doi:10.1126/scitranslmed.3000446
9. Martins A, Vieira H, Gaspar H, et al. Marketed marine natural products in the pharmaceutical and cosmeceutical industries: tips for success. *Mar Drugs.* 2014;12(2):1066–1101. doi:10.3390/md12021066
10. Taylor D. The pharmaceutical industry and the future of drug development. In: Hester RE, Harrison RM, eds. *Pharmaceuticals in the Environment.* The Royal Society of Chemistry; 2015:1–33.

1. Krause J, Tobin G. Discovery, development, and regulation of natural products. In: Kulka M, ed. *Using Old Solutions to New Problems: Natural Drug Discovery in the 21st Century.* InTech; 2013:3–35.

12. Dias DA, Urban S, Roessner U. A historical overview of natural products in drug discovery. *Metabolites.* 2012;2(2):303–336. doi:10.3390/metabo2020303

13. Clardy J, Walsh C. Lessons from natural molecules. *Nature.* 2004;432(7019):829–837. doi:10.1038/nature03194

14. Croteau R, Kutchan TM, Lewis NG. Natural products (secondary metabolites). In: Buchanan BB, Gruissem W, Jones RL, eds. *Biochemistry and Molecular Biology of Plants.* Wiley; 2000:1250–1319.

15. Paterson I, Anderson EA. Chemistry. The renaissance of natural products as drug candidates. *Science.* 2005;310(5747):451–453. doi:10.1126/science.1116364

16. Newman DJ, Cragg GM, Snader KM. The influence of natural products upon drug discovery. *Nat Prod Rep.* 2000;17(3):215–234. doi:10.1039/a902202c

17. Jones WP, Chin YW, Kinghorn AD. The role of pharmacognosy in modern medicine and pharmacy. *Curr Drug Targets.* 2006;7(3):247–264. doi:10.2174/138945006776054915

18. Patridge E, Gareiss P, Kinch MS, et al. An analysis of FDA-approved drugs: natural products and their derivatives. *Drug Discov Today.* 2016;21(2):204–207. doi:10.1016/j.drudis.2015.01.009

19. Butler MS. The role of natural product chemistry in drug discovery. *J Nat Prod.* 2004;67(12):2141–2153. doi:10.1021/np040106y

20. Cragg GM, Newman DJ. Natural products: a continuing source of novel drug leads. *Biochim Biophys Acta.* 2013;1830(6):3670–3695. doi:10.1016/j.bbagen.2013.02.008

21. Katz L, Baltz RH. Natural product discovery: past, present, and future. *J Ind Microbiol Biotechnol.* 2016;43(2/3):155–176. doi:10.1007/s10295-015-1723-5

22. Mahajan GB, Balachandran L. Antibacterial agents from actinomycetes—a review. *Front Biosci (Elite Ed).* 2012;4:240–453. doi:10.2741/373.

23. Nguyen J-T, Kiso Y. *Discovery of Peptide Drugs as Enzyme Inhibitors and Activators Peptide Chemistry and Drug Design.* John Wiley & Sons; 2015:157–201.

24. Calvo-Rojas G, Gómez-Outes A. Clinical drug development in thromboembolic diseases: regulatory and methodological approach. *Curr Drug Discov Technol.* 2012;9(2):105–118. doi:10.2174/1570163811209020105.

25. Freedman B. Equipoise and the ethics of clinical research. *N Engl J Med.* 1987;317(3):141–145. doi:10.1056/NEJM198707163170304

26. Lansimies-Antikainen H, Laitinen T, Rauramaa R, et al. Evaluation of informed consent in health research: a questionnaire survey. *Scand J Caring Sci.* 2010;24(1):56–64. doi:10.1111/j.1471-6712.2008.00684.x

27. Umscheid CA, Margolis DJ, Grossman CE. Key concepts of clinical trials: a narrative review. *Postgrad Med.* 2011;123(5):194–204. doi:10.3810/pgm.2011.09.2475

28. Govani SM, Higgins PD. How to read a clinical trial paper: a lesson in basic trial statistics. *Gastroenterol Hepatol (NY).* 2012;8(4):241–248. https://www.ncbi.nlm.nih.gov/pmc/articles/PMC3380258

29. Thomas DW, Burns J, Audette J, et al. *Clinical Development Success Rates 2006–2015.* Biomedtracker; 2016. https://www.bio.org/sites/default/files/legacy/bioorg/docs/Clinical%20Development%20Success%20Rates%202006-2015%20-%20BIO,%20Biomedtracker,%20Amplion%202016.pdf

30. Davit BM, Nwakama PE, Buehler GJ, et al. Comparing generic and innovator drugs: a review of 12 years of bioequivalence data from the United States Food and Drug Administration. *Ann Pharmacother.* 2009;43(10):1583–1597. doi:10.1345/aph.1M141

31. Schuirmann DJ. A comparison of the two one-sided tests procedure and the power approach for assessing the equivalence of average bioavailability. *J Pharmacokinet Biopharm.* 1987;15(6):657–680. doi:10.1007/BF01068419

32. Sabatini S, Ferguson RM, Helderman JH, et al. Drug substitution in transplantation: a National Kidney Foundation White Paper. *Am J Kidney Dis.* 1999;33(2):389–397. doi:10.1016/S0272-6386(99)70318-5

33. Reiffel JA. Formulation substitution and other pharmacokinetic variability: underappreciated variables affecting antiarrhythmic efficacy and safety in clinical practice. *Am J Cardiol.* 2000;85(10)(suppl 1):46–52. doi:10.1016/S0002-9149(00)00906-1

34. Meredith P. Bioequivalence and other unresolved issues in generic drug substitution. *Clin Ther.* 2003;25(11):2875–2890. doi:10.1016/S0149-2918(03)80340-5

35. Bialer M. Generic products of antiepileptic drugs (AEDs): is it an issue? *Epilepsia.* 2007;48(10):1825–1832. doi:10.1111/j.1528-1167.2007.01272.x

36. Liow K, Barkley GL, Pollard JR, et al. Position statement on the coverage of anticonvulsant drugs for the treatment of epilepsy. *Neurology.* 2007;68(16):1249–1250. doi:10.1212/01.wnl.0000259400.30539.cc

37. Gidal BE, Tomson T. Debate: substitution of generic drugs in epilepsy: is there cause for concern? *Epilepsia.* 2008;49(suppl 9):56–62. doi:10.1111/j.1528-1167.2008.01927.x

38. Straka RJ, Keohane DJ, Liu LZ. Potential clinical and economic impact of switching branded medications to generics. *Am J Ther.* 2017;24(3):e278–e289. doi:10.1097/MJT.0000000000000282

39. Berg MJ. What's the problem with generic antiepileptic drugs? A call to action. *Neurology.* 2007;68(16):1245–1246. doi:10.1212/01.wnl.0000262876.37269.8b

40. Halkin H, Shapiro J, Kurnik D, et al. Increased warfarin doses and decreased international normalized ratio response after nationwide generic switching. *Clin Pharmacol Ther.* 2003;74(3):215–221. doi:10.1016/S0009-9236(03)00166-8

41. Alloway RR, Isaacs R, Lake K, et al. Report of the American Society of Transplantation conference on immunosuppressive drugs and the use of generic immunosuppressants. *Am J Transplant.* 2003;3(10):1211–1215. doi:10.1046/j.1600-6143.2003.00212.x

42. Kaplan WA, Ritz LS, Vitello M, et al. Policies to promote use of generic medicines in low and middle income countries: a review of published literature, 2000–2010. *Health Policy.* 2012;106(3):211–224. doi:10.1016/j.healthpol.2012.04.015

43. Treur M, Heeg B, Moller HJ, et al. A pharmaco-economic analysis of patients with schizophrenia switching to generic risperidone involving a possible compliance loss. *BMC Health Serv Res.* 2009;9:32. doi:10.1186/1472-6963-9-32

44. Helmers SL, Paradis PE, Manjunath R, et al. Economic burden associated with the use of generic antiepileptic drugs in the United States. *Epilepsy Behav.* 2010;18(4):437–444. doi:10.1016/j.yebeh.2010.05.015

45. Andermann F, Duh MS, Gosselin A, et al. Compulsory generic switching of antiepileptic drugs: high switchback rates to branded compounds compared with other drug classes. *Epilepsia.* 2007;48(3):464–469. doi:10.1111/j.1528-1167.2007.01007.x

46. Consumer Healthcare Products Association. *FAQs about Rx-to-OTC switch.* Accessed December 19, 2019. https://www.chpa.org/about-consumer-healthcare/faqs/FAQs-rx-otc-switch

47. Chang J, Lizer A, Patel I, et al. Prescription to over-the-counter switches in the United States. *J Res Pharm Pract.* 2016;5:149–154. doi:10.4103/2279-042X.185706

48. Ann WH. Rx-to-OTC switch—the process and procedures. *SAGE J.* 1985;19:119–126. doi:10.1177/009286158501900207

49. Meadows M. *Promoting safe & effective drugs for 100 years. FDA Consumer.* Published 2006. https://www.fda.gov/AboutFDA/History/ProductRegulation/ucm2017809.htm

50. Consumer Healthcare Products Association. *Briefing information on the Rx-to-OTC switch process.* Published 2012. https://www.chpa.org/our-issues/otc-medicines/rx-otc-switch

51. OTC Drug Facts Rule, 64 Fed. Regist. 13254. Over-the-counter human drugs, Labeling Regulations, March 17, 1999 as codified at 21 CFR 201.66.

52. Newton G, Popovich NG, Pray WS. Rx-to-OTC switches: from prescription to self-care. *J Am Pharm Assoc (Wash).* 1996;36(8):488–495. doi:10.1016/s1086-5802(16)30103-6

53. Consumer Healthcare Products Association. *White paper: value of OTC medicines to the U.S. healthcare system.* Published March 18, 2019. http://overthecountervalue.org/white-paper/

54. Consumer Healthcare Products Association. *New study: over-the-counter (OTC) products used by millions of Americans saves healthcare system billions annually.* Published 2019. https://www.biospace.com/article/releases/new-study-over-the-counter-otc-products-used-by-millions-of-americans-saves-healthcare-system-billions-annually/

55. Juergens J. Over the counter (OTC) drug addiction, abuse, and treatment. Updated September 18, 2020. https://www.addictioncenter.com/drugs/over-the-counter-drugs/

Foundations of Prescription Writing

Brent Luu, Laura Van Auker, and David Grega

LEARNING OBJECTIVES

- List the classes of controlled substances as defined by the Drug Enforcement Agency (DEA).
- Identify medications that require a prescription under law.
- Interpret a written prescription using commonly accepted abbreviations.
- Compare the ethical principles of autonomy, beneficence, nonmaleficence, and justice as they relate to prescribing.
- Create a valid and acceptable prescription for a generic, brand-name, and brand-name preferred drug.
- Evaluate the ethics surrounding prescribing for self or family.

INTRODUCTION

Under U.S. laws and regulations, prescription drugs can be prescribed only by authorized prescribers. This practice became official following the introduction of the Durham–Humphrey Amendment of the Federal Food, Drug, and Cosmetic Act in the early 1950s. The amendment requires that drugs that are not safe for self-medication must bear a legend on the label that states: "Caution: Federal Law prohibits dispensing without a prescription." The amendment also holds pharmacists liable for prosecution if the category of drugs is sold "over the counter" without a *bona fide* prescription or oral authorization from an authorized licensed clinician.[1]

Licensed clinicians authorized by law to prescribe medications may be grouped into two broad categories: the physician and nonphysician prescribers. Each of these groups is subject to its own professional state board and federal regulations that define their scope of practice. For example, physician assistants (PAs) have been involved in prescribing medication since the first PA program at Duke University graduated a class of three PAs in 1967. Currently all 50 states and Washington, DC, authorize PA prescribing, and all but Kentucky allow some level of controlled substance prescriptive privileges. This authority followed several years of state legislature amendments and new regulations that required a robust lobby and advocacy by the pioneers of the PA profession.[2,3]

PAs are clinicians, licensed by individual states, and nationally board certified to practice medicine and prescribe medications on healthcare teams with physicians and other clinicians. Their scope of practice is determined by their education and experience, state laws and regulations, and individual policies of different facilities. Although PAs are dependent upon a collaborative relationship with a supervising physician, this supervision allows significant autonomy of practice, under a delegation of services agreement. All states require graduation from a PA Program accredited by the Accreditation Review Commission on Education of the Physician Assistant (ARC-PA) and successful completion of the Physician Assistant National Certifying Exam (PANCE), administered by the National Commission on Certification of Physician Assistants (NCCPA).

The history of nurses providing medication to patients in the United States extends back to 1893 in New York City and the founding of Mary Wald's Henry Street Visiting Nurses.[4] With the passage of the Food and Drug Act in 1906, boundaries of what constituted the practice of medicine were being defined, limiting the ability of nurses to provide medication to clients with limited healthcare access. Mary Wald responded by creating a medical advisory council that wrote standing medical orders allowing her home health nurses to continue serving the urban poor.[5]

The founding of the nurse practitioner (NP) role is credited to nurse Loretta Ford and her pediatrician colleague Dr. Henry Silver at the University of Colorado, Denver, in 1965.[6] The modern call for nurses to practice at their highest level was nationally introduced in the Institute of Medicine (IOM) report *The Future of Nursing: Leading Change, Advancing Health*. The IOM report recommended enhanced nursing education and removal of practice restrictions to improve national health. Lacking a common national policy, independent prescribing by advanced practice registered nurses (APRNs), considered "unrestricted" or "full scope of practice," has been addressed by individual states with considerable variation.[6]

The National Council of State Boards of Nursing (NCSBN) has developed an evidence-based consensus statement for standardized licensure, accreditation, certification, and education in an effort to provide state legislatures a blueprint for adoption to limited effect.[7] Within states, the various APRN roles—nurse practitioners (NP), certified nurse-midwives (CNM), clinical nurse specialists (CNS), and certified registered nurse anesthetists (CRNA)—may have varied prescriptive practice restrictions, at times based upon clinic type, inpatient care, or rural designation. Shortages of primary care clinicians across the United States have provided momentum for legislative change, particularly for underserved populations. The American Association of Nurse Practitioners (AANP) maintains a state-by-state resource site providing current regulatory information on NP prescriptive authority and scope of practice. The NCSBN with its consensus model for APRN practice advocates for a universal regulatory authority from a common national model.[7]

FEDERAL DRUG LAW AND REGULATIONS

Prescription medications did not officially exist until the late 1930s. Prior to this period, medications were available on the market without much restriction or regulation. The law did not require safety data for new drugs; in other words, selling drugs with toxic effects on the market was not illegal. The requirement of a prescription originated from an incident occurring in 1937 that involved the sale of *sulfanilamide elixir*.[8] Previously, the powder and tablet form of this medication had been used to treat streptococcal infections; however, despite increasing demand, the liquid form of the drug had not yet been developed. Subsequently, the liquid formulation of sulfanilamide was formulated by dissolving it in diethylene glycol, a solvent that is also known as an antifreeze. Shortly after the introduction of this elixir on the market, the product claimed more than 100 lives due to severe kidney damage and failure after ingestion.[2]

In response to the many reports of deaths that linked to the product, the U.S. Food and Drug Administration (FDA) immediately launched a full investigation, which eventually led to the enactment of the Federal Food, Drug, and Cosmetic Act of 1938.[9] This Act requires that new drugs must demonstrate safety before being placed on the market. Meanwhile, the FDA also states that dangerous drugs other than over-the-counter (OTC) products must be given under the direction of a medical expert, which officially began a new era of prescription-only (Rx-only) drugs. Since the first introduction of the federal law in 1938, the Durham–Humphrey Amendment was passed by Congress in 1951, which defines drugs that are unsafe without medical supervision.[10] This amendment has further clarified which drugs belong to the "Rx-only" group and limits the sale of these drugs according to the prescription from a medical professional. Meanwhile, all other drugs may be purchased without a precription.[10]

Since the introduction of these pivotal federal laws, many more laws and regulations have been passed at both the federal and state levels, aiming to protect the consumers and public health. The FDA has developed regulations based on the legal framework that has been established by these laws. FDA follows the procedures that have been set forth by the Administrative Procedure Act to develop regulations, which involves the process of "notice and comment rulemaking," allowing the public to provide feedback on a proposed regulation. Once a proposed regulation is finalized and becomes an official federal regulation, it will be published as a part of the Code of Federal Regulations (CFR), which consists of 50 different titles addressing different areas. Among these titles, the CFR Title 21 involves food and drugs that are further divided into nine volumes and three chapters. Volumes 1 through 8 are grouped to Chapter 1, which is comprised of Parts 1 through 1299 that are under jurisdiction of the FDA, Department of Health and Human Services. Additionally, Volume 9 is divided into Chapters 2 and 3, which cover parts 1300 to 1399 and parts 1400 to 1499, respectively. The Drug Enforcement Administration (DEA), under the Department of Justice (DOJ), is the regulatory entity of Chapter 2, while the Office of National Drug Control Policy oversees the regulations within Chapter 3 (**Table 8.1**).[11] Although these CFRs are considered part of federal laws, they are not part of the original Food, Drug, and Cosmetic Act.[12] Further details of each of the parts within a specific chapter can be found at the following website: www.ecfr.gov/cgi-bin/text-idx?SID=cf7b29df84f7d4ae9f1cc44ebca49b87&mc=true&tpl=/ecfrbrowse/Title21/21tab_02.tpl.

THE DRUG ENFORCEMENT ADMINISTRATION

The DEA under the DOJ defines and regulates all controlled substances. This agency was established in 1973 to enforce the federal Controlled Substance Act (CSA) of 1970. It has evolved from the Bureau of Narcotics

TABLE 8.1 Organization of the Code of Federal Regulations Title 21: Food and Drugs

Regulatory Entity	Volumes	Chapter	Parts
Food and Drug Administration, Department of Health and Human Services	1–8	I	1–1299
Drug Enforcement Agency, Department of Justice	9	II	1300–1399
Office of National Drug Control Policy	9	III	1400–1499

Source: Adapted from Electronic Code of Federal Regulation. 2018. Accessed October 29, 2018. https://www.ecfr.gov/cgi-bin/text-idx?SID=b08849a235a7ba4fb2a5647e8cc90668&mc=true&tpl=/ecfrbrowse/Title21/21tab_02.tpl

and Dangerous Drugs (BNDD), which resulted from the merger of the Bureau of Drug Abuse Control (BDAC) in the Department of Health, Education, and Welfare, together with the Bureau of Narcotics from the Treasury Department (**Figure 8.1**).[13] Its purpose is to prevent diversion and abuse of controlled substances, meanwhile, ensuring a sufficient, uninterrupted supply of these agents for legitimated medical and scientific needs.[14]

The law mandates that all transactions of controlled substances follow a "close system" distribution, which requires all legitimated handlers including manufacturers, distributors, pharmacies, prescribers, and researchers be registered with the DEA and have strict accountability of all distributions. Furthermore, the agency also classified all controlled substances into five schedules:

- **Schedule I Drugs:** Agents that currently have no acceptable medical use within the United States; therefore, they may not be prescribed, dispensed, nor administered for medical treatment.
- **Schedule II to V Drugs:** Agents considered to have acceptable medical use. Subsequently, they may be prescribed, dispensed, and administered for medical purposes. Examples of selected schedule I to V drugs are listed in **Table 8.2**. For a more complete list of drugs and their corresponding schedule, please visit the DEA website at: www.deadiversion.usdoj.gov/schedules/orangebook/c_cs_alpha.pdf.

To prescribe controlled substances, prescribers must register and apply for a DEA number using Form 224 for a new applicant (online or hard copy).[1] For further details, visit: www.deadiversion.usdoj.gov/drugreg/index.html. Under the CSA, all entities that handle controlled substances must register or be exempted from registration by the DEA. Registered clinicians may only engage in activities that are authorized by state or federal laws. When there are differences between the state and federal laws, the more stringent regulations of these laws would be applied. Consequently, clinicians should have a clear understanding of their practicing state laws and DEA regulations.

In the event of a "significant theft or loss" of controlled substances, clinicians or registrants are required to notify the Field Division Office of the Administration in the area and complete the DEA Form 106 to report such loss or theft "upon discovery," which has been interpreted as "immediately without delay."[1] The DEA field offices are organized into three broad divisions—Foreign Offices, Domestic Division, and Operational Division:

- **Foreign Offices:** 93 offices in 69 countries worldwide
- **Domestic Division:** 239 offices in 23 divisions spread throughout various cities across the United States (**Figure 8.2**).
- **Operational Division:** Houses both the Diversion Control Division and the Aviation Division. The mission of the Diversion Control Division is to prevent, detect, and investigate the diversion of controlled pharmaceuticals and listed chemicals from legitimate sources while ensuring an adequate and uninterrupted supply for legitimate medical, commercial, and scientific needs. Furthermore, the mission of the Aviation Division is to provide aviation support to operational and intelligence elements within DEA and the law enforcement community to detect, locate, identify, and assess illicit narcotics-related to trafficking activities.

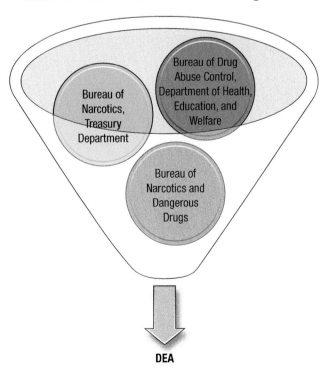

FIGURE 8.1 The emergence of the Drug Enforcement Administration (DEA).

TABLE 8.2 Examples of Controlled Substances and Their Corresponding Drug Enforcement Administration Schedule

Schedule	Agents
I	**Drugs that have no acceptable medical use in the United States:** Heroin; LSD; marijuana (cannabis); peyote; methaqualone; MDMA; "ecstasy"
II	**Drugs that have high risk for abuse and dependence:** *Analgesics:* Cocaine, methamphetamine, methadone, hydromorphone (Dilaudid®), meperidine (Demerol®), oxycodone (OxyContin®), fentanyl; combined products of hydrocodone containing fewer than 15 mg per unit dose (e.g., Vicodin®) *Stimulants:* Dextroamphetamine (Dexedrine®), amphetamine/dextroamphetamine (Adderall®), and methylphenidate (Ritalin®)
III	**Drugs that have moderate-to-low risk for abuse and dependence:** *Analgesics:* Products containing <90 mg of codeine per unit dose (e.g., Tylenol® with codeine), ketamine *Steroids:* Anabolic steroids, testosterone
IV	**Drugs that have low risk for abuse and dependence:** *Analgesics:* Pentazocine (Talwin®), tramadol (Ultram®) *Benzodiazepines:* Alprazolam (Xanax®), diazepam (Valium®), lorazepam (Ativan®) *Others:* carisoprodol (Soma®), zolpidem (Ambien®)
V	**Drugs that have lower risk for abuse than Schedule IV:** Antitussive preparations containing <200 mg of codeine or per 100 mL (e.g., Cheratussin AC®), loperamide (Lomotil®), pregabalin (Lyrica®), lacosamide (Vimpat®)

LSD, lysergic acid diethylamide; MDMA, 3,4-methylenedioxy-methamphetamine.

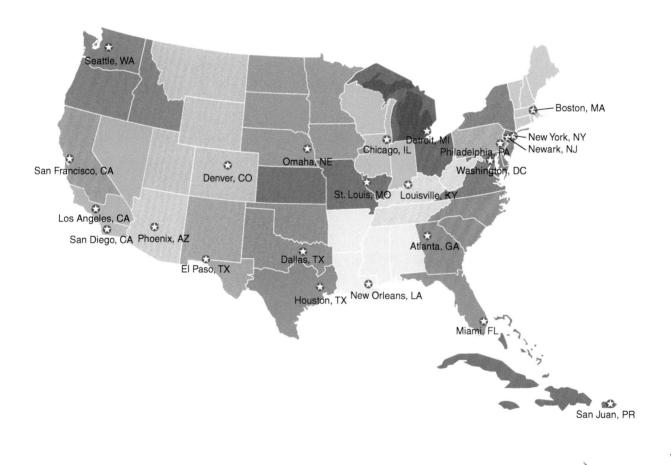

FIGURE 8.2 Domestic divisions of the Drug Enforcement Agency in the United States.

Source: Adapted from United States Drug Enforcement Administration. *Domestic divisions.* https://www.dea.gov/domestic-divisions

Although electronic prescribing has gained much popularity in recent years due to advances in computer technologies, physical paper prescriptions are the original mode of prescribing. Since the prescription blanks may be stolen and forged, the DEA has recommended approaches to prevent or mitigate theft and forgery of prescription pads (**Box 8.1**).

REQUIREMENTS OF A VALID PRESCRIPTION

According to federal laws, a prescription is an order of medication that is directly dispensed to a patient or an ultimate user. In other words, the drug order written by a prescriber in the outpatient setting and given directly to the end user (the patient) is a "prescription," whereas a drug order provided to a healthcare team member (e.g., nurse, a pharmacist, other clinician) in the *inpatient* setting or other facility for immediate administration to a patient is an "order."[1] The required information on a prescription may be grouped into three separate sections: information related to (a) the prescriber, (b) the patient, and (c) the drug (**Figure 8.3**).

PATIENT INFORMATION

The DEA requires that a prescription include the patient's full name and address.[1] Although the patient's gender, age, and date of birth (DOB) are not specifically required on a prescription by law, they are important data that will help other clinicians (e.g., pharmacists) evaluate the appropriateness of the prescription and ensure patient safety and accuracy. In fact, The Joint Commission (TJC), a national accreditation body of hospital and other healthcare facilities, has recommended using two patient identifiers as part of the National Patient Safety Goals (NPSG),[15] which may include "[i]nformation associated with an individual that reliably identifies the individual as the person for whom the service or treatment is intended."[16]

DRUG INFORMATION

The body of the prescription allows the prescriber to write the specific medication or device and provide the directions for use. It bears the "Rx" symbol, which is an abbreviation derived from the Latin term *recipe*, which means "to take."[17] Following the symbol are spaces for the prescriber to write either the full generic or brand name of the drug and its specific strength, which should be written in units that match the commercially available products (**Figure 8.4**).

GENERIC SUBSTITUTION

When a brand name of the product is written, prescribers should always make sure that generic substitution is permissible, unless the brand of the medication is ordered due to a patient's specific need. Brand-name drug products are usually protected by the U.S. Patent and Trademark Office when they are newly developed (see Chapter 7 for further details on drug approval and development processes). This protection gives them the exclusive right to be sold on the market. During this protective period, there are no generic products available since the patents prohibit generic companies from selling their versions of the drug. However, once the patents of the brand-name drugs expire, the generic drugs can gain full approval and access to the market.

Allowing "generic substitution" for a specified product will give the pharmacist the legal authority to substitute generic drugs that are therapeutically equivalent to the ordered product, providing cost savings to the patient under the coverage of the insurance company's formulary. The generic products of a medication are the same as the approved brand-name drugs in quality, safety,

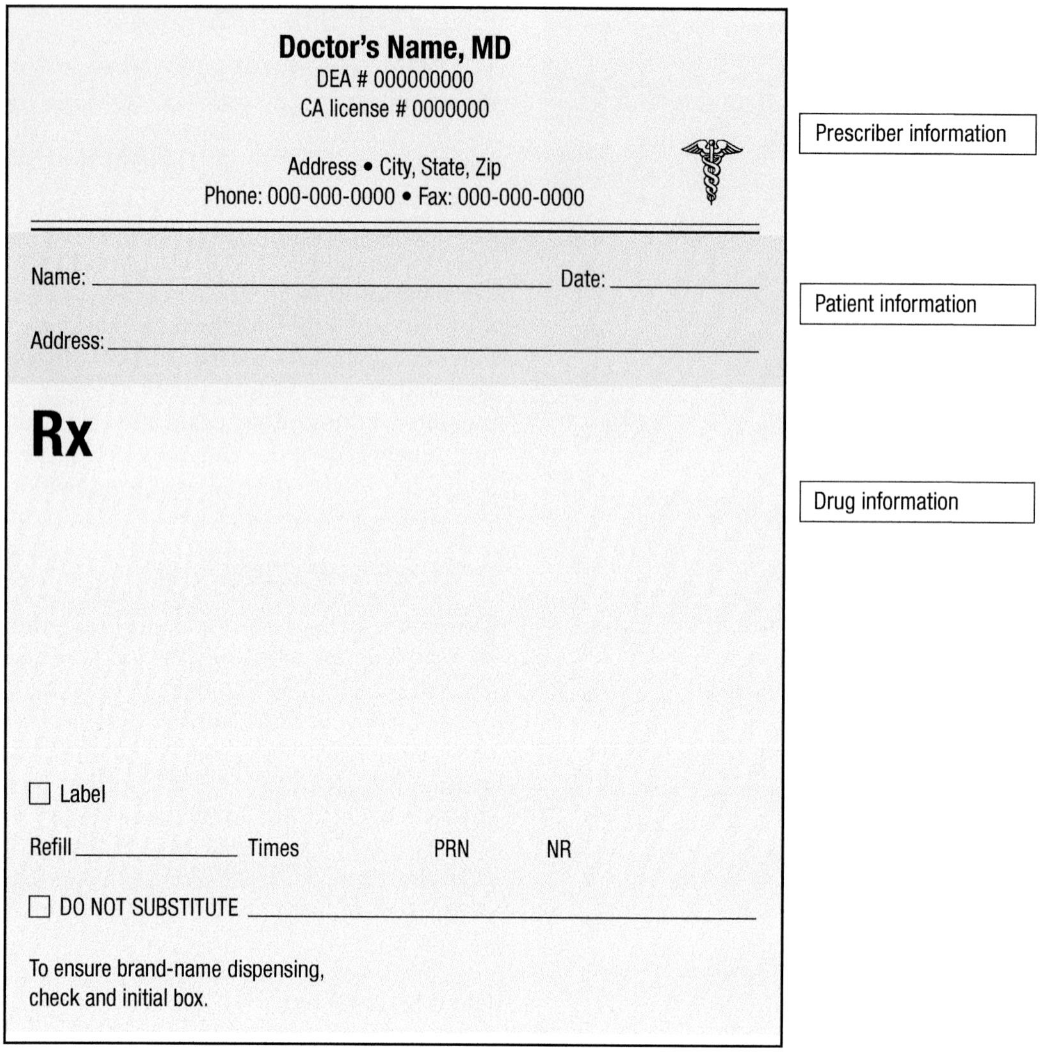

Doctor's Name, MD
DEA # 000000000
CA license # 0000000

Address • City, State, Zip
Phone: 000-000-0000 • Fax: 000-000-0000

Prescriber information

Name: _____ Date: _____

Address: _____

Patient information

Rx

Drug information

☐ Label

Refill _____ Times   PRN   NR

☐ DO NOT SUBSTITUTE _____

To ensure brand-name dispensing,
check and initial box.

FIGURE 8.3 An example of a general prescription.

form, and route of administration. All FDA-approved generic products are held to the same standards as their brand-name counterparts and are subject to the Abbreviated New Drug Application (ANDA) approval process before they can be widely marketed to the consumers. Generic products must have the same properties as their brand-name counterparts[18]:

- Same active ingredient
- Same indications for use, strength, dosage form, and route of administration
- Acceptable inactive ingredients
- Manufactured under the same strict standards
- Storage container and labeling appropriate for shipping and selling on the market

If a specific product of a prescription is requested with "no substitution allowed," the prescription will be noted by the prescriber as a DAW (Dispense as Written) or be marked "Do Not Substitute" on the prescription. When the substitution is not allowed, the pharmacist must dispense the ordered drug exactly as indicated on the prescription. The DAW measure is usually applied in cases where patients are taking drugs that have narrow therapeutic windows because it will help to minimize confusion that may lead to errors. Furthermore, any change in concentration of a drug with a narrow therapeutic window may put a patient at higher risk for undesirable outcomes; therefore, drug-level stability may be better maintained without the generic substitution. For example, warfarin is a common anticoagulant that is used for prevention of clot formation from various conditions. Although generic substitution of warfarin is widely accepted in clinical practice, close monitoring should be implemented when a brand of warfarin is switched to

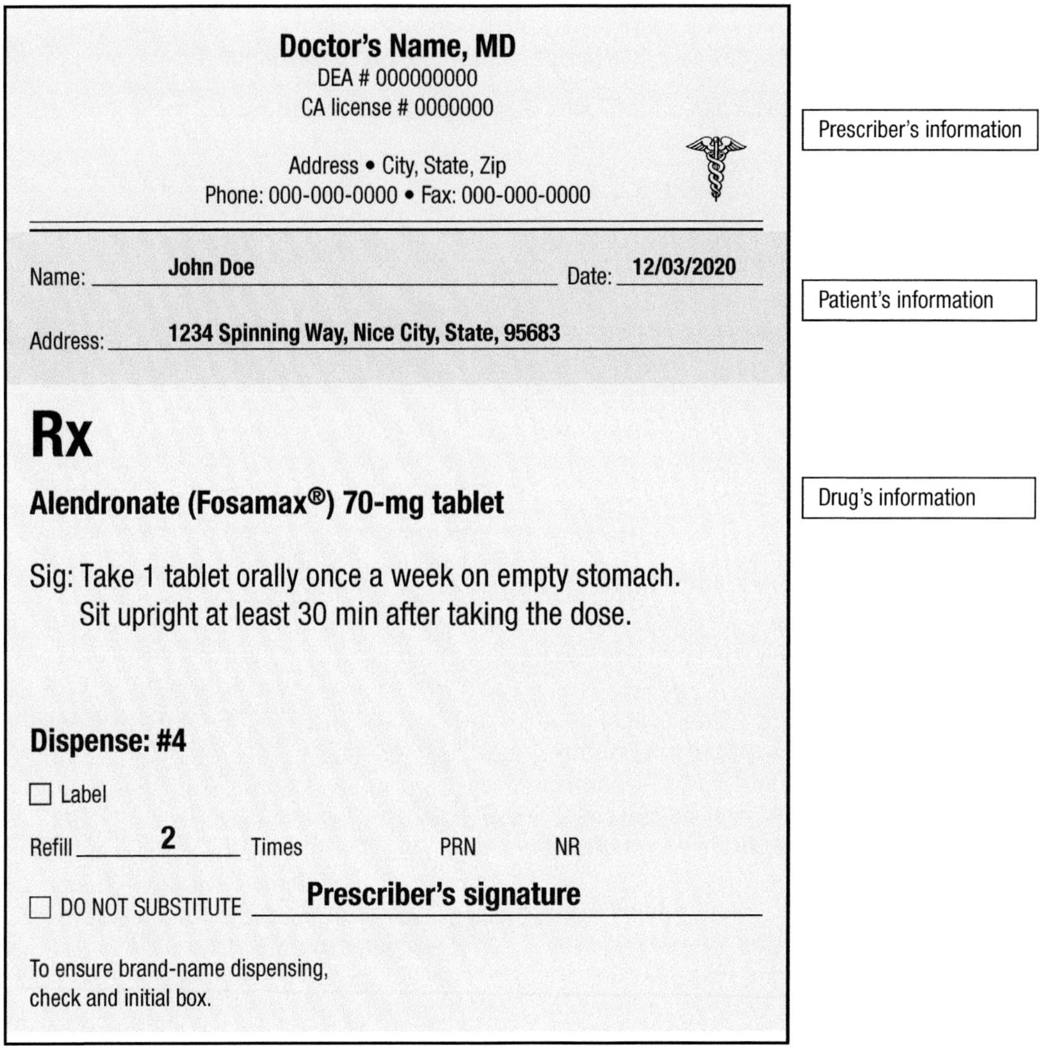

FIGURE 8.4 An example of an alendronate (Fosamax®) prescription for a patient.

the generic version or vice versa because there may be some variability on the individual level that may lead to toxicities.[19] Per the FDA definitions, the generic version of a drug must show bioequivalence to its brand-name counterpart. In other words, when generic substitution is allowed, there may be up to 20% of differences between the two products.

Following the name and strength of the ordered product is the *Sig*, derived from the Latin term *signo*, which means "mark." This is the area where the prescriber writes the instructions for the patient of how to take a prescribed medication. The specific dose with appropriate units and frequency of use are provided together with other clear specific instructions such as "take with or without foods" or "sit upright for at least 30 minutes after taking the dose." Many prescribers choose to use abbreviations while writing the prescription; however, errors may result from using ambiguous or illegible abbreviations, leading to misinterpretation

of the directions and serious undesirable outcomes. The TJC has developed a list of "Do Not Use" abbreviations, and the Institute for Safe Medication Practices (ISMP) has developed the "List of Error-Prone Abbreviations, Symbols, and Dose Designations." These recommendations aim to mitigate these problems.[16,20] For example, instead of simply writing the letter "u" or "U," prescribers should write the complete word "unit" while prescribing drugs that are dosed as such (e.g., insulins). The abbreviation "qd" or "QD" is often mistaken for "qid" or "QID"; therefore, prescribers should write "daily" or "every day" to prevent these avoidable mistakes (**Table 8.3**).

When writing numbers to indicate the medication's dose or strength, prescribers should always use a "leading zero" in front of decimal points and avoid using "trailing zero" after all whole numbers. For example, the strength of a prescription for digoxin should be written as 125 mcg (i.e., avoid trailing zero → 125.0 mcg) or

TABLE 8.3 Commonly Used Abbreviations and Recommendations to Prevent Errors

Abbreviations	Intended Meaning	Misinterpretation	Recommendations
μg	Microgram	Mistaken as "mg"	Write "mcg"
cc	Cubic centimeters	Mistaken as "u" (units)	Write "mL"
IN	Intranasal	Mistaken as "IM" or "IV"	Write "intranasal" or "NAS"
QD, q.d., qd	Every day	Mistaken as "q.i.d.," especially if the period after the "q" or the tail of the "q" is misunderstood as an "I"	Write "daily" or "every day"
QOD, Q.O.D., q.o.d, qod	Every other day	Period after the "Q" mistaken for "I" and the "O" mistaken for "I"	Write "every other day"
qhs	Nightly at bedtime	Mistaken as "qhr" or every hour	Write "nightly"
HCT	Hydrocortisone	Mistaken as hydrochlorothiazide	Write complete drug name
HCTZ	Hydrochlorothiazide	Mistaken as hydrocortisone (seen as HCT250 mg)	Write complete drug name
MS, MSO4	Morphine sulfate	Mistaken as magnesium sulfate	Write complete drug name

0.125 mg (i.e., avoid using simple "dot" for decimals → .125 mg). For other do-not-use or error-prone abbreviations, please refer to the TJC and ISMP websites: www.jointcommission.org/facts_about_do_not_use_list; www.ismp.org/recommendations/error-prone-abbreviations-list.

Once the instructions for the patient have been completed, the quantity or day of supply of the prescription must be provided. Topical products may be ordered and dispensed in the amounts of grams or ounces rounded off to the nearest commercially available size. Clinicians should not use "tube" as the ordered quantity since each product may have different-sized tubes, which can range from 15 to 80 g. The most commonly available tube sizes for topical products are 15, 30, 60, or 80 g, though there may be a few exceptions. For products that are available as liquid, the quantity may be ordered in ounces or milliliters (mL) to be dispensed at a sufficient amount to cover the whole duration of treatment. Please refer to Chapter 11 for further unit conversions. The quantity of tablets or capsules dispensed should also cover the whole duration of therapy. For example, a prescription of "prednisone 40 mg on day 1, 30 mg on day 2, 20 mg on day 3, 10 mg on day 4, then stop," should have an ordered quantity of 10 tablets of the 10-mg strength or 5 tablets of the 20-mg strength. In other words, the patient will need to take four tablets on the first day, three tablets on the second day, two tablets on third day, and one tablet on the fourth day of the 10-mg strength. However, the patient would need half the quantity for the same dose of prednisone when the 20-mg tablet strength is used.

ETHICAL ASPECTS OF PRESCRIBING

The clinical prescribing of medications in patient care is guided by ethical standards of practice relevant to all clinical decision-making.[21] The ethical principles of autonomy, beneficence, nonmaleficence, and justice have direct applications for clinical prescribing. The World Health Organization (WHO) has developed the "STEPS" approach, which encourages ethical prescriptive practice guidelines with patient-centered prescribing to include safety, tolerability, effectiveness, price, and simplicity of treatment and dosing.[22]

Autonomy is applied through informed consent to include patient education in treatment risks, benefits, and alternatives as well as use of shared patient decision-making guidelines.[23] Clinician responsibility for beneficence is advanced through maintenance of a well-informed and current understanding of new medications regarding their safety, efficacy, and mechanism of action.[24] Clinical compassion as beneficence is manifested through the process of identifying the correct diagnosis and selection of the best therapeutic treatment as well as patient considerations.

The FDA regulates pharmaceutical samples and dictates that in all cases it is illegal and unethical to sell samples intended for free distribution to patients. It may be appropriate in some clinical environments to dispense purchased medications and supplements obtained in bulk and provided with minimal profit where prescription cost or pharmacy distance are significant barriers to care.

Nonmaleficence, or "do no harm," is assured through appropriate history taking, identification of potential multidrug interactions, and treatment of side effects, as well as appropriate monitoring of treatment effect and potential for misuse or abuse.[25] When transfer of care must occur, assurance of transfer to another clinician is required to maintain essential therapies. Systematic use of clinical guidelines and consultation with appropriate clinical specialists and pharmacists reduce the risk of patient harm from prescribing errors or serious medication interactions and side effects. The ethical principle of justice is maintained by demonstrating dignity and respect for all patients through equal access to care and treatment in a stigma-free environment regardless of clinical diagnosis, social status, or personal preferences for treatment. The American Academy of Family Practice (AAFP) summarized the 2007 WHO "Guide to Good Prescribing" into a systematic eight-step approach to prescribing that encompasses the principles of ethical prescribing[22]:

1. Evaluate and clearly define the patient's problem.
2. Specify the therapeutic objective.
3. Select the appropriate drug therapy.
4. Initiate therapy with appropriate details and consider nonpharmacologic therapies.
5. Give information, instructions, and warnings (informed consent).
6. Evaluate therapy regularly.
7. Consider drug cost when prescribing.
8. Use computers and other tools to reduce prescribing errors.

STANDARD OF CARE FOR SPECIALTY POPULATIONS

With advancing standards of care in pediatrics and gerontology, clinicians must perform a vigilant self-assessment of personal skill and knowledge to meet appropriate standards of care. Age and size-specific dosing is critical in pediatrics and polypharmacy is common in geriatric patients.[26] Specialty care settings such as psychiatric-mental health or infectious disease may require additional certifications, mentorship, or continuing education to gain versatility in specialty therapeutics. It is the responsibility of the clinician to be aware of not only the regulatory requirements, but also the community standards established through peer practice and prescribing patterns. Additional training and regulations have recently been established for acute and chronic pain management, opioid prescribing, and rehabilitation environments. Clinicians who are new to a special population or specialty practice setting should seek additional peer and medical supervisory mentoring as well as focused continuing education. Resources for consult and referral should be clearly established for optimal patient care and to advance clinician expertise and confidence.

PRESCRIBING FOR SELF, FAMILY, AND NONPATIENTS

Regulations for prescribing for oneself, family members, or nonpatients vary by state for many clinicians. While prescribing noncontrolled medications informally may not be illegal, it is considered unethical by most professional medical standards except in limited noncomplex or emergent situations where alternatives are limited.[27] PAs prescribe through physician delegation and APRNs prescribe through collaborative agreements that require the patient to be within the clinicians' clinical practice. Prescribing controlled substances for oneself or a family member violates medical codes of ethics or state law in nearly all states. Doing so for self or a family member violates federal DEA licensure statutes, as does prescribing for a nonpatient.

Treating family and friends may involve conflicts of interest as well as loss of objectivity in the dual role of clinician and relative, friend, or colleague.[28,29] Limited or inappropriate evaluation, history taking, and physical examination are more likely. Coupled with inadequate documentation, the ethical standards for beneficence in patient care are not met. Informed consent may be limited or biased. Lack of autonomy creates the potential for withholding of highly sensitive information or inability by a family member to question or decline care prescribed.

While highly discouraged, it is recognized by most clinicians that, barring absolute legal contraindications, prescribing for oneself or a family member for nonnarcotic prescriptions remains a gray zone requiring critical consideration. In smaller and rural communities, the presence of family and social friends and coworkers within one's practice may be unavoidable.[29] Ethical prescribing calls for a clear assessment for alternatives and special consideration for providing care equal to office-based standards of care. Weighing circumstances and developing a clear vision of clinical boundaries around prescribing for oneself, family, and friends provides for the safest level of care and clinical practice.[28]

CONSCIENCE CLAUSE: PERSONAL BELIEF VERSUS PROFESSIONAL RESPONSIBILITY

In 2011, the Health and Human Services (HHS) Office for Civil Rights (OCR) instituted a policy intended to protect agencies and healthcare workers who refused to provide or participate in services they found counter to their personal religious beliefs or moral conscience.[30] This has extended to prescribing practices, which has led to some confusion about professional obligations to provide pharmaceuticals, services, or referrals that are counter to a clinician's religious beliefs or conscience. Some have advocated that patients' rights for services must prevail and have voiced concerns about the ethics of clinician refusals and guarantees that patients will maintain the autonomy required to receive care they seek.[31] In May 2019, the HHS OCR issued a Final Conscience Regulation providing protection from discrimination to clinicians and agencies declining participation in 25 identified federal conscience provisions, including prescribing of abortifacients, contraceptives, or medications for assisted suicide. A clinician refusing based upon conscience may refer to another clinician with an alternative view to assist the patient or not. Professional responsibility would dictate that a clinician not create an absolute barrier to a legally requested healthcare service.[31] Clinicians choosing to refuse prescribing based upon conscience have significant discrimination protections and may report to HHS OCR if violations are experienced in the workplace. In November 2019, the HHS Final Conscience Regulation was struck down by federal judges in the U.S. District Court of New York as unconstitutional.

OFF-LABEL DRUG USE

The prescribing of a medication in typical or different dosage or medication form outside of its FDA-approved indication for a disease or symptom is called off-label drug use (OLDU).[32] OLDU has become common practice in all specialties and is prompted by a dearth of medications in specialty populations such as pediatrics, geriatrics, psychiatry, or in pregnancy where pharmaceutical companies have avoided seeking FDA approval due to costly testing restrictions and related ethical issues. As the FDA does not regulate the practice of medicine, off-label prescribing is not illegal but does carry increased liability for the patient and clinician if careful consideration of the risk and benefits are not diligently considered. Consultation with a pharmacist provides a broader reference for current standards of practice as well as greater consideration of specific patient-related contraindications or potential adverse effects.[25] Pharmaceutical companies are banned from promoting drugs for indications not approved by the FDA. However, when asked, they may provide legitimate resources (e.g., peer-reviewed articles and data) regarding OLDU of their products.[32] In practice, OLDU has become commonplace for many medications, at times becoming a de facto standard of care. It is the ultimate responsibility of the clinician to self-educate about new or established patterns of medication prescribing and to weigh the ultimate risks and benefits in providing evidence-based and safe quality care for each individual patient.[25]

CASE EXEMPLAR: Patient With Antibiotic Treatment Failure

BR is an 8-year-old male following up for impetigo. His mother says that the rash is not clearing up the way the clinician indicated it would. His impetigo involves the right upper extremity and started after a fall from a bicycle. Following the accident, he was given a tetanus shot, his wound was cleaned in the clinic, and a prescription for dicloxacillin was provided. His mother picked up the antibiotic immediately after the appointment and has been giving BR the medicine as directed: "Once a day, just like the bottle says."

Past Medical History
- Usual childhood illnesses
- Current on vaccines

Medications
- Dicloxacillin, 250 mg four times per day for 10 days

Physical Examination
- Afebrile
- Large area of abrasion with secondary infection over the extensor aspect of the right elbow and wrist. Moderate honey-colored exudate with swelling.

Discussion Questions
1. The patient record shows that the clinician ordered the antibiotic to be given four times per day, yet the bottle says once per day. How could this happen?

CASE EXEMPLAR: Patient With Bronchitis

TL is a 42-year-old female nurse who works in the primary care setting. A clinician colleague has noticed that she has been coughing a lot over the past few days and suggested to her that it might be time to think about quitting smoking. Today she asks the clinician for a prescription for an antibiotic. She says, "a Z-Pak is usually all I need." She does not think she has a fever. She says that the clinician's partner, Dr. S, usually writes her a prescription when she wants one.

Past Medical History
- Unknown

Medications
- Unknown

Physical Examination
- Well-developed, well-nourished female in no acute distress
- Coughing frequently with apparen[t] way sounds
- No obvious cyanosis

Discussion Questions
1. The ethical principles of autonomy (she approached the clinician for help), beneficence (the clinician would be helping her), nonmaleficence (the clinician certainly is not hurting her), and justice (she wants to remain in the workforce) all seem to be met, so are there any concerns with providing the prescription that TL has requested?
2. How would the ethical issues change if the clinician were to bring TL into an examination room to perform a professional physical examination?
3. As a leader at the medical practice, what can the clinician do to protect herself and the staff against ethical dilemmas related to prescribing?

CLINICAL PEARLS

- In the event of a "significant theft or loss" of controlled substances, clinicians or registrants are required to notify the local field division office of the DEA to report such loss or theft "upon discovery," which has been interpreted as "immediately without delay."
- The required information on a prescription may be grouped into three separate sections: information related to (a) the prescriber, (b) the patient, and (c) the drug.
- When a brand name of the product is written, prescribers should always make sure that generic substitution is permissible, unless the brand of the medication is ordered due to the patient's specific need.
- All FDA-approved generic products are held to the same standards as their brand-name counterparts and are subject to the Abbreviated New Drug Application (ANDA) approval process before they can be widely marketed to consumers.
- TJC and ISMP have developed lists of abbreviations that should not be used to avoid the risk of error.
- The "STEPS" (safety, tolerability, effectiveness, price, and simplicity of treatment and dosing) approach to prescribing encourages ethical prescriptive practice guidelines with patient-centered prescribing.
- While prescribing noncontrolled medications informally for oneself, family members, or nonpatients may not be illegal, it is considered unethical by most professional medical standards except in limited noncomplex or emergent situations.

KEY TAKEAWAYS

- The Durham–Humphrey Amendment of the Federal Food, Drug, and Cosmetic Act holds pharmacists liable for prosecution if prescription drugs are sold without a *bona fide* prescription or oral authorization from an authorized licensed prescriber.
- The DEA's purpose is to prevent diversion and abuse of controlled substances while ensuring a sufficient, uninterrupted supply of these agents for legitimated medical and scientific needs.
- Allowing "generic substitution" for a specified product will give the pharmacist the legal authority to substitute generic drugs that are therapeutically equivalent to the ordered product.
- Per FDA definitions, the generic version of a drug must show bioequivalence to its

(*continued*)

brand-name counterpart, allowing up to 20% of differences between the two products.

- The clinical prescribing of medications in patient care is guided by ethical standards of practice: autonomy, beneficence, nonmaleficence, and justice.
- Prescribers who refuse to provide or participate in services they find counter to their personal religious beliefs or moral conscience are protected by law.
- As the FDA does not regulate the practice of medicine, the practice of off-label prescribing is not illegal but does carry increased liability.

REFERENCES

1. The Durham–Humphrey amendment. *JAMA*. 1952; 149(4):371. doi:10.1001/jama.1952.02930210055017
2. *PA prescribing*. American Academy of PAs. 2017. Accessed January 9, 2019. https://www.aapa.org/wp-content/uploads/2017/01/Prescribing_IB_2017_FINAL.pdf
3. *PA prescribing authority by state*. American Academy of PAs. 2016. Accessed January 9, 2019. https://www.aapa.org/wp-content/uploads/2016/12/PA_Prescribing_Chart.pdf
4. Keeling AW. Historical perspectives on an expanded role for nursing. *Online J Issues Nurs*. 2015;20(2):2. doi:10.3912/OJIN.Vol20No02Man02
5. Keeling A. *Nursing and the Privilege of Prescription: 1893–2000*. The Ohio State University; 2006:1–27.
6. Peterson ME. Barriers to practice and the impact on health care: a nurse practitioner focus. *J Adv Pract Oncol*. 2017;8(1):74–81. https://www.ncbi.nlm.nih.gov/pmc/articles/PMC5995533.
7. National Council of State Boards of Nursing. *Consensus Model for APRN Regulation: Licensure, Accreditation, Certification & Education*. National Council of State Boards of Nursing; 2015.
8. Wax PM. Elixirs, diluents, and the passage of the 1938 Federal Food, Drug and Cosmetic Act. *Ann Intern Med*. 1995;122(6):456–461. doi:10.7326/0003-4819-122-6-199503150-00009.
9. *A History of the FDA and Drug Regulation in the United States*. Published June 15, 2006. https://www.fda.gov/media/73549/download
10. Piemme TE, Sadler AM, Carter RD. *The Physician Assistant: An Illustrated History*. Acacia Publishing; 2013.
11. *Electronic Code of Federal Regulation*. 2018. Accessed October 29, 2018. https://www.ecfr.gov/cgi-bin/ECFR?SID=9b8d47d545f71b1e4d9ec389cb23854d&mc=true&page=browse
12. *What is the difference between the Federal Food, Drug, and Cosmetic Act (FD&C Act), FDA regulations, and FDA guidance?* Food and Drug Administration. Accessed October 24, 2018. https://www.fda.gov/aboutfda/transparency/basics/ucm194909.htm
13. Drug Enforcement Administration. *History*. Accessed December 5, 2018. https://www.dea.gov/history
14. Drug Enforcement Administration, Office of Diversion Control. *Practitioner's Manual: An Informational Outline of the Controlled Substances Act*. 2006 ed. United States Deparment of Justice; 2006.
15. The Joint Commission. *National patient safety goals effective January 2019*. https://www.jointcommission.org/-/media/tjc/documents/standards/national-patient-safety-goals/historical/npsg_chapter_ome_jan2019.pdf?db=web&hash=521A220C06E0BDF383D109DE9F378417, accessed 09/25/2019
16. The Joint Commission. *Two patient identifiers—understanding the requirements*. Updated April 16, 2020.https://www.jointcommission.org/standards/standard-faqs/home-care/national-patient-safety-goals-npsg/000001545
17. Shetty A, Shetty S, Dsouza O. Medical symbols in practice: myths vs reality. *J Clin Diagn Res*. 2014;8(8): PC12–PC14. doi:10.7860/JCDR/2014/10029.4730
18. *Generic drug facts*. U.S. Food and Drug Administration. Accessed September 4, 2019. https://www.fda.gov/drugs/generic-drugs/generic-drug-facts
19. Dentali F, Donadini MP, Clark N, et al. Brand name versus generic warfarin: a systematic review of the literature. *Pharmacotherapy*. 2011;31(4):386–393. doi:10.1592/phco.31.4.386
20. *List of error-prone abbreviations*. Institute of Safe Medication Practices. Published October 2, 2017. https://www.ismp.org/recommendations/error-prone-abbreviations-list
21. Jackson J. Exploring the ethics of prescribing medicines. *Emerg Nurs*. 2010;18(2):24–6. doi:10.7748/en2010.05.18.2.24.c7756
22. Pollock M, Bazaldua OV, Dobbie AE. Appropriate prescribing of medications: an eight-step approach. *Am Fam Physician*. 2007;75(2):231–236. https://www.aafp.org/afp/2007/0115/p231.html.
23. Stead U, Morant N, Ramon S. Shared decision-making in medication management: development of a training intervention. *BJPsych Bull*. 2017;41(4):221–227. doi:10.1192/pb.bp.116.053819
24. Mitchell A. Responsibility for ethical prescribing. *J Nurs Pract*. 2016;12(3):20. doi:10.1016/j.nurpra.2016.01.008
25. Basak R, McCaffrey DJ III. Hospital pharmacists' perceived beliefs and responsibilities in indication-based off-label prescribing. *Int J Clin Pharm*. 2018;40(1):36–40. doi:10.1007/s11096-017-0567-7
26. Davies EA, O'Mahony MS. Adverse drug reactions in special populations—the elderly. *Br J Clin Pharmacol*. 2015;80(4):796–807. doi:10.1111/bcp.12596
27. Buppert C. *Can NPs prescribe for family members or themselves?* Medscape Nurses. Published May 27, 2004. https://www.medscape.com/viewarticle/478418
28. Latessa R, Ray L. Should you treat yourself, family or friends? *Fam Pract Manag*. 2005;12(3):41–44. https://www.aafp.org/fpm/2005/0300/p41.html
29. Gold KJ, Goldman EB, Kamil LH, et al. No appointment necessary? Ethical challenges in treating friends and family. *N Engl J Med*. 2014;371(13):1254–1258. doi:10.1056/NEJMsb1402963

30. Department of Health and Human Services, Office for Civil Rights, Office of the Secretary. Protecting statutory conscience rights in health care; Delegations of authority. *Fed Regist.* 2019;84(98):23170–23272. https://www.govinfo.gov/content/pkg/FR-2019-05-21/pdf/2019-09667.pdf

31. Sonfield S. *Rights vs. Responsibilities: Professional Standards and Provider Refusals.* The Guttmacher Institute; 2005.

32. Wittich CM, Burkle CM, Lanier WL. Ten common questions (and their answers) about off-label drug use. *Mayo Clin Proc.* 2012;87(10):982–990. doi:10.1016/j.mayocp.2012.04.017

Responsible Controlled-Substance Prescribing

Vasco Deon Kidd, Andrew Lowe, Brent Luu, and Gerald Kayingo

LEARNING OBJECTIVES

- Define opioid abuse and addiction.
- Explain how opioid abuse presents in the healthcare setting.
- Identify patient factors that increase the risk for development of opioid use disorder.
- Demonstrate effective teaching techniques for patients using or requiring opioids for pain control.
- Design a pain management strategy for a patient that minimizes risk of opioid misuse and addresses the need to control pain.
- Assess patient behaviors that would prompt referral to a professional for substance addiction and abuse.

INTRODUCTION

A perfect storm of challenges led to America's opioid crisis, which continues to claim the lives of about 130 Americans each day.[1] The origins of the opioid epidemic are both complex and multifactorial. In 2018, the federal government declared a nationwide public health emergency to curb the opioid epidemic. Yet, despite a public outcry, opioid overdose rates are rapidly accelerating. According to the Centers for Disease Control and Prevention (CDC), about 40% of opioid-related deaths can be attributed to prescriptions of opioids.[1] Some populations are more affected than others.

For example, the Black community has experienced the largest surge in opioid overdose deaths among any racial and ethnic group.[2] Because of the highly addictive nature of opiates/opioids and their dangerous side effects, there appears to be a concerted effort by commercial health plans, pharmacy benefit managers, Centers for Medicare and Medicaid Services (CMS), and policy makers to decrease the use of opioid prescriptions. But has the national campaign on combating the opioid epidemic resulted in changing prescriber behavior? Despite growing awareness and several abuse-prevention initiatives, opioid prescriptions have not substantially declined from their peaks and remain one of the most prescribed drug classes in the United States.[3] This chapter provides effective strategies that promote responsible and conscientious controlled substance prescribing in the clinical setting.

BACKGROUND

The management of patients with acute and chronic nonmalignant pain represents a real challenge for practicing clinicians. The chronic use of opioids now carries an "addiction-related" stigma and concerns about efficacy and safety of opiates have been called into question. Overprescribing of opioids and opiates by clinicians in various disciplines remains a serious public health concern and a major contributor to the opioid epidemic. The largest prescribers of controlled substances are primary care clinicians. According to the 2013 Medicare Part D prescription drug coverage claims, family practice doctors issued slightly over

15 million prescriptions, while internal medicine physicians issued 12.8 million.[4] Excessive opioid prescribing may be in part due to significant limitations in medical education curricula and residency training around addiction and aberrant opioid use behavior.[5] Opioids are highly addictive, and the risk of long-term opioid use increases with subsequent prescriptions. For example, a second opioid prescription doubles the risk that a patient will continue to use opioids up to a year later.[6] Consequently, among patients taking a prescribed opioid for 90 days; at least 50% will still be taking opioids at 5 years.[7] In addition, opioid use can be a gateway toward substance use disorders, such as heroin addiction. Research showed that out of the estimated 2.4 million people who developed substance use disorders, nearly half a million suffer from heroin abuse.[8] Therefore, clinicians should consider adopting policies for opioid prescription during pain management that closely align with the current CDC guidelines. In addition, improving pain through effective communication strategies is critical when initiating opioid or nonopioid therapy.

OPIOID PRESCRIBING: ACUTE PAIN MANAGEMENT

The causes of acute pain are multifactorial and include surgery, infection, soft tissue injury, fractures, dental issues, and joint pain. When addressing pain symptoms, clinicians should solicit a thorough patient history, pain characteristics, quality of the pain, comorbidities that may exacerbate the pain, clinical efficacy of prior pain therapy, and any current *controlled substance agreement* with a prescribing clinician. The major goals in managing any pain are to provide sufficient analgesia to relieve pain and improve function. For example, patients with acute musculoskeletal pain from strains, sprains, contusions, dislocations, and simple fractures, unless contraindicated, can be treated with a short duration of acetaminophen or nonsteroidal anti-inflammatory drugs (NSAIDs) alone or in combination. See Chapter 22 for a discussion of acetaminophen and NSAIDs. In addition, overprescribing of controlled substances for acute pain may have far reaching legal implications.[9]

A synopsis of the literature shows that NSAIDs reduce concurrent opioid requirements and shorten hospital length of stay.[10] Furthermore, acetaminophen (Tylenol®) and NSAIDS have been shown to have good efficacy in improving both pain relief and function without interfering with fracture healing.[11,12] In one study of 60 patients with ankle fractures, researchers concluded that those who used nonopioid medications reported less pain than those who used opioids.[13] But if opioids are needed to address acute pain, clinicians should review a patient's prescribing history through a Prescription Drug Monitoring Program (PDMP) system prior to prescribing an opioid.[14] The CDC recommends that clinicians prescribe the lowest effective dose of immediate-release-opioids for 3 days for most patients and up to 7 days for patients with nontraumatic pain unrelated to major surgery.[14] Interestingly, major nationwide retail chains and health maintenance organizations (HMO) in the United States, such as Walmart, Sam's Club, and Kaiser Permanente, have aligned their pharmacy policies to coincide with the CDC recommendations and now restrict initial acute opioid prescriptions to no more than a 7-day supply. This trend will eventually be seen in other pharmacy corporations as time goes on and more clinicians are adopting these recommendations.

OPIOID PRESCRIBING: CHRONIC PAIN MANAGEMENT

Nonmalignant chronic pain is classified as persistent or recurrent pain lasting longer than 3 months.[15] According to the American Pain Foundation, nearly 50 million Americans are afflicted with chronic pain. The four most common causes of chronic pain are headaches, back, joint, and nerve pain.[16,17] Patients using long-term opioids to address chronic pain may report worsening pain as compared to those using other pain management modalities.[18] The utility of opioid therapy in chronic pain remains controversial. The CDC has issued guidelines to clinicians recommending nonopioid and nonpharmacologic treatments as the preferred treatment options for chronic pain.[14] Clinicians should be cautious in considering opioid analgesics for mechanical back pain, as well as hip and knee arthritis.[19,20] Research clearly demonstrates that chronic opioid consumption prior to total joint arthroplasty has been associated with worse outcomes, such as readmission, infection, stiffness, and aseptic revision.[21,22] In addition, studies have demonstrated that long-term opioid use for chronic pain was associated with higher healthcare utilization, lower activity levels, and worsening of the pain.[23,24] Furthermore, persistent use of controlled substances, especially schedule II agents, or the commonly prescribed tramadol (schedule IV), is a substantial risk factor for fracture nonunion.[25] Tramadol may also precipitate seizures and/or hyponatremia, especially in elderly patients.

Amid these growing concerns, the mainstay of nonmalignant chronic pain management should consist of nonopioid alternatives such as topical analgesics (e.g., diclofenac cream, capsaicin), acetaminophen, antispasmodics, targeted peripheral topical analgesic patches (e.g., lidocaine 5%), trigger-point injections, and NSAIDs.[14] Research seems to suggest that opioids are no more effective than acetaminophen in addressing chronic back and symptomatic osteoarthritis.[26] It should be noted that NSAIDs can cause dyspepsia and even peptic ulcer disease (see Chapter 22 for a discussion of NSAID prescribing). Additional nonpharmacologic approaches such as physical therapy (PT), home exercise programs, cognitive behavioral therapy, and sleep hygiene can also aid in the reduction of chronic pain. Lastly, patients for whom these and other nonopioid alternatives are ineffective should be referred to a pain management specialist for consideration of other modalities such as opioids, spinal cord and peripheral nerve stimulation, nerve blocks, and radiofrequency denervation.[27,28]

CONTROLLED SUBSTANCE PRESCRIBING: SAFETY IMPROVEMENT

Clinicians should avoid concurrent benzodiazepine and opioid prescribing as this elevates the risk of overdose. Patients requiring opioid therapy beyond 90-mg morphine equivalents should receive naloxone (opioid antagonist) to combat potential unintended consequences of opioid treatment.[14] Also, it is important to avoid prescribing opiate medications to a patient who has a signed *controlled substance agreement* with another prescriber. Patients who have signed such agreements have consented to having their pain relief needs met by one clinician (e.g., pain management specialist). Additionally, clinicians should exercise caution when prescribing opioid therapy to patients taking cannabinoids as it is unknown whether these products alter plasma opioid levels.

STRATEGIES TO MITIGATE CONTROLLED SUBSTANCE MISUSE

Research shows that 52% of Americans misused prescription drugs in 2017, which is unchanged from 2016.[29] Opioid misuse often occurs when prescription opioids are shared, stolen, obtained illegally, or sold for a profit. In addition, combining opioids with medications used to treat anxiety or sleep can also contribute to misuse and lead to respiratory depression. Furthermore, opioid misuse is associated with an increased risk of infectious disease transmission such as HIV and hepatitis C.[30]

There are various evidence-based strategies that clinicians can employ to prevent controlled substance misuse. One such strategy discussed earlier is the use of PDMPs. The PDMPs are state-run electronic databases used to combat opioid misuse by tracking the prescribing and dispensing of opioids. PDMPs differ in scope and design; for example, some PDMPs share data using prescriber "report cards," while others do not. The research on the impact of PDMPs is mixed, but in one study, the use of PDMPs in some states has been associated with reductions in opioid use among Medicare beneficiaries compared with states that do not have the program.[31] Certain states such as California require mandatory review of a PDMP before subsequently prescribing a controlled substance and every 4 months for patients with uninterrupted use of opioids for chronic pain.

The second strategy in preventing opioid misuse is patient education. Prescribers should inform patients about correct opioid usage, potential dangers of nonrecreational medication sharing, "doctor shopping," and mixing opioids with other drugs to enhance psychoactive effects. Additionally, to reduce diversion of controlled substances, patients should be counseled on proper storage and disposal of unused opioid medications. A third strategy involves increasing access to medication-assisted treatment (MAT) for those presenting with opioid use disorder. MAT is part of a comprehensive multimodal treatment consisting of medications, counseling, and behavioral therapies to address substance use disorders to curb opioid overdose rates. Clinicians should be familiar with how to identify opioid use disorder (as defined by the criteria of the *Diagnostic and Statistical Manual of Mental Disorders*, Fifth Edition). Clinicians should have protocols in place for when to refer patients for MAT. These and other prevention strategies may mitigate opioid misuse.[14]

IMPROVING PAIN MANAGEMENT THROUGH EFFECTIVE COMMUNICATION

Communication about pain and opioids can be quite challenging in today's healthcare environment. Clinicians may find it difficult to understand the individual pain needs of their patients and negotiate a plan of care. Patients and healthcare clinicians have differing goals, opinions, and biases concerning treatment options.[32] A 2017 study found that a majority (60,8%) of prescribers surveyed did not feel confident managing patients with chronic pain.[33]

Patients afflicted by acute or chronic pain should be treated with the upmost respect and never demonized or classified as drug seekers, especially during difficult encounters. Mitigating potential or challenging encounters when treating chronic pain patients requires effective communication, which has been linked to better patient outcomes, improved ability to manage pain, and reduction in disability and opioid use.[34,35] In addition, effective and empathic communication can improve pain and anxiety in patients with acute and chronic pain syndrome.[35] Patients should have an active part in shared decision-making concerning their pain relief needs.

Effective communication may include nonverbal strategies. Clinicians should pay attention to social cues, such as altered facial expressions or body posture, coping skills, and how patients react to their pain. When negotiating chronic pain syndromes, clinicians should focus treatment strategies on maintaining an acceptable quality of life for their patients. This involves a clinical assessment of the patient's psychological and physical health. Patients with chronic nonmalignant pain should be assessed and treated for concurrent psychiatric disorders, which can exacerbate and influence the expression of pain. In addition, patients with mental health problems may not always follow their treatment plans. Taking time to engage the chronic pain patient should lead to a healthy dialogue that improves treatment adherence. A multimodal treatment plan with ongoing follow-up is needed to improve chronic pain syndromes and health outcomes.[36]

In light of the ongoing opioid crisis, it is important to communicate and educate patients on the risks, benefits, and alternatives of opioid and nonopioid therapies. The benefits of nonopioid therapy as a first-line option in addressing acute and chronic pain have been supported by the literature. However, in some cases, a patient may require opioids for legitimate medical purposes; therefore, clinicians should identify and address any implicit or explicit biases they may hold regarding the use of prescription opioids. **Box 9.1** provides several strategies that can be used to facilitate empathic communication regarding pain symptoms and treatment plans.

These and other strategies can help prevent undertreatment of pain while improving physical and psychological outcomes. In addition, effective communication is the key to providing safe, satisfactory, high-quality healthcare.

CONCLUSION

Responsible controlled substances prescribing should be an expectation for all prescribers. Systemic opioid analgesics should only be used when indicated. Alter-

---

BOX 9.1
STRATEGIES TO FACILITATE EMPATHIC COMMUNICATION REGARDING PAIN

Use empathic statements, such as:
- "I would be just as frustrated as you."
- "I understand this isn't easy."
- "We're going to work on this together."
- "We can make gradual changes and see what works for you."
- "We may not need to make abrupt or drastic changes at this time."

Consider your nonverbal communication, such as:
- Making eye contact
- Having appropriate, caring facial expressions
- Using a caring tone and pace
- Being mindful of your body posture

Source: Centers for Disease Control and Prevention. *Module 3: Communicating With Patients: Applying CDC's Guideline for Prescribing Opioids.* March 26, 2020. https://www.cdc.gov/drugoverdose/training/communicating; Centers for Disease Control and Prevention. *Wide-Ranging Online Data for Epidemiologic Research (WONDER).* National Center for Health Statistics. 2017. http://wonder.cdc.gov

---

native therapies should always be considered in cases of acute and noncancer chronic pain. There is little evidence to support the use of opioids in the treatment of osteoarthritis, simple fractures, strains, sprains, contusions, or dislocations. Moreover, the use of opioids to treat patients with chronic noncancer pain remains controversial due to concerns about efficacy and safety. If opioids are required to treat nonterminal pain conditions, the lowest effective dose of immediate-release opioids should be given for a short duration. Given the vast array of pharmacological and nonpharmacological treatments on the market, it is important for clinicians to individualize pain treatment to the specific needs of their patients. This starts with effective communication strategies along with an honest assessment of the needs of the patient in addressing their acute and chronic pain based on the best practices and available evidence. The opioid-centric model of pain delivery has fallen out of favor. Prescribers should rethink how to best optimize communication and pain management strategies that improve the quality of patient care without jeopardizing pain treatment.

CASE EXEMPLAR: Patient With Traumatic Injury

MF is a 25-year-old graduate student who was involved in a motorcycle accident 2 days ago and sustained several injuries. He presented with a left femur fracture, multiple rib fractures bilaterally, and burst spine fractures at T4 and T5 levels. Upon arrival to the ED, his pain was 9/10 and marginally controlled with hydromorphone 1 mg every hour as needed. He had an episode of desaturation while in the ED; therefore, he was admitted to the ICU.

Past Medical History
- Significant for asthma since the age of 5

Family History
- Noncontributory

Social History
- Social alcohol use
- No tobacco use
- Occasional use of marijuana (legal in his state)
- Denies any other illicit drug use
- Occupation: Teaching assistant in the laboratory at the local pharmacy school

Physical Examination
- Blood pressure: 150/95; pulse: 95; respiration rate 18; temperature: 97.7 °F
- Well-developed, well-nourished male in moderate distress due to pain
- Respiratory effort is reduced due to pain associated with rib fractures
- Examination is benign except for decreased mobility due to injuries

Labs
- Within normal limits,
- Blood alcohol: 0.24 mg/dL
- Urine: Positive for methamphetamines and cannabinoids

Assessment
- A diagnosis of multiple fractures is made, and orthopedic surgery is planned to fix the injuries to the spine and left femur.
- Patient is complaining of severe pain "all over"; rates pain at 9/10. He describes pain as throbbing, sharp, with significant back spasm.
- Trauma surgeon started the patient on morphine by patient-controlled analgesia (PCA) with the following settings:
  ○ Morphine PCA dose, 2 mg
  ○ Lockout interval: 15 minutes
  ○ Maximum: Four doses/hour
  ○ Additional doses of morphine 4 mg were administered four times in the past 24 hours in response to the patient's loud complaints

Discussion Questions
1. What are the potential factors that may have contributed to the desaturation episode in the ED?
2. MF will more than likely become a patient with chronic pain after this incident. How should his chronic pain be managed after discharge? What are some strategies to mitigate the risk of opioid misuse?
3. What drug–drug interactions should a clinician avoid while considering an opioid as a pain reliever for this patient?
4. To proactively treat potential overdose of opioids, what medication should also be prescribed when opioids are prescribed or have escalated to this level?
5. What patient communication strategies should a clinician implement to optimize outcomes?

CASE EXEMPLAR: Patient With Osteoarthritis

SI is a 55-year-old female with advanced osteoarthritis of the right knee and left hip. She has mild osteoporosis as seen on plain films during evaluation of her joint pains. In years past, she was a competitive bodybuilder, but she has been unable to exercise because of her pain. She is contemplating total joint arthroplasty, initially for the hip and eventually for the knee. She ambulates with a cane.

Past Medical History
- Osteoarthritis
- Osteoporosis
- Hypothyroidism
- Depression
- Breast augmentation with abdominoplasty, complicated by prolonged postoperative pain
- Bunionectomy, complicated by prolonged postoperative pain
- Bilateral carpal tunnel release

Medications
- Levothyroxine, 100 mcg once daily
- Gabapentin, 600 mg TID
- Hydrocodone, 7.5 mg/acetaminophen 325 mg one to two tablets TID to QID
- Celecoxib, 400 mg once daily
- Bupropion, 300 mg once daily
- Calcium, vitamin D, multivitamins

Social History
- Smoker, half pack per day
- Alcohol, two to three glasses of wine per day
- Employed in retail; recently resigned because she could not climb the stairs to get to the time clock
- Married

Physical Examination
- Well-developed, well-nourished female in no distress
- Height: 66 inches; weight: 162 lbs.; blood pressure: 142/96; pulse: 80; respiration rate: 16; temperature 98.6 °F
- Knee with palpable osteophytic spurs, 1+ effusion, decreased range of motion

Labs and Imaging
- Blood count, electrolytes, coagulation studies, rheumatoid studies negative
- X-ray shows extensive degenerative joint disease of the knee with narrowing, subchondral cysts, osteophytic spurs

Discussion Questions
1. Assess SI's risks related to her upcoming surgery.
2. Assess SI's risks for opioid dependence and abuse.
3. What can be done preoperatively to reduce SI's risks of opioid dependence postoperatively?

CLINICAL PEARLS

- When addressing pain symptoms, clinicians should solicit a thorough patient history, pain characteristics, quality of the pain, comorbidities that may exacerbate the pain, clinical efficacy of prior pain therapy, and a current *controlled substance agreement* with a prescribing clinician. The CDC recommends that clinicians prescribe the lowest effective dose of immediate-release opioids for 3 days for most patients and up to 7 days for patients with nontraumatic pain unrelated to major surgery.
- Nonmalignant chronic pain is classified as persistent or recurrent pain lasting longer than 3 months.
- Chronic opioid use before or after major surgery is a risk factor for adverse surgical outcomes.
- A multimodal treatment plan with ongoing follow-up is needed to improve chronic pain syndromes and health outcomes.

KEY TAKEAWAYS

- The largest group of prescribers of controlled substances are primary care clinicians.
- If opioids are needed to address acute pain, clinicians should review a patient's prescribing history through a PDMP system prior to prescribing an opioid.
- The mainstay of nonmalignant chronic pain management should consist of nonopioid alternatives such as topical analgesics, acetaminophen, antispasmodics, targeted peripheral topical analgesic patches, trigger-point injections, and NSAIDs.
- When negotiating chronic pain syndromes, clinicians should focus treatment strategies on maintaining an acceptable quality of life for their patients, including a clinical assessment of the patient's psychological and physical health.

REFERENCES

1. Centers for Disease Control and Prevention. *Wide-ranging Online Data for Epidemiologic Research (WONDER)*. National Center for Health Statistics. 2017. http://wonder.cdc.gov

2. Scholl L, Seth P, Kariisa M, et al. Drug and opioid-involved overdose deaths—United States, 2013–2017. *MMWR Morb Mortal Wkly Rep*. 2018;67:1419–1427. https://www.ncbi.nlm.nih.gov/pmc/articles/PMC6334822/pdf/mm675152e1.pdf

3. Jeffery MM, Hooten WM, Henk HJ, et al. Trends in opioid use in commercially insured and Medicare Advantage populations in 2007–16: retrospective cohort study. *Br Med J*. 2018;362:k3537. doi:10.1136/bmj.k2833

4. Centers for Medicare and Medicaid Services. *Medicare Provider Utilization and Payment Data: Part D Prescriber*. 2019. https://www.cms.gov/Research-Statistics-Data-and-Systems/Statistics-Trends-and-Reports/Medicare-Provider-Charge-Data/Part-D-Prescriber.html

5. Khidir H, Weiner SG. A call for better opioid prescribing training and education. *West J Emerg Med*. 2016;17(6):686–689. doi:10.5811/westjem.2016.8.31204

6. Shah A, Hayes CJ, Martin BC. Characteristics of initial prescription episodes and likelihood of long-term opioid use—United States, 2006–2015. *MMWR Morb Mortal Wkly Rep*. 2017;66(10):265. doi:10.15585/mmwr.mm6610a1

7. Martin BC, Fan MY, Edlund MJ, Devries A, Braden JB, Sullivan MD. Long-term chronic opioid therapy discontinuation rates from the TROUP study. *J Gen Intern Med*. 2011;26(12):1450–1457. doi:10.1007/s11606-011-1771-0

8. Ahrnsbrak R, Bose J, Hedden SL, et al. *Key substance use and mental health indicators in the United States: results from the 2015 National Survey on Drug Use and Health*. Substance Abuse and Mental Health Services Administration; 2017. https://www.samhsa.gov/data/sites/default/files/NSDUH-FFR1-2016/NSDUH-FFR1-2016.htm

9. Dineen KK, DuBois JM. Between a rock and a hard place: can physicians prescribe opioids to treat pain adequately while avoiding legal sanction? *Am J Law Med*. 2016;42(1):7–52. doi:10.1177/0098858816644712

10. Solomon, DH. Nonselective NSAIDs: overview of adverse effects. In: Furst DE, Romain PL, eds. *UpToDate*. Updated March 5, 2020. https://www.uptodate.com/contents/nonselective-nsaids-overview-of-adverse-effects#H1

11. Dodwell ER, Latorre JG, Parisini E, et al. NSAID exposure and risk of nonunion: a meta-analysis of case–control and cohort studies. *Calcif Tissue Int*. 2010;87(3):193 doi:10.1007/s00223-010-9379-72.

12. Taylor IC, Lindblad AJ, Kolber MR. Fracture healing and NSAIDs. *Can Fam Physician*. 2014;60(9):817. https://www.ncbi.nlm.nih.gov/pmc/articles/PMC4162697.

13. Helmerhorst GT, Lindenhovius AL, Vrahas M, et al. Satisfaction with pain relief after operative treatment of an ankle fracture. *Injury*. 2012;43(11):1958–1961. doi:10.1016/j.injury.2012.08.018.

14. Dowell D, Haegerich TM, Chou R. CDC guideline for prescribing opioids for chronic pain—United States, 2016. *MMWR Recomm Rep*. 2016;65(No. RR-1):1–49. doi:10.15585/mmwr.rr6501e1

15. Merskey H, Bogduk N. *Classification of Chronic Pain*. 2nd ed. IASP Press; 1994:1.

16. Freburger JK, Holmes GM, Agans RP, et al. The rising prevalence of chronic low back pain. *Arch Intern Med*. 2009;169(3): 251–258. doi:10.1001/archinternmed.2008.543

17. Yawn BP, Wollan PC, Weingarten TN, et al. The prevalence of neuropathic pain: clinical evaluation compared with screening tools in a community population. *Pain Med*. 2009;10(3):586–593. doi:10.1111/j.1526-4637.2009.00588.x

18. U.S. Food and Drug Administration's Patient-Focused Drug Development Initiative. *The voice of the patient*. U.S. Food and Drug Administration; 2014. https://www.fda.gov/downloads/ForIndustry/UserFees/PrescriptionDrugUserFee/UCM513311.pdf

19. Abdel SC, Maher CG, Williams KA, et al. Efficacy, tolerability, and dose-dependent effects of opioid analgesics for low back pain: a systematic review and meta-analysis. *JAMA Intern Med*. 2016;176(7), 958–968. doi:10.1001/jamainternmed.2016.1251

20. van Laar M, Pergolizzi JV, Jr, Mellinghoff H-U, et al. Pain treatment in arthritis-related pain: beyond NSAIDs. *Open Rheumatol J*. 2012;6:320–330. doi:10.2174/1874312901206010320

21. Cancienne JM, Patel KJ, Browne JA, et al. Opioid use and total knee arthroplasty. *J Arthroplasty*. 2018;33(1):113–118. doi:10.1016/j.arth.2017.08.006

22. Hereford T, Cryar K, Edwards P, et al. Patients with hip or knee arthritis underreport narcotic usage. *J Arthroplasty*. 2018;33(10):3113–3117. doi:10.1016/j.arth.2018.05.032

23. Breivik H, Collett B, Ventafridda V, et al. Survey of chronic pain in Europe: prevalence, impact on daily life, and treatment. *Eur J Pain*. 2006;10:287–333. doi:10.1016/j.ejpain.2005.06.009

24. Eriksen J, Sjogren P, Bruera E, et al. Critical issues on opioids in chronic non-cancer pain: an epidemiological study. *Pain*. 2006;125:172–179. doi:10.1016/j.pain.2006.06.009

25. Buchheit T, Zura R, Wang Z, et al. Opioid exposure is associated with nonunion risk in a traumatically injured population: an inception cohort study. *Injury*. 2018;49(7):1266–1271. doi:10.1016/j.injury.2018.05.004

26. Krebs EE, Gravely A, Nugent S, et al. Effect of opioid vs nonopioid medications on pain-related function in patients with chronic back pain or hip or knee osteoarthritis pain: the SPACE randomized clinical trial. *JAMA*. 2018;319(9):872–882. doi:10.1001/jama.2018.0899

27. Kidd V. Opioid prescribing in orthopedic surgery: an evolving paradigm. *J Orthop Phys Assistants*. 2018;6(1):e4. doi:10.2106/JBJS.JOPA.17.00033

28. Kidd V. Radiofrequency genicular nerve ablation: a novel approach to symptomatic knee osteoarthritis. *J Orthop Phys Assistants*. 2018;6(1):e10. doi:10.2106/JBJS.JOPA.17.00039

29. Wohlgemuth J, Kaufman H. Quest diagnostics' health trends report on drug misuse in America. 2018. Accessed December 16, 2018. https://questdiagnostics.com/dms/Documents/drug-prescription-misuse/Health_Trends_Report_2018.pdf

30. Springer SA, Korthuis PT, del Rio C. Integrating treatment at the intersection of opioid use disorder and infectious disease epidemics in medical settings: a call for action after a National Academies of Sciences, Engineering, and Medicine workshop. *Ann Intern Med.* 2018;169:335–336. doi:10.7326/M18-1203

31. Moyo P, Simoni-Wastila L, Griffin BA, et al. Impact of prescription drug monitoring programs (PDMPs) on opioid utilization among Medicare beneficiaries in 10 US states. *Addiction.* 2017;112:1784–1796. doi:10.1111/add.13860

32. Frantsve LM, Kerns RD. Patient-provider interactions in the management of chronic pain: current findings within the context of shared medical decision making. *Pain Med.* 2007;8:25–35. doi:10.1111/j.1526-4637.2007.00250.x

33. Pearson AC, Moman RN, Moeschler SM, et al. Provider confidence in opioid prescribing and chronic pain management: results of the Opioid Therapy Provider Survey. *J Pain Res.* 2017;*10*:1395–1400. doi:10.2147/JPR.S136478

34. Sugai DY, Deptula PL, Parsa AA, et al. The importance of communication in the management of postoperative pain. *Hawaii J Med Public Health.* 2013;72(6):180–184. PubMed PMID: 23795326.

35. Burton AK, Waddell G, Tillotson M, et al. Information and advice to patients with back pain can have a positive effect: a randomized controlled trial of a novel educational booklet in primary care. *Spine.* 1999;24(23):2484–2491. doi:10.1097/00007632-199912010-00010

36. Howick J, Moscrop A, Mebius A, et al. Effects of empathic and positive communication in healthcare consultations: a systematic review and meta-analysis. *J R Soc Med.* 2018;111(7):240–252. https://doi.org/10.1177/0141076818769477

Antibiotic Stewardship

Lucy W. Kibe

LEARNING OBJECTIVES

- Describe the relationship between epidemiologic transition and the discovery and implementation of antibiotic therapy.
- Outline the progression and predicted outcomes of microbial resistance, including financial and mortality costs.
- Differentiate between the tenets of antibiotic stewardship among individual clinicians, the healthcare systems, health insurance, and pharmaceutical companies in preventing antibiotic misuse.
- Outline educational strategies to prevent antibiotic misuse for all clinicians and the patients they treat.
- Define the role of governmental agencies in supporting antibiotic stewardship and suggest how this role supports the goals of the Centers for Disease Control and Prevention (CDC).

INTRODUCTION

There is evidence that antimicrobial agents existed as early as 350 to 550 CE in Sudan, Egypt, and China. Hundreds of years later, the first agents were isolated, such as the arsenic-containing drug Salvarsan by Paul Ehrlich in 1909 for the treatment of syphilis, and the sulfonamide Prontosil by Bayer chemists Josef Klarer and Fritz Mietzsch in 1935.[1] However, the greatest medical milestone was in the mid-20th century when Alexander Fleming identified an unexpected contamination of mold, an antibiotic he later called *penicillin*. Subsequently, several new classes of antibiotics were developed and manufactured between the 1950s and 1970s for use in clinical and veterinary medicine. Following this "golden era" of discovery of novel antibiotics, the focus shifted from the development of new antibiotics to the modification of existing ones.[1] Today, several antibiotics are available to treat and prevent numerous types of infections, but few new antibiotics are in development.

Prior to the 20th century, infectious diseases were the leading cause of death, particularly cholera, diphtheria, pneumonia, smallpox, typhoid fever, and syphilis. In 1900, the average life expectancy at birth in the United States was 46 years for females and 48 years for males. In 2016, this had increased to 76 years for males and 81 years for females.[2] This is attributed to antibiotic therapy, immunizations, and improved sanitation and other public health practices. Developed countries experienced a dynamic shift in the leading causes of death from infectious diseases to chronic diseases such as cardiovascular disease, stroke, and cancer. This phenomenon, also known as *epidemiologic transition*, is a well-established, complex, dynamic phenomenon experienced by communities over time.[3] In developed countries, infectious diseases are largely a problem among hospitalized, immunocompromised, surgical, and elderly patients. Developing countries still record death from infectious diseases; however, they have also experienced considerable improvement since the advent of antibiotics.[4]

Without antibiotics, infectious diseases would be catastrophic. For example, before the antibiotic era, 90% of children with bacterial meningitis died, bacterial pharyngitis led to complications and was sometimes fatal, and otitis media had an increased risk of causing brain abscess.[5] Today, several fields of medicine rely on antibiotics, including surgery, cancer chemotherapy, acute and critical care, and dentistry.[6] In one study, antibiotic treatment of skin infections reduced mortality from 75% to 10%.[5]

While the human and economic benefits of antibiotics have been well appreciated for the last seven decades, a new era is looming. In the war between human innovations and bacterial resistance, the little bugs are quickly gaining the upper hand (**Box 10.1**).

THE BURDEN OF ANTIMICROBIAL RESISTANCE

Antimicrobial resistance is an evolutionary prodigy in which microbes mutate to withstand destruction from targeted antimicrobials. There is an endless war between microbes mutating to resist antibiotics and scientists discovering new antibiotics or modifying existing antibiotics to adapt to these mutations, which are dynamic across the entire ecosystem (**Exhibit 10.1**).

For many years, it was presumed that progressive scientific efforts would surpass antibiotic resistance. However, in recent years fewer new antimicrobials have been developed and drug resistance has become prolific (**Exhibit 10.2**). This has led to increasing difficulty in the treatment of antimicrobial-resistant infections.[7] A survey of infectious disease physicians in 2011 found that 63% had encountered a patient with an infection that was resistant to commonly available antibiotics.[8] Indeed, Sir Alexander Fleming had forewarned of the dangers of antimicrobial resistance. In his Nobel Prize lecture,[9] he said:

> The time may come when penicillin can be bought by anyone in the shops. Then there is the danger that the ignorant man may easily underdose himself and by exposing his microbes to nonlethal quantities of the drug make them resistant. Here is a hypothetical illustration. Mr. X. has a sore throat. He buys some penicillin and gives himself, not enough to kill the streptococci but enough to educate them to resist penicillin. He then infects his wife. Mrs. X gets pneumonia and is treated with penicillin. As the streptococci are now resistant to penicillin the treatment fails. Mrs. X dies. Who is primarily responsible for Mrs. X's death? Why Mr. X whose negligent use of penicillin changed the nature of the microbe. Moral: If you use penicillin, use enough.

As predicted, misuse of antibiotics has led to a rising number of infections caused by multiresistant drugs and pan-resistant bacteria. More importantly, common hospital-acquired and community-acquired infections, such as urinary tract infections, wound infections, bloodstream infections, and pneumonia, have developed high rates of resistance worldwide.[10] These resistant bacteria include methicillin-resistant *Staphylococcus aureus* (MRSA), penicillin-resistant *Streptococcus pneumoniae* (PRSP), vancomycin-resistant enterococci (VRE), and multidrug-resistant Gram-negative bacilli (MDRGNB).

MRSA is the most commonly identified multiresistant pathogen and has garnered intense media attention. *S. aureus*, discovered in 1880, was sufficiently treatable with the advent of penicillin. By the 1950s, strains of *S. aureus* resistant to penicillin had emerged; however, they were responsive to its modified form, methicillin. In 1961, scientists identified a strain of *S. aureus* that resisted methicillin. Subsequently, *S. aureus* could be treated only with beta-lactams and vancomycin, but by 2002, strains of *S. aureus* resistant to vancomycin were identified. MRSA infections led to significant mortality and morbidity and increased intensive care unit (ICU), hospital, and long-term care facility stays compared to methicillin-sensitive *S. aureus*.[11,12] It is estimated that MRSA infections alone lengthen hospital stays by an average of 10 days, have a 2.5-fold higher mortality rate, and carry a healthcare cost burden between $3.2 and $4.2 billion annually.[13]

Overall, in the United States, approximately 2 million infections occur from antibiotic resistance, contributing to the healthcare burden of increased hospitalizations and complications, as well as 23,000 deaths annually. The estimated cost of antibiotic resistance is $55 billion annually.[14] In the European Union and Thailand, antibiotic resistance leads to 25,000 deaths annually and an increase in hospital stays by 2.5 and 3.2 months, respectively. In India, resistant bacteria passed from mothers cause more than 58,000 infant deaths annually. World Health Or-

EXHIBIT 10.1 ANTIBIOTIC RESISTANCE-THREATS IN THE UNITED STATES

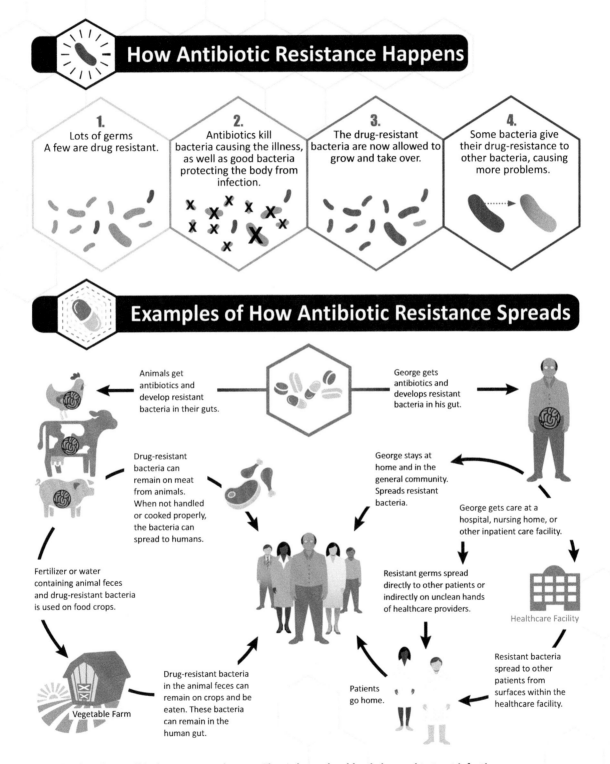

How Antibiotic Resistance Happens

1. Lots of germs A few are drug resistant.

2. Antibiotics kill bacteria causing the illness, as well as good bacteria protecting the body from infection.

3. The drug-resistant bacteria are now allowed to grow and take over.

4. Some bacteria give their drug-resistance to other bacteria, causing more problems.

Examples of How Antibiotic Resistance Spreads

Animals get antibiotics and develop resistant bacteria in their guts.

George gets antibiotics and develops resistant bacteria in his gut.

Drug-resistant bacteria can remain on meat from animals. When not handled or cooked properly, the bacteria can spread to humans.

George stays at home and in the general community. Spreads resistant bacteria.

George gets care at a hospital, nursing home, or other inpatient care facility.

Fertilizer or water containing animal feces and drug-resistant bacteria is used on food crops.

Resistant germs spread directly to other patients or indirectly on unclean hands of healthcare providers.

Healthcare Facility

Drug-resistant bacteria in the animal feces can remain on crops and be eaten. These bacteria can remain in the human gut.

Vegetable Farm

Patients go home.

Resistant bacteria spread to other patients from surfaces within the healthcare facility.

Simply using antibiotics creates resistance. These drugs should only be used to treat infections.

Source: From Centers for Disease Control and Prevention. *Antibiotic resistance threats in the United States.* 2013. https://www.cdc.gov/drugresistance/threat-report-2013/pdf/ar-threats-2013-508.pdf

EXHIBIT 10.2 TIMELINE OF ANTIBIOTIC-RESISTANCE THREATS IN THE UNITED STATES

Developing Resistance
Timeline of Key Antibiotic-Resistance Events

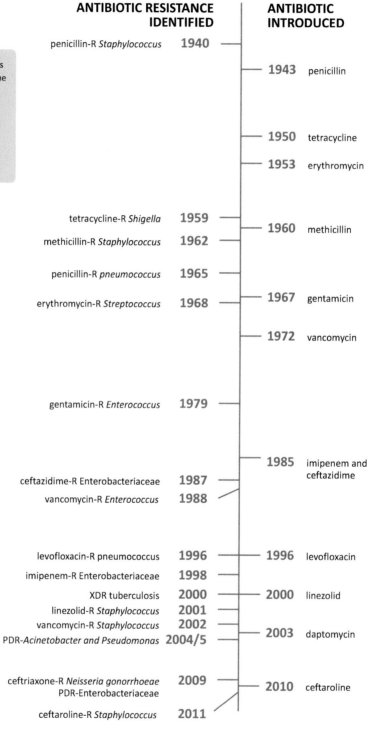

ANTIBIOTIC RESISTANCE IDENTIFIED		ANTIBIOTIC INTRODUCED	
penicillin-R *Staphylococcus*	1940		
		1943	penicillin
		1950	tetracycline
		1953	erythromycin
tetracycline-R *Shigella*	1959	1960	methicillin
methicillin-R *Staphylococcus*	1962		
penicillin-R *pneumococcus*	1965		
erythromycin-R *Streptococcus*	1968	1967	gentamicin
		1972	vancomycin
gentamicin-R *Enterococcus*	1979		
		1985	imipenem and ceftazidime
ceftazidime-R Enterobacteriaceae	1987		
vancomycin-R *Enterococcus*	1988		
levofloxacin-R pneumococcus	1996	1996	levofloxacin
imipenem-R Enterobacteriaceae	1998		
XDR tuberculosis	2000	2000	linezolid
linezolid-R *Staphylococcus*	2001		
vancomycin-R *Staphylococcus*	2002	2003	daptomycin
PDR-*Acinetobacter and Pseudomonas*	2004/5		
ceftriaxone-R *Neisseria gonorrhoeae*	2009	2010	ceftaroline
PDR-Enterobacteriaceae			
ceftaroline-R *Staphylococcus*	2011		

Dates are based upon early reports of resistance in the literature. In the case of pan drug-resistant (PDR)-*Acinetobacter* and *Pseudomonas,* the date is based upon reports of healthcare transmission or outbreaks. Note: Penicillin was in limited use prior to widespread population usage in 1943.

Source: From Centers for Disease Control and Prevention. *Antibiotic resistance threats in the United States.* 2013. https://www.cdc.gov/drugresistance/threat-report-2013/pdf/ar-threats-2013-508.pdf

ganization (WHO) data from several countries show similar trends in increasing individual, health system, and economic burdens due to antibiotic resistance, with resource-poor countries reporting the greatest burden.[15] This is even more consequential because resource-poor countries are more likely to have fewer restrictions on antibiotic availability to the public, such as not requiring a prescription for purchase. Moreover, a WHO survey of 12 countries found a lack of understanding of antibiotics and resistance among the general public.[16]

Recognizing the global burden of antibiotic resistance, the WHO proclaimed it the central focus of the World Health Day, April 7, 2011. Subsequently, a global action plan was endorsed by the WHO and the United Nations in 2015 and 2016, respectively, signaling a global and political commitment to address the antimicrobial crises across human and animal health and agriculture.[16]

ANTIBIOTIC STEWARDSHIP

It is estimated that up to 50% of antibiotic use in inpatient and outpatient settings is unnecessary or inappropriate.[17] Common causes of inappropriate use include treatment of nonbacterial infections, treatment of colonization or contamination, overuse of broad-spectrum therapy, and inappropriately short or long duration of use. Outpatient antibiotics are used more frequently in children and the elderly, with 50% to 60% used for upper respiratory infections that are largely self-limiting. In 2009, outpatient antibiotic expenditure in the United States totaled $10.7 billion, accounting for 60% of all antibiotic expenditure across all healthcare settings.[18] Approximately 50% of hospitalized patients received an antibiotic, 45% of which were treated with one of four antibiotics: vancomycin (14%), ceftriaxone (11%), piperacillin/tazobactam (10%), and levofloxacin (9%).[19]

In collaboration with the WHO, several regions and countries have taken steps to address the threat of antibiotic resistance to protect the public and avoid economic loss. On September 18, 2014, President Barack Obama issued an executive order to develop the National Action Plan.[20] This action plan included accelerating drug development, preventing the spread of resistant infections, developing better diagnostic tools, improving data collection and surveillance, educating stakeholders, and improving global coordination for antibiotic resistance concerns.

In fiscal years 2016, 2017, and 2018, the U.S. Congress allocated $160, $163, and $168 billion, respectively, for the CDC to implement the Antibiotic Resistance Solutions Initiative.[21] Specific goals of the National Action Plan that were to be achieved by 2020 are outlined in Box 10.2.

BOX 10.2
GOALS OF THE NATIONAL ACTION PLAN

1. For CDC-Recognized Urgent Threats:
   a. Reduce by 50% the overall incidence of *Clostridium difficile* infections compared to estimates from 2011.
   b. Reduce by 60% carbapenem-resistant *Enterobacteriaceae* infections acquired during hospitalization compared to estimates.
   c. Maintain the prevalence of ceftriaxone-resistant *Neisseria gonorrhoeae* below 2% compared to estimates from 2013.
2. For CDC-Recognized Serious Threats:
   a. Reduce by 35% multidrug-resistant *Pseudomonas* spp. infections acquired during hospitalization compared to estimates from 2011.
   b) Reduce by at least 50% overall methicillin-resistant *Staphylococcus aureus* bloodstream infections as compared to 2011.
   c) Reduce by 25% multidrug-resistant nontyphoidal Salmonella infections compared to estimates from 2010 to 2012. Reduce by 15% the number of multidrug-resistant tuberculosis infections.
   d) Reduce by at least 25% the rate of antibiotic-resistant invasive pneumococcal disease among less than 5-year-olds compared to estimates from 2008.
   e) Reduce by at least 25% the rate of antibiotic-resistant invasive pneumococcal disease among greater than 65-year-olds compared to estimates from 2008.

Source: Centers for Disease Control. *U.S. National Action Plan for Combating Antibiotic-Resistant Bacteria (National Action Plan).* Published March 2015, October 2020. https://www.cdc.gov/drugresistance/us-activities/national-action-plan.html

---

The reality is that the government cannot do this alone. Antibiotic stewardship is the responsibility of individual clinicians, healthcare systems, health insurance, and pharmaceutical companies, as well as researchers; local, national, and international policy makers; educators; and the general public. The following are the multidisciplinary tenets of antibiotic stewardship.[22,23]

TENETS OF MULTIDISCIPLINARY ANTIBIOTIC STEWARDSHIP

Responsibilities of Clinicians
- Use universal precautions to prevent bacterial transmission among and between patients and coworkers.
- Develop sound prescribing etiquette; avoid prescribing antibiotics for nonbacterial conditions "just in case."

- Follow current guidelines and policies to prescribe the appropriate antibiotic for the diagnosed condition.
- Avoid using broad-spectrum antibiotics unless indicated.
- Prescribe the right dose for the shortest duration required.
- Use diagnostic testing to initiate or adjust appropriate antibiotic regimens.
- Educate patients on proper use of antibiotics and about antibiotic resistance.
- Educate patients on harmful effects of antibiotics such as allergic reactions, *Clostridium difficile*, and candida infections.
- Educate patients on proper hygiene and sanitation practices.
- Ask patients if they have a history of *C. difficile* and prescribe appropriately.

Responsibilities of Healthcare Systems, Hospitals, Acute Care Facilities, Nursing Homes, and Clinics

- Minimize intrahospital *C. difficile* spread.
- Contain intrahospital MRSA, VRE, and MDRGNBs.
- Employ the use of antibiograms to ensure prompt point-of-care decision-making practices.
- Adopt and implement antibiotic stewardship programs using CDC's established framework (see **Box 10.3**).
- Make available prompt diagnostic testing prior to antibiotic use as often as possible.
- Set strict policies and guidelines in all practice settings.
- Appoint diverse teams to coordinate antibiotic stewardship processes and provide support from executive leadership.
- Educate all staff across the organization and patients visiting the facilities on principles of antibiotic stewardship.
- Develop continuous data collection and surveillance to track progress.

Responsibilities of Private Health Insurance Companies, Medicaid, and Medicare

- Reward individuals or facilities for successful implementation of antibiotic stewardship programs and practices.
- Use clinical performance data to provide timely feedback on judicious use of antibiotics.
- Control use of broad-spectrum antibiotics by requiring prior authorizations, but without interfering with access.

Responsibilities of Medical and Veterinary Pharmaceutical Companies

- Invest in research and development of new antibiotics, vaccines, diagnostics, and other tools.
- Provide clear instructions on appropriate guidelines and use of antibiotics.

BOX 10.3
SELECTED EXAMPLES OF GLOBAL ANTIBIOTIC STEWARDSHIP INITIATIVES

World Health Organization: https://www.who.int/antimicrobial-resistance/global-action-plan/en

United States: https://www.cdc.gov/antibiotic-use/healthcare/implementation/core-elements.html

Australia: https://www.safetyandquality.gov.au/wp-content/uploads/2018/04/AMSAH-Book-WEB-COMPLETE.pdf

Canada: http://www.phn-rsp.ca/pubs/anstew-gestan/pdf/pub-eng.pdf

Pharmacist Guide: https://www.ashp.org/Products-and-Meetings-Aliases/The-Pharmacists-Guide-to-Antimicrobial-Therapy-and-Stewardship

Multicontinent Collaboration: https://www.reactgroup.org

- Ensure that antibiotics given to animals under veterinary supervision are for disease treatment and not for growth promotion or disease prevention.
- Price antibiotics to ensure affordability of appropriate course of treatment for uninsured patients.
- Fund education and other public health initiatives that promote antibiotic stewardship.
- Issue warnings alongside advertisements in antibiotic marketing.
- Supply systems to ensure proper disposal of unused antibiotics.

Responsibilities of Clinician Education and Professional Organizations

- Incorporate antibiotic stewardship principles into medical, nursing, and physician assistant education curricula and competencies.
- Provide and/or require continuing medical education opportunities around antibiotic stewardship.
- Create and share clinical practice guidelines that include proper diagnosis and judicial antibiotic practice.
- Promote member participation in national, local, and regional initiatives on inappropriate antibiotic prescribing and use.
- Highlight new research and technologies in simplified formats to support antibiotic stewardship.

Responsibilities of Federal, State, and Local Health Agencies

- Set strict expectations for the development and implementation of antibiotic stewardship activities across the spectrum of healthcare.

- Increase surveillance of antibiotic-resistant infections and promptly disseminate findings.
- Provide accessible data and tools to help guide stewardship activities.
- Connect local stakeholders and coalitions.
- Develop and disseminate appropriate educational resources.
- Fund innovations and research that facilitate optimal antibiotic use.
- Control biosecurity in agriculture to prevent unnecessary infections.
- Regulate movement of plants and livestock across regions to prevent the spread of resistant bacteria.

Responsibilities of Patients and Families

- Discuss with clinicians about when antibiotics will and won't help; educate themselves about antibiotic resistance.
- Discuss with clinicians about how to relieve symptoms; do not demand antibiotics.
- Ask what infection an antibiotic is treating, how long antibiotics are needed, and what side effects can be expected.

- Obtain all recommended immunizations.
- Take antibiotics only when prescribed and exactly as prescribed.
- Do not save an antibiotic for later use or share the drugs with someone else.
- Practice good sanitation and general hygiene.
- Stay healthy and keep others healthy by washing hands, covering coughs, staying home when sick, and getting recommended vaccines.

CONCLUSION

Antibiotic resistance is not a looming risk; it is a present threat. The very antibiotics that revolutionized the history of medicine now threaten to paralyze medical innovations. Bacteria colonies, once defeated, are mutating to evade therapeutic techniques; they are rapidly winning a war against the human race. All stakeholders must urgently employ strategies to prevent defeat.

CASE EXEMPLAR: Patient With Earache

AG is a 5-year-old female who, according to her mother, has been complaining of her left ear hurting for the past 48 hours. The child did not sleep well the last two nights and has been crying about her ear this morning. The mother has brought her to the clinic for assessment and intervention.

Past Medical History
- History of otitis media 12 months prior
- Seasonal allergies to trees
- All immunizations current
- No known drug allergies
- Only other visits, routine annual evaluation
- No history of any injuries or hospitalizations

Medications
- Daily vitamins

Family History
- Normal labor and delivery

Physical Examination
- Pulse: 110; respiration rate: 22 (crying); temperature: 98.0 °F
- Chest clear to auscultation

- No drainage noted from ears
- Drainage from nose is clear
- Throat pink with no swelling or exudate
- Tympanic membrane pearly white with no budging

Assessment
- Inflammation of sinuses, with swelling, causing ear pain. Clinician suggests cetirizine or levocetirizine. Mother requests antibiotic therapy.

Discussion Questions
1. Since the clinician's physical assessment fails to confirm the need for antibiotic therapy, what should the clinician tell the mother about watchful waiting and the use of antihistamines?
2. If the mother insists on an antibiotic prescription, what should the clinician teach the mother about the impact of misuse and avoidance of antibiotic therapy unless indicated?
3. Define the role of patients and/or families in response to antibiotic stewardship.

CASE EXEMPLAR: Implementation of New Antibiotic Guidelines

JS is visiting the local free clinic with complaints of a bug bite on the left ankle with redness, swelling, and pain. The bite occurred 2 days ago, and he believes it was a spider bite but could not identify its color or size. He has been placing an over-the-counter antibiotic ointment on the bite and covering it with a bandage. Today he began to feel "bad" in general and thinks it is related to the bite.

Medications
- None
- No known drug allergies

Physical Examination
- Blood pressure: 136/82; pulse: 98; respiration rate: 82; temperature: 101.0 °F

- In addition to the redness and swelling around the "bite," the area is warm to the touch and red streaks are noted to extend up from the bite approximately 8 cm

Assessment
- Infected spider bite with cellulitis
- Consider cephalexin, 250 mg three times a day for 10 days

Discussion Questions
1. What findings from the assessment support the decision to prescribe an antibiotic?
2. What patient education regarding appropriate use of antibiotics should the clinician provide for this patient?

CLINICAL PEARLS

- The worldwide misuse of antibiotics has led to significant negative patient outcomes in which the bacteria are winning, requiring a multidisciplinary approach to antibiotic stewardship.
- The federal government and the CDC have outlined specific guidelines and actions for all components of the healthcare system to manage the problem.
- Sound prescribing etiquette must be developed and clinicians must avoid prescribing antibiotics "just in case." This involves the right dose for the shortest duration and the avoidance of the use of broad-spectrum drugs.
- To ensure appropriate antibiotic use throughout all populations—human and animal—antibiotic stewardship must be followed.
- Patient and clinician education is critical.

KEY TAKEAWAYS

- The initial discovery and ongoing development of antibiotic therapy had a greater positive impact on patient outcomes than any previous medical discoveries.
- Antibiotic resistance is real, and the resultant effects are widespread, costly to patients and systems, and require a multifaceted, multidisciplinary approach to manage and combat impact.
- Much of antibiotic resistance can be tied to the inappropriate use of antibiotic therapy throughout the world.
- Education for all entities who encounter and intervene with antibiotic therapy must address the current situation of antibiotic resistance.
- All entities must be ready and willing to implement and ensure adherence to proposed antibiotic use guidelines.

REFERENCES

1. Aminov RI. A brief history of the antibiotic era: lessons learned and challenges for the future. *Front Microbiol.* 2010;1:134. doi:10.3389/fmicb.2010.00134

2. National Center for Health Statistics. *Table 15. Life expectancy at birth, at age 65, and at age 75, by sex, race, and Hispanic origin: United States, selected years 1900–2016.* 2017. https://www.cdc.gov/nchs/data/hus/2017/015.pdf.

3. McKeown RE. The epidemiologic transition: changing patterns of mortality and population dynamics. *Am J Lifestyle Med.* 2009;3(suppl 1):19S–26S. doi:10.1177/1559827609335350

4. Adedeji WA. The treasure called antibiotics. *Ann Ib Postgrad Med.* 2016;14(2):56–57. https://www.ncbi.nlm.nih.gov/pmc/articles/PMC5354621.

5. Pfizer. *The Value of Antibiotics in Treating Infectious Diseases.* n.d. https://pfe-pfizercom-d8-prod.s3.amazonaws.com/health/VoM_Antibiotics_NOV2016.PDF

6. Infectious Disease Society of America. Combating antimicrobial resistance: policy recommendations to save lives. *Clin Infect Dis.* 2011;52(suppl 5):S397–S428. doi:10.1093/cid/cir153

7. Talbot GH, Bradley J, Edwards JE, et al. Bad bugs need drugs: an update on the development pipeline from the Antimicrobial Availability Task Force of the Infectious Diseases Society of America. *Clin Infect Dis.* 2006;42(5):657–668. doi:10.1086/499819

8. Hersh AL, Newland JG, Beekmann SE, Polgreen PM, Gilbert DN. Unmet medical need in infectious diseases. *Clin Infect Dis.* 2012;54(11):1677–1678. doi:10.1093/cid/cis275

9. Fleming A. Penicillin. Nobel Lecture, December 11, 1945. Accessed February 12, 2019. https://www.nobelprize.org/uploads/2018/06/fleming-lecture.pdf

10. World Health Organization. *Antimicrobial Resistance: Global Report on Surveillance.* World Health Organization; 2014. https://www.who.int/antimicrobial-resistance/publications/surveillancereport/en

11. Antonanzas F, Lozano C, Torres C. Economic features of antibiotic resistance: the case of methicillin-resistant *Staphylococcus aureus. Pharmacoeconomics.* 2015;33(4):285–325. doi:10.1007/s40273-014-0242-y

12. Oehler RL. *MRSA: Historical Perspective.* http://www.antimicrobe.org/h04c.files/history/MRSA-Oehler.pdf

13. Sampathkumar P. Methicillin-resistant *Staphylococcus aureus:* the latest health scare. *Mayo Clin Proc.* 2007;82(12):1463–1467. doi:10.1016/S0025-6196(11)61088-4

14. Wozniak TM, Barnsbee L, Lee XJ, et al. Using the best available data to estimate the cost of antimicrobial resistance: a systematic review. *Antimicrob Resist Infect Control.* 2019;8(1):26. doi:10.1186/s13756-019-0472-z

15. Laxminarayan R, Duse A, Wattal C, et al. Antibiotic resistance—the need for global solutions. *Lancet Infect Dis.* 2013;13(12):1057–1098. doi:10.1016/S1473-3099(13)70318-9

16. World Health Organization. *Antibiotic resistance.* Published July 31, 2020. https://www.who.int/news-room/fact-sheets/detail/antibiotic-resistance

17. Centers for Disease Control and Prevention. *Antibiotic resistance threats in the United States, 2013.* Published 2013. https://www.cdc.gov/drugresistance/threat-report-2013/pdf/ar-threats-2013-508.pdf

18. Suda KJ, Hicks LA, Roberts RM, et al. Antibiotic expenditures by medication, class, and healthcare setting in the United States, 2010–2015. *Clin Infect Dis.* 2018;66(2):185–190. doi:10.1093/cid/cix773

19. Magill SS, Edwards JR, Beldavs ZG, et al. Prevalence of antimicrobial use in US acute care hospitals, May–September 2011. *JAMA.* 2014;312(14):1438. doi:10.1001/jama.2014.12923

20. The White House. *Executive Order—Combating antibiotic-resistant bacteria.* Published 2014. https://obamawhitehouse.archives.gov/the-press-office/2014/09/18/executive-order-combating-antibiotic-resistant-bacteria

21. Centers for Disease Control. *U.S. National Action Plan for Combating Antibiotic-Resistant Bacteria (National Action Plan).* Published March 2015. Updated October 2020. https://www.cdc.gov/drugresistance/us-activities/national-action-plan.html

22. LaPlante K, Cunha CB, Morrill HJ, et al. *Antimicrobial Stewardship: Principles and Practice.* C.A.B.I. International; 2017.

23. World Health Organization. *Antibiotic Resistance: Multi-Country Public Awareness Survey.* World Health Organization; 2015. http://www.who.int/drugresistance/documents/baselinesurveynov2015/en

Applied Calculations for Prescribing

David S. Grega and Brent Luu

LEARNING OBJECTIVES

- Describe the use and relevance of the systems of measurement, equivalents, and system conversion in practice.
- Outline the calculations related to cardiac functioning.
- Discuss the calculations related to endocrine functioning.
- Discuss therapeutic ranges of drugs with narrow therapeutic windows.
- Illustrate other relevant calculations in various clinical settings while caring for patients.

INTRODUCTION

Clinical decisions regarding pharmacotherapeutics can often be challenging for busy clinicians. Having a reliable clinical reference source to help with this critical decision-making is essential. Clinical pharmacotherapeutic calculation specifics are often scattered throughout various chapters and hidden under different subheadings, making it difficult for clinicians to accomplish quick, efficient clinical practice decisions. This chapter will consolidate the most commonly used calculations in various settings to assist the pharmacotherapeutic decisions in everyday practice.

MEASUREMENT SYSTEMS, EQUIVALENTS, AND SYSTEM CONVERSIONS

The measurements of weight and volume in medicine are often based on the apothecary, household, or metric systems. Due to its ease of conversion, the metric system has been adopted worldwide as a standardized system. This system is also referred to as the International System of Units (SI Units) and can be multiplied or divided by multiples of 10, using a decimal point. The measurements of volumes are often expressed in liter (L), deciliter (dL), milliliter (mL), or microliter (mcL); and of weights are in kilogram (kg), gram (g), milligram (mg), microgram (mcg), or nanogram (ng); and of lengths are in meter (m), centimeter (cm), or millimeter (mm).

The apothecary system that began back in the early days of medicine and the Western English or "household" system have been used for centuries. It is mostly used for measurements of weight or volume and are known to be less accurate. Due to the inconsistency between the units of conversion and the high risk of errors during unit conversion, these systems of measurements are discouraged in most clinical settings. Many clinicians have adopted the metric system as their standard of practice; however, some medication labels and containers still use these systems. Consequently, clinicians should be aware and familiar with the conversion of these units to metric equivalents. For example, the expressions of liquid volumes are in ounces (oz) or fluid ounces, teaspoons, tablespoons, or drops. Meanwhile, the expressions of weights are in pounds, ounces, drams, or grains. A summary of the commonly used apothecary or household measurements and their metric equivalents is shown in **Table 11.1**.

BODY SURFACE AREA

Dosing per body surface area (BSA) is thought to be an accurate method of calculating medication dose because the body weight of obese or underweight patients may differ significantly from the average "normal" individual. This is particularly important with medications that have a very narrow therapeutic window with serious toxicities, such as chemotherapeutic

TABLE 11.1 Selected Common Household or Apothecary Quantities With Metric Equivalents

Common Household or Apothecary Measurements		Metric Equivalents
1 tsp		5 mL
1 tbsp	3 tsp	15 mL
1 oz	2 tbsp	30 mL
Measuring cup	8 oz	240 mL
Teacup	6 oz	180 mL
1 pt	16 oz	480 mL (~500 mL)
1 qt	2 pt	960 mL (~1,000 mL)
1 gallon	4 qt	3,840 mL (~4,000 mL)

oz, ounce; pt, liquid pint; qt, quart; tbsp, tablespoon; tsp, teaspoon.

Source: Toney-Butler TJ, Wilcox L. *Dose calculation desired over have formula method. [Updated April 6, 2020]. In: StatPearls [Internet]*. StatPearls Publishing; 2020. https://www.ncbi.nlm.nih.gov/books/NBK493162/?report=classic

agents. There are at least six different ways to calculate BSA developed throughout the years.[1,2] The most popular and user-friendly formula for practical application is the Masteller's formula.[1] Masteller's formula was found to be most consistent and accurate in both pediatric and adult populations. Other formulas such as the Du Bois may overestimate the BSA by 15% in 15% of cases. Meanwhile, it may underestimate up to 8% of infants, especially for patients with BSA less than 0.7 m[2].[1] The following are different forms of the Masteller's formula to calculate BSA:*

$$BSA = \sqrt{\frac{\text{Height (cm)} \times \text{Weight (kg)}}{3,600}}$$

or

$$BSA = \sqrt{\frac{\text{Height (in)} \times \text{Weight (lbs.)}}{3,131}}$$

Example: Calculate the BSA of a male, height 70 inches (178 cm), weight 180 lbs. (82 kg):

$$BSA = \sqrt{\frac{178 \text{ (cm)} \times 82 \text{ (kg)}}{3,600}} = 2.01 \text{ m}^2$$

or

$$BSA = \sqrt{\frac{70 \text{ (in)} \times 180 \text{ (lbs.)}}{3,131}} = 2.01 \text{ m}^2$$

BODY MASS INDEX

Body mass index (BMI) is a measurement that helps to determine if a person is underweight, normal weight, overweight, or obese.[3-5] It is calculated by taking the ratio of the person's weight in kilograms and the square of their height in meters. The higher the BMI, the more obese the person. This calculation has been used as a screening tool to determine other health risks of an individual. BMI may be expressed as follows:**

$$BMI = \frac{\text{Weight (kg)}}{(\text{Height [m]})^2}$$

or

$$BMI = \frac{\text{Weight (lb)}}{\text{Height (in)}^2} \times 703$$

Example: Calculate the BMI of a patient, height 70 inches (1.8 m), weight 180 lbs. (82 kg):

$$BMI = \frac{82 \text{ (kg)}}{(1.8 \text{ [m]})^2} = 25.3 \text{ kg/m}^2$$

or

$$BMI = \frac{180 \text{ (lb)}}{(70 \text{ [inches]})^2} \times 703 = 25.8 \text{ kg/m}^2$$

Since the normal BMI is defined as 18.5 to 24.9 kg/m[2], a patient with the above BMI would be considered as overweight (**Table 11.2**).

TABLE 11.2 BMI Classifications

BMI	Classification
<18.5	Underweight
18.5–24.9	Normal
25.0–29.9	Overweight
30–34.9	Obese I
35–39.9	Obese II
>40.0	Obese III

BMI, body mass index.

Sources: How fast should the drops drip? *Nurs Made Incred Easy*. 2004;2(4): 60–62. https://journals.lww.com/nursingmadeincrediblyeasy/Fulltext/2004/07000/How_fast_should_the_drops_drip_.12.aspx; https://www.cdc.gov/obesity/adult/defining.html#:~:text=Adult%20Body%20Mass%20Index%20(BMI)&text=If%20your%20BMI%20is%20less,falls%20within%20the%20obese%20range.

*Equation from Mosteller RD. Simplified calculation of body-surface area. *N Engl J Med*. 1987;317(17):1098. doi:10.1056/NEJM198710223171717
**Equation from Keys A, Fidanza F, Karvonen MJ, Kimura N, Taylor HL. Indices of relative weight and obesity. *Int J Epidemiol*. 2014;43(3): 655–665. doi:10.1093/ije/dyu058

ESTIMATION OF RENAL FUNCTION

Drug elimination may occur at multiple levels within the body, which may involve chemical reactions during hepatic metabolism. These modes of elimination are mostly responsible for the termination of drug actions. Drug metabolism accounts for many of the variations seen in therapeutic drug responses from one patient to another. Both internal and external factors may affect the rate or extent of drug metabolism. When a drug is metabolized, it usually forms water-soluble metabolites to be readily excreted by the kidneys. Some drugs may be excreted renally unchanged without undergoing metabolism. The process of renal elimination of either unchanged drugs or their metabolites involve glomerular filtration, which may be estimated by the creatinine clearance (CrCl). The clearance of a drug from the body is estimated by measuring how much volume of plasma containing the drug is being filtered by the kidneys per unit of time, which is expressed in milliliters per minute.[6] This rate of drug clearance is one of the important factors that determine the drug plasma half-life ($t^{1/2}$).

The Cockcroft–Gault (CG) equation is one of the most popular equations that provides an estimation of CrCl, which approximates the GFR. This equation uses serum creatinine as a surrogate marker to determine kidney function. An apparently minor increase in serum creatinine (SCr) can reflect a marked fall in GFR. For this reason, the calculation of CrCl using a validated formula such as CG equation is an essential tool to monitor the patient's kidneys function and determine the necessary dose adjustment for drugs that are renally excreted (**Table 11.3**).[6]

TABLE 11.3 Selected Common Medications and Recommended Renal Dose Adjustments

Drug	Dosage	Recommended Renal Dose Adjustments
Amoxicillin PO (IR)	500–875 mg PO q12h	Do not use 875 mg or ER tablet for CrCl <30 mL/minute CrCl 10–29 mL/minute: 250–500 mg q12h CrCl <10 mL/minute: 250–500 mg q24h
Amoxicillin/ clavulanate potassium	500/125–875/125 mg PO q12h	Do not use 875/125 mg or ER tablet for CrCl <30 mL/minute CrCl 10–29 mL/minute: 250/125–500/125 mg PO q12h CrCl <10 mL/minute: 250/125–500/125 mg PO q24h
Allopurinol	100–800 mg PO daily (max: 800 mg/day)	CrCl 10–20 mL/minute: 200 mg PO daily CrCl 3–10 mL/minute: Do not exceed 100 mg PO daily
Atenolol	25–100 mg PO daily (max: 100 mg/day)	CrCl 15–35 mL/minute: Do not exceed 50 mg PO once daily CrCl <15 mL/minute: Do not exceed 25 mg PO once daily
Alendronate sodium	10–40 mg PO daily or 70 mg/week PO	CrCl <35 mL/minute: Not recommended
Celecoxib	200 mg PO once daily or 100 mg PO qid	Renal impairment (severe): Not recommended
Gabapentin	300–1,200 mg PO tid (max: 3,600 mg/day)	CrCl ≥60 mL/minute: 1,800 mg/day CrCl 30–59 mL/minute: 600–1,800 mg/day CrCl <30 mL/minute: Do not administer
Lithium carbonate (capsules/ tablets)	IR: 300 mg PO tid; titrate by 300 mg PO every 3 days to goal serum levels ER: 1,800 mg/day PO in two to three divided doses	CrCl 30–89 mL/minute: Initiate at lower doses and titrate more slowly than usual dosage; frequently monitor CrCl <30 mL/minute: Not recommended

Levofloxacin	250–750 mg PO daily	For usual dose of 750 mg/day:
		  CrCl 20–49 mL/minute: 750 mg q48h
		  CrCl <20 mL/minute: 750 mg × 1, then 500 mg q48h
		For usual dose of 500 mg/day:
		  CrCl 20–49 mL/minute: 500 mg × 1, then 250 mg q24h
		  CrCl <20 mL/minute: 500 mg × 1, then 250 mg q48h
		For usual dose of 250 mg/day:
		  CrCl 10–19 mL/minute: 250 mg q48h
		  CrCl <10 mL/minute: Undefined

Naproxen	250 or 500 mg PO bid (max: 1,250 mg/day)	CrCl <30 mL/minute: Not recommended

bid, twice daily; CrCl, creatinine clearance; ER, extended-release; h, hour; IR, immediate-release; max, maximum; PO, orally; q, every; TID, three times daily.

Source: Dosing & therapeutic tools database (electronic version). Micromedex. 2019. https://www.micromedexsolutions.com/micromedex2/librarian/ssl/true

Cockcroft–Gault CrCl equation[7]:
In men:

$$CrCl \ (mL \ / \ minute) = \frac{(140 - Age) \times Weight \ (kg)}{Serum \ Creatinine \ (mg/dL) \times 72}$$

In women:

$$CrCl \ (mL \ / \ minute) = \frac{(140 - Age) \times Weight \ (kg)}{Serum \ Creatinine \ (mg/dL) \times 72} \times 0.85$$

PLASMA OSMOLALITY VERSUS OSMOLARITY

Osmolality refers to the number of active solutes per 1 kg of solvent, while *osmolarity* is defined as the number of active solutes per 1 L of solvent.[8] Since 1 L of water is equivalent to 1 kg at standard conditions, the values of both osmolality and osmolarity in biological systems that use water as the primary solvent are similar, but they carry different units (i.e., osmol/L vs. osmol/kg). Therefore, osmolality and osmolarity are often incorrectly used interchangeably. In addition, osmolarity is temperature dependent because the volume of solvent can expand at higher temperature. Meanwhile, osmolality is independent of temperature because the mass of the solvent is constant at any temperature.[8]

Serum osmolality is one of the important laboratory values that clinicians use to detect if other osmotically active molecules, such as ethanol, methanol, or ethylene glycol, are abnormally present in blood. The osmolality of blood depends on all the different solutes that exist in blood, including proteins, electrolytes, glucose, and others. To simplify the calculation, serum osmolality may be estimated by the contents of sodium, blood urea nitrogen (BUN), and glucose, which may be expressed as follows:*

$$Serum \ Osmolality \ (mOsm/kg) = 2[Na] + \frac{BUN}{2.8} + \frac{Glucose}{18}$$

where [Na] is the concentration of sodium in serum.

Since serum osmolality is primarily affected by sodium, BUN, or glucose, the elevation of these levels will also lead to an increase of blood osmolality.[9] In other words, if a patient develops hypernatremia, or an accumulation of BUN due to renal impairment, or hyperglycemia due to diabetes, the serum osmolality of this individual would also be high. Most laboratory studies reported the normal range of serum osmolality at 285 to 290 mOsm/kg; therefore, fluids that have osmolality lower than this normal range are considered hypotonic solutions; meanwhile, fluids that have higher osmolality in relation to this range would be considered as hypertonic solutions. Since osmosis is the movement of water across a select permeable membrane from an area of low to higher osmolality, the movement of water in and out of red blood cells may be significantly affected by the level of tonicity of the intravenous (IV) fluids.[10] In other words, when administering IV fluids, such as half normal saline (0.45% NS) or quarter normal saline (0.225% NS), which have osmolality lower than serum (e.g., hypotonic solutions), the red blood cells would increase in size due to osmosis. If the expansion of the red blood cells exceeds a viable capacity, hemolysis can occur, which may lead to a full cascade of other complications. On the contrary, when a hypertonic solution is administered, it could cause shrinkage of red blood cells, which also leads to its own set of complications (see **Figure 11.1**).

CALCULATING THE OSMOLALITY OF INTRAVENOUS FLUIDS

Commonly used bulk IV fluids in clinical practice consist of varying concentrations of sodium chloride, dextrose, or other electrolytes plus dextrose. Generally, the four popular concentrations of sodium chloride

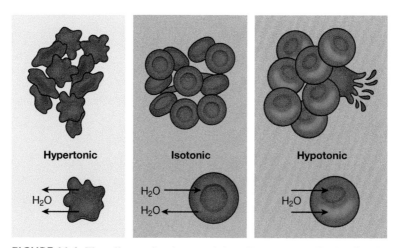

Hypertonic **Isotonic** **Hypotonic**

H_2O H_2O H_2O
 H_2O

FIGURE 11.1 The effects of various tonicity of intravenous fluids when in contact with red blood cells.

*Equation from Corenblum B, Flynn EA. Pituitary disorders. In: Sadrzadeh H, Kline G, eds. *Endocrine Biomarkers*. Elsevier; 2017:301–349.

TABLE 11.4 Osmolality of Commonly Used Intravenous Solutions

Intravenous Fluids	Calculated Osmolality
3% NaCl	953 mOsm/kg
0.9% NaCl	286 mOsm/kg
0.45% NaCl	143 mOsm/kg
0.225% NaCl	71.5 mOsm/kg
Dextrose 5%*	252 mOsm/kg
Dextrose 10%**	505 mOsm/kg
Lactated Ringers***	273 mOsm/kg

*Hospira. *5% dextrose injection, USP.* 2005. www.accessdata.fda.gov/drugsatfda_docs/label/2005/016367s178lbl.pdf

**Baxter International. *Dextrose injection, USP.* Food and Drug Administration. 2014. www.accessdata.fda.gov/drugsatfda_docs/label/2014/017521s068lbl.pdf

***Baxter International. *Lactated Ringer's injection.* 2019. www.baxterpi.com/pi-pdf/Lactated_Ringers_Injection_+Viaflex_PI.pdf

NaCl, sodium chloride.

that are used most contain: 0.225%, 0.45%, 0.9%, or 3%. From these concentrations, the osmolality of each IV fluid may be calculated as follows:

Osmolality of 0.9% NaCl:

$$= \frac{0.9 \text{ g NaCl}}{100 \text{ mL}} \times \frac{1{,}000 \text{ mL}}{1 \text{ kg}} \times \frac{1 \text{ mol NaCl}}{(23 \text{ g Na} + 35.5 \text{ g Cl})}$$

$$\times \frac{1{,}000 \text{ mmol}}{1 \text{ mol NaCl}} \times \frac{2 \text{ mOsm (active solutes)}}{1 \text{ mmol NaCl}}$$

$$\approx 308 \text{ mOsm/kg}$$

Since the osmotic coefficient (the factor that corrects for nonideal settings) of NaCl at physiologic conditions was determined at 0.93,[11] the corrected osmolality of NaCl 0.9% is 308 mOsm/kg × (0.93) = 286 mOsm/kg, which is within the normal range of plasma osmolality; therefore, it is an isotonic solution. **Table 11.4** summarizes the osmolality of the commonly used IV fluids.

FREE WATER VOLUME DEFICIT

The maintenance of body volume requires a balance of water and sodium. Automatic regulating systems such as the renin–angiotensin–aldosterone system (RAAS) and the antidiuretic hormone (ADH) help to maintain the balance of extracellular volume. This osmoregulation cascade may eventually lead to a change in sodium concentration in plasma; therefore, the rise of sodium concentration can be used to estimate the amount of volume loss in the extracellular space. To estimate the amount of volume deficit, the following formula may be used:

$$\text{Free Water Volume Deficit} = (\% \text{ of total body water})$$

$$\times \text{ Weight (kg)} \times \left(\frac{[\text{Na}^+]_{obs}}{140} - 1 \right)$$

where $[\text{Na}^+]_{obs}$ is the observed sodium concentration in plasma and the % of total body water is the fraction of body weight that represents the water content in the body, which varies with age.[12] The approximate body weight as water is 60% in an adult male. Meanwhile, for young females and elderly males, this fraction is estimated at 50% and elderly females at 45%.[13] When a person has water depletion due to dehydration, often the sodium level will rise in plasma. If this person weighs 70 kg and his plasma sodium concentration was measured at 150 mEq/L, then his calculated volume deficit would be as follows:

$$\text{Free Water Volume Deficit} =$$

$$(0.6) \times 70(\text{kg}) \times \left(\frac{150}{140} - 1 \right) = 3 \text{ L}$$

In other words, this patient has lost 3 L of his total body water, which is very significant and needs to be replaced appropriately. Refer to Chapter 21 for further details in fluid management strategies and hypernatremia correction.

SODIUM DEFICIT AND FRACTIONAL EXCRETION OF SODIUM

When patients develop hyponatremia due to sodium loss, the total deficit of sodium may be estimated with the following equation[14]

$$\text{Total Sodium Deficit} = (\% \text{ of total body water})$$

$$\times \text{ Weight (kg)} \times ([\text{Na}^+]_{desired} - [\text{Na}^+]_{actual})$$

where $[\text{Na}^+]_{desired}$ and $[\text{Na}^+]_{actual}$ are concentrations of sodium at desired and actual levels. For example, laboratory reports for a 70 kg adult male who has developed hyponatremia due to sodium loss will show the actual sodium level at 122 mEq/L. To calculate the sodium deficit, a desired level of sodium is often set at 140 mEq/L. As a result, the estimated total sodium loss for this patient would be as follows

$$\text{Total Sodium Deficit} = (0.6) \times 70(\text{kg})$$

$$\times (140 - 122 \text{ mEq/L}) = 756 \text{ mEq}$$

Since each liter of normal saline (i.e., 0.9% NaCl) provides about 154 mEq of sodium, this level of sodium deficit would need approximately 5 L of normal saline to completely replace the sodium loss. Please see Chapter 21 for strategies of correcting hyponatremia.

Most sodium in the body is present in the extracellular fluid (ECF) compartment, which is very effectively filtered by the kidneys. However, once sodium is filtered through the glomerulus, a majority of its content is reabsorbed throughout the nephrons, leading to less than 1% of fractional excretion of sodium (FENa) in most normal individuals. Nevertheless, this level may be elevated in individuals who have higher salt intake.[15] Additionally, in patients who develop prerenal azotemia due to volume depletion, the FENa continues to stay at this low level (i.e., <1%), implying that most of the nephrons are still able to reabsorb sodium. When this fractional excretion rises above 1%, it is often indicative of intrinsic renal injury.[15] In general, the values of fractional excretion of sodium may be interpreted as follows: (a) prerenal <1%; (b) intrinsic >1%; and (c) postrenal >4%.[14] As a result, it is a useful parameter in assisting in the diagnosis of various conditions that involve renal impairment. The estimation of FENa may be calculated as follows:

$$FENa = \left(\frac{S_{cr}}{U_{cr}} \times \frac{U_{Na}}{S_{Na}} \right) \times (100)$$

where S_{cr} and U_{cr} are the serum and urinary creatinine; meanwhile, U_{Na} and S_{Na} are urinary and serum sodium levels, respectively. If an individual has the following laboratory values:

- Plasma creatinine: 2.3 mg/dL
- 24-hour urinary creatinine: 500 mg/dL
- 24-hour urinary sodium: 500 mEq/L/day
- Plasma sodium: 145 mEq/L

Then

$$FENa = \left(\frac{2.3 \text{ mg/dL}}{500 \text{ mg/dL}} \times \frac{500 \text{ mEq/L}}{145 \text{ mEq/L}} \right) \times (100) = 1.6\%$$

Since the result of calculated FENa for this individual is greater than 1%, the clinician may interpret this finding as evidence that the patient is having an intrinsic kidney injury that has led to the observed laboratory values.

CALCULATIONS RELATED TO CARDIAC FUNCTION

CARDIAC OUTPUT AND CARDIAC INDEX

Reduction of cardiac output (CO), as in heart failure, may subsequently slow the delivery of medications to the liver, therefore delaying their metabolism. Renal function may also become compromised, and reduced GFR will affect elimination of a certain medication, prolonging its duration of action as expected in a patient with normal

cardiac output. In congestive heart failure (CHF), congestion of the portal system and gastrointestinal impairment of drug absorption may also occur. Because of these factors, medications that primarily require hepatic metabolization or renal excretion will often require reduced dosages. As a result, knowing how to calculate CO and cardiac index (CI) will assist clinicians assessing the clinical status of patients who develop cardiac insufficiency. The calculation of CO is determined by the product of the stroke volume (SV) of the left ventricle and the heart rate, which is shown in the following expression:

Cardiac Output (CO) = SV (stroke volume) × HR (heart rate)

Traditionally, CO or CI is directly determined by using a Swan–Ganz catheter; however, this is an invasive procedure. The pulmonary artery wedge pressure (PAWP) together with cardiac index (CI) may be used to stratify different subsets of patients who develop cardiac diseases. For example, **Table 11.5** shows the various hemodynamic subset classifications of heart failure.

The use of a Swan–Ganz catheter does not show survival benefits. In fact, according to the SUPPORT trial, the 30-day survival rate of critically ill patients managed by pulmonary artery catheter was less than the survival rate of those without the catheter.[16] As a result, noninvasive techniques are favorable in estimating cardiac output. Ultrasonography or echocardiography are often used to estimate the stroke volume. For example, if the heart rate of a 63 kg female with height 64 inches

TABLE 11.5 Classification of Heart Failure by Hemodynamic Subsets

1. PAWP = 18 mmHg with CI = 2.2 L/min/m²	Absence of heart failure; no pulmonary congestion; no peripheral hypoperfusion
2. PAWP >20 mmHg and CI <2 L/min/m²	Pulmonary congestion (i.e., wet); poor perfusion (i.e., cold)
3. PAWP <20 mmHg and CI <2 L/min/m²	No pulmonary congestion (i.e., dry); peripheral hypoperfusion (i.e., cold)
4. PAWP >20 mmHg and CI >2 L/min/m²	Pulmonary congestion (i.e., wet); no hypoperfusion (i.e., warm)
5. PAWP <20 mmHg and CI >2 L/min/m²	No pulmonary congestion (i.e., dry); no hypoperfusion (i.e., warm)

PAWP, pulmonary artery wedge pressure.

Source: Adams KF Jr, Giblin EM, Pearce N, Patterson JH. Integrating new pharmacologic agents into heart failure care: role of heart failure practice guidelines in meeting this challenge. *Pharmacotheraphy*. 2017;37(6):645–656. doi:10.1002/phar.1934; Cooper LB, Mentz RJ, Stevens SR, et al. Hemodynamic predictors of heart failure morbidity and mortality: fluid or flow? *J Card Fail*. 2016;22(3):182–189. doi:10.1016/j.cardfail.2015.11.012

was measured at 80 beats/minute and the SV was determined at 100 mL, then the CO may be calculated as:

Cardiac Output (CO) $= 100 \text{ mL} \times 80/\text{minute}$

$$= 8,000 \text{ mL/minute or } 8 \text{ L/minute}$$

The normal range of cardiac output is defined as 4 to 8 L/minute, though men tend to have slightly higher CO than women. Furthermore, during mental stress, CO may increase to 15 L/minute while physical exercise may increase CO up to 35 L/minute.[17] Since cardiac output is dependent on the size of the patient, cardiac index (CI) may be calculated to assess patients with critical illnesses or heart diseases. The expression of CI is as shown in the following expression:

$$\text{Cardiac Index (CI)} = \frac{CO \text{ (L/minute)}}{BSA \text{ (m}^2)}$$

Where CO is cardiac output measured in liters per minute and BSA is the body surface area measured in m².[18] Following the previous example, the patient's CI can be calculated once the BSA is determined. Since she weighs 63 kg and has a height of 64 inches, the BSA is estimated at:

$$BSA = \sqrt{\frac{64 \text{ (in)} \times 134 \text{ (lbs.)}}{3,131}} = 1.66 \text{ m}^2$$

As a result, her CI is:

$$\text{Cardiac Index (CI)} = \frac{8 \text{ (L/minute)}}{1.66 \text{ (m}^2)} = 4.8 \frac{L}{\text{minute} \times \text{m}^2}$$

CALCULATIONS RELATED TO THE ENDOCRINE SYSTEM

ESTIMATION OF HEMOGLOBIN A1C AND AVERAGE GLUCOSE

Hemoglobin A1C (A1C) is an important parameter in managing patients with diabetes. Hemoglobin A1C is formed by the glycosylation of hemoglobin in red blood cells due to chronic hyperglycemia. A1C is widely used as an indicator of the average blood glucose levels during the last 3 months.[19] In nondiabetic patients, the normal range for the hemoglobin A1C level is between 4% and 5.6%. When A1C exceeds this level, it is indicative that chronic hyperglycemia has developed. The relationship between A1C and estimated average glucose (eAG) may be expressed as:*

$$eAG = (28.7 \times A1C) - 46.7$$

To simplify this expression, all the constants may be rounded up to the nearest 10. As a result, the previous equation may be rewritten as:

$$eAG = (30 \times A1C) - 50$$

or

$$\text{Estimated A1C} = \frac{(eAG + 50)}{30}$$

With this simplification of the equation, an average blood glucose may be quickly determined if the A1C is obtained or vice versa. For example, a patient with an A1C of 7% would translate to an eAG of:

$$eAG = (30 \times 7\%) - 50 = 160 \text{ mg/dL}$$

Or a patient with an average blood glucose of 200 mg/dL would have an estimated A1C of:

$$\text{Estimated A1C} = \frac{(200 + 50)}{30} \simeq 8.3\%$$

INSULIN SENSITIVITY

The sensitivity of insulin varies significantly among patients diagnosed with diabetes. Various formulas and rules have been studied and applied; however, some rules are more user friendly and have therefore become more popular in clinical practice. Specifically, these are the 1500 rule and 1700 rule, as well as the 500 rule.[20,21] By applying these rules, a clinician can estimate the correction factors (CF) of an individual toward insulin or carbohydrates. In other words, these CFs approximate the sensitivity a patient may have developed toward insulin or carbohydrate when a total daily dose (TDD) of insulin is determined. The expressions of these rules are as follows:

1500 rule:

$$CF = \frac{1,500}{TDD}$$

1700 rule:

$$CF = \frac{1,700}{TDD}$$

500 rule:

$$CarbF = \frac{500}{TDD}$$

To apply these rules, a TDD of insulin needs to be determined, which can be obtained from the usage of the insulin pump or a sliding scale. For example, if the TDD of a patient is 25 units of insulin daily, the 1500 rule could be applied to provide the following results:

*Equation from Nathan DM, Kuenen J, Borg R, et al. Translating the A1C assay into estimated average glucose values. *Diabetes Care.* 2008;31(8):1473–1478. doi:10.2337/dc08-054

1500 rule:

$$CF = \frac{1,500}{25 \text{ units}} = 60 \text{ mg} / \text{dL}$$

The quotient obtained from applying the rule suggests that for each unit of insulin, the patient's blood glucose may drop by 60 mg/dL. Using the same TDD, if the 1700 rule is applied, the formula would provide a result of 68 mg/dL. In other words, if this patient is following the 1700 rule rather than the 1500 rule, the patient's blood glucose would have dropped by 68 mg/dL per unit of insulin. The higher the numerator, the more sensitive the patient is to insulin.

On the other hand, the 500 rule is applied to match insulin boluses with carbohydrate intake.[21] If it is applied to the same TDD of 25 units of insulin daily, the resulting carbohydrate factor (CarbF) would be at 20 g. In other words, for every 20 g of carbohydrate intake, the patient would need 1 unit of insulin to cover.[21]

DRUGS WITH NARROW THERAPEUTIC WINDOWS

THERAPEUTIC RANGES

Therapeutic ranges refer to drug levels that are high enough to exert their therapeutic effects with tolerable side effects but below the toxic levels. Some medications have very narrow therapeutic windows, which require close monitoring because the drug levels between the therapeutic and toxic effects are very similar. Selected examples of medications with narrow therapeutic windows are vancomycin, warfarin, digoxin, phenobarbital, phenytoin, valproic acid, and lithium.

Vancomycin

Vancomycin is a commonly used antibiotic in hospital settings, especially for methicillin-resistant *Staphylococcus aureus* (MRSA) infections or perioperative prophylaxis. The minimum therapeutic trough level should be maintained above 10 mcg/mL to avoid bacterial resistance. Furthermore, higher trough levels (e.g., 15–20 mcg/mL) should be targeted to generate a ratio of area under the curve to minimum inhibitory concentration (AUC:MIC) of 400 for pathogens that have MIC of 1 mcg/mL.[22] A loading dose of 25 to 30 mg/kg based on actual body weight may be used for complicated infections to rapidly attain the target trough.[22] In general, trough levels are drawn a half hour prior to the next dose once it is at steady state. Since the half-life of vancomycin is approximately 4 to 6 hours in patients with good renal function, 30 hours are typically needed for a patient to reach steady state following the initiation of therapy. The dosing frequency of vancomycin is usually every 12 hours for normal kidney function; therefore, trough level of steady state is often scheduled at half hour prior to the third or fourth dose. Furthermore, for patients who have excellent kidney function with dosing frequency of every 8 hours, trough level may be scheduled a half hour prior to the fifth dose.[22]

Warfarin

Warfarin is an oral anticoagulant that has been used for many decades to prevent clot formation caused by various disease states. The therapeutic levels of warfarin are measured by international normalizing ratio (INR), which depends on the specific indication. Most of the indications for warfarin require a therapeutic INR of 2 to 3, except in patients with mechanical heart valves (i.e., single-tilting disk and bi-leaflet valves) where an INR target of 2.5 to 3.5 is required.[23,24] Warfarin has a delayed onset of action, and peak anticoagulant effect may be delayed by 72 to 96 hours. It also has a terminal half-life of about a week.[25] As a result, monitoring INR lab tests are generally done every 3 days during the initial phase of the therapy until the INR is stabilized within the specified targeted therapeutic window.

Digoxin

Digoxin is an important and useful therapy for patients with atrial fibrillation and/or heart failure. Studies have shown that digoxin could reduce 30-day all-cause hospital readmission in heart failure, which is due in part to both its positive inotropic activity and negative chronotropic effects.[26] In adults, digitalization may be achieved by two general approaches, rapid or more gradual accumulation. Rapid digitalization may be achieved with a preferred intravenous (IV) or intramuscular (IM) loading dose (e.g., 8–12 mcg/kg) divided into 3 doses. Fifty percent of the loading dose may be given at first dose, then 25% at second and third dose separated by 6 to 8 hours' interval. This is followed by a maintenance dose, which may be titrated up every 2 weeks depending on the clinical response. A more gradual digitalization begins with an appropriate maintenance dose, then titrate every five half-lives to reach steady state. The therapeutic response may be achieved between 1 to 3 weeks for most patients since the elimination half-life of digoxin is 1.5 to 2 days in patients with normal renal function.[27] The therapeutic range for digoxin is generally reported at 0.8 to 2 ng/mL; however, a lower serum trough level at 0.5 to 1 ng/mL may be appropriate for some individuals. The collection of trough level should be scheduled at least 6 to 8 hours after the last oral dose and at least 4 hours after the IV dose to allow enough time for distribution and equilibration.[27]

Phenobarbital

Phenobarbital is primarily approved for seizure disorders with the exception of absence seizures. The generally accepted therapeutic range of phenobarbital is

15 to 40 mcg/mL; nevertheless, there are reports of patients who are seizure-free at a drug level of 10 mcg/mL. On the contrary, reports also claim that there are cases of refractory seizure while phenobarbital levels are within therapeutic range. As a result, many clinicians choose to rely on a patient's clinical response rather than a targeted drug level.[28]

Phenytoin

Phenytoin is also approved for seizure disorders; however, it has been used off-label as an antiarrhythmic to counteract arrhythmias that are induced by digoxin overdose.[29] The conventional therapeutic range of phenytoin is 10 to 20 mcg/mL. Studies have suggested that the antiseizure activity of phenytoin is dose related. In other words, the frequency of seizure control is poor at drug concentrations less than 10 mcg/mL and significantly improved when the concentrations are between 15 to 20 mcg/mL.[28] Several studies have also shown that levels greater than 20 mcg/mL may be optimal for certain individuals. Consequently, drug levels of phenytoin are not routinely monitored and instead are checked only when patients are experiencing break-through seizures or adverse effects.[28]

Phenytoin is highly protein bound and it is generally accepted that only the free phenytoin carries out its pharmacologic effects. As a result, patients with hypoalbuminemia are at risk for toxicities. In fact, albumin levels of less than 3.5 g/dL have been shown to contribute to phenytoin intoxication.[30] To correct total phenytoin levels for albumin, the Sheiner-Tozer equation is usually applied as follows:[30]

$$\text{Corrected Total Phenytoin} = \frac{\text{Total Phenytoin Observe (mcg / mL)}}{(0.2 \times \text{Albumin g/dL}) + 0.1}$$

From the previous equation, the free unbounded phenytoin level may be derived by multiplying the corrected total phenytoin by 0.1, since 90% of the phenytoin are protein bounded. Given the wide acceptance of the Sheiner-Tozer correction of phenytoin, reports have shown the calculated free phenytoin levels may not be suitable for patients with hypoalbuminemia. Therefore, routine monitoring of free concentrations of phenytoin should be performed.[30]

Valproic Acid

Valproic acid is another agent used for seizure control. It is also a candidate for therapeutic drug monitoring when there are potential drug–drug interactions, breakthrough seizures, or adverse reactions. It associates with nonlinear pharmacokinetics due to plasma protein binding, which results in large differences among individuals in dose-to-plasma concentration relationships. The current plasma reference range for valproic acid is 50 to 100 mcg/mL (or

TABLE 11.6 Summary of Common Narrow-Therapeutic Drugs

Drug	Starting Dose	Half-Life	Therapeutic Range	Precautions/ Contraindications	Therapeutic Drug Monitoring	Renal Dosing
Warfarin	2–10 mg PO daily	20–60 h (anticoagulant effect)	INR: 2.0–3.0 Mechanical valve: 2.5–3.5	Foods ↑ vitamin K; drug–drug interactions	INR: Daily or q3d until desired range	Consider starting at lower dose
Phenytoin	Loading: 10–15 mg/kg IV (max: 50 mg/ minute); maintenance: 100 mg PO/IV q6–8h	10–15 h IV	10–20 mcg/mL	Elderly, ethanol, CV, abrupt withdrawal, HLA-B*1502 positive, diabetes mellitus, thyroid disease	Phenytoin serum levels: obtain ≥5–7 half-lives (≥7–10 d) after treatment initiation, dosage change, addition or subtraction of another drug to the regimen	Do not give PO loading regimen
Valproic acid	10–15 mg/kg/d PO divided into two to three doses	9–16 h PO	50–100 mcg/mL	Abrupt discontinue, hepatic diseases, myelosuppression, bleeding risk	Within 2–4 d of first dose, draw trough before next dose until therapeutic	Hepatic monitoring
Phenobarbital	50–100 mg PO bid– tid (seizures)	53–118 h	15–40 mcg/mL	Elderly, abrupt withdrawal, hepatic impairment, reproductive potential in female patients, depression	Draw peak 4–12 h after dose, trough just before next dose	—

(continued)

TABLE 11.6 Summary of Common Narrow-Therapeutic Drugs (*continued*)

Drug	Starting Dose	Half-Life	Therapeutic Range	Precautions/ Contraindications	Therapeutic Drug Monitoring	Renal Dosing
Lithium	900–2,000 mg PO in divided doses BID-TID	18–36 h	0.6–1.2 mEq/L	Renal impairment, pregnancy, CV diseases, thyroid disorders, fever/infection, dehydration	Potential toxicity >1.5 mEq/L; levels 2 × weekly until stable, then at least every 6 months	CrCl 10–50 mL/minute: 50%–75% dose; CrCl <10 mL/minute: 25%–50% dose
Digoxin	Loading: 0.25 mg IV/PO q2h (max: 1.5 mg); maintenance: 0.125–0.375 mg IV/PO daily (AF guideline dosing)	36–48 h	0.5–2 ng/mL Toxic >2 ng/mL	CV: AV Block, WPW, electrical cardioversion, thyroid disorders	Monitor closely initially, then within 5–7 d after dose change	Renal impairment increases the risk of toxicity; monitoring and dosage adjustment recommended

AF, atrial fibrillation; AV, atrioventricular; bid, twice daily; CrCl, creatinine clearance; CV, cardiovascular; d, day; h, hour; INR, international normalized ratio; IV, intravenous; max, maximum; PO, orally; TID, three times daily; WPW, Wolff–Parkinson–White Syndrome.

4–15 mcg/mL unbounded). Reports claim that the risk of thrombocytopenia is significantly increased when the level is greater than or equal to 110 mcg/mL for females or greater than or equal to 135 mcg/mL for males.[28,31]

Lithium

Lithium is a commonly prescribed drug for bipolar disorders with a very narrow therapeutic window. The desired plasma trough level ranges from 0.6 to 1.2 mEq/L during long-term therapy. However, to prevent manic episodes in patients who are naïve to lithium, the targeted levels should be at 0.8 to 1.0 mEq/L.[32] Lithium can affect the kidneys' functions and limit their ability to concentrate urine. In addition, any conditions that could lead to drastic change of kidney functions (e.g., heart failure, hypotension, or severe dehydration) can lead to lithium toxicities. Often, lithium dose is given every 12-hours dosing; therefore, trough level should be scheduled approximately 12 hours post last dose. However, if dosing is every 24 hours, the trough level may be drawn 24 hours after the last dose.[33]

PARENTERAL ROUTES OF ADMINISTRATION AND RELATED CALCULATIONS

Parenteral medications are given by injection, which primarily include intradermal (ID), subcutaneous (SQ), intramuscular (IM), and intravenous (IV). Because parenteral routes can accelerate entry of an active drug into the body systems, it is imperative to review all the "Rights" during medication administration—the Right Patient, Right Drug, Right Dose, Right Route, Right Indication, and Right Time—for each of the medications to be administered.

INTRADERMAL INJECTIONS

In an ID injection, medication is injected into the dermis—the layer of skin right beneath the epidermis. This type of injection can be used to anesthetize the skin for invasive procedures and to test for allergies, tuberculosis, histoplasmosis, and other diseases. Injection volume is typically less than 0.5 mL. A 1 mL syringe, calibrated in 0.01 mL increments, is usually used, along with a 25- to 27-gauge (G) needle with length of 3/8 to 5/8 inches.

SUBCUTANEOUS INJECTIONS

In an SQ injection, the drug is injected into the subcutaneous tissue, which is beneath the dermis and above the muscle.[34] Because the SQ tissue has more capillaries, drugs are absorbed faster in this layer than in the dermis. Insulin, heparin, tetanus toxoid, and other ingredients such as opioid analgesics may be injected SQ. Typically, 0.5 to 1 mL of a drug can be injected SQ. The needles used for SQ injections are 23 to 28G and 1/2 to 5/8 inches long. Sites of SQ injection generally include the anterior aspect of the thighs, lateral areas of the upper arms and thighs, abdomen (above, below, and lateral to the umbilicus), and upper back. Local anesthetic injections with agents such as lidocaine can be directed SQ just under the dermis to provide local surface anesthesia, as in deeper wound preparation and closure.

INTRAMUSCULAR INJECTIONS

Medications may be administered by IM injection, which allows for quick absorption into the vasculature.[35] Complications such as abscess, cellulitis, bleeding, muscle fibrosis, or nerve or blood vessel injuries may develop if the technique of administration is inappropriately performed. Generally, IM volume of injections ranges from 0.5 to 5 mL. The choice of injection site depends on the patient's muscle mass, overlying tissue, and the volume of the injection. **Box 11.1** indicates the recommended maximum volume per site of injection. The needles are 1 to 3 inches long and are 18 to 23G in diameter. Pediatric IM injections are given most commonly in the lateralis of the thighs, often requiring dual bilateral injections to meet the dose requirements (**Table 11.7**).

CALCULATING DRIP RATES

Calculations to determine the *drip rate* are important in the administration of bulk IV solutions.[36] When a total volume of a certain bulk IV solution is already determined within a period of time, this drip rate can be calculated and set so that the patient is safely receiving the infusion over the intended time frame.[37] For example, if a patient requires 1,000 mL of normal saline be given within 4 hours, calculating the drip rate will determine the rate at which it should be administered within the desired time frame. To calculate the drip rate, the calibration for the selected IV tubing needs to be identified. Different IV tubing sets deliver fluids at varying amounts per drop. *The drop factor* refers to the number of drops per mL (cc) of solution calibrated for that set of tubing, which is listed on the package of the set. Typically, a

standard (macro-drip) comes with drop factors of 10, 15, or 20 gtt/mL (drops/mL), while a micro-drip (mini-drip) set is calibrated for 60 gtt/mL. These micro-drip sets are often used in slow infusion rates.[38] From the previous example, if the 10 gtt/mL set was selected, the following equation can be used to determine the drip rate:

$$\text{Drip Rate} = \frac{1,000 \text{ mL}}{4 \text{ hours}} \times \frac{1 \text{ hour}}{60 \text{ minutes}} \times \frac{10 \text{ gtt}}{1 \text{ mL}}$$
$$\approx 42 \text{ gtt/minute (42 drops/minute)}$$

Alternatively, one may be able to quickly determine a drip rate by following these three steps:

1. Determine the time in minutes:
   ○ If the drip is to be given over 2 hours, then it would be 120 minutes.
2. Divide the determined minutes by the drop factor selected:
   ○ If standard drop factor 20 gtt/mL IV tubing is selected, then 120 is divided by 20, producing 6.
3. Take the total volume to be delivered in mL divided by the result in step 2:
   ○ If the total volume is 500 mL, then 500 is divided by 6, producing 83 gtt/minute.

CONCLUSION

Clinical calculations, parenteral drug administration, and drug monitoring are important elements while caring for patients. They are helpful tools for clinicians to aid in decision-making and confirming a diagnosis. Prescribers should be familiar with these calculations to facilitate and promote patient safety. Notably, the results of many calculations are essentially estimations; therefore, the error rate may be high. New clinicians must always evaluate the results, ensure that they fit the clinical situation, and are being appropriately applied in each specific scenario. When in doubt, consider consulting a pharmacist or a more experienced colleague for further assistance.

BOX 11.1
MAXIMUM INJECTABLE VOLUMES PER SITE IN ADULTS

Recommended
- Ventrogluteal: 2.5 mL
- Vastus lateralis: 5 mL
- Deltoid: 1 mL
- Rectus femoris: 5 mL

TABLE 11.7 Intramuscular Injection Guidelines

Location of Injection	Patient Age	Needle Length (Inches)	Needle Gauge
Vas lateralis muscle (≤0.5 mL volume)	Infants (<18 months)	7/8–1	25–27 G
Deltoid muscle Ventrogluteal site Dorsogluteal site Vastus lateralis muscle	Children (>18 months and walking to 18 years) Dorsogluteal site: Contraindicated for children <3 years	7/8–1¼	22–25 G
Deltoid muscle, ventrogluteal site Dorsogluteal site Vastus lateralis muscle	Adults (>18 years); avoid in obese adults Deltoid muscle, ventrogluteal site: May be best for cachetic adults	1–1½ (up to 3 inches for large adults)	19–25 G

CASE EXEMPLAR: Calculating IV Fluid Intake

KL is a 22-year-old woman who is seen in the clinic with complaints of nausea, vomiting, and diarrhea. She has not been able to maintain any fluid intake. Her skin is dry and flushed. Dark circles surround her eyes.

Past Medical History
- Nonremarkable, healthy, 22-year-old female
- No known drug allergies

Medications
- Daily vitamin
- Ibuprofen for pain
- Birth control

Physical Examination
- Blood pressure: 92/62; pulse: 90; respiration rate: 22; temperature: 100.2 °F
- Dehydration notes
- Mucous membranes dry
- Lips dry and cracked

Labs
- Urinalysis:
  - Concentrated, dark yellow, obtained from catheter
  - Specific gravity: 1.032
- Sodium: 124 mEq/L
- Potassium: 5.3 mEq/L
- Chloride: 105 mEq/L

Discussion Questions

1. The infusion order is for 1 liter of saline over 2 hours. The IV setup tubing delivers 10 gtts/mL. Calculate the drip rate for this order in drops per minute.
2. The infusion rate is changed. Calculate the drip rate for the administration of 1,000 mL over 3 hours by using the same set of IV tubing.
3. To help control the patient's nausea, the clinician orders an IM injection of promethazine 25 mg. What needle size—length and gauge—should be used, and in what location should the injection be administered?

CASE EXEMPLAR: Calculating Body Surface Area and Sodium Deficit

FF is a 34-year-old male who was playing soccer when he collapsed on the field. He had been drinking water, but not much and no other fluids. A fellow player believed FF had possible heat stroke and brought him to the clinic.

Past Medical History
- Fracture of left arm at age 7
- Peptic ulcer, diagnosed 2 years ago

Medications
- Sucralfate, 1 g, four times daily
- Cimetidine, 800 mg at bedtime

Physical Examination
- Height: 75 inches; weight: 190 lbs.; blood pressure: 90/62; pulse: 130; respiration rate: 32; temperature: 103.4 °F
- Semi-alert male
- Breathing: Rapid and shallow
- Skin: Hot to the touch; tenting of skin
- Mucous membranes: Dry
- Urine output: Scant
- No vomiting

Labs
- Urinalysis:
  - Concentrated, dark yellow, obtained from catheter
  - Specific gravity: 1.026
- Sodium: 124 mEq/L
- Potassium: 4.9 mEq/L
- Chloride: 108.9 mEq/L
- Liver function: Normal

Discussion Questions

1. The clinician needs to determine FF's sodium level. What is FF's actual sodium deficit?
2. Now that FF's sodium deficit level is known, the clinician will administer an IV to replace the sodium. How should the required amount of replacement be calculated?
3. To administer additional medication, FF's body surface area (BSA) must be calculated. What is FF's BSA?

CLINICAL PEARLS

- The metric system has been adopted worldwide as a standardized system. However, some groups still use the apothecary or household systems, so clinicians should be familiar with the conversion of these units to metric equivalents.
- Important calculations relative to dosing include body surface area, BMI, and estimation of renal function.
- Knowing how to calculate CO and CI will assist prescribers assessing the clinical status of patients who developed cardiac insufficiency.
- The rise and fall of sodium concentration can be used to estimate the amount of volume loss in the extracellular space and the amount of sodium deficit.
- It is important to monitor hemoglobin A1C in patients with diabetes. A1C and average blood glucose may be quickly estimated by using the following equation during a clinic visit: eAG = (30 × A1C) − 50
- Medications with very narrow therapeutic windows require close monitoring because the levels between therapeutic and toxic effects are close to each other.

KEY TAKEAWAYS

- BSA calculation is critical in drugs with narrow therapeutic indices. The most popular and user-friendly formula for BSA is Masteller's formula; it is also the most consistent and accurate in both adult and pediatric populations.
- Examples of medications with narrow therapeutic windows are vancomycin, warfarin, digoxin phenobarbital, phenytoin, valproic acid, and lithium. The clinician must be familiar with the indices of these drugs.
- *Osmolality* and *osmolarity* are often incorrectly used interchangeably. *Osmolarity* is temperature dependent because the volume of solvent can expand at higher temperatures. *Osmolality* is independent of temperature since the mass of the solvent is constant at any temperature.
- In an intradermal injection, medication is injected into the dermis—the layer of skin right beneath the epidermis. In a subcutaneous injection, the drug is injected into the subcutaneous tissue, which is beneath the dermis and above the muscle. IM injections are injected intramuscularly.

- To calculate an IV drip rate, the calibration drop factor needs to be identified as this refers to the number of drops per mL set for that tubing.

REFERENCES

1. Hatahira H, Iguchi K, Sasaoka S, et al. Body surface area formulas for the calculation of the chemotherapy dosage [in Japanese]. *Gan To Kagaku Ryoho*. 2017;44(11):1011–1015. Pubmed PMID: 29138378.
2. Nafiu OO, Owusu-Bediako K, Chiravuri SD. Effect of body mass index category on body surface area calculation in children undergoing cardiac procedures. *Anesth Analg*. 2020;130(2):452–461. doi:10.1213/ANE.0000000000004016
3. El Edelbi R, Lindemalm S, Eksborg SJ. Estimation of body surface area in various childhood ages–Validation of the Mosteller formula. *Acta Pediatr*. 2012;101(5):540–544. doi:10.1111/j.1651-2227.2011.02580.x
4. Lee J-Y, Choi J-W, Kim HJ. Determination of body surface area and formulas to estimate body surface area using the alginate method. *J Physiol Anthropol*. 2008;27(2):71–82. doi:10.2114/jpa2.27.71
5. Verbraecken J, Van de Heyning P, De Backer W, Van Gaal L. Body surface area in normal-weight, overweight, and obese adults. A comparison study. *Metabolism*. 2006;55(4):515–524. doi:10.1016/j.metabol.2005.11.004
6. Shahbaz H, Gupta M. Creatinine clearance. [Updated September 2, 2020]. In: *StatPearls [Internet]*. StatPearls Publishing; 2020. https://www.ncbi.nlm.nih.gov/books/NBK544228.
7. Michels WM, Grootendorst DC, Verduijn M, et al. Performance of the Cockcroft-Gault, MDRD, and new CKD-EPI formulas in relation to GFR, age, and body size. *Clin J Am Soc Nephrol*. 2010;5(6):1003–1009. doi:10.2215/CJN.06870909
8. Koeppen BM, Stanton BA. Physiology of body fluids. In: Koeppen BM, Stanton BA. eds. *Renal Physiology*. 5th ed. Mosby; 2013:1–14.
9. Nikolova VL, Pattanaseri K, Hidalgo-Mazzei D, et al. Is lithium monitoring NICE? Lithium monitoring in a UK secondary care setting. *J Psychopharmacol*. 2018;32(4):408–41. doi:10.1177/0269881118760663
10. Goodhead LK, MacMillan FM. Measuring osmosis and hemolysis of red blood cells. *Adv Physiol Educ*. 2017;41(2):298–305. doi:10.1152/advan.00083.2016
11. Feher J. Osmosis and osmotic pressure. In: Feher J, ed. *Quantitative Human Physiology*. Academic Press; 2012:141–152.
12. Cheuvront SN, Kenefick RW, Sollanek KJ, et al. Water-deficit equation: systematic analysis and improvement. *Am J Clin Nutr*. 2013;97(1):79–85. doi:10.3945/ajcn.112.046839
13. Lunn KF, Johnson AS, James KM. Fluid therapy. In: Little SE, ed. *The Cat: Clinical Medicine and Management* W.B. Saunders; 2012:52–89.
14. Braun MM, Barstow CH, Pyzocha NJ. Diagnosis and management of sodium disorders: hyponatremia and

hypernatremia. *Am Fam Physician.* 2015;91(5):299–307. https://www.aafp.org/afp/2015/0301/p299.pdf

15. Steiner RW. Interpreting the fractional excretion of sodium. *Am J Med.* 1984;77(4):699–702. doi:10.1016/0002 -9343(84)90368-1

16. Babbs CF. Noninvasive measurement of cardiac stroke volume using pulse wave velocity and aortic dimensions: a simulation study. *Biomed Eng Online.* 2014;13:137. doi:10.1186/1475-925X-13-137

17. Bacon S. Cardiac output. In: Gellman MD, Turner JR, eds. *Encyclopedia of Behavioral Medicine.* Springer; 2013:332–333.

18. Carlsson M, Andersson R, Bloch KM, et al. Cardiac output and cardiac index measured with cardiovascular magnetic resonance in healthy subjects, elite athletes and patients with congestive heart failure. *J Cardiovasc Magn Res.* 2012;14(1):51. doi:10.1186/1532-429X-14-51

19. Arnhold J. Cell and tissue destruction in selected disorders. In: Arnhold J, ed. *Cell and Tissue Destruction.* Academic Press; 2020:249–287.

20. King AB, Armstrong DU. A prospective evaluation of insulin dosing recommendations in patients with type 1 diabetes at near normal glucose control: bolus dosing. *J Diabetes Sci Technol.* 2007;1(1):42–46. doi:10.1177/193229680700100107

21. Walsh J, Roberts R, Bailey T. Guidelines for insulin dosing in continuous subcutaneous insulin infusion using new formulas from a retrospective study of individuals with optimal glucose levels. *J Diabetes Sci Technol.* 2010;4(5):1174–1181. doi:10.1177/193229681000400516

22. Martin JH, Norris R, Barras M, et al. Therapeutic monitoring of vancomycin in adult patients: a consensus review of the American Society of Health-System Pharmacists, the Infectious Diseases Society of America, and the Society of Infectious Diseases Pharmacists. *Clin Biochem Rev.* 2010;31(1):21–24. https://www.ncbi.nlm .nih.gov/pmc/articles/PMC2826264

23. Harris C, Croce B, Cao C. Tissue and mechanical heart valves. *Ann Cardiothorac Surg.* 2015;4(4):399. doi:10.3978/j.issn.2225-319X.2015.07.01

24. Kamthornthanakarn I, Krittayaphong R. Optimal INR level for warfarin therapy after mechanical mitral valve replacement. *BMC Cardiovasc Disord.* 2019;19(1):97. doi:10.1186/s12872-019-1078-3

25. *Coumadin (warfarin) tablets: package insert.* 2011. https://www.accessdata.fda.gov/drugsatfda_docs/ label/2011/009218s107lbl.pdf

26. Ahmed A, Bourge RC, Fonarow GC, et al. Digoxin use and lower 30-day all-cause readmission for Medicare beneficiaries hospitalized for heart failure. *Am J Med.* 2014;127(1):61–70. doi:10.1016/j.amjmed.2013.08.027

27. *Lanoxin (digoxin): package insert.* 2011. https:// www.accessdata.fda.gov/drugsatfda_docs/label/2011/ 020405s006lbl.pdf

28. Greenberg RG, Melloni C, Wu H, et al. Therapeutic index estimation of antiepileptic drugs: a systematic literature review approach. *Clin Neuropharmacol.* 2016;39(5):232–240. doi:10.1097/WNF.0000000000000172

29. Rumack BH, Wolfe RR, Gilfrich H. Phenytoin (diphenyl-hydantoin) treatment of massive digoxin overdose. *Br Heart J.* 1974;36(4):405–408. doi:10.1136/hrt.36.4.405

30. Hong J-M, Choi Y-C, Kim W-J. Differences between the measured and calculated free serum phenytoin concentrations in epileptic patients. *Yonsei Med J.* 2009;50(4):517–520. doi:10.3349/ymj.2009.50.4.517

31. *Depakene (valproic acid).* 2011. https://www .accessdata.fda.gov/drugsatfda_docs/label/2011/018081 s046_18082s031lbl.pdf

32. Luu B, Rodway G. Lithium therapy for bipolar disorder. *J Nurse Pract.* 2018;14(2):93–99. doi:10.1016/j .nurpra.2017.09.025

33. Reddy DS, Reddy MS. Serum lithium levels: ideal time for sample collection! Are we doing it right? *Indian J Psychol Med.* 2014;36(3):346–347. doi:10.4103/0253-7176.135399

34. Shepherd E. Injection technique 2: administering drugs via the subcutaneous route. *Nursing Times.* 2018;114(9):55–57. https://insights.ovid.com/nurs-ing-times/nrtm/2018/09/000/injection-technique-adminis-tering-drugs-via/59/00006203

35. Shepherd E. Injection-technique 1 administering drugs via the intramuscular route. *Nursing Times.* 2018;114(8):3. https://cdn.ps.emap.com/wp-content/ uploads/sites/3/2018/07/180725-Injection-technique-1 -administering-drugs-via-the-intramuscular-route.pdf

36. Labus D, Hendler CB. *Dosage Calculations made Incredibly Easy!* Wolters Kluwer Health/Lippincott Williams & Wilkins; 2012.

37. Wilson KM. The nurse's quick guide to I.V. drug calculations. *Nursing Made Incredibly Easy.* 2013;11(2), 1–2. doi:10.1097/01.NME.0000426306.10980.65

38. How fast should the drops drip? *Nursing Made Incredibly Easy.* 2004;2(4):60–62. https://journals.lww.com/ nursingmadeincrediblyeasy/Fulltext/2004/07000/How _fast_should_the_drops_drip_.12.aspx

Promoting Adherence With Pharmacotherapy

Lisa M. O'Neal and Erin Lyden

LEARNING OBJECTIVES

- Outline the types of medication nonadherence and explain why this is a multifaceted problem.
- Define and discuss the two types of medication nonadherence.
- Discuss the factors that contribute to the development of self-stigma, the role self-stigma plays in medication nonadherence, and strategies the clinician can implement to minimize its effects.
- Summarize the role medication side effects play in medication nonadherence and identify strategies to lessen this response.
- Relate the concepts of health literacy and motivational interviewing to communication between the clinician and the patient to improve medication adherence.

INTRODUCTION

Medication adherence has been a long-standing problem for decades, with little to no advances in overall compliance.[1,2] *Adherence* is described as taking the prescribed medication as directed 80% or more of the time.[1] It is estimated that worldwide in developed countries medication adherence occurs only approximately 50% of the time.[1–3] This is a costly problem for the United States and other countries for several reasons:

- For the patient, it increases morbidity and mortality[1–3] while decreasing quality of life.[3]

- The financial burden of lack of adherence is estimated to be more than $100 billion annually in preventable healthcare costs.[1,4,5]
- Nonadherence-related hospitalizations are estimated to be 25% or more.[2,6]
- Nonadherence-related deaths are estimated to exceed 100,000 in the United States alone.[5,6]

These numbers are astounding. The lack of medication adherence, while prevalent, is often overlooked and frequently remains unaddressed by clinicians.[5] However, the reason we have seen so little advancement in medication adherence is because it is so multifaceted.[1,7] This chapter addresses the reasons why patients exhibit medical nonadherence.

BACKGROUND

Patients' lack of adherence can be classified as intentional, unintentional, or a combination of both. *Intentional nonadherence* is simply the decision of a patient to not adhere to the prescribed regimen. This can stem from beliefs or concerns about the disease or medication. *Unintentional nonadherence* occurs when a patient inadvertently or accidently does not follow the intended regimen. This type of nonadherence can stem from financial considerations, poor memory, or inability to open the bottle.[8,9] Remember that patients' situations change with time, and so this important question of medication adherence should be raised at each encounter.[9] Every clinician should use basic motivational interviewing to elicit why patients are noncompliant and educate them on the importance and value of adherence.[5]

INTENTIONAL NONADHERENCE

Intentional nonadherence can be a result of so many internal factors. Several studies have shown that if there are concerns about the medication, patients may dose reduce or stop. If the disease process and trajectory are not clearly understood, once adherent, a patient may become nonadherent when symptoms are under control.[8] Intentional nonadherence can stem from not only a lack of understanding but also fear—of stigma, side effects, and longevity of medication. Fear of stigma requires further research to modify but nonetheless should be identified by the prescriber.

THE ROLE OF SELF-STIGMA IN NONADHERENCE

Medication adherence has been found to be directly correlated with a patient's level of self-stigma.[10,11] To understand the concept of self-stigma, it is important to understand how self-stigmatization arises and how it is a barrier to pharmacological adherence. Stigma is a complex construct that arises from a variety of sources. *Social/perceived stigma* is the public disapproval of an individual who may differ from cultural norms.[11] To be stigmatized, one would be labeled as socially condemned or disgraced, and subsequently can be excluded or discriminated by society.[12] One example is a person with a mental illness.

Self-stigma arises when an individual takes on the label as part of their own identity and devalues themselves by internalizing the stereotype or negative connotations associated with a particular illness or disease. Nelson et al. found that self-stigma can be implicit; therefore, individuals affected with self-stigma may not have the willingness, awareness, or ability to disclose self-stigma.[13] As a result, it is of utmost importance that the clinician be cognizant of self-stigma when prescribing medications that treat socially stigmatized diseases, including depression, other mental disorders (e.g., schizophrenia), and substance use disorder.[14] Furthermore, the clinician must also consider the patients' willingness to seek treatment for their condition. Patients with socially stigmatized conditions must be motivated to treat their disease; otherwise, nonadherence is inevitable.[14] To determine whether or not a patient is motivated to treat their condition, the clinician must query the patient for the following:

- **Recognition of the problem:** A patient with drug or alcohol dependence may not believe they have a problem.
- **Willingness to obtain treatment:** A patient may say, "I want to stop or get better."
- **Past treatment history:** If the patient obtained treatment in the past, were they adherent?[14]

Additionally, studies have found that there is a negative correlation between the level of self-stigma and lower levels of education.[11] The presence of a live-in partner affects the levels of self-stigma that a patient may experience. More specifically, patients living without a partner have higher levels of self-stigma and lower levels of pharmacotherapy adherence.[11] Age and age of disease onset also play a significant role in the level of self-stigma one might experience. Kamaradova et al. found that the younger a patient is chronologically and the younger they are at diagnosis of disease, the lower their adherence to treatment.[11]

When working with patients with self-stigma, it is important for clinicians to convey a nonjudgmental acceptance of the patient and their condition, as it has been found to be "instrumental in overcoming negative emotions, self-stigma, and perceived social stigma associated with treatment."[14] Moreover, it is important to consider the aforementioned factors and how they correlate with the level of self-stigma that one may experience. Engaging in a thoughtful, systematic interview with the patient can provide the clinician with useful information that can help the clinician address the causes of self-stigma to improve their patients' adherence to treatment and/or medication.

THE ROLE OF SIDE EFFECTS IN NONADHERENCE

Medication side effects can interfere with daily activities and are a main reason for intentional nonadherence in patients.[15] Clinicians greatly underestimate side effects of medications used routinely in chronic illnesses.[16] The side effects that patients experience may result in patients lowering doses or stopping the medication altogether.[15–17] These side effects can be actual or previously held beliefs about the medication, causing the deviation from the prescribed regimen.[18] Clinicians must recognize when a side effect is not tolerable to a patient and discuss accordingly.

Patients should also be a part in the decision-making process in regard to medication options. For example, the clinician should discuss the risks and benefits of a medication or treatment with a patient. Together, they should come to an agreement on which medication will satisfy not only the treatment needs for the condition, but also the side effects the patient is willing to accept. This will help patients to be compliant with their treatment.[19]

THE ROLE OF HEALTH LITERACY IN NONADHERENCE

Health literacy can be defined as a person's knowledge, motivation, and ability to access, understand, evaluate, and utilize health information in order to make judgments and decisions in everyday life concerning healthcare, disease prevention, and health promotion to maintain or improve quality of life.[20,21] Studies have shown that people with low health literacy have a higher incidence of nonadherence to medication regimens/pharmacotherapies, inappropriate use of medications; decreased mental and physical health; noncompliance with prescribed orders; worse chronic illness control, which may lead to an increase in complications; less vocalization of health concerns; less involvement in decision-making about treatment; and overall poor communication with clinicians.[20–23] In addition to being a major cause of medication nonadherence, low health literacy has been shown to be directly related to an increase in emergency room visits and hospital utilization.[22,23]

This chapter will focus on health literacy and its effect on medication adherence and/or nonadherence. Nonadherence to pharmacotherapies is influenced by a variety of factors including: patients' lack of understanding of their disease and associated treatment, treatment demands, and lack of social support, to name a few. Patients of low socioeconomic status (SES) are most vulnerable to low health literacy due to poor education, increased likelihood of engagement in behaviors that lead to poor health (e.g., smoking, poor diet), and nonadherence to prescribed medication therapies/regimens.[22] Pharmacotherapies have an integral role in the treatment and management of myriad diseases and conditions. Failure to adhere to prescribed pharmacotherapies inevitably leads to poor health outcomes for the patient. Moreover, the cost of medication nonadherence is astounding. Improving health literacy, especially in patients of low SES, has been shown to significantly improve medication adherence.[24]

The elderly are also at a higher risk of low health literacy due to a decline in cognitive functioning as they age, which can lead to impairments in recollection and understanding. Decreased hearing and vision can contribute to difficulty reading and comprehending prescribed regimens of care. Lastly, a sense of shame or embarrassment for their lack of understanding contributes to the elderly population having less communication with their clinician regarding healthcare regimens.[25]

Currently, there is no standardized intervention(s) to improve health literacy among patients; however, there are interventions that can be utilized to improve health literacy. At the forefront, a quick health literacy screening should be completed at each clinical visit. Basic, easy-to-understand communication between clinician and patient is essential for improving health literacy. Strategies that can be implemented include utilization of culturally appropriate written and verbal information that is presented in plain, nonmedical language that patients can read and follow. Keep in mind that due to today's increasingly diverse patient population, these materials (e.g., handouts, pamphlets, educational software programs, online resources, audiovisual offerings) should be individualized for the patient's specific language and culture to be the most beneficial.[24] Con-

sciously incorporating effective communication with the patient to address the patient's concerns or questions is essential to improving health literacy. Helping the patient improve their health literacy will lead to improved healthcare decision-making, decreased healthcare system use, improved patient–clinician satisfaction, and increased adherence to prescribed pharmacotherapy.

Motivational Interviewing to Improve Health Literacy

Motivational interviewing (MI) has been shown to improve medication adherence and communication between clinician and patient.[26] MI is a form of counseling conducted by the clinician that is collaborative and patient-centered. It is used by the clinician to elicit the patient's motivation to change (e.g., behavior, commitment to adherence) by utilizing several core skills, including open-ended questions (**Table 12.1**).[27] The

TABLE 12.1 Core Motivational Interviewing Skills

Core Skills	Description
Open-ended questions	Used to establish acceptance and trust between the clinician interviewer and the patient or client; the client should be doing the majority of the talking, while the interviewer listens and encourages
Affirmations	This can be done in the manner of a compliment, highlighting an individual's strengths and efforts of behavioral change
Reflection: Simple	Repeat: Adds little to no meaning or emphasis to what the patient or client has said Rephrase: Slightly altering what a patient or client has said
Reflections: Complex	A clinician interviewer's reflection that adds additional or different meaning beyond what the patient has just said; a guess as to what the individual may have meant
Continuing the paragraph	A method of reflective listening in which the clinician offers what may be next (as yet unspoken) by the patient or client's paragraph
Amplified	Reflects back on what an individual has said in an amplified or exaggerated form—to state in an even more extreme fashion than the client or patient has done
Reflection of feeling	Emphasizing the emotional content of what the individual has said; guess about emotion(s) patient may be experiencing
Paraphrase	Speculation about what a patient or client means
Double-sided	Reflects both sides of an individual's ambivalence
Metaphor	Painting a picture that can clarify the patient or client's position

Note: Core skills of MI are patient-centered, strength-based, and authentic strategies that lead to patient activation and motivation to change.

Source: From Tucker S, Sheikholeslami D, Roberts H. Evidence-based therapeutic communication and motivational interview in health assessment. In: Gawlik KS, Melnyk BM, Teal AM, eds. *Evidence-Based Physical Examination: Best Practices for Health and Well-Being Assessment.* Springer Publishing Company; 2020: Table 25.1.

1. Assess beliefs, behavior, and knowledge about medication.
2. Advise medication behavior change.
3. Agree upon clear goals for medication use.
4. Assist in addressing barriers and securing social support.
5. Arrange follow-up meeting.[28]

purpose of this chapter is not to review all aspects of MI; rather, it is to highlight its importance and usefulness in assisting not only the clinician, but also the patient in identifying and recognizing their reasons for nonadherence.

"What ideas do you have that may be helpful for you to remember to take your birth control medication?" is an example of a MI question. Note that the question transfers the autonomy to the patient. MI has been shown to be a very effective tool for improving medication adherence if used from first contact with the patient and continually at each visit. For a more in-depth review of MI, please consult *Evidence-Based Physical Examination: Best Practices for Health and Well-Being Assessment.*[29]

Five A's Theory-Based Counseling Model

The five A's is a simple mnemonic that is used for patient counseling that promotes patient-centeredness and assists in medication- related discussion between the clinician and patient.[30,31] The five A's counseling has been associated with improved clinician–patient interaction and motivation for pharmacotherapy adherence.[32,33] See **Box 12.1** for the steps of the five A's counseling model. Utilization of the five A's is a quick and easily implemented tool that can assist the clinician in evaluating and implementing behavioral changes with the patient to address medication adherence.

UNINTENTIONAL NONADHERENCE

Unintentional nonadherence is inadvertent or accidental. Sometimes it stems from a cognitive issue or a simple misunderstanding; other times it stems from obstacles that are not preventable by the patient, such as cost or access.[9] The important thing to keep in mind with unintentional nonadherence is that the patient may or may not be aware of it, making its detection more difficult.

THE ROLE OF COST IN NONADHERENCE

Medication cost can deter patients from staying adherent to their medication regimens. A U.S. study showed that one in four elderly patients go without their medication because of cost.[3] At least one-quarter of U.S. citizens state they have problems paying medical bills.[33] Other studies have demonstrated that higher out-of-pocket payers were more likely to forego their prescriptions.[1,3,4,34–36] These statistics show that this one factor can have an enormous impact on adherence. And yet one retrospective study showed that discussion of cost was only mentioned in 30% of visits.[8]

Cost is more complex than just the simple price of a medication. Some patients may have different cost tiers with medication or a preferred medication for a specific diagnosis, while others may be self-pay. Some patients may have an initial out-of-pocket deductible that needs to be met before their insurance starts paying, while others may be dealing with additional circumstances. This is why asking about compliance and obstacles is so important. The clinician may be able to help in different ways based on why cost is an obstacle. Is there another medication that will work? Will a 90- versus 30-day supply save money? Do you have samples that you can give them? Is there an available generic formulation? Is there a local pharmacy that offers a discounted price for the prescribed drug or its generic version? Word of warning: When prescribing generics, inform the patients that the generic formulation contains the same active ingredients, although the color or shape may change. Patients sometimes feel that the generic is subpar to the brand name so advance discussion is advised.[1]

Simple probing as to why cost may be an issue has the potential to greatly impact adherence. If the patient understands the importance of the medication, a solution can often be found.

THE ROLE OF FORGETFULNESS IN NONADHERENCE

Even patients without cognitive decline forget to take their medications. After all, by prescribing a medication, the clinician is essentially asking the patient to perform a new behavioral change. Discussing the patient's daily routine and finding ways the medication regimen may fit into that routine will help to ensure adherence. Studies have shown that patients with strong routines score higher for both intentional and unintentional nonadherence. One example of how this might work is instructing an asthmatic patient to use their inhaler just before brushing their teeth. Keeping the inhaler near their toothbrush will help ensure the patient follows the new routine.[8]

Sometimes it is not possible to find a fit quite like the example. In those cases, there are a number of smartphone apps and automated home medication dispensers that have shown promise.[9,37] These solutions work best for patients without cognitive impairments.[9] A review of literature shows that for those with cognitive decline, frequent human communication is the best strategy.[38]

THE ROLE OF PATIENT EDUCATION IN NONADHERENCE

Treatment regimens can often be interpreted differently than the prescriber intended. One example is twice-a-day treatment. Some patients may interpret this directive as twice anytime in the day, such as before and after breakfast instead of morning and evening. Having the patient explain the treatment regimen back to the clinician can help ensure understanding and reduce occurrence of this type of nonadherence. The most effective method is to provide and review with the patient a patient-education form that includes the treatment plan and the times of day to take medications. The patient can take this form home and refer to it as needed.[9] The clinician should also ensure that the patient is aware of the chronicity and disease trajectory of their current health state so they fully understand the ill effects nonadherence might have on their overall health.

CONCLUSION

Adherence to pharmacotherapy is undoubtedly challenging for both the patient to achieve and for the clinician to detect. Nonadherence is as individualized as the patient themselves. The need for identification and change of nonadherence is imperative, as it affects both mortality and financial responsibility. As such, it is up to the clinician to create an environment of trust that is free of judgment and allows the patient to have a sense of empowerment about their disease management and treatment. Within this optimal environment, patients will be more willing to truthfully disclose their medication-taking behavior. Furthermore, utilization of motivational interviewing, the five A's, and observation of the patient condition can provide the clinician with clues to their adherence. Clinicians should be cognizant of the importance of health literacy and query patients accordingly to assess their health literacy. Being observant of missed appointments, poor progress in disease outcomes, missed refills, or increased hospital or outpatient clinic visits are all clues to nonadherence. Awareness of known barriers to adherence, such as complicated medication regimens, cost of medications, lack of access to medications, and low health literacy, are all elements that contribute to nonadherence. Being knowledgeable about these barriers is key to the success of patients and their improvement in pharmacotherapy adherence.

All clinicians want to see their patients as healthy as possible and prescribe regimens to this end. Remember this is a discussion, and, as such, the patient should be involved. Be sure the patient has the right information to understand the recommendation. The patient's adherence should be evaluated during every visit, even when they seem well controlled. Patients will sometimes take medications just before an appointment to give the appearance that things are controlled and they are adherent. Ensure that you have made evaluation of adherence an integral part of your exam (use the five A's). Be sure that the environment feels noncritical. If nonadherence is detected, thank the patient for their honesty and remind them that you are partners in their healthcare. Decide if the nonadherence is intentional, nonintentional, or a combination of the two, then use motivational interviewing to further uncover the root cause and assist in remedying the obstacle(s). Lastly, modify the treatment plan to what will work best for the patient.[39]

MO is a 45-year-old African American male with chronic asthma and obesity who presents with a chief complaint of knee pain. Additionally, he reports symptoms of depression. MO has been prescribed two medications for his asthma (one corticosteroid inhaler for long-term control and one bronchodilator, a rescue inhaler). He voluntarily reports that he is taking his medication exactly as prescribed. In addition to treating his chief complaint, the clinician tells MO that they will further evaluate his depressive symptoms and may be able to prescribe an antidepressant. MO discloses that his work situation is not consistent, and he has tried Prozac in the past and it didn't work.

The clinician queries, "Can you please tell me how you are taking your two asthma medications?" MO responds, "I take my Flovent HVA (long-term steroid inhaler) twice a day, and my Ventolin (beta-2 antagonist rescue inhaler) one inhalation a day when I feel wheezy." This provides an opportunity for the clinician to assess MO's health literacy by asking him to clarify what twice a day means for him.

MO responds, "I take two puffs in the morning of the Flovent." The clinician acknowledges what MO's interpretation of "twice a day" means to him; however, he clarifies in easy-to-understand terms that the Flovent should be taken two times a day, 12 hours apart. The clinician suggests, "You can take one inhalation first thing in the morning before you brush your teeth, and then again 12 hours later (usually at bedtime) before you brush your teeth."

The clinician then uses the same process to clarify the use of Ventolin and explain in layman's terms that the Ventolin is to be used only for an acute attack (not daily), one to two inhalations every 4 to 6 hours. The clinician asks MO to repeat this information to confirm understanding. MO discloses that it may be hard for him to remember to take his Flovent in the morning and before bedtime. This is an opportunity

for the clinician to utilize motivational interviewing. The clinician asks MO, "Can you think of some ideas that may help you take your Flovent medication as prescribed?" This allows MO to take autonomy of the situation and come up with a solution that best suits his lifestyle. MO suggests, "I can put the inhaler by my toothbrush because I brush my teeth in the morning and before bed, and I can put a note on my Ventolin to only use when I need it."

The clinician can now take the time to circle back to address MO's feelings of depression and past experience with Prozac, again utilizing the five A's. The clinician begins by assessing any barriers and beliefs to antidepressants by asking, "When you started taking Prozac, did you miss any doses?" This provides knowledge about how MO took the medication. The clinician can then review with MO that the antidepressant medication works best if taken at the same time every day, feelings of change in mood may not be immediate, and it can take up to 3 months to notice an effect. The clinician then continues with the remaining A's to not only promote patient centeredness, but also assist in MO's success for medication adherence. Additionally, the clinician uses this time to address and review possible side effects, investigate MO's financial situation by using nonjudgmental questions, and provide resources for access to either free or discounted medications.

Discussion Questions

1. How should the clinician classify MO's nonadherence, and what additional interventions should the clinician employ to assist this patient?
2. Outline anticipated interactions the clinician may have with this patient using the following three A's: Agree upon clear goals for medication use, assist in addressing barriers and securing social support, and arrange follow-up meeting.

CASE EXEMPLAR: Patient With Likely Unintentional Nonadherence

JS is a 75-year-old male who visits the clinic today for continued elevation of his blood pressure and for medication refills. Today his pressure is 170/110 in his left arm and 168/106 in his right arm. His wife is with him and asks if she could speak to you for a moment while JS is getting dressed. She relates that he still manages his medication by himself after she places them in the weekly pill holder at the beginning of each week. She is not certain he is taking his blood pressure medicine and is not totally sure about all of his meds.

Past Medical History
- History of hypertension 30+ years
- No known allergies
- Surgery 4 years ago for swallowed fish bone
- No history of any injuries or hospitalizations

Medications
- Simvastatin, 40 mg once daily
- Lisinopril, 40 mg once daily
- Daily iron tablet for chronic anemia

Family History
- Father and mother had a history of hypertension and elevated cholesterol.

Social History
- Smoked one pack of cigarettes per day; quit 15 years ago

Physical Examination
- Chest clear to auscultation
- Denies chest pain
- No dyspnea on exertion
- EKG: rsR, right bundle branch conduction abnormality (RBBB)

Discussion Questions
1. The clinician decides to have JS complete an initial health literacy screening. What does the clinician anticipate finding?
2. After visiting with JS, the clinician believes JS is unintentionally nonadherent. What factors would help the clinician come to this conclusion, especially given JS's age?
3. JS's wife fails to confirm there are any financial problems relative to medication acquisition. How could the clinician discuss this with JS's wife, and using the discussion regarding health literacy, how could the clinician assist this couple?

CLINICAL PEARLS

- Adherence is described as taking the prescribed medication as directed 80% or more of the time.
- The five A's can assist the clinician in intervening with nonadherence: (a) Assess beliefs, behavior, and knowledge about their medication; (b) Advise medication behavior change; (c) Agree upon clear goals for medication use; (d) Assist in addressing barriers and securing social support; and (e) Arrange follow-up meeting.
- It is important to take time to address the concern of the cost of medication and nonadherence.
- Determining the ways medication regimens fit with the patient's daily schedule will help with the success of adherence. Phone apps may also help significantly.
- Having patients explain treatment expectations back to you using their own words will identify areas that need clarification.
- Written treatment plans that include times of day to take medications is a proven method for supporting adherence.

KEY TAKEAWAYS

- It is estimated that medication adherence occurs only 50% of the time.
- Nonadherence is costly to all involved, both physically and fiscally, with the suggested financial burden estimated to be more than $100 billion annually. These costs are considered preventable.
- *Intentional nonadherence* is the decision of a patient to not adhere to the prescribed regimen. *Unintentional nonadherence* occurs when a patient inadvertently or accidently does not follow the intended regimen.
- Self-stigma arises when an individual takes on a negative label as part of their own identity. Patients with conditions that initiate self-stigma must be motivated to treat their disease.
- In most cases of self-stigma, nonadherence is inevitable.
- The clinician assists patients prone to nonadherence by encouraging them to admit they have a problem and that they are willing to treat it.

REFERENCES

1. Sanchez C, Farrell N, Lapp E. Generic drugs, cost, and medication adherence. *US Pharm.* 2015;6:14–19. https://www.uspharmacist.com/article/generic-drugs-cost-and-medication-adherence

2. Lam WL, Fresco P. Medication adherence measures: an overview. *Biomed Res Int.* 2015;2015:1–12. doi:10.1155/2015/217047

3. Aziz H, Hatah E, Makmor Bakry M, et al. How payment scheme affects patients' adherence to medications? A systematic review. *Patient Prefer Adherence.* 2016;10:837–850. doi:10.2147/PPA.S103057

4. Milan R, Vasiliadis HM, Gontijo Guerra S, et al. Out-of-pocket costs and adherence to antihypertensive agents among older adults covered by the public drug insurance plan in Quebec. *Patient Prefer Adherence.* 2017;11:1513–1522. doi:10.2147/PPA.S138364

5. Kleinsinger F. The unmet challenge of medication nonadherence. *Perm J.* 2018;22:18–33. doi:10.7812/TPP/18-033

6. Kim J, Combs K, Downs J, et al. Medication adherence: the elephant in the room. *US Pharm.* 2018;43:30–34. https://www.uspharmacist.com/article/medication-adherence-the-elephant-in-the-room

7. Zullig LL, Blalock DV, Dougherty S, et al. The new landscape of medication adherence improvement: where population health science meets precision medicine. *Patient Prefer Adherence.* 2018;12:1225–1230. doi:10.2147/PPA.S165404

8. Thorneloe RJ, Griffiths CEM, Emsley R, et al. Intentional and unintentional medication non–adherence in psoriasis: the role of patients' medication beliefs and habit strength. *J Invest Dermatol.* 2018;138(4):785–794. doi:10.1016/j.jid.2017.11.015

9. Usherwood T. Encouraging adherence to long-term medication. *Aust Prescr.* 2017;40(4):147–150. doi:10.18773/austprescr.2017.050

10. Cinculova A, Prasko J, Kamaradova D, et al. Adherence, self-stigma and discontinuation of pharmacotherapy in patients with anxiety disorders—Cross-sectional study. *Neuro Endocrinol Lett.* 2017;38(6):429–442. https://www.nel.edu/userfiles/articlesnew/38_6_Cinculova_429-436.pdf

11. Kamaradova D, Latalova K, Prasko J, et al. Connection between self-stigma, adherence to treatment, and discontinuation of medication. *Patient Prefer Adherence.* 2016;10:1289–1298. doi:10.2147/PPA.S99136

12. Feldhaus T, Falke S, von Gruchalla L, et al. The impact of self-stigmatization on medication attitude in schizophrenia patients. *Psychiatry Res.* 2018;261:391–399. doi:10.1016/j.psychres.2018.01.012

13. Nelson E, Werremeyer A, Kelly GA, et al. Self-stigma of antidepressant users through secondary analysis of photovoice data. *Ment Health Clin.* 2018;8(5):214–221. doi:10.9740/mhc.2018.09.214

14. Hammarlund R Crapanzano KA, Luce L, et al. Review of the effects of self-stigma and perceived social stigma on the treatment-seeking decisions of individuals with drug- and alcohol-use disorders. *Subst Abuse Rehabil.* 2018;9:115–136. doi:10.2147/SAR.S183256

15. Tedla YG, Bautista LE. Drug side effect symptoms and adherence to antihypertensive medication. *Am J Hypertens.* 2016;29(6):772–779. doi:10.1093/ajh/hpv185

16. Cooper V, Metcalf L, Versnel J, et al. Patient-reported side effects, concerns and adherence to corticosteroid treatment for asthma, and comparison with physician estimates of side-effect prevalence: a UK-wide, cross-sectional study. *NPJ Prim Care Respir Med.* 2015;25:15026. doi:10.1038/npjpcrm.2015.26

17. Morrison P, Meehan T, Stomski NJ. Living with antipsychotic medication side-effects. *Int J Ment Health Nurs.* 2015;24:253–261. doi:10.1111/inm.12110

18. Heller MK, Chapman SCE, Horne R. Beliefs about medication predict the misattribution of a common symptom as a medication side effect—Evidence from an analogue online study. *J Psychosom Res.* 2015;79(6):519–529. doi:10.1016/j.jpsychores.2015.10.003

19. Wykes T, Evans J, Paton C, et al. What side effects are problematic for patients prescribed antipsychotic medication? The Maudsley Side Effects (MSE) measure for antipsychotic medication. *Psychol Med.* 2017;47(13):2369–2378. doi:10.1017/S0033291717000903

20. Peerson A, Saunders M. Health literacy revisited: what do we mean and why does it matter? *Health Promot Int.* 2009;24(3):285–296. doi:10.1093/heapro/dap014

21. Kickbusch I, Pelikan JM, Apfel F, Tsouros AD, eds. *Health Literacy: The Solid Facts.* The World Health Organization, Regional Office for Europe; 2013. https://apps.who.int/iris/bitstream/handle/10665/128703/e96854.pdf

22. Jansen T, Rademakers J, Waverijin G, et al. The role of health literacy in explaining the association between educational attainment and the use of out-of-hours primary care services in chronically ill people: a survey study. *BMC Health Serv Res.* 2018;18(1):394. doi:10.1186/s12913-018-3197-4

23. Campbell ZC, Stevenson JK, McCaffery KJ, et al. Interventions for improving health literacy in people with chronic kidney disease. *Cochrane Database Syst Rev.* 2016;(2):CD012026. doi:10.1002/14651858.CD012026

24. Miller TA. Health literacy and adherence to medical treatment in chronic and acute illness: a meta-analysis. *Patient Educ Couns.* 2016;99(7):1079–1086. doi:10.1016/j.pec.2016.01.020

25. Chesser AK, Keene Woods N, Smothers K, et al. Health literacy and older adults: a systematic review. *Gerontol Geriatr Med.* 2016;2. doi:10.1177/2333721416630492

26. McKenzie K, Chang Y. The effect of nurse-led motivational interviewing on medication adherence in patients with bipolar disorder. *Perspect Psychiatr Care.* 2015;51(1):36–44. doi:10.1111/ppc.12060

27. Rosengren DB. *Building Motivational Skills: A Practitioner Workbook.* 2nd ed. The Guilford Press; 2018.

28. Vallis M, Piccinini-Vallis H, Sharma AM, et al. Clinical review: modified 5 A's: minimal intervention for obesity counseling in primary care. *Can Fam Physician.* 2013;59(1):27–31. https://www.cfp.ca/content/cfp/59/1/27.full.pdf

29. Tucker S, Sheikholeslami D, Roberts H. Evidence-based therapeutic communication and motivational interview in health assessment. In: Gawlik KS, Melnyk BM, Teal AM, eds. *Evidence-Based Physical Examination: Best Practices for Health and Well-Being Assessment.* Springer Publishing Company; 2020.

30. Franziska D, Stein J, Pabst A, et al. Five A's counseling in weight management of obese patients in primary care: a cluster-randomized controlled trial (INTERACT). *BMC Fam Pract.* 2018;19(1):97. doi:10.1186/s12875-018-0785-7

31. Pollak K, Tulsky JA, Bravender T, et al. Teaching primary care physicians the 5 A's for discussing weight with overweight and obese adolescents. *Patient Educ Couns.* 2016;99(10):1620–1625. doi:10.1016/j.pec.2016.05.007

32. Jay M, Gillespie C, Schlair S, et al. Physicians' use of the 5A's in counseling obese patients: is the quality of counseling associated with patients' motivation and intention to lose weight? *BMC Health Serv Res.* 2010;10:159. doi:10.1186/1472-6963-10-159

33. Hunter WG, Zhang CZ, Hesson A, et al. What strategies do physicians and patients discuss to reduce out-of-pocket costs? Analysis of cost-saving strategies in 1,755 outpatient clinic visits. *Med Decis Making.* 2016;36(7):900–910. doi:10.1177/0272989X15626384

34. Farias AJ, Du XL. Association between out-of-pocket costs, race/ethnicity, and adjuvant endocrine therapy adherence among Medicare patients with breast cancer. *J Clin Oncol.* 2016;35(1):86–95. doi:10.1200/JCO.2016.68.2807

35. Bibeau WS, Fu H, Taylor AD, et al. Impact of out-of-pocket pharmacy costs on branded medication adherence among patients with type 2 diabetes. *J Manag Care Spec Pharm.* 2016;22(11):1338–1347. doi:10.18553/jmcp.2016.22.11.1338

36. Kaul S, Avila JC, Mehta HB, et al. Cost-related medication nonadherence among adolescent and young adult cancer survivors. *Cancer.* 2017;123:2726–2734. doi:10.1002/cncr.30648

37. Hoffmann C, Schweighardt A, Conn K, et al. Enhanced adherence in patients using an automated home medication dispenser. *J Healthc Qual.* 2018;40(4):194–200. doi:10.1097/JHQ.0000000000000097

38. Costa E, Giardini A, Savin M, et al. Interventional tools to improve medication adherence: review of literature. *Patient Prefer Adherence.* 2015;9:1303–1314. doi:10.2147/PPA.S87551

39. Brown MT, Sinsky C. *Medication Adherence: Improve the Health of Your Patients and Reduce Overall Healthcare Costs.* American Medical Association Stepsforward. Published 2018. https://edhub.ama-assn.org/steps-forward/module/2702595?resultClick=1&bypassSolrId=J_2702595

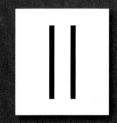

System-Specific and Patient-Focused Prescribing

Pharmacotherapy for Ear, Nose, Mouth, and Throat Conditions

Jaclyn K. Gaulden, Elizabeth F. Snyder, and Catherine C. Wilson

LEARNING OBJECTIVES

- Differentiate between acute otitis media (AOM) and acute otitis externa (AOE) according to etiology, signs and symptoms, and management.
- Describe the manifestation of cerumen impaction, identify populations at risk, and discuss management strategies.
- Describe the manifestation of allergic rhinitis and identify its treatment options.
- Differentiate between bacterial and viral rhinosinusitis in regard to symptoms and management.
- Outline the more common oral and dental disorders and identify appropriate management strategies.

INTRODUCTION

Among the most common reasons for patients to visit their primary care clinicians are ear, nose, mouth, and throat complaints.[1] Ophthalmic, nasal, and oral diseases and infections affect people of all ages. For example, newborn infants have an increased risk for candidiasis infections of the tongue and oral cavity, and small children are at greater risk for acute otitis media among other illnesses. Adolescents are at increased risk for infections such as mononucleosis and streptococcal pharyngitis, whereas, adults are at risk for work-related exposure to nasal irritants, and the elderly are at increased risk for cecum impaction, dental loss, and dry mouth. As a result, clinicians require an extensive

working knowledge of ophthalmic-, ototic-, nasal-, and oral-treatment medications. Clinicians must understand the implication of these medications, how they should be used in different patient populations, and the precautions (if any) they should take when prescribing these medications.

Before any treatment for ear, sinus, oral, or dental procedures is considered, the clinician should consider if all preventative measures have been taken and whether the patient has been properly educated for reduction of symptoms in the future. Current guidelines for treatment include recommendations to maximize patient care and are based upon the highest levels of evidence with consideration of the risk and benefit ratio.[2]

This chapter will examine the treatment of some of the most common diseases affecting the ear, nose, mouth, and throat. In addition, special considerations, such as renal dose modifications and age-related constraints needed for the medications, will also be addressed.

PHARMACOTHERAPY FOR COMMON EAR CONDITIONS

BACKGROUND

Human medicine has been studied for centuries but real progress in the understanding of bodily systems occurred only in relatively recent history. Draining ears from acute otitis media with rupture was so common that until the 17th century, it was considered normal. In the 17th century, scientists began to write about ear anatomy, but clear understanding of ototic ailments developed only after the invention of the otoscope by von Troeltsch in Germany in 1860.[3]

The ear consists of three general parts: Outer (external) ear, inner ear, and middle ear (**Figure 13.1**).

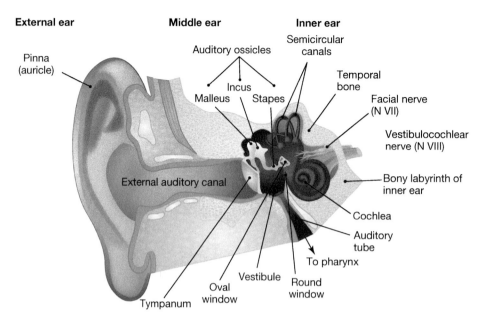

FIGURE 13.1 Anatomy of the ear.

Source: Colandrea M, Raynor E. Evidence-based assessment of the ears, nose, and throat. In: Gawlik KS, Melnyk BM, Teall AM, eds. *Evidence-Based Physical Examination: Best Practices for Health & Well-Being Assessment.* Springer Publishing Company; 2021: Fig. 13.2.

The function of the ear is to transmit airwaves and turn them into sound. The ear functions best under fairly dry conditions. If anything blocks the flow of air or pushes on the delicate parts of the middle and inner ear, hearing is affected and often pain results. The blockages can occur from cerumen, exudate, or swelling of the tissue alone or in combination.

ACUTE OTITIS MEDIA

Acute otitis media (AOM) is an infection of the middle ear that can also involve the rupture of the tympanic membrane. AOMs occur because of eustachian tube dysfunction. The eustachian tubes allow air and fluid to drain from the middle ear to equalize pressure. If the eustachian tubes do not function correctly, fluid can become trapped in the middle ear causing otitis media with effusion (OME; **Figure 13.2**). If bacteria is also trapped with the fluid, their growth causes AOM. The most common bacteria associated with AOM infections are *Streptococcus pneumoniae* (gram-positive), *Haemophilus influenza* (gram-negative), and *Moraxella catarrhalis* (gram-negative).

Children who are at increased risk for AOM include those who are bottle-fed or exposed to cigarette smoke, in day care, have a family history of AOM, use pacifiers, or have a history of gastroesophageal reflux.[4]

Like most ototic problems, the diagnosis for AOM is made from the history and physical examination of the patient. Patients with AOM will often have a history of acute upper respiratory infection either of viral or allergic etiology.[5] The patient will complain of pain, impaired hearing, fever, and purulent drainage if rupture

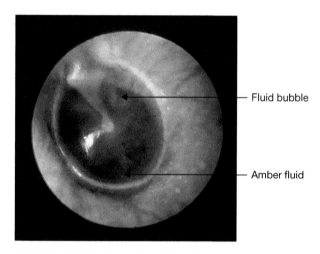

FIGURE 13.2 Otitis media with effusion.

Source: Colandrea M, Raynor E. Evidence-based assessment of the ears, nose, and throat. In: Gawlik KS, Melnyk BM, Teall AM, eds. *Evidence-Based Physical Examination: Best Practices for Health & Well-Being Assessment.* Springer Publishing Company; 2021: Fig. 13.34

of the tympanic membrane has occurred. On physical examination, the clinician will note an erythematous and bulging tympanic membrane. If rupture has occurred, the inner ear can be filled with purulent drainage, but the tragus will not be painful. If there is not much purulent drainage, the clinician may sometimes see a hole in the tympanic membrane.

Treatment for Acute Otitis Media

Prevention is still the best treatment. Advising parents to vaccinate children for *H. influenza*, influenza, and the conjugated pneumococcal vaccine has been shown to decrease the likelihood of AOM.[6–8] Like all ototic infections, treatment depends on the age and symptoms of the patient. For example, in children over 6 months of age and adults, watchful waiting is an option for AOM depending on the severity of symptoms[5]; however, it is important to treat the pain with analgesics. The standard of care for first-line antibiotics is high-dose amoxicillin if the patient has not been exposed to other antibiotics in the past 30 days, there is not concurrent purulent conjunctivitis, and there is no penicillin allergy. For patients with penicillin allergies, the first-line treatment is cefdinir.[5,9] There are, however, those who favor the guideline changes to first-line amoxicillin–clavulanate since "a significant proportion of otopathogens in the pneumococcal vaccine ear are not sensitive to amoxicillin."[10,11] The second-line antibiotic is either amoxicillin–clavulanate or clindamycin with or without ceftriaxone for patients with penicillin allergies.[9] See **Table 13.1** for treatment options for AOM.

ACUTE OTITIS EXTERNA

Acute otitis externa (AOE) is an infection or inflammation of the external auditory canal or inner ear, the pinna or outer ear, or both. This occurs when the delicate tissues of the ear are compromised by the introduction of bacteria, changes in pH, or mechanical damage. AOE is commonly called *swimmer's ear* since the exposure to water in the inner ear can cause maceration of the tissue and allow the growth of fungus or bacteria. The most common bacteria seen in AOE is *Pseudomonas aeruginosa* and *Staphylococcus aureus*.[12]

The risk factors for AOE include inner ear exposure to water, hairy ear canals, canal stenosis, use of ear plugs or hearing aids, and skin conditions such as eczema or psoriasis.[13]

Treatment for Acute Otitis Externa

Treatment for AOE depends on age and whether the tympanic membrane is intact. The primary focus of treatment is management of pain and, if possible, the removal of exudate in the inner ear.[14] AOE is treated with ear drops, but not all drops can be used in patients without an intact tympanic membrane. Nonantibiotic treatment for patients with an intact tympanic membrane include analgesics and over-the-counter (OTC) acetic acid drops.[14] Antibiotic drops that can be used in people without an intact tympanic membrane include ofloxacin 0.3%; ciprofloxacin 0.2% plus hydrocortisone 1.0%; or ciprofloxacin 0.3% plus dexamethasone 0.1%. See **Table 13.2** for treatment options for AOE.

Ciprofloxacin is much more expensive than ofloxacin, but the safety and efficacy of both antibiotics are generally not established for children less than 6 months of age. Neomycin, polymyxin B, and hydrocortisone are less expensive than ciprofloxacin; nevertheless, they can be used only with an intact tympanic membrane.[13] If there is a significant swelling, the clinician should place a wick in the inner ear to allow the distribution of the medication.

CERUMEN IMPACTION

Cerumen is a naturally occurring substance that protects and cleans the middle ear. If there is a buildup of cerumen, it can harden and totally or partially block the inner ear, which may cause pain and hearing loss. Cerumen impaction can occur at any age but is more common in older adults.[15] Cerumen impaction risk is

TABLE 13.1 Pharmacotherapy for Acute Otitis Media				
Medication	Dose/Frequency	Indications	Contraindications	Common Side Effects
Amoxicillin	Adult: 500–1,000 mg q12h Pediatric: 95 mg/kg divided q12h	First-line for AOM	Hypersensitivity to amoxicillin; concurrent purulent conjunctivitis; PCN allergy	Diarrhea
Erythromycin base/ sulfisoxazole	200/600 per 5 mL	First-line for AOM with PCN allergy	Hypersensitivity to erythromycin or sulfisoxazole	Diarrhea
Cefdinir	14 mg/kg/day in one to two doses	Second-line for AOM with PCN allergy	Hypersensitivity to cefdinir; slight potential for reaction with PCN allergy	Diarrhea, red-colored stools
Amoxicillin–clavulanate	Adult: 875 mg q12h Pediatric: 80–100 mg q12h	First- or second-line for AOM if multidrug-resistant *Streptococcus pneumoniae* is suspected	Hypersensitivity to amoxicillin or other component of medication; history of cholestatic jaundice	Diarrhea (>10%)

AOM, acute otitis media; PCN, penicillin; q12h, every 12 hours.

TABLE 13.2 Pharmacotherapy for Acute Otitis Externa

Medication	Dose/Frequency	Indications	Contraindications	Common Side Effects
Ciprofloxacin 0.3% and dexamethasone 0.1%	Four drops q12h	AOE with or without perforation in children 6–12 months of age	Hypersensitivity to any component of the medication	N/A
Ofloxacin otic 0.3%	Five drops bid	AOE with or without perforation in children >12 months of age	Hypersensitivity to any component of the medication	N/A
Neomycin and polymyxin B sulfates and hydrocortisone otic suspension	Four drops q6–8h	AOE without perforation	Hypersensitivity to any component of the medication	N/A

AOE, acute otitis externa; bid, twice daily; q6–8h, every six to eight hours; q12h, every 12 hours.

increased in children, persons with mental limitations, and the elderly, especially those in nursing homes. Approximately 10% of children, 33% of people with mental limitations, and 57% of elderly people living in nursing homes experience cerumen impaction.[15]

There is often a history of hearing loss or pain with cerumen impaction. Diagnosis of cerumen impaction is made by inspection of the inner ear. The clinician will note a large amount of cerumen in the ear canal and may not be able to visualize the tympanic membrane.

Treatment for Cerumen Impaction

Cerumen impaction is treated by the removal of the cerumen. This can be done at home with commercially available tools, such as Mack's ProRinse©. Other at-home ear wax removers, such as the Clinere Personal Ear Cleaners©, should not be used at home due to the risk of tympanic membrane perforation. Without the ability to view the inner ear, the patient cannot be sure that the wax has been removed. The patient should be advised not to use cotton swabs as these can push cerumen farther back in the canal, causing pain and worsening the impaction. The clinician can remove the wax using either the ear-wash method or direct removal of the wax. Uses of a product like carbamide peroxide can soften the cerumen prior to cerumen removal, allowing easier removal by a healthcare professional.[16]

PHARMACOTHERAPY FOR COMMON NASAL CONDITIONS

BACKGROUND

Dr. John Bostock was the first to describe hay fever in his paper read to the Medical and Chirurgical Society on March 16, 1819.[17] When exposed to an allergen, inflammatory cells such as mast cells, CD4-positive T cells, B cells, macrophages, and eosinophils infiltrate the lining of the nose. This results in arteriolar dilation due to the release of histamine and leukotrienes. See **Figure 13.3** for anatomy of the internal nasal cavity.

ALLERGIC RHINITIS

Allergic rhinitis, which is the most common type of chronic rhinitis, is a common disorder that is thought to affect up to 40% of the population and is defined as an inflammation of the nasal mucosa.[18] Contrary to prior thought, allergic rhinitis is not localized to the nose and passageways; instead, it involves the entire respiratory tract. Likewise, it was traditionally thought that allergic rhinitis was either seasonal or perennial; however, some patients do not fit into either of these categories. The Allergic Rhinitis and Its Impact on Asthma (ARIA) guidelines have classified allergic rhinitis in a different way[18]:

- **Intermittent allergic rhinitis:** Present in patients when symptoms occur fewer than 4 days/week or fewer than 4 consecutive weeks
- **Persistent allergic rhinitis:** Present in patients when symptoms occur more than 4 days a week or for more than 4 consecutive weeks
- **Symptoms:**
  - Mild: Does not impair sleep or activities of daily living
  - Moderate or severe: Significantly affects sleep or activities of daily living

Risk factors for allergic rhinitis include family history; birth during pollen season; early use of antibiotics; maternal smoking, particularly during the first year of life; first-born status; and presence of allergen-specific IgE.[19]

Allergic rhinitis generally presents with sneezing, rhinorrhea, nasal itching and obstruction, postnasal drip, cough, and, on occasion, itching of the palate and

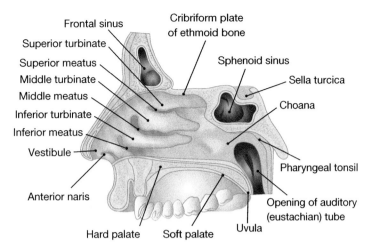

FIGURE 13.3 Anatomy of the internal nasal cavity.
Source: Colandrea M, Raynor E. Evidence-based assessment of the ears, nose, and throat. In: Gawlik KS, Melnyk BM, Teall AM, eds. *Evidence-Based Physical Examination: Best Practices for Health & Well-Being Assessment.* Springer Publishing Company; 2021:Fig. 13.11.

inner ear. In addition, some patients will have fatigue and general malaise. Physical findings include "allergic shiners," which are dark circles under the eyes that resemble bruises or "black eyes"; Dennie-Morgan line, a fold or line in the skin below the lower eyelid; and a transverse nasal crease. Physical examination will often show pale and boggy turbinates and clear rhinorrhea. "Cobblestoning" can often be found in the posterior pharynx, which is hyperplastic lymphoid tissue. Laboratory testing is usually normal in patients with allergic rhinitis. The diagnosis of allergic rhinitis can be made on the presence of the characteristic symptoms, history, and physical findings. Imaging is not usually performed.

In more difficult or complicated cases, patients can be referred for allergy testing to find the specific allergens causing the symptoms. Options for allergy testing include skin testing, serum testing, nasal cytology (helps to differentiate an allergy from an infection), and allergy challenge.[19]

Treatment for Allergic Rhinitis

Relief of symptoms is the goal in patients with allergic rhinitis. Therapeutic options include avoidance of allergens first, then nasal saline irrigation, oral antihistamines (second-generation are first-line), intranasal corticosteroids, combination intranasal corticosteroid/antihistamine sprays, leukotriene receptor antagonists, and allergen immunotherapy or a combination. Second-generation oral antihistamines include fexofenadine, desloratadine, loratadine, and cetirizine. Decongestants may be used short term only.

If symptoms persist, an allergist referral should be considered.[18] See **Table 13.3** for treatment options for allergic rhinitis.

PHARMACOTHERAPY FOR COMMON SINUS CONDITIONS

BACKGROUND

Ancient Egyptians first identified the paranasal sinuses, and there is indication that they were aware of the maxillary sinuses as early as 3700 to 1500 BCE due to medical writings dating back this far. Egyptians are thought to be the pioneers of sinus surgery because they used special instruments to remove the brain through the ethmoid cells.[20]

Humans have four sets of sinuses, which are all lined with pseudostratified columnar epithelium (**Figure 13.4**). The largest sinuses, which are located under the eyes in the maxillary bones, are the maxillary sinuses. The frontal sinuses are above the eyes within the frontal bone.[21] Only the maxillary and frontal sinuses can be indirectly examined. The ethmoid and sphenoid sinuses cannot be directly examined due to their position in the skull and their smaller size.[22] The ethmoid sinuses sit between the nose and the eyes while the sphenoid sinuses are located within the sphenoid bone. The sinuses play several roles including decreasing the weight of the skull, providing a buffer against facial trauma, heating and humidifying air, and providing an immunological defense against pathogens.[21]

TABLE 13.3 Pharmacotherapy for Allergic Rhinitis

Medication	Dose/Frequency	Indications	Contraindications	Side Effects
Cetirizine	Adult: 10 mg once daily 6–12 months: 2.5 mg once daily 1–2 years: 2.5 mg once daily; may increase to 2.5 mg q12h 2–5 years: 2.5 mg once daily; may increase to 2.5 mg q12h or 5 mg once daily	Allergic rhinitis	Hypersensitivity to cetirizine, hydroxyzine, or any component of the medication	Drowsiness, headache, insomnia, dizziness
Fexofenadine	Adult: 180 mg once daily 2–11 years: 30 mg q12h; max 60 mg/d	Allergic rhinitis	Allergic reaction to fexofenadine or any component of the medication	Headache, vomiting
Loratadine	Adult: 10 mg once daily 2–5 years: 5 mg once daily	Allergic rhinitis	Hypersensitivity to loratadine or any component of the medication	Headache, sedation, drowsiness, fatigue, nervousness, xerostomia
Fluticasone propionate	Adult: 2 sprays once daily or q12h (severe rhinitis) Pediatric: 1–2 sprays once daily	Allergic rhinitis	Hypersensitivity to fluticasone or any component of the medication	Headache, body pain, dizziness, weight gain
Fluticasone propionate/ azelastine hydrochloride	Adult: 1 spray bid <12 years: Not recommended	Allergic rhinitis	No contraindication in U.S. labeling	Headache, dysgeusia, epistaxis
Montelukast	Adult: 10 mg once daily Pediatric: Dependent upon seasonal vs. perennial allergic rhinitis	Allergic rhinitis	Hypersensitivity to montelukast or any component of the medication	Headache, dizziness, fatigue, atopic dermatitis

bid, twice daily; q12h, every 12 hours

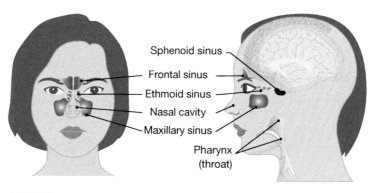

FIGURE 13.4 Paranasal sinuses.
Source: Colandrea M, Raynor E. Evidence-based assessment of the ears, nose, and throat. In: Gawlik KS, Melnyk BM, Teall AM, eds. *Evidence-Based Physical Examination: Best Practices for Health & Well-Being Assessment.* Springer Publishing Company; 2021: Fig. 13.12.

RHINOSINUSITIS

Acute rhinosinusitis (ARS) is the symptomatic inflammation of the paranasal sinusitis and the nasal cavity.[23] The most common etiology of ARS is viral, although bacterial infection does occur in 0.5% to 2% of cases.[24] The classification of ARS is based on symptom duration. Acute rhinosinusitis occurs with symptoms fewer than 4 weeks, subacute with symptoms for 4 to 12 weeks, chronic with symptoms greater than 12 weeks, and recurrent with four or more episodes per year.[25]

Acute viral rhinosinusitis (AVRS) is caused from a direct contact with the conjunctiva or nasal mucosa. Rhinovirus, influenza, and parainfluenza virus are the most common viral causes. Symptoms usually present the first day after inoculation. Acute bacterial rhinosinusitis (ABRS), which is the most common complication of a viral infection, occurs when bacteria infect an inflamed sinus cavity. ABRS can occur with other conditions that obstruct the nose, such as allergic rhinitis, dental infection, or immunodeficiency. The most common bacteria occurring with ABRS are *S. pneumoniae*, *H. influenza*, and *M. catarrhalis*.[23]

Risk factors for chronic rhinosinusitis include genetics, comorbid medical conditions, and demographic and environmental factors. Medical conditions that can put one at a higher risk for chronic rhinosinusitis are those that affect the airway, such as allergic rhinitis and asthma. Gastroesophageal reflux disease (GERD) has also been linked to chronic rhinosinusitis. Environmental exposures such as tobacco have been shown to increase rhinosinusitis.[26] Any patient with chronic rhinosinusitis should be assessed for modifying factors in addition to those already mentioned; these include allergy and immune testing, cystic fibrosis, immunocompromised status, and presence of nasal polyps or ciliary dyskinesia.[25]

Although the symptoms of AVRS and ABRS overlap and there is no validated clinical criteria to distinguish between them, they have different clinical courses. AVRS is similar in course to other upper viral respiratory infections and has partial or complete resolution within 7 to 10 days. If a fever is present, it is present early in the illness before respiratory symptoms become more prominent. Patients with ABRS generally have symptoms that last longer than 10 days and tend to have a biphasic pattern (worsening after a period of improvement). Symptoms of ARS include nasal congestion, purulent discharge, and sinus discomfort. Patients may also have symptoms of fever, fatigue, cough, headache, and ear pain.

Physical findings on examination may include tenderness over the cheeks or upper teeth, as well as edema or erythema and purulent drainage in the nose or posterior pharynx. The physical finding of pain or pressure with percussion of the sinuses is not diagnostic in isolation, and the sensitivity and specificity has not been fully established. In addition, transillumination of the maxillary and frontal sinuses does not have enough sensitivity or specificity for use in diagnosis. The diagnosis of ARS is based on clinical signs and symptoms and is diagnosed when a patient presents with nasal obstruction, facial pain/pressure, and fewer than 4 weeks of purulent nasal drainage. Secondary symptoms such as cough and headache support the diagnosis.[23] ABRS cannot be diagnosed based on nasal purulence, which is a sign of inflammation and not infection.[25]

Treatment for Rhinosinusitis

Patients with AVRS do not require antibiotic therapy and should be managed with symptomatic therapies. Symptomatic therapies for both AVRS and ABRS include OTC analgesics and antipyretics, saline irrigation, and intranasal glucocorticoids. A course of oral decongestants (3–5 days) can be considered when eustachian tube dysfunction is an issue along with the AVRS.[23] Oral decongestants should be cautioned in patients with certain medical conditions, including hypertension and anxiety.[25]

In patients with uncomplicated ABRS, 2015 guidelines recommend that they be managed symptomatically and observed in follow-up. Factors such as general health, age, and comorbidities must be taken into consideration when choosing this option. For patients who do not have good follow up or are at high risk, antibiotics should be started, whereas patients who are observed and seen in follow up require antibiotics if they worsen or fail to improve within 7 days.[23]

For patients without risk factors for pneumococcal resistance, amoxicillin two or three times daily can be prescribed. The other option is amoxicillin–clavulanate two or three times daily. Coverage for ampicillin-resistant *H. influenzae* and *M. catarrhalis* are improved with the addition of clavulanate to the amoxicillin. For patients with high risk factors, such as age ≥65 years, hospitalization in the last 5 days, antibiotic use within the past month, compromised immune system, multiple comorbidities, or severe infection for pneumococcal resistance, high-dose amoxicillin–clavulanate is recommended.

For patients with a penicillin allergy, doxycycline once or twice daily is recommended as initial therapy. Patients who are improving on therapy should be treated with antibiotic therapy for 5 to 7 days.[23] Most trials in patients with ARS are with antibiotic therapy for 10 days. Studies have shown more adverse events with the longer course of antibiotics (10 days compared to 5 days); therefore, shorter courses should be considered for patients with illness that is not as severe.[25] Although there is limited data regarding treatment failure and secondary options, patients who fail to improve or worsen on initial therapy should be treated with a broader spectrum drug and/or a drug in a different drug class than the first drug used. Options include amoxicillin–clavulanate, levofloxacin; or moxifloxacin. For the penicillin-allergic patient, treatment options include doxycycline and levofloxacin, or moxifloxacin. The fluoroquinolones should be used only when there are no other treatment options as the risks generally outweigh the benefits. Patients who fail a second course of antibiotic therapy should be referred for imaging and further evaluation. Likewise, a relapse after another treatment of 7 to 10 days should be referred for further evaluation.[23] See **Table 13.4** for treatment options for rhinosinusitis.

CT scan or MRI can be recommended in complicated cases, severe illnesses, and suspected complications such as intraocular infections. Sinus aspirate or endoscopic cultures can be done in patients with suspected intracranial involvement or other complications.[23]

TABLE 13.4 Pharmacotherapy for Rhinosinusitis

Medication	Dose/Frequency	Indications	Contraindications	Side Effects
Doxycycline	Adult: 100 mg bid or 200 mg once daily	Rhinosinusitis	Hypersensitivity to doxycycline, other tetracyclines, or any component of the medication	Hypertension, diarrhea
Levofloxacin	500–750 mg once daily	Rhinosinusitis	Hypersensitivity to levofloxacin, any component of the medication, or other quinolones; fluoroquinolones may prolong QTc interval	Black-Box Warning: Tendinitis and tendon rupture, peripheral neuropathy, CNS effects
Moxifloxacin	400 mg once daily	Rhinosinusitis	Hypersensitivity to levofloxacin, any component of the medication, or other quinolones; fluoroquinolones may prolong QTc interval	Black-Box Warning: Tendinitis and tendon rupture, peripheral neuropathy, CNS effects
Amoxicillin–clavulanate	Adult: 875 mg q12h Pediatric: 80–100 mg q12h	Acute rhinosinusitis	Hypersensitivity to amoxicillin or any other component of the medication; history of cholestatic jaundice	Diarrhea (>10%)

bid, twice daily; CNS, central nervous system; q12h, every 12 hours; qd, once daily.

PHARMACOTHERAPY FOR COMMON ORAL AND DENTAL CONDITIONS

BACKGROUND

Treatments for oral and dental conditions date back centuries with physicians typically treating medical conditions, and dentists working to extract teeth, create dentures, and drill and fill teeth. In 1880, American dentist Willoughby Miller studied oral bacteria at a microscopic level and concluded that mouth germs were a vector for all human suffering.[27] Thus, physicians in America and Britain were known to order dental extractions and tonsillectomies to treat a range of disorders, including hiccups, madness, cancers, phobias, and hypertension. Today, medicine continues to be specialized as dentists care for most oral-hygiene issues and physicians treat other medical conditions.

COMMON ORAL AND DENTAL CONDITIONS

Candida albicans is often an associated factor in infections involving the oral mucous membranes and is a common concern for patients who use antibiotics or inhaled corticosteroids. *Herpes labialis* is another infection involving the herpes simplex virus that is found around the lips, manifesting as a grouping of vesicles with an erythematous base. After an initial outbreak, the virus may remain dormant and replicate later due to environmental stimuli.

Acute pharyngitis, both viral and bacterial, is common in family practice and urgent care settings. Group A *Streptococcus* (GAS) is a treatable cause of the symptoms, while viral pharyngitis is often self limiting.[28] Proper identification of the causative factor for a sore throat is imperative in minimizing the overuse of antibiotic therapy for viral illnesses. Other common viruses that can cause pharyngitis symptoms include enteroviruses, influenza A and B, parainfluenza viruses, and respiratory syncytial virus.[28] Evaluation of pharyngeal disorders includes assessment of the more urgent concerns, such as edema of the posterior pharynx, uvula edema, difficulty swallowing, and maintenance of a patent airway.

Dental caries and periodontal disease (gingivitis and periodontitis) are two major chronic oral diseases that will not revert back to prior state even with treatment.[29] Dental caries tend to be genetically linked, contributing to approximately 60% of all cases.[30] With plaque being a known major contributor to oral hygiene, clinicians should advocate for healthy oral environments and hygiene whenever possible. Pulpitis, or inflammation of dental pulp, occurs when dental caries progress and the pulp is exposed, thus leading to pain and infection. Periodontal disease, while not painful, contributes to tooth loss and produces halitosis.[31]

Risk factors for many of the common oral, throat, and dental complaints may vary based upon age. In one quantitative study of 210 babies in a birth cohort noted to have upper respiratory infections, risk factors included winter season, nasopharyngeal colonization with *S. pneumoniae*, and occupation of caregiver.[32] In other populations, crowded living conditions, low socioeconomic status, and poor nutrition increase the risk of GAS infection, which can lead to more serious disorders such as acute rheumatic fever (ARF).[33] Proper education on the benefits of handwashing, avoiding droplet exposure from those who are ill, and adequate fluids and rest are important nonpharmacologic interventions to prevent the spread of common oral and upper respiratory disorders.

According to the World Health Organization (WHO), dental caries is the most widespread noncommunicable disease in the world.[34] Treatment is much more costly than simple cost-effective interventions, such as minimizing sugar intake from an early age and introduction of regular fluoride. Early childhood caries (ECC), or the presence of one or more decayed, filled, or missing tooth surfaces in children, can lead to dental pain, odontogenic infections, gastrointestinal disorders, malnutrition, and iron-deficient anemia, as well as other disorders.[35]

Diagnosing and treating oral concerns can present challenges due to the variety of oral lesions and disease processes in all ages. In elderly patients, more serious lesions (e.g., squamous cell carcinoma, leukoplakias, and melanomas) can be missed if the clinician is not adequately evaluating oral surfaces. In more common oral disorders like *Candida albicans*, the white patches in the mouth or on the tongue can be distinguished from the precancerous white patches of leukoplakia by carefully questioning recent antibiotic use or other risk factors versus the chronicity of the disorder and risk factors such as tobacco and alcohol use. Other lesions such as aphthous ulcers can be distinguished from a melanoma as melanoma exhibits asymmetry, irregular borders, and may have varying color changes or a persistent erosion, papule, or plaque of the oral cavity. A benign ulcer, or *canker sore*, is typically painful and round to oval with a greyish base and is much more common. Syphilis, which is less common, may present as a fissured papule in the oral commissure lines or corners of the mouth.

Adequate history taking can help to eliminate some causes and help facilitate appropriate treatment. Persistent lesions with certain risk factors should be biopsied to rule out cancerous causes. Cytologic testing along with histopathologic assessment are the most reliable ways to potentially discern if oral lesions are cancerous.[36] For more acute-onset lesions in the absence of immunosuppression, known HIV disease, or chronic tobacco and alcohol use, conservative pharmacologic and nonpharmacologic therapies should be considered first.

Diagnosis of dental issues in the primary care setting occurs when patients present with pain, swelling, or signs of infection. Assessment of the dental structures, risk for infection, and pain control, pending a dental consult, are the role of the primary care clinician. Dentists and oral surgeons are the primary clinicians ordering further diagnostic testing for dental disorders.

Treatment for Common Oral and Dental Conditions

Not all oral and dental lesions require prescription medications or pharmacologic therapies for treatment. Some oral ulcers are self limiting and may resolve with symptomatic care and avoidance of aggravating food and drink. For pulpitis, the treatment is often dental drilling into the tooth to remove the inflamed nerve, thus cleaning the root canal. Some clinicians may use a trial of antibiotics and an analgesic, but there is no evidence to support this as a preferred therapy.[31] Antibiotics for dental issues can serve to minimize the spread of infection, but should be reserved for fever, lymphadenopathy, or when surrounding-tissue swelling and irritation are present.[31] Due to the presence of beta-lactamase among oral anaerobes, treatment failure with penicillin (PCN) alone is well documented and thus PCN monotherapy is no longer recommended.[31] Amoxicillin and clavulanate is recommended, or in penicillin-allergic patients, consider clindamycin. See **Table 13.5** for treatment options for common oral and dental disorders.

In many settings, oral care can impact health outcomes and associated medical conditions. For example, in one study by Gomaa et al.,[37] the researchers looked at the effect of adoption of 0.12% chlorhexidine oral solution use on pediatric ventilated patients. The result of the study was an improved outcome in the intensive care unit for 50 patients. Another example is evidence-based measures to prevent dental caries starting at an early age, such as the application of fluoride varnish shortly after the first tooth eruption, as well as regular plaque removal.[38] Regardless of medical management, thermal changes with food and liquids can contribute to worsening pain when the nerve root is exposed.

CONCLUSION

When assessing and diagnosing any ear, nose, oral, or dental conditions in the primary or urgent care setting, the clinician must understand the anatomy of the ears, sinuses, and mouth and how to recognize which issues can be safely treated and which should be referred to a dentist; oral surgeon; or ears, nose, and throat (ENT) specialist.

TABLE 13.5 Pharmacotherapy for Common Oral and Dental Conditions

Medication	Dose/Frequency	Indications	Contraindications	Side Effects
Clotrimazole troche	10-mg troche dissolved in mouth 5× daily	*Candida albicans* in HIV seronegative patients or general population	Hypersensitivity to clotrimazole or any component of the medication	Abnormal liver functions, pruritus, nausea, vomiting
Miconazole buccal tablet	50-mg tablet applied to mucosal surface for 30 seconds once daily	*C. albicans* in HIV seronegative patients or general population	Hypersensitivity to miconazole, milk-protein concentrate, or any component of the medication	Headache, fatigue, pruritus, diarrhea, nausea, oral discomfort
Nystatin	400,000–600,000 units swished and swallowed qid	*C. albicans*	Hypersensitivity to nystatin or any component of the medication	Metallic taste; may cause dental caries when used for prolonged periods due to sugar content
Fluconazole	200-mg loading dose; 100–200 mg once daily until symptoms resolve	*C. albicans:* recommended for recurrent or hard-to-treat cases and for those at risk for esophageal candidiasis	CrCl ≤50 mL/minute (no dialysis) reduce dose by 50%; avoid with CYP3A4 substrates	Headache, mild dizziness, skin rash, nausea, abdominal pain
Triamcinolone oral paste 0.1%	Thin film applied to ulcer bid–tid	Recurrent aphthous stomatitis, oral inflammatory, and ulcerative lesions	Hypersensitivity to triamcinolone; fungal, viral, or bacterial infections of the mouth; may cause adrenal suppression in high doses over prolonged periods	Glandular, gritty sensation may not be palatable; localized burning
Fluocinonide gel 0.05%	Thin layer applied to ulcer bid–qid	Recurrent aphthous stomatitis, oral inflammatory and ulcerative lesions	Hypersensitivity to fluocinonide or any component of the medication	Intracranial hypertension, localized burning or irritation
Amoxicillin–clavulanate	Adult: 875 mg q12h Pediatric: 80–100 mg/kg/d (of amoxicillin)	Mild odontogenic infections, Group A streptococci infections	Hypersensitivity to amoxicillin or any other component of the medication; history of cholestatic jaundice	Diarrhea (>10%)
Clindamycin	450 mg q8h	Mild odontogenic infections with PCN allergy	Hypersensitivity to clindamycin, lincomycin, or any other component of the medication	Black-Box Warning: May cause severe and possibly fatal colitis; use with caution in patients with a history of GI disease
No medication; self-limited condition	N/A	Herpes simplex	N/A	N/A

bid, twice daily; CrCl, creatinine clearance; GI, gastrointestinal; PCN, penicillin; q8h, every 8 hours; q12h, every 12 hours; qid, four times daily.

CASE EXEMPLAR: Patient With Rhinorrhea

RH, a 49-year-old Black female, presents to the primary care clinician's office with a complaint of 5 days of purulent rhinorrhea and intermittent nasal congestion. RH reports that she is prone to seasonal allergies but states they flared only 5 days ago. Over-the-counter medications seldom work for her. RH is asking for a steroid injection and a Z-Pak (azithromycin), which her former clinician always prescribed. She is also asking for medication for a yeast infection, as she commonly gets one when she is treated with antibiotics.

Past Medical History
- Seasonal allergies
- Hypertension
- Chronic kidney disease, stage 3
- Hyperlipidemia

Allergies
- Codeine (itching)
- Penicillin (rash)

Medications
- Lisinopril, 10 mg once daily
- Simvastatin, 40 mg once at bedtime
- Acetylsalicylic acid (aspirin), 81 mg once daily

Family History
- Noncontributory

Social History
- Married
- Smoker
- Denies alcohol abuse

Physical Examination
- Weight: 195 lbs.; blood pressure: 160/80; pulse: 84; respiration rate: 16; oxygen saturation: 97%
- Ears: Tympanic membranes cloudy bilaterally
- Eyes: PERRLA (pupils, equal, round, reactive [to] light, accommodation); conjunctiva slightly injected; clear drainage
- Nose: Enlarged pale nasal turbinates; no frontal or maxillary sinus tenderness
- Mouth/oral: Cobblestoning of the posterior pharyngitis with clear postnasal discharge; tonsils nonenlarged; no exudate
- Neck: Supple; no adenopathy
- Lungs: Clear to auscultation anterior and posterior; no wheezing or rhonchi
- Heart: Regular rate and rhythm without murmur, gallop, or rub

Discussion Questions

1. Is a steroid injection an appropriate treatment for RH?
2. What over-the-counter allergy medications are evidence-based for nasal congestion and safe for RH (given her blood pressure)?
3. Is it appropriate to prescribe an antibiotic now? What do evidence-based guidelines state would be an appropriate presentation for the addition of an antibiotic?
4. Is it appropriate to prescribe a medication for a yeast infection now? If so, what is the most appropriate medication?

CR: Patient With Otitis Externa

...e who is brought to the clinic ...laints of acute left ear pain. ...d him up from a week-long ...ted his ear hurt so bad he ...nother looked at this ear, ...outside canal was very swollen. He could not even touch his ear. His mother states: "He is never sick, and he never cries."

Past Medical History
- All immunizations current
- No history of surgeries
- No history of allergies
- No history of significant illness

Medications
- Multivitamin, daily
- Occasional allergy medication with children's loratadine

Physical Examination
- Pulse: 100; respiration rate: 22; temperature: 100.2 °F data scan
- Left ear canal swollen; unable to access with otoscope to observe tympanic membrane
- Swelling noted in lymph nodes below ear
- Ear is red and warm to touch

Diagnosis
- External otitis

Discussion Questions

1. What factors in ZM's recent history should the clinician consider, and what additional questions should the clinician ask the mother?
2. What treatment options are indicated for ZM?
3. What patient teaching should the clinician provide?

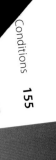

KEY TAKEAWAYS

- Clinicians require an extensive working knowledge of ophthalmic, ototic, nasal, and oral treatment medications and how they should be used in different patient populations and the precautions that need to be taken when prescribing.
- Before any treatment is considered, the clinician should determine if all preventative measures have been taken and whether the patient has been properly educated for reduction of symptoms in the future.
- In more difficult or complicated cases of allergies or sinusitis, patients can be referred for allergy testing, including skin testing, serum testing, nasal cytology, and allergy challenge.
- Diagnosing and treating oral concerns can present challenges due to the variety of oral lesions and disease processes in all ages. In elderly patients, more serious lesions such as squamous cell carcinoma, leukoplakias, and melanomas can be missed if the clinician does not adequately evaluate oral surfaces.
- In a more common oral disorder such as *C. albicans*, the white patches in the mouth or on the tongue can be distinguished from the precancerous white patches of leukoplakia by questioning of recent antibiotic use or other risk factors versus the chronicity of the

disorder and risk factors such as tobacco use and alcohol use.
- Antibiotics for dental issues can minimize the spread of infection but should be reserved for fever, lymphadenopathy, or when swelling and irritation are present in surrounding tissue.

REFERENCES

1. Finley CR, Chan DS, Garrison S, et al. What are the most common conditions in primary care? Systematic review. *Can Fam Physician*. 2018;64(11):832–840. https://www.ncbi.nlm.nih.gov/pmc/articles/PMC6234945

2. Hui C. Acute otitis externa. *Paediatr Child Health*. 2013;18(2):96–98. doi:10.1093/pch/18.2.96

3. Altemeier W. A brief history of otitis media. *Pediatr Ann*. 2000;29(10):559. doi:10.3928/0090-4481-20001001-03

4. Harmes K, Blackwood A, Burrows H, et al. Otitis media: diagnosis and treatment. *Am Fam Physician*. 2013;88(7):435–440. https://www.aafp.org/afp/2013/1001/p435.pdf

5. Donaldson J. Acute otitis media. In: Meyers AD, ed. *Medscape*. Updated September 25, 2019. https://emedicine.medscape.com/article/859316-overview

6. Kaur R, Morris M, Pichichero M. Epidemiology of acute otitis media in the postpneumococcal conjugate vaccine era. *Pediatrics*. 2017;140(3):e20170101. doi:10.1542/peds.2017-0181

7. Narhayati M, Ho J, Azman M. Influenza vaccine for preventing acute otitis media. *Cochrane Database Syst Rev*. 2017;(10):CD010089. doi:10.1002/14651858.CD010089.pub3

8. Sigurdsson S, Eythorsson E, Hrafnkelsson B, et al. Reduction in all-cause acute otitis media in children <3 years of age in primary care following vaccination with 10-valent pneumococcal *Haemophilus influenzae* protein-D conjugate vaccine: a whole-population study. *Clin Infect Dis.* 2018;67(8):1213–1219, doi:10.1093/cid/ciy233

9. Lieberthal A, Carroll A, Chonmaitree T, et al. The diagnosis and management of acute otitis media. *Pediatrics.* 2013;131(3):e964–e999. doi:10.1542/peds.2012-3488

10. Meissner H. Understanding otitis media in 2018. *AAP News.* Published June 26, 2018. https://www.aappublications.org/news/2018/06/26/idsnapshot062618

11. Pichicher M. Antibiotic choice for acute otitis media 2018. *Family Practice News.* Published January 25, 2018. https://www.mdedge.com/familypracticenews/article/157059/infectious-diseases/antibiotic-choice-acute-otitis-media-2018

12. Ghossaini S. Otitis externa. *BMJ Best Practice.* Updated October 23, 2019. https://bestpractice.bmj.com/topics/en-us/40

13. Rosenfeld R, Schwartz S, Cannon R, et al. Clinical practice guideline: acute otitis externa. *Otolaryngol Head Neck Surg.* 2014;150(1 suppl):S1–S24. doi:10.1177/0194599813517083

14. Waitzman A. Otitis externa. In: Elluru RG, ed. *Medscape.* Updated March 9, 2020. https://emedicine.medscape.com/article/994550-overview

15. Michaudet C, Malaty J. Cerumen impaction: diagnosis and management. *Am Fam Physician.* 2018;98(8):525–529. https://www.aafp.org/afp/2018/1015/p525.html

16. van Wyk F. Cerumen impaction removal. In Meyers AD, ed. *Medscape.* Updated May 9, 2018. https://emedicine.medscape.com/article/1413546-overview

17. Ramachandran M, Aronson JK. John Bostock's first description of hayfever. *JR Soc Med.* 2011;104(6):237–240. doi:10.1258/jrsm.2010.10k056

18. Small P, Keith PK, Kim H. Allergic rhinitis. *Allergy Asthma Clin Immunol.* 2018;14(suppl 2):51. doi:10.1186/s13223-018-0280-7

19. deShazo RD, Kemp SF. Allergic rhinitis: clinical manifestations, epidemiology, and diagnosis. In: Corren J, Feldweg AM, eds. *UpToDate.* Updated January 20, 2020. https://www.uptodate.com/contents/allergic-rhinitis-clinical-manifestations-epidemiology-and-diagnosis

20. Mavrodi A, Paraskevas G. Evolution of the paranasal sinuses' anatomy through the ages. *Anat Cell Biol.* 2013;46(4):235–238. doi:10.5115/acb.2013.46.4.235

21. Cappello ZJ, Minutello K, Dublin AB. Anatomy, head and neck, nose paranasal sinuses. [Updated September 20, 2020]. In: *StatPearls* [Internet]. StatPearls Publishing; 2020. https://www.ncbi.nlm.nih.gov/books/NBK499826

22. Rhoads J, Petersen SW. *Advanced Health Assessment and Diagnostic Reasoning.* 3rd ed. Jones & Bartlett Learning; 2018.

23. Patel ZM, Hwang PH. Acute sinusitis and rhinosinusitis in adults: clinical manifestations and diagnosis. In: Deschler DG, File TM Jr, Kunins L, eds. *UpToDate.* Updated September 3, 2020. https://www.uptodate.com/contents/acute-sinusitis-and-rhinosinusitis-in-adults-clinical-manifestations-and-diagnosis

24. Rosenfeld R. Acute sinusitis in adults. *N Engl J Med.* 2016;375(10):962–970. doi:10.1056/NEJMcp1601749

25. Rosenfeld RM, Piccirillo JF, Chandrasekhar SS, et al. Clinical practice guideline (update): adult sinusitis. *Otolaryngol Head Neck Surg.* 2015;152(suppl 2):S1–S39. doi:10.1177/0194599815572097

26. Min J, Tan BK. Risk factors for chronic rhinosinusitis. *Curr Opin Allergy Clin Immunol.* 2015;15(1):1–13. doi:10.1097/ACI.0000000000000128

27. Gutmann JL. The evolution of America's scientific advancements in dentistry in the past 50 years. *JADA.* 2009;140 (suppl 1):8S–15S. doi:10.14219/jada.archive.2009.0354

28. Chow AW, Doran S. Evaluation of acute pharyngitis in adults. In: Aronson MD, Bond S, eds. *UpToDate.* Updated September 21, 2020. https://uptodate.com/contents/evauation-of-acute-pharyngitis-in-adults

29. Jang Y-J, Kim N-S. Relationship of oral health behavior to subjective oral health status and the DMFT index in Korean adults. *J Korea Soc Dent Hyg.* 2011;11:499–509. http://www.jksdh.or.kr/view/jksdh-11-4-08.pdf

30. Shah PM, Vishnu Priya V, Gayathri R. Awareness of prevalence of dental caries among genetically related population. *Drug Intervent Today.* 2018;10(9):1781–1785. http://jprsolutions.info/files/final-file-5b669e49913772.07831089.pdf

31. Chow AW. Complications, diagnosis, and treatment of odontogenic infections. In: Durand ML, Bloom A, eds. *UpToDate.* Updated August 28, 2020. https://www.uptodate.com/contents/complications-diagnosis-and-treatment-of-odontogenic-infections

32. Rupa V, Isaac R, Manoharan A, et al. Risk factors for upper respiratory infection in the first year of life in a birth cohort. *Int J Pediatr Otorhinolaryngol.* 2012;76(12):1835–1839.

33. Coffee PM, Ralph AP, Krause VL. The role of social determinants of health in the risk and prevention of group A streptococcal infection, acute rheumatic fever and rheumatic heart disease: a systematic review. *PLoS Negl Trop Dis.* 2018;12(6):e0006577. doi:10.1371/journal.pntd.0006577

34. World Health Organization. *Sugars and Dental Caries.* World Health Organization; 2017. https://www.who.int/oral_health/publications/sugars-dental-caries-keyfacts/en

35. Wagner Y, Heinrich-Weltzien R. Risk factors for dental problems: recommendations for oral health in infancy. *Early Hum Dev.* 2017;114:16–21. doi:10.1016/j.earlhumdev.2017.09.009

36. Lingen MW, Tampi MP, Urquhart O, et al. Adjuncts for the evaluation of potentially malignant disorders in the oral cavity: diagnostic test accuracy systematic review and meta-analysis—A report of the American Dental Association. *J Am Dent Assoc.* 2017;148(11):797. doi:10.1016/j.adaj.2017.08.045

37. Gomaa MM, Wahba Y, El-Bayoumi MA. Pre versus post application of a 0.12% chlorhexidine based oral hygiene protocol in an Egyptian pediatric intensive

care unit: practice and effects. *Egypt J Crit Care Med.* 2017;5(3):587–591. doi:10.1016/j.ejccm.2017.11.002

38. *WHO Expert Consultation on Public Health Intervention Against Early Childhood Caries: Report of a meeting.* World Health Organization; 2017. https://www.who.int/publications/i/item/who-expert-consultation-on-public-health-intervention-against-early-childhood-caries

Pharmacotherapy for Eye Conditions

Tedi Begaj and Shlomit Schaal

LEARNING OBJECTIVES

- Differentiate between perforating and penetrating eye injuries and the corresponding treatment.
- Compare and contrast chalazion and hordeolum and the appropriate interventions for each.
- Discuss the management of various eye infections, including pre- and postseptal cellulitis, varicella, and the various organisms that lead to conjunctivitis.
- Outline the management of corneal abrasion.
- Describe the symptoms and etiology of glaucoma and outline the classifications of drugs and their methods of action used in its management.

INTRODUCTION

The eye is a complex organ with multiple unique cells, each serving various specific roles and functions. Due to the complexity of the various ocular physiologic processes, there is a profound range of disorders affecting both the eye and orbit. This chapter discusses various ocular diseases and their treatments, with particular emphasis on common conditions that present to urgent and emergent services in the community.

OCULAR PENETRATING AND PERFORATING INJURIES (OPEN GLOBE)

Injury from sharp or high-velocity objects or instruments can result in severe loss of vision as well as potential loss of the eye. By definition, penetrating injuries enter the eye but do not exit; perforating injuries have an entrance and exit wound. Careful examination is indicated in tandem with imaging. Imaging modalities include ultrasonography, MRI for injuries with a nonmetallic etiology, and CT scan in cases where suspicion is high for metallic intra-ocular foreign body. If an open globe seems likely, both immediate evaluation by ophthalmology and initiation of treatment are necessary. **Figure 14.1** details general treatment principles.

Antibiotic treatment aims to prophylactically reduce posttraumatic endophthalmitis by providing coverage against common organisms such as *Staphylococcus*, *Streptococcus*, *Bacillus*, and gram negatives.[1] Commonly used antibiotics are presented in **Table 14.1** along with suggested dose adjustments for patients with renal dysfunction.[2] Chapter 6 provides further information on dose reduction in patients with renal impairment. Antibiotics are generally continued for 48 hours.

Tabatabaei and colleagues found no difference between oral and intravenous administration in occurrence of endophthalmitis or visual acuity at 1 year.[3] Thus, in circumstances without capacity for intravenous medications or when transfer to an outside hospital might require several hours, initiation of an oral regimen may be appropriate.

EYELIDS AND ORBIT

PHARMACOTHERAPY FOR CHALAZION AND HORDEOLUM

Hordeola are acute infections of an oil gland located on the eyelid, which can be either internal or external depending on the involved gland. Staphylococcal bacterial are responsible for the majority of hordeola. Chalazia are a sterile inflammatory granulomatous response from an obstructed meibomian gland, commonly on

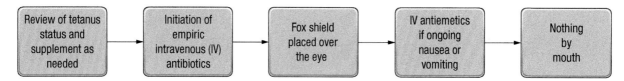

FIGURE 14.1 Open globe treatment algorithm.

TABLE 14.1 Antibiotic Prophylaxis in Open Globe Injury

Medication	Dosage	Impaired Renal Function
Vancomycin	1 g q8h	100% of dose every 12–24 hours[4]
Cephalosporins		
Cefepime	1–2 g q12h	50% of dose every 24 hours
Ceftazidime	1 g q8h	100% of dose every 12–24 hours

h, hour; q, every.

the upper eyelid. The clinician should rule out preseptal and orbital cellulitis as these conditions early on can mimic chalazia or hordeola.

A hot compress several times a day with lid massage is a conservative but effective approach for either hordeola or chalazia. Daily lid scrubbing and ensuring total removal of face and eye makeup before sleep helps in the acute phase but may also reduce the incidence of these conditions.

Internal Hordeolum

Topical antibiotics are not usually effective given the depth of infection.[5] Therefore, oral penicillinase-resistant penicillins (e.g., dicloxacillin) or macrolides (e.g., erythromycin, azithromycin) can hasten resolution.

External Hordeolum

Antibiotic ointment (e.g., bacitracin [alone or in combination with polymyxin B and/or neomycin], or erythromycin) applied four times a day may accelerate resolution.

Chalazion

Topical or oral antibiotics have minimal effect given the inflammatory but noninfectious cause of these lesions. The application of hot compresses with gentle massage is effective in only 40% of cases.[6] Therefore, chalazia that persist for several weeks or are recurrent should be referred to ophthalmology for further treatment including steroid injections or incision and curettage.[7]

PHARMACOTHERAPY FOR PRESEPTAL AND POSTSEPTAL CELLULITIS

Inflammation of tissue anterior to the orbital septum is known as preseptal cellulitis while posterior to the

septum is known as postseptal (orbital) cellulitis. Both conditions are most commonly due to infectious etiologies.[8] Current microbiologic data reports that *Staphylococcus aureus, Streptococcus pneumoniae,* other streptococci, and anaerobes are the most common agents.[9]

Oral Antibiotics

For the afebrile patient with a mild preseptal cellulitis (**Figure 14.2A**), with no changes in vision and no limitations of extraocular movement, oral antibiotics may be initiated with close monitoring (**Table 14.2**). If there is a history of a previous *methicillin-resistant S. aureus* (MRSA) infection or concern due to concomitant comorbidities (e.g., diabetes, immunosuppression), then empiric MRSA treatment is warranted.

Intravenous Antibiotics

For patients with severe preseptal cellulitis or orbital cellulitis (**Figure 14.2B**), broad-spectrum IV antibiotics are warranted to cover both MRSA and gram-negative agents (**Table 14.3**). These patients should be hospitalized if there is in-house ophthalmologic coverage or transferred to an outside hospital that encompasses such capabilities. If there is a history of a penetrating eyelid injury, then there is an increased risk of exposure to organic material. The antibiotic regimen should include metronidazole for superior anaerobic coverage.[10]

PHARMACOTHERAPY FOR VARICELLA ZOSTER

Primary varicella zoster (VZV) infection results in chickenpox, usually at a young age. After clinical resolution, VZV can remain dormant in the trigeminal and dorsal root ganglia for years before reactivation, which may present as a viral prodrome, with neuritis and a subsequent dermatomal distribution of a vesicular rash. Reactivation of VZV within the ophthalmic nerve (first division of trigeminal nerve [V1]) is known as herpes zoster ophthalmicus (HZO).

Cutaneous Reactivation

HZO affecting only the skin requires treatment with oral acyclovir, valacyclovir, or famciclovir.[11] Currently, there are no large trials to support efficacy of one medicine over another. Common doses are described in **Table 14.4.**

Acyclovir has poor bioavailability, necessitating a dosing frequency of five times daily. Two

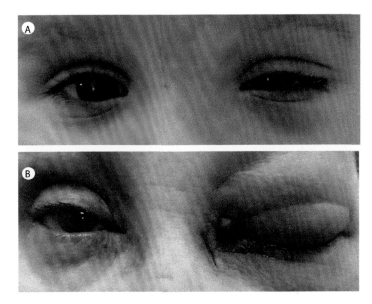

FIGURE 14.2 Periorbital cellulitis. **(A)** Preseptal cellulitis of the left eye: mild inferior and super periorbital erythema with minimal upper lid edema and no conjunctival injection or discharge; the patient had full range of extraocular movement. **(B)** Orbital (postseptal) cellulitis with significant erythema and edema, causing a mechanical ptosis; vision was decreased and extraocular movements were limited.

TABLE 14.2 Oral Antibiotics in Preseptal Cellulitis

Medication	Adult Dosing and Frequency
No Suspicion of MRSA	
Amoxicillin–clavulanic acid	875 mg bid
Cefpodoxime	400 mg bid
Previous MRSA Infection or High MRSA Suspicion Due to Comorbidities	
Trimethoprim–sulfamethoxazole	160–800 mg bid
Clindamycin	300 mg tid
Doxycycline	100 mg bid

bid, twice daily; MRSA, methicillin-resistant *Staphylococcus aureus*; tid, three times daily

TABLE 14.3 Intravenous Antibiotics in Orbital Cellulitis

Medication	Adult Dosing and Frequency
MRSA coverage Vancomycin	1 g q8h
Gram-negative coverage Piperacillin and tazobactam	3.375 g q6h–q8h
Ampicillin and sulbactam	3 g q6h
Cefepime	1–2 g q12h
Ceftazidime	1 g q12h
Penetrating Eyelid Injury and Exposure to Organic Material	
Metronidazole	500 mg q6h–q8h

h, hour; MRSA, methicillin-resistant *Staphylococcus aureus*; q, every.

TABLE 14.4 Anti-Herpetic Treatment

Medication	Adult Dosing and Frequency
Acyclovir	Oral 800 mg five times daily
Valacyclovir	Oral 1,000 mg tid
Famciclovir	Oral 500 mg tid

tid, three times daily.

meta-analyses[12,13] of several placebo-controlled trials demonstrated that oral acyclovir (800 mg, five times daily) accelerated resolution of acute neuritis at 3 and 6 months as well and additionally decreased risk of post-herpetic neuralgia by 46% at 6 months.

Valacyclovir has a superior bioavailability (three- to five-fold increase) as compared to acyclovir. A randomized, double blind, multicenter study comparing oral valacyclovir dosage of 1,000 mg three times daily for 7 to 14 days and oral acyclovir dosage of 800 mg five times daily for 7 days reported no differences in pain intensity or quality of life measures. There were also similar rates of cutaneous resolution in all groups.[14]

Ocular Involvement

HZO can cause conjunctivitis, keratitis (epithelial, stromal, or endothelial), uveitis, and retinitis.

Any patient with ocular irritation (e.g., conjunctival injection, discharge) or changes in vision (e.g., new floaters, flashing lights, or decreased visual acuity) needs prompt ophthalmologic evaluation to rule out ocular involvement.

CONJUNCTIVA

PHARMACOTHERAPY FOR CONJUNCTIVITIS

Conjunctivitis is characterized by dilation of the conjunctival vessels, resulting in edema and hyperemia usually associated with tearing or discharge. The majority of cases are due to viruses, bacteria, or allergic inflammation.

Viral Conjunctivitis

Most viral conjunctivitis cases are caused by adenoviruses while a small proportion are due to herpes viruses, mainly herpes simplex virus I (HSV-1). As these entities are quite contagious, care must be taken to avoid spread. This includes frequent hand washing in addition to avoidance of contact with communal objects, eyes, and the hands of others.

Supportive care is the mainstay of treatment: cold compresses and (refrigerated) artificial tears several times a day as needed. However, should there be a high suspicion for HSV conjunctivitis, empiric treatment with oral acyclovir or valacyclovir may be initiated with referral for a thorough ophthalmic evaluation.

Bacterial Conjunctivitis

Staphylococcal species, followed by *S. pneumoniae* and *Haemophilus influenzae*, are the most common pathogens for bacterial conjunctivitis. All broad-spectrum antibiotic drops appear to be effective, with no significant difference in achieving clinical cure[15]; topical medical therapy is shown in **Table 14.5**.

Chlamydial Conjunctivitis

In both the pediatric and adult patient, treatment of chlamydial conjunctivitis consists of a macrolide antibiotic drop four times daily in combination with an oral macrolide (e.g., Azithromycin 1 g, one time).[15] A thorough systemic evaluation is critical, and treatment may be further modified based on systemic involvement.

Gonococcal Conjunctivitis

Gonococcal conjunctivitis (GC) classically features purulent mucus discharge (**Figure 14.3A**), which should be irrigated and removed with a sterile solution. In addition to topical macrolides or fluoroquinolones, treatment consists of a one-time dose of 1 g of intramuscular ceftriaxone. Given the possible co-infection with chlamydia, dual therapy to cover chlamydia may be warranted. Unlike most other bacteria, however, GC can penetrate an intact cornea (**Figure 14.3B**), causing corneal thinning and intraocular inflammation. Therefore, a low suspicion coupled with a rapid diagnosis and treatment of GC is critical to prevent corneal melt and vision loss. Additionally, an evaluation for possible disseminated *Neisseria gonorrhoeae* should be performed as these patients may require hospitalization.

Allergic Conjunctivitis

Allergic conjunctivitis is an inflammatory response of the conjunctiva due to an antigen. Commonly, it may be part of a larger systemic reaction. Allergic conjunctivitis encompasses different categories of ocular allergy

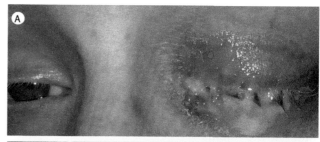
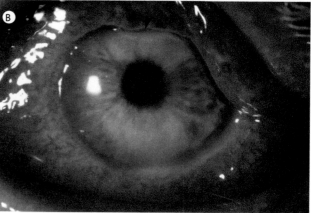

FIGURE 14.3 Gonococcal conjunctivitis. **(A)** Significant yellow-green mucopurulent discharge with mild periorbital erythema of the left eye. **(B)** After removal of purulent discharge, there is severe conjunctival injection and swelling (chemosis) with corneal thinning superiorly (*arrowhead*) and intraocular inflammation.

TABLE 14.5 Topical Ocular Antibiotics		
Drug Class	**Medication**	**Dosing and Frequency**
Aminoglycosides	Gentamicin 0.3% Tobramycin 0.3%	1 drop three to four times daily
Fluoroquinolones	Besifloxacin 0.6% Ciprofloxacin 0.3% Gatifloxacin 0.3% Levofloxacin 0.5% Moxifloxacin 0.5% Ofloxacin 0.3%	1 drop four times daily
Macrolides	Azithromycin 1% Erythromycin 0.5%	One drop two to four times daily
Combination	Trimethoprim/ polymyxin B	Two drops four times daily

with varying pathophysiology that are based on seasonal variation, involvement or sparing of the cornea, predisposition to atopic reactions, and soft contact lens wearers.

There are a multitude of topical medicines for allergic conjunctivitis, from over-the-counter (OTC) vasoconstrictors to antihistamine agents to mast cell stabilizers and finally to various dual-mechanism agents (Histamine H_1 receptor antagonist and mast cell stabilizers). **Table 14.6** lists the various options.

In general, OTC antihistamine/vasoconstriction topical medicines are utilized as first line agents given their low cost. Should the symptoms persist, combination drops such as olopatadine 0.1% or ketotifen are subsequently employed.[16] Mast cell stabilizers are usually employed if other classes have failed. Although topical corticosteroids are potent agents in relieving symptoms, they should not be used in an emergent setting in allergic conjunctivitis due to their potentially significant adverse effects.

CORNEA

PHARMACOTHERAPY FOR CORNEAL ABRASION

Corneal abrasions are defined as focal loss of the corneal epithelium due to mechanical trauma, significant ocular dryness, anesthetic abuse, or various other etiologies. Commonly used in clinics and the emergency department, fluorescein staining at a particular corneal location is obligatory for diagnosis.

Antibiotics

Topical antibiotics are used for corneal epithelial defects in order to prevent infection; corneal stem cells found at the limbus will migrate and regenerate the damaged epithelium. Similar to bacterial conjunctivitis, topical antibiotics (Table 14.5) should be used to treat corneal abrasions. In addition, ointment (either antibiotic or artificial tear gel) is also recommended as lubrication provides pain relief.

Contact lens wearers are at an increased risk of *Pseudomonas aeruginosa* infections, which necessitates the use of fluoroquinolone or aminoglycoside therapy.[17] In the United States, a retrospective study found that 100% of *P. aeruginosa* strains were sensitive to either ciprofloxacin or levofloxacin and ~94% were sensitive to gentamicin.[18]

Anesthetics

Topical anesthesia with proparacaine 0.5% or tetracaine 0.5% is commonly used in the emergency setting to provide temporary pain relief. The dangers of such medicines include delayed healing, decreased sensation leading to corneal thinning, and ulcer development, as well as direct toxicity to the epithelium. Even two drops of 0.5% proparacaine can decrease corneal thickness as early as 1 to 2 minutes after instillation.[19] It is therefore critical that topical anesthetics be employed diagnostically in the clinic or hospital setting and never provided or prescribed for patients.

Diluted topical anesthetic (e.g., 0.05% proparacaine) has been investigated previously[20,21] in an effort to provide analgesia but limit corneal toxicity. These studies are limited due to small study populations and inclusion criteria of only small, uncomplicated abrasions irrespective of mechanism. Thus, a large randomized placebo-controlled trial is needed to determine the safety of dilute anesthetics.

CHEMICAL EXPOSURE

Chemical (acid or alkali) injury to the eye requires immediate intervention. In general, alkali agents penetrate tissue more than acids due to their lipophilic composition. Damage to the cornea or conjunctiva can lead to significant visual impairment and even future blindness.

Irrigation Solutions

The eye must be irrigated until the pH returns to the normal physiologic range (7.0), which may require several liters of solution. A 2010 review found insufficient evidence to determine the optimal eye irrigation solution (e.g., normal saline, lactated Ringer's solution, or balanced saline solution).[22] Although there is debate about the ideal irrigating solution, early and aggressive irrigation is the only critical aspect to limit anterior segment destruction.

Topical Treatment

For mild injuries, topical broad-spectrum antibiotics (e.g., trimethoprim/polymyxin B) or fluoroquinolones

TABLE 14.6 Topical Agents for Allergic Conjunctivitis

Drug Class	Medication	Dosing and Frequency
Antihistamine	Azelastine 0.05% Emedastine 0.05%	One drop two to four times daily
Vasoconstrictors and antihistamine	Naphazoline/ pheniramine	One drop four times daily
Mast cell stabilizer	Cromolyn sodium 4% Lodoxamide 0.1% Nedocromil 2%	One drop two to four times daily
NSAID	Ketorolac 0.5%	One drop four times daily
Antihistamine and mast cell stabilizer	Ketotifen Olopatadine 0.1%	One drop two times daily

NSAID, nonsteroidal anti-inflammatory drug.

can be used four times daily. In addition, for alkali injuries, topical steroids (e.g., prednisolone acetate 1%) are added four times daily to reduce inflammation and tissue degradation.[23] The patient needs to be evaluated by ophthalmology as soon as possible.

For severe injury, urgent ophthalmologic evaluation is necessary as treatment might require placement of a large contact lens (Prokera) or surgical debridement in order to prevent symblepharon, a potentially sight-threatening consequence in which the bulbar conjunctiva adheres and fuses to the palpebral conjunctiva.

Oral Adjuvants

Ascorbic acid is a cofactor in collagen synthesis. Systemic administration of vitamin C (oral 500 mg, three times daily) helps promote collagen production and attenuates ulceration of the cornea by chemical injury.[24] Vitamin C should be avoided in patients with renal impairment as high levels may worsen renal function.[25]

Tetracyclines inhibit matrix metalloproteinases (MMPs), which can degrade collagen. Oral doxycycline 50 mg once or twice daily inhibits MMPs, collagenases, and attenuates ocular inflammation commonly seen after chemical exposure.[26]

GLAUCOMA

A common ocular chief complaint in the emergency department is eye pain. A subset of patients has conjunctival injection and blurry vision associated with a gnawing, constant, pressure like pain that may be due to elevated intra-ocular pressure (IOP). After confirmation of elevated pressure (normal ranging from 10 to 21 mmHg), several key topical medicines[27] are available to the clinician in order to decrease IOP. In general, a drug may either decrease production of aqueous or enhance outflow of aqueous. **Table 14.7** lists the current available medicines.

PHARMACOTHERAPY FOR REDUCED PRODUCTION OF AQUEOUS

Beta Blockers

Beta blockers reduce IOP by attenuating the sympathetic drive of the ciliary epithelium and thus decreasing aqueous humor production. Twice daily timolol is an effective agent at lowering IOP. Since serious adverse events include chronic obstructive pulmonary disease (COPD) exacerbation and bronchospasms, bradycardia, and arrhythmia,[28] careful individual consideration must be taken before use. Although the majority of beta blockers are nonselective (both beta 1 and beta 2 inhibition), betaxolol is beta 1 selective and thus carries decreased risk of adverse respiratory events.

Carbonic Anhydrase Inhibitors

Carbonic anhydrase inhibitors (CAIs) reduce IOP by decreasing bicarbonate production, which subsequently perturbs sodium and fluid transport, causing decreased aqueous production.[29] They are effective at lowering IOP when used two or three times a day. Although they are not contraindicated in patients with sulfa allergies, they should be avoided. Topical preparations commonly have limited side effects—mainly irritation and burning upon application—but rarely can cause the same systemic effects as oral CAIs, such as metabolic acidosis, hypokalemia, and gastrointestinal discomfort.

TABLE 14.7 Topical Anti-Glaucoma Agents		
Drug Class	**Medication**	**Dosing and Frequency**
Beta blockers	Timolol maleate solution 0.5% Timolol maleate gel 0.25, 0.5% Betaxolol HCl 0.25%, 0.5% Metipranolol 0.3%	One drop one to two times daily
Carbonic anhydrase inhibitors	Dorzolamide HCl 2% Brinzolamide 1%	One drop two times daily
Alpha agonist	Brimonidine tartrate 0.1% Apraclonidine HCl 0.5%, 1%	One drop three times daily
Prostaglandin analogs	Latanoprost 0.005% Travaprost 0.004% Bimatoprost 0.01%, 0.03% Latanoprostene bunod 0.024% Tafluprost ophthalmic solution 0.0015%	One drop nightly
Miotics	Pilocarpine HCl 1%, 2%, 4% Carbachol 0.75%, 1.5%, 3%	One drop four times daily

HCl, hydrochloride.

Alpha Agonist

Alpha 2 receptor agonists mainly decrease aqueous humor production but also may increase outflow drainage.[30] They are contraindicated in children under the age of 5 given a risk of central nervous system depression as well as patients taking monoamine oxidase inhibitors (MAOIs) due to the risk of triggering a hypertensive crisis. Otherwise, they tend to cause allergic like symptoms.

ENHANCEMENT OF OUTFLOW OF AQUEOUS

Prostaglandin Analogs

Prostaglandin analogs exert their effect by increasing the outflow of aqueous humor from the eye; a common regimen is one drop at night.[31] They are used with caution in patients with a history of uveitis or cystoid macular edema and are contraindicated in pregnant women. In addition, they may increase iris and periorbital pigmentation as well as lead to eyelash growth.

Cholinergic Agents

Miotics enhance outflow of aqueous by constricting the pupil. Frequently, clinicians start at the lowest concentration (1%) and build up to higher strengths (4%). They may cause accommodative spasms and are usually contraindicated in patients with retinal holes or risk for retinal detachment as they displace the lens-iris diaphragm forward.[32]

CASE EXEMPLAR: Patient With Eye Pain

AM is a 22-year-old man presenting to the local emergency department (ED) with acute onset of right eye pain. The pain started 6 hours prior and has not improved with artificial tears or oral acetaminophen. He reports the possibility of accidentally "scratching his right eye" when trying to remove his contact lens.

Past Medical History
- Wears soft contact lenses, replaces monthly
- Denies swimming or showering in contacts
- Occasionally sleeps in contacts

Physical Examination
- Visual acuity: right eye, 20/40; left eye, 20/20
- Right eye is diffusely injected, small pinpoint area of haze is noted in the periphery at 6 o'clock; region subsequently stains with fluorescein

Discussion Questions
1. What is the appropriate pharmacologic treatment for AM?
2. What is the appropriate follow up for AM?
3. How should AM be counseled regarding his contact lens use?

CASE EXEMPLAR: Patient With Eye Pain and Blurry Vision

DB is a 66-year-old male who presents to the clinic with significant pain in his left eye and blurring of vision. His symptoms started 5 hours ago and have progressively worsened. The pain is constant and "pressure like." He denies any history of trauma.

Past Medical History
- Hypertension
- Hyperlipidemia
- Has had several surgeries, including a total knee and cholecystectomy, both over 5 years ago
- No known drug allergies

Medications
- Irbesartan, 150 mg
- Simvastatin, 40 mg
- Aspirin, 81 mg

Physical Examination
- Visual acuity: Right eye, 20/40; left eye, only able to count fingers
- Right pupil brisk and reactive, left pupil sluggish and mid dilated
- Significant left conjunctival injection, with a cloudy cornea; no staining with fluorescein

Discussion Questions
1. The clinician measures the intra-ocular pressure (IOP). Why is assessment of IOP critical at this time?
2. DB's IOP on the right is 16 and 44 mmHg on the left. The clinician consults ophthalmology, who recommend multiple rounds of timolol, dorzolamide, and brimonidine. Are any of these medications contraindicated in this patient?
3. If the IOP cannot be reduced under 30 mmHg, what additional treatment is necessary?

KEY TAKEAWAYS

- Penetrating injuries enter the eye but do not exit, while perforating injuries have an entrance and exit wound. For either type of injury, careful examination, imaging, and intervention are critical. Antibiotic therapy is indicated.
- Several types of infections affect the eyelid or the orbital septum and require antibiotic therapy—either topical, oral, or, in some instances, intravenous. Viral infections can also occur.
- Conjunctivitis can be viral or bacterial. In addition, certain sexually transmitted diseases (e.g., gonorrhea or syphilis) can cause infection of the conjunctiva.
- Corneal abrasions are focal loss of the corneal epithelium by mechanical trauma, significant ocular dryness, or anesthetic abuse. Fluorescein staining at a particular corneal location is obligatory for diagnosis. Topical antibiotics (either antibiotic or artificial tear gel) should be used.
- Glaucoma, diagnosed by an increase in IOP greater than 21 mmHg, is treated either by a reduction in aqueous humor or an increase in its outflow.

REFERENCES

1. Chhabra S, Kunimoto DY, Kazi L, et al. Endophthalmitis after open globe injury: microbiologic spectrum and susceptibilities of isolates. *Am J Ophthalmol.* 2006;142(5):852–854. doi:10.1016/j.ajo.2006.05.024

2. Huang JM, Pansick AD, Blomquist PH. Use of intravenous vancomycin and cefepime in preventing endophthalmitis after open globe injury. *J Ocul Pharmacol Ther.* 2016;32(7):437–441. doi:10.1089/jop.2016.0051

3. Tabatabaei SA, Soleimani M, Behrooz MJ, et al. Systemic oral antibiotics as a prophylactic measure to prevent endophthalmitis in patients with open globe injuries in comparison with intravenous antibiotics. *Retina.* 2016;36(2):360–365. doi:10.1097/IAE.0000000000000727

4. Golightly LK, Teitelbaum I, Kiser TH, et al, eds. *Renal Pharmacotherapy.* Springer Science; 2013.

5. Marren SE BJ, Melore GG. Diseases of the eyelids. In: Bartlett JD, Jaanus SD, eds. *Clinical Ocular Pharmacology.* 4th ed. Butterworth-Heinemann; 2001:485–522.

6. Garrett GW, Gillespie ME, Mannix BC. Adrenocorticosteroid injection vs. conservative therapy in the treatment of chalazia. *Ann Ophthalmol.* 1988;20(5):196–198. PubMed PMID: 3408086.

7. Goawalla A, Lee V. A prospective randomized treatment study comparing three treatment options for chalazia: triamcinolone acetonide injections, incision and cu-

rettage and treatment with hot compresses. *Clin Exp Ophthalmol.* 2007;35(8):706–712. doi:10.1111/j.1442-9071.2007.01617.x.

8. American Academy of Ophthalmology. Orbital inflammatory and infectious diseases. In: Foster JA, ed. *2018-2019 Basic and Clinical Science Course (BCSC), Section 7: Orbit, Eyelids, and Lacrimal System.* American Academy of Ophthalmology; 2018.

9. Chaudhry IA, Shamsi FA, Elzaridi E, et al. Inpatient preseptal cellulitis: experience from a tertiary eye care centre. *Br J Ophthalmol.* 2008;92(10):1337–1341. doi:10.1136/bjo.2007.128975

10. Jedrzynski MS, Bullock JD, McGuire TW, et al. Anaerobic orbital cellulitis: a clinical and experimental study. *Trans Am Ophthalmol Soc.* 1991;89:313–347. https://www.ncbi.nlm.nih.gov/pmc/articles/PMC1298631

11. Gnann JW Jr, Whitley RJ. Clinical practice. Herpes zoster. *N Engl J Med.* 2002;347(5):340–346. doi:10.1056/NEJMcp013211

12. Jackson JL, Gibbons R, Meyer G, Inouye L. The effect of treating herpes zoster with oral acyclovir in preventing postherpetic neuralgia. A meta-analysis. *Arch Intern Med.* 1997;157(8):909–912. doi:10.1001/archinte.1997.00440290095010

13. Wood MJ, Kay R, Dworkin RH, et al. Oral acyclovir therapy accelerates pain resolution in patients with herpes zoster: a meta-analysis of placebo-controlled trials. *Clin Infect Dis.* 1996;22(2):341–347. doi:10.1093/clinids/22.2.341

14. Beutner KR, Friedman DJ, Forszpaniak C, et al. Valaciclovir compared with acyclovir for improved therapy for herpes zoster in immunocompetent adults. *Antimicrob Agents Chemother.* 1995;39(7):1546–1553. doi:10.1128/aac.39.7.1546

15. Azari AA, Barney NP. Conjunctivitis: a systematic review of diagnosis and treatment. *JAMA.* 2013;310(16):1721–1729. doi:10.1001/jama.2013.280318

16. La Rosa M, Lionetti E, Reibaldi M, et al. Allergic conjunctivitis: a comprehensive review of the literature. *Ital J Pediatr.* 2013;39:18. doi:10.1186/1824-7288-39-18

17. Willcox MD. Management and treatment of contact lens-related *Pseudomonas* keratitis. *Clin Ophthalmol.* 2012;6:919–924. doi:10.2147/OPTH.S25168

18. Pachigolla G, Blomquist P, Cavanagh HD. Microbial keratitis pathogens and antibiotic susceptibilities: a 5-year review of cases at an urban county hospital in north Texas. *Eye Contact Lens.* 2007;33(1):45–49. doi:10.1097/01.icl.0000234002.88643.d0

19. Herse P, Siu A. Short-term effects of proparacaine on human corneal thickness. *Acta Ophthalmol (Copenh).* 1992;70(6):740–744. doi:10.1111/j.1755-3768.1992.tb04879.x

20. Ball IM, Seabrook J, Desai N, et al. Dilute proparacaine for the management of acute corneal injuries in the emergency department. *CJEM.* 2010;12(5):389–396. doi:10.1017/s1481803500012537

21. Waldman N, Densie IK, Herbison P. Topical tetracaine used for 24 hours is safe and rated highly effective by patients for the treatment of pain caused by corneal abrasions: a double-blind, randomized clinical trial. *Acad Emerg Med.* 2014;21(4):374–382. doi:10.1111/acem.12346

22. Chau JP, Lee DT, Lo SH. Eye irrigation for patients with ocular chemical burns: a systematic review. *JBI Libr Syst Rev.* 2010;8(12):470–519. doi:10.1111/j.1741-6787.2011.00220

23. Dohlman CH, Cade F, Pfister R. Chemical burns to the eye: paradigm shifts in treatment. *Cornea.* 2011;30(6):613–614. doi:10.1097/ICO.0b013e3182012a4f

24. Brodovsky SC, McCarty CA, Snibson G, et al. Management of alkali burns: an 11-year retrospective review. *Ophthalmology.* 2000;107(10):1829–1835. doi:10.1016/s0161-6420(00)00289-x

25. Nankivell BJ, Murali KM. Images in clinical medicine. Renal failure from vitamin C after transplantation. *N Engl J Med.* 2008;358(4):e4. doi:10.1056/NEJMicm070984

26. Smith VA, Cook SD. Doxycycline—a role in ocular surface repair. *Br J Ophthalmol.* 2004;88(5):619–625. doi:10.1136/bjo.2003.025551

27. Dikopf MS, Vajaranant TS, Edward DP. Topical treatment of glaucoma: established and emerging pharmacology. *Expert Opin Pharmacother.* 2017;18(9):885–898. doi:10.1080/14656566.2017.1328498

28. Brooks AM, Gillies WE. Ocular beta-blockers in glaucoma management. Clinical pharmacological aspects. *Drugs Aging.* 1992;2(3):208–221. doi:10.2165/00002512-199202030-00005

29. Maren TH, Conroy CW. A new class of carbonic anhydrase inhibitor. *J Biol Chem.* 1993;268(35):26233–26239. https://www.jbc.org/content/268/35/26233.full.pdf

30. Toris CB, Camras CB, Yablonski ME. Acute versus chronic effects of brimonidine on aqueous humor dynamics in ocular hypertensive patients. *Am J Ophthalmol* 1999;128(1):8–14. doi:10.1016/s0002-9394(99)00076-8

31. Doucette LP, Walter MA. Prostaglandins in the eye: function, expression, and roles in glaucoma. *Ophthalmic Genet.* 2017;38(2):108–116. doi:10.3109/13816810.2016.1164193

32. Kobayashi H, Kobayashi K, Kiryu J, et al. Pilocarpine induces an increase in the anterior chamber angular width in eyes with narrow angles. *Br J Ophthalmol.* 1999;83(5):553–558. doi:10.1136/bjo.83.5.553

Pharmacotherapy for Skin Conditions

Steadman McPeters

ANATOMY OF THE SKIN

The human skin is the largest organ of the integumentary system and serves as the outer covering of the body. The skin has multiple layers of ectodermal tissue that protect the underlying internal organs, bones, ligaments, and muscles. The anatomy of the skin consists of three well-defined layers: the epidermis, dermis, and subcutaneous tissue. These layers and other features of the skin are illustrated in **Figure 15.1**.

EPIDERMIS

The epidermis is the outermost layer of the skin. As seen in Figure 15.1, the epidermis consists of several layers, beginning with the innermost and deepest basal layer or stratum germinativum; followed by the stratum spinosum, stratum granulosum, and stratum lucidum; and ending with the outermost later, the stratum corneum. Melanocytes and germinal cells are present in the epidermis. The melanocytes produce *melanin*, the pigmentation of skin color. Subsequently, melanin guards the skin against ultraviolent (UV) radiation.

DERMIS

The dermis is located below the epidermis. It forms the true skin that is made up of connective tissue, largely collagen. The dermis contains blood vessels and capillaries, nerve endings, muscle, sebaceous glands, and hair follicles. The major function of the dermis is to provide nourishment to and support for the epidermis.

SUBCUTANEOUS TISSUE

The subcutaneous tissue is the innermost layer of the skin and is primarily composed of fat. This layer of the skin provides insulation to help regulate body temperature, as well as protection of the outer skin layers. Furthermore, the fat that is stored serves as a reservoir origin of calories.

TOPICAL PREPARATIONS

Topical preparations are most often applied directly to the body surfaces of skin and/or mucous membranes to treat various skin conditions. Topical preparations can be found in creams, lotions, ointments, foams, gels, pastes, and powders. **Table 15.1** defines the most common topical preparation forms.

TOPICAL GLUCOCORTICOIDS

Topical glucocorticoids are prescribed to treat and relieve inflammation and pruritus associated with dermatological conditions such as insect bites, eczema, and dermatitis.

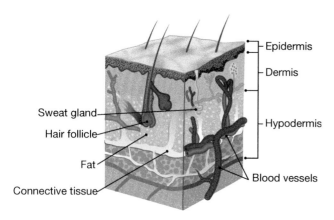

FIGURE 15.1 Anatomy of the skin.
Source: Reproduced from Gawlik KS, Melnyk BM, Teall AM, eds. *Evidence-based physical examination.* Springer Publishing Company; 2021:228, Figure 9.1.

They can be dispensed in a cream, ointment, or gel that penetrates to the origin of action, achieving a therapeutic response. Subsequently, topical glucocorticoids can benefit the skin by acting as an emollient or drying agent.

It is important to note that topical glucocorticoids can be absorbed in the systemic circulation. The absorption extent is based on the duration of use and the amount applied to the affected surface area. An occlusive dressing can enhance the absorption of the glucocorticoid.

Adverse effects can occur with the use of topical glucocorticoids and present either locally or systemically. Localized reactions include skin irritation, infection, atrophy of the dermis and epidermis, acne, and hypertrichosis. Systemic toxicity can present when extreme amounts of a high-potency glucocorticoid are used in a large area (generally covered by an occlusive dressing) over a long period of time. Effects of systemic toxicity include a growth delay in children and adrenal suppression in all age groups.

KERATOLYTIC AGENTS

Keratolytic agents are used to promote "shedding" of the horny layer of the skin. The horny layer of the skin is the outermost layer of the epidermis, which contains dead cells that are shed regularly in a process known as desquamation. These agents are used in areas where there is an overgrowth or thickening of the skin (e.g., calluses, warts). Salicylic acid, sulfur, and benzoyl peroxide are keratolytic agents used to treat these types of skin conditions discussed.

TABLE 15.1 Topical Preparation Forms	
Dosage Form	**Description**
Creams	Oil and water emulsion Ratio of water to oil affects the thickness of their consistency and how oily or sticky it feels to the skin Not as thick as ointment, but thicker than lotions Good for inflamed skin and dry sensitive skin More appropriate for intertriginous regions
Lotions	Water-based, nongreasy and tend to promote patient satisfaction Some contain acids or alcohol which can cause a burning sensation Little if any oil resulting in a lighter feel than creams Easy to spread; good choice for large or hairy areas
Ointments	Thick and greasy (i.e., oil or petroleum jelly base); little to no water Provide the highest medication absorption of all formulations Useful in the management of conditions with thickened skin or inflammation Provides an occlusive film that retains moisture; not a good choice for weeping or oozing skin conditions or areas of heavy sweating Excellent choice for dry skin conditions
Foams	Aerated solutions Spread easily and dry quickly Good choice for oily skin and large or hairy areas
Gels	Transparent preparations that contain cellulose with a water or alcohol base Liquefy on skin contact and have a cooling effect as it dries Nongreasy and good choice for oily skin Spread easily; good for covering large or hairy areas Good for facial regions because they dry clear and invisible
Pastes	Mixtures of an ointment and a powder; addition of powder increases adherence to the skin Powder disrupts the occlusive nature of an ointment allowing for air to reach the covered skin Pastes can be used in areas that are occluded (e.g., diaper rash paste beneath a diaper)
Powders	Talc or cornstarch base Dry with a silky feel that reduces friction between surfaces Useful between skin folds Good choice when applied to regions that tend to sweat (e.g., feet or axillae)

Salicylic Acid

Salicylic acid is readily absorbed through the skin and causes desquamation by breaking down the cement that binds scales to the horny layer of the skin. This affect is achieved with concentrations between 3% and 6%. Concentrations greater than 6% can result in tissue injury. Concentrations between 3% and 6% are used to treat acne, psoriasis, and dandruff. Concentrations up to 40% are used to treat and remove warts, calluses, and corns.[1]

Sulfur

Sulfur produces peeling and drying of the skin and is used to treat skin conditions such as acne and seborrheic dermatitis. Sulfur can be distributed in shampoos, gels, or lotions. For additive effects, sulfur can be combined with salicylic acid. The concentrations range from 2% to 10%.[2]

Benzoyl Peroxide

Benzoyl peroxide can produce drying and peeling of the skin. It is considered the first-line treatment for mild-to-moderate acne. Benzoyl peroxide is classified both as a keratolytic agent and an antibiotic. Its keratolytic component releases active oxygen, subsequently resulting in a reduction of inflammation by peeling the horny layer of the epidermis. Serious hypersensitivity reactions have been reported in patients with asthma.

SYSTEMIC PREPARATIONS

Systemic preparations are used in treating widespread infections such as, but not limited to, superficial fungal infections of the skin, hair, or nails, or when topical preparation has been ineffective. Other skin conditions that benefit from systemic preparations include extensive allergic contact dermatitis, infections of the hair and nails, widespread dermatophytosis, and chronic nonresponsive yeast infections. When a skin condition affects a large surface area of the skin, systemic administration is advantageous, as these widespread infection and inflammatory conditions may be difficult to manage and treat with a topical preparation.

DERMATITIS

INTRODUCTION

Dermatitis is a skin rash caused by a disruption in skin responsiveness triggered by an external vehicle. The term *eczema* is often used in substitution for dermatitis. Eczema typically refers to atopic dermatitis. When "eczematous" is used, it generally describes crusting and oozing in contrast to solely erythema. The term *dermatitis* is used to qualify a skin disorder (e.g., contact dermatitis).

Contact dermatitis accounts for 5.7 million visits to clinicians each year. Atopic dermatitis (i.e., eczema) affects between 5% and 10% of the U.S. population.[3] This particular dermatitis begins in childhood.

BACKGROUND

Contact Dermatitis

Contact dermatitis describes any dermatitis that is caused by an exposure to a substance or an external agent. This can take place through single or multiple exposures to an allergen. The result is typically an inflammatory process.

There are two types of contact dermatitis: irritant and allergic dermatitis. Toxic effects on the skin result in irritant contact dermatitis. Allergic dermatitis is caused by an exposure to an antigen that develops an immunologic response.

Irritant contact dermatitis (ICD) is not an allergic response. The water–protein–lipid matrix of the epidermis becomes damaged, resulting in irritant contact dermatitis. The affected area is erythematous and presents with scaly eruptions that are the result of an exposure to a thermal injury or chemical. The duration of the exposure and potency of the irritant, as well as the skin condition, affect the severity of the reaction.

Allergic Contact Dermatitis

Allergic contact dermatitis (ACD) is an immunological response to an antigen. Multiple phases occur during this response. The initial stage is the sensitization phase where the host is immunized to the antigen. When re-exposure occurs, a fast and more potent immune response of a secondary nature occurs. T-cells are the hallmark mediatory bodies of the reaction. During activation, T-cells release cells of the immune system which cause stimulation of local blood vessels, immune cell recruitment, and sensitization response amplification. Evidence of response can be visualized approximately 1 week following exposure to an antigen.

Atopic Dermatitis

The term *atopic dermatitis* (AD) is often used interchangeably with *eczema*. AD is an inflammatory skin disease that presents with dry and pruritic skin that is erythematous and is the result of cutaneous hyperreactivity to environmental stimuli. AD is a response to an allergen or antigen. With AD, high concentrations of serum immunoglobulin (Ig)E—immunoregulatory T cells—are decreased, the antibody-dependent cellular cytotoxicity is defective, and cell-mediated immunity is decreased. Genetic factors, skin barrier defects, and immune dysregulation constitute the pathogenesis of AD. Subsequently, filaggrin (FLG) is a protein that is necessary to the normal functioning of the skin. An eficiency in FLG may contribute, and predispose patients, to AD by increasing transepidermal water loss, infection, and inflammation.

RISK FACTORS FOR DERMATITIS

Multiple risk factors are related to dermatitis. The most common risk factors include, but are not limited to:

- Age
- Allergies and asthma
- Occupation
- Health conditions

Dermatitis can occur from infancy to geriatrics; however, atopic dermatitis (i.e., eczema) often develops in infancy and childhood. Individuals who have a personal and familial history of eczema and asthma are typically predisposed to the development of AD. An individual's occupation plays a role in the development of dermatitis. Certain jobs expose one to metals or chemicals that can increase the risk of dermatitis. Healthcare workers commonly develop dermatitis of the hands. Health conditions such as congestive heart failure, Parkinson's disease, and HIV pose an increased risk for the development of dermatitis.

DIAGNOSIS OF DERMATITIS

Both ICD and ACD present with papules, vesicles, and blisters that are linear in formation. An individual will describe the lesions to be pruritic. The ICD lesions are typically found only in the area of exposure whereas the ACD lesions are more diffuse in nature. The hallmark presentation of AD includes pruritus, severe dry skin, and hyperreactivity of the cutaneous layer of skin. The clinical presentation varies from red, weeping, scaly, and crusted lesions to lichenified plaques in a flexural arrangement over the wrist, ankles, and neck. Facial dermatitis and eyelid eczema are most often seen in older adults.

Diagnosis is typically made through a thorough familial and onset history and physical examination. Patch testing is the gold standard for contact allergen identification; however, it is not recommended to be an indicator for ICD.

PHARMACOTHERAPY FOR DERMATITIS

Initiating drug therapy for individuals with dermatitis is appropriate; however, prevention is the most effective

form of treatment for contact dermatitis. Patients must be educated to recognize the triggers that cause dermatitis and develop a plan of avoidance.

The goals of drug therapy for dermatitis are as follows:

- Restore normal epidermal barrier
- Treat the inflamed skin
- Control itching

Topical steroids are the therapy of choice for dermatitis. Topical immunosuppressants can be used if available and systemic corticosteroids are the treatment of choice for widespread areas and symptoms. Antihistamines are used to treat the pruritus. **Table 15.2** summarizes common medications used to treat dermatitis.

DERMATOPHYTE INFECTIONS OF THE SKIN

INTRODUCTION

Dermatophyte infections are the causes of fungal infections of the skin and are common across the world. The hair and nails can also be affected. Tinea or dermatophytosis lead to various clinical manifestations on different parts of the body.

BACKGROUND

The varieties of tinea infections are defined by their location: head (tinea capitis), body (tinea corporis), hand (tinea manus), foot (tinea pedis), groin (tinea cruris), and nails (tinea unguium—onychomycosis). Tinea capitis most commonly affects children aged 3 to 9 years and usually presents simultaneously with tinea corporis. Tinea pedis is seen mostly in the adolescent population and young adulthood. Tinea unguium is caused by yeast, fungi, and mold.

RISK FACTORS FOR DERMATOPHYTE INFECTIONS

Areas of the skin more susceptible to fungal infections include those that are warm and moist, such as interdigital areas of the toes. Individuals with cancer or other immunocompromised patients are more susceptible to dermatophytosis. Subsequently, family history can also predispose one to fungal infections. The infection is typically spread from person to person by cats and dogs, as well as other animals and inanimate objects.

DIAGNOSIS OF DERMATOPHYTE INFECTIONS

Individuals present with burning and pruritus, as well as stinging of the scalp or skin. Microscopic

TABLE 15.2 Pharmacotherapy for Contact Dermatitis

Medication	Dose/Frequency	Side Effects	Contraindications and Other Considerations
Low-Potency Medications			
Alclometasone dipropionate 0.05% (c, o) Fluocinolone acetonide 0.01% (s) Hydrocortisone base or acetate 0.5% (c) Hydrocortisone base or acetate 1% or 2.5% (o, c) Triamcinolone acetonide 0.025% (c, l, o)	Adult: Apply bid × 14 days Pediatric: Apply bid × 7 days	Acneiform lesions, burning erythema, folliculitis, irritation, pruritus, skin atrophy, skin irritation, striae	Fluocinolone acetonide: <6 years not recommended Hydrocortisone base or acetate: <12 years not recommended First-line treatment for contact dermatitis Can be taken with oral antihistamines for symptom relief Apply to moist skin surface; occlusive dressing is helpful
Intermediate-Potency Medications			
Betamethasone valerate 0.12% (f) Desonide 0.12% (c, l, o) Desoximetasone 0.05% (ec) Fluocinolone acetonide 0.025% (c, o) Flurandrenolide 0.025% or 0.05% (c, o) Fluticasone propionate 0.005% or 0.05% (c, o) Hydrocortisone butyrate 0.1% (c, o, s) Hydrocortisone valerate 0.2% (c, o) Mometasone furoate 0.1% (c, o, l) Prednicarbate 0.1% (ec) Triamcinolone acetonide 0.1% (c, o) or 0.2% (a)	Adult: Apply bid × 14 days Pediatric: Apply bid × 7 days	Acneiform lesions, burning, erythema, folliculitis, irritation, pruritus, skin atrophy, skin irritation, striae	Desonide: <3 months not recommended As second-line treatment for contact dermatitis, increase potency of topical corticosteroid Avoid using moderate- or high-potency topical corticosteroids on face or intertriginous areas
High-Potency Medications			
Amcinonide 0.1% (c, l, o) Betamethasone dipropionate augmented 0.05% (ec) Desoximetasone 0.05% (g) Desoximetasone 0.25% (ec, o) Diflorasone diacetate 0.05% (o, c) Fluocinonide 0.05% (c, g, o, s, ec) Halcinonide 0.1% (c, o, s, ec) Triamcinolone acetonide 0.5% (c, o)	Adult and pediatric: Apply bid × 7–14 days	Acneiform lesions, burning, erythema, folliculitis, irritation, pruritus, skin atrophy, skin irritation, striae	As second-line treatment for contact dermatitis, increase potency of topical corticosteroid Avoid using moderate- or high-potency topical corticosteroids on face or intertriginous areas
Very High-Potency Medications			
Betamethasone dipropionate augmented 0.05% (o, g) Clobetasol propionate 0.05% (c, g, o, sp, ec) Diflorasone diacetate 0.05% (o) Fluocinonide 0.1% (c) Flurandrenolide 4 mcg/sq (c) Halobetasol propionate 0.05% (c, o)	Adult and pediatric: Apply bid × 7–14 days	Acneiform lesions, burning, erythema, folliculitis, irritation, pruritus, skin atrophy, skin irritation, striae	As second-line treatment for contact dermatitis, increase potency of topical corticosteroid. Avoid using moderate- or high-potency topical corticosteroids on face or intertriginous areas
Topical Immunosuppressants			
Pimecrolimus 1% (o)	1 mg/kg once daily, decreased by 5 mg every 2 days for 2 weeks	Burning, erythema, flu-like symptoms, pruritus	Third-line treatment for contact dermatitis If dermatitis flares up, consider increasing dose; then taper as noted
Tacrolimus 0.03%, 0.1% (o)	Apply light layer bid	Burning, erythema, flu-like symptoms, pruritus	Not recommended for children <2 years

a, aerosol; bid, two times daily; c, cream; ec, emollient cream; f, foam; g, gel; l, lotion; o, ointment; s, solution; sp, scalp preparation.

evaluation, fungal cultures, and the use of a Wood lamp are diagnostic measures a clinician can take to diagnose a fungal infection of the scalp or skin. The Wood lamp is specifically used in the diagnosis of microsporum.

Tinea Capitis

Tinea capitis is spread from human to human, animals, and other organisms. It is highly contagious and most commonly seen in African American prepubertal children. *Trichophyton tonsurans* is the causative agent in 90% of cases. *Microsporum audouinii* and *Microsporum canis* can also be responsible organisms of infection. The presentation of tinea capitis consists of inflammatory nodules and broken hairs (e.g., alopecia) that result in seborrheic dermatitis (e.g., "cradle cap" in an infant) with impetigo features, including crusting, scaling, and pustular lesions. Approximately 15% of individuals have a cross-infection with tinea corporis.[4]

Tinea Corporis

Tinea corporis is a fungal infection that can involve the face, limbs, or trunk and is commonly referred to as "ringworm." The typical presentation is an erythemic ring-shaped lesion that is scaly with demarcated margins. It is transmitted by human-to-human contact, animals, and infected mats from gyms. *Trichophyton rubrum* is the most common cause; *M. canis* and *Trichophyton mentagrophytes* can also be the responsible organisms.

Tinea Cruris

Tinea cruris is more common in men than women and is commonly referred to as "jock itch." Risk factors include copious sweating, obesity, diabetes, and immunodeficiency. This infection presents as lesions in the groin area that are erythemic, macular, and can be quite large. Tinea cruris is commonly seen in the inguinal folds versus the scrotum. Key symptoms of tinea cruris include a burning sensation and pruritis. The most common causative dermatophyte is *T. rubrum*; *Epidermophyton floccosum* is also a responsible organism. Subsequently, a fungal infection of the feet can be present as well.

Tinea Pedis

Tinea pedis is commonly referred to as "athlete's foot." It presents as scaling, burning, and itching between the spacing of the toes. It is typically seen in young athletic men. *T. rubrum* and *T. mentagrophytes* are the responsible organisms. There are three types of tinea pedis: interdigital (between the toes), plantar (soles and entire plantar surface), and acute vesicular (sole of the foot, great toe, and instep).

Tinea Manus

Tinea manus is a fungal infection of the hand that presents with diffuse scaling and vesicles of the palms and fingernails. This infection is typically unilateral. Subsequently, tinea pedis is most always associated with tinea manus.

Tinea Unguium

Tinea unguium is a fungal infection of the nail that most commonly affects the toenails. This results in a thick and scaly nail bed. A yellowish discoloration is often seen. If untreated, the nail can become thicker and turn more of a yellowish-brown color. *E. floccosum*, *T. rubrum*, *T. mentagrophytes*, *Candida albicans*, *Aspergillus*, *Fusarium*, and *Scopulariopsis* are the responsible organisms.

PHARMACOTHERAPY FOR DERMATOPHYTE INFECTIONS

Pharmacological treatment is used to treat and defend the site against a fungal infection. Treatment can be systemic or topical, dependent upon the location of the lesion. Topical therapy is usually the treatment of choice unless otherwise contraindicated. **Table 15.3** summarizes common medications for fungal infections.

VIRAL SKIN INFECTIONS

INTRODUCTION

Herpes virus and papillomaviruses are two common virus-producing skin diseases. In the United States, 20% of the adult population is affected with the herpes virus and papillomaviruses, and the two are evenly distributed.[5] These viruses belong to the deoxyribonucleic acid (DNA) family.

The human papillomavirus (HPV) is responsible for the production of warts (verrucae). HPV infects the epithelial tissues of the skin and mucous membranes. Approximately 20% of children have one or more warts.[5]

BACKGROUND

Viral infections of the skin are obligate intracellular parasites. They contain a nucleic acid core that is encapsulated by proteins. A host cell is required for replication. In return, DNA viruses replicate by their own specific means. Viral infections are highly contagious and are spread via direct contact with the skin or mucous membranes. Herpes simplex virus 1 (HSV-1) infection most often involves the face and skin above the waist while herpes simplex virus 2 (HSV-2) is typically

TABLE 15.3 Pharmacotherapy for Fungal Infections of the Skin

Medication	Dose/Frequency	Contraindications	Side Effects	Other Considerations
Topical Agents				
Clotrimazole (o, p)	Apply ointment gently to affected and surrounding skin areas bid × 4 weeks (1 week past clinical cure); powder as needed	Pregnancy or lactation; exercise caution in patients with hepatocellular failure	Erythema, irritation, stinging, pruritus	May be purchased OTC
Miconazole	Cover affected areas with cream lotion or powder bid × 2–4 weeks (1 week past clinical cure)	Pregnancy or lactation	Irritation, maceration	Avoid applying near eyes
Ketoconazole	Apply to affected and surrounding areas once daily × 2–4 weeks (1 week past clinical cure)	Pregnancy or lactation, asthma, sulfite sensitivity; not recommended for children	Irritation, stinging, pruritus	—
Oxiconazole	Apply to affected and surrounding areas once or twice daily × 2–4 weeks (1 week past clinical cure)	Pregnancy or lactation	Pruritus, burning	Avoid applying near eyes or mucous membranes
Sulconazole	Apply to affected and surrounding areas bid × 4 weeks (1 week past clinical cure)	Pregnancy or lactation; not recommended for children	Pruritus, burning sensation, erythema	Avoid contact with eyes
Ciclopirox	Apply to affected area bid × 4 weeks	Not recommended for children <10 years	Pruritus, burning sensation	Avoid occlusive dressing; lotion formulation good for nails
Naftifine	Apply to affected area once daily × 4 weeks	Not recommended for children	Burning, stinging, dryness, erythema, itching	Avoid occlusive dressing; avoid contact with mucous membranes
Terbinafine	Apply to affected area bid × 4 weeks	Not recommended for children	Burning, irritation, skin exfoliation, dryness	Avoid occlusive dressing; avoid contact with mucous membranes
Tolnaftate	Apply small amount bid × 4 weeks	Not recommended for children <2 years	Stinging, burning, irritation	
Selenium sulfide, 1% (OTC), 2.5%	Massage into affected area, rest 15 minutes, rinse thoroughly		Irritation, hair loss	Use if lesions are resistant or widespread
Nystatin, 100,000 units/mL	Infants: 1 mL each side of mouth Adults: 2–3 mL each side of mouth		GI upset, oral irritation	Continue use for at least 48 hours after clinical cure; keep in mouth as long as possible before swallowing
Oral Agents				
Griseofulvin	Microsize: Adult: 500–1,000 mg/kg once daily × ≥8 weeks; pediatric: 10–15 mg/kg once daily × ≥8 weeks Ultramicrosize: Adult: 330–660 mg/kg once daily × ≥8 weeks; pediatric: 10 mg/kg once daily × ≥8 weeks	Pregnancy, porphyria, hepatic failure; prescribe with caution to patients sensitive to penicillin; antagonizes oral contraceptives and warfarin; antagonized by barbiturates	Headache, nausea, vomiting, diarrhea, photosensitivity	Most effective when taken with a high-fat meal; avoid alcohol; monitor CBC and LFT with long-term use; may aggravate lupus erythematosus
Ketoconazole	200 mg once daily	Not recommended for children; do not use with other drugs metabolized by CYP3A	Nausea, vomiting, abdominal pain, urticaria, pruritus	—

(continued)

TABLE 15.3 Pharmacotherapy for Fungal Infections of the Skin *(continued)*				
Medication	Dose/Frequency	Contraindications	Side Effects	Other Considerations
Oral Agents *(continued)*				
Itraconazole	200 mg once daily × 12 weeks	Not recommended for children; do not use with other drugs metabolized by CYP3A	GI upset, rash, fatigue, headache, dizziness, edema	May use pulse dosing; ingestion of food increases absorption
Terbinafine	62.5–250 mg once daily	Liver or renal disease; not recommended for children	GI disturbance, LFT abnormalities, urticaria, pruritus	—
Fluconazole	Adult: 100–200 mg once daily Pediatric: 3–6 mg/kg once daily	Potentiates warfarin, theophylline, oral hypoglycemics; may increase serum levels of phenytoin, cyclosporine; thiazides increase levels; may decrease effect of oral contraceptives	GI upset, headache, rash, hepatotoxicity	Decrease dose if creatine clearance <50 mL/min

bid, twice daily; CBC, complete blood count; CYP3A, cytochrome P450 enzyme 3A; GI, gastrointestinal; LFT, liver function tests; o, ointment; OTC, over the counter; p, powder.

associated with infection of the genital area. Herpes zoster, commonly known as shingles, and varicella (i.e., chicken pox) are results of the varicella-zoster virus (VZV). Plantar warts (*verrucae plantaris*) are typically associated with HPV-1; however, common warts (*Verruca vulgaris*) are generally caused by HPV-2. Warts that are flat and present on the face, neck, back, and chest are often associated with HPV-3.

RISK FACTORS FOR VIRAL SKIN INFECTIONS

Risk factors for herpes viruses include the female gender, human immunodeficiency virus (HIV), cancer, and aging. In general, patients who are immunocompromised are at risk as well. Infected mothers who give birth through the vaginal canal also put the infant at risk for transmitting the herpes virus. Similarly, intake of steroids, chemotherapy agents, pregnancy, and handling raw meat, fish, or other animal matter are risk factors of HPV.

DIAGNOSIS OF VIRAL SKIN INFECTIONS

HSV-1 and HSV-2 present with vesicular eruptions that are painful and typically recur. HSV-1 can be present in the mouth, pharynx, lips, or face. The VZV infections have similar symptoms. Varicella can present with fever in addition to the vesicular eruptions. VZV can be reactivated in the nerve root ganglion, which can be brought on by stressors. This reactivation of VZV is herpes zoster, which presents with a unilateral erythema that follows a nerve line. It is very painful and produces itching. Diagnosis is typically made via patient history, familial history, and physical assessment.

Warts are often flesh-colored and are raised on the skin. They can also be brownish in color and contain hyperkeratotic matter. Diagnosis is made frequently via physical assessment.

PHARMACOTHERAPY FOR VIRAL SKIN INFECTIONS

Nonpharmacologic approaches such as salt-water rinses and Burrow's solution can be used for HSV-1 infections; however, topical agents are the primary treatment. Oral lesions can be treated with a 1:1 dose of Maalox®. Benadryl® can be used as a mouth wash four times a day for comfort. Systemic therapies are used for VZV infections and should be initiated within 72 hours of the presenting disease. The goal of therapy is to reduce pain and promote comfort while stopping the reproduction of the viral disease. **Table 15.4** summarizes common medications for the treatment of herpes virus infections.

Aggressive therapy may be needed for wart treatment; however, some warts will resolve spontaneously with one treatment. Salicylic acid is the recommended first-line treatment for nonanogenital infection with HPV. If pharmacological treatment is not effective, surgical consultation by a dermatologist may be warranted.

TABLE 15.4 Pharmacotherapy for Herpes Virus Infections of the Skin

Medication	Dose/Frequency	Indications and Contraindications	Side Effects	Other Considerations
Acyclovir 5%	Apply q3h × 7 days	Indications: First-line for HSV-1; begin at earliest sign of outbreak	Pruritus, pain on application	Must use glove or finger cot for application; do not use on mucous membranes or near eyes
Penciclovir 1%	Apply q2h × 4 days	Indications: First-line for HSV-1; begin at earliest sign of outbreak Contraindications: Renal impairment	Headache, mild skin irritation	—
Acyclovir	VZV: adult—200 mg 5 × / day × 7 days; pediatric—20 mg/kg once daily × 5 days HSV-1: Initial outbreak—200 mg 5 × / day × 10 days; recurrence—200 mg 5 × / day × 5 days	Indications: First-line for VSV; second-line for HSV-1 Contraindications: Renal impairment	Nausea, vomiting, headache, CNS disturbance, rash, malaise	Do not exceed maximum dose
Famciclovir	VZV: 500 mg tid × 7 days HSV-1: Initial outbreak—250 mg tid × 10 days; recurrence—125 mg tid or 1,000 mg bid × 1 day	Indications: First-line for VSV; second-line for HSV-1 Contraindications: Renal impairment	Headache, GI upset, paresthesias	May be affected by drugs metabolized by aldehyde oxidase
Valacyclovir	VZV: 1 g tid × 7 days HSV-1: Initial outbreak—1 g bid × 10 days; recurrence—2,000 mg bid × 1 day	Indications: First-line for VSV; second-line for HSV-1 Contraindications: Renal impairment, HIV	GI upset, headache, dizziness, abdominal pain	Potential for renal or CNS toxicity with nephrotoxic drugs

bid, twice daily; CNS, central nervous system; GI, gastrointestinal; HIV, human immunodeficiency virus; tid, three times daily.

BACTERIAL SKIN INFECTIONS

INTRODUCTION

Bacterial infections present in a variety of cases ranging from minor to severe and sometimes life-threatening. Less-invasive bacterial infections are typically treated with antibiotic therapy and wound care management. Cellulitis and necrotizing fasciitis are two common bacterial infections of the skin.

The reported incidence of cellulitis is 200 cases per 100,000 patient-years.[6] Most cases of cellulitis in adults are caused by group A beta-hemolytic streptococci.[7] Cellulitis is very common in children and the most common causative organism is *Staphylococcus aureus*.[8] It is also often seen in the middle-aged and geriatric populations. Cellulitis can develop in healthy individuals without any predisposing factors, which leads to its consideration as a seasonal disease that is typically seen in the warmer months.

Necrotizing fasciitis is a severe bacterial infection of the subcutaneous tissue that is indicative of systemic activity and mortality. Studies have shown the mortality rate was at 24% to 34% but may exceed 50% in individuals with a vascular disease.[9] The incident rate is 0.3 to 15 cases per 100,000 population.[10]

BACKGROUND

Group A *Streptococcus* (GAS) and/or *S. aureus* are the responsible organisms for the development of cellulitis. Several microbials are responsible for necrotizing fasciitis, including *Streptococcus pyogenes*, *S. aureus*, *Bacteroides fragilis*, and *Peptostreptococci*. Cellulitis can lead to the development of an abscess if left untreated. Individuals diagnosed with necrotizing fasciitis are extremely ill and demand intensive critical care. Surgery is typically consulted for debridement and IV antibiotic therapy is warranted.

RISK FACTORS FOR BACTERIAL SKIN INFECTIONS

Individuals with predisposing factors and those who are exposed to community-associated methicillin-resistant *S. aureus* (CA-MRSA) are at risk for developing cellulitis. For this reason, healthy individuals can acquire cellulitis. Individuals with conditions such as diabetes and atherosclerotic disease are at risk for necrotizing fasciitis and have a poor prognosis. If development of necrotizing fasciitis begins in an extremity and progresses to the back, chest wall, or buttock area, very poor outcomes are expected. Both cellulitis and necrotizing fasciitis can lead to death if untreated.

DIAGNOSIS OF BACTERIAL SKIN INFECTIONS

Cellulitis can begin from a localized area of trauma. In children, cellulitis most often results from an insect or animal bite. The affected area becomes erythemic, warm, and tender to palpation. Swelling, induration, and pus can develop as well as fever. In severe cases, excruciating pain may develop at the affected area. Individuals with necrotizing fasciitis require intensive care and treatment by various clinicians and specialists. Tissue destruction and "hardness" occur with or without antibiotic therapy. Drainage of pus can be present while sepsis, instability of hematology, and multiorgan dysfunction can also occur.

PHARMACOTHERAPY FOR BACTERIAL SKIN INFECTIONS

Choosing the appropriate drug for bacterial skin infections can be challenging due to antibiotic resistance. Good hygiene such as frequent hand washing, cleansing of skin twice daily with soap and water, avoidance of scratching, and avoidance of tight clothing are all measures to prevent the development of a bacterial infection. **Table 15.5** provides an overview of selected antibiotics for bacterial infections of the skin.

The treatment of choice for individuals with the diagnosis of mild cellulitis can most often be followed on an outpatient level with oral antibiotic therapy. Severe

TABLE 15.5 Pharmacotherapy for Bacterial Skin Infections

Medication	Dose/Frequency	Contraindications	Side Effects	Other Considerations
Broad-Spectrum Penicillins				
Amoxicillin-clavulanate	Adult: 500–875 mg q12h or 250–500 mg q8h Pediatric: 22.5 mg/kg q12h or 13.3 mg/kg q8h	Penicillin allergy; use caution in patients with severe renal disease or less severe allergy to cephalosporins	Nausea, vomiting, diarrhea, rash, allergic reactions, fungal infections, Pseudomembranous colitis, seizures (high doses)	Taking with food may decrease GI symptoms Drug interactions: Warfarin, oral contraceptive
Dicloxacillin	Adult: 125–250 mg q6h Pediatric: 3.125–6.25 mg/kg q6h	Penicillin allergy; use caution in patients with severe renal or hepatic disease, pregnancy, lactation	Nausea, vomiting, diarrhea, rash, allergic reactions, fungal infections, Pseudomembranous colitis, seizures (high doses), drug-induced hepatitis	Taking with food may decrease GI symptoms Drug interactions: warfarin
First-Generation Cephalosporins				
Cephalexin Cefazolin	Cephalexin: Adults: 500 mg q12h Pediatric: 12.5–25 mg/kg q12h Cefazolin: Adult: 500 mg q12h or 1 g q6–8h (IV) Pediatric: 25–50 mg/kg divided into three or four equal doses	Penicillin allergy, allergy to cephalosporins; use caution in patients with renal disease, pregnancy, lactation	Nausea, vomiting, diarrhea, rash, allergic reactions, fungal infections, Pseudomembranous colitis, seizures (high doses), Stevens–Johnson syndrome, hemolytic anemia	Taking with food may decrease GI symptoms
Second-Generation Cephalosporins				
Cefaclor Cefprozil Cefuroxime	Cefaclor: Adult: 250–500 mg q8h or 375–500 mg q12h (ER) Pediatric: 6.7–13.3 mg/kg q8h, not to exceed 1 g/d Cefprozil: Adult: 250–500 mg q12h or 500 mg q24h Pediatric: 20 mg/kg q24h Cefuroxime: Adult: 250–500 mg q12h Pediatric: 15 mg/kg q12h	Serious penicillin allergy, allergy to cephalosporins; use caution in patients with renal disease, pregnancy, lactation	Nausea, vomiting, diarrhea, rash, allergic reactions, fungal infections, Pseudomembranous colitis, seizures (high doses), Stevens–Johnson syndrome, hemolytic anemia	Taking with food may decrease GI symptoms

(continued)

TABLE 15.5 Pharmacotherapy for Bacterial Skin Infections (continued)

Medication	Dose/Frequency	Contraindications	Side Effects	Other Considerations
Third-Generation Cephalosporins				
Cefpodoxime	Adult: 400 mg q12h	Serious penicillin allergy, allergy to cephalosporins; use caution in patients with renal disease, pregnancy, lactation	Nausea, vomiting, diarrhea, rash, allergic reactions, fungal infections, Pseudomembranous colitis, seizures (high doses), Steven–Johnson syndrome, hemolytic anemia	Taking with food may decrease GI symptoms
Ceftriaxone	Adult: 0.5–1.0 g q12h (IM or IV) or 1–2 g q24h (IM or IV) Pediatric: 50–75 mg/kg q24 (IM or IV), not to exceed 2 g	Serious penicillin allergy, allergy to cephalosporins; use caution in patients with renal disease, pregnancy, lactation	Nausea, vomiting, diarrhea, rash, allergic reactions, fungal infections, Pseudomembranous colitis, seizures (high doses), Steven–Johnson syndrome, hemolytic anemia	IM: Dilute with lidocaine to reduce pain at injection site
Fluoroquinolones				
Ciprofloxacin	Adult: 500–750 mg q12h	Fluoroquinolone allergy, pregnancy; use caution in patients with renal disease, CNS disease, elderly, lactation; not approved for children <18 years	Nausea, diarrhea, altered taste, dizziness, drowsiness, headache, insomnia, agitation, confusion, Pseudomembranous colitis, Stevens-Johnson syndrome	Drug interactions: Antacids, zinc, sucralfate, iron, theophylline, warfarin, probenecid, foscarnet, glucocorticoids, didanosine
Levofloxacin	500–750 mg once daily	Not approved for children	Nausea, diarrhea, altered taste, dizziness, drowsiness, headache, insomnia, agitation, confusion, Pseudomembranous colitis, Stevens-Johnson syndrome	—
Moxifloxacin	400 mg once daily	—	—	—
Other Medications				
Clindamycin	Adult: 150–450 mg q6h Pediatric: 2–5 mg/kg q6h or 2.7–6.7 mg/kg q8h	Allergy, history of Pseudomembranous colitis, severe hepatic disease	Nausea, vomiting, diarrhea, rash, allergic reaction, fungal infections, Pseudomembranous colitis	Take with full glass of water Drug interactions: Kaolin
Daptomycin	4 mg/kg once daily (IV)	Daptomycin allergy; not approved for children <18 years	CPK elevation with or without myopathy (reversible)	Monitor for CPK elevations, especially in patients receiving HMG-CoA reductase inhibitors
Linezolid	Adult: 600 mg (IV) or q12h (po) Pediatric: 10 mg/kg q8h	Allergy, uncontrolled hypertension	Bone marrow suppression, rare optic neuritis, or peripheral neuropathy with long-term use	Drug interaction: SSRIs, MAOIs
Tigecycline	100 mg × 1 dose, then 50 mg q12h	Tigecycline allergy; use caution in patients with tetracycline allergies	Nausea and vomiting are common	Adjust dose for severe hepatic impairment
Trimethoprim–sulfamethoxazole	Adult: 1–2 double-strength tablets q12h Pediatric: 8 mg/kg divided q12h	Sulfonamide or trimethoprim allergy, at-term pregnancy, lactation	Bone marrow suppression, rash, nausea, vomiting	Not to be used to treat infections caused by group A streptococcus
Vancomycin	Adult: 15 mg/kg q12h (IV) Pediatric: 10 mg/kg q6h (IV)	Vancomycin allergy	Infusion-related reactions, phlebitis, renal impairment	Monitor serum concentrations

CNS, central nervous system; CPK, creatinine phosphokinase; ER, extended-release; h, hour; IM, intramuscularly; IV, intravenously; MAOI, monoamine oxidase inhibitor; q, every; SSRI, selective serotonin reuptake inhibitor.

cases may require hospitalization with IV antibiotic therapy. For patients with mild-to-moderate cellulitis, penicillin VK and amoxicillin–clavulanate are drugs of choice and are prescribed for 7 to 10 days. These antibiotics treat against GAS; however, in severe cases of cellulitis, the selected regimen of antibiotic should also cover CA-MRSA. Cellulitis that has developed into an abscess requires sulfamethoxazole (Bactrim) or clindamycin. Surgical intervention is the expected need for an individual diagnosed with necrotizing fasciitis. Combination empiric antibiotic therapy has been used, which may include clindamycin, vancomycin, and/or piperacillin–tazobactam. The drugs and dosages are outlined in Table 15.5.

PSORIASIS

INTRODUCTION

Psoriasis is a common inflammatory disease of the skin that is noted for recurrent exacerbations as well as remission. Approximately 3% of the U.S. population is affected by this condition, while each year 150,000 new cases are diagnosed.[11] According to a population-based study in the United States, 2.5% of Caucasians and 1.3% of African Americans are affected.[12] The prevalence occurs equally among males and females; nevertheless, psoriasis is a familial disease with more than 20% of patients reporting a family history.[13] Up to 30% of patients with psoriasis may develop psoriatic arthritis.[14] The peak ages of onset follow a bimodal pattern at age 16 for females and 22 for males and at age 60 for females and 57 for males.[15] As a result, this is a disorder that can affect patients across the life span.

BACKGROUND

Psoriasis is an autoimmune disease that is led by T-cell activation. In this process, neutrophils are activated, which is responsible for the inflammatory process of the disease. It is a disease of emotion, often presenting in patients who experience severe depression and suicidality.

RISK FACTORS FOR PSORIASIS

Genetics plays a key role in the development of psoriasis. It attracts individuals who are monozygotic twins. Smoking, obesity, infections, alcohol, vitamin D deficiency, drugs (e.g., systemic corticosteroids, lithium carbonate, beta-blockers) and stress are all common risk factors to the disease.

DIAGNOSIS OF PSORIASIS

A diagnosis of psoriasis is usually made through history and physical examination. Typical clinical manifestations include:

- Well-demarcated, erythematous papules or plaques surrounded by silvery or whitish scales most often on the scalp, ears, elbows, knees, umbilicus, or nails
- Symmetric lesions
- Small scattered teardrop-shaped papules and plaques

PHARMACOTHERAPY FOR PSORIASIS

Psoriasis is a chronic disease that can have an impact on one's quality of life. Therefore, prior to treatment, an individualized screening for any risk factors (e.g., smoking) should be implemented. Goals of therapy include decreasing the impact of the clinical manifestations and increasing the overall quality of life, reducing pruritis, achieving remission, and facilitating minimal side effects from treatment. **Table 15.6** summarizes selected agents for the treatment of psoriasis.

ACNE VULGARIS

INTRODUCTION

Acne vulgaris is a common skin disorder seen in up to 90% of the adolescent population. In adult populations, 30% to 50% will report having acne.[16] Individuals with acne can experience psychological effects depending on the extent and severity of this disorder. These effects can include anxiety, embarrassment, and impaired social contact. Multiple over-the-counter (OTC) and prescription drugs are available and clinicians should individualize treatment interventions.

BACKGROUND

Acne usually presents during the pubertal stage of life and is seen more often in males than females. Lesions can appear on the face, neck, chest, shoulders, and back. Individuals can experience *open comedones* (i.e., blackheads) with mild acne and *closed comedones* (i.e., whiteheads) when the pores become blocked and scales form across the skin surface. Acne typically improves during a patient's early 20s; however, it can also be a chronic skin disorder that can extend over decades.

Acne begins in individuals when there is an increased androgen production that causes a corresponding increase in sebum production and follicular epithelial cells. The overall result is the clogging of pores. Sebum is then converted into irritant fatty acids by *Propionibacterium acnes* that promote inflammation.

RISK FACTORS FOR ACNE VULGARIS

Oily skin and genetic predisposition are risk factors to the development of acne. Foods, stress, and dirt can exacerbate acne as well. Drugs such as corticosteroids,

TABLE 15.6 Pharmacotherapy for Psoriasis

Medication	Dose/Frequency	Contraindications	Side Effects	Other Considerations
Emollients	Apply to affected skin tid–qid	—	Folliculitis, maceration, miliaria	Avoid application near eyes
Tar preparations	Coal tar: Apply qhs and allow to remain on skin Emulsion: 15–25 mL dissolved in bath water, immerse affected area for 10–20 minutes 3–7 times / week Shampoo: Massage into scalp and rinse, apply a second time, let rest for 5 minutes	Open or infected lesions	Irritation, photoreactions, unpleasant odor, folliculitis	May stain skin and clothing
Anthralin (antipsoriatic)	Apply for 30–60 minutes, remove	Renal disease, acute psoriasis	Irritation	May stain skin, towels, sinks, tub; avoid contact with eyes, mucous membranes; avoid irritation by applying emollients to unaffected skin
Calcipotriene (vitamin D analog)	Apply bid	Hypercalcemia, vitamin D toxicity	Burning, stinging, skin peeling, rash	Do not use on face
Tazarotene (vitamin A derivative)	Apply qhs	—	Pruritus, erythema	Avoid vitamin A
Hydrocortisone (topical corticosteroid)	Apply bid–qid	Primary bacterial infections or fungal infections	Burning, folliculitis, hypothalamic–pituitary–adrenal axis suppression	Use lowest effective dose; avoid prolonged use; use occlusive dressing
Apremilast	Day 1: 10 mg once daily Day 2: 10 mg bid Day 3: 10 mg a.m.; 20 mg p.m. Day 4: 20 mg bid Day 5: 20 mg a.m.; 30 mg p.m. Maintenance: 30 mg bid	Known hypersensitivity	GI upset, diarrhea	Starter kit to minimize side effects
Cyclosporine	Initial dose: 1.25 mg/kg orally bid for ≥4 weeks; increase by 0.5 mg/kg/day at 2-week intervals based on patient response Maximum dose: 2–5 mg/kg once daily	Pregnancy, lactation; use caution in patients with impaired renal and hepatic function	Tremor, gingival hyperplasia, GI upset, hypertension, renal dysfunction, acne	Increased risk of digoxin toxicity; decreased therapeutic effect with use of hydantoins, rifampin, sulfonamides Drug interactions:Lovastatin, diltiazem, ketoconazole
Methotrexate	12.5–25 mg/kg/week	Pregnancy, lactation; use caution in patients with impaired renal and hepatic function, leukopenia	Headache, blurred vision, fatigue, malaise, GI upset, gingivitis, hepatotoxicity, bone marrow depression, rash, alopecia, fever	Decreased level of digoxin; increased risk of toxicity with salicylates, phenytoin, sulfonamides; take folic acid 1 mg on nontreatment days
Adalimumab	80 mg SC initially, then 40 mg every other week	Concurrent live vaccine, active infection; use caution with pregnant patients	Headache, nausea, rash, reaction at injection site	—
Etanercept	50 mg twice a week × 3 months, then 40 mg weekly SC	Concurrent live vaccine, active infection; use caution with pregnant patients, patients with impaired renal function, asthma, blood dyscrasia, CNS demyelinating disease, history of recurrent infections	Infection, injection site pain, localized erythema, rash, URI, abdominal pain, vomiting	Maximum of 25 mg can be given in each site, requiring two injections
Infliximab	5 mg/kg IV	Concurrent live vaccine, severe CHF, infection, malignancy	GI upset, headache, fatigue, cough, nasopharyngitis, URI	

bid, two times a day; CHF, congestive heart failure; CNS, central nervous system; GI, gastrointestinal; qhs, before bed; qid, four times a day; SC, subcutaneously; tid, three times a day; URI, upper respiratory infection.

isoniazid, lithium, and phenytoin can also contribute to acne. Women with polycystic ovary syndrome (PCOS) or a history of menstrual irregularities are at risk for the development of acne.

DIAGNOSIS OF ACNE VULGARIS

Diagnosis of acne is made by a patient history and physical assessment. Acne is classified and treated according to the severity as previously mentioned.

TREATMENT FOR ACNE VULGARIS

Treatment of acne can be prolonged due to its potential as a chronic skin disease. Individuals with mild-to-moderate acne typically respond well to therapy. Appropriate and effective treatment will prevent scarring, shorten the length of the disease process, and decrease the psychological impact.

Nonpharmacologic therapies include removal of excess oil by using a gentle cleanser with a nonirritant soap twice daily. It is essential to educate patients not to perform vigorous scrubbing of the face. It is best to refrain from oil-based make up or moisturizing products.

Topical and oral drugs are used to treat acne. These treatments may be divided into two subgroups: antimicrobial agents and retinoids. **Table 15.7** summarizes common drug therapies and dosages for the treatment of acne.

TABLE 15.7 Pharmacotherapy for Acne Vulgaris

Medication	Dose/Frequency	Contraindications	Side Effects	Other Considerations
Tretinoin (c, g)	Apply once daily, increase strength as tolerated	Eczema, sunburn; pregnancy category C	Erythema, local skin irritation, photosensitivity	If not tolerated, apply to dry skin for shorter periods, alternate days; avoid products with alcohol, astringents, spices, lime
Benzoyl peroxide 2.5%–5.0%	Apply once daily; increase to bid–tid	—	Irritation	May bleach fabrics; alternate with other topical medications
Azelaic acid 20% cream	Apply bid	—	Pruritis, irritation	Hypopigmentation in dark-skinned individuals
Erythromycin 2%–3%	Apply bid	Erythromycin allergy	Irritation	—
Tazarotene 0.05%, 0.1% (g, c)	Apply once daily	Pregnancy category X	Irritation, photosensitivity	Obtain negative pregnancy test, use contraception
Tetracycline	500–1,000 mg daily divided bid–qid; taper to 250 mg once daily after improvement; discontinue after 4–6 months of therapy	Children <12 years; pregnancy category D	Photosensitivity, GI upset, decreased effectiveness of oral contraceptives	May increase serum digoxin levels; absorption reduced if taken with antacids, iron, zinc, dairy products; may increase blood urea nitrogen values if renal system impaired
Erythromycin	500–1,000 mg daily divided bid–qid	Erythromycin or macrolide allergy; not recommended for children <2 months	Nausea, vomiting, diarrhea, rash, allergic reactions, fungal infection, hepatitis, ototoxicity	Take 1 hour before or 2 hours after meal
Isotretinoin	0.5–1.0 mg/kg once daily	Adolescents before cessation of growth; pregnancy category X	Increased cholesterol and triglyceride levels, dry skin and mucous membranes, depression; aggressive, violent behaviors; back pain; arthralgias in pediatric patients	Female patients of childbearing age must have two negative pregnancy tests prior to therapy initiation, monthly negative pregnancy tests while on therapy; monitor cholesterol and triglyceride levels, CBC, LFTs before therapy, at 4 weeks, and as indicated
Ethinyl estradiol with norgestimate	One tablet once daily	Premenarchal girls, male patients	—	Women who smoke should avoid use of oral contraceptives

bid, two times a day; c, cream; CBC, complete blood count; g, gel; LFT, liver function test; tid, three times a day.

CONCLUSION

Skin conditions may be caused by noninfectious or infectious sources. Infections that cause various patterns of skin eruptions may be due to parasites, virus, or bacteria. Noninfectious sources of skin eruptions may result from the activation of immune responses. It is prudent for clinicians to make accurate diagnoses when assessing various skin conditions. The treatment of skin disorders may be systemic, topical, or a combination of both formulations. Understanding the root causes of the skin disorders and targeting the appropriate common pathogens related to various skin infections will assist prescribers to effectively treat the patients and improve outcomes.

CASE EXEMPLAR: Patient With Painful Rash

HZ is a 75-year-old male who complains of a painful rash on his upper back. The rash has been present for the past 5 to 7 days and is only on the right side. He feels some tenderness around the right front of his chest but does not see a rash. HZ recently recovered from a COVID-19 infection that put him in the hospital for 4 weeks. He believes he picked up the rash from the hospital bed linens or gowns.

Past Medical History
- Hypertension
- Osteoarthritis of the knees

Medications
- Hydrochlorothiazide, 25 mg daily
- Lisinopril, 20 mg daily
- Naproxen, 500 mg twice daily

Physical Examination
- Height: 70 inches; weight: 168 lbs.; blood pressure: 152/94; pulse: 82; respiration rate: 16; temperature: 97.2 °F

- Well-developed, underweight elderly male in no distress
- Lungs: Scattered rhonchi
- Heart: Regular rate and rhythm, no murmurs
- Skin: Right upper posterior thorax with nearly confluent vesicular rash on an erythematous base over right fourth thoracic dermatome

Labs
- None

Discussion Questions

1. What is the diagnosis for HZ, and what are the goals of pharmacologic management?
2. What pharmacologic interventions are available to help HZ?
3. What special considerations need to be taken in HZ's treatment?

CASE EXEMPLAR: Patient With Lump on His Head

TC is a 6-year-old African American male presenting with a lump on his head. He denies trauma. The lump is mildly uncomfortable but more itchy than painful. It has been growing in size for the past 2 to 3 weeks, and he seems to be losing some of his hair over the lump.

Past Medical History
- Usual childhood illnesses
- Current on vaccines

Medications
- None

Physical Examination
- Height: 45 inches; weight: 45 lbs.; pulse: 84; respiration rate: 12; temperature: 98.6 °F
- Well-developed, well-nourished African American male child in no distress

- Scalp with 5-cm diameter round boggy mass over the right occiput with overlying hair loss; scaliness of the skin; no exudate; nontender

Labs
- Skin scraping: Fungal elements on potassium hydroxide (KOH) preparation

Discussion Questions

1. What are the pharmacotherapeutic goals for TC?
2. What drug therapy should the clinician recommend for TC?
3. What special precautions are required for the medications prescribed?

TAKEAWAYS

- al glucocorticoids are prescribed to treat relieve inflammation and pruritus associated with dermatological conditions such as insect bites, eczema, and dermatitis.
- Keratolytic agents are used to promote "shedding" of the horny layer of the skin.
- Systemic preparations are used in treating widespread infections such as superficial fungal infections of the skin, hair, or nails or when topical preparation has been ineffective.
- The goals of drug therapy for dermatitis are to restore the normal epidermal barrier, treat the inflamed skin, and control itching.
- Dermatophyte infections are the causes of fungal infections of the skin and are highly contagious.
- Psoriasis is an autoimmune disease that is led by T-cell activation; risk factors include genetic predisposition, smoking, obesity, infection, alcohol, vitamin D deficiency, drugs (e.g., systemic corticosteroids, lithium carbonate, beta-blockers), and stress.

REFERENCES

1. Salicylic acid. In: *IBM Micromedex® DRUGDEX®* (electronic version). IBM Watson Health. Accessed November 2020. https://www.micromedexsolutions.com/micromedex2/librarian/CS/297F33/ND_PR/evidencexpert/ND_P/evidencexpert/DUPLICATIONSHIELDSYNC/DE7A02/ND_PG/evidencexpert/ND_B/evidencexpert/ND_AppProduct/evidencexpert/ND_T/evidencexpert/PFActionId/evidencexpert.IntermediateToDocumentLink?docId=529100&contentSetId=100&title=Salicylic+Acid&servicesTitle=Salicylic+Acid#

2. Sulfur. In: *IBM Micromedex® DRUGDEX®* (electronic version). IBM Watson Health. Accessed November 2020. https://www.micromedexsolutions.com/micromedex2/librarian/CS/1C9A05/ND_PR/evidencexpert/ND_P/evidencexpert/DUPLICATIONSHIELDSYNC/5DC3B5/ND_PG/evidencexpert/ND_B/evidencexpert/ND_AppProduct/evidencexpert/ND_T/evidencexpert/PFActionId/evidencexpert.IntermediateToDocumentLink?docId=1138&contentSetId=31&title=SULFUR&servicesTitle=SULFUR#

3. Arcangelo VP. Contact dermatitis. In: Arcangelo VP, Peterson AM, Wilbur V, Reinhold JA eds. *Pharmacotherapeutics for Advanced Practice.* 4th ed. Wolters Kluwer; 2017:155–162.

4. Arcangelo VP. Fungal infections of the skin. In: Arcangelo VP, Peterson AM, Wilbur V, Reinhold JA, eds. *Pharmacotherapeutics for Advanced Practice.* 4th ed. Wolters Kluwer; 2017:163–172.

5. Arcangelo VP. Viral infections of the skin. In: Arcangelo VP, Peterson AM, Wilbur V, Reinhold JA eds. *Pharmacotherapeutics for Advanced Practice.* 4th ed. Wolters Kluwer; 2017:173–180.

6. Spelman D, Baddour LM. Cellulitis and skin abscess: epidemiology, microbiology, clinical manifestations, and diagnosis. In: Lowy FD, Kaplan SL, Baron EL, eds. *UpToDate.* Updated October 7, 2020. https://www.uptodate.com/contents/cellulitis-and-skin-abscess-clinical-manifestations-and-diagnosis/print

7. Talbot E, Shevy LE. Cellulitis. In: Buttaro T, Trybulski J, Polgar-Bailey P, Sandberg-Cook J, eds., *Primary Care: A Collaborative Practice.* 5th ed. Elsevier; 2017:260.

8. Wathen D, Halloran DR. Blood culture associations in children with a diagnosis of cellulitis in the era of methicillin-resistant *Staphylococcus aureus. Hosp Pediatr.* 2013;3(2):103–107. doi:10.1542/hpeds.2012-009

9. Jabbour G, El-Menyar A, Peralta R, et al. Pattern and predictors of mortality in necrotizing fasciitis patients in a single tertiary hospital. *World J Emerg Surg.* 2016;11:40 doi:10.1186/s13017-016-0097-y

10. Stevens DL, Baddour LM. Necrotizing soft tissue infections. In Wessels MR, Edwards MS, Baron EL, eds. *UpToDate.* 2018. Updated November 3, 2020. https://www.uptodate.com/contents/necrotizing-soft-tissue-infections/print

11. Feldman SR, Goffe B, Rice G, et al. The challenge of managing psoriasis: unmet medical needs and stakeholder perspectives. *Am Health Drug Benefits.* 2016;9(9):504–513. https://www.ncbi.nlm.nih.gov/pmc/articles/PMC5394561

12. Alexis AF, Blackcloud P. Psoriasis in skin of color: epidemiology, genetics, clinical presentation, and treatment nuances. *J Clin Aesthet Dermatol.* 2014;7(11):16–24. https://www.ncbi.nlm.nih.gov/pmc/articles/PMC4255694

13. Ran D, Cai M, Zhang X. Genetics of psoriasis: a basis for precision medicine. *Precis Clin Med.* 2019;2(2):120–130. doi:10.1093/pcmedi/pbz011

14. Cather JC, Young M, Bergman MJ. Psoriasis and psoriatic arthritis. *J Clin Aesthet Dermatol.* 2017;10(3):S16–S25. Pubmed PMID: 28360971.

15. Singh S, Kalb RE, de Jong EMGJ, et al. Effect of age of onset of psoriasis on clinical outcomes with systemic treatment in the Psoriasis Longitudinal Assessment and Registry (PSOLAR). *Am J Clin Dermatol.* 2018;19:879–886. doi:10.1007/s40257-018-0388-z

16. Carre MD. Acne vulgaris and rosacea. In: Arcangelo VP, Peterson AM, Wilbur V, Reinhold JA, eds. *Pharmacotherapeutics for Advanced Practice.* 4th ed. Wolters Kluwer; 2017:207–218.

Pharmacotherapy for Neurologic Conditions

Alan H. Yee, Kwan L. Ng, Katherine Park, Alexandra (Sasha) Duffy, Doris Chen, and Tyrell Simkins

LEARNING OBJECTIVES

- Describe the pathophysiology underlying epilepsy, outline the clinical manifestations associated with that pathophysiology, and define treatment options.
- Describe the pathophysiology underlying dementia, associated clinical manifestations, and treatment options.
- Differentiate between multiple sclerosis, myasthenia gravis, and Guillain-Barre syndrome; recognize the clinical manifestations and underlying pathophysiology; and outline treatment options.
- Differentiate between the types of stroke, including etiology, clinical manifestations, and treatment options.
- Describe the pathophysiology underlying Parkinson's disease, including the clinical manifestations associated with that pathophysiology, and outline treatment options.

EPILEPSY

INTRODUCTION

Epilepsy is the fourth most common neurologic disorder. One in 26 people will develop epilepsy in their lifetime, and approximately 50 million people worldwide suffer from the condition.[1] Epilepsy affects people of all ages though it is most often diagnosed in younger children and older adults. Epilepsy is a chronic disorder characterized by recurrent, unprovoked seizures that occur as a result of abnormal electrical activity within the brain. The cerebral neurons undergo complex chemical changes that contribute to electrical activity homeostasis. For normal electrophysiological response, a balance must be established between excitatory and inhibitory neuronal signals. When imbalanced, surges of abnormal electrical firing result in seizures. Epilepsy is diagnosed when one experiences two or more unprovoked seizures that occur more than 1 day apart, or when a patient has an unprovoked seizure with high risk of recurrence. Descriptions of epilepsy may be based on the abnormal brain region involved. In other words, focal epilepsy describes the occurrence of seizures that arise from a discrete cerebral location whereas generalized (or "entire brain") epilepsy describes abnormal seizure activity resulting from whole-brain electrical dysfunction.[2]

RISK FACTORS FOR EPILEPSY

Perinatal complications, developmental delay, childhood febrile convulsions, family history of epilepsy, prior central nervous system infection, traumatic brain injury, stroke, brain tumor, or prior intracranial surgery are considered risk factors for developing epilepsy.

DIAGNOSIS OF EPILEPSY

The diagnosis of epilepsy is based on a thorough history and physical examination in combination with supportive diagnostic studies that include EEG and neuroimaging (e.g., MRI, CT). The role of imaging aids in identification of a seizure nidus such as tumors, stroke, trauma, infection, or an autoimmune process.

Epileptiform activity captured on EEG is present in nearly half of patients with epilepsy who undergo a routine study.[3,4] The diagnostic yield of electrophysiologic testing increases with frequency of testing, longer duration of continuous recording, and testing performed at shorter intervals from the actual seizure event. Abnormal epileptiform activity is rare in healthy individuals and is seen in up to 0.5%.[5] However, epileptiform discharges are captured in 2% to 2.6% of adults with underlying neurologic or psychiatric diseases.[6] Prolonged inpatient or outpatient (continuous) EEG monitoring improves the diagnostic yield in capturing epileptiform discharges as well as examining patients with unexplained recurrent paroxysmal events.

Seizures may have protean manifestations depending on the brain region involved and are classified as either focal or generalized.[7] Focal seizures begin in one brain region or involve a single group of neurons in one cerebral hemisphere. Further subcategorization of focal seizures is based on whether impairment in consciousness occurred. In other words, alertness is not impaired in *focal aware seizures* (known previously as "simple partial seizures"), while alertness is impaired in *focal impaired awareness seizures* (known previously as "complex partial seizures"). Additional characterization incorporates abnormal motor activity (e.g., automatisms, muscle spasm, and clonic, tonic, atonic, myoclonic, or hyperkinetic behavior) and nonmotor symptoms (e.g., behavioral arrest or emotional, cognitive, sensory, or autonomic symptoms).

Generalized seizures begin simultaneously in both hemispheres and are further classified based on the presence of accompanying abnormal motor activity. Patients who develop "staring spells" without the development of motor symptoms experience seizures referred to as *absence seizures*. One-sided focal seizures that spread to involve the contralateral hemisphere are referred to as *secondary generalization*, and oftentimes manifest as abnormal unilateral or bilateral tonic–clonic activity.

Numerous nonepileptic conditions can mimic seizures. Convulsive syncope, transient ischemic attacks, transient global amnesia, movement disorders, migraines, panic disorder, psychogenic nonepileptic events, and sleep disorders are common conditions often mistaken for seizures. Most seizures are typically stereotyped—exhibit similar clinical behavior—and last up to 2 minutes. Diagnostic confirmation and determination of seizure type are key to the management of epilepsy.

TREATMENT OF EPILEPSY

Preventative anticonvulsant treatment should be considered following seizure diagnosis. Targeted drug therapy is based on seizure type, comorbidities, drug interactions (e.g., warfarin or hormonal replacement), and, importantly, family planning. According to the National Institute for Health and Care Excellence (NICE), the first-line therapies for focal seizure are levetiracetam, carbamazepine, oxcarbazepine, zonisamide, gabapentin, and lamotrigine. Meanwhile, for generalized tonic–clonic seizures, lamotrigine, valproate, carbamazepine, or oxcarbazepine are considered as first-line therapies. For generalized absence seizures, ethosuximide and valproate are agents to be considered first. Lastly, for generalized myoclonic seizures, levetiracetam, lamotrigine, and valproate as well as topiramate are considered as first-line therapies.[8,9] **Table 16.1** summarizes common seizure disorders and recommended first-line therapies.

Nearly half of all patients are seizure-free following initiation of a well-tolerated first anticonvulsant. In those who experience breakthrough episodes, a

---

TABLE 16.1 Classification of Common Seizure Disorders and Recommended First-Line Therapy

Seizure Classification With Definition and Characteristics	First-Line Monotherapy Based on Level of Evidence*	
	Pediatric (<16 years)	Adult
Focal (partial) Originates within networks limited to one hemisphere; characterized by subjective (aura), motor, autonomic, and dyscognitive features	Level A: Oxcarbazepine Level B: None Level C: Carbamazepine, phenobarbital, phenytoin, topiramate, valproic acid, vigabatrin Level D: Clobazam, clonazepam, lamotrigine (Lamictal), zonisamide	**Younger adults (16–59 years)** Level A: Carbamazepine, levetiracetam, phenytoin, zonisamide Level B: Valproic acid Level C: Gabapentin, lamotrigine, oxcarbazepine, phenobarbital, topiramate, vigabatrin Level D: Clonazepam, primidone **Older adults (≥60 years)** Level A: Gabapentin, lamotrigine Level B: None Level C: Carbamazepine Level D: Topiramate, valproic acid

(continued)

TABLE 16.1 Classification of Common Seizure Disorders and Recommended First-Line Therapy *(continued)*

Seizure Classification With Definition and Characteristics	First-Line Monotherapy Based on Level of Evidence*	
	Pediatric (<16 years)	**Adult**
Generalized *Convulsive:* Typically bilateral and symmetric; variants with asymmetry, including head and eye deviation possible *Atonic:* Loss or diminution of muscle tone without apparent preceding myoclonic or tonic features; very brief (<2 seconds); may involve the head, trunk, or limbs *Tonic:* Bilaterally increased tone of the limbs, typically lasts seconds to 1 minute; often occurs while awake and in sequences of varying intensity of tonic stiffening *Myoclonic:* Level of awareness varies, ranging from complete loss of awareness to retained awareness; rhythmic myoclonic jerks of the shoulders and arms with tonic abduction that results in progressive lifting of the arms during the seizure; bilateral, unilateral, or asymmetric; perioral myoclonia, rhythmic jerks of the head and legs may occur; seizures last 10–60 seconds, typically occur daily; myoclonic status epilepticus is ongoing (>30 minutes) irregular jerking, often with partially retained awareness *Negative myoclonic:* Background muscle tone undergoes brief cessation lasting <500 ms; may have initial loss of posture caused by negative myoclonus, followed by subsequent voluntary and compensatory movement to restore posture *Myoclonic–atonic:* Myoclonic seizure occurs, followed by an atonic seizure; a series of myoclonic jerks may occur before atonia and may be hard to detect; patients typically experience a sudden fall because the seizure affects the head and limbs	Level A: None Level B: None Level C: Carbamazepine, phenobarbital, phenytoin, topiramate, valproic acid Level D: Oxcarbazepine, topiramate, valproic acid	Level A: None Level B: None Level C: Carbamazepine, lamotrigine, oxcarbazepine, phenobarbital, phenytoin, topiramate, valproic acid Level D: Gabapentin, levetiracetam, vigabatrin
Absence *Typical:* Onset and offset of altered awareness occurs abruptly; myoclonus of limbs is rare; oral and manual automatisms common; severity varies; clonic movements of facial parts may occur; behaviors before seizure onset may extend repeatedly *Atypical:* Onset and offset of loss of awareness is less than abrupt; often associated with other features (e.g., loss of muscle tone of the head, trunk, limbs; subtle myoclonic jerks) *Eyelid myoclonia:* Awareness retained; absence seizures associated with brief, repetitive, and often rhythmic, fast (4–6 Hz) myoclonic jerks of the eyelids with simultaneous upward deviation of the eyeballs and extension of the head; typically very brief (<6 seconds), occurs multiple times daily *Myoclonic absence:* Causes rhythmic myoclonic jerks of the shoulders and arms; results in progressive lifting of the arms during the seizure due to tonic abduction; myoclonic jerks typically bilateral, but may be unilateral or asymmetric; perioral myoclonia and rhythmic jerks of the head, legs may occur; seizures last 10–60 seconds, typically occur daily; level of awareness varies	Level A: Ethosuximide (Zarontin), valproic acid Level B: None Level C: Lamotrigine Level D: None	Level A: None Level B: None Level C: Carbamazepine, lamotrigine, oxcarbazepine, phenobarbital, phenytoin, topiramate, valproic acid Level D: Gabapentin, levetiracetam, vigabatrin
Focal/generalized *Epileptic spasms:* May be focal or generalized; sudden flexion, extension, or mixed flexion–extension of proximal and truncal muscles lasting longer than a myoclonic jerk (which lasts milliseconds), but not as long as a tonic seizure (which lasts >2 seconds); occur in a series, usually on wakening; subtle forms may occur with only chin movement, grimacing, head nodding; may be bilaterally symmetric, asymmetric, or unilateral	Optimal treatment not well defined and patients should be treated based on whether seizure activity is focal or generalized using the previously listed drugs	

*Choice of drug should be individualized. Levels of evidence are based on the quality of the supporting trials. For initial monotherapy, level A indicates that the antiepileptic drug (AED) is known to be efficacious or effective; level B indicates that the AED is probably efficacious or effective; level C indicates that the AED is possibly efficacious or effective; and level D indicates that the AED is potentially efficacious or effective.

Source: With permission from Liu G, Slater N, Perkins A. Epilepsy: treatment options. *Am Fam Physician.* 2017;96(2):87–96. https://www.aafp.org/afp/2017/0715/p87.html

second additional medication can be preventative in up to an additional 13% of patients. Patients who continue to experience seizures despite two medications are considered refractory and are unlikely to derive sustainable benefit following the addition of a third agent.[10] Those with medically refractory epilepsy—a failure of two or more medications—should be referred to a comprehensive epilepsy center for other abortive treatment options. Surgical intervention is an effective method to prevent and/or minimize recurrence in these cases. Treatments include partial surgical resection, transection, ablation to implantation of vagal nerve stimulation, and other deep brain stimulator devices. Carbohydrate restriction diets (e.g., ketogenic diet) or the modified Atkin's diet may provide some relief in seizure freedom. **Table 16.2** provides a summary of currently available antiepileptic drugs and their indications, toxicities, and mechanism of actions.

DEMENTIA

INTRODUCTION

Dementia affects an estimated 50 million people worldwide. They are typically over the age of 65. As the population ages and life expectancy increases, the prevalence of dementia will continue to rise. The most common cause of dementia is Alzheimer's disease (AD). Types of dementia include vascular dementia, frontotemporal dementia (FTD), dementia with Lewy bodies (DLB), and Parkinson's disease dementia (PDD).[11–15]

The pathophysiology of dementia is thought to be due to overproduction and impaired clearance of specific proteins in the brain. Abnormal tau tangle proteins (also known as neurofibrillary tangles) are seen in both AD and FTD, but beta-amyloid plaques (also known as amyloid plaques or senile plaques) are seen only in AD.[16] The neurofibrillary tangles are found intracellularly and are derived from damaged microtubules within the neurons. These tau protein aggregates form tangles that block the neuronal transporting system, subsequently disrupting the communication between neurons.[17] On the contrary, beta-amyloid plaques are found in the extracellular space nearby blood vessels of the central nervous system. These plaques are derived from the amyloid precursor proteins (APP), which are membrane glycoproteins that participate in a wide range of neuronal activities such as development, signaling, intracellular transport, and maintenance of neuronal homeostasis.[18] The alpha-synuclein aggregates are detected in both DLB and PDD. These pathological proteins have a predilection for different cerebral regions and lead to variable degrees of cerebral atrophy. The mechanisms in which these proteins impair neuronal function are not well understood.[12]

RISK FACTORS FOR DEMENTIA

Age confers the greatest risk of developing dementia followed by relation to a first-degree relative with the condition. The 10% to 30% increased risk due to kinship is not synonymous with forms of genetically inherited dementia.[19] Numerous modifiable risk factors have been identified and include those seen in patients with cardiovascular and cerebrovascular disease (e.g., hypertension, diabetes, hyperlipidemia) as well as brain trauma, lower educational level, physical activity, and diet. However, none of these have been definitive. Aerobic exercise, healthy dieting, social interaction, and adequate sleep have been linked to lower cognitive decline risks.

DIAGNOSIS OF DEMENTIA

Ante mortem diagnosis of dementia is based on clinical assessment. Dementia is defined as cognitive or behavioral impairment in two or more cognitive domains that lead to functional decline. The most commonly affected domain is memory, typically short-term episodic memory. Other domains include language (e.g., word finding difficulties), visuospatial abilities (e.g., getting lost), executive functioning (e.g., handling finances), and personality and behavior.

Quick screening tools for dementia include the Mini-Cog and General Practitioner Assessment of Cognition. However, if time allows, the Mini Mental Status Exam (MMSE) and Montreal Cognitive Assessment (MoCA) may be more informative. The MoCA is available in several languages and is culturally tailored. In-depth neuropsychological testing is best at delineating the most affected cognitive domains and can be pursued if the pattern of presentation is unclear. Insidious, progressive dementia is likely a result of a neurodegenerative process. Dramatic impairment of cognitive function can frequently be seen in the setting of illness, surgery, or hospitalization.

Workup primarily focuses on evaluating for non-neurodegenerative etiologies for cognitive decline. Screening for depression, vitamin B12 deficiency, and abnormal thyroid function should be completed in all patients. In specific patients, testing for syphilis, HIV, heavy metals, and other vitamin deficiencies, as well as cerebrospinal fluid (CSF) studies, may be considered. The American Academy of Neurology (AAN) recommends that all patients obtain brain imaging, either noncontrast MRI or CT. These studies can reveal masses, subdural hematomas, strokes, and evidence of normal pressure hydrocephalus. Characteristic imaging patterns can also be seen such as asymmetrical parietal lobe and hippocampal atrophy in AD or of the frontal and temporal lobes in FTD. Fluorodeoxyglucose (FDG)–positron emission tomography (PET) imaging can help differentiate

TABLE 16.2 Pharmacotherapy for Epilepsy

Medication	Therapeutic Spectrum	Dosage	Mechanism of Action	Enzyme Induction/ Inhibition	Side Effects, Contraindications/ Warnings	Comments
Levetiracetam*	Focal + generalized	Initial: 500 mg bid; increase by 500 mg/dose every 1–2 weeks (max: 1,500 mg bid, although higher doses frequently used as tolerated)	Precise mechanism unknown, potential action on calcium, potassium channels and involvement in GABAergic inhibitory transmission; also acts on synaptic vesicle protein 2A	None	Mood-related side effects, irritability, agitation, fatigue Rare: SJS/TEN, psychosis, pancytopenia	Often the first agent tried given low rate of side effects and lack of known drug–drug interactions
Lamotrigine	Focal + generalized	Weeks 1–2: 25 mg once daily; weeks 3–4: 50 mg once daily; week 5 +: increase by 50 mg daily every 1–2 weeks Maintenance: 225–375 mg/d in 2 divided doses Titration to be adjusted if patient on enzyme inducer or inhibitor.	Blocks sodium channels and inhibits release of glutamate	May induce its own metabolism by UGT-glucuronidation (minor)	Dizziness, diplopia, tremor, rash (SJS) Rare: SJS/TEN, aseptic meningitis Black-Box Warning: Serious skin rash/SJS	May worsen myoclonic seizures
Valproate	Focal + generalized	Initial: 10–15 mg/kg/d; increase by 5–10 mg/kg/d on a weekly basis Maximum recommended dose: 60 mg/kg/d	Increases GABAergic inhibitory pathway, acts on sodium and calcium channels	Induces CYP2C9	Tremor, dizziness, weight gain, hair loss Rare: SJS/TEN, agranulocytosis, aplastic anemia, hepatic failure, pancreatitis, PCOS Contraindicated in severe hepatic disease; pregnancy Black-Box Warning: Hepatic failure, pancreatitis, neurometabolic disorders, congenital malformations/neural tube defects with in-utero exposure	
Topiramate	Focal + generalized	Initial: 25 mg bid; increase by 50 mg/d on a weekly basis (max: 200 mg bid)	Blocks sodium channels while enhancing GABAergic inhibitory pathway and antagonizing excitatory AMPA/glutamate receptors; also weak carbonic anhydrase inhibitor	Inhibits CYP2C19 (minor) Induces CYP3A4 (minor)	Fatigue, word finding difficulty, difficulty concentrating, anorexia, anxiety, tremor, paresthesia Rare: Acute angle glaucoma, renal stones Extended-release form contraindicated in recent alcohol use or concomitant use of metformin in patient with metabolic acidosis	
Zonisamide	Focal + generalized	Initial: 100 mg once a day; increase by 100 mg/d every 2 weeks (max: 400 mg once daily)	Blocks sodium and calcium channels; also weak carbonic anhydrase inhibitor	None	Fatigue, difficulty concentrating, anorexia Rare: SJS/TEN, aplastic anemia, renal stones Avoid in sulfonamide allergy	
Perampanel	Focal + generalized	Initial: 2 mg qhs; increase by 2 mg/d on weekly basis (max: 12 mg qhs)	Noncompetitive inhibitor of AMPA receptor on postsynaptic neurons	Appears to induce metabolism of progestin-containing hormonal contraceptives	Irritability, somnolence, gait disturbance, aggression, mood-related side effects, weight gain Rare: Severe psychosis Black-Box Warning: Dose-related serious or life-threatening neuropsychiatric events	

TABLE 16.2 Pharmacotherapy for Epilepsy *(continued)*

Medication	Therapeutic Spectrum	Dosage	Mechanism of Action	Enzyme Induction/ Inhibition	Side Effects, Contraindications/ Warnings	Comments
Brivaracetam	Focal + generalized	Initial: 50 mg bid (max: 200 mg bid)	Acts on synaptic vesicle protein 2A in the brain	Inhibits CYP2C19 (minor) Inhibits epoxide hydroxylase	Headache, dizziness, ataxia, nystagmus Rare: Angioedema, bronchospasm, neutropenia, psychosis	
Clobazam	Focal + generalized	Initial: 10 mg/d (max: 40 mg bid)	Binds to GABA-A receptors of postsynaptic neurons	Inhibits CYP2D6 (moderate)	Somnolence, aggression, irritability Rare: SJS, respiratory depression Black-Box Warning: Concomitant use of benzodiazepines and opioids may result in profound sedation, respiratory depression, coma, death	
Felbamate	Focal + generalized	Initial: 1,200 mg/d in 3–4 divided doses; increase by 1,200 mg/d on weekly basis (max: 3,600 mg/d in 3–4 divided doses)	Binds to ion channels of NMDA receptors, thereby decreasing excitatory transmission; weak effect on GABA receptor; also may act on sodium and calcium channels	Inhibits CYP2C19 (minor)	Insomnia, dizziness, ataxia, weight loss Rare: Aplastic anemia, liver failure Black-Box Warning: Aplastic anemia, hepatic failure	
Rufinamide	Focal + generalized	Initial: 200–400 mg bid; increase by 400–800 mg/d every other day (max: 1,600 mg/d)	Prolongs inactive state of sodium channels	Induces CYP3A4 (minor) Inhibits CYP2E1 (minor)	Dizziness, somnolence, headache, fatigue Rare: SJS/TEN, shorted QT interval Contraindication: Familial short QT syndrome	
Carbamazepine	Focal	Initial: 400 mg/d in 2–4 divided doses; increase by 200 mg/d on a weekly basis (max: 1,600 mg/d)	Blocks voltage-gated sodium channels	Potent and broad-spectrum inducer of CYP, UGT-glucuronidation, and P-gp	Drowsiness, double vision, headache, rash, hyponatremia Rare: Agranulocytosis, aplastic anemia, SJS/TEN, hepatic failure, pancreatitis US Boxed Warning: Serious dermatologic reactions such as SJS/TEN; risk increases with presence of HLA-B*1502 allele; aplastic anemia, agranulocytosis	May worsen generalized onset seizures
Eslicarbazepine	Focal	Initial: 400 mg/d; increase by 400–600 mg/d on weekly basis	Blocks voltage-gated sodium channels	Induces CYP3A4 and UGT1A1 glucuronidation (weak) but does not induce its own metabolism Inhibits CYP2C19 (moderate)	Drowsiness, double vision, headache, rash, ataxia, hyponatremia Rare: Prolonged PR interval, AV block, SJS/TEN Hypersensitivity to oxcarbazepine	May worsen generalized onset seizures
Oxcarbazepine	Focal	Initial: 300 mg bid; increase by 600 mg/d on a weekly basis (max: 600 mg bid)	Blocks voltage-gated sodium channels and modulates activity of voltage activated calcium channels	Induces CYP3A4 (moderate to severe) and UGT-glucuronidation but does not induce its own metabolism	Drowsiness, double vision, ataxia, headache, rash, hyponatremia Rare: SJS/TEN, agranulocytosis, pancytopenia	May worsen generalized onset seizures
Lacosamide	Focal	Initial: 50 mg bid; increase by 50 mg/dose on weekly basis (max: 200 mg bid)	Enhances slow inactivation of sodium channels	Inhibits CYP2C19 (minor)	Ataxia, dizziness, double vision, fatigue, Rare: PR interval prolongation, AV block, ventricular arrhythmias, neutropenia Hypersensitivity to eslicarbazepine	

(continued)

TABLE 16.2 Pharmacotherapy for Epilepsy (continued)

Medication	Therapeutic Spectrum	Dosage	Mechanism of Action	Enzyme Induction/ Inhibition	Side Effects, Contraindications/ Warnings	Comments
Phenytoin	Focal	Initial: 100 mg tid; increase intervals no sooner than 7–10 d; dosing should be individualized Maintenance: 300–600 mg/d	Blocks voltage-gated sodium channels	Potent and broad-spectrum inducer of CYP and UGT-glucuronidation	Confusion, double vision, ataxia, slurred speech, gingival hypertrophy, rash Rare: SJS/TEN, agranulocytosis, hepatic failure, dermatitis, adenopathy hirsutism IV injections avoided in sinus bradycardia, sinoatrial block, AV block Black-Box Warning: IV phenytoin must be administered slowly	May worsen Generalized onset seizures Follows nonlinear kinetics, and thus has a narrow therapeutic window; drug levels should be monitored closely; serum level should be corrected based on albumin level
Phenobarbital	Focal	Initial: 2 mg/kg/d in divided doses; dosing should be individualized based on clinical response	Enhances GABAergic inhibitory pathway. Also decreases calcium current	Potent and broad-spectrum inducer of CYP and UGT-glucuronidation	Somnolence, dizziness, lethargy, ataxia, development of tolerance Rare: SJS/TEN, agranulocytosis, connective tissue contractures, respiratory depression Contraindicated in hepatic impairment, dyspnea, airway obstruction	May worsen generalized onset seizures
Pregabalin	Focal	Initial: 150 mg/d in 2–3 divided doses; increase at weekly intervals (max: 600 mg/d)	Binds to alpha-2-delta subunit of presynaptic voltage-gated calcium channels, thereby inhibiting release of excitatory transmitters	None	Dizziness, somnolence, ataxia, weight gain, edema Rare: Angioedema, rhabdomyolysis	Renal dosing required in renal failure
Gabapentin	Focal	Initial: 100–300 mg tid (max: 1,200 mg tid)	Binds to alpha-2-delta subunit of presynaptic voltage-gated calcium channels, thereby inhibiting release of excitatory transmitters	None	Somnolence, dizziness, edema Rare: Multiorgan hypersensitivity	May worsen generalized onset seizures Renal dosing required in renal failure
Tiagabine	Focal	Initial: 4 mg once daily; increase by 4–8 mg/d on weekly basis (max: 32–56 mg/d in 2–4 divided doses)	Inhibits uptake of GABA into presynaptic neurons	None	Dizziness, fatigue, somnolence Rare: SJS/TEN, nonconvulsive status epilepticus	May worsen generalized onset seizures
Vigabatrin	Focal	Initial: 500 mg bid; increase by 500 mg/d on weekly basis (max: 1,500 mg bid.)	Irreversible inhibition of GABA-transaminase, thus increasing GABA at the synaptic cleft	Induces CYP2C9	Dizziness, fatigue, vision loss Rare: Depression, MRI abnormalities Black-Box Warning: Permanent vision loss	May worsen generalized onset seizures
Ethosuximide	Generalized absence	Initial: 500 mg/d; increase by increments ≤250 mg every 4–7 days (max: 1,500 mg/d); can be given in 2–3 divided doses	Reduces T-type calcium currents in the thalamus	None	Anorexia, nausea, abdominal pain, hyperactivity, drowsiness Rare: SJS/TEN, agranulocytosis Hypersensitivity to succinimides	Monitor CBC, liver enzymes

AV, atrioventricular; bid, twice daily; CBC, complete blood count; d, day; max: maximum dose; PCOS, polycystic ovary syndrome; qhs, every night at bedtime; SJS, Stevens-Johnson syndrome; TEN, toxic epidermal necrolysis; tid, three times a day.

between AD and FTD. PET amyloid scan and CSF analysis of amyloid-to-tau ratio are on the horizon as acceptable biomarkers to support diagnosis. Routine testing for apolipoprotein E4 (APOE4), which is the most prevalent genetic risk factor of AD, is not recommended.[20]

TREATMENT OF DEMENTIA

Nonpharmacological Therapies

Nonpharmacological therapies include practical tools for day-to-day living (e.g., memory aids and reminders) and sensory aids (e.g., glasses and hearing aids). Important assessments of patient safety include the ability to drive, manage finances, and to live alone. Patients with dementia do better when keeping to a schedule and are prone to delirium in unfamiliar surroundings. Recognizing the challenging emotional states for patients and caregivers, as well as pursuing proactive future planning, are important pillars of dementia care.

Pharmacological Therapies

Pharmacological therapies approved for dementia—predominantly AD—include donepezil, rivastigmine, galantamine, and memantine. Though these medications do not stop or slow the underlying neurodegenerative process, they may offer some symptomatic improvement in memory and concentration. Donepezil, rivastigmine, and galantamine are all acetylcholinesterase inhibitors (AChEI), which prevent breakdown of acetylcholine. Degeneration of the nucleus basalis in AD results in decreased acetylcholine projections to the hippocampus and neocortex. Although all three are approved for use in mild-to-moderate disease, only donepezil is approved for patients with severe AD. Rivastigmine requires additional approval in those with PDD and is available as a transdermal patch. AChEI may improve cognitive symptoms, apathy, and non-emergency hallucinations and delusions in DLB, as well as the cognitive symptoms in vascular dementia. However, AChEI provide no benefit in FTD and may worsen behavioral symptoms.

AChEI can lead to bradycardia and heart block; thus, caution should be exercised in patients with cardiac conduction dysfunction as well as in those taking PR interval prolonging agents (e.g., beta-blockers). Prescribers should also be aware that these agents may lower seizure threshold. Common side effects include gastrointestinal (GI) symptoms such as nausea and vomiting, diarrhea, and drowsiness. Vivid dreams may occur when donepezil is taken at night; therefore, earlier daytime administration may be preferred. If taking an initial agent leads to side effects, taking an alternative AChEI is a reasonable approach.

Memantine is a N-methyl-D-aspartate (NMDA) receptor antagonist that leads to reduction in glutamatergic excitotoxicity. Its use is approved for moderate-to-severe AD and it has been shown to provide modest improvement in cognition and behavior. It is frequently prescribed as adjunctive therapy to AChEI. Memantine may improve agitation that develops in those with FTD. Although side effects (e.g., dizziness, confusion) are uncommon, discretionary use in patients with cardiovascular and seizure disorders must be considered. **Table 16.3** lists drug therapies that are currently used to treat various subtypes of dementia.

Patients with DLB and PDD are at increased risk of drug-induced Parkinsonism, somnolence, orthostatic hypotension, and neuroleptic malignant syndrome, and should avoid dopamine antagonists (e.g., haloperidol, risperidone, and olanzapine).

IMMUNE-MEDIATED NEUROLOGIC DISORDERS

INTRODUCTION

Significant advancements in the diagnosis and treatment of autoimmune neurologic conditions have occurred over the past decade. Abnormal immune-mediated responses are now recognized as the primary mechanism leading to diseases such as multiple sclerosis (MS), myasthenia gravis (MG), Guillain-Barre syndrome (GBS), and limbic encephalitis. MS remains the prototypical and most studied neuroimmunologic disorder with greater than 2.2 million people affected worldwide.[21]

Interactions between the central nervous system (CNS) and immune system are tightly regulated. Abnormal access of circulating immune components to the CNS can wreak havoc on function and lead to specific neuroimmunologic disorders. The biology of the most well-described CNS autoimmune neurologic condition (MS) results from abnormal T-cell attacks on CNS myelin. Self-directed T-lymphocyte invasion leads to a pathological cascade of events culminating in inflammatory cell recruitment and damage to myelin sheaths.[22] All other neuroimmunologic diseases have similar mechanistic themes but differ by the neuroanatomical substrate targeted. For instance, MG is an autoimmune disorder caused by inappropriate targeting and destruction of the neuromuscular junction. Autoantibodies bind to nicotinic receptors and cause complement-mediated destruction resulting in weakness due to inability to activate muscle contraction.[23]

TABLE 16.3 Pharmacotherapy for Dementia

Medication*	Dose/Frequency	Other Indications	Side Effects	Caution
Donepezil	Start 5 mg daily; increase to 10 mg daily after 4–6 weeks; after 3 months, increase to 23 mg daily	Vascular dementia DLB cognitive symptoms and apathy DLB/PPD nonemergency visual hallucinations and delusions	Nausea, vomiting, diarrhea, drowsiness Donepezil: Vivid dreams with nighttime dosing	Cardiac conduction abnormalities, bradycardia/heart block, seizure disorder
Rivastigmine	4.6 mg/24 h patch once daily; may increase to 9.6 mg/24 h patch, then 13.3 mg/24 h patch in 4-week intervals			
Galantamine	4 mg bid × 4 weeks; increase to 8 mg bid; can further increase to 12 mg bid in 4 weeks			
Memantine	Start 5 mg daily × 1 week; increase to 5 mg bid × 1 week, then increase to 10 mg/5 mg × 1 week, then 10 mg bid	FTD behavior	Rarely confusion and dizziness	Cardiovascular disease, seizure disorder, hepatic and/or renal impairment

AD, Alzheimer's disease; bid, twice daily; DLB, dementia with Lewy bodies; FTD, frontotemporal dementia; h, hour; PPD, Parkinson's disease dementia.

*Approved indications: All medications approved for mild-to-moderate AD; donepezil and memantine are approved for severe AD; rivastigmine is approved for PDD.

RISK FACTORS FOR IMMUNE-MEDIATED NEUROLOGIC DISORDERS

A family history of autoimmune disease remains the most widely recognized risk factor for future development of a neuroimmunologic condition. However, each disease carries a unique risk factor profile. Epstein-Barr virus exposure, female gender, smoking, low ultraviolet light exposure, and low vitamin D levels are risk factors for MS.[22] In MG, younger women and older men are affected more often as well as those with a thymoma or thymic hyperplasia.[23] Antecedent bacterial (e.g., *Campylobacter jejuni*) and viral infections (e.g., cytomegalovirus, influenza A) are commonly associated with the development of GBS.[24]

DIAGNOSIS OF IMMUNE-MEDIATED NEUROLOGIC DISORDERS

A detailed clinical history and examination remain the cornerstone of diagnosis. A hallmark feature of MS is repeated "attacks" (e.g., recurrent focal neurologic symptoms and signs) at various times affecting different neurologic functions. Specialized criteria known as the MacDonald Criteria incorporate clinical information with appropriate testing (e.g., MRI, spinal fluid analysis) and are used to make the diagnosis.[25] Characteristic muscle weakness patterns seen in MG

and GBS should prompt specialized testing for presence of unique autoantibodies—acetylcholine receptor antibodies in MG and ganglioside antibodies in GBS. Diagnosing specific neuroimmunologic conditions is challenging and relies on diagnostic constructs that integrate history and physical examination with complex testing.

TREATMENT OF IMMUNE-MEDIATED NEUROLOGIC DISORDERS

Treatment of neuroimmunologic diseases is centered on establishing control of the immune system and is divided into two therapeutic categories: acute versus long-term therapy. Acute clinical attacks are halted by nonspecific immunosuppressive agents such as glucocorticoids like methylprednisolone.[26] This is followed by long-term disease-modifying treatment (DMT). Of the many neurologic conditions, MS-related therapy has seen the greatest advancement. There are now more than 15 U.S. Food and Drug Administration (FDA)-approved agents, each with unique biological mechanisms of action.[27] These drugs were designed to prevent ongoing CNS attacks, but may also minimize permanent CNS injury. **Tables 16.4 to 16.6 summarize the current available treatment options for MS.**

TABLE 16.4 FDA-Approved Disease-Modifying Therapies for Multiple Sclerosis

Medication	Target/Composition	Mechanism of Action
First-Line Therapy		
Beta-Interferon	Binds IFN receptor	Multifactorial: Induces T_{reg} and suppressive B cells
Glatiramer acetate	Random polymers of four amino acids	Induces a shift from TH1 to TH2 type immunity
Dimethyl fumarate	Small molecule activator of Nrf2 pathway	Incompletely understood; increases antioxidant functions in response to inflammation/injury
Teriflunomide	Inhibits pyrimidine synthesis	Reduces inflammation and T cell activation
Second-Line Therapy		
Fingolimod	Sphinosine-1-phosphate receptor antagonist	Sequesters lymphocytes in lymph nodes.
Alemtuzumab	Humanized monoclonal anti-CD52 antibody	Depletes all lymphocytes
Natalizumab	Humanized monoclonal antibody against alpha-4 integrin	Prevents egress of lymphocytes from the circulation into CNS
Ocrelizumab	Humanized monoclonal anti-CD20 antibody	Reduces B cells participating in antigen presentation

CNS, central nervous system; INF, interferon.

TABLE 16.5 FDA-Approved Therapies for Multiple Sclerosis

Medication	Dose/Frequency	Main Side Effects
Beta-interferon	IM; qod, tiw, weekly, or every 2 weeks	Injection reactions, flu-like symptoms, depression
Glatiramer acetate	IM; daily or tiw	Injection reactions
Dimethyl fumarate	PO; twice daily	GI symptoms, flushing, LFT abnormalities, lymphopenia, infections
Teriflunomide	PO; daily	GI symptoms, LFT abnormalities, alopecia
Fingolimod	PO; daily	Bradycardia, AV node block, macular edema, infections, lymphopenia, LFT abnormalities
Alemtuzumab	IV; annually	Infusion reactions, cytopenia, secondary autoimmunity (thyroid, renal, platelet reduction)
Natalizumab	IV; monthly	Infusion reactions, infections, PML, LFT abnormalities
Ocrelizumab	IV; every 6 months	Infusion reactions, infections, malignancy

AV, atrioventricular; GI, gastrointestinal; IM, intramuscular; IV, intravenous; LFT, liver function test; PML, progressive multifocal leukoencephalopathy; PO, orally; qod, every other day; tiw, three times weekly.

TABLE 16.6 Other Therapies Used for Neuroimmunologic Disorders

Medication	Mechanism of Action	FDA-Approved Indications	Off-Label Uses
Methylprednisolone	Reduces inflammation acutely and chronically inhibits lymphocyte function	Acute anti-inflammatory or immunosuppressive need, MS exacerbation	N/A
Prednisone	Reduces inflammation acutely and chronically inhibits lymphocyte function	MS exacerbation	MG, long-term immunosuppression
Intravenous immunoglobulin	Complex immunomodulation	Chronic demyelinating inflammatory polyneuropathy, multifocal motor neuropathy	GBS, MG, MS, autoimmune encephalitis
Rituximab	Reduces B cells	None	NMO, MG, autoimmune encephalitis
Mycophenolate mofetil	Cytostatic on all lymphocytes	None	MG, steroid-sparing agent

FDA, Food and Drug Administration; GB, Guillain–Barre syndrome; MG, myasthenia gravis; MS, multiple sclerosis; NMO, neuromyelitis optica.

CEREBROVASCULAR DISORDERS AND RELATED NEUROLOGIC EMERGENCIES

INTRODUCTION

Stroke is a leading cause of disability in the United States and is a devastating disease some fear more than death.[28] One new stroke occurs every 40 seconds, and approximately 795,000 strokes occur annually.[29] Gender, race, and advanced age are nonmodifiable factors associated with higher risks. Stroke incidence and mortality have declined in recent decades, corresponding with increasing statin and antihypertensive medication use.[30] Despite this nationwide reduction, racial and geographic disparities persist with the greatest disease burden and mortality occurring within the southeast region of the United States, which is referred to as the "Stroke Belt."[29]

Stroke is a sudden unexpected neurologic disability caused by acute cerebral ischemia (e.g., arterial blockage) or hemorrhage (e.g., arterial rupture). The majority of strokes result from ischemic infarction (87%) while a minority are due to both intraparenchymal and aneurysmal subarachnoid hemorrhage (10% and 3%, respectively).[29] Traditional cardiovascular risk factors, in particular hypertension, contribute to progressive lipohyalinosis of cerebral small arterial beds and large artery atherosclerosis. As opposed to acute arterial thrombosis and occlusion that leads to tissue infarction, hemorrhage within the brain parenchyma or overlying subarachnoid space from a ruptured cerebral aneurysm can be a consequence of longstanding hypertension. Despite cerebral hemorrhage representing the minority of stroke subtypes, it is responsible for a nearly four-fold greater number of deaths within the initial weeks following brain injury when compared to ischemic infarction.[31]

Excess mortality seen in ischemic and hemorrhagic stroke is often due to progressive, secondary mass effect seen within the initial days following injury. Space-occupying strokes cause dangerous compression onto other critical structures, such as the brainstem, and may lead to death if left untreated. Up to one in four patients will have neurologic decline within the first hours of hospital presentation following acute cerebral hemorrhage. In contrast, maximal brain swelling from damaged tissue following ischemic stroke ensues within days to the first week in those with large hemispheric infarction.[32,33]

RISK FACTORS FOR CEREBROVASCULAR DISEASE

Hypertension, diabetes, tobacco use, and atrial fibrillation remain powerful, but modifiable, risk factors for cerebrovascular disease.[29] Although both stroke subtypes have similar risk profiles, tobacco and alcohol abuse are more strongly associated with hemorrhagic stroke as opposed to other factors (e.g., atrial fibrillation, prior myocardial infarction, diabetes) more commonly linked to brain ischemia.[31] Tobacco cessation, dietary modification, and physical activity are nonpharmacologic strategies that may improve stroke prevention.[34,35]

DIAGNOSIS OF CEREBROVASCULAR DISORDERS

Abrupt onset, focal neurologic disability is the hallmark feature of stroke. Unilateral weakness, sensory loss, speech difficulty, and visual disturbance are common presenting symptoms with corresponding abnormal neurologic exam findings. Ischemic and hemorrhagic stroke present similarly; therefore, urgent cranial imaging is required to discriminate between the two. CT is the initial test of choice as it quickly identifies the presence or absence of blood. However, MRI is more sensitive at identifying small or subtle infarction. The temporal profile of symptom onset aids in differentiating stroke from other causes of neurologic spells, such as seizures, hemodynamic disturbances, metabolic derangements, and psychiatric manifestations. These other conditions can mimic stroke in up to 43% of emergency room visits and should remain diagnoses of exclusion.[36]

TREATMENT OF CEREBROVASCULAR DISORDERS

Acute Ischemic Stroke

Emergent treatment is predicated on timely reperfusion of the causative vessel occlusion via thrombolysis with intravenous (IV) recombinant tissue plasminogen activator (r-tPA), alteplase, and/or mechanical thrombectomy. Rapid reperfusion reduces cerebral infarct volume, limiting the degree of disability and risk of death. Alteplase must be administered within 4.5 hours from clearly defined symptom onset in patients who fulfill inclusion/exclusion criteria.[37] Early time-dependent treatment yields the greatest benefit. Thirty-three percent of patients have good outcomes when treated within the first 3 hours. In other words, 10 patients treated acutely within the earlier time frame leads to one patient achieving functional recovery, compared to 20 patients treated within the accepted 3- to 4.5-hour time-window leading to a similar outcome.[38] The most feared complication—symptomatic intracranial hemorrhage (sICH)—occurred in 6% of those treated with thrombolysis. Recent landmark clinical trials conclusively demonstrate the benefit of emergency mechanical thrombectomy up to 24 hours from symptomatic onset in patients with the most severe stroke types that result from occlusion of a major intracranial artery.[37]

Secondary Prevention of Ischemic Stroke

Atherothrombosis of both large and small arteries and cardiogenic cerebral emboli are the most common causes of stroke. Antiplatelet agents reduce thrombosis, remaining the mainstay of therapy for acute stroke patients who are ineligible for thrombolysis as well as for long-term secondary prevention. The most widely studied antiplatelet drug, aspirin, can reduce recurrent events when administered within 48 hours of stroke and lowers risk by 15% even at low doses (e.g., 50 mg daily).[37,39] Other commonly prescribed antiplatelet agents include clopidogrel and the combination of aspirin–dipyridamole (25 mg/200 mg extended-release)—the former prevented vascular events more often than aspirin in the CAPRIE (Clopidogrel versus Aspirin in Patients at Risk of Ischemic Events) trial but was of equal efficacy in stroke prevention compared to the latter agent in PROFESS (Prevention Regimen for Effectively Avoiding Second Strokes).[40] Aspirin–dipyridamole notoriously causes headaches and may lead to noncompliance.

Nonvalvular atrial fibrillation (NVAF) causes embolic stroke and represents 15% of all ischemic subtypes. Anticoagulation is the treatment of choice of which warfarin, a vitamin K antagonist, remains the prototypical agent. Although effective, maintenance of anticoagulation within the narrow international normalized ratio (INR) range between 2 and 3 is challenging due to dietary and drug-drug interactions.[40] Anticoagulation with direct oral anticoagulants (DOAC) have similar or lower rates of stroke and bleeding complications compared to adjusted-dose warfarin (INR 2.0–3.0).[40] The DOACs offer several advantages: lower risk of intracerebral hemorrhage, routine laboratory testing is not required, no dietary interactions, and markedly reduced susceptibility to drug interactions.

Hemorrhagic Stroke

Patients presenting with acute intracerebral cerebral hemorrhage (ICH) are frequently critically ill. Diagnosis is straightforward following identification of blood product on brain imaging. Urgent control of hypertension, correction of coagulopathy, and identification of those who may benefit from surgical intervention are vital during the initial phase of acute ICH care. Specialized neurologic intensive care monitoring is often mandatory for signs of clinical deterioration from hematoma expansion, progressive cerebral edema, obstructive hydrocephalus, and airway compromise.

Raised Intracranial Pressure From Ischemic and Hemorrhagic Stroke

Severe intracranial pressure (ICP) can develop early following large space-occupying strokes, typically within the first week after the event. Emergent surgical decompression may be required in some cases;

however, early administration of hyperosmolar therapy should be trialed to reduce brain water content by augmenting the tissue–intravascular osmolarity gradient. Mannitol (a sugar alcohol) acts by reducing intravascular water, dehydrates tissues, and causes systemic diuresis.[41] Peak ICP reduction is reached within 15 to 35 minutes of administration and is sustained for several hours before redosing is required.[42] Hypertonic saline, a hyperosmolar solution administered as a 3% to 23.4% sodium chloride concentrate, generates a rapid osmolar gradient between brain tissue and the vasculature. Although use of these medications is commonplace in neurocritical care, the long-term outcome benefits remain uncertain.[43–45] Subsequent dosing and ceiling drug effect are dependent upon the degree of serum osmolarity and hypernatremia.

Table 16.7 summarizes common ischemic stroke prevention drugs and treatments recommended for related neurologic emergencies.

MOVEMENT DISORDERS: TREMOR SYNDROMES

INTRODUCTION

Tremor is the most commonly encountered movement disorder characterized by involuntary rhythmic oscillations of a body part. The body region affected by oscillatory movement is classified as being present while at rest (*resting tremor*), in motion (*kinetic tremor*), or when the limb is outstretched and stationary (*postural tremor*). Although tremor is seen in numerous conditions, it is seen most often in essential tremor (ET) and PD. Higher tremor frequency of 10 Hz or greater is seen in orthostatic tremor and enhanced physiological tremor as opposed to the characteristic slower frequency tremor seen in ET and PD.

Tremor results from dysfunction of key cerebral structures and related neurotransmitters that involve the basal ganglia, cerebelli, and interconnected circuitry. Both essential and Parkinsonian tremor are associated with increased activity within the cerebellothalamocortical circuit. That is, abnormally increased activation of the globus pallidus, a component of the basal ganglia, results from dysfunction of its dopaminergic pathway. In addition, the GABAergic (inhibitory neurotransmitter) dysfunction within specific cerebellar and brainstem centers may also contribute to the tremor seen in these conditions.[46] Hallmark histologic features seen in PD are the loss of dopamine-secreting neurons within the basal ganglia along with the presence of Lewy bodies whereas the disease underpinnings of ET are less well understood.[47]

The overall prevalence of ET is 0.9% for all ages, increasing by five-fold in those aged 65 and older.

TABLE 16.7 Selected Prevention Drugs and Treatments for Ischemic Stroke and Related Neurologic Emergencies

Medication	Mechanism of Action	Dose/Frequency	Side Effects	Contraindications
Ischemic Stroke Prevention				
Antiplatelets				
Aspirin	Irreversibly inhibits platelet cyclooxygenase-1 by blocking formation of thromboxane A2 (a potent vasoconstrictor and platelet aggregation)	81–325 mg PO daily	Bleeding diathesis, GI ulcer, tinnitus, thrombocytopenia hypersensitivity	Hypersensitivity, GI ulcer, bleeding diathesis
Clopidogrel	Prodrug metabolized by CYP450 to produce the active metabolite; selectively inhibits the binding of ADP to its platelet P2Y12 receptor and subsequent ADP-mediated activation of the glycoprotein GPIIb/IIIa complex, thereby inhibiting platelet aggregation	75 mg PO daily	Bleeding diathesis, GI ulcer, TTP	Bleeding diathesis, GI ulcer Black-Box Warning: Diminished antiplatelet effect in CYP2C19 poor metabolizers
Aspirin-dipyridamole	Dipyridamole inhibits the activity of adenosine deaminase and phosphodiesterase, which lead to inhibition of platelet aggregation and may cause vasodilation.	25 mg/200 mg PO bid	Headaches, GI ulcer, bleeding diathesis, thrombocytopenia	Hypersensitivity, GI ulcer, bleeding diathesis
Anticoagulants				
Warfarin	Inhibits vitamin K epoxide reductase complex 1 (VKORC1) depleting vitamin K–dependent coagulation factors (II, VII, IX, and X)	2–12 mg PO daily; dosing varies based on INR	Major hemorrhage, GI symptoms, purple-toe syndrome	Hypersensitivity, bleeding diathesis, acute kidney injury Black-Box Warning: Risk of major or fatal bleeding
Apixaban	Direct, selective, and reversible inhibition of free and clot-bound factor Xa	5 mg bid	Major hemorrhage, GI symptoms, thrombocytopenia	Hypersensitivity, bleeding diathesis, mechanical valve Black-Box Warning: Risk of thrombotic event when discontinued; epidural/spinal hematoma risk
Rivaroxaban	Direct, selective, and reversible inhibition of free and clot-bound factor Xa	20 mg daily	Major hemorrhage, GI symptoms, thrombocytopenia	Hypersensitivity, bleeding diathesis, mechanical valve Black-Box Warning: Risk of thrombotic event when discontinued; epidural/spinal hematoma risk
Dabigatran	A specific, reversible, direct thrombin inhibitor	150 mg bid	Major hemorrhage, GI symptoms, thrombocytopenia	Hypersensitivity, bleeding diathesis, mechanical valve Black-Box Warning: Risk of thrombotic event when discontinued; epidural/spinal hematoma risk
Acute Ischemic Stroke Reperfusion Therapy				
Thrombolytic Agents				
Alteplase	Promotes initiation of fibrinolysis by binding to fibrin and converting plasminogen to plasmin	0.9 mg/kg (max: 90 mg); load with 10% of 0.9 mg/kg dose as an IV bolus over 1 minute, followed by remaining dose as a continuous infusion over 60 minutes	Severe bleeding (including intracranial), hypersensitivity	Stroke inclusion/exclusion criteria

(continued)

TABLE 16.7 Selected Prevention Drugs and Treatments for Ischemic Stroke and Related Neurologic Emergencies (*continued*)

Acute Ischemic Stroke Reperfusion Therapy

Thrombolytic Agents

Tenecteplase	Promotes initiation of fibrinolysis by binding to fibrin and converting plasminogen to plasmin	Dosing not established for treatment of stroke	Severe bleeding (including intracranial), hypersensitivity	Currently not FDA approved for treatment of stroke

Cerebral Edema

Hyperosmolar Agents

Mannitol	Reduces intravascular water, dehydrates tissues, and causes systemic diuresis.	20% solution; initial bolus 0.25–1 g/kg, repeat dosing q6–8 h if serum mOsm <320 mOsm/L	Renal failure at high serum osmolality, skin sloughing (IV infiltration), hypotension, electrolyte disturbances	Serum Osmol >320 mOsml (relative contraindication), renal failure, severe hypotension
Hypertonic saline	Generates a rapid osmolar gradient	3%–23.4% NaCl IV infusion*	Hypotension (with rapid infusion), osmotic demyelination syndrome (rapid sodium fluctuations), electrolyte disturbances	Volume overload

*23.4% routinely administered through central venous access.

ADP, adenosine diphosphate; bid, twice daily; GI, gastrointestinal; h, hour; INR, international normalized ratio; max, maximum total dose; NaCl, sodium chloride; PO, orally; q, every; TTP, thrombocytopenic purpura.

Males are affected more often; however, ET has no clear ethnic predilection.[48] Additionally, PD is the second most common progressive neurodegenerative disease worldwide, affecting 1% of those aged 60 and older. Men are affected slightly more often than women with an average age of onset of 60.[47] Interestingly, growing evidence suggests an overlapping existence of ET and PD as the concurrent presence of both in individuals appears more frequently than chance alone.[49]

RISK FACTORS FOR TREMOR SYNDROMES

Increased age is associated with the development of ET and is the greatest risk factor in men with PD. Although no specific gene has been linked to ET, familial heritability has demonstrated incomplete penetrance (30%–70%) in an autosomal dominance pattern in those with relatives who have the disease.[50] Head injury, pesticide exposure, nonsmoking, family history, and low daily caffeine consumption have been linked to PD; however, the vast majority of cases remain idiopathic and only 10% are hereditary.[47,51] Genetic and environmental factors are suspected to be contributors to the development of both ET and PD.

DIAGNOSIS OF TREMOR SYNDROMES

Specific clinical criteria remain the gold standard for diagnosing ET and PD as no confirmatory biomarker or imaging test has been identified. ET is characterized by an action tremor affecting mostly the arms but can involve the head, neck, or voice. A moderate 5- to 10-Hz tremor frequency is classic with predominantly symmetrical limb involvement of flexion–extension movements. The tremor can decrease (i.e., "improve") following alcohol consumption, and an additional characteristic seen in advanced stages includes impaired balance. The Parkinson's tremor occurs at rest, oftentimes unilateral when it begins, and can become bilateral over time with preservation of tremor intensity asymmetry. A slower 4- to 6-Hz frequency is expected, and the tremor is described as a "pill-rolling" supination–pronation movement. The lip, jaw, chin, and legs can be affected while some patients report the addition of an "internal tremor." Additional hallmark characteristics accompanying the rest tremor include bradykinesia (slow movements), rigidity, and postural instability. A prodrome of abnormal rapid eye movement (REM) behavior sleep, olfactory dysfunction, and constipation may be nonmotor symptoms that precede the diagnosis.[46,47,52,53]

TREATMENT OF TREMOR SYNDROMES

Initiation of therapy is based on the impact the tremor has on quality of life and daily function. Nonpharmacological interventions for PD include exercise and tailored therapies, which are effective in disease management. Surgical treatments such as lesioning and deep brain stimulation are optional.

Various first-line drugs are available for the treatment of ET (**Table 16.8**). Propranolol is a nonselective beta-adrenergic blocker that reduces tremor by 50% to 60% with lasting effects observed in up to 50% of patients. Primidone, an anticonvulsant, offers similar effectiveness reducing tremor by 60% and provides benefit in nearly half of those who take it. Symptomatic response from either drug is not predictable, nor does it appear to correlate with serum concentrations. Other drugs that likely confer some benefit include topiramate and gabapentin.[53]

Repletion of dopamine in PD is the primary aim of pharmacotherapy and is tailored to specific symptoms. Potent treatments, such as dopamine agonists and levodopa, and less-intensive options, such as monoamine oxidase type B inhibitors (MAOI-B), are available. Adjunctive therapy prohibiting degradation of levodopa and dopamine include catechol-*O*-methyltransferase (COMT) inhibitors and MAOI-B, often prolonging the pharmacological effects. Rasagiline (an MAOI-B) may provide some disease-modifying effects; however, subsequent data have been inconclusive.[47]

TABLE 16.8 Pharmacotherapy for Essential Tremor and Parkinson's Disease

Drug Class	Medication	Dose/Frequency	Side Effects
Essential Tremor			
Nonselective beta-adrenergic blocker	Propranolol	30–60 to 60–240 mg in one to two doses	Bradycardia, syncope, fatigue, erectile dysfunction
Anticonvulsant	Primidone	12.5–25 to 150–750 mg/d in two to three divided doses	Nausea, sedation, malaise, ataxia, dizziness, confusion
Anticonvulsant	Topiramate	25–50 to 150–300 mg/d in two divided doses	Weight loss, anorexia, extremity paresthesia, trouble concentrating, memory disturbance, increase risk of kidney stones
Anticonvulsant	Gabapentin	300–900 mg/d to 1,200–3,600 mg/d in two divided doses	Dizziness, sedation, ataxia, weight gain, nausea
Parkinson's Disease			
Levodopa-carbidopa	Levodopa	Titrate to initial dose of 100/25 mg tid to 1,500/375 mg/d or more based on symptoms	Nausea, orthostatic hypotension, dyskinesia, hallucinations
Dopamine agonists	Pramipexole (ER)	Start 0.125 to 0.5–1.5 mg tid (0.375 up to 4.5 mg/d)	Nausea, orthostatic hypotension, hallucinations, impulse-control disorders, peripheral edema, sleepiness, sleep attacks
	Ropinirole (ER)	Start 0.25 mg tid, max 24 mg/d (6–24 mg once daily)	Nausea, orthostatic hypotension, hallucinations, impulse-control disorders, peripheral edema, sleepiness, sleep attacks
	Rotigotine patch	Start 2 mg/24 h, max 16 mg/24 h	Nausea, orthostatic hypotension, hallucinations, impulse-control disorders, peripheral edema, sleepiness, sleep attacks
MAO-B inhibitors	Rasagiline	1 mg daily	Headache, arthralgia, dyspepsia, depression, flu-like symptoms, exacerbation of levodopa side effects
	Selegiline	2.5–5 mg bid	Stimulant effect, dizziness, headache, confusion, exacerbation of levodopa side effects
COMT Inhibitors	Entacapone	200 mg with selected or each dose of levodopa	Dark-colored urine, explosive diarrhea, exacerbation of levodopa side effects

bid, twice daily; COMT, catechol-*O*-methyltransferase; d, day; h, hour; MAO-B, monoamine oxidase-B; tid, three times daily.

CASE EXEMPLAR: Patient With Epilepsy

LS is a 31-year-old woman who presents after a first time seizure. The patient recalls experiencing an unusual rising sensation in the abdomen accompanied by an unpleasant, brief, metallic taste before losing awareness. Bystanders observed her to develop leftward head turning followed by stiffening and rhythmic jerking of her limbs. She appeared disoriented for 15 minutes following the event but steadily recovered to baseline functioning.

Past Medical History

- Febrile convulsion in childhood following pneumonia at the age of 10
- No birth-related or developmental complications

Medications

- Fluoxetine, 40 mg once daily

Family History

- Uncle with alcohol-associated withdrawal seizures

Labs

- Electrolytes: Normal
- Blood glucose level: Normal
- Urine toxicology screening: Negative

Discussion Questions

1. What is an important risk factor that might have contributed to LS's epilepsy?
2. Initial workup reveals normal electrolytes, normal blood glucose level, and negative urine toxicology screening. Which diagnostic studies should be obtained to further understand the risk of recurrent unprovoked seizures?
3. An EEG is obtained and shows epileptiform discharges over the right temporal head region. What is the best next course of action in terms of antiseizure therapy?

CASE EXEMPLAR: Patient With Face Drooping and Slurred Speech

JS is a 62-year-old male brought urgently into clinic by his wife who reports "something is just not right with J." She says he is walking and leaning to one side, his face looks odd, and his words are slurred. She thinks he is having a stroke.

Past Medical History

- Hypertension
- Hypercholesteremia
- Anemia

Medications

- Spironolactone, 50 mg daily
- Losartan, 50 mg daily
- Simvastatin, 40 mg daily
- Ibuprofen for pain

Family History

- Father deceased, liver failure due to alcoholism
- Mother alive, hypertension

Social History

- Smoker
- Plays poker at a senior citizens' center
- Little physical activity

Physical Examination

- Height: 70 inches; weight: 250 lbs.; blood pressure: 188/94; pulse: 110; respiration rate: 24
- Obesity
- Droop to right side of face
- Difficulty forming words
- Sluggish mental response

Labs and Imaging

- Electrocardiogram: Atrial fibrillation with slowed ventricular response
- Potassium: 4.5 mEq/L
- Sodium: 142 mEq/L
- Liver function: Normal

Discussion Questions

1. What factors in JS's history place him at risk for stroke?
2. The clinician determines that JS needs additional intervention that is beyond the scope of the clinic, so he is transferred by ambulance to the nearest emergency department. After initial tests, an ischemic stroke is confirmed. Treatment will begin with alteplase. Why is time important in the administration of alteplase? What is the intended outcome of this intervention and what short- and long-term side effects may JS experience?
3. What pharmacological and nonpharmacological treatments will JS continue at home?

KEY TAKEAWAYS

- Epilepsy is diagnosed when two or more unprovoked seizures occur more than one day apart or when a patient has an unprovoked seizure with risk of recurrence. Risk factors include perinatal complications, developmental delay, childhood febrile convulsions, family history of epilepsy, and prior CNS alterations.
- Diagnosis of epilepsy is based on history, examination, EEG, and neuroimaging (e.g., MRI and CT). Targeted drug therapy is based on seizure type, comorbidities, existing drug therapy, and family planning.
- The most common cause of dementia is AD, and age underpins the greatest risk of development. It is thought to be due to overproduction and impaired clearance of specific proteins in the brain. Diagnosis is based on clinical assessment. Treatment includes donepezil, rivastigmine, galantamine, and memantine.
- Abnormal immune-mediated responses are the primary mechanisms leading to diseases such as MS, MG, GBS, and limbic encephalitis. Family history is the greatest risk factor. Treatment centers on control of the immune system.
- Stroke is caused by acute cerebral ischemia (e.g., arterial blockage) or hemorrhage (e.g., arterial rupture). Immediate recognition and intervention to restore oxygen to the affected area of the brain is key to reduction of complications and recovery.
- PD is the result of a lack of dopamine in the brain and is manifested by tremor and bradykinesia. It is managed by dopamine replacement and symptom management.

REFERENCES

1. World Health Organization. *Epilepsy: A Public Health Imperative*. World Health Organization; 2019.
2. Scheffer IE, Berkovic S, Capovilla G, et al. ILAE classification of the epilepsies: position paper of the ILAE Commission for Classification and Terminology. *Epilepsia*. 2017;58:512–521. doi:10.1111/epi.13709
3. Baldin E, Hauser WA, Buchhalter JR, et al. Yield of epileptiform electroencephalogram abnormalities in incident unprovoked seizures: a population-based study. *Epilepsia*. 2014;55:1389–1398. doi:10.1111/epi.12720
4. Paliwal P, Benjamin RB, Leonard LY, et al. Early electroencephalography in patients with emergency room diagnoses of suspected new-onset seizures: diagnostic yield and impact on clinical decision-making. *Seizure*. 2015;31:22–26. doi:10.1016/j.seizure.2015.06.013
5. Gregory RP, Oates T, Merry RT. Electroencephalogram epileptiform abnormalities in candidates for aircrew training. *Electroencephalogr Clin Neurophysiol*. 1993;86:75–77. doi:10.1016/0013-4694(93)90069-8
6. Zivin L, Marsan CA. Incidence and prognostic significance of "epileptiform" activity in the EEG of non-epileptic subjects. *Brain*. 1968;91(4):751–778. doi:10.1093/brain/91.4.751
7. Fisher RS, Cross JH, French JA, et al. Operational classification of seizure types by the International League Against Epilepsy: position paper of the ILAE Commission for Classification and Terminology. *Epilepsia*. 2017;58:522–530. doi:10.1111/epi.13670
8. Conway JM. Epilepsy. *J Am Coll Clin Pharm*. 2019;2(3):314–318. doi:10.1002/jac5.1123
9. Liu G, Slater N, Perkins A. Epilepsy: treatment options. *Am Fam Physician*. 2017;96(2):87–96. https://www.aafp.org/afp/2017/0715/p87.html
10. Kwan P, Brodie M. Early identification of refractory epilepsy. *N Engl J Med*. 2000;342:314–319. doi:10.1056/NEJM200002033420503
11. Finger EC. Frontotemporal dementias. *Continuum (Minneap Minn)*. 2016;22(2):464–489. doi:10.1212/CON.0000000000000300
12. Gomperts SN. Lewy body dementias: dementia with Lewy bodies and Parkinson disease dementia. *Continuum (Minneap Minn)*. 2016;22(2);435–463. doi:10.1212/CON.0000000000000309
13. World Alzheimer Report. 2018: *The State of the Art of Dementia Research: New Frontiers*. Alzheimer's Disease International; 2018. https://www.alz.co.uk/worldreport2018
14. World Alzheimer Report. 2019: *Attitudes to Dementia*. Alzheimer's Disease International; 2019. https://www.alz.co.uk/research/WorldAlzheimerReport2019.pdf.
15. Centers for Disease Control and Prevention. *Alzheimer's Disease and Healthy Aging*. Centers for Disease Control and Prevention; 2020. https://www.cdc.gov/aging/aginginfo/alzheimers.htm#anchor_1489431553
16. Apostolova LG. Alzheimer disease. *Continuum (Minneap Minn)*. 2016;22(2):419–434. doi:10.1212/CON.0000000000000307
17. Guo T, Noble W, Hanger DP. Roles of tau protein in health and disease. *Acta Neuropathol*. 2017;133(5):665–704. doi:10.1007/s00401-017-1707-9
18. Chen G, Xu T, Yan Y. et al. Amyloid beta: structure, biology and structure-based therapeutic development. *Acta Pharmacol Sin*. 2017;38:1205–1235. doi:10.1038/aps.2017.28
19. Loy CL, Schofield PR, Turner AM, et al. Genetics of dementia. *Lancet*. 2014;383(9919):P828–P840. doi:10.1016/S0140-6736(13)60630-3
20. Safieh M, Korczyn AD, Michaelson DM. ApoE4: an emerging therapeutic target for Alzheimer's disease. *BMC Med*. 2019;17:64. doi:10.1186/s12916-019-1299-4
21. Wallin MT, Culpepper WJ, Nichols E, et al. Global, regional, and national burden of multiple sclerosis 1990–2016: a systematic analysis for the Global Burden of Disease Study 2016. *Lancet Neurol*. 2019;18(3):269–285. doi:10.1016/S1474-4422(18)30443-5
22. Dobson R, Giovannoni G. Multiple sclerosis–a review. *Eur J Neurol*. 2019;26(1):27–40. doi:10.1111/ene.13819
23. Binks S, Vincent A, Palace J. Myasthenia gravis: a clinical-immunological update. *J Neurol*. 2016;263(4):826–834. doi:10.1007/s00415-015-7963-5

24. Willison HJ, Jacobs BC, Van Doorn PA. Guillain-Barré syndrome. *Lancet*. 2016;388(10045):717–727. doi:10.1016/S0140-6736(16)00339-1

25. Thompson AJ, Banwell BL, Barkhof F, et al. Diagnosis of multiple sclerosis: 2017 revisions of the McDonald criteria. *Lancet Neurol*. 2018;17(2):162–173. doi:10.1016/S1474-4422(17)30470-2

26. Vandewalle J, Luypaert A, De Bosscher K, et al. Therapeutic mechanisms of glucocorticoids. *Trend Endocrinol Metab*. 2018;29(1):42–54. doi:10.1016/j.tem.2017.10.010

27. Rommer PS, Milo R, Han MH, et al. Immunological aspects of approved MS therapeutics. *Front Immunol*. 2019;10:1564. doi:10.3389/fimmu.2019.01564

28. Solomon NA, Glick HA, Russo CJ, et al. Patient preferences for stroke outcomes. *Stroke*. 1994;25(9):1721–1725. doi:10.1161/01.STR.25.9.1721

29. Mozaffarian D, Benjamin EJ, Go AS, et al. Heart disease and stroke statistics—2016 update. *Circulation*. 2016;133(4):e38–e360. doi:10.1161/CIR.0000000000000350

30. Fang MC, Coca Perraillon M, Ghosh K, et al. Trends in stroke rates, risk, and outcomes in the United States, 1988 to 2008. *Am J Med*. 2014;127(7):608–615. doi:10.1016/j.amjmed.2014.03.017

31. Andersen KK, Olsen TS, Dehlendorff C, et al. Hemorrhagic and ischemic strokes compared: stroke severity, mortality, and risk factors. *Stroke*. 2009;40(6):2068–2072. doi:10.1161/STROKEAHA.108.540112

32. Fan JS, Huang HH, Chen YC, et al. Emergency department neurologic deterioration in patients with spontaneous intracerebral hemorrhage: incidence, predictors, and prognostic significance. *Acad Emerg Med*. 2012;19(2):133–138. doi:10.1111/j.1553-2712.2011.01285.x

33. Brott T, Broderick J, Kothari R, et al. Early hemorrhage growth in patients with intracerebral hemorrhage. *Stroke*. 1997;28(1):1–5. doi:10.1161/01.STR.28.1.1

34. Estruch R, Ros E, Salas-Salvadó J, et al. Primary prevention of cardiovascular disease with a Mediterranean diet supplemented with extra-virgin olive oil or nuts. *N Engl J Med*. 2018;378(25):e34. doi:10.1056/NEJMoa1800389

35. Lee CD, Folsom AR, Blair SN. Physical activity and stroke risk: a meta-analysis. *Stroke*. 2003;34(10):2475–2481. doi:10.1161/01.STR.0000091843.02517.9D

36. Neves Briard J, Zewude RT, Kate MP, et al. Stroke mimics transported by emergency medical services to a comprehensive stroke center: the magnitude of the problem. *J Stroke Cerebrovasc Dis*. 2018;27(10):2738–2745. doi:10.1016/j.jstrokecerebrovasdis.2018.05.046

37. Powers WJ, Rabinstein AA, Ackerson T, et al. 2018 guidelines for the early management of patients with acute ischemic stroke: a guideline for healthcare professionals from the American Heart Association/American Stroke Association. *Stroke*. 2018;49(3):e46–e110. doi:10.1161/STR.0000000000000158

38. Emberson J, Lees KR, Lyden P, et al. Effect of treatment delay, age, and stroke severity on the effects of intravenous thrombolysis with alteplase for acute ischaemic stroke: a meta-analysis of individual patient data from randomised trials. *Lancet*. 2014;384(9958):1929–1935. doi:10.1016/S0140-6736(14)60584-5

39. Johnson ES, Lanes SF, Wentworth CE, et al. A metaregression analysis of the dose-response effect of aspirin on stroke. *Arch Intern Med*. 1999;159(11):1248–1253. doi:10.1001/archinte.159.11.1248

40. Kernan WN, Ovbiagele B, Black HR, et al. Guidelines for the prevention of stroke in patients with stroke and transient ischemic attack: a guideline for healthcare professionals from the American Heart Association/American Stroke Association. *Stroke*. 2014;45(7):2160–2236. doi:10.1161/STR.0000000000000024

41. Videen TO, Zazulia AR, Manno EM, et al. Mannitol bolus preferentially shrinks non-infarcted brain in patients with ischemic stroke. *Neurology*. 2001;57(11):2120–2122. doi:10.1212/WNL.57.11.2120

42. Wise BL, Chater N. The value of hypertonic mannitol solution in decreasing brain mass and lowering cerebrospinal-fluid pressure. *J Neurosurg*. 1962;19(12):1038–1043. doi:10.3171/jns.1962.19.12.1038

43. Hemphill JC, Greenberg SM, Anderson CS, et al. Guidelines for the management of spontaneous intracerebral hemorrhage: a guideline for healthcare professionals from the American Heart Association/American Stroke Association. *Stroke*. 2015;46(7):2032–2060. doi:10.1161/STR.0000000000000069

44. Wijdicks EFM, Sheth KN, Carter BS, et al. Recommendations for the management of cerebral and cerebellar infarction with swelling: a statement for healthcare professionals from the American Heart Association/American Stroke Association. *Stroke*. 2014;45(4):1222–1238. doi:10.1161/01.str.0000441965.15164.d6

45. Oddo M, Poole D, Helbok R, et al. Fluid therapy in neurointensive care patients: ESICM consensus and clinical practice recommendations. *Intensive Care Med*. 2018;44(4):449–463. doi:10.1007/s00134-018-5086-z

46. Helmich RC, Toni I, Deuschl G, et al. The pathophysiology of essential tremor and Parkinson's tremor. *Curr Neurol Neurosci Rep*. 2013;13(9):378. doi:10.1007/s11910-013-0378-8

47. Connolly BS, Lang AE. Pharmacological treatment of Parkinson disease: a review. *JAMA*. 2014;311(16):1670. doi:10.1001/jama.2014.3654

48. Louis ED, Ferreira JJ. How common is the most common adult movement disorder? Update on the worldwide prevalence of essential tremor. *Mov Disord*. 2010;25(5):534–541. doi:10.1002/mds.22838

49. Fekete R, Jankovic J. Revisiting the relationship between essential tremor and Parkinson's disease: relationship between ET and PD. *Mov Disord*. 2011;26(3):391–398. doi:10.1002/mds.23512

50. Clark LN, Louis ED. Challenges in essential tremor genetics. *Rev Neurol*. 2015;171(6–7):466–474. doi:10.1016/j.neurol.2015.02.015

51. Noyce AJ, Bestwick JP, Silveira-Moriyama L, et al. Meta-analysis of early nonmotor features and risk factors for Parkinson disease. *Ann Neurol*. 2012;72(6):893–901. doi:10.1002/ana.23687

52. Jankovic J. Parkinson's disease: clinical features and diagnosis. *J Neurol Neurosurg Psychiatry*. 2008;79(4):v–376. doi:10.1136/jnnp.2007.131045

53. Deuschl G, Raethjen J, Hellriegel H, et al. Treatment of patients with essential tremor. *Lancet Neurol*. 2011;10(2):148–161. doi:10.1016/S1474-4422(10)70322-7

Pharmacotherapy for Cardiovascular Conditions

Sandhya Venugopal, Manoj Kesarwani, Nipavan Chiamvimonvat, Martin Cadeiras, and Ezra A. Amsterdam

LEARNING OBJECTIVES

- List the medications used in the treatment of acute coronary syndrome, angina pectoris, hypertension, hyperlipidemia, dysrhythmia, atrial fibrillation, and congestive heart failure.
- Classify drugs used in the treatment of cardiovascular disease by their mechanism of action.
- Customize a treatment protocol based on underlying pathophysiology and comorbidities.
- Explain the indications and contraindications for classes of drugs used to treat cardiovascular disease.
- Employ the guidelines published by consensus organizations to create treatment approaches.

INTRODUCTION

Cardiovascular disease is a major cause of disability and premature death throughout the world and contributes substantially to the escalating costs of health care. Acute coronary events frequently occur suddenly and are often fatal before medical care can be given. Modification of risk factors has been shown to reduce mortality and morbidity in people with diagnosed or undiagnosed cardiovascular disease. The landscape of cardiovascular pharmacotherapy has significantly evolved with many new medications approved by the Food and Drug Administration (FDA) within the last decade and several guideline updates recently published. This chapter aims to provide guidance on medications used for the treatment of cardiovascular diseases and a focused update on selected cardiovascular medications and drug classes.

PHARMACOTHERAPY FOR ACUTE CORONARY SYNDROME

The acute coronary syndromes (ACS) include unstable angina, non-ST-segment-elevation myocardial infarction (NSTEMI), and ST-segment elevation myocardial infarction (STEMI). ACS is characterized by acute myocardial ischemia and/or injury, which may not always result in the presence of pathologic Q-waves on the electrocardiogram. The pathogenesis of ACS is complex and results in coronary thrombosis and immediate myocardial oxygen supply/demand imbalance.[1] Antiplatelet therapy, anticoagulation, angiotensin-converting enzyme inhibitors (ACEI) *or* angiotensin receptor blockers (ARBs), beta-adrenergic blockers, calcium-channel antagonists, nitrates, and high-intensity statins are standard medical therapy during early hospital care in ACS.[1] ACEI, ARBs, beta-adrenergic blockers, calcium-channel antagonists, nitrates, and statins are discussed elsewhere in this chapter. The focus here is on antiplatelet and anticoagulation therapy, as represented in **Table 17.1**. Fibrinolytic therapy is not included in this discussion but is an important alternative to revascularization for STEMI when percutaneous coronary intervention (PCI) is not an option or will be delayed, and coronary artery bypass graft surgery is not a viable alternative.

Beta-adrenergic blockers in the first 24 hours of hospitalization for acute MI reinfarction decreases malignant arrhythmias and limits infarct size in anterior STEMI; however, they have no benefit on short-term mortality in the setting of primary PCI.[2,3]

TABLE 17.1 Antiplatelet and Anticoagulant Therapy in Acute Coronary Syndromes

Drug/Class	Mechanism of Action	Dosing	Special Considerations
Antiplatelet Therapy			
Aspirin	Irreversibly reduces platelet aggregation by inhibiting the cyclooxygenase enzyme	162–325-mg (non-enteric-coated) loading dose, then 81 mg/day (oral)	First-line therapy in ACS
Clopidogrel	Irreversibly inhibits the P_2Y_{12} (adenosine diphosphate) receptor, thereby reducing platelet activation and aggregation	300–600-mg loading dose, then 75 mg/day (oral)	Thienopyridine prodrug that requires two-step process by the CYP450 system to form active metabolite
Prasugrel	Irreversibly inhibits the P_2Y_{12} (adenosine diphosphate) receptor, thereby reducing platelet activation and aggregation	60-mg loading dose, then 10 mg/day (oral)	Indicated in ACS only when coronary anatomy is predefined; requires step process by the CYP450 system to form active metabolite
Ticagrelor	Reversibly and directly inhibits the P_2Y_{12} receptor, thereby reducing platelet activation and aggregation	180-mg loading dose, then 90 mg twice daily (oral)	Relatively short $t_{1/2}$, but superior to clopidogrel in terms of efficacy with more consistent inhibition of platelet activity
Cangrelor	Reversibly and directly inhibits the P_2Y_{12} receptor, thereby reducing platelet activation and aggregation	Weight-based (IV) dosing: 30 mcg/kg, then 4 mcg/kg/min for at least 2 hours or duration of PCI, whichever is longer	Adjunctive therapy for PCI to further ↓ ischemic events when combined with aspirin and clopidogrel
Glycoprotein IIb/IIIa inhibitors	Bind platelet glycoprotein IIb/IIIa receptors to reduce platelet aggregation	Dosing is specific to whether abciximab, eptifibatide, or tirofiban are used	Primarily an adjunctive therapy for PCI; typically used in high-risk ACS
Parenteral Anticoagulant Therapy			
Unfractionated heparin	Binds to antithrombin III, resulting in inactivation of thrombin and other clotting factors	60-units/kg (up to 4,000-units) loading dose, then 12 units/kg/hour	Activates platelets; should be administered for 48 hours or until PCI is performed; can be combined with GP IIb/IIIa inhibitors
Low-molecular-weight heparin/enoxaparin	Binds to antithrombin III to increase activity and cause inactivation of thrombin and factor Xa	1 mg/kg subcutaneously every 12 hours (dose needs to be adjusted for renal impairment)	Additional 0.3 mg/kg dose should be given if last dose >8 hours before PCI or only 1 subcutaneous dose given; ↑ risk of bleeding relative to UH
Bivalirudin	Direct thrombin inhibitor	0.75-mg/kg loading dose, then 1.75 mg/kg/hour (dose needs to be adjusted for renal impairment)	Lower rate of bleeding relative to UH/LMWH; can be monitored by activated clotting time
Fondaparinux	Selective synthetic factor Xa inhibitor	2.5 mg subcutaneously daily	Not recommended as sole anticoagulant during PCI

ACS, acute coronary syndrome; GP, glycoprotein; IV, intravenous; LMWH, low-molecular-weight heparin; PCI, percutaneous coronary intervention; UH, unfractionated heparin.

↑ increase; ↓ decrease

Source: Adapted from Amsterdam EA, Wenger NK, Brindis RG, et al. 2014 AHA/ACC guideline for the management of patients with non-ST-elevation acute coronary syndromes: a report of the American College of Cardiology/American Heart Association Task Force on Practice Guidelines. *J Am Coll Cardiol.* 2014;64: e139–e228. doi:10.1016/j.jacc.2014.09.017

PHARMACOTHERAPY FOR ANGINA PECTORIS

Myocardial ischemia is a state of inadequate oxygen supply to cardiac muscle, typically caused by obstructive atherosclerotic coronary artery disease (CAD). An imbalance in myocardial oxygen supply-demand underlies ischemia and angina pectoris. Antianginal pharmacologic agents alleviate ischemia by decreasing one or more of the major determinants of myocardial oxygen demand (heart rate, systolic blood pressure [BP], contractility, and left ventricular dimension) and improve myocardial oxygen supply-demand balance (**Table 17.2**).[1]

TABLE 17.2 Hemodynamic Effects of Antianginal Drugs

Drug	Heart Rate	Systolic Blood Pressure	Contractility	Left-Ventricular Volume
Nitrates	↑	↓	↔	↓
Beta-blockers*	↓	↓	↓	↔, ↑
Calcium Channel Blockers				
Diltiazem	↓	↓	↓	↔
Verapamil	↓	↓	↓↓	↔
Amlodipine	↔	↓	↔	↔
Nifedipine	↔	↓	↔	↔
Ranolazine	No significant hemodynamic effects			

*Potential bronchospasm.

↑ increase; ↓ decrease; ↔ no significant effect at usual doses in patients with adequate left ventricular function

Source: Adapted from Amsterdam EA, Wenger NK, Brindis RG, et al. 2014 AHA/ACC guideline for the management of patients with non-ST-elevation acute coronary syndromes: a report of the American College of Cardiology/American Heart Association Task Force on Practice Guidelines. *J Am Coll Cardiol.* 2014;64:e139–e228. doi:10.1016/j.jacc.2014.09.017; Divakaran S, Loscalzo J. The role of nitroglycerin and other nitrogen oxides in cardiovascular therapeutics. *J Am Coll Cardiol.* 2017;70(19):2393–2410. doi:10.1016/j.jacc.2017.09.1064; Pascual I, Moris C, Avanzas P. Beta-blockers and calcium channel blockers: first line agents. *Cardiovasc Drugs Ther.* 2016;30(4):357–365; doi:10.1007/s10557-016-6682-1; Richards JR. *Beta-Blockers: Physiological, Pharmacological and Therapeutic Implications. Nova Science Publishers; 2018.*

The *nitrates* (nitroglycerine, isosorbide dinitrate, and isosorbide mononitrate) relax vascular smooth muscle, causing arterial and veno-dilation. Venous return to the right heart is reduced, lowering ventricular dimensions. Blood pressure also falls, and myocardial oxygen demand is reduced. The decrease in blood pressure results in a baroreceptor-mediated reflex tachycardia that can be prevented by adding a beta-blocker or rate-limiting calcium blocker. The sublingual form of nitroglycerine is taken to abort anginal episodes. Long-acting nitrates (isosorbide dinitrate and mononitrate) are used prophylactically to prevent angina. In the event of coronary artery spasm, nitrates can dilate these vessels.[4] See Table 17.2 for adverse effects of antianginal medications.

Beta-adrenergic blocking agents (BB) reduce myocardial oxygen demand by decreasing heart rate, blood pressure, and myocardial contractility by competitive inhibition of the actions of endogenous catecholamines on myocardial beta-1 receptors. Combining a nitrate with a BB can provide comprehensive reduction of myocardial oxygen demand; the BB prevents nitrate-associated tachycardia and the nitrate mitigates potential BB-induced increase in ventricular volume due to decreased contractility.[3]

Calcium channel blockers (CCBs) include rate-limiting preparations (diltiazem and verapamil) and the dihydropyridines (nifedipine and amlodipine). The rate-limiting CCBs relieve ischemia by attenuating heart rate, blood pressure, and myocardial contractility. The dihydropyridines have more potent vasodilating and antihypertensive actions than the rate-limiting CCBs. Both categories of CCBs are effective in relieving coronary artery spasm.[5]

Ranolazine is unique among the antianginal agents in that its mechanism of action is not dependent on influencing the determinants of myocardial oxygen demand. Its mechanism of action appears to be inhibition of the late phase of the ventricle's inward sodium current (INa +) which is heightened during ischemia. Because ranolazine does not negatively impact hemodynamic function, it can be utilized in angina patients with marginal cardiac functional status.[6]

PHARMACOTHERAPY FOR HYPERTENSION

Hypertension (HTN) is a leading cause of mortality and morbidity. Most patients with HTN are responsive to lifestyle modification and a broad array of pharmacologic agents.[7-9] The pathogenesis of essential HTN, the diagnosis in ~90% of patients with the disease, involves abnormal function of regulatory mechanisms that control the metabolism of salt, water, and vascular resistance. Current pharmacologic antihypertensive therapy targets one or more of these factors. In 2017, the American College of Cardiology/American Heart Association (ACC/AHA) revised their guideline for the management of HTN.[7] Categories of BP were updated (**Table 17.3**) based on the relation of BP to cardiovascular events.

Accurate patient BP determination comprises the average of two to three measurements obtained over several months. The foundation of BP treatment is nonpharmacologic intervention: weight loss, increased physical activity, reduction in sodium intake, and moderation in alcohol consumption (**Table 17.4**).[8] Further recommendations include: antihypertensive medication for patients with stage 1 HTN and cardiovascular

TABLE 17.3 Categories of Blood Pressure

Category	Blood Pressure Range
Normal BP	<120/80 mmHg
Elevated BP	Systolic BP 120–129 *and* diastolic BP <80 mmHg
Stage 1 HTN	Systolic BP 130–139 *or* diastolic BP 80–89 mmHg
Stage 2 HTN	Systolic BP ≥140 *or* diastolic BP ≥90 mmHg

BP, blood pressure; HTN, hypertension.

Source: Adapted from Whelton PK, Carey RM, Aronow WS, et al. 2017 ACC/AHA/AAPA/ABC/ACPM/AGS/APhA/ASH/ASPC/NMA/PCNA guideline for the prevention, detection, evaluation, and management of high blood pressure in adults: a report of the American College of Cardiology/American Heart Association Task Force on Clinical Practice Guidelines. *J Am Coll Cardiol.* 2018;71(19):e127–e248. doi:10.1161/HYP.0000000000000075

TABLE 17.4 Efficacy of Lifestyle Modification on Blood Pressure

Lifestyle Modification	Blood Pressure Decrease (mmHg)
Decreased salt intake	2–8
Weight loss	5–20
DASH diet*	8–14
Increased physical activity	4–9
Less excessive alcohol intake	2–4

*The Dietary Approaches to Stop Hypertension (DASH) diet is rich in fruits, vegetables, whole grains, and low-fat dairy foods. It includes meat, fish, poultry, nuts, and beans, and is limited in sugar-sweetened foods and beverages, red meat, and added fats. Vegetarian variations of the DASH diet are available (https://dashdiet.org/what-is-the-dash-diet.html).

Source: Chobanian AV, Bakris GL, Black HR, et al. The seventh report of the Joint National Committee on Prevention, Detection, Evaluation, and Treatment of High Blood Pressure: the JNC 7 report. *JAMA.* 2003;289(19):2560–2572. doi:10.1001/jama.289.19.2560

disease or a greater than or equal to 10% 10-year risk of arteriosclerotic cardiovascular disease (ASCVD) as well as for those with stage 2 HTN. For stage 2, two BP-lowering medications in addition to healthy lifestyle changes are recommended.[8]

DRUG CLASSES USED IN THE TREATMENT OF HYPERTENSION

Thiazide Diuretics

Thiazide diuretics (chlorthalidone, hydrochlorothiazide) are used as monotherapy or can be administered adjunctively with other antihypertensive agents. Thiazides inhibit renal reabsorption of sodium and chloride through inhibition of Na-Cl cotransporters in the distal convoluted tubule of the kidney.[10] As a result, thiazide diuretics increase sodium delivery to the late distal tubule, which increases potassium loss via stimulation of the aldosterone-sensitive sodium pump to increase sodium reabsorption in exchange for potassium and hydrogen ions. Hypokalemia and metabolic alkalosis may result. Additional side effects of thiazides include hypovolemia due to overdiuresis and hyperglycemia associated with decreased insulin sensitivity, which appears to be proportional to the duration of therapy. The mechanism for decreased insulin sensitivity is not fully understood.[11]

Angiotensin-Converting Enzyme Inhibitors

ACEIs are the treatment of choice in patients with hypertension and chronic kidney disease with proteinuria. ACEIs prevent the conversion of angiotensin I to angiotensin II (a powerful vasoconstrictor) and inhibit degradation of bradykinin, thought to be the cause of cough and angioedema caused by ACEIs. ACEIs are contraindicated in pregnancy.[10]

Angiotensin Receptor Blockers

ARBs are used for patients who cannot tolerate ACEIs. ARBs competitively block binding of angiotensin-II to angiotensin type I (AT_1) receptors, thereby reducing effects of angiotensin II–induced vasoconstriction, sodium retention, and aldosterone release. The breakdown of bradykinin is not inhibited, precluding cough related to increased bradykinin.[10]

Calcium Channel Blockers

Calcium channel blockers (CCBs) are potent arterial dilators by which they lower BP. The dihydropyridines achieve this effect by binding to L-type calcium channels in vascular smooth muscle, resulting in vasodilation and decreased blood pressure. Non-dihydropyridines lower BP by their negative inotropic actions and vasodilator effects; they also are negative chronotropic agents.[10]

Beta-Blockers and Beta-1 Selective Blockers

Beta-blockers are generally not recommended as first-line agents for the treatment of hypertension; however, they are suitable alternatives in the presence of a compelling indication (e.g., heart failure [HF], myocardial infarction, ischemic heart disease). Selective beta-blockers cause relatively specific antagonism of beta-1 receptors and are preferred in patients with bronchospastic airway disease who require a beta-blocker. Bisoprolol and metoprolol succinate are preferred in patients with HF with reduced ejection fraction (HFrEF).[12]

Other Drug Classes

Other drug classes to consider in the treatment of severe or treatment-resistant HTN include direct vasodilators (hydralazine, minoxidil), which relax vascular smooth muscle and thereby decrease peripheral resistance and improve BP. These agents are associated with reflex tachycardia and sodium and water retention; they should be used with a beta-blocker and a diuretic.[12] Centrally acting alpha2-agonists (methyldopa, clonidine) stimulate presynaptic alpha2-adrenergic receptors in the brainstem, which reduces sympathetic nervous activity. These drugs may trigger hypertensive crisis if stopped abruptly, and are associated with significant central nervous system (CNS) side effects (e.g., dizziness, sedation, fatigue), especially in the elderly. As a result, they are reserved as last-line agents.[12]

In Black patients without HF or nephropathy, initial treatment favors a thiazide diuretic or calcium channel blocker over an ACEI or ARB.[8] Combination therapy with two or more drugs may be necessary to achieve BP goals.[8] For patients with stage 2 HTN, initiation of drug therapy with two agents is recommended.[8] Numerous two- and three-drug combinations are available as fixed-dose combinations. Avoid prescribing drugs with similar mechanisms of action or clinical effects.

PHARMACOTHERAPY FOR DYSLIPIDEMIA

Although the basis of lipid-lowering therapy is favorable lifestyle alterations, a majority of patients require pharmacologic therapy to achieve recommended lipid targets. For primary prevention of cardiovascular disease, recommendations are based upon 10-year ASCVD risk (Table 17.5). ASCVD risk for adults aged 20 to 79 can be calculated using the ASCVD Risk Estimator Plus (http://tools.acc.org/ASCVD-Risk-Estimator-Plus/#!/calculate/estimate). For secondary prevention in patients who have had a major cardiovascular event or procedure, the 2018 Guideline on Management of Blood Cholesterol recommends initiation of high-intensity statin therapy.[13]

The most effective lipid-lowering drugs are the statins and the PCSK-9 inhibitors (Table 17.6). These two drug classes have demonstrated outstanding efficacy in reducing serum low-density lipoprotein cholesterol (LDL-C) and decreasing cardiovascular events while maintaining safety. The statins have compiled an excellent record of effectiveness and safety over several decades. Other lipid-lowering agents are also helpful in management of dyslipidemia as adjunctive drugs or when the latter are not well tolerated (see Table 17.6).[13]

Depending on the specific drug and dose, *statins* decrease serum LDL-C by 20% to 50% (see Table 17.6). They also increase HDL-C modestly and have a variable and moderate lowering effect on triglycerides. Adverse effects are primarily elevated serum transaminase and myopathy. Myopathy occurs as myalgia in up to 20% of patients. Myositis is extremely rare, and hepatotoxicity

---

TABLE 17.5 Guideline-Directed Cholesterol Management for Primary Prevention Based Upon 10-Year Arteriosclerotic Cardiovascular Disease Risk

10-Year ASCVD Risk*	Recommended Intervention
Low (<5%)	Discuss ASCVD risk Emphasize healthy lifestyle and risk-factor reduction
Borderline (5%–<7.5%)	Assess for risk-enhancing factors**; consider moderate-intensity statin if present Consider obtaining CAC score to guide decisions about statin use

Intermediate (7.5%–<20%)	Consider moderate- to high-intensity statin therapy
	For patients who need aggressive LDL-C lowering who do not tolerate high-intensity statins, consider moderate-intensity statin PLUS a nonstatin lipid-lowering drug
	Consider obtaining CAC score to guide decisions about statin use:
	    CAC score = 0, withhold statin and reassess in 5–10 years if no higher risk comorbidities
	    CAC score 1–99, begin statin for patients aged 55 and older
	    CAC score ≥100 or ≥75th percentile, start statin therapy

High (≥20%)	In high-risk patients with multiple clinical risk factors, begin statin with goal to reduce LDL-C by ≥50% (likely high-intensity statin)

* Calculated using the ASCVD Risk Estimator Plus (http://tools.acc.org/ASCVD-Risk-Estimator-Plus/#!/calculate/estimate/).

** Risk-enhancing factors: FH early ASCVD; current LDL-C 160–189 mg/dL, non-HDL-C 190–219 mg/dL; metabolic syndrome; CKD; chronic inflammatory disease; PMH preeclampsia or early menopause, high-risk ethnicity; high lipid biomarkers (TG ≥175 mg/dL); HS-CRP ≥2.0 mg/dL; lipoprotein (a) ≥50 mg/dL; apolipoprotein B ≥130 mg/dL; ABI <0.9.

ABI, ankle-brachial index; ASCVD, arteriosclerotic cardiovascular disease; CAC, coronary artery calcium; CKD, chronic kidney disease; FH, family history; HDL-C, high-density lipoprotein cholesterol; HS-CRP, high-sensitivity C-reactive protein; LDL-C, low-density lipoprotein cholesterol; PMH, past medical history; TG, triglycerides.

Source: Adapted from American College of Cardiology. ASCVD risk estimator plus. Accessed May 14, 2020. http://tools.acc.org/ASCVD-Risk-Estimator-Plus/#!/calculate/estimate

TABLE 17.6 Comparison of Efficacy and Side Effects of Lipid-Lowering Agents

Drug Class	LDL-C Reduction	HDL-C Change	Triglycerides	Side Effects
Statins Fluvastatin* Lovastatin* Pravastatin** Simvastatin** Atorvastatin*** Rosuvastatin***	~25% ~30% 34% 40% 50% 50%	Small, variable increase	10%–20% increase	Class effects: Myopathy, transaminitis
PCSK-9 Inhibitors Alirocumab Evolocumab	50%–60% reduction with statin			Local irritation at injection site, rhinitis, flu-like symptoms
Inhibitor of Cholesterol Absorption Ezetimibe	18%		5% reduction	Rare
Bile–acid resins Cholestyramine Colestipol Colesevelam	15%–30%	≤5% increase	May increase	Gastrointestinal: Bloating, constipation
Fibrates Gemfibrozil Fenofibrate	10%–20%	10%–20% increase	20%–50% reduction	Nausea, cholelithiasis, myopathy (more likely with gemfibrozil)

* Low-intensity statin.

** Moderate-intensity statin.

*** High-intensity statin.

HDL-C, high-density lipoprotein cholesterol; LDL-C, low-density lipoprotein cholesterol.

Source: Adapted from American College of Cardiology. ASCVD risk estimator plus. Accessed May 14, 2020. http://tools.acc.org/ASCVD-Risk-Estimator-Plus/#!/calculate/estimate

is rare and short-lived after discontinuation of statin, but increased in patients with excessive alcohol intake and concomitant use of niacin, fibrates, macrolide antibiotics, certain antifungal agents, and HIV protease inhibitors.[13]

The recently available PCSK-9 inhibitors are the most potent LDL-C–lowering drugs. Their mechanism of LDL-C lowering is based on inhibition of the recycling pathway of hepatic LDL-C receptors by which the latter are degraded. Administration of the PCSK-9 inhibitors is by subcutaneous self-injection twice monthly. Extensive analysis of safety data has revealed rhinitis and local irritation at injection sites as the most important side effects. Although the high cost of these drugs has been prohibitive, this drawback has been partially alleviated by industry and insurance firms.[13]

Ezetimibe inhibits absorption of cholesterol in the small intestine. As monotherapy, it lowers LDL-C by up to 20%. One of the most frequent uses of ezetimibe has been in combination with a statin, in which LDL-C lowering is augmented by 15% to 30% without an increase in myopathy or significant elevation of transaminase.[13]

The most important application of the *fibric acid derivatives* (fenofibrate and gemfibrozil) is reduction of elevated serum triglycerides by as much as 50%; HDL may increase by up to 20%.[13] Because they are metabolized by the liver and excreted in the urine, the fibric acid derivatives should be used at lower doses and with caution in patients with abnormal liver or kidney function. Side effects include myopathy, cholelithiasis, and gastrointestinal symptoms. Studies demonstrate the efficacy and safety of combination atorvastatin–fenofibrate therapy in the treatment of mixed lipidemia, including use of lower dose atorvastatin plus fenofibrate and alternate-day regimens.[14,15] The combination of a fibric acid derivative with a statin increases the possibility of rhabdomyolysis, though this adverse effect is more likely when combined with gemfibrozil rather than fenofibrate. Nevertheless, creatine kinase should be monitored at baseline and periodically (every 6 months and if complaints of myalgias) in this setting.[16]

The *bile acid sequestrants* (cholestyramine, colestipol, and colesevelam) bind intestinal bile acids, thereby reducing their reabsorption to the liver through the enterohepatic circulation. Because of their modest cholesterol-lowering potency and adverse effects, these drugs are second-line agents for cholesterol lowering. Side effects are constipation and nausea, and these drugs hinder absorption of fat-soluble vitamins and drugs such as warfarin and thyroid.[13]

TABLE 17.7 Classification of Antiarrhythmic Drugs

Vaughn Williams Class	Updated Class	Pharmacological Targets	Examples of Drugs	Clinical Applications
	0	Blockade of pacemaker current	Ivabradine	Stable angina and chronic heart failure with heart rate ≥70 bpm
I	Ia	Na+ channel blocker (moderate)	Quinidine Ajmaline Disopyramide	SQTS, Brugada Syndrome
	Ib	Na+ channel blocker (weak)	Lidocaine Mexiletine	VT after myocardial infarction (lidocaine), LQTS (mexiletine)
	Ic	Na+ channel blocker (marked)	Propafenone Flecainide	SVT and VT in patients without structural heart disease
	Id	Blockade of the late Na+ current	Ranolazine	Stable angina; a potential new class of drugs for tachyarrhythmias
II		Beta-blockers	Nonselective beta-blockers (carvedilol, propranolol, nadolol) Selective beta1-blockers (atenolol, bisoprolol, esmolol, metoprolol)	Sinus tachycardia, rate controlled for AF and atrial flutter, LQTS (atenolol, propranolol, and nadolol), CPVT (nadolol)
		Adenosine A1 receptor activators	Adenosine	Reduction in AVN conduction, AVNRT
III		Nonselective K+ channel blockers	Amiodarone Dronedarone Ambasilide	AF, VT, tachyarrhythmias with WPW
		hERG (K_v11.1) channel blockers	Dofetilide Ibutilide Sotalol	AF and VT in patients without structural heart disease
		Ultrarapid K+ channel (K_v1.5, I_{Kur}) blockers	Vernakalant	Immediate conversion of AF <2 days in duration
IV	IVa	Ca2+ channel blockers	Verapamil Diltiazem	Reduction in AVN conduction
	IVb	Intracellular Ca2+ channel blocker	Flecainide Propafenone	CPVT

AVN, atrioventricular node; AVNRT, AVN reentrant tachycardia; CPVT, catecholaminergic polymorphic ventricular tachycardia; LQTS, long QT syndrome; SQTS, short QT syndrome; SVT, supraventricular tachycardia; VT, ventricular tachycardia.

Source: Vaughan Williams EM. Classification of antidysrhythmic drugs. *Pharmacol Ther B.* 1975;1:115–138. doi:10.1016/0306-039x(75)90019-7

PHARMACOTHERAPY OF DYSRHYTHMIAS AND ANTICOAGULATION IN ATRIAL FIBRILLATION

DRUGS FOR DYSRHYTHMIAS

The landmark classification of antiarrhythmic drugs (AADs) is based on their mechanisms of action in blocking cardiac ion channels: Na (Class I), K+ (Class III), Ca2+ (Class IV), and adrenergic activities (Class II) were proposed by Vaughan Williams more than three decades ago (**Table 17.7**).[17] Multiple exceptions exist within the classification but it has provided important insights into the effects of AADs on cardiac action potentials and their antiarrhythmic activities. An updated version published in 2018 extended subcategories within each existing class and added a new class of drugs acting on sinoatrial automaticity (Class 0).[18] Two additional classes were also proposed for emerging areas of therapeutics: Class V, drugs acting on mechanosensitive channels, and Class VI, drugs acting on connexin-associated channels. These last two investigational classes are not discussed here.

ANTIARRHYTHMIC DRUGS FOR CHRONIC VENTRICULAR ARRHYTHMIAS

Ventricular arrhythmias in patients with structural heart disease and reduced ejection fraction are associated with an increased risk of sudden cardiac death. Implantable cardioverter defibrillators (ICDs) are first-line therapy in high-risk patients with structural heart disease, while

TABLE 17.8 Amiodarone-Related Adverse Drug Reactions: Incidence, Findings, and Management (in Descending Order of Frequency by System)

Adverse Reaction	Incidence (%)	Signs/Symptoms or Diagnosis	Management*
Ocular	>90	Photophobia, blurred vision, corneal microdeposits	Corneal deposits confirm drug adherence; do not require discontinuation
	<5	Halo vision	Common; does not require discontinuation
	≤1	Optic neuropathy	Discontinue drug; consult ophthalmologist
Skin	25–75	Photosensitivity	Avoid prolonged sun exposure, use sunblock; consider dose reduction
	<10	Blue discoloration	Reassurance; decrease dose
Gastrointestinal	30	Nausea, anorexia, constipation	Consider dose reduction (may ↓ symptoms)
	15–30	ALT or AST >2× normal	Exclude other causes of elevated LFTs; consider drug discontinuation if a reversible cause not found
	<3	Hepatitis and cirrhosis	Consider drug discontinuation if hepatitis present; GI consult, consider liver biopsy to evaluate for cirrhosis
Nervous System	3–30	Ataxia, paresthesias, tremor, peripheral polyneuropathy, insomnia, impaired memory	Frequently dose related; may improve or resolve with dose adjustment
Thyroid	4–22	Hypothyroid	Treat with L-thyroxine; may resolve with discontinuation of amiodarone
	2–12	Hyperthyroidism	Endocrinology consultation, treatment targeted at underlying etiology (PTU, MTZ, +/- prednisone); may need to discontinue amiodarone
Cardiac	5	Bradycardia and AV block	Cardiology consultation; may need permanent pacemaker
	<1	Ventricular proarrhythmia	Cardiology/electrophysiology consultation; usually discontinue drug.
Pulmonary	2	Cough or dyspnea or both, especially with focal or diffuse opacities on high-resolution CT scan and decrease in DLCO from baseline	Pulmonary consultation, consider corticosteroids (severe cases); usually discontinue drug; may consider continuing if drug levels high and abnormalities resolve with lower dosage; rarely, continue if no effective alternative
Genitourinary	<1	Epididymitis and ED	Pain may resolve spontaneously; urology consultation for ED treatment options

*Amiodarone has a very long half-life (mean 58 days, range 15 to 142 days); therefore, drug effects last for months and dose adjustment or discontinuation will not result in immediate symptom improvement.

ALT, alanine aminotransferase; AST, aspartate aminotransferase; AV, atrioventricular; CT, computed tomography; D$_L$CO, diffusion capacity of carbon monoxide; ED, erectile dysfunction; GI, gastrointestinal; MTZ, methimazole; PTU, propylthiouracil.

Source: Adapted with permission from Vamos M, Hohnloser SH. Amiodarone and dronedarone: an update. *Trends Cardiovasc Med.* 2016;26(7): 597–602. doi:10.1016/j.tcm.2016.03.014

AADs and catheter ablation serve as adjunctive therapy. A combination of amiodarone and beta-blockers can be used to reduce the incidence of ICD shocks, although sotalol and mexiletine can also be considered.[19,20]

ANTIARRHYTHMIC DRUGS FOR ATRIAL FIBRILLATION

Three strategies are considered for treatment of atrial fibrillation (AF): Rhythm control, rate control, and stroke prevention.[21] Despite the availability of a large number of

AADs, the choices in patients with heart disease are limited due to proarrhythmic effects of these medications. Amiodarone remains the most effective and widely used pharmacotherapy for AF, even though it is fraught with multiple extra-cardiac side effects (**Table 17.8**).[21–23]

Because the adverse effects of amiodarone may be severe and potentially life-threatening, careful monitoring of the patients taking amiodarone is essential. Assessment of amiodarone-related symptoms (**Table 17.9**), recurrence of arrhythmia, and need for drug titration or changes should be assessed every

TABLE 17.9 Recommended Baseline and Monitoring Diagnostic Tests for Patients Receiving Chronic Amiodarone Therapy

Diagnostic Test	Timing of Test*
Liver function tests	Baseline and every 6 months
Thyroid function tests	TSH, free T4, and total or free T3 at baseline; follow-up TSH every 6 months
Chest x-ray (CXR)	Baseline, then annually
Electrocardiogram	Baseline and when clinically relevant
Ophthalmologic evaluation	Baseline if visual impairment, then age-appropriate interval for routine screening
Pulmonary function tests (with D_LCO)	Baseline and for unexplained or persistent cough or dyspnea, abnormalities on annual follow-up CXR, or if clinical suspicion of pulmonary toxicity
High-resolution chest CT scan	If clinical suspicion of pulmonary toxicity

*Recommended intervals; more frequent follow-up needed if clinically indicated.

D_LCO, diffusion capacity of carbon monoxide; T3, triiodothyronine; T4, thyroxine.

Source: Adapted with permission from Vamos M, Hohnloser SH. Amiodarone and dronedarone: an update. *Trends Cardiovasc Med.* 2016;26(7): 597–602. doi:10.1016/j.tcm.2016.03.014

TABLE 17.10 Indications for Specialty Consultation in Suspected Amiodarone Toxicity

Specialty to Consult	Indications for Consultation
Electrophysiologist	Worsening or new arrhythmia symptoms Amiodarone toxicity requires changes in drug dosing or drug discontinuation New amiodarone therapy in patient with an ICD (for EPS and defibrillation threshold testing) Pregnant patient who requires amiodarone Pediatric patient who requires amiodarone
Endocrinologist	Any symptoms of hyperthyroidism Acutely ill patient where interpretation of TFTs is difficult When considering treating subclinical hypothyroidism
Gastroenterologist	LFTs increase to >2× normal
Pulmonologist*	Abnormal CXR at baseline or follow-up Abnormal PFT value (especially FVC or D_LCO) at baseline or follow-up New cough or dyspnea, especially if unexplained

*Obtain PFT and high-resolution chest CT if not previously completed.

CT, computed tomography; CXR, chest x-ray; D_LCO, diffusion capacity of carbon monoxide; EPS, electrophysiology testing; FVC, forced vital capacity; ICD, implantable cardioverter-defibrillator; TFT, thyroid function test.

Source: Adapted with permission from Vamos M, Hohnloser SH. Amiodarone and dronedarone: an update. *Trends Cardiovasc Med.* 2016;26(7): 597–602. doi:10.1016/j.tcm.2016.03.014

3 to 6 months in the first year, then every 6 months for the duration of therapy.[23] Recommended diagnostic follow-up to evaluate for amiodarone-related toxicity is outlined in Table 17.9. Indications for referral to a specialist for evaluation of suspected toxicity and alternative therapy options are noted in **Table 17.10**.

Other options for selected cases of AF include sotalol and dronedarone.[21,22] Vernakalant has been superior to amiodarone for cardioversion of recent-onset AF (<2 days), but not for long-term rhythm or rate control.[24] Optimizing function with guideline-directed medical therapy is critical.

PREVENTION OF STROKE IN PATIENTS WITH ATRIAL FIBRILLATION

Because of the risk of stroke that AF confers, anticoagulation therapy should be considered in all patients with this arrhythmia unless patients are low risk based on validated scores (e.g., CHA_2DS_2-VASc score of 0 in males, 1 in females).[25] Vitamin K antagonists (VKAs; e.g., warfarin) reduce systemic thromboembolism by greater than 60% and all-cause mortality by greater than 25% versus placebo; novel or non-vitamin K antagonist oral anticoagulants (NOACs) provide additional reductions of 10% to 19%.[26] Bleeding risk should be assessed (e.g., HAS-BLED score[27]).

NOVEL ORAL ANTICOAGULANTS

Novel oral anticoagulants (NOACs) comprise direct factor Xa inhibitors (apixaban, rivaroxaban, darexaban, edoxaban), direct thrombin inhibitors (dabigatran), and PAR-1 antagonists (vorapaxar, atopaxar) and are the preferred therapy for nonvalvular AF. They have more stable pharmacological profiles, no

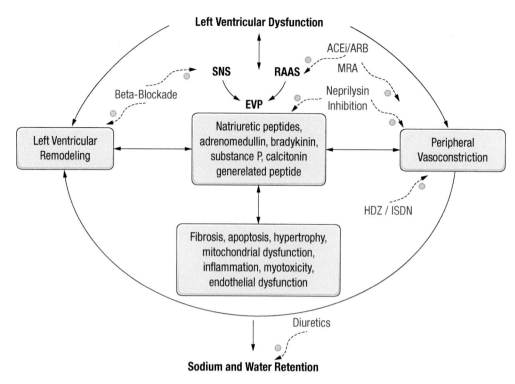

FIGURE 17.1 Pathophysiology of Heart Failure: Multiple causes lead to left ventricular dysfunction, producing alterations in cardiovascular physiology which activate many compensatory mechanisms including activation of the renin angiotensin aldosterone system (RAAS) and the sympathetic nervous system (SNS) to maintain cardiac output through salt and water retention, vasoconstriction and increased contractility. Activation of natriuretic peptides, vasodilatory prostaglandins, nitric oxide (NO), and other EVP (endogenous vasoactive peptides) lead to vasodilation, natriuresis and diuresis, lowering blood pressure, sympathetic tone, and aldosterone levels. EVP are degraded by neprilysin, which is also responsible for the breakdown of bradykin and angiotensin II. Gradual introduction of angiotensin-converting enzyme (ACE) inhibitors, angiotensin receptor blockers (ARB), mineralocorticoid antagonists (MRA) and beta-blockers are well-established counteractive therapies. Neprilysin is inhibited by sacubitril, which prevents metabolism of natriuretic peptides, prolonging duration of their favorable effects. As a result, sacubitril is used together with ARB for its dual effects (i.e., inhibiting the degradation of natriuretic peptides and facilitating the breakdown of angiotensin II). The combination of hydralazine and isosorbide induces direct vasorelaxation through the NO related pathway. Diuretics are the cornerstone of therapy to maintain fluid homeostasis.

significant interference from diet, and less risk of intracranial bleeding than warfarin.[21] NOACs have rapid onset and offset of action so that bridging with parenteral anticoagulant therapy is not necessary during initiation or brief interruption of therapy for surgical procedures. However, these drugs are renally excreted so dose adjustment may be necessary in chronic renal disease. For patients with severe kidney disease, mechanical heart valves, or mitral stenosis, warfarin remains the drug of choice.[21] The mnemonic ABCDE can be used when considering a particular NOAC: Abnormally low weight (dose reduction might be needed), bleeding risk, creatinine clearance, drug interactions (e.g., P-glycoprotein inhibitors), and elderly (dose reduction might be needed).[21]

PHARMACOTHERAPY FOR HEART FAILURE

Mortality associated with HF is about 50% at 5 years across the entire spectrum of patients, including those with severely reduced, mid-range, or preserved ejection fraction.[28] For HFrEF, neurohormonal blockade therapy of the angiotensin, neprilysin, adrenergic, and aldosterone pathways is the foundation of therapy. Figure 17.1 illustrates the pathophysiology of HF and the associated points of therapeutic intervention. Concomitant therapies include heart rate control with ivabradine, enhancing contractility with digoxin, and symptom relief with diuretics (Table 17.11).[29]

ANGIOTENSIN-CONVERTING ENZYME INHIBITORS AND ANGIOTENSIN RECEPTOR BLOCKERS

ACEI therapy has been associated with reduced sympathetic activity, increased vasodilatory kinins, improved endothelial function, and improved survival, as documented in multiple studies.[30–32] ARBs inhibit binding of angiotensin II (ATII) to the ATII receptor and do not affect kinin metabolism. ARBs have also

TABLE 17.11 Pharmacotherapy for Heart Failure

Drug	Dose Range	Indication	Outcomes	Comments
Angiotensin-Converting Enzyme Inhibitors				
Captopril Enalapril Lisinopril Ramipril	6.25–50 mg tid 2.5–20 mg bid 2.5–40 mg daily 1.25–10 mg daily	NYHA Class I–IV	17% reduction in mortality (NNT = 26), 31% reduction in HF hospitalizations	Captopril may be easier to manage to start ACE titration in patients with low blood pressure
Angiotensin Receptor Blockers				
Candesartan Losartan Valsartan	4–32 mg daily 25–150 mg daily 20–160 mg bid	NYHA Class I–IV	23% reduction cardiovascular death or HF hospitalization	Alternative for patients ACE intolerant; may be added to ACE if intolerant to aldosterone antagonist
Beta-Blockers				
Bisoprolol Carvedilol Carvedilol CR Metoprolol	1.25–10 mg daily 3.125–50 mg bid 10–80 mg daily 12.5–200 mg daily	NYHA Class I–IV	34% reduction in mortality (NNT 9), 41% reduction in HF hospitalization	Safe when started in NYHA IV; avoid discontinuation if possible
Angiotensin Receptor Neprilysin Inhibitors				
Sacubitril/valsartan	24/26–97/103 mg bid (sacubitril/ valsartan)	NYHA Class II–IV	20% reduction mortality and HF hospitalization (NNT 35), 16% reduction all-cause mortality	Switch, stable patients on ACE (36hs washout) contraindicated if history of angioedema
Aldosterone Antagonists				
Spironolactone Eplerenone	12.5–50 mg daily 25–50 mg daily	NYHA Class II–IV	30% reduction in mortality (NNT 6), 35% reduction in hospitalization	Risk of hyperkalemia; contraindicated if Cr >2.5 (male) or 2.0 mg/dL (women)
Nitric Oxide Enrichment Therapy				
Isosorbide dinitrate/hydralazine	20 mg ISDN/37.5 mg Hydralazine–40 mg ISDN/100 mg HDZ tid	African American NYHA Class III–IV	43% relative reduction in mortality (NNT 7), 33% relative reduction HF hospitalization	Likely effective in non-African American intolerant to ACEI, ARB, or ARNI
Sinus Node Modulator				
Ivabradine	2.5 mg BID–7.5 mg bid	HR >70 NYHA Class II–III	18% relative reduction HF hospitalization	Patients in NSR, titrate to HR 50–60

ACE, angiotensin-converting enzyme; ACEI, angiotensin-converting enzyme inhibitor; ARB, angiotensin receptor blocker; ARNI, angiotensin receptor neprilysin inhibitor; bid, twice daily; Cr, creatinine; HDZ, hydralazine; HF, heart failure; HR, heart rate; ISDN, isosorbide dinitrate; IV, intravenous; NNT, number needed to treat; NSR, normal sinus rhythm; NYHA, New York Heart Association; TID, thrice daily.

Source: Adapted from Packer M, Coats AJ, Fowler MB, et al. Effect of carvedilol on survival in severe chronic heart failure. *N Engl J Med.* 2001;344(22):1651–1658. doi:10.1056/NEJM200105313442201

improved clinical status and survival in patients with HFrEF and are excellent agents for patients intolerant to ACEIs.[32]

Beta-Blockers

Beta-adrenergic blockade to attenuate the deleterious effects of excessive myocardial stimulation by endogenous catecholamines in patients with HFrEF can reduce mortality. This property has been proven for three beta-blockers: Metoprolol succinate,[33] carvedilol,[34,35] and bisoprolol.[36]

Angiotensin Receptor Neprilysin Inhibitors

Compared to ACE inhibition with enalapril, co-inhibition of neprilysin and angiotensin receptor with sacubitril/valsartan (LCZ696) is associated with reduced cardiovascular death or HF hospitalization.[36] Sacubitril/valsartan should replace an ACEI or ARB in symptomatic patients with HFrEF and systolic blood pressure greater than 95 mmHg. Specific contraindications include angioedema, hyperkalemia, and pregnancy. Switching from ACEI to angiotensin receptor neprilysin inhibitors (ARNI) should allow for a 36-hour drug-free period to minimize risk of angioedema.[37,38]

Aldosterone Antagonists

Antagonism of aldosterone with potassium-sparing diuretic spironolactone has demonstrated reduction in mortality, hospitalizations, and sudden death when compared to conventional therapy in patients with HFrEF with NYHA functional Class II, III and IV.[39] Because of its affinity for progesterone and androgen receptors, spironolactone is associated with dose- and therapy-duration-dependent endocrine-mediated side effects (e.g., hirsutism, gynecomastia, increased vaginal bleeding, change in libido).[40] For patients who are intolerant of spironolactone, eplerenone, a significantly more selective aldosterone blocker, is an option.[41] Contraindications to aldosterone antagonists are hyperkalemia or serum creatinine greater than 2.5 mg/dL in men or 2.0 mg/dL in women.[29]

Hydralazine/Nitrates

Randomized evaluation of the combination of hydralazine with isosorbide dinitrate *added* to standard therapy for African Americans with Class III to IV HF demonstrated improved survival.[42] Therefore, the addition of this combination therapy is recommended in all African American–descent patients with HFrEF who have persistent symptoms despite optimal standard therapy.[38] It also remains a potential option for HF patients of other races or ethnicity[39] who remain NYHA Class III or IV despite optimal standard therapy.[38,42]

Ivabradine

The cardiac effects of ivabradine are specific to the sinoatrial node; the drug has no effect on BP, intracardiac conduction, myocardial contractility, or ventricular repolarization. In patients with HFrEF, with sinus resting heart rate greater than 70 bpm despite maximally tolerated titration of a beta-blocker, further heart rate control by addition of ivabradine reduced the risk of the combined endpoint of hospitalization for worsening HF or cardiovascular death and is indicated in patients with these criteria.[43]

Symptomatic Treatments

Loop diuretics remain the first option to alleviate fluid overload. Similar outcomes resulted with intravenous bolus versus continuous infusion of loop diuretics for patients admitted with acute decompensated heart failure. Addition of a thiazide such as metolazone as needed alleviates congestion. Lower doses of diuretics and single-agent diuretic regimens may be associated with more favorable clinical outcomes. Digoxin, the oldest positive inotropic drug, reduces HF hospitalizations and may be helpful for rate control in patients with HF and atrial fibrillation.[38]

CONCLUSION

This chapter has reviewed the major pharmacotherapy for cardiovascular disease, which remains a major cause of disability and premature death globally. Modification of risk factors through both lifestyle and pharmacological interventions has been shown to reduce mortality and morbidity in people with diagnosed or undiagnosed cardiovascular disease. Cardiovascular pharmacotherapy has advanced notably over the last decade, with many new medications that target newly understood mechanisms of disease and with ongoing research in these areas. Additionally, updates to guidelines for the management of many aspects of cardiovascular disease have been published within the last 5 years. This chapter provided a focused update on selected medications and guidelines used for the treatment of cardiovascular diseases.

 CASE EXEMPLAR: Patient With Hypertension

MP is a 58-year-old man who presents for his annual visit with his clinician. He has no complaints of chest pain, palpitations, syncope, dyspnea, or lightheadedness. His only exercise is golf once a week; however, he uses a cart to navigate the course.

Past Medical History
- Known hypertension

Medications
- None

Family History
- Father died of "heart problems" at the age of 52

Social History
- Smokes one pack of cigarettes per day
- Consumes two to three cocktails per night to "settle [his] nerves"

Physical Examination
- Height: 67 inches; weight: 176 lbs; body mass index: 27.6; blood pressure: 162/94 (consistent with prior readings); respiration rate: 16; oxygen saturation on room air: 97%; temperature: 98.4 °F
- Cardiovascular examination: Regular rhythm; S1 best heard at the apex; S2 best heard in the right

(continued)

2nd intercostal space and left parasternal border; no murmurs; carotid pulses 2/4 bilaterally
- Pulmonary examination: Lungs clear to percussion and auscultation
- Abdominal examination: Negative
- Extremities: Warm with 2/4 pedal pulses; no peripheral edema

Labs and Imaging
- Hs-Troponin: Negative (<14 ng/L)
- Creatinine: 0.9 mg/dL (0.8–1.3 mg/dL)
- Triglycerides: 200 mg/dL (<150 mg/dL)
- High-density lipoproteins: 30 mg/dL (>40 mg/dL)
- Low-density lipoproteins: 150 mg/dL (<100 mg/dL)
- Total cholesterol: 230 mg/dL (<200 mg/dL)
- Random glucose: 126 mg/dL (654 ng/L)
- Creatinine: 0.9 mg/dL (0.8–110 mg/dL)
- Resting ECG shown in the graph that follows:

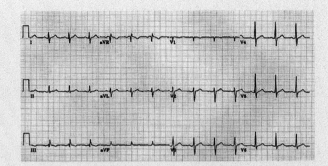

Discussion Questions

1. Based on American College of Cardiology/American Heart Association 2017 Hypertension guidelines, how would you manage MP's blood pressure?
2. How would a clinician address MP's lipid values during this visit?

CASE EXEMPLAR: Patient With Radiating Chest Pain

CP is a 64-year-old male who presents to the emergency department (ED) via ambulance for chest pain. He was out shoveling snow from his driveway when he developed left anterior chest pain, pressure-type, radiating to his jaw and shoulder. Despite the cold weather, he was sweating. He also noted palpitations and shortness of breath, although he thought it was just because he was "a little out of shape." He was afraid that something was definitely wrong, so he asked his wife to call 911.

Past Medical History
- Hypertension
- Hyperlipidemia
- Diabetes mellitus
- Gout

Medications
- Hydrochlorothiazide, 25 mg once daily
- Allopurinol, 300 mg once daily

Social History
- Retired factory worker
- Smokes one pack of cigarettes per day
- Drinks about six beers per day (sometimes more)

Physical Examination
- Well-developed obese man in moderate distress
- Height: 69 inches; weight: 252 lbs.; blood pressure: 172/110; pulse: 92; respiration rate: 16; temperature: 98.7 °F
- Lungs: Scattered bilateral wheezes
- Heart: Regular with grade II/VI systolic murmur
- Extremities: No edema

Labs and Imaging
- Complete blood count with mild leukocytosis (WBC 12.9k)
- Potassium: Low at 2.9 mEq/L
- Glucose: 252 mg/dL
- Troponin I: 1.7 ng/L
- Uric acid: 11.1 mg/dL
- EKG: ST segment depression with T-wave inversion over lateral leads; no pathologic Q waves

Next Steps
- CP's admitting diagnoses are non-ST segment elevation acute coronary syndrome, hypertension, diabetes mellitus, obesity, alcohol abuse, hyperuricemia, and smoker

Discussion Questions

1. What medications should be instituted for CP?
2. What medications should be continued after discharge?
3. What lifestyle modifications can be recommended for CP?

KEY TAKEAWAYS

- The following are among the medications that may be used in the management of ACS: Antiplatelet therapy, anticoagulation, angiotensin-converting enzyme inhibitors (ACE-inhibitors) *or* angiotensin receptor blockers (ARBs), beta-adrenergic blockers, calcium-channel antagonists, nitrates, and high-intensity statins.
- Antianginal pharmacologic agents alleviate ischemia by decreasing one or more of the major determinants of myocardial oxygen demand (heart rate, systolic blood pressure, contractility, and left ventricular dimension) and improve myocardial oxygen supply-demand balance.
- The foundation of BP treatment is nonpharmacologic intervention, including weight loss, increased physical activity, reduction in sodium intake, and moderation in alcohol consumption.
- Although the basis of lipid-lowering therapy is favorable lifestyle alterations, a majority of patients require pharmacologic therapy to achieve recommended lipid targets.
- The landmark classification of AADs is based on their mechanisms of action: Sodium channel blockers (Class I), K$^+$ (Class III), calcium channel blockers (Class IV), adrenergic activities (Class II), a new class of drugs acting on sinoatrial automaticity (Class 0), drugs that act on mechanosensitive channels (Class V), and drugs acting on connexin-associated channels (Class VI).
- For HFrEF, neurohormonal blockade therapy of the angiotensin, neprilysin, adrenergic, and aldosterone pathways is the foundation of therapy, along with digoxin and diuretics.

REFERENCES

1. Amsterdam EA, Wenger NK, Brindis RG, et al. 2014 AHA/ACC guideline for the management of patients with non-ST-elevation acute coronary syndromes: a report of the American College of Cardiology/American Heart Association Task Force on Practice Guidelines. *J Am Coll Cardiol*. 2014;64:e139–e228. doi:10.1016/j.jacc.2014.09.017

2. O'Gara PT, Kushner FG, Ascheim DD, et al. 2013 ACCF/AHA guideline for the management of ST-elevation myocardial infarction. A report of the American College of Cardiology Foundation/American Heart Association Task Force on Practice Guidelines. *J Am Coll Cardiol*. 2013;61(4):e78–e140. doi:10.1016/j.jacc.2012.11.019

3. Richards JR. *Beta-blockers: Physiological, Pharmacological and Therapeutic Implications*. Nova Science Publishers; 2018.

4. Divakaran S, Loscalzo J. The role of nitroglycerin and other nitrogen oxides in cardiovascular therapeutics. *J Am Coll Cardiol*. 2017;70(19):2393–2410. doi:10.1016/j.jacc.2017.09.1064

5. Pascual I, Moris C, Avanzas P. Beta-blockers and calcium channel blockers: first line agents. *Cardiovasc Drugs Ther*. 2016;30(4):357–365. doi:10.1007/s10557-016-6682-1

6. Rosano GMC, Vitale C, Volterrani M. Pharmacological management of chronic stable angina: focus on ranolazine. *Cardiovasc Drugs Ther*. 2016;30(4):393C–398C. doi:10.1007/s10557-016-6674-1

7. Benjamin EJ, Blaha MJ, Chiuve SE, et al. Heart disease and stroke statistics—2017 update: a report from the American Heart Association. *Circulation*. 2017;135(10):e146–e603. doi:10.1161/CIR.0000000000000491

8. Whelton PK, Carey RM, Aronow WS, et al. 2017 ACC/AHA/AAPA/ABC/ACPM/AGS/APhA/ASH/ASPC/NMA/PCNA guideline for the prevention, detection, evaluation, and management of high blood pressure in adults: a report of the American College of Cardiology/American Heart Association Task Force on Clinical Practice Guidelines. *J Am Coll Cardiol*. 2018;71(19):e127–e248. doi:10.1161/HYP.0000000000000075

9. Chobanian AV, Bakris GL, Black HR, et al. The seventh report of the Joint National Committee on Prevention, Detection, Evaluation, and Treatment of High Blood Pressure: the JNC 7 report. *JAMA*. 2003;289(19):2560–2572. doi:10.1001/jama.289.19.2560

10. Laurent S. Antihypertensive drugs. *Pharmacol Res*. 2017;124:116–125. doi:10.1016/j.phrs.2017.07.026

11. Lithell H, Berne C. Diabetogenic drugs. *Pharmacol Diabetes: Present Pract Future Perspect*. 2019;57–64. doi:10.1515/9783110850321-007

12. Reboussin DM, Allen NB, Griswold ME, et al. Systematic review for the 2017 ACC/AHA/AAPA/ABC/ACPM/AGS/APhA/ASH/ASPC/NMA/PCNA guideline for the prevention, detection, evaluation, and management of high blood pressure in adults. *J Am Coll Cardiol*. 2018;71(19):2176–2198. doi:10.1016/j.jacc.2017.11.004

13. Grundy SM, Stone NJ, Bailey AL, et al. 2018 AHA/ACC/AACVPR/AAPA/ABC/ACPM/ADA/AGS/APhA/ASPC/NLA/PCNA guideline on the management of blood cholesterol: a report of the American College of Cardiology/American Heart Association Task Force on Clinical Practice Guidelines. *J Am Coll Cardiol*. 2019;73(24):e285–e350. doi:10.1016/j.jacc.2018.11.003

14. Kiortsis DN, Millionis H, Bairaktari E, et al. Efficacy of combination of atorvastatin and micronised fenofibrate in the treatment of severe mixed hyperlipidemia. *Eur J Clin Pharmacol*. 2000;56(9–10):631–635. doi:10.1007/s002280000213

15. Harivenkatesh N, David DC, Haribalaji N, et al. Efficacy and safety of alternate day therapy with atorvastatin and fenofibrate combination in mixed dyslipidemia: a randomized controlled trial. *J Cardiovasc Pharmacol Ther*. 2014;19(3):296–303. doi:10.1177/1074248413518968

16. Wiklund O, Pirazzi C, Romeo S. Monitoring of lipids, enzymes, and creatine kinase in patients on

lipid-lowering drug therapy. *Curr Cardiol Rep.* 2013;15(9):397. doi:10.1007/s11886-013-0397-8

17. Vaughan Williams EM. Classification of antidys-rhythmic drugs. *Pharmacol Ther B.* 1975;1:115–138. doi:10.1016/0306-039x(75)90019-7

18. Lei M, Wu L, Terrar DA, et al. Modernized classification of cardiac antiarrhythmic drugs. *Circulation.* 2018;138:1879–1896. doi:10.1161/CIRCULATIONAHA.118.035455

19. Cardiac Arrhythmia Suppression Trial Investigators. Preliminary report: effect of encainide and flecainide on mortality in a randomized trial of arrhythmia suppression after myocardial infarction. *N Engl J Med.* 1989;321:406–412. doi:10.1056/NEJM198908103210629

20. Markman TM, Nazarian S. Treatment of ventricular arrhythmias: what's new? *Trends Cardiovasc Med.* 2019;29(5):249–261. doi:10.1016/j.tcm.2018.09.014

21. January CT, Wann LS, Alpert JS, et al. 2014 AHA/ACC/HRS guideline for the management of patients with atrial fibrillation: a report of the American College of Cardiology/American Heart Association Task Force on Practice Guidelines and the Heart Rhythm Society. *J Am Coll Cardiol.* 2014;64:e1–e76. doi:10.1016/j.jacc.2014.03.022

22. Vamos M, Hohnloser SH. Amiodarone and dronedarone: an update. *Trends Cardiovasc Med.* 2016;26(7):597–602. doi:10.1016/j.tcm.2016.03.014

23. Epstein AE, Olshansky B, Naccarelli GV, et al. Practical management guide for clinicians who treat patients with amiodarone. *Am J Med.* 2016;129(5):468–475. doi:10.1016/j.amjmed.2015.08.039

24. Tsuji Y, Dobrev D. Safety and efficacy of vernakalant for acute cardioversion of atrial fibrillation: an update. *Vasc Health Risk Manage.* 2013;9:165. doi:10.2147/VHRM.S43720

25. Lip GY, Nieuwlaat R, Pisters R, et al. Refining clinical risk stratification for predicting stroke and thromboembolism in atrial fibrillation using a novel risk factor-based approach: the Euro Heart Survey on atrial fibrillation. *Chest.* 2010;137:263–272. doi:10.1378/chest.09-1584

26. Freedman B, Potpara TS, Lip GY. Stroke prevention in atrial fibrillation. *Lancet.* 2016;388:806–817. doi:10.1016/S0140-6736(16)31257-0

27. Pisters R, Lane DA, Nieuwlaat R, et al. A novel user-friendly score (HAS-BLED) to assess 1-year risk of major bleeding in patients with atrial fibrillation: the Euro Heart Survey. *Chest.* 2010;138:1093–1100. doi:10.1378/chest.10-0134

28. Shah KS, Xu H, Matsouaka RA, et al. Heart failure with preserved, borderline, and reduced ejection fraction: 5-year outcomes. *J Am Coll Cardiol.* 2017;70:2476–2486. doi:10.1016/j.jacc.2017.08.074

29. Yancy C, Jessup M, Bozkurt B, et al. 2017 ACC/AHA/HFSA focused update of the 2013 ACCF/AHA guideline for the management of heart failure: a report of the American College of Cardiology/American Heart Association Task Force on Clinical Practice Guidelines and the Heart Failure Society of America. *Circulation.* 2017;136:e137–e161. doi:10.1161/CIR.0000000000000509

30. SOLVD Investigators, Yusuf S, Pitt B, et al. Effect of enalapril on survival in patients with reduced left ventricular ejection fractions and congestive heart failure. *N Engl J Med.* 1991;325:293–302. doi:10.1056/NEJM199108013250501

31. SOLVD Investigators, Yusuf S, Pitt B, et al. Effect of enalapril on mortality and the development of heart failure in asymptomatic patients with reduced left ventricular ejection fractions. *N Engl J Med.* 1992;327(10):685–691. doi:10.1056/NEJM199209033271003

32. Cohn JN, Tognoni G, Valsartan Heart Failure Trial Investigators. A randomized trial of the angiotensin-receptor blocker valsartan in chronic heart failure. *N Engl J Med.* 2001;345(23):1667–1675. doi:10.1056/NEJMoa010713

33. Hjalmarson A, Goldstein S, Fagerberg B, et al. Effects of controlled-release metoprolol on total mortality, hospitalizations, and well-being in patients with heart failure. The metoprolol CR/XL randomized intervention trial in congestive heart failure (MERIT-HF). *JAMA.* 2000;283(10):1295–1302. doi:10.1001/jama.283.10.1295

34. Packer M, Coats AJ, Fowler MB, et al. Effect of carvedilol on survival in severe chronic heart failure. *N Engl J Med.* 2001;344(22):1651–1658. doi:10.1056/NEJM200105313442201

35. Poole-Wilson PA, Swedberg K, Cleland JG, et al. Comparison of carvedilol and metoprolol on clinical outcomes in patients with chronic heart failure in the Carvedilol or Metoprolol European Trial (COMET): randomised controlled trial. *Lancet.* 2003;362(9377):7–13. doi:10.1016/S0140-6736(03)13800-7

36. The Cardiac Insufficiency Bisoprolol Study II (CIBIS-II): a randomised trial. *Lancet.* 1999;353(9146):9–13. doi:10.1016/S0140-6736(98)11181-9

37. McMurray JJ, Packer M, Desai AS, et al. Angiotensin-neprilysin inhibition versus enalapril in heart failure. *N Engl J Med.* 2014;371:993–1004. doi:10.1056/NEJMoa1409077

38. Yancy CW, Januzzi JL Jr, Allen LA, et al. 2017 ACC expert consensus decision pathway for optimization of heart failure treatment: answers to 10 pivotal issues about heart failure with reduced ejection fraction: a report of the American College of Cardiology Task Force on expert consensus decision pathways. *J Am Coll Cardiol.* 2018;71(2):201–230. doi:10.1016/j.jacc.2017.11.025

39. Pitt B, Zannad F, Remme WJ, et al. The effect of spironolactone on morbidity and mortality in patients with severe heart failure. Randomized Aldactone Evaluation Study Investigators. *N Engl J Med.* 1999;341(10):709–717. doi:10.1056/NEJM199909023411001.

40. Zannad F, McMurray JJ, Krum H, et al. Eplerenone in patients with systolic heart failure and mild symptoms. *N Engl J Med.* 2011;364:11–21. doi:10.1056/NEJMoa1009492

41. Garthwaite SM, McMahon EG. The evolution of aldosterone antagonists. *Mol Cell Endocrinol.* 2004;*217* (1–2):27–31. doi:10.1016/j.mce.2003.10.005

42. Taylor AL, Ziesche S, Yancy C, et al. Combination of isosorbide dinitrate and hydralazine in Blacks with heart failure. *N Engl J Med.* 2004;351(20):2049–2057. doi:10.1056/NEJMoa042934

43. Swedberg K, Komajda M, Böhm M, et al. Ivabradine and outcomes in chronic heart failure (SHIFT): a randomised placebo-controlled study. *Lancet.* 2010;376(9744):875–885. doi:10.1016/S0140-6736(10)61198-1

Pharmacotherapy for Respiratory Conditions

Jennifer Kuretski

LEARNING OBJECTIVES

- Outline the pathophysiology of asthma and chronic obstructive pulmonary disease (COPD).
- Outline the contributing factors and manifestations of asthma and COPD and their relationship to the diagnosis of the disease.
- Describe nonpharmacologic management of asthma and COPD.
- Discuss each of the classes of medications available to treat COPD and asthma and their expected outcomes.
- Discuss the pathophysiology, diagnosis, and management of cough and viral upper respiratory disorders.
- Define the use of oxygen in the management of asthma, COPD, and other oxygen-deficient disorders.

ASTHMA AND CHRONIC OBSTRUCTIVE PULMONARY DISEASE

INTRODUCTION

According to the most current report from the World Health Organization (WHO), approximately 339 million people worldwide suffered from asthma in 2016.[1] In the United States, approximately 1 in 12 adults and 1 in 10 children have asthma.[2] It is estimated that approximately 65 million people have moderate-to-severe chronic obstructive pulmonary disease (COPD).[3] Of the 65 million people across the world with COPD, approximately 24% live in the United States. It is estimated that 15.7 million Americans have been diagnosed with COPD; however, these numbers may be lower than actual prevalence.[4]

Each year, asthma costs about $3,300 per person in healthcare-related expenses.[2] In 2008, more than half of all children with asthma and more than one-third of adults with asthma missed school or work due to an asthma attack.[2]

In 2014, COPD was the third leading cause of death in the United States.[5] In 2018, a report from the Centers for Disease Control (CDC) indicated that chronic lower respiratory disease is the fourth leading cause of death in the United States.[6] Although the death rates have declined through the years (a 2.9% reduction from 2017 to 2018) for chronic lower respiratory diseases (40.9% in 2017 to 39.7% in 2018), the death rates for males and females per 100,000 population reported in 2018 in the United States were 855 and 611, respectively.

There are racial differences in people affected by asthma. About one in nine non-Hispanic Black people of all ages are diagnosed with asthma. This statistic is strongly influenced by age, as one in six non-Hispanic Black children are diagnosed with asthma.[2]

Patients meeting any of the following characteristics were more likely to report COPD: 65 to 74 years of age or older than age 75; American Indians or Alaska Natives; women; individuals who were unemployed, retired, or unable to work; individuals with less than a high school education, divorced, widowed, or separated; current or former smokers; and those with a history of asthma.[4]

BACKGROUND

Sir William Osler described asthma as a spasm of the bronchial muscles, swelling of the bronchial mucous membrane, and inflammation of the smaller bronchioles. He also described a similarity to "hay fever" and observed that asthma symptoms were typically presented in childhood and often occurred in multiple members of a family.[7] In the 1980s, allergens were described as triggers of the inflammatory response, including mobilization of mast cells, eosinophils, basophils, and mononuclear cells.[8] These descriptions are in line with the pathophysiology of asthma as it is known today with the exception of a few extra phenotypes (allergic asthma, nonallergic asthma, late-onset asthma, and asthma with obesity).[9]

Descriptions of COPD date back to the 1600s when lungs were described as "voluminous" by Bonet. In 1814, Badham described the chronic bronchitis component of COPD as "catarrh" or chronic cough with hypersecretion of mucus. Emphysema was defined by Laennec in 1821 as lung hyperinflation that "did not empty well." Charles Fletcher recognized the association between smoking and the rate of decline in FEV1 in 1976.[10] Over the years, there have been few changes in the definitions of COPD, whether emphysema or chronic bronchitis.

PHYSIOLOGY AND PATHOPHYSIOLOGY

Homeostasis of the respiratory system is a balance between gas exchange in the lungs and regulation of the blood pH. The gas exchange takes place between the alveoli of the lungs and capillaries, where carbon dioxide is eliminated and oxygen is taken in. Oxygen passively diffuses through to the capillaries to be delivered to other necessary locations, including organs, tissues, and cells.[11]

Smooth muscle in the bronchioles permits air flow to move through the lungs to facilitate that gas exchange process. Elasticity of the alveoli increases the surface area available for gas exchange. These normal physiologic processes constitute the respiratory system and any disturbance along these key areas can cause disease.[11]

The development of asthma depends upon the environmental factors as well as the clinical presentation of the patient. For example, allergic asthma begins with an allergic trigger, which signals the inflammatory cascade and the release of inflammatory mediators, such as mast cells and eosinophils, whereas patients with nonallergic asthma or asthma with obesity have respiratory symptoms of asthma without the eosinophilic airway inflammation.[9] Mucus hypersecretion, resulting in a chronic cough, is characteristic for chronic bronchitis, whereas inflammation and narrowing of the airways leads to a decrease in FEV1 and parenchymal destruction contributes to decreased gas exchange in emphysema.[12]

RISK FACTORS

There are several risk factors for asthma and COPD. According to the American Lung Association,[13] if a parent has asthma, a child is three to six times more likely to develop asthma than a child whose parents do not have

asthma. The presence of other allergic conditions, such as atopic dermatitis and/or allergic rhinitis, is also a risk factor for asthma, as is obesity, due to the possible low-grade inflammation associated with excess weight.

Smoking is a risk factor for both asthma and COPD; however, approximately 85% to 90% of cases of COPD are thought to be caused by cigarette smoke. Other risk factors for COPD include long-term exposure to air pollution, secondhand smoke and other harmful chemicals in the environment, and alpha-1 antitrypsin deficiency, which specifically can cause emphysema.[14]

Several factors contribute to the development of asthma. One of the most clearly understood relationships is between genetics and asthma. More specifically, certain interleukins and HLA-DQB1 have been identified as specific risk factors for the development of asthma. Some variations in genes for beta-2 adrenergic receptors have also been linked to treatment responsiveness in patients diagnosed with asthma.

The relationship between obesity and asthma should not be overlooked. The relationship is thought to be due to the inflammatory state associated with obesity, the effects of excess weight on lung function, and increased prevalence of other comorbidities.

Additional risk factors are considered environmental factors. These consist of allergens (e.g., dust mites and mold), occupational exposures (e.g., wood dusts and painting or cleaning chemicals), and infections (e.g., respiratory syncytial virus [RSV]). Approximately 40% of children admitted to a hospital for an RSV infection developed asthma later in life. Poverty, stress (specifically lower cortisol levels), and tobacco smoke are also risk factors for asthma.[15]

Age is also a risk factor for COPD. As individuals age, the risk for COPD increases due to a decrease in FEV1. Like asthma, environmental factors, such as occupational exposures and poverty, are additional risk factors for COPD.[16]

DIAGNOSIS OF ASTHMA AND CHRONIC OBSTRUCTIVE PULMONARY DISEASE

Wheezing, shortness of breath, cough, and/or chest tightness are possible symptoms of asthma; however, it is not uncommon for patients to lack symptoms. If a patient does have symptoms of asthma, they are more likely to be worse at nighttime or in the morning, vary in intensity over time, and may be triggered by other factors such as respiratory infections or environmental changes. Wheezing is the most common symptom associated with asthma in children aged 5 years and younger. Environmental changes include allergen exposures or changes in weather. If any of the previous symptoms present alone, it is not likely due to asthma.[15]

The most characteristic symptom of COPD is progressive dyspnea. Cough and sputum production are two other symptoms of COPD. Often a chronic cough is the first symptom of COPD; however, this is often overlooked as a cough can be a presenting symptom for many conditions. Like symptoms of asthma, all symptoms of COPD may vary in intensity over time.[17]

Signs and symptoms of asthma and/or COPD may be confused with a variety of differential diagnoses, including one another. Onset of symptoms, including timing and frequency, chest x-ray findings, and findings on pulmonary function tests, help to elucidate differences between confounding diagnoses listed in the text that follows as differential diagnoses.

Differential Diagnoses

Differential diagnoses for asthma and/or COPD include asthma and/or COPD as they have similar symptoms; however, a characteristic difference is time of presentation. Patients with COPD usually have an onset of the disease during the mid-life period, whereas patients with asthma are usually diagnosed early in life, during childhood.

Other differential diagnoses are upper respiratory infections, congestive heart failure, bronchiectasis, and tuberculosis. Upper respiratory illnesses can happen at any age and usually yield consistent symptoms for a short period of time, whereas symptoms of asthma and/or COPD wax and wane over extended periods of time. Additionally, COPD is more prevalent in older age groups.[18] Patients with congestive heart failure also have shortness of breath due to cardiac abnormalities, such as cardiomegaly or valvular dysfunction. Furthermore, congestive heart failure is a condition typically seen most frequently in older age groups. Pulmonary function tests demonstrate volume restriction, not airflow limitation. Bronchiectasis is similar in presentation due to significant amounts of purulent sputum; however, this sputum is often associated with bacterial infection. Lastly, tuberculosis is possible at all ages, and not uncommonly hemoptysis can be found in patients with tuberculosis.[16]

Diagnostic Tests

Diagnostic tests for the diagnosis of asthma and/or COPD include physical examination and spirometry. Although physical examination is a standard part of assessment for a patient presenting with asthma and/or COPD, the physical examination has low sensitivity and specificity. Signs and symptoms are rarely discovered on physical examination and other tests, such as diagnostic spirometry, are used for diagnostic confirmation.[16]

Standard diagnostic spirometry, used to measure airflow obstruction, has a sensitivity of 0.89 and a specificity of 0.98.[19] Handheld spirometry devices usually have a lower sensitivity and/or specificity, but it appears their results are still sufficient for measurement of airflow obstruction.[20]

Diagnostic spirometry is useful as it is a "reproducible and objective measurement of airflow limitation."[16] Results from diagnostic spirometry are necessary as it is a component of the diagnostic algorithms for both asthma and COPD.[15,16]

Currently, there are no standardized screening recommendations for asthma and/or COPD. Screening spirometry is not recommended by the United States Preventive Services Task Force (USPSTF).

TREATMENT OF ASTHMA AND CHRONIC OBSTRUCTIVE PULMONARY DISEASE

The overall goal of asthma treatment includes achieving control of symptoms while minimizing exacerbations. Control and minimal exacerbations can help the patient to maintain normal activities of daily living. Treatment goals consist of both nonpharmacologic and pharmacologic strategies.[15]

Likewise, the overall goal of COPD treatment includes a reduction of symptoms and risks associated with exacerbations. This strategy also helps patients to restore desired levels of activities of daily living. Treatment goals for COPD also consist of both nonpharmacologic and pharmacologic strategies.[16]

Nonpharmacologic and Pharmacologic Therapy

Nonpharmacologic therapy for COPD begins with smoking cessation. Smoking cessation is imperative for the long-term treatment of COPD. Smoking cessation can be achieved through behavioral changes or pharmacologic interventions, including nicotine replacement therapy. In addition to smoking cessation, vaccinations for secondary prevention are essential. Vaccinations include, but are not limited to, influenza and pneumococcus.[16]

Nonpharmacologic therapy for asthma may begin with allergen immunotherapy, either through subcutaneous immunotherapy or sublingual immunotherapy, if allergies are a contributing factor to their asthma. Similar to COPD, vaccinations are an essential component of the management plan for asthma. Vaccinations for influenza and pneumococcus are recommended for this population. Lifestyle modifications including smoking cessation, participation in physical activity, and avoidance of occupational exposures are other comanagement strategies for patients with asthma. If obesity is a contributing factor to asthma, weight reduction strategies are also encouraged.[15]

Pharmacologic therapy for asthma and COPD focuses on bronchodilation and reductions in inflammation. This can be achieved through the use of a variety of pharmacologic agents, in line with current treatment guidelines. Pharmacologic agents for the treatment of asthma are divided into two categories: controller medications and rescue medications. Controller medications include inhaled corticosteroids (ICS), ICS/long-acting beta agonist (LABA) combination medications, leukotriene modifiers, nedocromil sodium, systemic corticosteroids, anti-immunoglobulin E, and anti-interleukin-5. Rescue medications include short-acting inhaled beta-2-agonists (SABA) and short-acting anticholinergics. Other medications include theophylline.[15]

Various classes of medications are also used to treat COPD. These include bronchodilators, such as beta-2 agonists and anti-inflammatory medications such as antimuscarinic drugs; methylxanthines, such as theophylline; ICS; oral glucocorticoids; phosphodiesterase-4 inhibitors; and mucolytic agents. Prescribed combinations of medications are used based on current treatment guidelines.[16]

Treatment Guidelines

The Global Initiative for Chronic Obstructive Lung Disease (GOLD)[16] and the Global Initiative for Asthma[15] provide standardized guidelines for the diagnosis, management, and prevention of COPD and asthma.

Initial pharmacologic treatment of asthma is based on a stepwise approach to treatment which begins with an assessment of symptoms and a review of the response to treatment. Asthma control medication is adjusted for symptom control and can be stepped down if asthma control can be maintained for 2 to 3 months. Asthma treatment begins with the prescription of a rescue medication, such as a beta-2 agonist or bronchodilator.[15]

Initial controller treatment for adults and adolescents begins when a patient has infrequent asthma symptoms but they have at least one risk factor for exacerbation, including but not limited to frequent SABA use, low FEV1 (less than 60% of predicted), environmental exposures such as smoking and allergens or comorbidities such as obesity, or have asthma symptoms or the need for a SABA between two times a month and two times a week (or if the patient wakes during the night due to asthma at least once a month). In these instances, low-dose ICS should be added as the initial controller treatment. In addition, if a patient has asthma symptoms or the need to use a SABA more than twice a week, a low-dose ICS should also be used.[15]

If a patient has asthma symptoms most days of the week or wakes due to asthma more than once a week, a medium- or high-dose ICS or low-dose ICS/LABA combination should be used. Other options for controller treatment include leukotriene receptor antagonists, theophylline, or tiotropium.[15]

Initial pharmacologic treatment of COPD is based on individualized assessments of symptoms in combination with exacerbation risks. The decision for initial pharmacologic treatment is based on an ABCD assessment algorithm (**Figure 18.1**).[16]

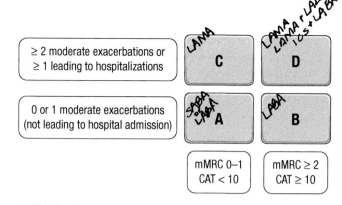

FIGURE 18.1 ABCD assessment algorithm, guiding the initial pharmacologic treatment of chronic obstructive pulmonary disease.

Source: Global Initiative for Chronic Obstructive Lung Disease. *Global Strategy for the Diagnosis, Management and Prevention of Chronic Obstructive Pulmonary Disease (2020 Report).* Global Initiative for Chronic Obstructive Lung Disease; 2020. https://goldcopd.org/wp-content/uploads/2019/12/GOLD-2020-FINAL-ver1.2-03Dec19_WMV.pdf

The algorithm utilizes information obtained from patients to determine pharmacologic treatment. Exacerbation history combined with mMRC or CAT scores point prescribers in the direction of appropriate pharmacologic treatment. The modified Medical Research Council (mMRC) dyspnea scale is a one question tool which asks the patient to match their shortness of breath with a grade (or description). The COPD Assessment Test (CAT) is an eight-question assessment about signs and symptoms of COPD. Scores from either one of these tools are used to determine the appropriate level of treatment for patients with COPD.[16]

Patients in category "A" should be treated with either short- or long-acting bronchodilator therapy. Patients in category "B" should begin with long-acting bronchodilators (LABA). If assigned to category "C," a long-acting muscarinic agent (LAMA) should be considered. Lastly, patients in category "D" should be started on a LAMA, LAMA + LABA, or an ICS plus a LABA.[16]

Although the algorithm is used for initial pharmacologic treatment, follow up pharmacological management should also be based on a review of symptoms. If a patient under pharmacologic treatment presents with complaints of dyspnea, the use of two bronchodilators is recommended. If a patient presents with dyspnea, while taking a LABA/ICS combination treatment, a LAMA can be added for better control of breathlessness.[16]

In a review of symptoms, if a patient presents with persistent COPD exacerbations, who is already taking a LABA, consider the addition of LAMA or ICS. If a patient still experiences exacerbations and has severe or very severe COPD, roflumilast should be considered as an option.[16]

The mechanisms of action of classes of drugs used to treat asthma and/or COPD will be reviewed in the text that follows.

Beta-2 Agonists

Bronchodilators, such as SABAs or LABAs, are used to increase FEV1 and improve airflow through the airways. SABAs, but not LABA, are the treatment choice in the setting of bronchospasm. Examples of SABAs include levalbuterol and albuterol. LABAs include formoterol, salmeterol, and vilanterol. Beta-2 agonists work through activation of the beta-2 adrenergic receptors, which leads to relaxation of smooth muscle in the lungs with resultant dilation of the airways. This relaxation of the smooth muscles of the bronchioles leads to improved airflow and a reduction in limitation of airflow, a concern in both asthma and COPD.[15]

Anticholinergics (and Anti-Muscarinic Agents)

Anticholinergics such as tiotropium (long-acting muscarinic agent [LAMA]) and ipratropium (short-acting muscarinic agent [SAMA]) work through binding to muscarinic receptors, preventing the increase in intracellular calcium in bronchial smooth muscle and blocking the action of acetylcholine. Similar to beta-2 agonists, anticholinergic (or anti-muscarinic) agents also work on bronchoconstriction through relaxation of the bronchial smooth muscle, although through a different mechanism as previously described. This class of medication also works to improve morbidity and mortality of patients with asthma and/or COPD through improved airflow.[15]

Inhaled Corticosteroids

ICS provide effective anti-inflammatory effects for both asthma and COPD. Administration technique is essential to the effective delivery of the OCS to the site of action. A reduction in inflammation is imperative for long-term improvement in morbidity and/or mortality associated with these disease states.[15]

Leukotriene Receptor Antagonist

Leukotriene receptor antagonists (LTRAs), such as montelukast, block the binding of leukotriene to its receptor and therefore prevent the associated inflammatory process. Similar to the anti-inflammatory effects of ICS, LTRAs work to improve inflammation associated with asthma.[15]

Roflumilast

Roflumilast, a phosphodieasterase-4 (PDE4) inhibitor, reduces inflammation through inhibition of the breakdown of intracellular cyclic AMP, which subsequently induces smooth muscles to relax and bronchial dilation.[16]

Theophylline

Theophylline, a methylxanthine, has demonstrated moderate bronchodilator effects in patients with COPD when theophylline serum levels are between 8 and 12 mcg/mL.[21,22] It has also demonstrated weak bronchodilator activity but modest anti-inflammatory properties in patients with asthma when theophylline peak concentrations are between 10 and 20 mg/L.[22,23]

Dosing, Side Effects, and Contraindications

Beta-2 Agonists

Dosing for albuterol begins with one to two inhalations of 90 mcg every 4 to 6 hours as needed for bronchospasm and/or shortness of breath. Possible side effects of albuterol include throat irritation, cough, and tachycardia. Albuterol is contraindicated in patients with a history of hypersensitivity to albuterol.[24]

Levalbuterol dosing begins with one to two inhalations of 45 mcg of levalbuterol every 4 to 6 hours as needed for bronchospasm. Possible side effects include dizziness, bronchitis, pharyngitis, rhinitis, and vomiting. Contraindications to the use of levalbuterol include hypersensitivity to levalbuterol.[25]

Formoterol dosing begins with inhalations of 20 mcg of formoterol every 12 hours as prescribed for maintenance treatment of COPD. Possible side effects include diarrhea, nausea, nasopharyngitis, dry mouth, and insomnia. Contraindications to the use of formoterol include use in patients with asthma, without the use of long-term asthma control medication.[26]

Salmeterol dosing begins with inhalations of 50 mcg of salmeterol every 12 hours in addition to concomitant treatment with an ICS. Possible side effects include headache. Contraindications to the use of salmeterol include severe hypersensitivity to milk protein.[27]

Anticholinergics (and Anti-Muscarinic Agents)

Tiotropium, a long-acting anticholinergic medication, should be taken as two inhalations of 18 mcg once daily. The most common side effects are upper respiratory infections, dry mouth, sinusitis, pharyngitis, nonspecific chest pain, and rhinitis. Contraindications to the use of tiotropium include hypersensitivity to ipratropium or tiotropium.[28]

Ipratropium, a short-acting anticholinergic medication, should be taken as two inhalations of 17 mcg, four times a day, not to exceed 12 inhalations in 24 hours. The most common side effects were bronchitis, COPD exacerbation, dyspnea, and headache. Contraindications to the use to ipratropium include hypersensitivity to the agent itself or concurrent use with atropine.[29]

Inhaled Corticosteroids

The dosing of ICS varies depending on the severity of the disease and each individual potency of the steroid. For example, beclomethasone dipropionate (HFA) dosing ranges of 100 mcg to 200 mcg are considered as low daily doses. Meanwhile, dosing at 400 mcg or greater are high daily dose. Budesonide (DPI) at 200 mcg to 400 mcg are low doses and 800 mcg or greater are high daily doses. ICS, when combined with a LABA, are more effective than each individual agent alone in improving lung function and preventing exacerbation. Unfortunately, regular use of ICS may increase risk of pneumonia, especially in patients with severe disease. Triple therapy of ICS together with a LAMA and a LABA may be necessary for a certain subset of patients to improve lung functions and exacerbations when compared to dual- or mono-therapy.[15]

Local adverse effects from ICS are oropharyngeal candidiasis and dysphonia.[15]

Leukotriene Receptor Antagonist

Montelukast dosing should be considered as "add-on" therapy and may reduce the dose of ICS in patients with moderate to severe asthma. Montelukast should be prescribed at 10 mg by mouth once daily, in the evening. The most common side effect of montelukast is headache.[30]

Other

Roflumilast dosing is one 500 mcg tablet per day, with or without food. Common side effects include diarrhea, weight decrease, nausea, headache, back pain, influenza, insomnia, dizziness, and decreased appetite. Contraindications to the use of roflumilast include moderate to severe liver impairment (either Child-Pugh class B or C).[31]

Theophylline dosing varies among patients depending on theophylline concentrations in serum. Possible side effects of theophylline include nausea, vomiting, headache, and insomnia. If theophylline concentrations are above 20 mcg/mL, persistent vomiting, cardiac arrhythmias, and intractable seizures are possible. Contraindications to the use of theophylline include history of hypersensitivity to theophylline.[32]

See **Table 18.1** for a summary of drugs discussed in the previous text.

COUGH AND VIRAL UPPER RESPIRATORY ILLNESS

INTRODUCTION

The etiology of most upper respiratory illnesses (URIs) are viral in origin. Over 200 viruses have been identified as causes of viral upper respiratory illnesses. Examples of these viruses include rhinoviruses, coronaviruses, adenoviruses, and coxsackieviruses. Although it is possible for URIs to occur at any time, most URIs occur in fall and winter in the United States. Despite the seasonal variations in prevalence of URIs, there are no racial differences in URIs.[33] Compared to other viruses that cause infections, rhinoviruses are the most common causative organism of viral URIs.[34]

Upper respiratory illnesses are one of the most common diagnoses for office visits in the outpatient setting. They are also one of the leading causes of missed days of work and/or school.[35]

There are differences in URIs based on sex. For example, nasopharyngitis, a type of URI, frequently occurs in women, ages 20 to 30 years of age.[33] This is believed to be due to exposure to young children who may also have URIs. Children are estimated to have about six to 10 colds per year.

BACKGROUND

In the United States, viral upper respiratory illnesses most often begin in August/September and increase throughout fall and winter and dwindle down in March and April. Over time, a variety of viruses have been identified as significant contributors to URIs. Rhinoviruses cause 30% to 35% of all adult upper respiratory illnesses, and approximately 10% to 15% of all adult colds are caused by other viruses such as adenoviruses, coxsackieviruses, and respiratory syncytial virus (RSV). This leaves about 35% to 50% of adult colds caused by other unidentified viruses.[33]

PHYSIOLOGY AND PATHOPHYSIOLOGY

The upper respiratory tract is made up of several body parts including, but not limited to, the external nose, vestibule, and nasal turbinates. The external nose serves as the entry point for air, or pathogens, to enter the upper portion of the respiratory tract. The vestibule contains stratified squamous epithelium and pseudostratified columnar epithelium, which secretes serous mucus and houses thick hairs, helping to keep large particles out of the respiratory system. The lower turbinate helps to protect the entry of any foreign particles into the lower respiratory system and therefore contribute to the maintenance of homeostasis.[36]

Viral URIs are usually self-limiting and typically present with symptoms such as a nasal congestion, runny nose, fever, cough, pharyngitis, and sneezing. Exposure to the respiratory viruses is the most common mechanism of transmission.[37]

Respiratory viruses are commonly spread through three mechanisms: hand contact, small particle droplets (from sneezing or coughing), or large particle droplet (from close contact).[34]

TABLE 18.1 Pharmacotherapy for the Treatment of Asthma and Chronic Obstructive Pulmonary Disease

Medication	Dose and Frequency	Side Effects
Short-Acting Beta-2 Agonists		
Albuterol	<4 years: Safety and efficacy not established for metered-dose inhaler >4 years: 122 inhalations of 90 mcg q4–6h prn	Throat irritation, cough, tachycardia
Levalbuterol	<4 years: Safety and efficacy not established for metered-dose inhaler >4 years: 1–2 inhalations of 45 mcg q4–6h as needed	Dizziness, bronchitis, pharyngitis, rhinitis, vomiting
Long-Acting Beta-2 Agonists		
Formoterol	Pediatrics: Safety and efficacy not established Adults: Inhalation of 20 mcg q12h	Diarrhea, nausea, nasopharyngitis, dry mouth, insomnia
Salmeterol	<4 years: Safety and efficacy not established for metered-dose inhaler >4 years: Inhalation of 50 mcg of salmeterol q12h	Headache
Anticholinergics		
Tiotropium	≥6 years: 2 Inhalations of 18 mcg once daily	Upper respiratory infections, dry mouth, sinusitis, pharyngitis, nonspecific chest pain, rhinitis
Ipratropium	Adults: 2 Inhalations of 17 mcg qid; not to exceed 12 inhalations in 24h	Bronchitis, COPD exacerbation, dyspnea, headache
Inhaled Corticosteroids		
Beclomethasone dipropionate (40 mcg/puff or 80 mcg/puff)	<4 years: Safety and efficacy not established 4–11 years: 40 mcg inhaled bid 12–17 years: 40–80 mcg inhaled bid Adult: 1–4 puffs inhaled orally q12hrs; max = 640 mcg/day 100–200 mcg/day, low dose; >400 mcg/day, high dose	Oropharyngeal candidiasis, dysphonia
Budesonide (90 mcg/puff or 180 mcg/puff)	Adult: 2 puffs inhaled po bid; max = 1,440 mcg/day; 200–400 mcg/day, low dose; >800 mcg/day, high dose	Oropharyngeal candidiasis, dysphonia
Fluticasone propionate (44 mcg/puff, 110 mcg/puff, or 220 mcg/puff)	<4 years: Safety and efficacy not established 4–12 years: 88 mcg bid Adults: 2–4 puffs inhaled bid; max = 1,760 mcg/day; 100–250 mcg/day, low dose; >500 mcg/day, high dose	Oropharyngeal candidiasis, dysphonia
Mometasone furoate (HFA: 50 mcg/puff, 100 mcg/puff, or 200 mcg/puff; Twisthaler DPI [dry powder inhaler]: 110 mcg/puff or 220 mcg/puff)	Adult: 1–2 puffs inhaled po once daily–bid; max = 800 mcg/day; 110–220 mcg/day, low dose; >440 mcg/day, high dose	Oropharyngeal candidiasis, dysphonia
Leukotriene Receptor Antagonists		
Montelukast	<12 months: Safety and efficacy not established 1–6 years: 4 mg po once daily 6–15 years: 5 mg po once daily >15 years: 10 mg po once daily	Headache
Other		
Roflumilast	Adult: 500-mcg tablet once daily, with or without food	Diarrhea, weight decrease, nausea, headache, back pain, influenza, insomnia, dizziness, decreased appetite
Theophylline*	Adult: 300–600 mg/day po once daily–bid	Nausea, vomiting, headache, insomnia; if theophylline concentrations >20 mcg/mL, persistent vomiting, cardiac arrhythmias, and intractable seizures possible

bid, twice daily; COPD, chronic obstructive pulmonary disease; h, hour; HFA, hydrofluoroalkane; po, by mouth; q, every; qid, four times daily.
*Pediatrics and adults: Dosing varies based on serum theophylline concentrations.

RISK FACTORS

Risk factors for viral URIs include children in day care, psychological stress, lack of adequate sleep, underlying chronic diseases, malnutrition, congenital immunodeficiency disorders, and cigarette smoking.[34]

Specific Risks and Disease Processes

Underlying chronic diseases may impair a high functioning immune system and therefore is strongly associated with acquisition of a viral URI. Additionally, malnutrition, cigarette smoking, and congenital immunodeficiency disorders present with similar risks and therefore association with viral URIs.[34]

Day care attendance is another risk factor for viral URI as children may have frequent viral URIs in a 1-year period and therefore attendance increases the potential exposure of children to the viral pathogen itself.[34]

The risk factors discussed previously can be managed through primary prevention strategies such as adequate rest, vaccination, and hand washing. Vaccinations, such as influenza vaccination, also provide a nonpharmacologic approach to reduce risk for the acquisition of viral URIs. Hand washing has demonstrated to be an effective strategy to prevent the spread of viral URIs.[38]

DIAGNOSIS

Symptoms of a viral upper respiratory illness, such as the common cold, start 48 to 72 hours after exposure to the virus. These symptoms include mucus, nasal congestion, sneezing, pharyngitis, cough, and headache. Fever is not very common in adults; however, it can be as high as 102 °F in children. Most symptoms last 2 to 14 days;[33] however, the cough may last for more than 3 weeks.[39]

Symptoms of a viral URI may be confused with other illnesses. For example, cough can be a symptom of a respiratory process, either upper or lower, of the gastrointestinal tract, or even caused by medication. There are a variety of respiratory differential diagnoses (to be discussed in the text that follows). Gastroesophageal reflux disease (GERD) may also present with cough, whereas a potential adverse effect of ACE inhibitors is also cough. It is important to assess for these other disease processes which may be the cause of a chief complaint of cough.

Differential Diagnoses

Differential diagnoses for viral URIs include otitis media, pneumonia, bronchitis, epiglottitis, whooping cough, croup, COVID-19, and bronchiolitis. Patients with otitis media typically present with an ear-related complaint. Signs and symptoms of pneumonia include symptoms of a viral URI; however, it may also include pleuritic chest pain or other lung-related signs, such as rhonchi. Patients presenting with epiglottitis usually have a swollen, erythematous epiglottis with resultant drooling and possible stridor. Whooping cough is a vaccine-preventable illness; thus, an assessment should revolve around possible exposure to the pathogen. Barking or a "seal cough" along with inspiratory stridor are concerning for croup. Influenza is another differential diagnosis that usually presents with high fever and symptoms such as myalgia which happen very suddenly. Lastly, bronchiolitis also involves inflammation of the bronchioles, which may present as wheezing in patients.[39]

Diagnostic Tests and Their Sensitivity and Specificity

Viral URIs are a clinical diagnosis and do not require confirmatory testing; however, there is a growing body of research regarding the use of procalcitonin and c-reactive protein levels, which are used to identify bacterial infections. The use of the biomarkers may be helpful in reducing inappropriate antibiotic prescriptions.[40]

No diagnostic tests are indicated for the diagnosis of URIs, including radiologic studies or viral/bacterial cultures from nasal swabs or washings.[34]

Routine screening for URIs is not indicated according to the USPSTF.

TREATMENT

General treatment strategies for URIs include fever reduction, if present, and symptom improvement through providing comfort measures.[39] Most treatment strategies revolve around nonpharmacologic therapies such as nasal suction for infants and children, steam inhalation, nasal irrigation, and rest. Over-the-counter (OTC) medications can also be used for symptomatic treatment, including fever reduction and cough suppression.

Nonpharmacologic and Pharmacologic Therapy

Nonpharmacologic therapy includes nasal suction, steam inhalation, nasal irrigation, honey, vapor rubs, and rest. Nasal suction is generally recommended for infants and children to provide relief of nasal congestion. Steam inhalation has been recommended for years by healthcare providers, although systematic reviews raise doubt regarding the clear clinical benefit of this treatment strategy.[39,41] Benefits and risks of this method of nonpharmacologic therapy should be discussed and considered with patients.

Nasal irrigation helps to loosen nasal mucus and clear the nasal passageway. Saline should be the solution of choice as the FDA warns against the use of tap water due to concern regarding infection risks.[39]

Honey has shown to reduce symptoms of the common cold,[42] though honey should not be used in children under the age of 1 due to risk of botulism.[39]

Vapor rubs also help to improve symptomatic congestion in patients with viral URIs.[43]

Lastly, rest is an important nonpharmacologic therapeutic recommendation for patients with viral URIs.[39]

Pharmacologic therapy revolves around symptomatic improvement, from nasal congestion relief to fever reduction and cough suppression. A variety of medications can be used, as described in current guidelines that follow.

Treatment Guidelines

Treatment strategy recommendations are divided based on severity of symptoms. Patients with mild symptoms generally do not require symptomatic treatment; however, patients with moderate to severe symptoms may benefit from the following therapeutic classes: analgesics, antihistamine/decongestant combinations, intranasal cromolyn, and intranasal ipratropium. Other considerations for treatment include dextromethorphan, decongestants, and expectorants[44]; however, these medications have demonstrated minimal or uncertain benefit for the use of viral upper respiratory illnesses.

Analgesics, such as acetaminophen and nonsteroidal anti-inflammatory drugs (NSAIDs), have been demonstrated to be equally efficacious and generally well-tolerated.[45]

Antihistamine/decongestant combinations may provide better symptomatic relief when prescribed together, but may produce more adverse effects, such as drowsiness or dry mouth.[44]

Intranasal cromolyn has demonstrated quicker resolution of symptoms, such as rhinorrhea, throat pain, and cough, compared to placebo.[44]

Intranasal ipratropium can also improve rhinorrhea and sneezing associated with viral upper respiratory illnesses.[44]

If cough is a presenting complaint, several agents are available for use, such as dextromethorphan, codeine, and benzonatate. These agents are nonspecific pharmacologic options used for cough suppression. Dextromethorphan, a commonly used OTC medication, has unreliably reduced cough severity. Codeine, an opioid cough suppressant, is another option; however, there is concern regarding its addictive potential and possible side effects. Lastly, benzonatate is approved for the specific indication of cough and works specifically on anesthetizing respiratory passages to suppress cough.[44,46]

Although the exact mechanism of antipyretic properties of acetaminophen is not well defined, acetaminophen is commonly used for fever reduction.[47] NSAID mechanism of action begins with inhibition of cyclooxygenase, which in turn impairs the synthesis of prostaglandin, a compound that has a role in inflammation.[48] Acetaminophen and NSAIDs are often used to improve inflammation and fever associated with viral upper respiratory illnesses.

Antihistamines work through blocking the action of histamine. Histamine can cause dilation of capillaries, with fluid leakage. Antihistamine use can improve symptoms associated with the fluid leakage, such as runny nose.[49] Decongestants are often co-administered with antihistamines for the improvement of symptoms associated with viral upper respiratory illnesses. Decongestants serve as alpha-adrenergic agonists of receptors present in respiratory mucosa. This causes vasoconstriction and therefore blockage of fluid leakage, such as in the case of a runny nose.[50]

Cromolyn's mechanism of action includes the inhibition of inflammatory mediator's release, such as mast cell degranulation.[51] Ipratropium works through antagonizing the action of acetylcholine, thus leading to anticholinergic effects.[29]

Dextromethorphan desensitizes the cough receptors and depresses the medullary cough center in the brain.[52] Codeine works in a similar mechanism to dextromethorphan; however, it belongs to the opioid analgesic class of medication.[53]

Medications such as guaifenesin are also used to thin bronchial secretions and loosen mucus for expectoration.[54]

Lastly, benzonatate anesthetizes the respiratory tract stretch receptors, therefore reducing the cough reflex. This contrasts with dextromethorphan and codeine, which work on the central medullary center.[55]

Dosing, Side Effects, and Contraindications

Acetaminophen is administered 325 to 650 mg by mouth every 4 hours, as needed. Potential side effects include angioedema, dizziness, rash, urticaria, and hepatotoxicity. Contraindications to the use of acetaminophen include, but are not limited to, hypersensitivity to it or related medications and severe active liver disease.[47]

NSAIDs include, but are not limited to, ibuprofen and naproxen. Ibuprofen is dosed 200 to 400 mg every 4 to 6 hours, as needed. Higher doses of ibuprofen can be considered, up to 3,200 mg per day, although the smallest effective dose should be taken to relieve symptoms associated with upper respiratory illnesses. Side effects include dizziness, epigastric pain, heartburn, constipation, nausea, rash, and tinnitus.[56] Naproxen is dosed 225 mg every 12 hours by mouth, as needed. If prescribed, naproxen is dosed 500 mg (or 550 mg naproxen sodium) by mouth every 12 hours, as needed. Side effects of naproxen include abdominal pain, constipation, dizziness, drowsiness, headache, heartburn, nausea, and edema.

Black-Box Warnings for NSAIDs include a potential for an increase in the risk of serious cardiovascular thrombotic events, myocardial infarction, and stroke and gastrointestinal events such as gastrointestinal bleeding, ulceration, and perforation. NSAIDs are contraindicated for perioperative pain after coronary artery bypass graft (CABG) surgery.[56,57]

Antihistamines may include, but are not limited to, loratadine, cetirizine, diphenhydramine, hydroxyzine, and fexofenadine. Loratadine is administered 10 mg by mouth once daily. Potential side effects include headache, somnolence, drowsiness, nervousness, fatigue, and dry mouth. Loratadine is contraindicated in those patients who have documented hypersensitivity to it or related compounds.[58] Cetirizine is dosed 5 to 10 mg by mouth once daily. Potential side effects include somnolence, headache, fatigue, dry mouth, and dizziness. Cetirizine is contraindicated in those patients who have documented hypersensitivity to it or hydroxyzine.[59] Diphenhydramine's dose is 25 to 50 mg by mouth every 4 hours, as needed. Side effects include, but are not limited to, sedation, sleepiness, dizziness, epigastric distress, and thickening of bronchial secretions. Contraindications include documented hypersensitivity or use in nursing mothers, premature infants, or neonates.[60] Lastly, fexofenadine is dosed 180 mg by mouth daily. Side effects include headache, vomiting, cough, and diarrhea. Contraindications to the use of fexofenadine include, but are not limited to, hypersensitivity to it or related medications.[61]

Decongestants consist of pseudoephedrine, phenylephrine, and oxymetazoline. Pseudoephedrine is prepared as immediate and extended release formulations. The immediate release formulation is dosed 60 mg by mouth every 4 to 6 hours as needed. The extended release formulation is dosed 120 mg by mouth every 12 hours or 240 mg by mouth every 24 hours. Potential side effects of pseudoephedrine include tremor, restlessness, insomnia, nausea, vomiting, nervousness, and hypertension. Contraindications to the use to pseudoephedrine include hypersensitivity, severe hypertension, severe coronary artery disease, and administration within 14 days of MAO inhibitor therapy.[62] Phenylephrine 0.25% nasal spray is administered two to three sprays every 4 hours, as needed, but not to exceed 3 days. Potential side effects include stinging, dryness, rebound congestion, sneezing, and burning. Contraindications include cardiac disease, including hypertension and palpitations, and the use of nonselective MAO inhibitor.[63] Lastly, oxymetazoline is an intranasal spray administered twice daily for 3 days. Dosing should not extend past this dosing window to avoid rebound congestion.[64]

Cromolyn intranasal spray (5.2 mg/spray) is administered one spray each nostril every 6 to 8 hours. Potential side effects include headache, unpleasant taste, hoarseness, cough, and epistaxis. Contraindication to use include documented hypersensitivity to cromolyn.[51]

Ipratropium 0.06% nasal spray is administered two sprays (0.42 mcg/spray) per nostril every 6 hours. Adverse effects may include headache, upper respiratory illness, epistaxis, pharyngitis, nasal dryness, taste disturbance, nausea, and xerostomia. Contraindications include documented hypersensitivity to it.[29]

Dextromethorphan syrup is dosed 30 mg by mouth every 6 to 8 hours, as needed, in adults and children over the age of 12. Children ages 6 to 12 years should be administered 5 to 10 mg every 4 hours or 15 mg every 6 to 8 hours, as needed. Children ages 4 and 6 years of age should be given 2.5 to 5 mg every 4 hours or 7.5 mg every 6 to 8 hours, as needed. Dextromethorphan should not be administered to children under the age of 4. Potential side effects include nausea, vomiting, constipation, drowsiness, dizziness, sedation, confusion, and nervousness.[65]

Codeine can be given off-label for cough, dosed at 7.5 to 30 mg by mouth every 4 to 6 hours, as needed, for adults. Potential side effects include constipation and drowsiness. Contraindications to use include respiratory depression, children younger than 12 years, and hypersensitivity to codeine.[53]

Common dosing of benzonatate for adults is 100 to 200 mg by mouth every 8 hours, not to exceed 600 mg daily. Potential side effects include sedation, headache, nausea, pruritus, and dizziness. Benzonatate is contraindicated in those patients who have documented hypersensitivity to it or related compounds.[55]

Table 18.2 summarizes the drugs discussed in the previous text.

OXYGEN DISORDERS

INTRODUCTION

Oxygen disorders are more prevalent in patients with COPD disease, morbid obesity, cystic fibrosis, chest wall deformities, and bronchiectasis.[66]

More than 3 million people die each year from COPD and 235 million people suffer from asthma.[67] Specific statistics on oxygenation disorders are lacking.

Patients with the following disease states may require supplemental oxygen at some point in their lives: COPD, pulmonary fibrosis, pneumonia, severe asthma attack, cystic fibrosis, and sleep apnea.[68]

BACKGROUND

Disturbances in oxygen use or supply can lead to a variety of diseases processes, from disorders of the respiratory tract to alterations in red blood cells.

PHYSIOLOGY AND PATHOPHYSIOLOGY

The normal physiologic process of oxygenation consists of a balance between oxygen consumption and oxygen delivery and extraction. Oxygen is taken in through the respiratory tract and moves from the alveoli to the capillary beds and eventually into the blood. Once in the blood, oxygen mostly binds itself

TABLE 18.2 Pharmacotherapy for the Treatment of Upper Respiratory Tract Infections

Medication	Dose and Frequency	Side Effects
Acetaminophen	325–650 mg po qid prn	Angioedema, dizziness, rash, urticaria, hepatotoxicity
NSAIDs		
Ibuprofen	200–400 mg po qid prn	Dizziness, epigastric pain, heartburn, constipation, nausea, rash, tinnitus
Naproxen	OTC: 220 mg po q12h prn Rx: 500 mg (or 550 mg naproxen sodium) po q12h prn	Abdominal pain constipation, dizziness, drowsiness, headache, heartburn, nausea, edema
Antihistamines		
Loratadine	10 mg po daily	Headache, somnolence, drowsiness, nervousness, fatigue, dry mouth
Cetirizine	5–10 mg po once daily	Somnolence, headache, fatigue, dry mouth, dizziness
Diphenhydramine	25–50 mg po q4h prn	Sedation, sleepiness, dizziness, epigastric distress, thickening of bronchial secretions
Fexofenadine	180 mg po daily	Vomiting, headache, cough, diarrhea
Decongestants		
Pseudoephedrine	Immediate-release: 60 mg po q4–6h prn Extended-release: 120 mg po q12h or 240 mg po q24h prn	Tremor, restlessness, insomnia, nausea, vomiting, nervousness, hypertension
Phenylephrine	0.25% nasal spray administered 2–3 sprays q4h prn; not to exceed 3 days	Stinging, dryness, rebound congestion, sneezing, burning
Miscellaneous		
Cromolyn sodium	Intranasal spray (5.2 mg/spray) is administered one spray each nostril q6–8h	Headache, unpleasant taste, hoarseness, cough, epistaxis
Ipratropium	0.06% nasal spray administered two sprays (0.42 mcg/spray) per nostril q6h	Headache, upper respiratory illness, epistaxis, pharyngitis, nasal dryness, taste disturbance, nausea, xerostomia
Dextromethorphan (immediate release)	<4 years: Do not administer 4–6 years: 2.5–5 mg q4h or 7.5 mg q6–8h prn 6–12 years: 5–10 mg q4h or 15 mg q6–8h prn >12 years: 30 mg po q6–8h prn	Nausea, vomiting, constipation, drowsiness, dizziness, sedation, confusion, nervousness
Codeine	7.5–30 mg po q4–6h prn	Constipation, drowsiness
Benzonatate	100–200 mg by mouth q8h; not to exceed 600 mg daily	Sedation, headache, nausea, pruritus, dizziness

bid, twice daily; h, hour; HFA, hydrofluoroalkane; NSAID, nonsteroidal anti-inflammatory drug; OTC, over the counter; po, by mouth; prn, as needed; q, every; qid, four times daily.

to hemoglobin, where it can be transported to essential tissues that require oxygen. Oxygen delivery and oxygen extraction are inversely related to each other. While resting, oxygen consumption is constant, despite changes in oxygen delivery due to oxygen extraction or the ability of the body to extract oxygen for use. When the demand for oxygen increases, such in cases of exercise or other metabolically demanding activities, oxygen consumption increases in response.[69] It is through this intrinsic process that the body maintains oxygenation homeostasis.

Changes in oxygen delivery or demand can be caused by a variety of disease processes. Exercise is an example of an increased oxygen demand that does not indicate the presence of a disease but, rather, is responsive to an increase in metabolic demands. Disease processes that may increase metabolic demand and therefore the need for oxygen include those which are found in critically ill patients in sepsis or septic shock.[69]

In contrast, disorders of the respiratory tract, heart, or hematologic abnormalities may decrease oxygen delivery. Respiratory tract diseases, such as asthma, COPD, and pneumonia, are examples of diseases that may decrease oxygen delivery. Abnormalities of the heart, such as decreased cardiac output, may be related to cardiac disease or hypovolemia, and can lead to decreased oxygen delivery. Lastly, reduced levels of hemoglobin, such as in the setting of anemia, may also decrease the ability of the body to deliver oxygen.[69]

RISK FACTORS

Risk factors for impaired oxygenation include those discussed in the previous text and those factors that put a patient at risk for each of those individual disease states. Common causes of hypoxemia also include anemia, acute respiratory distress syndrome, asthma, congenital heart defects, interstitial lung disease, medications such as narcotics and anesthetics, pneumothorax, pulmonary edema, pulmonary embolism, pulmonary fibrosis, and sleep apnea.[70]

DIAGNOSIS

Symptoms of hypoxemia include, but are not limited to, headache, shortness of breath, tachycardia, cough, wheezing, confusion, and bluish discoloration of skin, fingernails, and lips;[71] however, in the beginning stages of oxygenation abnormalities, patients may be asymptomatic.

Most of the symptoms associated with hypoxemia may be associated with other disease processes discussed in the text that follows as differential diagnoses.

Differential diagnoses for hypoxemia include a variety of causes of the hypoxemia as hypoxemia itself rarely occurs without a precipitating disease state. Differential diagnoses include hypovolemic shock, sepsis, septic shock, carbon monoxide poisoning, acute asthma attack, pneumonia, pneumothorax, pleural effusions, pulmonary embolism, and anemia.[66]

A chest x-ray can differentiate between pneumonia, pneumothorax, and pleural effusions. Sputum cultures can also be used to confirm a bacterial cause of pneumonia. Computed tomography (CT) scans of the chest can identify pulmonary embolism, in addition to the use of a d-dimer assay.[72] Hypovolemic shock and septic shock are differentiated by presence of an infectious cause. Carbon monoxide poisoning can be ruled in or out by testing for carbon monoxide. Lastly, anemia can be identified through collection and interpretation of a complete blood count (CBC).

Diagnostic Tests and Their Sensitivity and Specificity

Pulse oximetry is one method available to test for oxygenation levels. The sensitivity and specificity of pulse oximetry is 74% to 92% and 84% to 90%, respectively.[73]

Arterial blood gases are another diagnostic test available to test for oxygen levels. Sensitivity and specificity of arterial blood gases depends on the disease state for which the oxygen level is being analyzed; however, in studies in patients with COPD, during exercise, pulse oximetry was significantly lower than arterial oxygen levels by 0.7% on average.[74]

As previously discussed, pulse oximetry and arterial blood gases can be used to identify an alteration in oxygenation; however, in order to determine the cause of the alteration in oxygenation, further assessments should be completed to consider all relevant differential diagnoses.

Screening for alterations in oxygenation are generally not routinely recommended.

TREATMENT

Oxygenation treatment can either be prescribed for acute scenarios in the hospital or for continuous long-term therapy. Effective oxygen delivery is essential for a patient critically ill in the hospital setting. Oxygen can be administered through several methods. The "blow by" method is generally not recommended as it may not reliably deliver oxygen. Nasal cannula provides oxygen through two soft prongs inserted into the patient's nares. Low- and high-flow oxygen can be administered through nasal cannula. Masks, the most common method to administer oxygen, fit over the patient's nose and mouth. Venturi masks are the simplest type of mask and can facilitate administration of 6 to 10 L of oxygen per minute. Partial rebreathing masks are similar to the Venturi mask but also have an attached reservoir that can facilitate administration of oxygen at rates of 10 to 12 L/min. Lastly, nonrebreathing masks facilitate oxygenation rates of 10 to 15 L/min. These nonrebreathing masks create a "seal" to prevent the escape of oxygen.[75]

For purposes of the remainder of this discussion, indications and considerations for continuous long-term therapy will be discussed.

Indications for continuous long-term oxygen therapy for patients with chronic lung disease include an arterial oxygen level of 55 mmHg or less (or a pulse oximetry reading of 88% or less). If the patient has evidence of right-sided heart failure or erythrocytosis (hematocrit greater than 55%), indications for continuous long-term oxygen therapy are an arterial oxygen level of 59 mmHg or less or a pulse oximetry reading of 89% or less.[76]

Dosing, Side Effects, and Contraindications

Considerations for dosing of oxygen begin with a determination of the need for oxygen therapy. Oxygen should only be prescribed when persistent hypoxemia is present. Acute treatment with oxygen can be administered for patients who are clinically unstable; however, in order to receive continuous long-term oxygen therapy, patients should be clinically stable and on an optimized medical management plan.[76] Oxygen should be prescribed with a target oxygen saturation of 94%

to 98% in acutely ill patients, patients in hypercapnic respiratory failure being an exception. Patients with hypercapnic respiratory failure should have a pulse oximetry between 88% and 92%.[66]

Oxygen dosing begins 1 L/min for patients with arterial oxygen levels (on room air) of 50 mmHg. Two L of oxygen per minute are recommended for patients with arterial oxygen levels (on room air) of 45 mmHg. If a patient's arterial oxygen level is 35 or 40 mmHg, oxygen should be prescribed at 4 and 3 L/min, respectively.[76]

When administered at expected concentrations, oxygen has few adverse effects. Facial and upper respiratory tract burns are potential complications of continuous long-term oxygen therapy.[76]

CASE EXEMPLAR: Patient With Chronic Cough

TS, a 46-year-old Caucasian, non-Hispanic male, presents to the primary care office with complaints of productive cough. He states that this has been ongoing for several months, maybe even a year; however, it is concerning to him so he would like to discuss this with you.

Past Medical History
- Denies any significant medical history

Physical Examination
- Height: 70 inches; weight: 230 lbs

Social History
- Smokes one pack of cigarettes per day for the past 15 to 20 years
- Unsuccessful prior attempts at smoking cessation due to work-related stress

Labs
- Forced expiratory volume in one second/forced vital capacity (FEV1/FVC): 68 (range 76.5–88)
- Forced vital capacity (FVC): 4.09 (range 2.4–4.1)
- GOLD staging: Stage 1 chronic obstructive pulmonary disorder (COPD; mild)
- COPD assessment test (CAT) score: 7

Discussion Questions
1. Which risk factors for COPD are modifiable versus non-modifiable for TS?
2. What nonpharmacologic treatment strategies for TS should be addressed at this visit?
3. Based on current treatment guidelines, what classification is TS's COPD?
4. Based on this classification, what is the recommended pharmacologic treatment for TS?
5. What is the clinician's follow up plan for TS?

CASE EXEMPLAR: Patient With Acute Cough

YG, a 32-year-old Hispanic female, presents to the primary care office with complaints of productive cough. She states that it started 2 to 3 days ago. She reports concomitant low-grade fever and chills in addition to nasal congestion and discharge. Her daughter, who is 8 months old, recently had an upper respiratory illness. YG is afraid that she contracted these symptoms from her daughter. At this visit, her daughter is asymptomatic, and the upper respiratory illness had resolved.

Physical Examination
- Nasal congestion of bilateral nares with yellowish-white nasal discharge
- HEENT assessment otherwise normal
- Lungs: Clear bilaterally

Discussion Questions
1. What are the most common causes of viral upper respiratory illnesses?
2. What nonpharmacologic treatment strategies for YG should be addressed today?
3. What pharmacologic treatment should the clinician recommend for YG?
4. What teaching points should the clinician provide along with the recommended pharmacologic treatment plan?

- Allergic asthma begins with an allergic trigger, whereas nonallergic asthma occurs without the eosinophilic airway inflammation.
- Mucus hypersecretion is a characteristic of chronic bronchitis, whereas inflammation and narrowing of the airways are characteristics of COPD.
- Genetics, obesity, cellular, and environmental (e.g., smoking) factors contribute to the etiology of asthma and COPD.
- The overall goal of asthma and COPD treatment includes achieving control of symptoms while minimizing exacerbations.
- Pharmacologic agents for asthma and COPD focus on bronchodilation and reductions in inflammation and are divided into two categories: controller medications and rescue medications.
- The Global Initiative for Chronic Obstructive Lung Disease (GOLD) and the Global Initiative for Asthma provide standardized guidelines and algorithms for the diagnosis, management, and prevention of COPD and asthma, and the decision for initial pharmacologic treatment is based on an ABCD assessment algorithm.
- The etiology of most upper respiratory illnesses (URIs) is viral in origin. Viral URIs are usually self-limiting and typically present with symptoms such as nasal congestion, runny nose, fever, cough, pharyngitis, and sneezing.
- Treatment for viral infection includes analgesics (e.g., acetaminophen and NSAIDs), antihistamine/decongestant combinations, intranasal cromolyn, intranasal ipratropium, and dextromethorphan.
- Patients with COPD, pulmonary fibrosis, pneumonia, a severe asthma attack, cystic fibrosis, or sleep apnea may require supplemental oxygen at some point in their lives.
- Pulse oximetry or ABGs are tools to indicate the need for oxygen therapy. Oxygenation treatment can either be prescribed for acute scenarios in the hospital or for continuous long-term therapy.

REFERENCES

1. World Health Organization. *Asthma: key facts*. Published May 20, 2020. https://www.who.int/news-room/fact-sheets/detail/asthma
2. Centers for Disease Control and Prevention. *Asthma in the US*. 2011. https://www.cdc.gov/vitalsigns/asthma/index.html
3. World Health Organization. *Chronic respiratory diseases: burden of COPD*. 2018. https://www.who.int/respiratory/copd/burden/en
4. Wheaton AG, Cunningham TJ, Ford ES, Croft JB. Employment and activity limitations among adults with chronic obstructive pulmonary disease—United States, 2013. *Morb Mortal Wkly Rep*. 2015;65(11):290–295. https://www.cdc.gov/mmwr/preview/mmwrhtml/mm6411a1.htm
5. U.S. Department of Health and Human Services. *Health, United States 2015 With Special Feature on Racial and Ethnic Health Disparities*. National Center for Health Statistics; 2016. https://www.cdc.gov/nchs/data/hus/hus15.pdf
6. Xu J, Murphy SL, Kochanek KD, Arias E. *Mortality in the United States, 2018*. NCHS Data Brief, no 355. National Center for Health Statistics; 2020. https://www.cdc.gov/nchs/data/databriefs/db355-h.pdf
7. Osler W. *The Principles and Practice of Medicine*. D. Appleton & Company; 1892.
8. Durham SR, Carroll M, Walsh GM, et al. Leukocyte activation in allergen-induced late-phase asthmatic reactions. *N Engl J Med*. 1984;311:1398–1402. doi:10.1056/NEJM198411293112202
9. Bel EH. Clinical phenotypes of asthma. *Curr Opin Pulm Med*. 2004;10:44–50. doi:10.1097/00063198-200401000-00008
10. Petty TL. The history of COPD. *Int J Chron Obstruct Pulmon Dis*. 2006;1(1):3–14. doi:10.2147/copd.2006.1.1.3
11. Van De Graaff KM. *Human Anatomy*. McGraw Hill; 2002.
12. McDonough JE, Yuan R, Suzuki M, et al. Small-airway obstruction and emphysema in chronic obstructive pulmonary disease. *N Engl J Med*. 2011. 365(17):1567–1575. doi:10.1056/NEJMoa11069514
13. American Lung Association. *Asthma risk factors*. Updated October 23, 2020. https://www.lung.org/lung-health-diseases/lung-disease-lookup/asthma/asthma-symptoms-causes-risk-factors/asthma-risk-factors
14. American Lung Association. *COPD causes and risk factors*. Updated October 23, 2020. https://www.lung.org/lung-health-and-diseases/lung-disease-lookup/copd/symptoms-causes-risk-factors/what-causes-copd.htm15
15. Global Initiative for Asthma. *Online appendix: global strategy for asthma management and prevention*. Updated 2018. https://ginasthma.org/wp-content/uploads/2018/03/WMS-FINAL-GINA-2018-Appendix_v1.3.pd16
16. Global Initiative for Chronic Obstructive Lung Disease. *Global Strategy for the Diagnosis, Management and Prevention of Chronic Obstructive Pulmonary Disease (2020 Report)*. Global Initiative for Chronic Obstructive Lung Disease; 2020. https://goldcopd.org/wp-content/uploads/2019/12/GOLD-2020-FINAL-ver1.2-03Dec19_WMV.pdf
17. Kessler R, Partridge MR, Miravitlles M, et al. Symptom variability in patients with severe COPD: a pan-European cross-sectional study. *Eur Respir J*. 2011;37(2):264–272. doi:10.1183/09031936.000511118
18. Akinbami LJ, Liu X. *Chronic obstructive pulmonary disease among adults aged 18 and over in the United States, 1998–2009*. NCHS Data Brief 63. National Center for Health Statistics; 20119.

19. Jing JY, Huang TC, Cui W, et al. Should FEV1/FEV6 replace FEV1/FVC ratio to detect airway obstruction? A metaanalysis. *Chest.* 2009;135:991–998. doi:10.1378/chest.08-07220

20. Haroon S, Jordan R, Takwoingi Y, et al. Diagnostic accuracy of screening tests for COPD: a systematic review and meta-analysis. *BMJ Open.* 2015;5:1–10. doi:10.1136/bmjopen-2015-0082133

21. Kobayashi M, Nasuhara Y, Betsuyaku T, et al. Effect of low-dose theophylline on airway inflammation in COPD. *Respirology.* 2004;9(2):249–254. doi:10.1111/j.1440-1843.2004.00573.x

22. Hospira. *Theophylline: package insert.* Updated July 2008. https://www.accessdata.fda.gov/drugsatfda_docs/label/2009/019211s042lbl.pdf

23. Barnes PJ. Theophylline. *Am J Respir Crit Care Med.* 2013;188:901–906. doi:10.1164/rccm.201302-0388P22

24. GlaxoSmithKline. *Ventolin HFA: package insert.* Updated January 2020. https://www.gsksource.com/pharma/content/dam/GlaxoSmithKline/US/en/Prescribing_Information/Ventolin_HFA/pdf/VENTOLIN-HFA-PI-PIL.PDF

25. Sunovion. *Xopenex HFA: package insert.* Updated February 2017 https://www.xopenexhfa.com/XOPENEX-HFA-Prescribing-Information.pdf

26. Dey Pharma. *Performist: package insert.* Updated May 2010. https://www.accessdata.fda.gov/drugsatfda_docs/label/2010/022007s004lbl.pdf

27. GlaxoSmithKline. *Serevent Diskus: package insert.* Updated January 2020. https://www.gsksource.com/pharma/content/dam/GlaxoSmithKline/US/en/Prescribing_Information/Serevent_Diskus/pdf/SEREVENT-DISKUS-PI-MG-IFU.PDF

28. Boehringer Ingelheim Pharmaceuticals. *Spiriva HandiHaler: package insert.* Updated December 2009. https://www.accessdata.fda.gov/drugsatfda_docs/label/2009/021395s029lbl.pdf

29. Boehringer Ingelheim. *Ipratropium: package insert.* Updated 2012. https://www.accessdata.fda.gov/drugsatfda_docs/label/2012/021527s021lbl.pdf

30. Merck & Co. *Singulair: package insert.* Updated April 2020. https://www.merck.com/product/usa/pi_circulars/s/singulair/singulair_pi.pdf

31. Forest Laboratories. *Daliresp: package insert.* Updated August 2013. https://www.accessdata.fda.gov/drugsatfda_docs/label/2013/022522s003lbl.pdf

32. Endo Pharmaceuticals. *Theophylline: package insert.* Updated August 2017. http://www.endo.com/File%20Library/Products/Prescribing%20Information/Theo-24_prescribing_information.html#endoanchor-4

33. National Institute of Allergy and Infectious Diseases. The common cold. *Health Matters.* 2004;15(2):79–88. doi:10.1016/j.ejim.2004.01.006

34. Sexton DJ, McClain MT. The common cold in adults: diagnosis and clinical features. In: Kunins L, ed. *UpToDate.* Updated December 27 2019. https://www.uptodate.com/contents/the-common-cold-in-adults-diagnosis-and-clinical-features

35. United States Department of Health and Human Services. National ambulatory medical care survey: 2006 summary. *Natl Health Stat Report.* 2008;3:1–40. https://www.cdc.gov/nchs/data/nhsr/nhsr003.pdf

36. Sahin-Yilmaz A, Naclerio RM. Anatomy and physiology of the upper airway. *Proc Am Thor Soc* 2011;8:31–39. doi:10.1513/pats.201007-050RN

37. Zoorob R, Sidani MA, Fremont RD, Kihlberg C. Antibiotic use in acute upper-respiratory tract infections. *Am Fam Physician.* 2012;86:817–822. https://www.aafp.org/afp/2012/1101/p817.html.

38. Jefferson T, Del Mar C, Dooley L, et al. Physical interventions to interrupt or reduce the spread of respiratory viruses. *Cochrane Database Syst Rev.* 2010;1:CD006207. doi:10.1002/14651858.CD006207.pub3

39. Short S, Bashir H, Marshall P, et al. *Diagnosis and treatment of respiratory illness in children and adults.* Institute for Clinical Systems Improvement; 2017. https://www.icsi.org/wp-content/uploads/2019/01/RespIllness.pdf

40. Aabenhus R, Jensen JU, Jorgensen KJ, et al. Biomarkers as point-of-care tests to guide prescription of antibiotics in patients with acute respiratory infections in primary care. *Cochrane Database Syst Rev.* 2014;11:CD010130. doi:10.1002/14651858.CD010130.pub2

41. Singh M, Singh M. Heated, humidified air for the common cold. *Cochrane Database Syst Rev.* 2013;6:CD001728. doi:10.1002/14651858.CD001728.pub6

42. Waris A, Macharia M, Njeru EK, Essajee F. Randomised double blind study to compare effectiveness of honey, salbutamol and placebo in treatment of cough in children with common cold. *East Afr Med J.* 2014;91(2):50–56. https://www.ajol.info/index.php/eamj/article/view/109140

43. Paul IM, Beiler JS, King TS, et al. Vapor rub, petrolatum and no treatment for children with nocturnal cough and cold symptoms. *Pediatrics.* 2010;126:1092–1999. doi:10.1542/peds.2010-1601

44. Sexton DJ, McClain MT. The common cold in adults: treatment and prevention. In: Kunins L, ed. *UpToDate.* Updated March 24, 2020. https://www.uptodate.com/contents/the-common-cold-in-adults-treatment-and-prevention

45. Little P, Moore M, Kelly J, et al. Ibuprofen, paracetamol and steam for patients with respiratory tract infections in primary care: pragmatic randomized factorial trial. *Br Med J.* 2013;2013(347):1–13. doi:10.1136/bmj.f6041

46. Pfizer. *Tessalon (benzonatate, USP): package insert.* Updated December 2015. https://www.pfizer.com/files/products/uspi_tessalon.pdf

47. Fresenius. *Acetaminophen: package insert.* Updated October 2015. https://www.accessdata.fda.gov/drugsatfda_docs/label/2015/204767s000lbl.pdf

48. Solomon DH. NSAIDs: pharmacology and mechanism of action. In: Furst D, ed. *UpToDate.* Updated July 19, 2019. https://www.uptodate.com/contents/nsaids-pharmacology-and-mechanism-of-action

49. British Medical Journal. Today's drugs: antihistamines: mechanism of action. *BMJ.* 1963;2(5375):1642–1644. doi:10.1136/bmj.2.5373.1642

50. Corboz MR, Rivelli MA, Mingo GG, et al. Mechanism of decongestant activity of alpha 2-adrenoceptor agonists. *Pulm Pharmacol Ther.* 2008;21(3):449–454. doi:10.1016/j.pupt.2007.06.007

51. Aventis Pharmaceuticals. *Cromolyn sodium: package insert.* Published 2003. https://www.accessdata.fda.gov/drugsatfda_docs/label/2004/18596slr030_intal_lbl.pdf

52. Rosenbaum C, Boyer EW. Dextromethorphan abuse and poisoning: clinical features and diagnosis. In: Burns M, Traub S, eds. *UpToDate.* Updated March 20, 2019. https://www.uptodate.com/contents/dextromethorphan-abuse-and-poisoning-clinical-features-and-diagnosis

53. RLI. *Codeine sulfate: package insert.* Updated April 2013. https://www.accessdata.fda.gov/drugsatfda_docs/label/2013/022402s006lbl.pdf

54. Albrecht HH, Dicpinigaitis PV, Guenin EP. Role of guaifenesin in the management of chronic bronchitis and upper respiratory tract infections. *Multidiscip Respir Med.* 2017;12(31):1–11. doi:10.1186/s40248-017-0113-4

55. Pfizer. *Benzonatate: package insert.* Updated December 2015 https://www.accessdata.fda.gov/drugsatfda_docs/label/2011/011210s053lbl.pdf

56. Pfizer. *Ibuprofen: package insert.* Published 2007. https://www.accessdata.fda.gov/drugsatfda_docs/label/2007/017463s105lbl.pdf

57. Pediapharm. *Naproxen: package insert.* Updated May 2016. https://www.accessdata.fda.gov/drugsatfda_docs/label/2016/018965s022s023lbl.pdf

58. Bayer. *Claritin, loratadine product monograph.* Updated May 16, 2019. https://www.bayer.ca/omr/online/claritin-pm-en.pdf

59. Pfizer. *Cetirizine: package insert.* Published 2002. https://www.accessdata.fda.gov/drugsatfda_docs/label/2002/19835s15,%2020346s8lbl.pdf

60. BD Rx Inc. *Diphenhydramine: package insert.* Updated December 2012. https://www.accessdata.fda.gov/drugsatfda_docs/label/2013/091526lbl.pdf

61. Sanofi-Aventis. *Allegra: package insert.* Updated July 2007. https://www.accessdata.fda.gov/drugsatfda_docs/label/2008/020872s018,021963s002lbl.pdf

62. Sanofi-Aventis. *Pseudoephedrine: package insert.* Updated February 7, 2019. http://products.sanofi.ca/en/eltor.pdf

63. Kaiser Permanente. *Neo-synephrine (phenylephrine) 0.25% nasal spray.* Updated May 2020. https://healthy.kaiserpermanente.org/health-wellness/drug-encyclopedia/drug.neo-synephrine-phenylephrine-0-25-nasal-spray.448913

64. Bayer Healthcare. *Oxymetazoline hydrochloride spray: package insert.* Updated December 12, 2019. https://dailymed.nlm.nih.gov/dailymed/drugInfo.cfm?setid=65bf1556-f234-9439-e053-2a91aa0a3194

65. Mayo Clinic. *Drugs and supplements: dextromethorphan (oral route).* Updated October 1, 2020. https://www.mayoclinic.org/drugs-supplements/dextromethorphan-oral-route/precautions/drg-20068661

66. O'Driscoll BR, Howrad LS, Earis J, et al. British thoracic society guideline for oxygen use in adults in healthcare and emergency settings. *BMJ Open Respir Res.* 2017;4:1–20. doi:10.1136/bmjresp-2016-000170

67. World Health Organization. *Chronic respiratory diseases.* Accessed January 13, 2019. https://www.who.int/respiratory/en

68. American Lung Association. *Asthma risk factors.* Updated October 23, 2020. https://www.lung.org/lung-health-and-diseases/lung-disease-lookup/asthma/asthma-symptoms-causes-risk-factors/asthma-risk-factors.html

69. Rosen IM, Manaker S. Oxygen delivery and consumption. In: Parsons P, ed. *UpToDate.* Updated May 9, 2019 https://www.uptodate.com/contents/oxygen-delivery-and-consumption

70. Mayo Clinic. *Hypoxemia causes.* Published December 1, 2018. https://www.mayoclinic.org/symptoms/hypoxemia/basics/causes/sym-20050930

71. Samuel J, Franklin C. Hypoxemia and hypoxia. In: Myers JA, Millikan KW, Saclarides TJ, eds. *Common Surgical Diseases.* Springer; 2008.

72. Kranidis AI, Triantafyllou KA, Manolis AS. Pulmonary embolism: clinical features and diagnosis. *Hosp Chron.* 2006;1(2):69–73. http://www.hospitalchronicles.gr/index.php/hchr/article/view/9

73. Lee WW, Mayberry K, Crapo R, et al. The accuracy of pulse oximetry in the emergency department. *Am J Emerg Med.* 2000;18(4):427–431. doi:10.1053/ajem.2000.7330

74. Razi E, Akbari H. A comparison of arterial oxygen saturation measured by both pulse oximeter and arterial blood gas analyzer in hypoxemic and non-hypoxemic pulmonary diseases. *Turk Respir J.* 2006;7(2):43–47. https://www.semanticscholar.org/paper/A-Comparison-of-Arterial-Oxygen-Saturation-Measured-Razi-Akbari/088abb5bc4daccc7a5818e96cdea145a011c8fe2

75. Torrey SB. Continuous oxygen delivery systems for the acute care of infants, children, and adults. In: Parsons P, ed. *UpToDate.* Updated July 15, 2019. https://www.uptodate.com/contents/continuous-oxygen-delivery-systems-for-infants-children-and-adults

76. Tiep BL, Carter R. Long-term supplemental oxygen therapy. In: Stoller JK, ed. *UpToDate.* 2018. Updated May 8, 2019. https://www.uptodate.com/contents/long-term-supplemental-oxygen-therapy

Pharmacotherapy for Gastrointestinal Conditions and Conditions Requiring Nutritional Support

Ragan Johnson, Angela Richard-Eaglin, and Ricketta Clark

NAUSEA

INTRODUCTION

Nausea affects more than 50% of the adult population, with women reporting three times more episodes than men.[1] Nausea is a commonly occurring symptom described as an unpleasant sensation of queasiness and often involves the urge to vomit. Nausea and vomiting are induced by visceral, vestibular, and chemoreceptor trigger zone stimuli, which are mediated by serotonin, dopamine, histamine, and acetylcholine. Generally, there are no true risk factors; however, there are multiple causes including illness, emotions, motion sickness, medications, and vertigo. There is a gap in the literature related to recent and more extensive epidemiological data on nausea.

DIAGNOSIS OF NAUSEA

Nausea is a symptom of many underlying diseases and/or physiological imbalances. Determining the cause of nausea may be challenging at times because the spectrum of differential diagnoses is wide. Lab testing that may be useful for evaluating the causes of nausea include metabolic profiles, liver function tests, pancreatic enzymes, and pregnancy tests. Radiography, such as abdominal X-rays and CT scans, are first-line diagnostic tests for suspected mechanical obstruction. Following routine evaluation of unexplained chronic nausea and vomiting, esophagogastroduodenoscopy (EGD) is recommended to assess for the presence of ulcer, masses, gastric obstruction, or other disorders.

TREATMENT OF NAUSEA

In general, treatment is guided by the severity and characteristics of nausea, including whether it is acute or chronic. Acute nausea is usually self-limiting and does not require specific treatment. Prevention of dehydration is the primary focus in acute nausea. Nonpharmacological supportive measures for controlling nausea and vomiting include the following:

- **Food and beverages:** consumption of light, bland foods (e.g., saltine crackers, plain bread); consumption of clear or ice-cold drinks; practice of drinking beverages slowly; avoidance of greasy, fried, and sweet foods; and avoidance of mixing hot and cold foods
- **Other:** avoidance of activity after meals; avoidance of teeth brushing after meals

Pharmacological treatment is aimed at either: (a) nausea suppression and prevention of vomiting or (b) modulation of gastrointestinal (GI) motility. Many drug classes may be used to target various receptor sites to relieve nausea. The following drug classes are commonly used for treatment of nausea and vomiting (**Table 19.1**).

Anticholinergics

Anticholinergics (e.g., scopolamine) treat nausea by inhibiting acetylcholine at cholinergic sites in smooth muscles, secretory glands, and the central nervous system (CNS). These drugs also block histamine and serotonin while increasing cardiac output and inducing dryness. Anticholinergics can block cardiac muscarinic receptors at the sinoatrial node, therefore inducing tachycardia. Other common side effects are confusion, constipation, urinary retention, and blurred vision. This class of medication is contraindicated in patients with narrow-angle glaucoma, chronic lung disease, and those who have hypersensitivity to scopolamine and other belladonna alkaloids.[2]

Antihistamines

Antihistamines (e.g., meclizine and dimenhydrinate) treat nausea by binding to H1 receptors at the vestibular nucleus, which communicate with the vomiting center in the medulla of the central nervous system (CNS). Antihistamines that can cross the blood–brain barrier (BBB) also have anticholinergic properties that block muscarinic receptors in the CNS, thereby contributing to their anti-nausea effects.[3] Common side effects of antihistamines are very similar to those of anticholinergics and include drowsiness, confusion, blurred vision, constipation, and urinary retention. Contraindications of antihistamines include closed angle glaucoma, hyperthyroidism, asthma, hypertension, gastrointestinal obstruction, and prostatic hypertrophy.

Benzamides

Benzamides (e.g., metoclopramide and trimethobenzamide) block dopamine receptors and serotonin receptors in the chemoreceptor trigger zone (CTZ) of the CNS. Additionally, they enhance motility in the GI tract without stimulating gastric, biliary, or pancreatic secretions. Benzamides also increase sphincter tone in the lower esophagus. Adverse effects include sedation, sleep disruption, mood disturbances, anxiety, dystonic reactions, tardive dyskinesia, galactorrhea, and sexual dysfunction. This drug class is contraindicated in patients with hypersensitivity to benzamides or any of its components. Other contraindications include pheochromocytoma or other catecholamine-releasing paragangliomas, seizure disorder, history of tardive dyskinesia, or dystonic reaction to benzamides.[4] Concomitant use of benzamides with other agents blocking dopaminergic pathways is also likely to increase the risk of extrapyramidal reactions.

Benzodiazepines

The action of antiemetic effects of benzodiazepines (e.g., lorazepam) has not been clearly described. Nevertheless, benzodiazepines are found binding to the postsynaptic gamma-aminobutyric acid (GABA) receptors and facilitate the binding of GABA to those receptor sites. This action subsequently enhances the inhibitory effects of GABA, thereby slowing down the nerve impulses. This drug class may also be used as an antianxiety or antiseizure medication. The common side effects include dizziness, drowsiness, dysarthria, fatigue, ataxia, cognitive dysfunction, depression, irritability, and memory impairment.[5] Contraindications for benzodiazepines include hypersensitivity to the drug or components of the medication, sleep apnea, CNS depression, and history of severe alcohol or substance use disorders.

Cannabinoids

The antiemetic effects of cannabinoids are a result of their stimulation at the cannabinoid-1 (CB_1) receptors. They may also decrease nausea by reducing the GI motility. Studies have shown cannabinoids may even be useful for anticipatory nausea in patients receiving chemotherapies.[6] Nabilone (Cesamet®) is one of the first cannabinoids approved for nausea and vomiting induced by chemotherapy. Following this agent, dronabinol (Marinol®) was approved by the Food and Drug Administration (FDA) as an antiemetic and an appetite stimulant during the mid-1980s and early 1990s. Both nabilone and dronabinol are synthetic analogs of tetrahydrocannabinol (THC), which is primarily found in the cannabis plants. Since these agents are derived from the psychoactive compound THC, they may exacerbate mania, depression, or schizophrenia. Other adverse effects include cognitive impairment and altered mental state, abdominal pain, dizziness, and paradoxical nausea and vomiting. Patients can also experience euphoria, paranoid reaction, and somnolence while taking these medications. Meanwhile, amnesia, anxiety, nervousness, ataxia, confusion, and hallucination may also be precipitated. Contraindications of these agents in-

TABLE 19.1 Pharmacotherapy For Nausea

Drug Class	Drug/Dose	Contraindications	Side Effects
Anticholinergics	Scopolamine (SL, IV, IM, transdermal): 0.3–0.6 mg q24h	Hypersensitivity to scopolamine, other belladonna alkaloids, or any of its components; narrow-angle glaucoma; chronic lung disease	Tachycardia, confusion, dry mouth, constipation, urinary retention, blurred vision
Antihistamines	Meclizine (oral): 25–50 mg q24h Diphenhydramine (oral, IM, IV): 25–50 mg q6–8h Cinnarizine (oral): 25–75 mg q8h Cyclizine (oral): 25–50 mg q4–6h Hydroxyzine (oral, IM): 25–100 mg q6–8h	Closed-angle glaucoma, hyperthyroidism, asthma, hypertension, GI obstruction, prostatic hypertrophy	Drowsiness, confusion, blurred vision, constipation, urinary retention
Benzamides	Metoclopramide (oral, IM, IV): 10–20 mg q6–8h Trimethobenzamide (Tigan; oral, IM): 300 mg po tid–qid or 200 mg IM tid–qid	Hypersensitivity to benzamides or any of its components, situations where stimulation of GI motility may be dangerous, pheochromocytoma or other catecholamine-releasing paragangliomas, seizure disorder, history of tardive dyskinesia or dystonic reaction to benzamides, concomitant use with other agents likely to increase extrapyramidal reactions	Sedation, sleep disruption, mood disturbances, anxiety, dystonic reactions, tardive dyskinesia, galactorrhea, sexual dysfunction
Benzodiazepines	Lorazepam (oral, SL, IM, IV): 0.5–2 mg Alprazolam (oral): 0.25–1 mg	Hypersensitivity to the drug or components of the medication, sleep apnea, CNS depression, history of severe alcohol- or drug-use disorders	Dizziness, drowsiness, dysarthria, fatigue, ataxia, cognitive dysfunction, depression, irritability, memory impairment, sedation
Cannabinoids	Dronabinol (oral): 2.5–10 mg q6–8h Nabilone (oral): 1–2 mg q8–12h	Hypersensitivity to cannabinoids or any of its components (dronabinol: Capsules, sesame oil; oral solution, alcohol; receiving or have recently received disulfiram- or metronidazole-containing products within 14 days)	Dizziness, paranoia, palpitations, vasodilation/flushing, tachycardia, euphoria, abnormal thinking, hallucinations, visual changes, depersonalization
Corticosteroids	Dexamethasone (oral, IM, IV): 4–8 mg q4–6h	Hypersensitivity to dexamethasone or any of its components; systemic fungal infections	Bruising, acne, emotional instability, hyperglycemia, adrenal suppression, Cushing's syndrome
5-HT3 receptor antagonists	Ondansetron (oral, IV): 4–8 mg q4–8h, max: 16 mg/dose Dolasetron (oral): 100 mg po × 1 within 1 h prior to chemotherapy, max: 100 mg/dose; IV: 12.5 mg × 1 at onset of nausea/vomiting Granisetron (oral, IV): 1–2 mg q24h; transdermal: 3.1 mg/24 h patch × 7 days Palonosetron (IV): 0.075–0.25 mg q24h	Hypersensitivity to 5-HT3 receptor blockers or any of its components; concomitant use with apomorphine Note: Granisetron is sensitive to sunlight. Direct exposure of the medication to natural or artificial sunlight could compromise the effectiveness of the drug. Patch should be protected from sunlight while wearing. Skin area should also be covered for another 10 days after the patch is removed.	Headache, malaise, fatigue, constipation
NK-1 receptor antagonists	Aprepitant (oral capsule or suspension): 125 mg on day 1, then 80 mg q24h on day 2–3 (for chemo-related nausea/vomiting); Cinvanti® IV: 130-mg IV × 1 on day 1 of chemotherapy (for moderate–severe emetogenic drugs) 100-mg IV × 1 on day 1, then 80 mg po on days 2–3 (for moderately emetogenic drugs) Fosaprepitant (IV): 150-mg IV × 1 (for chemo-related N/V) Rolapitant (oral): 180 mg po × 1; IV: 166.5-mg IV × 1 Netupitant/palonosetron (oral): 300/0.5-mg capsule × 1 Fosnetupitant/palonosetron (IV): 235/0.25 mg IV × 1	Hypersensitivity to aprepitant or any of its components; concurrent use of aprepitant with pimozide	Fatigue, constipation, hiccups, hypotension, dehydration, neutropenia, and elevation of liver enzymes
Phenothiazines	Prochlorperazine (oral, IM, IV, rectal): 5–10 mg q6–8h Promethazine (oral, IM, IV, rectal): 12.5–25 mg q4–6h Chlorpromazine (oral, IM, IV): 10–25 mg q4–6h Perphenazine (oral): 4–8 mg q8–12h	Contraindications: *Drugs induce EPS or NMS, i.e., antipsychotics* Black-Box Warnings: None	Extrapyramidal side effects, tardive dyskinesias, neuroleptic malignant syndrome, hyperprolactinemia, prolonged QT

CNS, central nervous system; GI, gastrointestinal; IM, intramuscular; IV, intravenous; h, hour; N&V, nausea and vomiting; po, by mouth; q, every; qid, four times daily; tid, thrice daily.

Source: Data from Lexicomp. Accessed February 13, 2019. http://online.lexi.com.proxy.lib.duke.edu/lco/action/search?q=nausea&t=name&va=nausea; Singh P, Yoon SS, Kuo B. Nausea: a review of pathophysiology and therapeutics. *Therap Adv Gastroenterol.* 2016;9(1):98–112. doi:10.1177/1756283X15618131

clude hypersensitivity to the active cannabinoids or inactive ingredients of the capsule, such as sesame oil present in the dronabinol capsule.[7,8]

Corticosteroids

The antiemetic activity of the corticosteroid (e.g., dexamethasone) is unclear. According to a Cochrane review in 2017, there is very low quality of evidence that corticosteroid is effective in use for nausea and vomiting unrelated to surgery, chemotherapy, or radiotherapy in patients with advanced cancer.[9] The results showed that patients who received dexamethasone had lower rates of nausea as compared to placebo. The mean difference of nausea rate after 8 days of therapy between the treatment and placebo groups was reported at 0.48 on a scale of 0 to 10, with 10 being the worst nausea. Although the mean difference was lowered in the treatment group, it was not statistically significant.[9] Consequently, current data neither support nor refute the use of steroid in this scenario.

Side effects of corticosteroids include increased glucose intolerance, hyperglycemia, glycosuria, development of cushingoid state, hirsutism, and hypertrichosis. In addition, they can cause bradycardia, congestive heart failure, cardiac arrhythmias, fat embolism, or hypertension. Other effects such as euphoria, depression, emotional instability, muscle weakness, osteoporosis, headache, abnormal fat deposits, infection, hiccups, malaise, moon face, or weight gain may also develop. Contraindications of steroids are the development of hypersensitivity with the drug and systemic fungal infections.[10]

5-HT3 Antagonists

5-HT3 antagonists (e.g., ondansetron) inhibit serotonin peripherally, on vagal nerve terminals, and centrally in the chemoreceptor trigger zone. This is one of the most popular drug classes that is prescribed for nausea and vomiting. They are available in different formulations, including oral tablet or solution, oral disintegrated tablet (ODT), intravenous solution, or transdermal patch (e.g., granisetron, Sancuso®). In general, the agents within this drug class have short half-lives ranging from 4 to 8 hours, except palonosetron (Aloxi®), which has a half-life of approximately 40 hours.[11] The common adverse effects of 5-HT3 antagonists may involve constipation, diarrhea, headache, and fatigue. Less common side effects include extrapyramidal reactions, elevation of liver function tests (e.g., aspartate aminotransferase [AST] and alanine aminotransferase [ALT]), tachycardia, bradycardia, QTc prolongation, bronchospasm, angina, and hypokalemia.[11,12] The contraindications of 5-HT3 antagonists generally involve hypersensitivity of the active or inactive ingredients within the drug formu-

lation. Nevertheless, ondansetron is contraindicated when used together with apomorphine, a medication approved for Parkinson's disease. Concomitant use of these two medications may result in profound hypotension and loss of consciousness.[12]

Neurokinin-1 Receptor Antagonists

The neurokinin-1 (NK-1) receptor antagonists (e.g., aprepitant) inhibit the binding of substance P to the neurokinin-1 (NK-1) receptors, which are found on the vagal afferent neurons, gastrointestinal tract, and the brain. They are effective in preventing both acute and delayed vomiting. They also potentiate the antiemetic activity of corticosteroids and 5-HT3 receptor antagonists to prevent chemotherapy-induced emesis.[13] These drugs are available as oral capsule, tablet, powder suspension, or injection. The side effects of NK-1 antagonists include diarrhea, constipation, dyspepsia, abdominal pain, and hiccups. Other serious side effects may also include hypotension, dehydration, neutropenia, and elevation of liver enzymes. Since aprepitant is a substrate of the cytochrome 3A4 enzyme, it may interact with multiple medications that are inducers (e.g., rifampin, phenobarbital, or phenytoin) or inhibitors (e.g., ketoconazole, itraconazole, or erythromycin) of this enzyme.

Phenothiazines

Phenothiazines (e.g., prochlorperazine) provide their anti-nausea effects by inhibiting dopamine, muscarinic, and histamine (H1) receptors in the vomiting center and chemoreceptor trigger zone. Because of the blocking effects of these receptor types (e.g., dopamine, muscarinic, and H1 receptors), the side effects of this drug class are broad. They may cause extrapyramidal side effects, tardive dyskinesias, neuroleptic malignant syndrome (NMS), hyperprolactinemia, prolonged QT, and anticholinergic effects, as well as antihistaminic effects. Phenothiazines are contraindicated for patients who develop hypersensitivity with phenothiazines or those who have severe CNS suppression. Precautions must be implemented for patients who have higher risk of tardive dyskinesia, especially older adults, because this reaction may be irreversible.[14] In addition, concomitant use of phenothiazines with drugs that could precipitate NMS such as antipsychotics could also increase risk of this toxicity; therefore, they should be avoided when possible.

DIARRHEA

INTRODUCTION

Diarrhea is defined as loose, watery stools occurring three or more times a day. It is classified as either acute, persistent, or chronic. Acute diarrhea is defined as having less than 2 weeks of decrease in stool consistency. Meanwhile, persistent diarrhea refers to a decrease in stool consistency that lasts between 2 and 4 weeks. Diarrhea that lasts longer than 4 weeks or 1 month is classified as chronic diarrhea.[15] Acute diarrhea is the most common reason for outpatient visits. It is self-limiting and lasts 1 or 2 days. A physiological imbalance in the normal absorption of ions, organic substrates, and water creates an increase in the water content of stools and produces diarrhea. Prolonged diarrhea may lead to dehydration, malabsorption, and malnourishment. According to the Centers for Disease Control and Prevention (CDC), approximately 47.8 million cases of diarrhea occur annually in the United States.[16]

Diarrhea can be a result of several factors, including fructose, artificial sweeteners, viruses, bacteria, parasites, medication side effects, lactose intolerance, and digestive disorders such as irritable bowel syndrome, Crohn's disease, ulcerative colitis, microscopic colitis, and celiac disease.

DIAGNOSIS OF DIARRHEA

The diagnosis of diarrhea is generally clinical, based on the patient's presenting signs and symptoms as well as medical history. The causative factors may come from either infectious or noninfectious sources. Differential diagnoses will be based on whether diarrheal symptoms are acute, persistent, or chronic. Diagnostic testing for diarrhea is indicated only in patients with severe diarrhea, suspected nosocomial infection, persistent fever, bloody stools, or immunosuppression. Fecal occult blood tests contribute to diagnosis of inflammatory diarrhea with 71% sensitivity and 79% specificity.[17] Bacterial infections can be detected by lactoferrin stool testing with 67% to 91% sensitivity and 90% to 100% specificity.[18] Stool cultures are most effective when used for patients with blood in the stool, severe dehydration, or signs of inflammatory disease. They are also appropriate for patients who have immunosuppression or symptoms lasting more than 3 to 7 days. Furthermore, clostridium difficile testing for toxins A and B is recommended for the following patients: hospitalized patients with unexplained diarrhea after 3 days, or patients with unexplained diarrhea during antibiotic use or within 3 months after discontinuing antibiotics. Meanwhile, ova and parasite testing are recommended for patients with persistent diarrhea for greater than 7 days. Endoscopy can aid in determining noninfectious causes of acute diarrhea, including inflammatory bowel disease, NSAID-induced enteropathy, ischemic colitis, and cancer.[17]

TREATMENT OF DIARRHEA

Nonpharmacological approaches to the prevention and management of diarrhea include: (a) avoidance of trigger factors, (b) meticulous hand hygiene, and (c) fluid replacement. Treatment of diarrhea is largely related to the cause. Onset, duration, severity, presence of dehydration, vital signs, and physical examination will guide treatment considerations. In cases of dehydration, fluid replacement is the hallmark of treatment. Antibiotics are the treatment of choice for bacterial infections. Current American College of Gastroenterology (ACG) guidelines[19] for treatment of acute diarrhea include fluid replacement with electrolyte rehydration, water, juices, sports drinks, and saltine crackers (moderate level of evidence). The ACG also recommends prebiotics or probiotics (moderate level of evidence) for diarrhea cases associated with antibiotics. Bismuth subsalicylates is recommended for travelers with mild to moderate diarrhea (high level of evidence). It is also recommended to use adjunctive loperamide therapy for patients taking antibiotics to treat travelers' diarrhea (moderate level of evidence). Empiric antibiotic therapy should only be used in cases of travelers' diarrhea with a high probability of a bacterial cause (high level of evidence). Due to the increased likelihood of a viral cause, treatment of community-acquired diarrhea with antibiotics is discouraged (very low level of evidence).

Mechanism of Action of Antidiarrheal Medications

Antimotility agents such as loperamide or the opiate derivatives (i.e., diphenoxylate or opium tincture) can reduce the frequency of bowel movements by binding to opioid receptors on the intestinal smooth muscles leading to decrease in GI motility. These agents inhibit peristalsis and prolong transit time, thereby increasing stool viscosity, decreasing fecal volume, fluid, and electrolyte loss. Adsorbents such as attapulgite (magnesium aluminum phyllosilicate) decrease GI motility, adsorb fluids, and bind toxins from bacteria. Medicinal use of attapulgite is no longer available in the United States but it is available elsewhere outside the United States. Other adsorbents that are still available in the United States as over-the-counter (OTC) products are calcium polycarbophil, psyllium, and methylcellulose. Antisecretory agents such as bismuth subsalicylate (Pepto-Bismol) decrease GI motility and minimally absorb from the GI tract. The bismuth component of the drug is responsible for the local antimicrobial action against bacterial and viral GI pathogens; meanwhile, the anti-inflammatory properties are due to the salicylic acid.[20] Table 19.2 summarizes the selected antidiarrheal medications that are commonly used in clinical practice.

TABLE 19.2 Pharmacotherapy for Diarrhea

Drug/Dose	Contraindications	Side Effects
Loperamide hydrochloride Acute diarrhea—oral: 4-mg initial dose, then 2 mg after each loose stool (max: 16 mg/day) Chronic diarrhea—oral: 4-mg initial dose, then 2 mg after each loose stool (max: 16 mg/day); maintenance dose: 4–8 mg/day as a single dose or in divided doses (max: 16 mg/day); slowly titrate dose downward to minimum necessary for symptom control Travelers' diarrhea—oral: 4 mg after first loose stool, then 2 mg after each subsequent stool (max dose: 16 mg/day [OTC: 8 mg/day]) ≤48 hours); moderate-to-severe illness: loperamide recommended as adjunctive therapy with antibiotics	Hypersensitivity to loperamide or any of its components; abdominal pain without diarrhea; <2 years of age; acute dysentery; acute ulcerative colitis; bacterial enterocolitis resulting from *Salmonella*, *Shigella*, and *Campylobacter*; broad-spectrum antibiotic–induced pseudomembranous colitis	Dizziness, nausea, constipation, abdominal cramps
Diphenoxylate hydrochloride and atropine sulfate Oral: Initial dose of 5 mg qid until control achieved (max: 20 mg/day); reduce dose once control achieved	Hypersensitivity to diphenoxylate, atropine, or any of its components; obstructive jaundice; pseudomembranous enterocolitis, *Clostridioides*, or other enterotoxin-producing bacteria; patients <6 years old (tablets only)	Flushing, tachycardia, confusion, depression, dizziness, drowsiness, euphoria, hallucination, headache, hyperthermia, lethargy, malaise, numbness, restlessness, sedation, pruritus, urticaria, abdominal distress, anorexia, gingival swelling, nausea, pancreatitis, paralytic ileus, toxic megacolon, vomiting, xerostomia, urinary retention, anaphylaxis, angioedema
Camphorated tincture of opium Oral: 5–10 mL once daily–qid	Hypersensitivity to morphine or any of its components, poison-induced diarrhea (until the toxic components have been eliminated from the GI tract), convulsive states	Anorexia, biliary tract spasm, constipation, nausea, stomach cramps, vomiting, hypotension, peripheral vasodilation, CNS depression, depression, dizziness, drowsiness, physical and psychological drug dependence, dysphoria, euphoria, headache, increased intracranial pressure, insomnia, malaise, restlessness, sedation, decreased urine output, ureteral spasm, increased liver enzymes, respiratory depression, miosis
Tincture of opium Oral (undiluted opium tincture): 6 mg (0.6 mL) of 10 mg/mL formulation qid	Use in children, poison-induced diarrhea (until the toxic components have been eliminated from the GI tract)	Same as paregoric
Bismuth subsalicylate Oral: 524 mg q30–60m or 1,050 mg q60m prn for up to 2 days (max: eight doses of regular strength; four doses of maximum strength q24h)	Allergic to salicylates or are taking other salicylates, GI ulcer, bleeding or bloody/black stool	Anxiety, confusion, depression, headache, slurred speech, grayish black feces, impaction in infants and debilitated individuals), tongue darkening

CNS, central nervous system; GI, gastrointestinal; h, hour; N&V, nausea and vomiting; prn, as needed; q, every; qid, four times daily.

Source: Data from Barr W, Smith A. Acute diarrhea in adults. *Am Fam Physician.* 2014;89(3):180–189. https://www.aafp.org/afp/2014/0201/p180.html; Data from Lexicomp. Accessed February 13, 2019. http://online.lexi.com.proxy.lib.duke.edu/lco/action/search?q=nausea&t=name&va=nausea

CONSTIPATION

INTRODUCTION

Constipation is classified as a symptom—rather than a disease of the bowel—that is associated with the difficulty or infrequent passage of stool or a feeling of incomplete evacuation.[21] The episodes may occur chronically or in isolation and result from primary or secondary causes. The primary causes are often associated with defecatory disorders, which are characterized by impaired rectal evacuation with either slow or normal colonic transit.[21] Secondary causes of constipation may result from drug toxicities, metabolic conditions such as diabetes, hyperthyroidism, and hypercalcemia, or neuropathies such as Parkinson's disease or multiple sclerosis. The incidence of constipation in women to men is reported at a ratio of approximately 2:1.[21,22] The prevalence increases during pregnancy, after childbirth, and in adults older than 65 years of age. Most studies have shown that the prevalence of constipation is higher in nonWhite Americans than in White Americans.[21] Nonetheless, the incidence of constipation reported in the adult population from a review of 50 epidemiological studies was estimated as high as 35%.[23]

The general definition of constipation is fewer than three bowel movements per week. It may be categorized into three different categories: (a) normal-transit constipation (NTC), (b) slow-transit constipation (STC), and (c) pelvic floor dysfunction. In NTC, the most common type of constipation, the stool passes through the colon at a normal rate, but bowel evacuation is difficult. STC is a result of impaired phasic colonic motor activity, leading to bowel movement infrequency, decreased urgency, or straining to defecate. Pelvic floor dysfunction is characterized by impairments in pelvic floor or anal sphincter function due to poor coordination, causing prolonged or excessive straining, incomplete evacuation, use of perineal or vaginal pressure to evacuate bowels, or the need to digitally evacuate stool.[24] The risks for constipation include sex, age greater than 65 years, dehydration, low-fiber diet, low caloric intake, sedentary lifestyle, depression, eating disorders, and medications such as narcotics, sedatives, certain antidepressants, and some antihypertensives. Controllable risks can be managed by adequate fluid, fiber, and calorie intake, along with increasing physical activity.

DIAGNOSIS OF CONSTIPATION

Diagnosis of constipation is based on the Rome IV criteria, which states the symptoms should have started 6 months prior to the diagnosis and been present within the previous 3 months. Patients must have at least two of the following symptoms, which occur in at least 25% of defecations: less than three unassisted bowel movements per week, straining, lumpy or hard stools, sensation of incomplete evacuation, sensation of anorectal obstruction or blockage, and reliance on manual maneuvers to promote defecation.[25,26] Differential diagnoses to consider include colorectal cancer, large bowel obstruction, colonic ileus, and irritable bowel syndrome (IBS). Nonetheless, when a patient has family history of colorectal cancer or hematochezia, rectal bleeding, changes in stool character, anemia, and weight loss, screening should be conducted to rule out colorectal cancer as these are strong indicators for cancer.

Diagnostic testing for constipation is indicated for evaluation of metabolic or other pathologic causes. Laboratory tests aid in identifying anemia or endocrine causes of constipation such as diabetes mellitus, hypothyroidism, and hyperparathyroidism. Imaging studies could aid in evaluation of acute causes (e.g., sepsis) or chronic causes (e.g., ileus); however, the sensitivity and specificity of these imaging studies specific to evaluating constipation is limited.

TREATMENT OF CONSTIPATION

The general approach to treatment of constipation is diet modification and laxative use. The American Society of Colon and Rectal Surgeons' (ASCRS') clinical practice guidelines[27] recommendations for nonsurgical management of constipation include the following:

1. Dietary modification, including fiber and fiber supplements for initial management of symptomatic constipation (moderate-quality evidence)
2. Osmotic laxatives, such as polyethylene glycol and lactulose, for chronic constipation (moderate-quality evidence)
3. Stimulant laxatives, such as bisacodyl, for short-term second-line treatment of chronic constipation (moderate-quality evidence)
4. Newer agents, such as lubiprostone and linaclotide, when dietary modification and osmotic and/or stimulant laxatives failed (moderate-quality evidence)

Mechanism of Action for Laxatives

Laxatives increase colonic fluid retention, act on the colonic mucosa to decrease luminal water absorption, or increase intestinal motility. Types of laxatives include osmotic, stimulant, saline, bulk-forming, stool softeners, lubricant, and miscellaneous (**Table 19.1**).

Osmotic Laxatives

Osmotic laxatives are nonabsorbable solutions that are metabolized to form lactic acid, acetic acid, formic acid, and carbon dioxide. Through osmosis, these substances attract water to the bowel to equalize osmotic pressure and increase peristalsis within the colon. An example of this drug class is glycerin suppositories, which act through hyper-osmosis, local irritation to promote peristalsis, and lubrication.

Stimulant Laxatives

Stimulant or irritant laxatives increase peristalsis through the stimulation of the myenteric plexus. In addition, they directly act on the intestinal mucosa, and alter secretion of water and electrolytes, leading to shorter overall colonic transit time while increasing the water content in the GI lumen.[28]

Saline Laxatives

Saline laxatives increase intraluminal pressure in the small intestine and colon by attracting and retaining water. They also work by induction of contractions and stimulating cholecystokinin release, which increases intestinal secretion and stimulates transit.

Bulk-Forming Laxatives

Bulk-forming laxatives hold water and bulk in the stool, which softens the stool and stimulates peristalsis.

Additionally, they induce mechanical distention of the colon and further stimulate peristalsis.

Stool Softeners

Stool softeners soften stool by allowing penetration of fluids in fecal matter and by facilitating the mixture of fat and water. They also inhibit reabsorption of fluid and electrolytes.

Lubricants

Lubricants act by lubricating the intestines, slowing absorption of water in the colon, and softening stool.

Miscellaneous Laxatives

Miscellaneous laxatives work by increasing intestinal fluids and decrease transit time.

TABLE 19.3 Laxatives

Drug	Dose	Contraindications	Side Effects
Osmotic Laxatives			
Glycerin suppository	Rectal: One suppository once daily prn or as directed	None	Abdominal cramps, rectal irritation, tenesmus
Lactulose	Oral: 10–20 g (15–30 mL; 1–2 packets) daily; may increase to 40 g (60 mL; 2–4 packets) daily prn	Low-galactose diet	Dehydration, hypernatremia, hypokalemia, abdominal cramps, abdominal distention, abdominal distress, diarrhea (excessive dose), eructation, flatulence, nausea, vomiting
Polyethylene glycol 3350	Oral: 17 g dissolved in 4–8 ounces of beverage once daily or as directed	Hypersensitivity to polyethylene glycol or any of its components; known or suspected bowel obstruction	Loose stools, flatulence, abdominal pain, dyspepsia, abdominal distention, eructation, rectal hemorrhage, nausea
Sorbitol	Oral: 30–45 mL (70% solution); rectal enema: 120 mL (25%–30% solution)	None	Abdominal distress, nausea, vomiting, diarrhea, xerostomia, edema, electrolyte depletion, hyperglycemia, hypovolemia, lactic acidosis
Stimulant Laxatives			
Bisacodyl	Oral: 5–15 mg once daily; rectal (enema, suppository): 10 mg (one enema or suppository) once daily	None	Mild abdominal cramps, nausea, vomiting, rectal burning, vertigo, electrolyte disturbance
Senna	Syrup: 10–15 mL once daily (max: 15 mL bid) Tablets: 8.6 mg: Two tabs once daily; (max: four tablets bid) 15 mg: Two tabs once daily–bid 17.2 mg: One tab once daily (max: two tabs bid) 25 mg: Two tabs once daily–bid	None	Nausea, vomiting, abdominal cramps, diarrhea
Castor oil	Oral: 15–60 mL as a single dose	None	Abdominal cramps, diarrhea, nausea, hypotension, dizziness, pelvic congestion syndrome, electrolyte disturbance
Saline Laxatives			
Magnesium hydroxide	Liquid: 400 mg/5 mL: 30–60 mL once daily at bedtime or in divided doses 800 mg/5 mL: 15–30 mL once daily at bedtime or in divided doses 1,200 mg/5 mL: 10–20 mL once daily at bedtime or in divided doses Chewable tablet: 311 mg/tablet: Eight tabs once daily at bedtime or in divided doses	None	Abdominal cramps, upset stomach, vomiting, diarrhea

(continued)

TABLE 19.3 Laxatives *(continued)*

Drug	Dose	Contraindications	Side Effects
Saline Laxatives			
Sodium phosphates	Oral solution: 15 mL as a single dose (max single daily dose: 45 mL) Rectal (Fleet Enema): Entire contents of one 4.5-oz enema as a single dose	Hypersensitivity to sodium phosphate salts or any component of the formulation; tablets: acute phosphate nephropathy, bowel obstruction, bowel perforation, gastric bypass or stapling surgery, toxic colitis, toxic megacolon; oral solution: dehydration, heart failure, renal impairment, electrolyte abnormalities; use in children <5 years of age for bowel cleansing	Bloating, nausea, abdominal pain, vomiting, aphthous stomatitis, hyperphosphatemia
Magnesium citrate	Oral solution: 195–300 mL once or in divided doses	Low-salt diet	Abdominal pain, diarrhea, flatulence, nausea, vomiting
Bulk-Forming Laxatives			
Methylcellulose	Tablet: Two tablets prn up to six times/day (max: 12 caplets/day) Powder: 2 g (1 heaping tablespoon) in 8 oz (240 mL) of cold water; increase prn by 1 heaping tablespoon up to 3 × daily	None	Impaction above strictures, fluid overload, gas, bloating
Psyllium	Oral: 2.5–30 g/day in divided doses	Hypersensitivity to psyllium or any of its components; fecal impaction; GI obstruction	Anaphylaxis, abdominal cramps, constipation, diarrhea, esophageal obstruction, intestinal obstruction, allergic conjunctivitis, bronchospasm
Wheat dextrin	Oral: 1–3 caplets (1 g fiber/caplet) or 2 teaspoons (1.5 g fiber/teaspoon) up to three times per day	None	Bloating, flatulence, gastrointestinal distress
Stool Softeners			
Docusate/senna	Oral: Two tablets (17.2-mg sennosides plus 100-mg docusate) once daily (max: Four tabs bid)	Presence of abdominal pain, nausea, vomiting; concurrent use of mineral oil	Abdominal cramps, nausea, vomiting, diarrhea, red/brown, urine discoloration
Docusate calcium	Oral: 240 mg once daily	Acute abdominal pain, nausea, vomiting, or other symptoms of appendicitis or undiagnosed abdominal pain; concomitantly with mineral oil	Throat irritation
Docusate sodium	Oral: 50–360 mg once daily or in divided doses	Acute abdominal pain, nausea, vomiting, or other symptoms of appendicitis or undiagnosed abdominal pain; concomitantly with mineral oil	Throat irritation
Miscellaneous			
Linaclotide	Oral: 145 mcg once daily; 72 mcg once daily may be used based on patient presentation or tolerability	Patient <6 years old; known or suspected mechanical gastrointestinal obstruction	Diarrhea, headache, fatigue, dehydration, abdominal pain, flatulence, abdominal distention, viral gastroenteritis, dyspepsia, fecal incontinence, GERD, vomiting, upper respiratory tract, infection, sinusitis
Lubiprostone	Oral: 24 mcg bid	Known or suspected mechanical GI obstruction	Nausea, vomiting, diarrhea, loose stools, abdominal pain, flatulence, abdominal distention, abdominal distress, dyspepsia

bid, twice daily; GERD, gastroesophageal reflux disease; GI, gastrointestinal; prn, as needed; qid, four times daily; tid, thrice daily.

Source: Data from Lexicomp. Accessed February 13, 2019. http://online.lexi.com.proxy.lib.duke.edu/lco/action/search?q=laxatives&t=name&va=laxatives

IRRITABLE BOWEL SYNDROME

INTRODUCTION

IBS is a chronic condition characterized by the hallmark symptoms of abdominal pain and altered bowel movements without the presence of organic disease. IBS most often occurs in individuals 20 to 40 years of age and can persist for decades. The prevalence in females is significantly higher than in males.[29] It is estimated that $21 billion is spent annually due to indirect healthcare costs, decreased work productivity, and absenteeism.[30] Studies have shown that abdominal symptoms are one of the top 10 reasons patients seek care in the primary care setting.[31] More than 60% of sufferers experience psychological disturbances or chronic pain syndromes.

The symptoms of IBS can impact physical, emotional, and social well-being. In addition to the hallmark symptoms of abdominal pain and altered bowel movements, changes to stool form are also indicative. Biochemical and structural abnormalities are not associated with symptoms of IBS; however, signs of IBS are associated with issues with motility, visceral hypersensitivity, infection, and stress. Bloating, straining with defecation, urgency, incomplete evacuation, and mucoid stools are also symptoms that can be seen with IBS.[32] Four different subtypes classify this condition based on symptoms (**Table 19.4**). Some symptoms are cause for heightened concern and are considered "red flags" (**Box 19.1**). They indicate that the etiology of the symptoms may not be IBS and that an organic disease should be contemplated.[33]

DIAGNOSIS OF IRRITABLE BOWEL SYNDROME

There are no screening procedures for IBS; however, a diagnosis is made by history and evaluation of symptoms. The Rome IV criteria are widely used in diagnosing IBS.[34] Based on these criteria, IBS is diagnosed in patients with recurrent abdominal pain that occurs on an average of at

TABLE 19.4 Subtypes of Irritable Bowel Syndrome

Subtype	Symptoms
IBS with predominant constipation	Hard stools >25% of the time; loose stools <25% of the time
IBS with predominant diarrhea	Loose stools >25% of the time; hard stools <25% of the time
IBS-mixed	Hard stools >25% of the time; loose stools >25% of the time
Unclassified IBS	Neither loose nor hard stools >25% of the time

IBS, irritable bowel syndrome.

BOX 19.1
ALARM SYMPTOMS OF IRRITABLE BOWEL SYNDROME

Age >50
Short duration of symptoms
Weight loss
Nocturnal symptoms
Male sex
Family history of colorectal cancer
Anemia
Hematochezia
Recent antibiotic use

TABLE 19.5 Diagnostic Testing and Differential Diagnoses for Irritable Bowel Syndrome

Laboratory Findings	Diagnostic Procedures	Differential Diagnosis
Complete blood count	Colonoscopy	IBS-D:
Thyroid-stimulating hormone	Abdominal x-ray (IBS-C)	Celiac disease
Celiac disease serology (IgA especially)	Anorectal manometry	Microscopic colitis
Fecal occult blood		Small intestinal bacterial overgrowth
C-reactive protein (IBS-D)		Inflammatory bowel disease
		IBS-C:
		Organic disease
		Dyssynergic defecation
		Slow colonic transit

IBS-C, irritable bowel syndrome with predominant constipation; IBS-D, irritable bowel syndrome with predominant diarrhea.

---

least 1 day/week over the prior 3 months and is accompanied by two or more of the following symptoms:

- Defecation
- Change in stool frequency
- Stool form (appearance)

In addition to evaluating symptoms, physical examination, laboratory findings, and diagnostic procedures are used in differentiating IBS from other differential diagnoses (**Table 19.5**).

TREATMENT OF IRRITABLE BOWEL SYNDROME

Nonpharmacological Treatment

Dietary measures are the initial approach to treating IBS. Individuals with mild-to-moderate symptoms are urged to avoid gas-producing foods; fermentable oligo-, di-, and monosaccharides, or polyols (FODMAPs); lactose; and gluten foods.[32,35]

Pharmacological Treatment

For individuals who have mild-to-moderate symptoms that fail initial nonpharmacological management and those who have moderate-to-severe symptoms, pharmacological actions such as adjunctive therapy are necessary to improve symptoms and quality of life.[32,35] **Table 19.6** lists drug regimens to address common symptomatic control of IBS. Just as there are various symptoms and subtypes of IBS, the mechanisms of action of the medications used to treat this condition vary as well (see **Table 19.7**).

TABLE 19.6 Pharmacotherapy for Irritable Bowel Syndrome Symptoms

Symptoms	Treatment
Constipation	Psyllium, 3.4 g bid with meals, then adjust Lubiprostone, 8 mcg bid Linaclotide, 290 mcg once daily Polyethylene glycol 3350, 17 g of powder dissolved in 8 ounces of water once daily; titrate up or down to effect Tegaserod, 6 mg bid before meals
Diarrhea	Loperamide, 2–4 mg prn (maximum 12 mg/day) Eluxadoline, 100 mg bid Cholestyramine, 4 g with meals Alosetron, 0.5–1 mg bid (for severe symptoms in women) Rifaximin, 550 mg tid × 14 days
IBS with abdominal pain/bloating	Dicyclomine, 20 mg po qid prn Hyoscyamine, 0.125–0.25 mg orally or sublingually tid–qid prn Sustained-release hyoscyamine, 0.375–0.75 mg po q12h Amitriptyline, nortriptyline, and imipramine can be started at a dose of 10–25 mg at bedtime Desipramine should be started at a dose of 12.5–25 mg at bedtime Probiotics

bid, twice daily; h, hour; IBS, irritable bowel syndrome; po, by mouth; prn, as needed; q, every; qid, four times daily; tid, thrice daily.

TABLE 19.7 Mechanisms of Action for Drugs Used to Treat Irritable Bowel Syndrome

Drug Class	Mechanism of Action	Medications
Fiber	Increase gut motility, increasing stool output Create bulk in the stool Dilute colonic content Change metabolism of minerals, nitrogen, and bile acids	Psyllium Benefiber Metamucil Citrucel
Osmotic laxatives	Causes intestinal water secretion Increases stool frequency	Polyethylene glycol 3350 MiraLAX GoLYTELY
Antidiarrheals	Impedes peristalsis Lengthens transit time Decreases fecal volume	Loperamide Eluxadoline
Bile acid sequestrants	Binds bile salts, decreasing down diarrhea	Cholestyramine
5-Hydroxytryptamine (serotonin) 3 receptor antagonists	Modulates visceral afferent activity from the gastrointestinal tract Decreases colonic motility and secretion Improves abdominal pain	Alosetron
Antispasmodics	Acts via their anticholinergic or antimuscarinic properties Affects intestinal smooth muscle relaxation	Dicyclomine Hyoscyamine Sustained-release hyoscyamine
Antidepressants (tricyclic)	Slows transient time due to anticholinergic properties May provide benefit in diarrhea-predominant IBS due to anticholinergic effect	Imipramine Nortriptyline Amitriptyline Desipramine
Antibiotics	Inhibits bacterial RNA synthesis by binding to bacterial DNA-dependent RNA polymerase	Rifaximin
Chloride channel activators	Acts locally on the apical membrane of the gastrointestinal tract to increase fluid secretion in the intestines; thus, improving fecal transit	Lubiprostone
Guanylate cyclase-C (GC-C) agonists	Causes chloride and bicarbonate secretion to enter the intestinal lumen.	Linaclotide

DNA, deoxyribonucleic acid; IBS, irritable bowel syndrome; RNA, ribonucleic acid.

INFLAMMATORY BOWEL DISEASE

INTRODUCTION

Inflammatory bowel disease (IBD) is an idiopathic chronic inflammatory condition affecting the GI system. IBD is comprised of two conditions: Crohn's disease (CD) and ulcerative colitis (UC). While some of the symptoms of both conditions may overlap, these two conditions are distinct in many ways. There are many gastrointestinal complications associated with IBD based on disease type, location, severity, and duration. Also, extraintestinal symptoms and complications can occur with IBD. With longstanding disease, colorectal cancer can be seen.[36]

Crohn's disease is a condition that may affect the entire GI tract, from the mouth to the perianal areas. It is characterized by transmural inflammation of the intestines with patchy skip lesions. Because of this, fibrosis, structuring, and obstruction can potentially occur. The transmural inflammation can produce sinus tracts, therefore causing micro-perforations and fistulae.[37,38]

Ulcerative colitis is characterized as a chronic inflammatory condition of the colon that has periods of relapse and remission and is limited to the mucosal layer of the colon. The rectum is most often initially affected by the disease, but it may spread to other portions of the colon.[38]

IBD often occurs during adolescence with the median age of UC and CD happening in the third and fourth decades of life, respectively. While the etiology of IBD remains a mystery, genetic, microbial, and immunologic factors do play a role in the condition and there are several risk factors associated with this illness (**Table 19.8**).

While the symptoms of CD and UC overlap in many ways, they are distinctly different. These symptoms can be debilitating at times and decrease quality of life. The clinical manifestations of both illnesses can be insidious. Crohn's disease has an array of symptoms that may be intra-intestinal, systemic, and extraintestinal (**Table 19.9**).

Due to inflammation, UC presents with small frequent bowel movements, which are often bloody diarrhea. Colicky abdominal pain, urgency, tenesmus, and incontinence of stool are common

TABLE 19.8 Risk Factors for Inflammatory Bowel Disease

Risk Factors	Description
Age and sex	15–40 years of age; slight female predominance in CD; slight male predominance in UC
Race and ethnicity	UC and CD more common in Jews; incidence of IBD lower in Black and Hispanic populations compared to Caucasians
Genetic susceptibility	10%–25% of patients with IBD also have a first-degree relative with either CD or UC.
Smoking	Nicotine-containing products and/or smoking may have direct effect on mucosal lining of the intestines, affecting immune responses, smooth muscle tone, gut permeability, and microvasculature.
Diet	"Western"-style diet (e.g., processed, fried, sugary foods) increases risk of developing CD and possibly UC.
NSAIDs	Cyclooxygenase-mediated disturbance of the intestinal epithelial barrier associated with use of aspirin or other NSAIDs can affect the function between the gut microbiome and immune cells in the intestine lining. NSAIDs and aspirin work to alter platelet aggregation, release inflammatory mediators, and give a microvascular response to stress, which are key events in the pathogenesis of IBD.
Psychosocial factors	Inconsistent results in determining if psychological factors affect IBD; stress may have a role in the exacerbation of symptoms in patients with established IBD.

CD, Crohn's disease; IBD, inflammatory bowel disease; NSAID, nonsteroidal anti-inflammatory drug; UC, ulcerative colitis.

TABLE 19.9 Symptoms Associated With Crohn's Disease

Symptom	Description
Abdominal pain	Crampy
Diarrhea	Fluctuates over a long period of time
Bleeding	Microscopic levels of blood
Fistulas	Inflammation associated with the development of sinus tracts
Phlegmon/abscess	Sinus tracts may present as a phlegmon that may be palpable on physical examination; some sinus tracts lead to abscess formation
Perianal disease	Perianal pain and drainage from large skin tags, anal fissures, perirectal abscesses, and anorectal fistulas
Bile salt malabsorption	Occurs when >50–60 cm of terminal ileum is diseased or resected
Systemic symptoms	Fatigue; weight loss often related to decreased oral intake
Extraintestinal manifestations	Arthritis, eye involvement, skin disorders, primary sclerosing cholangitis, secondary amyloidosis, venous and arterial thromboembolism, renal stones, bone loss and osteoporosis, vitamin B12 deficiency, pulmonary involvement

TABLE 19.10 Laboratory and Diagnostic Studies for Inflammatory Bowel Disease

Condition	Laboratory Testing	Diagnostic Studies
Crohn's disease	CBC CMP CRP ESR Vitamin B12, D, and folate Stool studies (*C. difficile*/Ova and parasites) pANCA and ASCA	Abdominal plain films Small bowel follow through CT scan of abdomen and pelvis CT enterography Magnetic resonance enterography Colonoscopy Capsule ("pill") endoscopy
Ulcerative colitis	CBC CMP CRP ESR Vitamin B12, D, and folate Stool studies (*Clostridium difficile*/Ova and parasites) pANCA and ASCA	Plain films of the abdomen CT scan of abdomen Flexible sigmoidoscopy Colonoscopy

ASCA, antisaccharomyces cerevisiae antibodies; CBC, complete blood count; CMP, comprehensive metabolic profile; CRP, C-reactive protein; ESR, erythrocyte sedimentation rate; pANCA, antineutrophil cytoplasmic antibodies.

symptoms of UC with abdominal pain and tenesmus being most prevalent. The extent and the degree of inflammation correlates directly with the symptoms that are experienced. Less frequently, constipation can be seen in some patients who have distal bowel disease, thus producing symptoms of passing blood and mucus in the stool. Similar to Crohn's disease, signs of malnutrition and other systemic features may be present.[39]

DIAGNOSIS OF INFLAMMATORY BOWEL DISEASE

No single definitive symptom defines CD or UC as there are many varying manifestations of the illness. However, disease diagnosis is based on history, physical examination, laboratory, radiographic, endoscopic, and histological findings (**Table 19.10**).

TREATMENT OF INFLAMMATORY BOWEL DISEASE

Pharmacologic Treatment

The mainstay of treating CD and UC includes 5-aminosalicylates, steroids, antibiotics, and immunomodulators. The goal of treatment in treating both conditions is to relieve clinical symptoms and to cause induction of remission endoscopically, histologically, and clinically.[36,38] Based on the degree and severity of symptoms, location, and severity of disease, drug selections vary. Severe disease states and symptoms require more aggressive therapy, whereas milder symptoms and disease states require less potent medications. Surgical intervention may also be necessary with CD based on clinical signs, diagnostic studies, endoscopic findings, and histology.

Table 19.11 summarizes the drug treatments of IBD, their mechanism of actions, and common side effects.

GASTROESOPHAGEAL REFLUX DISEASE AND PEPTIC ULCER DISEASE

INTRODUCTION

Gastroesophageal reflux disease (GERD) is one of the most common diseases affecting the gastrointestinal system. The overall prevalence of GERD has increased over the last 25 years. This trend has shown that changes in dietary habits and subsequent increases in obesity among the pediatric and young-adult populations have led to an increase in the number of young people diagnosed with GERD. The prevalence of GERD is estimated at 10% to 20% of the general population and 25% to 40% of Americans develop GERD symptoms within their lifetime. Of those, about 7% to 10% report daily symptoms. GERD occurs in all age groups; however, the incidence increases in persons aged 40 and older. Men and women are equally affected.[40]

Each year, approximately 4.5 million individuals in the United States are affected by peptic ulcer disease (PUD). *Helicobacter pylori* (*H. pylori*) infections increase the lifetime prevalence of PUD by about 20%. Overall prevalence of PUD is 0.1% to 1.5%, annually. The approximate lifetime occurrence in men is 11% to 14%; and in women, the estimated occurrence over the life span is 8% to 11%. The rate of occurrence in younger men has shown a steady decline, while rates in older women are increasing. Occurrence and complications related to PUD have decreased in developed countries over the last several decades.[40]

TABLE 19.11 Pharmacotherapy for Inflammatory Bowel Disease

Drug Class	Medication/Dose	Mechanism of Action	Side Effects

5-Aminosalicylates	Crohn's disease and ulcerative colitis:
	  Sulfasalazine, 1–4 g/day divided bid
	  Asacol, 2.4–4.8 g/day divided tid
	  Lialda, 2.4–4.8 g/day once daily
	  Rowasa enema, 1–4 g/day
	  Canasa supplement, 1 g/day
		Unclear; may decrease colonic inflammation	Nausea, vomiting, dyspepsia, headache, malaise

Antibiotics	Crohn's disease:
	  Ciprofloxacin, 500 mg bid
	  Metronidazole, 1–1.5 g/day
		Inhibits DNA-gyrase in susceptible organisms; inhibits relaxation of supercoiled DNA and promotes breakage of double-stranded DNA; interacts with DNA to cause a loss of helical DNA structure and strand breakage resulting in inhibition of protein synthesis and cell death in susceptible organisms	Refer to Chapter 30, "Antimicrobial Pharmacotherapy"

Corticosteroids	Crohn's disease and ulcerative colitis:
	  Prednisone, 40–60 mg/day
	  IV methylprednisolone, 40–60 mg/day
		Decreases inflammation by suppression of migration of polymorphonuclear leukocytes and reversal of increased capillary permeability; regulates gene expression subsequent to binding specific intracellular receptors and translocation into the nucleus	Bradycardia, cardiac arrest, cardiac arrhythmia, cardiac failure, hypertension, arachnoiditis, depression, emotional lability, euphoria, headache, increased intracranial pressure, myasthenia, psychiatric disturbance, infection

Budesonide	Crohn's disease: Budesonide, 9 mg/day (typical dose)	Oral corticosteroid with significant first-pass hepatic metabolism; offers therapy to the gut with reduced systemic effect	Headache, acne vulgaris, moon face, nausea, respiratory tract infection, chest pain, hypertension, viral infection
Thiopurines	Crohn's disease and ulcerative colitis: Azathioprine, 1.5–2.5 mg/kg/day	Derivative of mercaptopurine; metabolites incorporated into replicating DNA and halt replication; blocks the pathway for purine synthesis	Malaise, nausea and vomiting, diarrhea, leukopenia, neoplasia, thrombocytopenia, hepatotoxicity, increased susceptibility to infection

Anti-TNF agents	Crohn's disease and ulcerative colitis:
	  Infliximab IV, 5 mg/kg at 0, 2, and 6 weeks, followed by 5 mg/kg every 8 weeks thereafter
	Ulcerative colitis:
	  Adalimumab, 160 mg (given on day 1 or split and given over 2 consecutive days), then 80 mg 2 weeks later (day 15)
		Chimeric monoclonal antibody that binds to human tumor necrosis factor alpha (TNFα), interfering with endogenous TNFα activity
		Recombinant monoclonal antibody that binds to human (TNFα), interfering with binding to TNFα receptor sites and subsequent cytokine-driven inflammatory processes
			Anemia, increased serum alanine aminotransferase, upper respiratory tract infection, headache, positive antinuclear antibodies titer
			Headache, positive antinuclear antibodies titer, infection, injection site reaction, hypertension, atrial fibrillation, cardiac arrhythmia, nausea, abdominal pain, cholecystitis, increased serum alanine aminotransferase

bid, twice daily; tid, thrice daily.

Intermittent gastroesophageal reflux, or backflow of gastric acid into the esophagus, is a normal physiologic response. However, when excessive backflow occurs, the esophageal lining becomes irritated, resulting in GERD. Normally, the esophagus, the lower esophageal sphincter (LES), and the stomach work in concert to limit the amount and length of time of exposure of acid in the esophagus. Each of the following physiologic dysfunctions may lead to GERD: (a) delayed clearance of gastric acids as a result of decreased esophageal motility, (b) LES malfunctions leading to

large amounts of gastric juice backflow (reflux) into the esophagus, and (c) an increase in the volume and pressure of gastric contents in the stomach due to delayed gastric emptying.

There are two types of peptic ulcer: gastric and duodenal. Gastric ulcers occur in the stomach and duodenal ulcers occur inside the duodenum, which is the upper portion of the small intestine. Normally, there is a physiologic balance between secretion of gastric acids and gastroduodenal mucosa. The superficial layer of this mucosa forms a protective layer that prevents permeation of acid and pepsin, both of which can compromise this defense mechanism.

In addition to this protective layer, some gastroduodenal cells buffer acid in the mucosa by secreting bicarbonate. When these defense mechanisms become compromised, mucosal injury may occur and lead to ulcer formation, and consequently cause PUD. Mucosal compromise may be induced by the following: *H. pylori* infection, nonsteroidal anti-inflammatory drugs (NSAIDs), alcohol consumption, bile salts, gastric acid, and pepsin.

RISK FACTORS OF GASTROESOPHAGEAL REFLUX DISEASE AND PEPTIC ULCER DISEASE

Risk factors for GERD include obesity, hiatal hernia, pregnancy, and delayed stomach emptying. Obesity, a preventable risk factor, can often be managed with lifestyle changes. Hiatal hernia impairs the normal function of the LES, leading to trapped gastric contents and reflux. During pregnancy, hormones may induce relaxation of the LES, which causes reflux of gastric acids into the esophagus. Additionally, uterine enlargement during pregnancy decreases the abdominal space and may cause reflux.

Nonpharmacologic approaches to managing these risk factors include weight loss, eating slowly, eating several small meals each day, avoiding lying down directly after eating, avoiding foods that trigger relaxation of the LES, wearing loose-fitting clothing, elevating the head of the bed, or sleeping on more than one pillow at bedtime.

Risk factors for PUD include previous history of disease, *H. pylori* infection, NSAIDs, concurrent medication use (NSAIDs, antacids, or oral steroids), alcohol or tobacco use, stress, genetics, anemia, and depression. Most cases of PUD are caused by *H. pylori* and NSAID use. *H. pylori* affects approximately half of the population and may not produce symptoms. NSAID-induced PUD risk can be reduced by using the minimum dose necessary and by advising patients to take this medication with food. Genetics and physiologic factors such as increased gastric acid production and stress are also strongly associated with PUD. Nonpharmacologic approaches to lowering the risk of PUD development associated with stress should be individualized based on triggers. These may include stress-reduction techniques and mental health counseling. Determining related causes of increased gastric acid production will guide nonpharmacologic management.

DIAGNOSIS OF GASTROESOPHAGEAL REFLUX DISEASE AND PEPTIC ULCER DISEASE

Gastroesophageal Reflux Disease

The signs and symptoms of GERD can be classified as typical and atypical. The most reported symptom of GERD is heartburn, usually occurring after meals,

when bending over, or when lying down. Heartburn is often worse at night. Regurgitation of food or bitter gastric liquids is another typical symptom of GERD. Overlapping symptoms between GERD and other disease processes may also exist. For example, atypical symptoms include noncardiac chest pain, which may mimic symptoms of ischemic myocardial infarction (MI). Cough and/or wheezing, dysphagia, soreness, or burning in the throat may also be recognized as upper respiratory infections and asthma. Additionally, other atypical symptoms may involve otitis media, hoarseness, epigastric pain and/or discomfort, dyspepsia, hiccups, nausea, and vomiting. Therefore, it is incumbent upon clinicians to obtain a comprehensive health history and include all relevant systems in the review of systems (ROS) and physical examination in order to differentiate between typical symptoms, atypical symptoms signaling GERD complications, and other secondary gastrointestinal diseases. One of the secondary conditions is gastroparesis, which is characterized by abdominal pain, bloating, nausea, vomiting, regurgitation, and constipation. While there is still controversy surrounding whether GERD and eosinophilic esophagitis (EoE) are mutually exclusive conditions, it is important to consider EoE in patients presenting with signs and symptoms of GERD, as the two often coexist. These considerations would aid in accuracy of diagnosis and prevent unnecessary diagnostic testing. **Table 19.12** provides a summary of differential diagnosis for GERD and its differentiating factors, and **Table 19.13** provides diagnostic testing.

Screening for Gastroesophageal Reflux Disease
Screening for GERD is highly dependent on obtaining a history. The most common symptoms consistent with a diagnosis of GERD are heartburn and regurgitation. Initial screening and confirmation for cases of uncomplicated GERD can be achieved by using a combination of clinical presentation and monitoring the patient's response to a medication trial. Patients who respond favorably to the medication often do not require objective testing. For persistent symptoms and/or complicated GERD, diagnostic screening is warranted. In general, routine screening for GERD is not recommended; however, in complicated cases such as Barrett's esophagus, the American Gastroenterological Association (AGA) recommends routine screening.[41]

Peptic Ulcer Disease

The most common symptom of PUD is epigastric pain that is typically characterized as burning. Other symptoms include feeling of fullness, bloating, abdominal pain, and discomfort in the upper abdomen. Pain is often worse after meals and at night. Gastric ulcer pain typically occurs soon after eating; with duodenal ulcers, the pain occurs a few hours after eating. An-

TABLE 19.12 Differential Diagnoses for Gastroesophageal Reflux Disease

Differential Diagnosis	Differentiating Factors
Peptic ulcer disease	Abdominal discomfort: Epigastric pain, burning or gnawing sensation Dyspepsia: Bloating, belching, gas, borborygmus, acidic taste Symptoms of anemia: Fatigue, dyspnea, arrhythmias, weakness
H. pylori infection	Abdominal aches and burning pain; increased pain on empty stomach Nausea Anorexia Dyspepsia Unintentional weight loss
Achalasia	Dysphagia (most common) Weight loss Regurgitation Associated with primary esophageal motility disorder; functional obstruction at the gastroesophageal junction
Dyspepsia	Bloating Belching and gas Borborygmus Acidic taste
Cholelithiasis	Pain: Postprandial; epigastric or right upper quadrant (RUQ), may radiate to the tip of the right scapula; constant; not relieved by antacids or positional changes. Dyspepsia Fat intolerance
Hiatal hernia	Most often asymptomatic Symptomatic patients may experience dysphagia, dyspnea, hematemesis, melena
Acute gastritis	History of previous mucosal injury Epigastric discomfort that worsens or improves with eating May be accompanied by nausea and/or vomiting Often occurs in people who eat raw fish
Chronic gastritis	Usually asymptomatic Symptomatic patients may experience epigastric pain, nausea and/or vomiting, anorexia, early satiety, weight loss
Angina pectoris	Retrosternal chest discomfort: Pressure, heaviness, squeezing, burning, or choking sensation Pain: Epigastric, jaw, neck, shoulders, or back Precipitating factors: Exertion, emotional stress, eating, cold exposure Lasts for approximately 1–5 minutes; position change, cough, and respirations do not change intensity Relieved by rest or nitroglycerin
Eosinophilic esophagitis	Dysphagia (most common) Regurgitation Occurs predominantly in males Most common in children and young adults
Gastroparesis	Regurgitation Bitter, sour taste Nausea Vomiting Early satiety Postprandial fullness Abdominal distention and bloating Abdominal pain Constipation

other distinguishing factor is that the pain from duodenal ulcers may be relieved with antacids or food but patients with gastric ulcers achieve minimal to no relief. Tables 19.14 and 19.15 provide a summary of differential diagnoses, their differentiating factors, and selected diagnostic tests for PUD.

Screening for Peptic Ulcer Disease

Currently, there are no recommendations for routine screening for PUD. Methods and frequency of screening are based on clinical presentation, relevant past medical history, and history of the present illness. Screening for PUD should be guided by the following: (a) symp-

TABLE 19.13 Diagnostic Tests for Gastroesophageal Reflux Disease

Diagnostic Test	Sensitivity/Specificity	Usefulness of Results
Esophagogastroduodenoscopy	62%/97%	Provides anatomical views Confirms GERD diagnosis with combination of history and biopsy specimen analysis Allows identification of presence and degree of existing complications, including strictures, erosive esophagitis, and Barrett's esophagus Provides exclusion data for distinguishing GERD from diseases with similar clinical presentations
Esophageal manometry	84%/89%	Allows assessment of LES function and the esophageal body Detects mechanical esophageal sphincter deficiencies Aids in accurate positioning of probe for 24-hour pH monitoring
Ambulatory 24-hour pH monitoring	96%/95%	Measures the degree of reflux Correlates reflux symptoms and reflux episodes

GERD, gastroesophageal reflux disease; pH, power of hydrogen.

TABLE 19.14 Differential Diagnoses for Peptic Ulcer Disease

Differential Diagnosis	Differentiating Factors
Gastroesophageal reflux disease	Epigastric pain may or may not be present Dyspepsia is an atypical symptom Not associated with anemia No signs of ulcers or esophageal erosions on endoscopic exam
Esophageal or stomach cancer	Family history Lymphadenopathy Weight loss Dysphagia Vomiting Early satiety Bleeding Anemia Dyspepsia onset after age 65 Mass or irregular ulcer on endoscopy Jaundice Palpable mass
Gastroparesis	Regurgitation Bitter, sour taste Nausea Vomiting Early satiety Postprandial fullness Abdominal distention and bloating Abdominal pain Constipation
Irritable bowel syndrome	Irregular bowel habits (diarrhea, constipation, or both) Abdominal pain (may be difficult to distinguish from peptic ulcer disease) Bloating
Functional dyspepsia	Bloating Belching and gas Borborygmus Acidic taste If endoscopic exam normal, then this is a diagnosis of exclusion
Biliary colic	Right upper quadrant pain occurring approximately 30 minutes after meals Pain comes and goes Pain may last minutes to hours at a time Gallstones present with CT or ultrasound inspection
Acute pancreatitis	Sudden onset epigastric pain radiating to the back Nausea Vomiting History of gallstones History of alcohol abuse

TABLE 19.15 Diagnostic Tests for Peptic Ulcer Disease

Diagnostic Test	Sensitivity/Specificity	Usefulness of Results
H. pylori testing: Serum Urea breath test Monoclonal antigen stool tests 　Enzyme immunoassay 　Immunochromatography 　Antibody tests	N/A 97%/100% 92%/94% 69%–87%/87%–93% 76%–84%/79%–80%	Does not distinguish between active and previous infection; Detects only active infection Aids in initial diagnosis and test of cure Detects only active infection Allows for point of care testing and rapid diagnosis Detects only active infection
Esophagogastroduodenoscopy	90%/no data	Provides anatomical views for analysis of the small intestine and stomach Allows for biopsy and cytologic brushing specimen collection to differentiate benign and malignant ulcers Allows antral biopsy for rapid urea and histopathology analysis for detecting *H. pylori* infection

Source: Data from Anand BS. Peptic ulcer disease workup. In: Katz PO, ed. *Medscape.* Updated December 21, 2018. Accessed January 31, 2019. https://emedicine.medscape.com/article/181753-workup#c7; Fashner J, Gitu AC. Diagnosis and treatment of peptic ulcer disease and *H. pylori* infection. *Am Fam Physician.* 2015;91(4):236–242. https://www.aafp.org/afp/2015/0215/afp20150215p236.pdf

toms suggestive of *H. pylori* infection, (b) signs and symptoms of PUD, (c) smokers, and (d) patients who are taking NSAIDs, especially in large quantities.

TREATMENT OF GASTROESOPHAGEAL REFLUX DISEASE AND PEPTIC ULCER DISEASE

The goal of GERD treatment is symptom management, reversing esophagitis, and preventing recurrence and associated complications. The degree of impairment on quality of life determines classification of symptoms as mild or moderate to severe. GERD symptoms occurring less than two times per week are considered intermittent and symptoms occurring two or more times per week are considered frequent. Treatment requires a systematic approach, which can be guided by the frequency and severity of symptoms, impact on quality of life, and the presence of esophageal and/or extra-esophageal complications such as erosive esophagitis or Barrett's esophagus.[41]

The ACG guidelines for the diagnosis and management of GERD include a combination of lifestyle modifications (evidence: conditional; low to moderate) and pharmacological treatment with proton-pump inhibitors (PPIs; evidence: strong, moderate to high), H_2-receptor antagonist (H$_2$RA; evidence: conditional, low to moderate), antacids, surface agents, and alginates (**Table 19.16**). Strength of recommendation ranges from "strong" (desirable outcomes greater than undesirable) to "conditional" (uncertainty regarding trade-offs). Level of evidence is classified as "high" (further research not likely to change confidence in expected outcomes), "moderate" (further research likely to change confidence in expected outcomes), and "low" (further research expected to significantly impact confidence in estimated outcomes and likely to change the expected outcome).

The general approach to management of PUD is to determine and treat the cause and to prevent complications and recurrence. Nonpharmacological management involves discontinuing drugs such as NSAIDs or avoiding and removing triggers such as spicy foods that contribute to PUD symptoms. Pharmacological therapy involves eradication of *H. pylori* with empiric antibiotic treatment based on bacterial resistance patterns. Recommended treatment options are standard triple therapy (only when clarithromycin resistance is low), levofloxacin-based triple therapy, sequential therapy, and quadruple therapy.[42]

The ACG guidelines recommend that dyspepsia be managed with the test-and-treat method in the absence of gastric-cancer alarm symptoms for patients who are younger than 60 years of age. All other patients should be diagnosed with endoscopy and treatment should be based on the diagnostic test results. Test of cure for *H. pylori* eradication is recommended after therapy for *H. pylori*-induced ulcers, ongoing dyspepsia, mucosal lymphoid tissue lymphoma, and gastric cancer resection. While other methods of treatment may be used for *H. pylori*, nonbismuth–based quadruple therapy has the highest rate of success. The ACG recommends the following regarding NSAID use: (a) avoid use in patients at high risk for gastric ulcer, (b) may be used in patients with low risk of GI-related complications, and (c) may be used in conjunction with a PPI or misoprostol in patients with moderate ulcer risk.[42]

Mechanism of Action of Drugs Used to Treat Gastroesophageal Reflux Disease and Peptic Ulcer Disease

Proton-Pump Inhibitors

PPIs inhibit gastric acid secretion in active proton pumps by blocking the gastric enzyme H$^+$/K$^+$-ATPase. As a result,

TABLE 19.16 Pharmacotherapy for Gastroesophageal Reflux Disease and Peptic Ulcer Disease

Drug Class	Drug Name and Dose	Side Effects and Contraindications
PPIs	**Dexlansoprazole (oral)** GERD: 30 mg once daily × 4 weeks **Esomeprazole (oral)** GERD: 20 mg once daily × 14 days (maximum: 20 mg/day); if needed, may repeat treatment after 4 months PUD: 40 mg once daily for up to 8 weeks *Helicobacter pylori* eradiation: *Clarithromycin triple regimen:* 20–40 mg bid in combination with clarithromycin 500 mg bid and either amoxicillin 1 g bid or metronidazole 500 mg tid; continue regimen × 14 days. **Note:** Do not use this regimen in patients with existing macrolide-resistance risk factors: Previous macrolide use, local clarithromycin resistance rates ≥15%, cure rates with clarithromycin-based regimens ≤85% *Bismuth quadruple regimen:* 20 mg bid in combination with tetracycline 500 mg qid, metronidazole 250 mg qid or 500 mg tid–qid, and either bismuth subcitrate 120–300 mg qid or bismuth subsalicylate 300 mg qid; continue regimen × 14 days *Concomitant regimen:* 20 mg bid in combination with amoxicillin 1 g bid, clarithromycin 500 mg bid, and either metronidazole or tinidazole 500 mg bid; continue regimen × 10–14 days *Sequential regimen:* 20 mg bid plus amoxicillin 1 g bid × 5–7 days; then continue esomeprazole along with clarithromycin 500 mg bid, and either metronidazole or tinidazole 500 mg bid × 5–7 days *Hybrid regimen:* 20 mg bid plus amoxicillin 1 g bid × 7 days; then continue esomeprazole and amoxicillin along with clarithromycin 500 mg bid, and either metronidazole or tinidazole 500 mg bid × 7 days *Levofloxacin triple regimen:* 20 mg bid in combination with amoxicillin 1 g bid and levofloxacin 500 mg once daily; continue regimen × 10–14 days **Lansoprazole (oral)** GERD: Short-term treatment—15 mg once daily × ≤8 weeks Duodenal ulcer: Short-term treatment—15 mg once daily × 4 weeks; maintenance therapy—15 mg once daily Dyspepsia (off-label use): 15 or 30 mg once daily × ≤8 weeks Gastric ulcer: Short-term treatment—30 mg once daily × ≤8 weeks *H. pylori* eradication: 30 mg tid administered with amoxicillin 1,000 mg tid × 14 days *or* 30 mg bid administered with amoxicillin 1,000 mg *and* clarithromycin 500 mg bid × 10–14 days *Clarithromycin triple regimen:* 30–60 mg bid in combination with clarithromycin 500 mg bid and either amoxicillin 1 g bid or metronidazole 500 mg tid × 14 days *Sequential regimen:* 30 mg bid plus amoxicillin 1 g bid × 5–7 days; then follow with clarithromycin 500 mg bid, either metronidazole or tinidazole 500 mg bid, and lansoprazole 30 mg bid × 5–7 days *Levofloxacin triple regimen:* 30 mg bid in combination with amoxicillin 1 g bid and levofloxacin 500 mg once daily × 10–14 days *Bismuth quadruple regimen:* 30 mg bid in combination with tetracycline 500 mg qid, metronidazole 250 mg qid or 500 mg tid–qid, and either bismuth subcitrate 120–300 mg qid or bismuth subsalicylate 300 mg qid × 10–14 days	**Side effects:** Headache, diarrhea, constipation, abdominal pain, flatulence, fever, nausea, vomiting, rash, angina, arrhythmias **Contraindications:** Known hypersensitivity to PPIs or any component of the formulation; concomitant use with products containing rilpivirine

(continued)

TABLE 19.16 Pharmacotherapy for Gastroesophageal Reflux Disease and Peptic Ulcer Disease *(continued)*

Drug Class	Drug Name and Dose	Side Effects and Contraindications
	Concomitant regimen: 30 mg bid in combination with amoxicillin 1 g bid, clarithromycin 500 mg bid, and either metronidazole or tinidazole 500 mg bid × 10–14 days	
	Hybrid regimen: 30 mg bid plus amoxicillin 1 g bid × 7 days; then follow with amoxicillin 1 g bid, clarithromycin 500 mg bid, either metronidazole or tinidazole 500 mg bid, and lansoprazole 30 mg bid × 7 days	
	Omeprazole (oral)	
	GERD: 20 mg once daily × ≤4 weeks	
	Duodenal ulcer: 20 mg once daily × 4 weeks; if needed, may be used an additional 4 weeks; ≤40 mg once daily may be used in patients with ulcers refractive to other therapies	
	Gastric ulcers: 40 mg once daily × 4–8 weeks	
	H. pylori eradication:	
	Clarithromycin triple regimen: 20–40 mg bid in combination with clarithromycin 500 mg bid and either amoxicillin 1 g bid or metronidazole 500 mg tid; continue regimen × 14 days	
	Bismuth quadruple regimen: 20 mg bid in combination with tetracycline 500 mg qid, metronidazole 250 mg qid or 500 mg tid–qid, and either bismuth subcitrate 120–300 mg qid or bismuth subsalicylate 300 mg qid; continue regimen × 10–14 days	
	Concomitant regimen: 20 mg bid in combination with amoxicillin 1 g bid, clarithromycin 500 mg bid, and either metronidazole or tinidazole 500 mg bid; continue regimen × 10–14 days	
	Sequential regimen: 20 mg bid plus amoxicillin 1 g bid × 5–7 days; then continue omeprazole along with clarithromycin 500 mg bid, and either metronidazole or tinidazole 500 mg bid × 5–7 days	
	Hybrid regimen: 20 mg bid plus amoxicillin 1 g bid × 7 days; then continue omeprazole and amoxicillin along with clarithromycin 500 mg bid, and either metronidazole or tinidazole 500 mg bid × 7 days	
	Levofloxacin triple regimen: 20 mg bid in combination with amoxicillin 1 g bid and levofloxacin 500 mg once daily; continue regimen × 10–14 days	
	Pantoprazole (oral)	
	GERD (mild): 20 mg once daily	
	GERD-associated esophagitis: 40 mg once daily × ≤8 weeks; may be used for an additional 8 weeks if healing has not occurred; maintenance therapy: 20–40 mg once daily	
	PUD: All regimens are for off-label use	
	Rabeprazole (oral)	
	GERD (nonerosive, symptomatic): 20 mg once daily × ≤4 weeks; may repeat for an additional 4 weeks	
	GERD (erosive or ulcerative): 20 mg once daily × 4–8 weeks; may repeat × ≤8 additional weeks; maintenance therapy: 20 mg once daily	
	Duodenal ulcer: 20 mg once daily × ≤4 weeks	
	H. pylori eradication:	
	Clarithromycin triple regimen: 20–40 mg bid in combination with clarithromycin 500 mg bid and either amoxicillin 1 g bid or metronidazole 500 mg tid; continue regimen × 14 days	
	Bismuth quadruple regimen: 20 mg bid in combination with tetracycline 500 mg qid, metronidazole 250 mg qid or 500 mg tid–qid, and either bismuth subcitrate 120–300 mg qid or bismuth subsalicylate 300 mg qid; continue regimen × 10–14 days	
	Concomitant regimen: 20 mg bid in combination with amoxicillin 1 g bid, clarithromycin 500 mg bid, and either metronidazole or tinidazole 500 mg bid; continue regimen × 10–14 days	
	Sequential regimen: 20 mg bid plus amoxicillin 1 g bid × 5–7 days; then continue rabeprazole along with clarithromycin 500 mg bid, and either metronidazole or tinidazole 500 mg bid × 5–7 days	
	Hybrid regimen: 20 mg bid plus amoxicillin 1 g bid × 7 days; then continue rabeprazole and amoxicillin along with clarithromycin 500 mg bid, and either metronidazole or tinidazole 500 mg bid × 7 days	
	Levofloxacin triple regimen: 20 mg bid in combination with amoxicillin 1 g bid and levofloxacin 500 mg once daily; continue × 10–14 days	

H2RAs	**Nizatidine (oral)** GERD: 150 mg bid × ≤12 weeks Duodenal ulcer: 300 mg once daily at bedtime or 150 mg bid × ≤8 weeks; maintenance therapy: 150 mg once daily at bedtime Gastric ulcer: 150 mg bid or 300 mg once daily bedtime × ≤8 weeks **Famotidine (oral)** GERD: 20 mg bid × ≤6 weeks GERD-associated esophagitis: 20 cr 40 mg bid × ≤12 weeks Duodenal ulcer: 40 mg once daily at bedtime or 20 mg t bid × ≤4–8 weeks; maintenance therapy: 20 mg once daily at bedtime × 1 year or as clinically indicated Gastric ulcer (acute therapy): 40 mg once daily at bedtime × ≤8 weeks **Cimetidine (oral)** GERD: 400 mg qid or 800 mg bid × 12 weeks Duodenal ulcer (active): 300 mg qid or 800 mg at bedtime or 400 mg bid × ≤8 weeks Duodenal ulcer (prophylaxis): 400 mg at bedtime Gastric ulcer (active): 300 mg qid or 800 mg at bedtime × ≤8 weeks **Ranitidine (oral)** GERD: 150 mg bid Duodenal ulcer: 150 mg bid or 300 mg once daily after evening meal or at bedtime; maintenance therapy: 150 mg once daily at bedtime Gastric ulcer: 150 mg bid; maintenance therapy: 150 mg once daily at bedtime	**Side effects:** Headache, drowsiness, fatigue, abdominal pain, constipation, diarrhea **CNS effects:** Delirium, confusion, hallucinations, slurred speech. **Contraindications:** None
Antacids	Alamag®, Alamag® Plus; Alka-Mints®, Alka-Seltzer® Gold Effervescent Antacid; Almacone®, Almacone® II Hi-Potency; AlternaGEL ®, Alu-Cap®, Alu-Tab®, Amphojel®, Antacid Double Strength®, Basaljel®, Calcium Carbonate Suspension; Calcium Carbonate Tablets; Chooz®, Citrocarbonate® Granules; Di-Gel®, Gaviscon®, Gaviscon® Extra Strength; Gaviscon® Liquid; Genaton®; Genaton® Liquid; Kudrox®, Lowsium®; Lowsium® Plus; Maalox Advanced Maximum Strength®; Maalox Advanced Regular Strength®, Maalox®, Maalox® Antacid/Anti-Gas Maximum Strength; Maalox® Max® Quick Dissolve Chewables Antacid/Antigas Maximum Strength; Maalox® Quick Dissolve® Chewables; Maalox® Quick Dissolve® Chewables Maximum Strength; Maalox® TC; Mag-Al®, Mag-Al® Plus; Mag-Al® XS; Mag-Ox® 400; Magnesium Oxide Tablets; Marblen®, Milk of Magnesia; Milk of Magnesia Concentrate; Mygel®, Mygel® II; Mylanta® Children's Upset Stomach Relief; Mylanta® Fast-Acting; Mylanta® Fast-Acting Double Strength; Mylanta® Fast-Acting Maximum Strength; Mylanta® Gelcaps®, Mylanta® Supreme Fast Acting; Pepcid® Complete; Phillips'® Milk of Magnesia; Phillips'® Milk of Magnesia Concentrate; Riopan Plus®, Riopan Plus® Double Strength; Rolaids® Antacid; Rulox®, Rulox® #1; Sodium Bicarbonate Tablets; Tempo®, Titralac® Extra Strength; Titralac® Plus; Titralac® Regular; Tums® Antacid/Calcium Supplement; Tums® E-X Antacid/Calcium Supplement; Tums® Ultra Antacid/Calcium Supplement; Uro-Mag® *All are available OTC and should be used according to package labeling* GERD (mild): Use as directed for relief of meal-induced heartburn PUD: Used as adjunct to other medications	**Side effects:** Nausea, constipation, diarrhea, headaches **Contraindications:** Hypersensitivity to any component of the formulation
Surface agents	**Aluminum sucrose sulfate (oral)** GERD: Used only to treat GERD in pregnancy Duodenal ulcer (active): 1 g qid × 4–8 weeks: maintenance therapy: 1 g bid	**Side effects:** Constipation **Contraindications:** Hypersensitivity to sucralfate or any component of the formulation

bid, twice daily; GERD, gastroesophageal reflux disease; H2RA, H2 receptor antagonist; PPI, proton-pump inhibitor; PUD, peptic ulcer disease; qid, four times daily; tid, thrice daily.

Source: Data from Lexicomp. Accessed February 13, 2019. http://online.lexi.com.proxy.lib.duke.edu/lco/action/search?q=gerd&t=name&va=gerd; Nugent CC, Terrell JM. *H2 Blockers.* StatPearls Publishing. Published January 2018. Updated October 27, 2018. https://www.ncbi.nlm.nih.gov/books/NBK525994

daytime, nocturnal, and meal-stimulated acid secretion is suppressed. All proton pumps are not simultaneously active; therefore, PPIs must be taken for at least 5 to 7 days to achieve a steady state. Inhibition of gastric acid secretion enables healing of GERD, PUD, Barrett's esophagus, and eradicates of *H. pylori* when used in combination with the recommended regimens. PPIs should be administered 30 to 60 minutes before meals. Common side effects include abdominal pain, diarrhea, vomiting, flatulence, headache, constipation, and nausea.

H2-Receptors Antagonists

H₂RAs suppress gastric acid secretion by blocking H₂ receptors on parietal cells. Under normal physiologic conditions, histamine is being released and stimulates the H₂ receptors, which subsequently promotes basal gastric acid secretion. When a H₂RA is administered, it would inhibit the histamine from binding to these receptor sites, causing a reduction of acid release. Symptom relief from H₂RAs occurs in approximately 1 hour and may last 4 to 10 hours, which proves useful for on-demand treatment of intermittent GI symptoms.

Antacids

Antacids decrease esophageal mucosa exposure to gastric acids during reflux episodes by neutralizing gastric pH. Use of antacids is limited to symptomatic and on-demand use in cases of mild GERD because they do not prevent recurrence of GERD. Heartburn relief occurs within 5 minutes but only lasts for 30 to 60 minutes.

Surface Agents and Alginates

Surface agents, such as sucralfate, bind to the gastroduodenal mucosa and, in effect, adhere to duodenal and gastric ulcers and gastric erosions to promote healing. Other mechanisms of action of surface agents include inhibition of pepsin, buffering gastric acids, and bile salt absorption. Efficacy of surface agents is limited due to their short duration of action and use is limited to GERD management in pregnant women. Alginates neutralize postprandial gastric acid and are useful in relieving symptoms after meals for treatment of mild GERD and as an adjuvant to treat refractory GERD.

VIRAL HEPATITIS

INTRODUCTION

Viral hepatitis is the inflammation of the liver, caused by a virus. It encompasses hepatitis A, B, C, D, and E viruses; however, the most common forms are A, B, and C.

Hepatitis A virus (HAV), discovered in 1963, is clinically described as a self-limiting acute illness with viral symptoms and is a member of the genus Hepatovirus.[43] Unlike hepatitis B and C, this disease does not result in chronicity. Because of its asymptomatic presentation, many cases of HAV go undetected and therefore underreported.[44]

Hepatitis B virus (HBV) is a liver infection that occurs when infected blood, semen, or other bodily fluids enter the bloodstream of a noninfected individual. Belonging to the hepadnaviruses, HBV molecularly is a double-stranded DNA virus. Over 250 million people are carriers of HBV worldwide. An estimated 600,000 die every year worldwide from HBV-related liver complications, making this a global public health concern.[45] Due to the increase in intravenous drug use, approximately 20,900 newly acute cases of HBV were diagnosed in the United States in 2016.[46] Hepatitis B can be acute or chronic. Chronic HBV risks decrease with increasing age of onset. The prevalence of new HBV infections has declined from 1990 to 2014 with the most significant decline occurring in children born after 1991 when the recommendation of routine vaccinations was introduced.

Hepatitis C virus (HCV) is a form of viral hepatitis that is blood borne. HCV is a single-stranded RNA virus that originates from the genus Hepacivirus and encompasses six major HCV genotypes. It can be acute or chronic with 70% to 85% of cases becoming chronic, thus leading to cirrhosis, hepatocellular carcinoma, and the need for liver transplantation. It is currently the leading cause of liver transplantation in the United States.[43]

The remaining forms of viral hepatitis are not commonly seen in the United States. Hepatitis D, also known as "delta hepatitis," is only seen in individuals who have HBV as it is an incomplete virus with an inability to stand alone. Hepatitis E is self-limiting in its presentation, thereby avoiding chronicity.

SCREENING FOR VIRAL HEPATITIS

Screening guidelines have been established for hepatitis B and C. For hepatitis B, the screening involves testing for the HBV surface antigen (HBsAg) which has greater than 98% specificity and sensitivity. Further testing for the antibodies to the hepatitis B surface antigen (anti-HBs) and hepatitis B core antigen (anti-HBc) should also be done to differentiate between active infection and immunity. When a person has negative results of both HBsAg and anti-HBs, it is indicative of susceptibility. In other words, the patient has neither been exposed to HBV nor develops antibodies against the virus. Furthermore, if the HBsAg result is negative while anti-HBs and anti-HBc are positive, these results may be interpreted as immunity due to natural infection. On the other hand, if HBsAg and anti-HBc are negative, but anti-HBs is positive, these results imply that the patient has developed immunity due to vaccination. While no guidelines on proper screening intervals exist, periodic screening is recommended for those at risk and who are not immunized.[47]

For individuals who were born between 1945 and 1965, those with continued risks for HCV (IV drug abusers, hemodialysis), and those who have received blood transfusions or organ transplantation prior to universal blood screenings, it is recommended that they receive HCV screening using the highly sensitive (>90%) anti-HCV antibody test followed by confirmatory polymerase chain reaction (PCR) testing[48] (**Figure 19.1**).

DIAGNOSIS OF VIRAL HEPATITIS

Because viral hepatitis is a viral illness, it can be confused with many other diseases ranging from a viremia to a more chronic debilitating condition. Laboratory values, x-ray studies, and biopsies are used to make a definitive diagnosis (**Table 19.17**) and to assess the degree of damage occurring due to the disease process.

TREATMENT OF VIRAL HEPATITIS

Nonpharmacological Treatment

Because HAV and acute HEV are self-limiting, supportive care is the mainstay of treatment. Medications that could be hepatotoxic or metabolized by the liver should be used with caution in these individuals. Nonpharmacological interventions can be used to treat some of the symptoms that accompany viral hepatitis; however, with hepatitis B, C, D, and E (chronic) medications are needed to achieve a sustained virological response.

Pharmacological Treatment

The pharmacological treatment of viral hepatitis can range from supportive measures to the use of antiviral medications due to the presence of viremia. With hepatitis B, C, D, and E in its chronic state, antivirals are used to suppress and eradicate the virus, thus preventing the long-term effects of these conditions (**Table 19.18**). According to the American Association for the Study of Liver Diseases (AASLD) 2018 guidelines,[49] the preferred treatments for chronic HBV are Peg-IFN-2a for adult, and Peg-IFN-2b for children. In addition, oral therapies such as entecavir, tenofovir disoproxil fumarate (TDF), or tenofovir alafenamide (TAF), are also considered as first-line agents. Meanwhile, lamivudine and adefovir are less favorable due to high risk of resistance.[49]

The selection of drug treatment for chronic HCV is dependent on whether the patient is treatment naïve or experienced. Furthermore, the viral genotype as well as the status of liver cirrhosis also aids

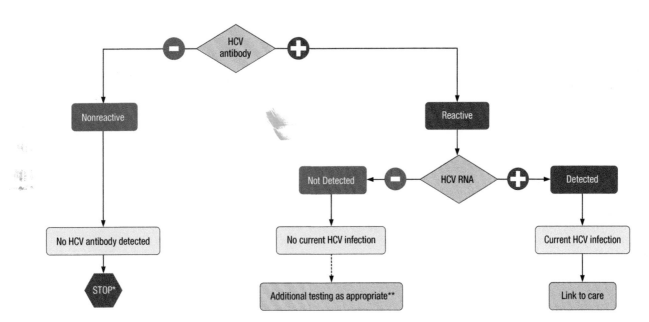

FIGURE 19.1 Recommended testing sequence for hepatitis C virus (HCV).

*For persons who might have been exposed to HCV within the past 6 months, testing for HCV RNA or follow-up testing for HCV antibody is recommended. For persons who are immunocompromised, testing for HCV RNA can be considered.

**To differentiate past, resolved HCV infection from biologic false positivity for HCV antibody, testing with another HCV antibody assay can be considered. Repeat HCV RNA testing if the person tested is suspected to have had HCV exposure within the past 6 months or has clinical evidence of HCV disease, or if there is concern regarding the handling or storage of the test specimen.

Source: With permission from Centers for Disease Control and Prevention. Testing for HCV infection: an update of guidance for clinicians and laboratories. *MMWR Morb Mortal Wkly Rep.* 2013;62(18):362–365. https://www.cdc.gov/mmwr/preview/mmwrhtml/mm6218a5.htm

TABLE 19.17 Differential Diagnoses and Diagnostic Tests for Viral Hepatitis

Type	Differential Diagnoses	Laboratory Tests	Diagnostic Tests
Hepatitis A	Adenovirus Hepatitis B, C, D, E Cytomegalovirus Herpes simplex virus Epstein-Barr Acute HIV infection Drug-induced hypersensitivity reactions	IgM anti-HAV Anti-HAV IgG Transaminase	None
Hepatitis B	Hepatitis A, C, D, E HIV STI Alcohol hepatitis Autoimmune hepatitis Cholangitis Hemochromatosis Wilson disease	HBsAg Anti-HBs HBeAg Anti-HBc Immunoglobulin IgM Hepatitis B DNA quantitative/qualitative Transaminase study	None
Hepatitis C	Hepatitis A, C, D, E Autoimmune hepatitis Cholangitis	Hepatitis C antibody (anti-HCV) Hepatitis C RNA antibody (HCV RNA quantitative/qualitative) Transaminase study	Liver biopsy Ultrasound elastography Magnetic resonance elastography Fibrosure or fibrotest
Hepatitis D	Alcoholic hepatitis Autoimmune hepatitis Budd–Chiari syndrome Cholangitis Cholecystitis Hepatitis A, B, C, E Liver abscess	HDAg Anti-HDV HDV RNA Quantitative	None
Hepatitis E	Hepatitis A, B, C, D HIV CMV Acute drug-induced liver injury Drug-induced hypersensitivity reactions Budd–Chiari syndrome	Anti-HEV IgM HEV RNA	None

anti-HBc, antibody to hepatitis B core antigen; anti-HBs, antibody to hepatitis B surface antigen; anti-HDV, antibody to hepatitis D virus; anti-HEV IgM, anti-hepatitis E virus immunoglobulin G; HBeAg, hepatitis B e antigen; HBsAg, hepatitis B surface antigen; HBV, hepatitis B virus; HDAg, hepatitis D antigen; HDV RNA, hepatitis D ribonucleic acid quantitative virus; HEV RN, hepatitis E virus ribonucleic acid quantitative virus.

the selection of therapy. In general, the duration of therapy is recommended for 12 weeks, except glecaprevir (300 mg)/pibrentasvir (120 mg), which is recommended for 8 weeks with or without compensated cirrhosis for all viral genotypes (i.e., genotype 1–6). The treatment of HCV is continuously evolving as new and effective therapies become available; therefore, it is prudent for clinicians to follow updates recommended from the AASLD and Infectious Diseases Society of America (IDSA).[50] For further details of the current guidelines of HCV treatments, visit www.hcvguidelines.org.

The only treatment of hepatitis D virus (HDV) during the last three decades is interferon-alfa (IFN-alfa). Since the pegylated form of IFN-alfa was shown to associate with higher response rate than the standard IFN-alfa, it is considered as a first-line agent. Further, the course of the therapy is usually offered for 1 year to patients who are treatment naïve or nonresponsive to the standard IFN-alfa.[51] There are a few studies of HDV treatments that target different mechanisms of actions such as the sodium taurocholate cotransporting polypeptide (NTCP) inhibitors, farnesyltransferase inhibitors (FTIs), and nucleic acid polymers (NAPs). However, all of these agents are still under clinical investigations.[51]

The primary treatment of hepatitis E viral infection is supportive care. Though oral ribavirin therapy has been used in recipients of solid organ transplant with chronic hepatitis E, the therapy is approved by the FDA only for chronic hepatitis C.[52,53] Refer to Table 19.18 for further details of ribavirin.

TABLE 19.18 Pharmacotherapy for Viral Hepatitis

Type	Drug/Dose	Side Effects	Comments
Hepatitis B[20]	Peg-IFN-2a (adult) 180 mcg SC weekly	Flu-like symptoms, fatigue, mood disturbances, cytopenias, autoimmune disorders	BBW: Can cause fatal or life-threatening neuropsychiatric, autoimmune, ischemic, and infectious disorders Peg-IFN-2: Hypersensitivity reactions to peginterferon alfa-2a, other alfa interferons; autoimmune hepatitis; hepatic decompensation, cirrhosis, HIV CrCl <30 mL/minute → 135 mcg SC weekly
	Entecavir 0.5 or 1.0 mg po daily	Lactic acidosis	Hypersensitivity to entecavir or any component of the formulation CrCl = 30–49 → 0.5 mg po q48h CrCl = 10–29 → 0.5 mg po q72h CrCl <10 → 0.5 mg po every week
	Tenofovir disoproxil fumarate (TDF) 300 mg PO daily Tenofovir alafenamide (TAF) 25 mg po daily	Nephropathy, Fanconi syndrome, osteomalacia, lactic acidosis	CrCl <10 mL/min → avoid use Avoid with cobicistat if CrCl <70 mL/minute
	Lamivudine 100 mg po daily	Pancreatitis, lactic acidosis	Hypersensitivity to lamivudine or any component of the formulation CrCl = 30–49 mL/min → 100 mg × 1, then 50 mg (solution) po daily CrCl = 15–29 mL/min → 100 mg × 1, then 25 mg (solution) po daily
	Adefovir 10 mg po daily	Acute renal failure, Fanconi syndrome, nephrogenic diabetes insipidus, lactic acidosis	Hypersensitivity to adefovir or any component of the formulation CrCl = 30–49 → give q48h CrCl = 10–29 → give q72h

Available Direct-Acting Antiviral Agents and Their Targets

Hepatitis C[21]	NS3/4 (Protease Inhibitors)	NS 5A	NS 5B (RNA Polymerase Inhibitors)
	Simeprevir Paritaprevir Grazoprevir Glecaprevir	• Ledipasvir • Ombitasvir • Velpatasvir • Elbasvir • Pibrentasvir	Nonnucleotide: Dasabuvir Nucleotide: Sofosbuvir

Combination Products

Drug/Dose	Side Effects	Comments
Ledipasvir–sofosbuvir 90/400 mg one tab po daily	Fatigue, headache, nausea, insomnia	Severe renal impairment: not defined Mild to moderate renal impairment: no adjustment
Glecaprevir 100 mg and pibrentasvir 40 mg three tabs po daily	Headache, fatigue, aminotransferase, bilirubin	Child-Pugh class B or C cirrhosis: Contraindicated Renal impairment: No adjustment
Elbasvir 50 mg and grazoprevir 100 mg po once daily	Headache, fatigue, nausea, aminotransferase elevations	Child-Pugh class B or C cirrhosis: contraindicated

(continued)

TABLE 19.18 Pharmacotherapy for Viral Hepatitis *(continued)*

Type	Drug/Dose	Side Effects	Comments
	Velpatasvir 100 mg and sofosbuvir 400 mg PO once daily	Headache, fatigue, nausea, nasopharyngitis, and insomnia	When co-administered with ribavirin, combination regimen
	Ombitasvir 12.5 mg/paritaprevir 75 mg/ritonavir 50 mg two tabs po qam + dasabuvir 250 mg one tab po bid	Fatigue, insomnia, hyperbilirubinemia, elevation of ALT, hepatic decompensation	Moderate to severe hepatic impairment: Contraindicated
	Velpatasvir 100 mg, sofosbuvir 400 mg, voxilaprevir 100 mg one tab PO daily	Headache, insomnia, diarrhea, elevation of CK, bradycardia, HBV reactivation, angioedema	Child-Pugh Class B or C: Contraindicated
Single Active Ingredient Products[a]			
	Sofosbuvir 400 mg po daily	Fatigue, headache, insomnia, nausea, diarrhea, elevation of bilirubin and CK, bradycardia, angioedema, HBV reactivation	Black-Box Warning: Screen for HBV infection before initiating due to HBV reactivation; monitor for hepatitis flare and hepatic failure. Peginterferon alfa 2b and daclatasvir: No longer available in United States
	Ribavirin 400–700 mg po bid or 600–1,000 mg po daily	Headache, insomnia, dizziness, rash, depression, hemolytic anemia, fever/rigors, alopecia, diarrhea, thrombocytopenia, pancreatitis	Child-Pugh Class B or C or autoimmune hepatitis: Contraindicated
Hepatitis D[22]	Pegylated interferon alfa 180 mcg weekly (Peg-intron)	Flu-like symptoms, hepatic, hematologic, respiratory, skin, genitourinary, cardiovascular, thyroid disturbances, dental and visual disorders, injection site reactions, psychiatric effects, hemorrhagic colitis, pancreatitis	Hepatitis decompensation before or during treatment, autoimmune hepatitis. Combination with ribavirin contraindicated in pregnancy, men with pregnant partners, hemoglobinopathies and CrCl <50 mL/minute
Hepatitis E	Ribavirin 600–1,000 mg daily	Anemia, flu-like symptoms, cardiac and pulmonary events, psychiatric effects, dizziness, nausea and vomiting, alopecia, rash, pruritis, diabetes, fatigue, headache myalgia, pancreatitis, dental and periodontal disorders	Contraindications: Autoimmune hepatitis, hemoglobinopathies, renal impairment, male partners of pregnant women. Pregnancy (e.g., birth defects or fetal death). Concomitant with didanosine

[a] Available in United States.

AASLD, American Association for the Study of Liver Diseases; ALT, alanine aminotransferase; CK, creatine kinase; CrCl, creatinine clearance; HBV, hepatitis B virus; IDSA, Infectious Diseases Society of America; po, by mouth; qam, every morning; SC, subcutaneous.

NUTRACEUTICALS

Nutraceuticals are nutritional products that have pharmaceutical activity beyond its nutritional value in the United States. They are often used to prevent and treat various conditions. Popular nutraceuticals include echinacea, omega-3, and folic acid. Other formulas—such as probiotics or live bacteria—are also often discussed with nutraceuticals. Meanwhile, prebiotics are specialized plant fibers that enhance the body's "good" bacteria in the gut. Bioactive plant compounds and probiotic bacteria interact with host cells and alter intracellular signal transduction pathways, resulting in a specific mediated host response. Probiotics are thought to either block adhesion of pathogenic bacteria to the intestinal lining, enhance intestinal immune response, repair intestinal permeability, bind to gram-negative bacteria to suppress growth of pathogenic bacteria, or increase intestinal absorption of electrolytes. The most common probiotics are *Lactobacillus* (*L. rhamnosus, L. acidophilus*), *Bifidobacterium*, and *Saccharomyces boulardii*; for example, the common over-the-counter (OTC) products such as Culturelle contains (*L. rhamnosus* GG), Align (*Bifidobacterium*), and Activia (*Bifidobacterium*). Probiotics have shown benefits when used in patients with GI complaints (see **Table 19.19**). Potential risks associated with the use of nutraceuticals include allergy to compounds, toxicity, endogenous/exogenous contaminants, or possible secondary contaminants. Most probiotics are generally safe; however, common side effects may include constipation, flatulence, hiccups, nausea, infection, and rash.[54]

A Cochrane review found that a dosage of 5 billion colony-forming units (CFUs) or greater per day was significantly more effective than a lower dosage.[54] There is a lack of clear guidelines for dosing and treatment length for prescribing probiotics. Probiotic species and brands vary in available CFUs and recommended length of treatment. Table 19.19 provides a summary of the current available evidence and selected treatments of various GI conditions.

TABLE 19.19 Probiotic Drugs for Select Gastrointestinal Conditions

Condition	Selected Treatments		Results	Evidence Rating
Helicobacter pylori infection	*Bacillus clausii, coagulans* *Bifidobacterium animalis subsp lactis, bifidum, breve, longum* *Clostridium butyricum* *Lactobacillus acidophilus, casei, rhamnosus, rhamnosus GG*	10 billion colony forming units per day Adjunct to antibiotics	Inhibits extracellular, intracellular, and antibiotic-resistant strains; prevents benzopyrene-induced gastric tumors; inhibits gastric mucosal adhesion	N/A
Irritable bowel syndrome	*Bifidobacterium animalis subsp lactis, bifidum, breve, longum* *Enterococcus faecalis* *Escherichia coli* (Nissle) *Lactobacillus acidophilus, casei, rhamnosus, rhamnosus GG*	Unknown	Improved abdominal pain in children and adults	B
Ulcerative colitis	*Bifidobacterium animalis subsp lactis, bifidum, breve, longum* *Escherichia coli* (Nissle) *Lactobacillus acidophilus, casei, rhamnosus, rhamnosus GG*	High-dose products with several species of *Bifidobacterium* preferred	Increased remission rates	A
Acute infectious diarrhea	*Lactobacillus rhamnosus, acidophilus* *Saccharomyces boulardii*	—	Reduced severity and duration of illness	NA
Clostridium difficile-associated diarrhea	*Bifidobacterium animalis subsp lactis, bifidum, breve, longum* *Clostridium butyricum* *Lactobacillus acidophilus, casei, rhamnosus GG*	—	Typically with duration of antibiotics or up to 5 days after	B

Evidence Ratings: A, consistent, good-quality evidence; B, inconsistent or limited quality patient-oriented evidence; C, consensus, disease-oriented evidence, usual practice, expert opinion, or case series.

Source: Data from Wilkins T, Sequoia J. Probiotics for gastrointestinal conditions: a summary of the evidence. *Am Fam Physician*. 2017;96(3):170–178A. https://www.aafp.org/afp/2017/0801/p170.html

ENTERAL/PARENTERAL NUTRITION

Enteral or parenteral delivery of calories, protein, electrolytes, vitamins, minerals, and fluids may be necessary for a certain condition and chronic illnesses. When patients do not obtain enough nutrients through the normal oral diets or have impaired GI functions, they may need nutritional supplementation via enteral or parenteral route. Examples of conditions that require nutritional support are intestinal failure or short bowel syndrome. Although short bowel syndrome is a relatively rare condition that equally affects both males and females, the disorder is usually acquired as a complication of Crohn's disease and requires a surgical removal of a significant section or all of the small intestines. Congenital causes of the disorder are very rare with the most common etiology being necrotizing enterocolitis.[55]

Treatment involves a coordinated team of specialists. Specific therapies vary depending on the patient's specific nutritional requirements, the severity of symptoms, and the extent of the small intestine and/or colon involvement. Once it has been determined that a patient requires nutrition support, individualized nutritional requirements must be determined (**Table 19.20**). Current guidelines recommend enteral supplementation as the preferred route of nutrition delivery when feasible.[56]

NUTRIENT-DRUG INTERACTIONS

The increasing popularity of food supplements and herbal products to deliver health-enhancing macro- and micronutrients has led to an increased risk of adverse interactions between prescribed drugs and these potentially bioactive compounds. Drug-nutrient interactions (DNI) are classified as "any food, herbal medicine, or dietary supplement induced changes in the oral bioavailability leading to changes in drug availability that may affect efficacy and/or toxicity."[57] DNIs can be viewed as either pharmaceutic, pharmacodynamic, or pharmacokinetic (**Table 19.21**). The small intestines contain a high amount of cytochrome (CYP) P450 and is the first step of the first-pass effect for drugs taken orally. Well-known risk factors for drug-nutrient interactions (DNI) are age, malnutrition, malabsorption, chronic liver disease, kidney failure, and polymedication. Common DNIs are listed in **Table 19.22**.

TABLE 19.20 Total Parenteral Nutrition and Home Nutrition Dosing and Side Effects

Dosing	Therapy	Side Effects
Dosing weight*= IBW + 0.4(ABW−IBW) Dosing weight = 1.1 * IBW **Calories** Start: 8–10 kcal/kg/day Goal: 25–35 kcal/kg/day **Protein** Mild-to-moderate illness: 0.8–1.2 g/kg protein per day Critically ill: 1.2–1.5 g/kg/day	Enteral nutrition	Aspiration Diarrhea Hyperglycemia Micronutrient deficiencies Constipation Fluid/water deficiency Refeeding syndrome
	Parenteral nutrition	Catheter-related sepsis Hyperglycemia Serum electrolyte imbalance Macro- or micronutrient excess or deficiency Hepatic dysfunction Refeeding syndrome

*For patients who are underweight, recommendations are to use current weight as dosing weight to prevent refeeding syndrome.

ABW, actual body weight; IBW, ideal body weight.

Source: Data from Pironi L, Arends J, Bozzetti F, et al. ESPEN guidelines on chronic intestinal failure in adults. *Clin Nutr.* 2016;35(2):247–307. doi:10.1016/j.clnu.2016.01.020

TABLE 19.21 Nutrient–Drug Interaction Classifications

Type of Interaction	Mechanism of Interaction	Example
Pharmaceutic	Physiochemical reactions taking place in a delivery device such as an enteral feeding tube or the gastrointestinal lumen	Ciprofloxacin absorption reduced due to chelation with enteral nutrition formula
Pharmacodynamic	Drugs' clinical effect; nutrients' physiological effect	Antagonistic: Warfarin and vitamin K results in decreased international normalized ratio Additive: Warfarin and vitamin E increases bleeding risk
Pharmacokinetic	Changes in bioavailability, clearance, distribution volume	Grapefruit juice inhibits CYP3A4, leading to higher blood concentrations of the nonmetabolized form of drug

TABLE 19.22 Selected Drug–Nutrient Interactions

Nutrient	Prescribed Drug	Clinical Manifestation
Grapefruit juice	CYP3A4 pathway drugs: Calcium channel blockers Amiodarone, apixaban, eplerenone, quinidine Antiinfectives (erythromycin, primaquine) Clopidogrel Buspirone, dextromethorphan, ketamine Simvastatin, atorvastatin	CYP3A4 inhibition: Severe hypotension, weakness, lower-limb edema Torsades de pointe, GI bleeding, cardiac arrhythmia Torsades de pointe, bone marrow suppression Decreased efficacy Hallucination, dizziness, increased sedation, drowsiness Rhabdomyolysis
Gingko biloba	Vitamin K antagonists (aspirin, NSAIDs) Sodium valproate	Increased bleeding Decreased efficacy
Ginseng	Oral antidiabetic agents	Increased risk of hypoglycemia
Saint John's wort	Digoxin, nifedipine, verapamil, oral contraceptives, oral anticoagulants, benzodiazepines, amitriptyline, buspirone, methadone, sertraline, phenytoin, simvastatin, atorvastatin, cimetidine, omeprazole Oral contraceptives Clozapine Insulin detemir Metronidazole	Decreased efficacy Menorrhagia Psychotic disorder Blood glucose fluctuation Confusion, flu-like illness, increased body temperature
Fish oil	Lithium	Potential drug interaction
Fish oil tablets	Enalapril	Hypertension
Folic acid; vitamin B6	Phenprocoumon	Increased international normalized ratio
Vitamin C	Nicotine	Myocardial infarction

GI, gastrointestinal.

Source: Data from de Boer A, van Hunsel F, Bast A. Adverse food–drug interactions. *Regul Toxicol Pharmacol.* 2015;73(3):859–865. doi:10.1016/j.yrtph.2015.10.009

CASE EXEMPLAR: Patient With Sudden Onset of Intermittent Mid-Epigastric Pain

PR is a 35-year-old female who presents with a sudden onset of intermittent mid-epigastric pain that started 4 weeks ago. Pain is 6/10 on the pain scale and described as burning that worsens after she eats Mexican food and when she is lying down. She has never experienced this before. PR reports that she has been taking over-the-counter (OTC) antacids that seemed to help at first, but now they provide no relief. She reports associated regurgitation and feeling of fullness all the time and this morning she had a sore throat.

Past Medical History
- Anaphylactic reaction to penicillin

Medications
- OTC antacids

Family History
- Noncontributory

Social History
- Occupation: Elementary school teacher (10 years)
- Nonsmoker
- Denies illicit drug use
- Consumes wine two to three times per month
- Regular exercise

Physical Examination
- Weight: 145 lbs.; blood pressure: 128/72; pulse: 80; respiration rate: 18; temperature: 98.7 °F
- General: Calm, cooperative, in no apparent distress
- Eyes: Pupils equal, round, reactive to light
- Ears: Tympanic membranes clear
- Nares: Without nasal septal deviation; pharyngeal mucosa pink and moist
- Throat: Oropharynx without edema, erythema, tonsillar enlargement, lesions
- Abdomen: Nondistended, soft, round, non-tender; normoactive bowel sounds in all quadrants

Discussion Questions

1. What are the top three differential diagnoses for PR?
2. What diagnostic tests, if any, are required for PR?
3. What pharmacological, nonpharmacological, and/or nutraceutical therapies should be prescribed for PR?
4. The results from PR's *H. pylori* test returned positive. What treatment should be added to her plan of care?

CASE EXEMPLAR: Patient With Diarrhea

CD is a 72-year-old male who presents with a complaint of diarrhea. He had recently been hospitalized for confirmed COVID-19 and was released on broad-spectrum antibiotics for concomitant pneumonia. He left the hospital on oral medications 4 days ago and his diarrhea started 2 days ago. He also complains of nausea, pain in the abdomen, and a low-grade fever. He has not seen blood in the stool. His appetite is poor, and he is not urinating much. His cough has resolved.

Past Medical History
- Status post COVID-19 infection
- Recent bacterial pneumonia, organism unknown
- Coronary artery disease with a previous drug-eluting stent

Medications
- Lisinopril, 20 mg daily
- Verapamil, 120 mg twice daily
- Amoxicillin/clavulanate, 875 mg/125 mg twice daily
- Multivitamin

Physical Examination
- Height: 70 inches; weight: 172 lbs.; blood pressure: 132/58; pulse: 90; respiration rate: 16; temperature: 100.4 °F

- Well-developed, underweight man in no distress
- Poor skin turgor
- Lungs: Scattered rhonchi in bases
- Heart: Regular rate and rhythm, grade II/VI systolic ejection murmur
- Abdomen: Soft, hyperactive bowel sounds, diffuse mild tenderness without guarding or rebound, no masses
- Rectal exam: Prostate 3+ enlarged, liquid stool, hemoccult positive

Labs and Imaging
- Complete blood count significant for leukocytosis: WBC 15.1×10^9/L, leukocytes $14,000 \times 10^9$/L
- Sodium: 150 mEq/L
- Potassium: 2.8 mEq/L
- Chest x-ray: clear
- Abdominal x-ray: Significant air in the GI tract; no ileus; no free air

Discussion Questions
1. What are the top three presumptive diagnoses for CD?
2. Why did CD develop diarrhea?
3. How should CD's diarrhea be managed?

KEY TAKEAWAYS

- Anticholinergics—such as scopolamine—treat nausea by inhibiting acetylcholine at cholinergic sites in smooth muscles, secretory glands, and the central nervous system (CNS). Benzamides block dopamine receptors and serotonin receptors in the chemoreceptor trigger zone (CTZ) of the CNS and enhance motility in the GI tract without stimulating gastric, biliary, or pancreatic secretions.
- Cannabinoids block nausea as a result of their stimulation at the cannabinoid-1 (CB_1) receptors and decrease GI motility, showing promise in nausea in patients receiving chemotherapies; 5-HT3 antagonists—such as ondansetron—inhibit serotonin peripherally on vagal nerve terminals and centrally in the chemoreceptor trigger zone.
- Loperamide and opioids reduce the frequency of bowel movement by binding to opioid receptors on the intestinal smooth muscles, leading to a decrease in GI motility. These agents slow peristalsis and prolong transit time, leading to increased stool viscosity. Laxatives increase colonic fluid retention, act on the colonic mucosa to decrease luminal water absorption, or increase intestinal motility.
- The mainstays of treating Crohn's disease and ulcerative colitis include 5-aminosalicylates, steroids, antibiotics, and immunomodulators.
- ACG guidelines for diagnosing and managing GERD and peptic ulcer disease include a combination of lifestyle modifications and pharmacologic treatment with PPIs, H_2RAs, antacids, surface agents, and alginates.
- The pharmacological treatment of viral hepatitis ranges from supportive measures to the use of antiviral medications based on the presence of viremia with the goal of suppressing and eradicating the virus to prevent the long-term effects of these conditions.
- Probiotics are thought to either block adhesion of pathogenic bacteria to the intestinal lining, enhance intestinal immune response, repair intestinal permeability, bind to gram-negative bacteria to suppress growth of pathogenic bacteria, or increase intestinal absorption of electrolytes.

REFERENCES

1. Singh P, Yoon SS, Kuo B. Nausea: a review of patho-physiology and therapeutics. *Therap Adv Gastroenterol. 2016*;9(1):98–112. doi.10.1177/1756283X15618131

2. Novartis Consumer Health. *Transderm scop (scopolamine)* [package insert]. U.S. Food and Drug Administration website. Updated April 2013. https:// www.accessdata .fda.gov/drugsatfda_docs/label/2013/017874s038lbl.pdf

3. Schaefer TS, Zito PM. Antiemetic histamine H1 receptor blockers. In: *StatsPearls* [Internet] StatPearls Publishing. Updated September 29, 2020. https:// www.ncbi.nlm.nih .gov/books/NBK533003

4. ANI Pharmaceutical. *Reglan (metoclopramide)* [package insert]. U.S. Food and Drug Administration website. Updated August 2017. https://www.accessdata.fda.gov/drugsatfda_docs/label/2017/017854s062lbl.pdf

5. MEDA Manufacturing GmbH. *Ativan (lorazepam)* [package insert]. U.S. Food and Drug Administration website. Published September 2016. https://www.accessdata.fda .gov/drugsatfda_docs/label/2016/017794s044lbl.pdf

6. Parker LA, Rock EM, Limebeer CL. Regulation of nausea and vomiting by cannabinoids. *Br J Pharmacol*. 2011;163(7):1411–1422. doi:10.1111/j.1476 -5381.2010.01176.x

7. AbbVie. *Marinol (dronabinol)* [package insert]. U.S. Food and Drug Administration website. Updated August 2017. https://www.accessdata.fda.gov/drugsatfda_docs/label/2017/018651s029lbl.pdf

8. Valeant Pharmaceuticals International. *Cesamet (nabilone)* [package insert]. U.S. Food and Drug Administration website. Updated May 2006. https://www.accessdata .fda.gov/drugsatfda_docs/label/2006/018677s011lbl.pdf

9. Vayne-Bossert P, Haywood A, Good P, et al. Corticosteroids for adult patients with advanced cancer who have nausea and vomiting (not related to chemotherapy, radiotherapy, or surgery). *Cochrane Database Syst Rev*. 2017;(7):CD012002. doi:10.1002/14651858.CD012002 .pub2

10. Merck & Co. *Decadron (dexamethasone)* [package insert]. U.S. Food and Drug Administration website. Accessed May 14, 2020. https://www.accessdata.fda.gov/drugs atfda_docs/label/2004/11664slr062_decadron_lbl.pdf

11. Fresenius Kabi. *Aloxi (polanosetron)* [package insert]. U.S. Food and Drug Administration website. Updated December 2018. https://www.accessdata.fda .gov/drugsatfda_docs/label/2018/208109s001lbl.pdf

12. GlaxoSmithKline. *Zofran (ondansetron)* [package insert]. U.S. Food and Drug Administration website. Updated October 2016. https:// www.accessdata.fda.gov/ drugsatfda_docs/ label/2016/020103s035_020605s019_020 781s019lbl.pdf

13. Merck & Co., Inc. *Emend (aprepitant)* [package insert]. U.S. Food and Drug Administration website. Updated December 2015. https://www.accessdata.fda .gov/drugsatfda_docs/label/2015/207865lbl.pdf

14. GlaxoSmithKline. *Compazine (prochlorperazine)* [package insert]. U.S. Food and Drug Administration website. Published July 2004. https://www.accessdata .fda.gov/drugsatfda_docs/label/2005/010571s096lbl.pdf

15. Ochoa B, Surawicz CM. *Diarrheal disease—acute and chronic*. University of Washington School of Medicine. Published October 2002. Updated December 2012. https://gi.org/topics/diarrhea-acute-and-chronic

16. DuPont HL. Persistent diarrhea: a clinical review. *JAMA*. 2016;315(24):2712–2723. doi:10.1001/jama.2016.7833

17. Barr W, Smith A. Acute diarrhea in adults. *Am Fam Physician*. 2014;89(3):180–189. https://www.aafp.org/afp/2014/0201/p180.html

18. Lamb CA, Mansfield JC. Measurement of faecal calprotectin and lactoferrin in inflammatory bowel disease. *Frontline Gastroenterol*. 2011;2:13–18. doi:10.1136/fg.2010.001362

19. Riddle MS, DuPont HL, Conner BA. ACG clinical guideline: diagnosis, treatment, and prevention of acute diarrheal infections in adults. *Am J Gastroenterol*. 2016;111:602–622. doi:10.1038/ajg.2016.126

20. National Center for Biotechnology Information. PubChem compound summary for CID 16682734, bismuth subsalicylate. Accessed May 16, 2020. https://pubchem .ncbi.nlm.nih.gov/compound/Bismuth-subsalicylate

21. Bharucha AE, Pemberton JH, Locke GR, 3rd. American Gastroenterological Association technical review on constipation. *Gastroenterology*. 2013;144(1):218–238. doi:10.1053/j.gastro.2012.10.028

22. Tamura A, Tomita T, Oshima T, et al. Prevalence and self-recognition of chronic constipation: results of an internet survey. *J Neurogastroenterol Motil*. 2016;22(4):677–685. doi:10.5056/jnm15187

23. Werth BL, Williams KA, Fisher MJ, Pont LG. Defining constipation to estimate its prevalence in the community: results from a national survey. *BMC Gastroenterol*. 2019;19:75. doi:10.1186/s12876-019-0994-0

24. Tack J, Müller-Lissner S, Stanghellini V, et al. Diagnosis and treatment of chronic constipation—a European perspective. *Neurogastroenterol Motil*. 2011;23(8):697–710. doi:10.1111/j.1365-2982.2011.01709.x

25. Sobrado CW, Neto IJFC, Pintoa RA, et al. Diagnosis and treatment of constipation: a clinical update based on the Rome IV criteria. *J Coloproctol (Rio J)*. 2018;38(2):137–144. doi:10.1016/J.JCOL.2018.02.003

26. Sanchez MI, Bercik P. Epidemiology and burden of chronic constipation. *Can J Gastroenterol*. 2011;25(suppl B):11B–15B. doi:10.1155/2011/974573

27. Paquette IM, Varma M, Ternent C, et al. The American Society of Colon and Rectal Surgeons' clinical practice guideline for the evaluation and management of constipation. *Dis Colon Rectum*. 2016;59(6):479–495. doi:10.1097/DCR.0000000000000599

28. Lawrensia S, Raja A. *Bisacodyl*. StatPearls Publishing. Published January 2020. Updated February 21, 2020. https://www.ncbi.nlm.nih.gov/books/NBK547733

29. Ikechi R, Fischer BD, DeSipio J, et al. Irritable bowel syndrome: clinical manifestations, dietary influences, and management. *Healthcare*. 2017;5(2):21. doi:10.3390/healthcare5020021

30. Cong X, Perry M, Bernier KM, et al. Effects of self-management interventions in patients with irritable bowel syndrome: systematic review. *West J Nurs Res*. 2018;40(11):1698–1720. doi:10.1177/0193945917727705

31. Finley CR, Chan DS, Garrison S, et al. What are the most common conditions in primary care? Systematic review. *Can Fam Physician*. 2018;64(11):832–840. https://www .cfp.ca/content/64/11/832

32. Ford AC, Lacy BE, Talley NJ. Irritable bowel syndrome. *N Engl J Med.* 2017;376(26):2566–2578. doi:10.1056/NEJMra1607547

33. Friedman S. Irritable bowel syndrome. In: Greenberger NJ, ed. *Current Diagnosis and Treatment: Gastroenterology, Hepatology and Endoscopy.* 3rd ed. McGraw-Hill; 2016:Chapter 24.

34. Kosako M, Akiho H, Miwa H, et al. Influence of the requirement for abdominal pain in the diagnosis of irritable bowel syndrome with constipation (IBS-C) under the Rome IV criteria using data from a large Japanese population-based internet survey. *BioPsychoSoc Med.* 2018;12:18. doi:10.1186/s13030-018-0137-9

35. Defrees D, Bailey J. Irritable bowel syndrome: epidemiology, pathophysiology, diagnosis, and treatment. *Prim Care.* 2017;44(4):655–671. doi:10.1016/j.pop.2017.07.009

36. Greenberger NJ, Blumberg RS, Burakoff, R, eds. *Current Diagnosis & Treatment: Gastroenterology, Hepatology, & Endoscopy.* 3rd ed. McGraw-Hill Education; 2016.

37. Feuerstein JD, Cheifetz AS. Crohn disease: epidemiology, diagnosis, and management. *Mayo Clin Proc.* 2017;92(7):1088–1103. doi:10.1016/j.mayocp.2017.04.010

38. Sairenji T, Collins KL, Evans, DV. An update on inflammatory bowel disease. *Prim Care.* 2017;44(4):673–692. doi:10.1016/j.pop.2017.07.010

39. Ungaro R, Mehandru S, Allen PB, et al. Ulcerative colitis. *Lancet.* 2017;389(10080):1756–1770. doi:10.1016/S0140-6736(16)32126-2

40. Richter JE, Rubenstein J. Presentation and epidemiology of gastroesophageal reflux disease. *Gastroenterology.* 2018;154(2):267–276. doi:10.1053/j.gastro.2017.07.045

41. Katz PO, Gerson LB, Vela MF. Guidelines for the diagnosis and management of gastroesophageal reflux disease. *Am J Gastroenterol.* 2013;108:302–328. doi:10.1038/ajg.2012.444

42. Chey WD, Leontiadis GI, Howden CW, Moss SF. ACG clinical guideline: treatment of *Helicobacter pylori* infection. *Am J Gastroenterol.* 2017;112(2):212–239. doi:10.1038/ajg.2016.563

43. Rutherford A, Dienstag JL. Viral hepatitis. In: Greenberger NJ, ed. *Current Diagnosis and Treatment: Gastroenterology, Hepatology and Endoscopy.* 3rd ed. McGraw-Hill Education; 2016:Chapter 40.

44. Centers for Disease Control and Prevention. Viral hepatitis. Viral hepatitis. Accessed December 28, 2018. https://www.cdc.gov/hepatitis/index.html

45. Centers for Disease Control and Prevention. *Hepatits B.* https://www.cdc.gov/vaccines/pubs/pinkbook/hepb.html

46. Centers for Disease Control and Prevention. *Surveillance for viral hepatitis—United States* 2016. https://www.cdc.gov/hepatitis/statistics/2016surveillance/index.htm

47. LeFevre ML. Screening for hepatitis B virus infection in nonpregnant adolescents and adults: U.S. Preventive Services Task Force recommendation statement. *Ann Inter Med.* 2014;161(1):58–66. doi:10.7326/M14-1018

48. Moyer VA. Screening for hepatitis C virus infection in adults: U.S. Preventive Services Task Force recommendation statement. *Ann Intern Med.* 2013;159(5):349–357. doi:10.7326/0003-4819-159-5-201309030-00672

49. Terrault NA, Lok ASF, McMahon BJ, et al. Update on prevention, diagnosis, and treatment of chronic hepatitis B: AASLD 2018 hepatitis B guidance. *Hepatology.* 2018;67(4):1560–1599. doi:10.1002/hep.29800

50. Ghany MG, Morgan TR, AASLD-IDSA Hepatitis C Guidance Panel. Hepatitis C guidance 2019 update: American Association for the Study of Liver Diseases–Infectious Diseases Society of America recommendations for testing, managing, and treating hepatitis C virus infection. *Hepatology.* 2020;71(2):686–721. doi:10.1002/hep.31060

51. Farci P, Anna Niro G. Current and future management of chronic hepatitis D. *Gastroenterol Hepatol.* 2018;14(6):342–351. https://www.ncbi.nlm.nih.gov/pmc/articles/PMC6111511

52. Teshale EH. Travel-related infectious diseases: hepatitis E. In: Centers for Disease Control and Prevention, ed. *CDC Yellow Book 2020.* https://wwwnc.cdc.gov/travel/yellowbook/2020/travel-related-infectious-diseases/hepatitis-e

53. Hoffmann-La Roche. *Copegus (ribavirin)* [package insert]. U.S. Food and Drug Administration website. Revised August 2011. https://www.accessdata.fda.gov/drugsatfda_docs/label/2011/021511s023lbl.pdf

54. Parker EA, Roy T, D'Adamo CR, et al. Probiotics and gastrointestinal conditions: an overview of evidence from the Cochrane Collaboration. *Nutrition.* 2018;45:125–134.e111. doi:10.1016/j.nut.2017.06.024

55. Coggins SA, Wynn JL, Weitkamp J-H. Infectious causes of necrotizing enterocolitis. *Clin Perinatol.* 2015;42:133–154. doi:10.1016/j.clp.2014.10.012

56. Pironi L, Arends J, Bozzetti F, et al. ESPEN guidelines on chronic intestinal failure in adults. *Clin Nutr.* 2016;35(2):247–307. doi:10.1016/j.clnu.2016.01.020

57. Mouly S, Lloret-Linares C, Sellier P-O, et al. Is the clinical relevance of drug-food and drug-herb interactions limited to grapefruit juice and Saint-John's wort? *Pharmacol Res.* 2017;118:82–92. doi:10.1016/j.phrs.2016.09.038

Pharmacotherapy for Genitourinary Conditions

Jon E. Siiteri

INTRODUCTION

Voiding disorders include overactive bladder, urinary incontinence, interstitial cystitis/bladder pain syndrome (IC/BPS), and chronic urinary retention. Estimates of the prevalence of voiding disorders based on population studies in the United States, Canada, Europe, and Korea range from 7% to 27% in men, and 9% to 43% in women for overactive bladder symptoms in the absence of infection or other causative factors. Overactive bladder symptoms increase in frequency with age, affecting between 70% and 80% of people by the age of 80.[1,2] Approximately 33% of patients have both overactive bladder symptoms and urge urinary incontinence.[3,4] Symptoms of overactive bladder include urinary frequency, urgency, and nocturia. For women, overactive bladder symptoms generally appear after menopause and are associated with multiparity.[5] In men, overactive bladder symptoms are most often associated with lower urinary tract symptoms of benign prostatic hyperplasia (BPH; see Chapter 28). The main symptom for the IC/BPS is painful urination with a female-to-male prevalence of about 9:1 in the United States.[6,7]

DEFINITIONS

The International Continence Society (ICS) uses the following definitions to describe lower urinary tract symptoms (LUTS) that are caused by conditions or diseases affecting the bladder and the urethra[5,8]:

- **Stress urinary incontinence:** Urine leakage associated with physical exertion such as coughing, laughing, running, and rising from a seated position.
- **Urge urinary incontinence:** Urine leakage associated with the sudden and compelling desire to void.
- **Mixed urge urinary incontinence:** A combination of stress urinary and urge urinary incontinence.
- **Overactive bladder:** Urgency (with or without urge incontinence), usually with frequency and nocturia, in the absence of other pathologic or metabolic conditions that might explain the symptoms. The American Urological Association (AUA) uses the term *overactive bladder* (OAB) as "a clinical diagnosis characterized by the presence of bothersome urinary symptoms" based on ICS definitions.[9]
- **Urgency:** A sudden and compelling desire to pass urine that is difficult to defer.
- **Nocturia:** Waking one or more times per night to void urine.
- **Underactive bladder:** Slow urinary stream, hesitancy, and straining to void with or without a feeling of incomplete bladder emptying, sometimes with storage symptoms.[10]
- **IC/BPS:** Defined by the Society of Urodynamics, Female Pelvic Medicine, and Urogenital Reconstruction

(SUFU) as "an unpleasant sensation (pain, pressure, discomfort) perceived to be related to the urinary bladder, associated with lower urinary tract symptoms of more than 6 weeks of duration, in the absence of infection or other identifiable causes."[7] The AUA expanded the definition of IC/PBS as "a complex (that) includes a large group of patients with bladder and/or urethral and/or pelvic pain, lower urinary tract symptoms, and sterile urine cultures, many with specific identifiable causes. IC/BPS comprises a part of this complex."[7]

NORMAL VOIDING PHYSIOLOGY

The two functions of the bladder are to store and empty urine. Storage of urine occurs at low bladder pressure with a rapid increase in bladder pressure as the volume approaches the total capacity of the bladder. The smooth muscle and connective tissue components of the urinary sphincter maintain continence by way of sympathetic and peripheral nerve input to the urethral and pelvic floor muscles surrounding the rectum, respectively. In the central nervous system (CNS), the midbrain pontine micturition center (PMC) integrates responses to bladder wall pressure sensation and pain/temperature conveyed by afferent A fibers and C fibers, respectively, as signals from the peripheral nervous system (PNS). The result is maintenance of continence via a small group of motor neurons in the ventral horn of the sacral S1–S4 spinal cord motor neurons.[11]

Multiple signaling factors are involved in mediating bladder sensation. Those identified currently include acetylcholine, norepinephrine, epinephrine, adenosine, nitrous oxide, and inflammatory cytokines. Dynamic stretching of the bladder wall during bladder filling activates afferent peripheral sensory nerves. Spontaneous detrusor activity during filling is inhibited by adrenergic sympathetic innervation. At the same time, bladder wall relaxation during filling is mediated by beta-3 adrenergic innervation.

Detrusor contractility is primarily under parasympathetic control. Acetylcholine released from parasympathetic efferent terminals within the detrusor activates M3 muscarinic receptors, resulting in a cyclic AMP-dependent process, causing an increase in intracellular calcium and subsequent activation of actin/myosin complexes.

Normal bladder emptying (micturition) is a complex interaction of the CNS, PNS, skeletal, and smooth muscle components. In a highly coordinated sequence of events mediated by the PMC, relaxation of the striated muscles of the detrusor sphincter under conscious control of the PNS combined with inhibition of sympathetic tone to the smooth muscle components of the sphincter is followed by reflex contraction of the detrusor mediated by the parasympathetic nervous system.

Storage of urine during the filling phase distends the bladder, which results in low-level afferent nerve stimulation. This increases outflow of sympathetic nerve stimulation to the base of the bladder and the urethra with simultaneous peripheral nerve stimulation via the pudendal nerve to the external urethral sphincter. These responses are mediated by spinal reflex pathways and are considered "guarding reflexes" that promote continence. Sympathetic nerve firing also inhibits detrusor muscle contractility via bladder ganglia.

Micturition begins with intense afferent input from a distended bladder to the brainstem micturition center, resulting in inhibition of the guarding reflexes. The PMC stimulates parasympathetic outflow to the bladder and internal sphincter muscle. This causes simultaneous detrusor contraction and relaxation of the sphincter. Maintenance of the voiding reflex is mediated by ascending afferent pathways to the PMC.

Considering the complexity of normal bladder function, there could be multiple causes of incontinence that involve any one or more of the regulatory functions described. These include impaired function of the detrusor muscle, the detrusor sphincter, the muscles of the perineum, and neurologic dysfunction at the level of the peripheral, autonomic, or central nervous systems.

PATHOPHYSIOLOGY OF URINARY INCONTINENCE

Causes of urinary incontinence may generally be considered to have three anatomic or physiologic origins. These are urge incontinence, overflow incontinence, and stress urinary incontinence.

URGE INCONTINENCE

Urge incontinence is associated with detrusor overactivity of non-neurogenic origin, detrusor overactivity of neurogenic origin, or poor bladder compliance. Urinary incontinence is two to three times more common in women than men due to the shorter length of the urethra in women, as well as the connective tissue, muscle, and nerve injury associated with childbirth. Individuals with a history of nervous system disorders such as Parkinson's disease, stroke, dementia, multiple sclerosis, and spinal cord injury are at increased risk for urge urinary incontinence.

OVERFLOW INCONTINENCE

Overflow incontinence is a result of chronic urinary retention, which is due to either an underactive bladder or bladder outlet obstruction in patients with non-neurogenic causes. Overflow incontinence is a less common form of incontinence due to impaired ability of the detrusor to contract. This condition, variously termed *underactive bladder, detrusor underactivity,* or *non-neurogenic chronic urine retention,* arises due to chronic outlet obstruction, as with BPH in men, or by voluntary suppression of the urge to urinate. Clinical diagnostic criteria have not been established, but the AUA has used a post-void residual urine volume >300 mL, either with or without symptoms, as an objective cut-off parameter.[12]

Certain occupations seem to predispose patients to this condition—for example, elementary school teachers, hospital floor nurses, and long-haul truck drivers (personal observation). Unfortunately, no pharmacotherapy treatments have proven to be effective for this type of incontinence as it requires some form of catheterization for emptying the bladder.

STRESS URINARY INCONTINENCE

Stress urinary incontinence occurs as a result of anatomic deficiencies due to hypermobility of the bladder neck or intrinsic sphincter deficiency (due to bladder neck dysfunction). In men treated for prostate cancer with either surgery or radiation therapy, incontinence rates were 23% and 12%, respectively, whereas men who received both treatments had incontinence rates of 52%.[13] Pharmacotherapy plays a limited role in addressing stress urinary incontinence and referral to a specialty clinic is advised. For the purposes of this chapter, only pharmacotherapies for urge urinary incontinence with detrusor overactivity of non-neurogenic origin or poor bladder compliance will be reviewed.

PATHOPHYSIOLOGY OF INTERSTITIAL CYSTITIS/BLADDER PAIN SYNDROME

The cause of IC/BPS is unknown, but the underlying pathophysiology is due to an inflammatory response of the urothelium with proliferation and activation of mast cells, a decrease in the thickness of the protective mucus lining of the bladder wall, and stimulation of afferent sensory nerves mediating pain perception.

Discomfort, pressure sensation, suprapubic tenderness, or pain in the bladder, lower abdomen, and the pelvis are symptoms of IBPS. This chronic condition is distinguished from urinary tract infection (UTI) symptoms by the severity and chronicity of symptoms. Urinalysis reveals absence of bacteria but commonly pyuria, and often microscopic hematuria. Although not routinely performed, definitive diagnosis is made by cystoscopy and bladder biopsy. Patients present with a wide spectrum of symptoms with no consistent findings on physical exam or clinical diagnostic responses. The AUA guideline on IC/BPS

advises diagnosis that is based on clinical principles or expert opinion.[7] The essentials of diagnosis require a careful history, physical examination, and laboratory tests to characterize the patient's complaint and to exclude infections or other causes of symptoms. The patient's complaint should occur for at least 6 weeks. A bladder diary is useful in distinguishing overactive bladder from IC/BPS. Characterization of the pain, onset, duration, and severity of symptoms, as well as the localization of symptoms, are items to obtain in the history. It is important to rule out other causes for symptoms, including vaginitis, urethritis, prostatitis, dyspareunia, ejaculatory pain in men, and pain with menstruation. Recording daily times of voiding and voiding volumes is important to establish the characteristic low volume of urination that is associated with IC/BPS.

IC/BPS usually presents in the fourth decade of life. Because the symptoms consist of pain in multiple locations without clear anatomic and physiologic correlates, it is considered by some to be part of a constellation of chronic pain syndromes, including fibromyalgia, irritable bowel syndrome (IBS), chronic fatigue syndrome, and may indeed coexist with them. Not entirely exclusive, but more commonly found in women, is sexual dysfunction, including dyspareunia, vulvodynia, and bowel symptoms (e.g., constipation and straining). IC/BPS is highly correlated with symptoms of depression and anxiety, perhaps indicating a common biological mechanism underlying these disorders.

Direct visualization of the bladder wall by cystoscopy in a small subset of patients (5%–20%) with IC/BPS symptoms reveals well-defined reddened mucosal areas with small vessels radiating toward a central scar called *Hunner's lesions.* Histologic analysis of these lesions identified acute and chronic inflammatory changes consistent with an inflammatory process underlying the pathophysiology in this subset of patients. This led to the leaky epithelium hypothesis for the pathophysiologic basis of IC/BPS. This hypothesis proposes that either disruption or increased permeability of the mucus lining of the bladder wall to the normal components of urine allows a chronic inflammatory response that yields the symptoms of pain, urinary frequency, and urgency identified with IC/BPS.[14]

PATHOPHYSIOLOGY OF CHRONIC URINARY RETENTION

Chronic urinary retention (CUR) can be caused by either neurogenic or non-neurogenic factors. For the purpose of reviewing pharmacotherapy for urinary disorders, this section will discuss only non-neurogenic causes of urinary retention. As with IC/BPS, there is a lack of consensus on the criteria that define chronic urinary retention. An objective determination that is generally accepted is a post-void residual urine volume >300 mL.[10] The two common causes of CUR are from either chronic outlet obstruction or underactive bladder.

CUR in men is most commonly a result of BPH. Other anatomical causes include urethral or bladder neck stricture, urethral stones, or tumors; in women, CUR is a result of high-grade pelvic floor prolapse or urethral diverticula. Prior surgical procedures for incontinence or vaginal vault prolapse may precede CUR.

Medications that can cause urinary retention due to obstruction include long-term use of antihistamines, adrenergic agonists, and antipsychotic medications. Poor bladder contractility can also be due to long-standing outlet obstruction. Medications used over a long time that impair bladder contractility include anticholinergic or antispasmodic medications, tricyclic antidepressants (TCAs), beta adrenergic agonists, calcium channel blockers, nonsteroidal anti-inflammatory drugs (NSAIDs), opioids, benzodiazepines, and antipsychotics.[9]

It is important to identify clinical sequelae that may result from CUR. Patients who are at high risk for morbidity due to CUR are those who have recurrent culture-proven UTIs requiring antibiotic treatment, culture-proven urosepsis, or stage III kidney disease with eGFR 30 to 59 mL/minute. Other high-risk criteria include radiologic evidence of hydronephrosis or hydroureter.[12]

The physical, social, psychological, and medical impact of these disorders is significant, leading to multiple functional disabilities and reduced quality of life.

PHARMACOTHERAPEUTIC AGENTS

URGE URINARY INCONTINENCE

Antimuscarinic Agents

The initial medications used for overactive bladder symptoms, including urinary frequency, urgency, and nocturia, were developed based on the understanding that contraction of the detrusor was mediated via muscarinic cholinergic receptors. The first drug used for this purpose was oxybutynin. It is a competitive antagonist for M1, M2, and M3 muscarinic acetylcholine receptors. This drug was first approved for use in the United States in 1993.

The significant adverse side-effect profile of oxybutynin, a secondary amine, includes dry mouth, dry eyes, constipation, blurred vision, dyspepsia, UTI secondary to urinary retention, and altered mental status in patients 60 years of age and older. Tertiary amine anticholinergics, demonstrated to have less permeability across the blood–brain barrier in animal studies, were developed with potentially less adverse CNS effects. These include darifenacin, fesoterodine, solifenacin, tolterodine, and trospium.[15] Comprehensive reviews of randomized clinical trials with placebo control groups demonstrate no evidence of superiority of one antimuscarinic drug over another.[9] Qualitative analysis of patient responses to anticholinergic medications, such as change in 24-hour urinary frequency, urgency, and urge incontinence, indicated patients with more severe symptoms, on average, experienced greater symptom relief.[9]

Beta-3 Agonist

Identification and elucidation of the role of beta-adrenoceptors in the detrusor and urothelium in 1989 led to the development of a unique beta-3 agonist indicated for the treatment of OAB.[16] The beta-3 adrenoreceptor subtype was shown to be the predominant adrenoceptor in the bladder. Norepinephrine-mediated stimulation of beta-3 receptors results in detrusor relaxation in humans and can increase bladder capacity. Additionally, afferent input to micturition centers in the midbrain is decreased, thus reducing symptoms of OAB. The mechanism of action is either via voltage-gated potassium channels or stimulation of adenylyl cyclase with subsequent formation of cyclic adenosine monophosphate (cAMP).

TREATMENT OF INTERSTITIAL CYSTITIS/ BLADDER PAIN SYNDROME

NONPHARMACOLOGIC TREATMENT

All patients are initially advised to adopt an elimination diet. Recommendations include avoiding tomato and tomato-based sauces, spices (e.g., pepper, curry powder, hot peppers, horseradish paste), high-potassium foods, citrus fruits and juices, caffeine, alcohol, and highly acidic foods such as pickles, mustard, and vinegar-based salad dressings.[14] In the context of chronic pain syndromes, IC/BPS patients are reported to receive benefit from stress reduction strategies.[7]

PHARMACOLOGIC TREATMENT

Chronic pain treatments that have shown some efficacy include tricyclic amines such as amitriptyline. The mechanism of action is unknown; however, in animal studies, amitriptyline is shown to have central and peripheral anticholinergic properties. In addition to inhibition of norepinephrine and serotonin reuptake, and because of mild sedative action, it is presumed to have centrally based action with antihistamine properties.[7] Clinical trials show demonstrable efficacy better than placebo. Typical adverse effects include dry mouth, dry eyes, nausea, headache, or somnolence.

Antihistamines that address the underlying inflammatory response, such as cimetidine and hydroxyzine, have shown some efficacy. The mechanism of action of these agents is based on inhibition of mast cell degranulation within the bladder wall and probable inhibition of histamine release. Fatigue, dizziness, dry mouth, constipation, and somnolence are known adverse effects.[7]

A synthetic polysaccharide heparin-like compound, pentosan polysulfate sodium (PPS), was approved in 1996 for the specific indication of treatment for IC/BPS.[17] This medication was demonstrated to increase the thickness of the proteoglycan layer lining the bladder in animal models. The adverse-effect profile is generally minimal and includes mild dyspepsia, nausea, and anorexia. Dosage is 100 mg orally three times daily.

Well-designed randomized clinical trials comparing PPS to placebo treatment showed mixed results in the reduction of IC/BPS symptoms.[18] In a multicenter, double-blind, randomized, placebo-controlled study of 368 adults with IC/BPS, PPS was no better than placebo with a preset standard of at least 30% improvement in symptoms.[7]

Intravesical Treatment

Intravesical treatment options in the urology setting include hydrodistention of the bladder under anesthesia and bladder installation of dimethyl sulfoxide, heparin, methylprednisolone, or lidocaine, often in a combination of several of these agents.

Onabotulinumtoxin A (Botox®) intravesical injection is proven to be effective in reducing irritative urinary symptoms such as urgency, frequency, and pain in some but not all patients. Proposed mechanisms of action for Botox injections include the inhibition of both afferent and efferent pathways based on evidence that Botox inhibits the release of neurotransmitters from the urothelium and nerve fibers, including acetylcholine, norepinephrine, adenosine triphosphate, and substance P. Intravesical injection of triamcinolone has also been shown to reduce pre- and postoperative pelvic pain and the irritative urinary symptoms described.[7]

CASE EXEMPLAR: Patient With Incontinence

MP is a 55-year-old woman who presents with complaint of inability to hold urine. She describes incidents where laughing or coughing results in a small to moderate release of urine. She has started wearing Peri Pads to avoid embarrassment.

Past Medical History
- Six vaginal deliveries, all to full term
- Osteoarthritis
- Postmenopausal

Medications
- Boniva, 150 mg once a month
- Calcium, 500 mg daily
- Vitamin D3, one daily

Family History
- Mother, alive and well; hypertension, type 2 diabetes
- Father, deceased; cardiovascular disease, myocardial infarction at age 77

Social History
- No alcohol intake
- Previous smoker
- Walks 2 miles/day

Physical Examination
- Vital signs normal
- Palpation of uterus suggests enlargement

Labs
- Liver function: Normal

Discussion Questions

1. What factors in MP's history would help support a diagnosis of overactive bladder?
2. The clinician prescribes oxybutynin 10 mg (extended-release). What does MP need to know about this drug?
3. If oxybutynin is ineffective, the clinician could use mirabegron, a beta-3 agonist. What does MP need to know about this new drug?

CASE EXEMPLAR: Patient With Urinary Retention

NN is a 66-year-old female who is seen in the clinic today with complaints that she cannot empty her bladder fully. She does not experience pain but does experience dribbling.

Past Medical History
- Surgery for vaginal prolapse 18 months ago
- Hypertension
- Urinary tract infections in the past
- Asthma controlled with medication

Medications
- Motrin, 800 mg for arthritic pain
- Hydrocodone for severe pain
- Procardia, 10 mg daily
- Albuterol inhaler, as needed
- Tiotropium bromide inhaler, two puffs each morning

Family History
- Unremarkable

Social History
- Elementary school teacher, 30 years

Physical Examination
- Blood pressure: 140/88; pulse: 80; respiration rate: 20

Labs
- Post-void residual urine volume: 400 mL

Discussion Questions

1. The clinician is considering a diagnosis of overflow incontinence or chronic urinary obstruction. What factors in NN's history would help support a diagnosis of chronic urinary obstruction?
2. What factors would support a diagnosis of overflow incontinence?
3. If overflow incontinence is the diagnosis, what treatment options are available for NN?

KEY TAKEAWAYS

- Voiding disorders include OAB, urinary incontinence, IC/BPS, and CUR.
- Symptoms of OAB include urinary frequency, urgency, and nocturia. For women, symptoms appear after menopause and are associated with multiparity. In men, symptoms are associated with BPH.
- The main symptom for IC/BP is painful urination and absence of bacteria in the urine.
- Oxybutynin and other anticholinergics are used to treat OAB. Side effects include dry mouth, dry eyes, constipation, blurred vision, dyspepsia, and altered mental status in patients 60 years of age and older.
- Patients with IC/BPS are advised to adopt an elimination diet. Chronic pain treatments have shown some efficacy. Onabotulinumtoxin A intravesical injection is effective in reducing irritative urinary symptoms, such as urgency, frequency, and pain.

REFERENCES

1. Coyne KS, Kvasz M, Ireland AM, et al. Urinary incontinence and its relationship to mental health and health-related quality of life in men and women in Sweden, the United Kingdom, and the United States. *Eur Urol.* 2012;61(1):88–95. doi:10.1016/j.eururo.2011.07.049
2. Zhang L, Zhu L, Xu T, et al. A population-based survey of the prevalence, potential risk factors, and symptom-specific bother of lower urinary tract symptoms in adult Chinese women. *Eur Urol.* 2015;68(1):97–112. doi:10.1016/j.eururo.2014.12.012
3. de Ridder D, Roumeguère T, Kaufman L. Overactive bladder symptoms, stress urinary incontinence and associated bother in women aged 40 and above; a Belgian epidemiological survey. *Int J Clin Pract.* 2013;67(3):198–204. doi:10.1111/ijcp.12015
4. Haylen BT, de Ridder D, Freeman RM, et al. An International Urogynecological Association (IUGA)/International Continence Society (ICS) joint report on the terminology for female pelvic floor dysfunction. *Neurourol Urodyn.* 2010;29:4–20. doi:10.1002/nau.20798
5. International Continence Society. *International Continence Society fact sheets: a background to urinary and faecal incontinence.* August 2015. https://www.ics.org
6. Hanno P, Dmochowski R. Status of international consensus on interstitial cystitis/bladder pain syndrome/painful

bladder syndrome: 2008 snapshot. *Neurourol Urodyn.* 2009;28:274. doi:10.1002/nau.20687

7. Hanno P, Burks DA, Clemens JQ, et al. *Diagnosis and Treatment of Interstitial Cystitis/Bladder Pain Syndrome.* American Urological Association Guideline; 2014:1–45.

8. Abrams P, Cardozo L, Fall M, et al. The standardisation of terminology of lower urinary tract function: report from the Standardisation Sub-committee of the International Continence Society. *Neurourol Urodyn.* 2002;21: 167–178. doi:10.1002/nau.10052.

9. Gormley EA, Lightner DJ, Burgio KL, et al. Diagnosis and treatment of overactive bladder (non-neurogenic) in adults. *J Urol.* 2012;188(6 suppl):2455–2463. doi:10.1016/j.juro.2012.09.079

10. Tarcan T, Rademakers K, Arlandis S, et al. Do the definitions of the underactive bladder and detrusor underactivity help in managing patients: International Consultation on Incontinence Research Society (ICI-RS) Think Tank 2017. *Neurourol Urodyn.* 2018;37:(S4)S60–S68. doi:10.1002/nau.23570

11. Stoffel, J. Detrusor sphincter dyssynergia: a review of physiology, diagnosis, and treatment strategies. *Transl Androl Urol.* 2016;5(1):127–135. doi:10.3978/j.issn.2223-4683.2016.01.08

12. Stoffel J, Lightner D, Peterson A, et al. *Non-Neurogenic Chronic Urinary Retention: Consensus Definition, management Strategies, and Future Opportunities.* Published 2016. https://www.auanet.org/guidelines/chronic-urinary-retention

13. Daugherty M, Chelluri R, Bratslavsky G, et al. Are we underestimating the rates of incontinence after prostate cancer treatment. *Int Urol Nephrol.* 2017;49(10): 1715–1721. doi:10.1007/s11255-017-1660-5

14. Han E, Nguyen L, Sirls L, et al. Current best practice management of interstitial cystitis/bladder pain syndrome. *Ther Adv Urol.* 2018;10(7):197–211. doi:10.1177/1756287218761574

15. Wishart DS, Knox C, Guo AC, et al. Drugbank: a comprehensive resource for in silico drug discovery and exploration. *Nucleic Acids Res.* 2006;34 (Database issue):D668–D672. doi:10.1093/nar/gkj067

16. Warren K, Burden H, Abrams P. Mirabegron in overactive bladder patients: efficacy review and update on drug safety. *Adv Ther Drug Saf.* 2016;7(5):204–216. doi:10.1177/2042098616659412

17. Sant GR, Propert KJ, Hanno PM, et al. A pilot clinical trial of oral pentosan polysulfate and oral hydroxyzine in patients with interstitial cystitis. *J Urol.* 2015;193(3): 857–862. doi:10.1097/01.ju.0000083020.06212.3d

18. Nickel JC, Herschorn S, Whitmore KE, et al. Pentosan polysulfate sodium for treatment of interstitial cystitis/bladder pain syndrome: insights from a randomized, double-blind, placebo controlled study. *J Urol.* 2003;170(3):810–815. doi:10.1016/j.juro.2014.09.036

Pharmacotherapy for Renal, Acid–Base, Fluid, and Electrolyte Disorders

Niti Madan, Vishwa C. Sheth, and Brian Y. Young

LEARNING OBJECTIVES

- Differentiate between the pathophysiology of acute tubular necrosis and acute interstitial nephritis and describe how each relates to acute kidney injury.
- Describe the management of acute kidney injury.
- Outline the etiology and management of chronic kidney disease.
- Compare and contrast volume depletion and volume overload including fluid management strategies.
- Define each of the acid–base disorders by etiology, laboratory data, patient manifestations, and expected pharmacology and fluid management.
- Define each of the electrolyte disorders by etiology, laboratory data, patient manifestations, and expected pharmacology and fluid management.

INTRODUCTION: GENERAL APPROACH TO RENAL DISORDERS

ACUTE KIDNEY INJURY

Acute kidney injury (AKI) is an important clinical problem, which is seen in upwards of 10% of hospitalized patients and up to 50% to 60% of patients in ICUs.[1,2] The most frequent causes of AKI are prerenal disease and acute tubular necrosis (ATN), with obstruction, glomerular disease, and interstitial nephritis being less common. Nephrotoxicity from drugs may account for 8% to 60% of hospital-acquired AKI,[3] and can occur from both prescribed and over-the-counter medications. Risk factors for drug-induced AKI include age, duration and intensity of drug therapy, multiple nephrotoxic exposure, shock, comorbidities (e.g., diabetes), and preexisting kidney disease.

Multiple mechanisms of AKI exist and vary according to the type of drug exposure. The mechanisms can be classified into those affecting the tubulointerstitial, vascular, and less commonly the glomerular compartments (Table 21.1).

Acute Tubular Necrosis

ATN may result from direct cytotoxic effects of the offending medication on renal tubules, though tubular obstruction, or reduction in renal medullary blood flow. ATN is accompanied by an increase in serum creatinine and variable degrees of urine output (oliguric [<400 mL urine/day] vs. nonoliguric [>400 mL urine/day]). Examination of the urine sediment may demonstrate renal tubular epithelial cells and muddy brown casts. Fractional excretion of sodium will typically be greater than 1%, with fractional excretion of urea greater than 40%.[6–8] Management of ATN is withdrawal of the offending agent, avoidance of further nephrotoxic insults, and supportive care.

Acute Interstitial Nephritis

Early reports frequently attributed drug-induced acute interstitial nephritis (AIN) to beta-lactam antibiotics. However, multiple other drugs, including nonantimicrobials, have been recognized as potential causes.

TABLE 21.1 Examples of Drugs That Induce Acute Kidney Injury According to Mechanism of Injury

Mechanism of Kidney Injury	Injury Subtype	Select Examples
Tubulointerstitial	Acute tubular necrosis	Antimicrobial agents (aminoglycosides, vancomycin, tenofovir, polymixins, amphotericin b, pentamidine, foscarnet) Chemotherapy agents (platins, ifosfamide, pemetrexed) Iodinated contrast NSAIDs Zoledronic acid
	Crystalline injury	Antiviral agents (acyclovir, atazanavir, indinavir) Antibacterial agents (sulfonamides, ciprofloxacin) Osmotic agents (mannitol, sucrose, hydroxyethyl starch, dextran) Methotrexate Triamterene Ascorbic acid Ethylene glycol Sodium–phosphate laxatives
	Interstitial nephritis	Antimicrobial agents (β-lactams, sulfonamides, fluoroquinolones, rifampin) NSAIDs Proton-pump inhibitors Allopurinol Diuretics 5-ASA Immune checkpoint inhibitors
Vascular	Afferent arteriolar vasoconstriction	NSAIDs Calcineurin inhibitors (i.e., cyclosporine, tacrolimus)[4]
	Efferent arteriolar vasodilation	Angiotensin-converting enzyme inhibitors Angiotensin receptor blockers
	Thrombotic microangiopathy	Chemotherapeutic agents (antiVEGF inhibitors, gemcitabine, mitomycin C) Interferon Calcineurin inhibitors mTOR inhibitors (i.e., rapamycin or sirolimus)[5] Thienopyridines (i.e., ticlopidine, clopidogrel) Quinine Oxymorphone
	Vasculitis	Propylthiouracil Hydralazine Cocaine laced with levamisole Infliximab
Glomerular	Minimal change	NSAIDs Lithium Interferon Pamidronate Vaccinations
	Focal segmental glomerulosclerosis	Anabolic steroids Heroin Lithium Interferon Pamidronate Sirolimus Vaccinations
	Membranous	NSAIDs Gold Penicillamine
	Lupus nephritis	Hydralazine Procainamide Quinidine Methyldopa

5-ASA, aminosalicylic acids; mTOR, mammalian target of rapamycin; NSAID, nonsteroidal anti-inflammatory drug; VEGF, vascular endothelial growth factor.

A kidney biopsy, if done, will reveal an inflammatory infiltrate of T lymphocytes, monocytes, and occasionally eosinophils in the interstitium. The time of onset is variable, ranging from a few days after exposure to several months. Patients may report signs or symptoms of a drug allergy; however, such findings may be less common than previously thought. For example, approximately 10% of patients have the full triad of rash, fever, and eosinophilia.[9] Urine sediment will most often show pyuria, and occasionally urine eosinophils and white cell casts will be present; thus, the diagnostic accuracy of urine eosinophils is limited. Definitive diagnosis is made with kidney biopsy. Management of AIN is withdrawal of the offending agent and consideration of corticosteroids depending on the severity and duration of injury.

The consequences of less common causes of drug-induced AKI (as shown in Table 21.1) can be just as serious as AKI from ATN or AIN. In all cases, the primary management is to withdraw the causative drug. In crystalline-induced injury, fluid hydration may help flush obstructed kidney tubules. In certain cases, specific agents may help prevent urinary crystallization. For example, fomepizole is used to limit the conversion of ethylene glycol to oxalate, a nephrotoxic metabolite that combines with calcium to form obstructing crystals and stones in the urine.

Thrombotic microangiopathy, vasculitis, and glomerulonephritis are rare manifestations of drug-induced AKI. Their presentation may be variable, some presenting insidiously with abnormal urinary sediment and slowly rising creatinine, some explosively with sufficient severity to require acute dialysis. These disorders may be accompanied by extrarenal manifestations such as a rash, cough, hemoptysis, or arthritis. In addition to removal of the inciting agent, interventions may include immunosuppressive agents and plasmapheresis depending on the underlying pathophysiology.

Management of Acute Kidney Injury

The management of AKI involves objective assessment of vital signs, physical examination, and hemodynamic monitoring, which may help determine volume status. Urine studies, such as fractional excretion of sodium, fractional excretion of urea, and urine microscopy to assess for cells and casts, can provide critical diagnostic information (see Chapter 11 for detailed calculation). In patients with suspected obstruction, kidney imaging is also recommended.

Care for patients with prerenal disease is focused on achieving adequate kidney perfusion. IV isotonic fluids should be used in patients with volume depletion. Crystalloid therapy is appropriate and cost-effective in the majority of patients. As discussed later in the section "Types of Fluids," a randomized trial of normal saline versus albumin colloid in ICU patients showed no kidney or mortality benefit to albumin.[10] One clinical scenario for which albumin may be most useful is that of the patient with cirrhosis with concern for hepatorenal dysfunction, where there may be low baseline serum albumin levels due to poor synthetic function. Given the lack of clear benefit over crystalloids, the regular use of synthetic colloids is not indicated for prerenal disease. Furthermore, colloids based on hydroxyethyl starch can cause kidney damage from osmotic nephrosis and are thus contraindicated in AKI.

ATN accounts for approximately half of the cases of AKI in hospitalized patients. The most common causes of ATN include renal ischemia, sepsis, and, as discussed previously, nephrotoxic drug exposure. In all cases of ATN, hypotension can result in continued kidney damage, and thus judicious use of isotonic fluids and vasopressors is needed to maintain adequate blood pressure. Loop diuretics can be effective in oliguric ATN for managing volume overload, though they do not improve kidney outcomes or mortality in ATN. However, loop diuretic challenge may be useful for prognostication, with poor urine output after a furosemide dose of 1 to 1.5 mg/kg predicting risk of progression of AKI and need for dialysis.[11] Unfortunately, no pharmacological interventions are known at this time to aid recovery from ATN. Examples of studied agents that have failed to improve outcomes include atrial natriuretic peptide, calcium channel blockers, diuretics, dopamine, fenoldopam, N-acetylcysteine, and statins.

CHRONIC KIDNEY DISEASE

Chronic kidney disease (CKD) is defined by the presence of decreased kidney function (GFR <60 mL/min/1.73 m^2) or kidney damage (e.g., albuminuria, active urinary sediment, pathological findings, or imaging abnormalities) for greater than 3 months.[12] In the United States, the prevalence of CKD is estimated at approximately 15% of adults, or 37 million people.[13] CKD is associated with an increased risk of mortality, especially cardiovascular death. Progression of CKD to end-stage renal disease (ESRD) eventually necessitates dialysis or kidneys transplantation; therefore, controlling of the underlying etiology that led to CKD is paramount to slowing the progression. However, other major risk factors exist, such as hypertension, that can cause worsening kidney function irrespective of the initial cause of CKD. These risk factors often result in intraglomerular hypertension and glomerular hypertrophy, leading to glomerulosclerosis. Proteinuria is a consequence of hyperfiltration and glomerular injury, especially true for diabetic kidney disease, the most common cause of ESRD in the United States and many other countries. General efforts to reduce CKD progression focus on blood pressure control, typically to less than 130/80 mmHg, and proteinuria reduction to less than 1 g/day. Thus, in patients with CKD and proteinuria, an angiotensin-converting enzyme (ACE) inhibitor (ACEi) or angiotensin receptor blocker (ARB) is the preferred agent due to its beneficial effects on glomerular hemodynamics. Multiple studies of diabetic kidney disease have clearly shown a marked reduction in CKD progression and incident dialysis when one of these agents is used. On the other hand, dual ACEi and ARB combination therapy should be avoided as there is a higher risk of adverse events, including hyperkalemia and AKI.[14] Finally, there is some limited data that mod-

erate dietary protein restriction and correction of metabolic acidosis with alkali therapy can have an additive effect in slowing CKD progression.

Multiple complications can result from the loss of kidney function.[12,15,16] These disorders include abnormalities in volume status, potassium, acid–base balance, red blood cell formation, and bone and mineral metabolism. It is important to manage each of these issues, as they affect the overall health of the patient and uncorrected derangements are associated with worse outcomes. **Table 21.2** summarizes the treatments of various complications which may result from CKD.

TABLE 21.2 Pathologic Consequences and Treatment Considerations for Complications of Chronic Kidney Disease

Complication	Pathophysiology in CKD	Treatment Considerations
Volume overload and edema	Sodium and water retention	Low-sodium diet Diuretics (loop diuretics are more effective than thiazide diuretics if GFR <30 mL/min/1.73 m²)
Hyperkalemia	Low renal excretion of dietary potassium may occur when GFR is <20 mL/min/1.73 m², though other risk factors may cause hyperkalemia to manifest earlier (e.g., ACEi, ARB, type IV RTA).	See "Potassium" section of text Low potassium diet Avoid nonselective beta blockers which may inhibit transcellular shifts of potassium Diuretic use may allow continuation of an ACEi or ARB in patients with hypertension and proteinuria Potassium-binding agents (SPS, patiromer, ZS9) enhance GI excretion, though side effects may preclude and there is a risk of poor absorption of other prescribed medications taken too close in timing Mineralocorticoid agonists such as fludrocortisone may assist urine excretion, though they are rarely used due to risk of hypertension and fluid overload
Metabolic acidosis	Urinary acid excretion declines in CKD. Renal ammonium production begins to fall at GFR <40–50 mL/min/1.73 m². Potential consequences of metabolic acidosis include increased bone resorption, muscle catabolism, diminished cardiovascular function, and increased rate of CKD progression.	Low phosphate and moderate protein restrictive diet Alkali therapy with sodium bicarbonate or sodium citrate; avoid potassium citrate due to risk of hyperkalemia If sodium citrate is used, avoid aluminum containing medications due to increased aluminum absorption and risk of toxicity
Anemia	Reduced production of erythropoietin by the diseased kidney, shortened RBC life span from increased fragility. Anemia may become evident as GFR drops <60 mL/min/1.73 m². Consequences may include fatigue, poor exercise tolerance, reduced cardiac function, and increased association with mortality.	Nutritional deficiencies of iron and other vitamins should be evaluated for prior to institution of ESAs ESAs available in the United States include epoetin alfa and longer acting darbepoetin ESAs may be given subcutaneously (i.e., predialysis or peritoneal dialysis patients) or intravenously (i.e., hemodialysis) Adverse events of ESAs may include headache, hypertension, and seizure risk High doses of ESAs targeting a normal hemoglobin goal are associated with increased risk of dialysis access thrombosis, cardiovascular events, and mortality Hemoglobin goal of 10–11 g/dL is recommended ESA use in patients with active cancer may be associated with increased thromboembolic events, accelerated cancer growth, and mortality

(continued)

TABLE 21.2 Pathologic Consequences and Treatment Considerations for Complications of Chronic Kidney Disease *(continued)*

Complication	Pathophysiology in CKD	Treatment Considerations
Hyperphosphatemia	Diminished renal excretion of phosphate may occur with GFR <40 mL/min/1.73 m². Elevated phosphate may be associated with increased risk of vascular calcification and mortality.	Low phosphate diet Phosphate binders are given with meals to reduce ingested phosphate absorption Options include calcium-containing binders (calcium carbonate and calcium acetate) and noncalcium-containing binders (sevelamer, lanthanum, and iron salts) No binder has clearly proven to be more effective at reducing mortality over another, though some experts avoid calcium-containing binders due to the concern for increased vascular calcification Except in cases of short-term therapy, aluminum-based binders are avoided due to risk of aluminum toxicity resulting in osteomalacia, microcytic anemia, and/or dialysis-associated dementia
Secondary hyperparathyroidism	Secondary hyperparathyroidism occurs due largely to the combination of phosphate retention, reduced kidney production of 1,25-dihydroxy vitamin D (calcitriol), and hypocalcemia that occurs in CKD. Each of these factors stimulates PTH secretion, which increases bone turnover. Consequences of chronically high PTH secretion include abnormal bone health, leading to increased risk of fractures.	Phosphate control as per above Correct nutritional deficiency of 25-hydroxy vitamin D to allow the kidneys an opportunity to produce endogenous calcitriol If 25-hydroxy vitamin D replete, consider supplementation with calcitriol or a synthetic analog (paricalcitol, doxercalciferol) Side effects of vitamin D analogs may include hypercalcemia and hyperphosphatemia In patients prone to hypercalcemia, calcimimetic therapy is an option to signal the calcium sensing receptor on parathyroid glands to reduce PTH production Calcimimetics can be administered orally (cinacalcet) or intravenously (etelcalcetide); side effects include nausea, hypocalcemia, and increased urinary calcium excretion

ACEi, angiotensin-converting enzyme inhibitors; ARB, angiotensin receptor blocker; CKD, chronic kidney disease; ESA, erythropoiesis-stimulating agent; GFR, glomerular filtration rate; GI, gastrointestinal; PTH, parathyroid hormone; RTA, renal tubular acidosis; SPS, sodium polystyrene sulfonate.

DRUGS FOR MANAGEMENT OF VOLUME DISORDERS

Sodium and water balance disorders are common. Hypovolemia represents loss of sodium and water; meanwhile, edema develops due to salt and water retention. Plasma sodium concentration is regulated by changes in water intake and excretion and not by sodium balance. Suppression of antidiuretic hormone (ADH) protects against water retention and development of hyponatremia. Thirst is the protective mechanism against water loss and hypernatremia development. Persistent ADH secretion causes impairment of water excretion, and results in hyponatremia as seen in reduced effective arterial volume and syndrome of inappropriate ADH secretion (SIADH).

Total body water (TBW) constitutes 50% and 60% of lean body weight in healthy adult women and men, respectively. The intracellular fluid (ICF) represents fluid within the cells and is approximately two-thirds of TBW. The extracellular fluid (ECF) is fluid outside the cell and accounts for one-third of TBW. ECF is subdivided into two compartments: interstitial and intravascular fluid or "plasma." The interstitial fluid (ISF) accounts for three-fourths of the ECF, while the other one-fourth is present as the intravascular fluid (IVF; **Figure 21.1**).

VOLUME DEPLETION

The term "volume" is used to describe extracellular fluid. The term "volume depletion" reflects deficiency in both total body sodium and water. The term "dehydration" suggests water deficit. Dehydration alone can lead to hypernatremia. Effective arterial blood volume is the volume of blood that can be mobilized to perfuse the tissues. Volume depletion results in reduced effective arterial blood volume that activates the renin-angiotensin-aldosterone system (RAS) and the sympathetic nervous system, causing sodium and water retention. Low effective arterial blood volume can occur even in edematous states—for example, patients with severe cardiac dysfunction may have an increase in extracellular fluid volume but poor effective perfusion to tissues, and patients with cirrhosis of the liver and edema may have poor effective perfusion because of splanchnic dilation. See the text that follows

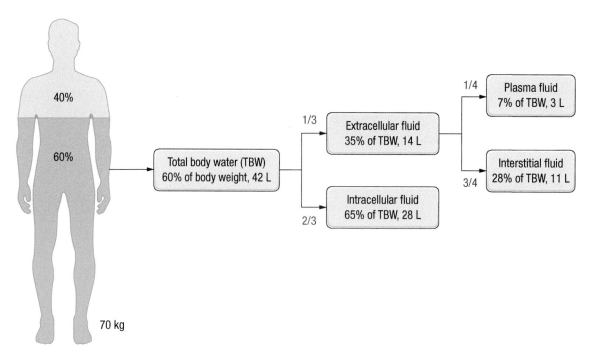

FIGURE 21.1 Distribution of water within a healthy adult.

for further discussion of volume overload and its pharmacologic treatment. Common causes of volume depletion include gastrointestinal losses such as vomiting and diarrhea, as well as excessive diuresis.

TYPES OF FLUIDS

Crystalloids

Therapeutic IV fluids include crystalloid and colloid solutions. Crystalloids are composed of water and electrolytes, all of which can pass freely through semipermeable membranes. These solutions correct electrolyte imbalances but result in smaller hemodynamic changes.

Crystalloids are classified according to their tonicity, which is directly related to sodium concentration. Isotonic solutions like normal saline have a tonicity equal to that of ICF and do not shift the distribution of water between the ECF and the ICF. Hypertonic solutions will draw water from ICF to ECF, while hypotonic fluids will result in shift of water from ECF to ICF. Various crystalloids are normal saline (0.9% NaCl), half normal saline (0.45% NaCl), 5% Dextrose/Half-Normal saline, hypertonic saline (3% NaCl), Lactate Ringer's, and Plasma-lyte.

Buffered Crystalloid Versus Isotonic Saline

Large volume resuscitation using isotonic saline may cause hyperchloremic metabolic acidosis. Isotonic fluids with lower chloride concentration (also known as "buffered" or "balanced" crystalloids), including Lactated Ringer's, Lactated Hartmann's solution, or Plasma-Lyte, may be used instead of isotonic saline for large volume resuscitation. For massive volume replacement, Lactated Ringer's reduces the likelihood of dilutional acidosis, but it contains lactate, which can increase the risk of alkalosis as well as lactic acidosis in the setting of liver failure. Controlled trials comparing 0.9% NaCl and Lactate Ringer's have not shown differences in mortality[17,18]; therefore, the choice between balanced solutions and normal saline should be individualized based on patient needs.

Colloids

Colloids do not dissolve into a true solution and therefore do not pass readily across semipermeable membranes. Colloids effectively remain in the intravascular space and increase the oncotic pressure of the plasma and shift fluids from the interstitial into the intravascular compartment. Therapeutic benefits are short-lived though as colloidal proteins and/or sugars are metabolized. Various colloids are 5% albumin, 25% albumin, the dextrans, hetastarch, and fresh-frozen plasma (FFP).

Albumin is a protein derived from fractionating human plasma and can be used for acute volume expansion. Compared to isotonic saline, albumin expands the plasma volume more rapidly and carries less risk of pulmonary edema. However, randomized trials and meta-analyses have failed to demonstrate added benefits from the use of 4% albumin. The Saline versus Albumin Fluid Evaluation (SAFE) trial found similar mortality with both therapies. Evidence-based indications for albumin include plasmapheresis/apheresis, large volume paracentesis greater than 4 L, spontaneous bacterial peritonitis, hypotension in hemodialysis patients with edema, and diuresis in hypoalbuminemic and/or hypotensive patients.[19]

Hyperoncotic hydroxyethyl starch (HES) solutions are starch and electrolyte solutions, including Hetastarch, Voluven, and Hextend. Low-molecular and high-molecular dextran solutions are polysaccharide plasma expanders. Colloid solutions are expensive and may cause hypersensitivity reactions, acute renal failure from osmotic nephrosis, and bleeding complications. These fluids should be avoided when renal dysfunction is present. Randomized controlled trials comparing HES and isotonic saline failed to show a difference in 90-day mortality but more patients in the HES group required renal replacement therapy.[20] Colloid solutions induce bleeding through platelet inhibition and possibly through dilution of clotting factors.

FLUID MANAGEMENT STRATEGIES

If patients have impaired tissue perfusion, the immediate therapeutic goal is to increase the intravascular volume with isotonic solutions and restore tissue perfusion. In severe cases, colloid or blood transfusion may be indicated to increase oncotic pressure within the vascular space. Once euvolemic, the IV fluid can be replaced by a more hypotonic maintenance solution at a rate that delivers estimated daily needs. Patients with septic shock need "early goal-directed therapy," but a more conservative approach is fluid administration 6 to 12 hours after presentation potentially to reduce the number of ventilator-days and ICU-days in patients with acute respiratory distress syndrome (ARDS).[21] While replenishing volume, one should be particularly cautious with patients at risk of fluid overload, such as those with kidney failure, cardiac failure, hepatic failure, or the elderly.

VOLUME OVERLOAD

Volume overload can result from primary renal salt retention or congestive heart failure, liver cirrhosis, and nephrotic syndrome. Iatrogenic volume overload occurs when a patient is hospitalized and receives massive quantities of intravenous fluids. Physical examination helps in determining volume overload. Point-of-care ultrasound has become increasingly popular in the emergency department (ED) and ICU to help identify volume overload by looking for "B-lines" in pulmonary venous congestion or by assessing the caliber of the inferior vena cava. Treatment for volume overload includes limiting dietary sodium intake to 2 g/day and the use of diuretics.

DIURETICS

Diuretics inhibit sodium reabsorption and can enhance urinary sodium chloride excretion, up to 25% to 30% of the filtered load. They are classified according to the segment of the nephron where they inhibit sodium or bicarbonate reabsorption.

Carbonic Anhydrase Inhibitors

Carbonic anhydrase inhibitors are mild in their potency, increase urine sodium excretion by 5% to 6%, and are useful in treating glaucoma and preventing altitude sickness. Acetazolamide inhibits the activity of carbonic anhydrase in the proximal convoluted tubules and prevents reabsorption of bicarbonate, resulting in an osmotic diuresis. It causes a metabolic acidosis and may be useful when metabolic alkalosis is present from other diuretics.

Thiazide Diuretics

Thiazide diuretics (hydrochlorothiazide, chlorthalidone, metolazone, indapamide) are intermediate in their potency and act on sodium-chloride cotransporter in the distal convoluted tubule. They cause a 5% to 13% increase in urine sodium excretion. Potential side effects are hypokalemia, hyponatremia, metabolic alkalosis, hypercalcemia, hyperuricemia, gout, hyperlipidemia, hyperglycemia, and pancreatitis. Hyponatremia can occur in the absence of volume depletion, as thiazide diuretics prevent maximal dilution of the urine. Chlorothiazide is the only thiazide diuretic available for intravenous use.

Loop Diuretics

Loop diuretics (furosemide, torsemide, bumetanide, ethacrynic acid) are the most potent diuretics, accounting for close to 30% of urine sodium excretion. They act from the tubular lumen to inhibit the sodium-potassium-2chloride cotransporter in the thick ascending limb of the loop of Henle. Loop diuretics are highly protein bound and enter the tubular lumen not by glomerular filtration but through tubular secretion, accomplished by organic anion transporters located in the proximal renal tubule. In edematous states, gut edema may reduce gastrointestinal absorption and reduce their bioavailability. Side effects are hypokalemia, metabolic alkalosis, ototoxicity at very high serum levels, and increased urinary calcium excretion.

Potassium-Sparing Diuretics

Potassium-sparing diuretics (spironolactone, eplerenone, amiloride, triamterene) act on the late distal tubule and collecting duct to increase urine sodium excretion by 3% to 5%. Amiloride and triamterene are weakly natriuretic and directly block the epithelial Na channel (ENaC). The competitive aldosterone antagonists, spironolactone and eplerenone, block the ability of aldosterone to stimulate ENaC and the Na/K ATPase pump. As the name implies, this class of diuretics is used to reduce the incidence of hypokalemia and to augment the effects of the loop diuretics. In addition, spironolactone is the preferred diuretic in patients with ascites from liver disease. Its side effects are hyperkalemia and metabolic acidosis. Spironolactone can also cause gynecomastia.

Osmotic Diuretics

Mannitol is the prototypical osmotic diuretic, while urea and glycerin are rarely used. These agents are freely filtered at the glomerulus but poorly reabsorbed by the renal tubule; the resulting increase in lumen osmolality reduces water reabsorption. Mannitol also reduces intracranial pressure and intraocular pressure (in glaucoma) through this osmotic effect. Movement of water from the intracellular to the extracellular compartment may cause hyponatremia and pulmonary edema.

DIURETIC RESISTANCE

Inadequate response to loop diuretics may be due to increased dietary salt intake, noncompliance with diuretics, use of medications like nonsteroidal anti-inflammatory drugs (NSAIDs), and/or enhanced sodium reabsorption in other portions of the renal tubule. Patients on a 2-g sodium restriction should have a 24-hour urine sodium less than 100 mmol/day:

In resistant cases, consider more frequent diuretic dosing, higher dose of diuretics, intravenous administration, or sequential blockade of the renal tubule with two diuretics from different classes (typically combining loop diuretic with either a thiazide or potassium-sparing diuretic).[22] Continuous intravenous infusion and bolus intermittent intravenous dosing of loop diuretics are two different intravenous options, and randomized controlled trials have shown no difference in outcome between the two strategies.[23]

Pure ultrafiltration using a dialysis machine or a special machine designed for aquapheresis should be considered only if kidney failure is present in a patient with volume overload that is refractory to diuretics. Randomized trials comparing continuous intravenous administration of furosemide with preemptive pure ultrafiltration to treat patients with decompensated congestive heart failure demonstrated equivalent outcomes, with more frequent adverse effects in the pure ultrafiltration group.[24]

PHARMACOTHERAPY FOR MANAGEMENT OF ACID–BASE DISORDERS

Acid–base physiology is adaptation in hydrogen ion concentration. Normal pH ranges from 7.35 to 7.45, which is needed for oxygen delivery to tissue,

maintaining protein structure and cell function. Any changes in acid–base homeostasis can have crucial pathophysiologic consequences, and extremes changes in pH can potentially be life threatening.[25–27]

APPROACH TO ACID–BASE DISORDERS

Diagnosing acid–base disorders can be a daunting and arduous task. Following a step-wise approach can be helpful:

Step 1: Identify primary acid–base disorder
- Use pH to identify acidemia (pH <7.4) or alkalemia (pH >7.4)
- Then assess HCO_3 and CO_2 to establish whether it is a metabolic or respiratory disorder:
  - Metabolic acidosis—Low HCO_3 (<24 mEq/L)
  - Metabolic alkalosis—High HCO_3 (>24 mEq/L)
  - Respiratory acidosis—High pCO_2 (>40 mmHg)
  - Respiratory alkalosis—Low pCO_2 (<40 mmHg)

Step 2: Calculate compensation
- Metabolic acidosis
  - Winter's formula: $pCO_{2(expected)} = [(1.5 \times HCO_3) + 8 (+2)]$, or
  - $\Delta pCO_2 = 1.2 \times (\Delta HCO_3)$
    - For every 1-mEq/L decrease in HCO_3, pCO_2 decreases by 1.2 mmHg
- Metabolic alkalosis
  - $pCO_{2(expected)} = [(0.7 \times HCO_3) + 20 (+5)]$, or
  - $\Delta pCO_2 = 0.7 \times \Delta HCO_3$
    - For every 1 mEq/L increase in HCO_3, pCO_2 increases by 0.7 mmHg
- Respiratory acidosis
  - Acute respiratory acidosis:
    - $\Delta pCO_2 = 10 \times HCO_3$
      - For every 10 mmHg increase in pCO_2, HCO_3 increases by 1 mEq/L
  - Chronic respiratory acidosis:
    - For every 10 mmHg increase in pCO_2, HCO_3 increases by 4 mEq/L
- Respiratory alkalosis
  - Acute respiratory alkalosis:
    - For every 10 mmHg decrease in pCO_2, HCO_3 decreases by 2 mEq/L
  - Chronic respiratory alkalosis:
    - For every 10 mmHg decrease in pCO_2, HCO_3 decreases by 5 mEq/L

Step 3: Calculate the anion gap (AG) if the primary acid-base disorder is a metabolic disorder
- Differentiate between high AG metabolic acidosis (AGMA) and nonAGMA.
  - $AG = \{[Na] - ([Cl] + [HCO_3])\}$, where Na is sodium, Cl is chloride, and HCO_3 is bicarbonate
  - Normal AG is less than 12

Step 4: Determine the ΔAG to ΔHCO3 ratio if AGMA is present

- Calculate the change in AG (ΔAG):

$$\Delta AG = AG_{(calculated)} - 12$$

- Calculate the change in HCO₃ (ΔHCO₃):

$$\Delta HCO_3 = 24 - HCO_{3\,(measured)}$$

- If $\Delta AG/\Delta HCO_3 > 2 \rightarrow$ then metabolic alkalosis is also present
- If $\Delta AG/\Delta HCO3 < 1 \rightarrow$ then AGMA is also present

Step 5: If a nonAGMA is present and the primary differential diagnosis is between a distal renal tubular acidosis (RTA) or gastrointestinal (GI) loss of HCO₃, determining the urine AG can help determine the etiology. The urine AG is not helpful in distinguishing GI losses from proximal or hyperkalemic (type IV) RTAs.

- Urine AG = Urine Sodium (U Na) + Urine Potassium (U K) – Urine Chloride (U Cl)
  - A positive urine AG, indicating the absence of an unmeasured cation or ammonium (NH_4^+), supports a distal RTA diagnosis.
  - A negative urine AG, indicating the presence of NH_4^+, indicates that GI loss is responsible.

CAUSES AND TREATMENT OF ACID–BASE DISORDERS

Metabolic Acidosis

Metabolic acidosis is a disorder that occurs as a result of either addition of protons or the loss of base, resulting in a decrease in serum HCO_3 levels and a decrease in extracellular pH. The low HCO_3 and pH trigger a compensatory increase in ventilation to reduce pCO_2 and bring pH back towards normal. Metabolic acidosis is classified as anion gap[28] versus nonanion gap, helping to narrow the search for potential causes (**Tables 21.3 and 21.4**, respectively).

Anion Gap Metabolic Acidosis
Alcohol Poisoning (Methanol, Ethylene Glycol, and Propylene Glycol)

Methanol and ethylene glycol (EG) are often found in antifreeze, windshield wiper fluids, radiator coolants, and solvents. Ingestion of methanol and EG leads to a high AGMA and a high osmolal gap. Propylene glycol (PG) is used as a vehicle for certain IV medications such as propofol, lorazepam, and diazepam, and may cause a high AGMA when the infusion is prolonged and/or administered in large doses.

Treatment includes elimination of or cessation of offending agents. Ethanol has greater affinity for alcohol dehydrogenase (ALDH) and has been used as a traditional treatment for EG poisoning. It is administered

TABLE 21.3 Causes of Anion Gap Metabolic Acidosis (Mnemonic)

G	Glycols (ethylene glycol and propylene glycol)
O	Oxoproline (acetaminophen ingestion in malnourished patients; mechanism not well understood)
L	L-Lactate
D	D-Lactate
M	Methanol
A	Aspirin
R	Renal Failure
K	Ketoacidosis

TABLE 21.4 Causes of Non-Anion Gap Metabolic Acidosis

Proximal Renal Tubular Acidosis (Type II)	Distal Renal Tubular Acidosis With Hypokalemia (Type I)	Distal Renal Tubular Acidosis With Hyperkalemia (Type IV)
Acetazolamide	Amphotericin	Diabetic nephropathy
Topiramate	Toluene	ACE inhibitors
Ifosfamide	Lithium	ARBs
Tenofovir	Ibuprofen	Heparin
Aminoglycosides	Ifosfamide	NSAIDs
AL amyloidosis	Sjogren syndrome	Calcineurin inhibitors
Multiple myeloma	Familial	Amiloride
Lead	Idiopathic	Trimethoprim
Copper		Triamterene
		Pentamidine
		Sickle cell anemia
		Lupus nephritis

ACE, angiotensin-converting enzyme; AL, amyloid light-chain; ARB, angiotensin-receptor blocker; NSAID, nonsteroidal anti-inflammatory drug.

as a 10% solution in 5% dextrose water (D5W). Loading dose of 0.8 to 1.0 g/kg followed by an infusion of 100 mg/kg/hour is suggested. Fomepizole is a potent competitive inhibitor of ALDH. Initial loading dose is 15 mg/kg followed by 10 mg/kg every 12 hours for four doses, then 15 mg/kg every 12 hours thereafter until EG level is less than 20 and the patient is asymptomatic with a normal blood pH. In severe cases, hemodialysis is recommended.

Lactic Acidosis

Lactic acidosis is further divided into three categories: type A lactic acidosis, type B lactic acidosis, and d-lactic acidosis.

Type A lactic acidosis is caused by a state of hypoperfusion or in conditions with inadequate oxygen delivery. Common causes of type A lactic acidosis include shock, severe hypoxemia, extreme exercise, and carbon monoxide poisoning. Treatment of type A lactic acidosis includes IV fluids, restoration of oxygen, vasopressors to ensure adequate tissue perfusion, and other supportive measures.

Type B lactic acidosis is caused by various drugs and toxins, such as metformin, linezolid, propofol, isoniazid, niacin, and salicylate. Treatment is cessation of the offending agent and supportive measures. In the case of metformin overdose with impaired kidney function, hemodialysis may be indicated.

Common causes of D-lactic acidosis include short bowel syndrome with bacterial overgrowth. Treatment includes oral fasting with IV nutrition and restoration of normal gut flora.

Ketoacidosis

Common causes of ketoacidosis include diabetic ketoacidosis (DKA), starvation ketoacidosis, and alcoholic ketoacidosis (AKA). Treatment for DKA includes IV fluid, electrolyte replacements, and IV insulin given as a bolus of 0.1 unit/kg followed by a continuous infusion of 0.1 unit/kg/hour. AKA and starvation ketoacidosis are treated with administration of IV fluids and glucose, taking care to administer thiamine before glucose to reduce the risk for Wernicke's encephalopathy.

Salicylate Toxicity

Treatment includes supportive measures such as IV fluid administration, charcoal lavage, and alkalization of the urine with IV sodium bicarbonate. In severe cases of overdose, hemodialysis may be required.

Renal Failure

The recommended treatment is to initiate sodium bicarbonate tablets 650 mg (~8 mEq) orally three times a day and titrate up the dose as needed, targeting a serum HCO_3 level of about 22 mEq/L.

Nonanion Gap Metabolic Acidosis

Proximal Renal Tubular Acidosis (Type II)

The recommended treatment is to administer 10 to 15 mEq of base per kg in two to three divided doses per day to overcome urinary bicarbonate losses and raise serum bicarbonate level. Potassium citrate or potassium and sodium citrate combination is preferred since type II RTA is often associated with hypokalemia.

Distal Renal Tubular Acidosis (Type I)

The recommended treatment is 1 to 2 mEq of base per kg in two to three divided doses per day. Sodium bicarbonate or sodium citrate is preferred, as serum potassium levels are either normal or only slightly low.

Distal Renal Tubular Acidosis With Hyperkalemia (Type IV)

Treatment includes stopping any offending agent that causes or exacerbates the underlying type IV RTA, dietary potassium restriction, and the use of potassium-binding agents and loop diuretics to increase potassium elimination. Fludrocortisone, an aldosterone agonist, 0.1 to 0.2 mg daily dose can also be considered but may exacerbate volume overload.

Metabolic Alkalosis

Causes of metabolic alkalosis can be divided into two groups: chloride-responsive alkalosis and chloride-resistant alkalosis. Each of these two groups can be further divided into normotensive and hypertensive causes (**Table 21.5**).

Chloride-Responsive Metabolic Alkalosis

Patients with chloride-responsive metabolic alkalosis, also known as "contraction alkalosis," are usually volume depleted from vomiting, gastric suctioning, or high nasogastric tube output. Treatment is removing the underlying etiology and volume repletion with IV isotonic fluids such as 0.9% NaCl, Plasma-Lyte, and Lactated Ringer's, along with correction of hypokalemia, if present, with potassium chloride. Although the initial phase of diuretic use is classified under chloride-resistance, treatment is the same as described here because the mechanism for alkalosis is also volume depletion, but the concurrent use of diuretics prevents renal conservation of chloride.

Chloride-Resistant Metabolic Alkalosis

Treatment for these disorders depends on the underlying etiology. For primary hyperaldosteronism, aldosterone antagonist (e.g., spironolactone, eplerenone) or potassium-sparing diuretics (e.g., amiloride, triamterene) can be used. Potassium-sparing diuretics

TABLE 21.5 Causes of Metabolic Alkalosis	
Chloride-Responsive Metabolic Alkalosis (Urinary Chloride <20 mEq)	**Chloride-Resistant Metabolic Alkalosis (Urinary Chloride >20 mEq)**
Normotensive	**Hypertensive**
Vomiting	Primary hyperaldosteronism
High nasogastric tube output	Cushing syndrome or disease
Gastric suctioning	Apparent mineralocorticoid
Chronic laxative abuse	excess (e.g., licorice ingestion)
Diuretics (remote use or over-diuresis)	Glucocorticoid-remedial hypertension
	Liddle syndrome
	Normotensive
	Diuretic (initial phase)
	Bartter syndrome
	Gitelman syndrome

are also useful for treating the metabolic alkalosis in Cushing's syndrome. Definitive treatment for primary hyperaldosteronism, Cushing's, and licorice-induced metabolic alkalosis is correction or removal of the underlying cause, if possible. For glucocorticoid-remediable hypertension (GRH), a genetic form of hypertension, resulting from a crossover event that places aldosterone synthesis under the control of adrenocorticotropic hormone (ACTH), treatment is to administer corticosteroids to suppress ACTH production. For Bartter and Gitelman syndrome, treatment focuses on potassium and magnesium replacement, with a potential role for inhibitors of distal tubular sodium–potassium exchange (e.g., spironolactone, eplerenone, amiloride, and triamterene) and drugs that reduce prostaglandin levels (i.e., NSAIDs). Liddle syndrome is treated with amiloride or triamterene to block the overactive epithelial sodium channel; aldosterone antagonists are not effective.

Respiratory Disorders

Table 21.6 summarizes the potential causes of both respiratory acidosis and alkalosis. Treatment of respiratory acid–base disorders consists of addressing the underlying causes, such as symptomatic treatment for pain, fever, or anxiety, and removing any drugs potentially responsible for the respiratory acid–base disorder. Depending on the etiology and the acuity of the underlying etiology, supplemental oxygen, noninvasive ventilation (e.g., BiPAP or CPAP), or mechanical ventilatory support may be required.

TABLE 21.6 Causes of Respiratory Disorders

Respiratory Acidosis	Respiratory Alkalosis
Central nervous system depression: general anesthesia, sedative overdose, head trauma, brain tumor, central sleep apnea Neuromuscular impairment: Guillain-Barre syndrome, status epilepticus, myasthenia gravis, amyotrophic lateral sclerosis, muscular dystrophy Upper airway obstruction: aspiration, obstructive sleep apnea, laryngospasm, angioedema, tonsillar hypertrophy, tumor of the vocal cords or larynx Lower airway obstruction: severe asthma, chronic obstructive lung disease, acute respiratory distress syndrome	Central nervous system stimulation: anxiety, fever, pain, psychosis, cerebrovascular accident, tumor Pulmonary: pneumonia, asthma, acute respiratory distress syndrome, interstitial lung disease, pulmonary embolism, congestive heart failure Drugs: salicylate, progesterone, nicotine

PHARMACOTHERAPY FOR MANAGEMENT OF ELECTROLYTE DISORDERS

Serum electrolytes reflect the stores of ECF electrolytes rather than that of ICF. In the ECF, sodium is the most common cation and chloride is the most abundant anion. In the ICF, potassium is the most common cation while phosphate is the main anion. Other ions of interest are the magnesium and calcium cations and the bicarbonate anion.

SODIUM

Normal serum sodium concentration ranges from 135 to 145 mEq/L. The plasma sodium concentration is regulated by changes in water intake and excretion, not by changes in sodium balance. Hyponatremia is due primarily to water that cannot be excreted, and hypernatremia is due primarily to loss of water that has not been replaced. Sodium balance disorders are hypovolemia and edema, which involve problems with both sodium and water handling. Hypovolemia results from loss of sodium and water (e.g., excessive sweating, diarrhea, over-diuresis). Ingestion of higher amounts of sodium may cause expansion of ECF with resulting edema and can exacerbate hypertension.

Hyponatremia

Hyponatremia is the most common electrolyte disturbance and is defined as serum sodium concentration below 135 mEq/L. Clinical symptoms appear at serum sodium concentration below 120 mEq/L and typically consist of irritability, mental slowing, unstable gait/falls, headache, and nausea. With profound (severe) hyponatremia (sodium concentration <110 mEq/L), confusion, seizure, stupor, coma, and respiratory arrest can be seen. Hyponatremia is classified based on the serum osmolality and volume status:

1. **Hypertonic hyponatremia:** Hypertonic hyponatremia, or translocational or redistributive hyponatremia, is usually seen with hyperglycemia and administration of mannitol. Glucose and mannitol are osmotically active agents, which will shift water from ICF to ECF but have little effect on total body sodium, thus lowering sodium concentration. For every 100 mg/dL increase in serum glucose above 200 mg/dL, serum sodium concentration is expected to decrease by 1 mEq/L.
2. **Isotonic hyponatremia**: Isotonic hyponatremia, or pseudo-hyponatremia, is due to the presence of hyperlipidemia (hypertriglyceridemia or high cholesterol levels) or increase in plasma proteins (paraproteinemia) in conditions like multiple myeloma and Waldenstrom's macroglobulinemia. In normal subjects, plasma water accounts for 93%

of the plasma volume, and fats and proteins the remaining 7%. Plasma water fraction can fall below 80% when lipids or protein levels are high. Though the plasma water sodium concentration and plasma osmolality are unchanged, the measured sodium concentration in the total plasma volume is reduced since the specimen contains less plasma water.

3. **Hypotonic (low-serum osmolality) hyponatremia**: Hypotonic (low-serum osmolality) hyponatremia is classified based on the clinical assessment of volume (i.e., ECF) status:

   a) *Hypovolemic hyponatremia:* In hypovolemic hyponatremia, ECF volume is decreased. These patients usually have a deficit of both total body sodium and TBW, but the sodium deficit exceeds TBW deficit. The volume depletion, when profound, leads to physiologic release of antidiuretic hormone (ADH), enhancing absorption of water by the kidneys. Common causes include profuse sweating, diarrhea or vomiting, over-diuresis, and burns. Treatment includes giving IV fluids to replace sodium and water and to restore effective perfusion, which will "turn off" ADH and allow the kidneys to excrete the excess water.

   b) *Hypervolemic hyponatremia:* Although ECF volume is increased and these patients have edema, effective arteriolar perfusion is reduced, leading to physiologic ADH release and water retention. Prototypical diseases are congestive heart failure, where perfusion is impaired because of myocardial dysfunction, and cirrhosis of the liver, in which liver dysfunction leads to splanchnic dilation and decreased perfusion. These patients have an excess of total body sodium and TBW, but TBW excess is greater than total body sodium. Treatment includes sodium and water restriction as well as use of diuretics. Additional treatment for congestive heart failure may include use of inotropic agents and afterload reducing medications (see Chapter 17).

   c) *Euvolemic hyponatremia:* Patients with euvolemic hyponatremia have a normal ECF volume and total body sodium, but an excess of TBW because of nonphysiologic stimulation of ADH release. Syndrome of inappropriate ADH release (SIADH) can be seen with lung cancer, pulmonary disease, central nervous system disorders, some medications such as antidepressants, hypothyroidism, adrenal insufficiency, stress, pain, and nausea. Acute management includes fluid restriction, and hypertonic saline (3% NaCl) if the patient has severe hyponatremia (Na <110 mEq/L) and/or severe symptoms (profound altered mental status, seizures, coma). Conivaptan (intravenous ADH antagonist) may be used in hospitalized patients to treat euvolemic or hypervolemic hyponatremia.

If the underlying etiology for SIADH is not reversible, long-term treatment options for euvolemic hyponatremia are fluid restriction, loop diuretics to reduce urine osmolality (effectively increasing free water excretion), salt tablets or urea to provide additional solutes to aid in free water excretion, demeclocycline, lithium, and tolvaptan. Demeclocycline is given at a dose of 600 to 1,200 mg/day. Its clinical effect is seen after a few days as it is thought to reduce aquaporin expression. Demeclocycline can cause nephrotoxicity. Tolvaptan is an oral ADH antagonist and may be used to treat symptomatic euvolemic (Na <125 mEq/L) hyponatremia or hypervolemic hyponatremia from congestive heart failure. The starting dose is 15 mg daily and maximum tolerated dose is 60 mg/day. Avoid concurrent use of tolvaptan with CYP 3A4 inhibitors like ketoconazole, grapefruit juice, diltiazem, verapamil, fluconazole, and clarithromycin. Two additional causes of euvolemic hyponatremia that do not involve ADH release are water intoxication and use of thiazide diuretics. In water intoxication, the rate of water ingestion exceeds the ability of the kidneys to eliminate the excess water. Treatment is to reduce water intake. Thiazide diuretics impair the ability of the kidneys to excrete water by preventing maximal dilution of the urine and, when combined with reduced solute intake, may cause hyponatremia.

The choice of fluids to treat hyponatremia depends upon the severity of the hyponatremia and the volume status of the patient. Patients with volume depletion and hyponatremia can be managed with normal saline. In SIADH patients, normal saline will often worsen the hyponatremia as urine osmolality is typically significantly higher than the osmolality of normal saline (308 mOsm/kg). In these patients, salt tablets or hypertonic saline will be required. If hyponatremia is severe (Na <120 mEq/L) and accompanied by neurological symptoms, 100 mL of 3% NaCl is given over 10 minutes and may be repeated up to two more times for persistent neurologic symptoms. When milder symptoms are present, 3% NaCl may be administered at a rate of 0.5 to 2 mL/kg/hour. The goal of correction is no faster than 6 to 8 mEq/L rise in sodium concentration in 24 hours.[29] The rate of correction should be less than 0.5 mEq/L/hour. Overly aggressive correction of symptomatic hyponatremia (>8 mEq/L) in 24 hours can result in osmotic demyelination (ODS).

Hypernatremia

Hypernatremia is present when the serum sodium concentration exceeds 145 mEq/L. Causes of hypernatremia include hypotonic fluid losses (e.g., sweating, fever, diarrhea), markedly decreased water intake, osmotic diuresis, central diabetes insipidus from low ADH levels (as seen in brain injury and toxic phenytoin levels), and nephrogenic diabetes insipidus from poor response to ADH (from chronic tubulointerstitial nephritis or drugs like lithium). Even when the above causes are present, an intact thirst mechanism and ability to obtain water mitigates the risk for developing hypernatremia, as patients are able to replete ongoing water losses through water intake. Therefore, hypernatremia typically occurs in patients with mental status changes or who have reduced or no access to water. Hypernatremia in hospitalized patients is frequently iatrogenic and results from resuscitation with hypertonic fluids or inappropriate fluid management in patients with ongoing water losses. Signs and symptoms usually are present when serum sodium concentration is greater than 160 mEq/L and consist of thirst, mental slowing, dry mucous membranes, acute weight loss, seizure, and/or coma. Treatment of hypernatremia involves calculating the TBW deficit and correcting with hypotonic fluids over 48 to 72 hours. The rate of correction should not exceed 0.5 mEq/L/hour. Half the calculated TBW deficit should be replaced in the first 12 to 24 hours and the remainder in the subsequent 24 to 48 hours. Rapid correction can result in cerebral edema and death.

Antidiuretic Hormone Agonists and Antagonists

Arginine vasopressin (AVP) and desmopressin are antidiuretic hormone (ADH) agonists, which reduce urine volume and increase urine concentration (urine osmolality). They are useful in treating central diabetes insipidus and are sometimes effective in treating patients with partial nephrogenic diabetes insipidus, as pharmacologic doses of ADH agonists may overcome tubular resistance to ADH. When the rate of correction of hyponatremia is too rapid, ADH agonists can be used to slow down the rate of correction.

Vasopressin receptor antagonists or the "vaptans" oppose the actions of ADH and other naturally occurring peptides that act on the same V2 receptor to produce a selective water diuresis (aquaresis) without affecting sodium and potassium excretion. The ensuing loss of electrolyte-free water will tend to raise the serum sodium concentration in patients with SIADH.[30] In addition to their use in selected SIADH patients, ADH receptor antagonists may be used off label to treat hyponatremia in selected patients with congestive heart failure. These drugs should be avoided in patients with liver failure because of the potential for hepatotoxicity. Conivaptan is an intravenous vasopressin antagonist[31] and tolvaptan is an oral formulation.

POTASSIUM

The body's normal daily potassium requirement is 40 to 80 mEq to maintain a serum potassium concentration of 3.5 to 5.0 mEq/L. Potassium homeostasis may be affected by acid–base balance of the body; acidemia (reduced pH) may cause hyperkalemia through translocation of potassium from the ICF to the ECF. Potassium regulation is primarily by the kidneys, and excess dietary potassium is excreted in the urine.

Hypokalemia

"Hypokalemia" is defined as a serum potassium less than 3.5 mEq/L and, when mild, is generally asymptomatic. Severe hypokalemia and mild hypokalemia in susceptible individuals may result in cramps, muscle weakness, polyuria, electrocardiogram changes (flattened T waves and presence of U waves), and cardiac arrhythmias (bradycardia, heart block, atrial flutter, premature ventricular contraction, ventricular fibrillation). Causes of hypokalemia include: inadequate potassium intake, kidney losses (in the setting of hypomagnesemia, hyperaldosteronism, use of thiazide and loop diuretics, use of corticosteroids, vomiting or nasogastric suctioning), gastrointestinal losses (e.g., diarrhea), and cellular redistribution from the ECF to the ICF (albuterol, insulin, and, to a lesser extent, alkalosis). Although vomiting and nasogastric suctioning are gastrointestinal losses of fluids, potassium loss actually occurs in the kidneys because of hypovolemia-induced secondary hyperaldosteronism. Medications such as foscarnet, amphotericin B, and cisplatin can cause hypokalemia through depletion of magnesium.

Hypomagnesemia induces kidney potassium wasting. The mechanism of hypokalemia in magnesium deficiency, however, remains unexplained. Potassium secretion from the cell into the lumen by the cells of the connecting tubule and cortical collecting tubule is mediated by the luminal renal outer medullary potassium (ROMK) channels, a process that is inhibited by intracellular magnesium. Hypomagnesemia is associated with a reduction in the intracellular magnesium concentration, which stimulates ROMK channels to cause potassium secretion. Given the very high cell potassium concentration, this would promote potassium secretion from the cell into the lumen and enhanced urinary losses. The hypokalemia in this setting is refractory to potassium supplementation and requires correction of the magnesium deficit first or concurrently with potassium repletion. Hypokalemia is an important risk factor for digoxin toxicity. Every 1 mEq/L decline of serum potassium reflects about 200 mEq of total body potassium loss in the adult. A 24-hour urine potassium excretion of more than 25 to 30 mEq/day or a urine potassium to urine creatinine ratio of greater than 13 mEq/g suggests renal wasting of potassium.

Treatment consists of oral potassium replacement: potassium chloride is preferred in most patients and especially in patients with hypokalemia and alkalosis, while potassium bicarbonate and its precursors (potassium acetate and potassium citrate) and potassium gluconate are preferred in patients with acidosis and hypokalemia. Potassium chloride will correct hypokalemia more quickly because chloride is excluded from the ICF, keeping more of the infused potassium in the ECF. Intravenous replacement is needed when serum potassium is below 2.5 mEq/L or at any level of potassium when associated with electrocardiographic changes. IV infusions in premixed solutions are available for potassium chloride and acetate (10–20 mEq diluted in 100 mL of normal saline). Potassium infusion at rates exceeding 10 mEq/L requires cardiac monitoring and central venous access for administration because of the risk of cardiac arrhythmias, vein irritation, and thrombophlebitis when infused peripherally.

Hyperkalemia

Hyperkalemia is present when serum potassium concentration exceeds 5 mEq/L. Clinical manifestations include muscle weakness, paresthesia, hypotension, electrocardiogram (ECG) changes (peaked T waves, shortened QT intervals, and progressive widening of PR intervals and QRS complexes), cardiac arrhythmias, and potentially acidemia through suppression of ammonia production (a required buffer for renal tubular proton elimination). Causes of hyperkalemia include:

- Increased potassium intake from excessive dietary potassium and/or excess potassium supplements
- Decreased potassium excretion from: (a) use of potassium-sparing diuretics (aldosterone antagonists such as spironolactone and eplerenone, and epithelial sodium channel blockers such as triamterene and amiloride); (b) drugs or disease states that block or reduce aldosterone production (e.g., cyclosporine, heparin, nonsteroidal anti-inflammatory agents, Addison disease); (c) other drugs that block the epithelial sodium channel (pentamidine, trimethoprim); and (d) impaired nephron function in acute kidney injury or chronic kidney disease
- Potassium release from the intracellular space, as seen in tissue breakdown and/or cell lysis from surgery, trauma, hemolysis, rhabdomyolysis, blood transfusion reaction, and tumor lysis syndrome, as well as translocation from the ICF to ECF in hyperosmolal states, insulinopenia, and certain types of metabolic acidosis

Management of hyperkalemia includes:

1. Agents to "stabilize" the cell membrane and antagonize the proarrhythmic effects of hyperkalemia. If serum potassium is greater than 7 mEq/L and/or hyperkalemic ECG changes are present, then IV calcium chloride is given to "stabilize" the myocytes. Calcium chloride 1 g is administered by direct IV injection or diluted in 50 mL of D5W and given IV over 15 minutes. Clinical effects are seen in 1 to 2 minutes and the effect persists for 10 to 30 minutes. This infusion can be repeated as necessary with close monitoring of serum calcium or ionized calcium. Calcium administration is a temporizing measure to allow time for definitive removal of potassium.

2. Agents to shift potassium into the intracellular space, acutely lowering serum potassium—such as insulin and beta-2-agonists. Insulin is typically given at the same time as IV calcium therapy, at a dose of 10 units IV, preceded by 25 g of dextrose 50% (25 g in 50 mL) to prevent hypoglycemia. Alternatively, 20 units of regular insulin with dextrose 10% can be given by continuous IV infusion over 1 to 2 hours. Onset of action is 30 minutes and clinical effects last 2 to 6 hours. Monitoring of blood glucose levels to detect hypoglycemia is important after insulin administration, especially in patients without diabetes. High-dose inhaled beta-2 agonists (e.g., albuterol) also may be used to acutely shift potassium into the intracellular space. Sodium bicarbonate may be used if metabolic acidosis is present, though its utility in lowering potassium levels is questioned. As with calcium, these agents are temporizing measures to control hyperkalemia until potassium can be eliminated.

3. Definitive therapy that lowers total body potassium content by increasing potassium excretion:
   a) **Loop diuretics** increase potassium excretion in urine in patients with intact kidney function but are less useful in patients on dialysis or with advanced kidney disease.
   b) **Dialysis** (hemodialysis or hemofiltration)
   c) **Potassium-binding agents** bind potassium in the gastrointestinal tract and enhance its excretion in feces. Sodium polystyrene sulfonate (SPS or Kayexalate) can be given orally, by nasogastric tube, or as a retention enema. Concurrent administration of sorbitol is no longer recommended because of an increased risk of colonic necrosis, ischemic colitis, bleeding, and colonic perforation, attributed to the sorbitol, though recent studies suggest that SPS itself may be the culprit. Oral doses of kayexalate are 15 g to 30 g given once to four times a day, and rectal doses 30 g to 50 g up to every 6 hours, until effect. Onset of action is greater than 2 hours. Because of the risk for bowel complications, SPS should be given only when life-threatening hyperkalemia is present, hemodialysis and other cation exchange resins are not readily available, and other measures to reduce potassium have failed. Newer agents such as sodium zirconium cyclosilicate (SZC or Lokelma)[32,33] and patiromer (Veltassa)[34] are preferred. Both come in a powder form and need to be mixed with water before oral administration. Neither are absorbed systemically. SZC exchanges sodium and hydrogen counterions for potassium in the gastrointestinal tract. Dose is 10 g orally three times a day for 48 hours initially, followed by 5 g to 15 g daily for maintenance.

Patiromer is a polymer that contains calcium-sorbitol counterion, with exchange of calcium for potassium. It is given orally at a dose of 8.4 g to 25.2 g daily. Both patiromer and SZC should be administered at least 2 to 3 hours apart from other oral medications to avoid reduced bioavailability of the other medications. Hypomagnesemia and GI side effects are common with patiromer.

MAGNESIUM

Serum magnesium concentration is a relatively poor measure of total body magnesium stores. The body requires 300 to 350 mg of dietary magnesium a day to maintain a normal serum magnesium concentration of 1.5 to 2.2 mg/dL. Magnesium maintains neuromuscular stability and is involved in myocardial contraction.

Hypomagnesemia

Serum magnesium levels less than 1.5 mg/dL can occur in the setting of poor nutritional intake, alcoholism, and dependency on total parenteral nutrition. Additional risk factors for gastrointestinal loss of magnesium include malabsorption, inadequate absorption from steatorrhea, diarrhea, and use of laxatives and proton pump inhibitors. Increased urinary losses of magnesium are seen with primary hyperaldosteronism, renal tubular disorders, diabetic ketoacidosis, and medications such as aminoglycosides, amphotericin B, cisplatin, cyclosporine, insulin, and loop and thiazide diuretics. Obtaining a 24-hour urine to determine daily magnesium excretion will differentiate between renal wasting (>10–30 mg/day) and extra-renal losses (<10 mg/day) of magnesium. Hypocalcemia and hypokalemia are often observed with hypomagnesemia, and magnesium repletion is necessary for reversing the low calcium and potassium levels. Symptoms of low magnesium levels include muscle weakness, cramps, agitation, confusion, tremor, seizures, and ECG changes with increased PR and QT intervals and widened QRS interval.

Treatment for mild asymptomatic magnesium deficiencies is increased dietary magnesium intake or oral replacement with magnesium oxide or magnesium chloride. Diarrhea from magnesium supplements is a common side effect and limits the dose. Sustained-release preparations include magnesium chloride and magnesium L-lactate, which cause less diarrhea, are slowly absorbed, and minimize renal excretion of the administered magnesium. In severe magnesium deficiency (<1 mEq/L), 1 to 2 g of magnesium sulfate is given intravenously over 2 to 15 minutes. One gram of magnesium sulfate contains 98 mg or 8 mEq of elemental magnesium. Repeated infusions of magnesium sulfate over a few days may be necessary for repletion as up to 50% of an administered intravenous magnesium dose may be excreted in the urine. Serum magnesium levels in patients with reduced kidney function must be monitored closely as the risk for toxicity is high. Underlying etiology for magnesium deficiency should be addressed. Patients with hypomagnesemia due to renal losses may benefit from potassium-sparing diuretic like amiloride.

Hypermagnesemia

Hypermagnesemia is usually iatrogenic and is seen in patients with kidney failure on medications rich in magnesium (antacids, laxatives, magnesium supplements), lithium therapy, and in women with preeclampsia treated with magnesium. Hypermagnesemia is present when serum magnesium levels exceed 2.5 mg/dL and is further classified as mild (2.5–4 mg/dL), moderate (4–12 mg/dL), and severe (>13 mg/dL). Milder symptoms are nausea, vomiting, bradycardia, hyporeflexia, and somnolence. More serious symptoms include muscle paralysis, complete heart block, asystole, respiratory failure, and refractory hypotension. Treatment involves intravenous normal saline and diuretics to enhance renal elimination and IV calcium gluconate to reverse the neuromuscular and cardiovascular effects. Hemodialysis may be necessary when hypermagnesemia is severe and/or kidney function is compromised.

CALCIUM

Calcium is found mainly in bones with only 1% in the ECF and ICF. Ionized calcium is critical for the conduction of nerve impulses, myocardial contractions, skeletal muscle contraction, and the formation of bones and teeth. Normal serum calcium levels range from 8.6 to 10.2 mg/dL and correspond to total serum calcium. Serum calcium and phosphorous levels have a reciprocal relationship and are regulated by complex interactions between parathyroid hormone, vitamin D, calcitonin, and fibroblast growth factor 23. About half of the serum calcium is bound to plasma proteins, predominantly albumin, and the remainder exists as ionized calcium, the physiologically important component. Consequently, ionized calcium levels remain normal despite a low total serum calcium level in hypoalbuminemia and a high total serum calcium level in hyperalbuminemia. An increase or decrease in serum albumin level of 1 g/dL from normal will result in a respective increase or decrease in total serum calcium level of 0.8 mg/dL, resulting in the following equation to calculate corrected calcium level:

Corrected calcium (mg/dL) = Measured calcium mg/dL + (0.8 [4 – measured albumin g/dL])

Changes in acid–base status may also influence the degree of protein binding, rendering total serum calcium levels a less useful indicator of ionized calcium levels. In these settings, ionized calcium levels should be measured directly.

Hypocalcemia

Common causes of hypocalcemia include vitamin D deficiency (primary or due to chronic kidney disease), poor dietary calcium intake, hypoparathyroidism (primary or as a result of hypo- or hypermagnesemia), altered binding intravascularly (hypoalbuminemia and metabolic alkalosis described previously, and massive blood product infusion with chelation of calcium by citrate), and tissue calcium deposition (in the setting of hyperphosphatemia and pancreatitis). Medications that can cause hypocalcemia include phosphorous binders, loop diuretics, phenytoin, phenobarbital, corticosteroids, aminoglycosides, and acetazolamide, through a variety of mechanisms. Clinically, symptoms and signs are seen when total serum calcium is less than 6.5 mg/dL (ionized calcium <1.12 mmol/L) and include numbness, tingling, perioral tingling, muscle spasms, hypoactive reflexes, anxiety, hallucinations, hypotension, seizures, myocardial infarction, lethargy, stupor, Trousseau's sign, and Chvostek's sign. Asymptomatic mild hypocalcemia is managed with oral calcium supplementation with calcium carbonate or Tums and calcium acetate. Acute symptomatic hypocalcemia requires IV calcium replacement with calcium chloride or calcium gluconate. Calcium chloride should be administered via a central venous catheter because of venous irritation and extravasation. Ten milliliters of calcium gluconate contains 90 mg of elemental calcium while 10 mL of calcium chloride contains 270 mg of elemental calcium. Rate of intravenous infusion must not exceed 30 to 60 mg of elemental calcium per minute because of the risk of bradycardia, hypotension, or cardiac asystole with rapid administration. Concurrent vitamin D deficiency should be corrected as well, and potential underlying cause for hypocalcemia removed.

Hypercalcemia

"Hypercalcemia" is defined as a total serum calcium concentration greater than 10.2 mg/dL and is classified as mild (10.3–12 mg/dL), moderate (12.1–13 mg/dL) and severe (>13 mg/dL). Causes include hyperparathyroidism, malignancy, Paget's disease, immobilization, granulomatous diseases, hyperthyroidism, acidosis, and milk-alkali syndrome. Various medications can cause hypercalcemia through a variety of different mechanisms: thiazide diuretics, lithium, vitamin A, vitamin D, tamoxifen, estrogens, and calcium supplements. Evaluation of hypercalcemia starts with measuring intact parathyroid hormone (iPTH) level, which is high in primary hyperparathyroidism. If iPTH is low, additional diagnostic evaluation include PTH related protein (PTHrp—seen in malignancies), vitamin D metabolites (vitamin D intoxication or granulomatous diseases), Vitamin A levels, thyroid-stimulating hormone (TSH), serum protein electrophoresis and urine protein electrophoresis (multiple myeloma). All patients with hypercalcemia should be treated aggressively with IV normal saline (0.9% NaCl) at a rate of 200 to 300 mL/hour, with close monitoring of volume status and potential use of loop diuretics in patients with renal insufficiency or heart failure to prevent fluid overload. The resultant natriuresis will increase urinary calcium excretion. Other treatments include bisphosphonates, calcitonin, hydrocortisone, and gallium. Denosumab is an option in patients with hypercalcemia refractory to bisphosphonates or with contraindications to bisphosphonates such as kidney failure. Close monitoring of serum calcium is necessary because of the risk of hypocalcemia. Calcimimetics such as cinacalcet and etelcalcetide may be used to reduce serum calcium levels in patients with parathyroid cancer, secondary hyperparathyroidism due to chronic kidney disease, and elevated calcium-phosphorous product (Ca × Pi).[35] Emergent hemodialysis is indicated in hypercalcemia refractory to the above treatments and in patients with kidney failure.

PHOSPHOROUS

Phosphorous is found primarily in bone (80%–85%), with the remainder distributed mainly in the ICF (15%–20%) and less than 1% in the ECF. Normal serum phosphorous levels are 2.7 to 4.5 mg/dL.

Hypophosphatemia

Mild-to-moderate hypophosphatemia is present when serum levels are less than 2.5 mg/dL but greater than 1 mg/dL. Severe hypophosphatemia (<1 mg/dL) can cause respiratory failure through impairment of diaphragmatic contractility and acute hemolysis and rhabdomyolysis through disruption of processes that maintain cell membrane integrity.

Causes for low phosphorous are:

- **Increased redistribution to ICF:** malnutrition during refeeding, hyperglycemia, insulin therapy, acute respiratory alkalosis, and hungry bone syndrome
- **Poor gastrointestinal absorption and/or loss:** aluminum-based antacids, sucralfate, starvation, vitamin D deficiency, alcoholism, phosphate binders, diarrhea, or laxative abuse
- **Increased renal losses:** diuretic use, alcohol abuse, diabetic ketoacidosis, hyperparathyroidism. A 24-hour urine phosphorous level greater than 100 mg and/or a fractional excretion of phosphorous more than 5% suggest renal wasting of phosphorous
- **Spurious hypophosphatemia:** can be caused by paraproteins interfering with the phosphate assay

Signs and symptoms of hypophosphatemia include paresthesia, muscle weakness, myalgias, bone pain, anorexia, nausea, hemolysis, rhabdomyolysis, acute respiratory failure, seizures, and coma. Dietary intake of phosphorous-rich foods, such as dairy products, eggs, animal proteins, whole grains, and nuts, should be encouraged for patients with mild hypophosphatemia. Oral repletion with sodium or potassium phosphate is indicated if serum phosphate is less than 2.0 mg/dL. Intravenous formulations are used for severe hypophosphatemia (serum levels <1.0 mg/dL) at a dose of 1 mmol/kg given slowly over 4 to 12 hours to reduce the risk of tissue calcium and phosphate deposits. Sodium-based are preferred over potassium-based formulations unless concurrent hypokalemia is present.

Hyperphosphatemia

"Hyperphosphatemia" is defined as a serum concentration greater than 4.5 mg/dL. Clinical manifestations are similar to those of hypocalcemia and include paresthesia, ECG changes, and metastatic calcifications. Causes for high phosphorous include:

- **Acute phosphate load:** from an endogenous source such as tumor lysis syndrome, hemolysis, and rhabdomyolysis; or exogenously from the administration of phosphorous containing laxatives and enemas, transfusion of stored blood, and, rarely, fosphenytoin
- **Redistribution of phosphorous from the ICF to the ECF:** acid–base imbalance, lactic acidosis, and diabetic ketoacidosis

- **Increased proximal tubular phosphate reabsorption or reduced renal clearance:** Increased tubular phosphate reabsorption occurs in hypoparathyroidism or during treatment with bisphosphonates or Vitamin D therapy. Reduced renal clearance of phosphorus occurs in acute and chronic renal failure.
- **Pseudo-hyperphosphatemia:** Conditions such as hyperglobulinemia, hyperlipidemia, hemolysis, high dose liposomal amphotericin B, heparin and hyperbilirubinemia may interfere with the analytical methods used to measure phosphorus levels.

Management includes dietary protein and phosphorus restriction and administration of phosphorous binders with meals to prevent phosphorus absorption. Many classes of phosphorus binders are now available: aluminum-based antacids, calcium-based binders (calcium carbonate and calcium acetate), non-calcium-based binders (e.g., sevelamer hydrochloride, sevelamer carbonate, lanthanum carbonate), and iron-based binders (e.g., sucroferric oxyhydroxide [Velphoro] and ferric citrate [Auryxia]). Intravenous calcium should be avoided because of risk for metastatic calcification unless symptoms of hypocalcemia are present.

CASE EXEMPLAR: Patient With Acute Tubular Necrosis Secondary to Vancomycin

JS is a 56-year-old patient in the Critical Care Unit (CCU) with a diagnosis of acute tubular necrosis (ATN). He was moved to the unit 24 hours ago with flank pain and "just not feeling well." He has been nauseous and unable to eat much. He had a laparoscopic cholecystectomy 8 days ago. He developed a wound infection and was admitted to the facility and began receiving vancomycin for the past 48 hours. Lab tests confirm an increase in serum creatinine. Urine output for the past 24 hours has been 800 mL.

Past Medical History
- Hypertension
- Gallbladder disease
- Laparoscopic cholecystectomy 8 days ago. Developed significant wound infection. Culture and sensitivity (antibiogram) indicated vancomycin as drug of choice.

Medications
- Vancomycin

Physical Examination
- Blood pressure: 172/100; pulse: 98; respiration rate: 24; temperature: 100.2 °F

Labs
- Serum creatinine (SCr): 2.0 mg/dL
- ABGs:
  - pH = 7.30
  - $PaCO_2$ = 31
  - HCO_3^- = 28
- Liver function: normal
- Serum Electrolytes:
  - Potassium: 5.9 mEq
  - Sodium 135 mEq/L

Discussion Questions

1. What factor in the JS's history would be considered a contributing factor to the development of acute tubular necrosis (ATN)? What current signs and symptoms help confirm ATN?
2. Given the findings from the laboratory data, what type of acid–base imbalance is present, what leads to this interpretation, and what treatment plan should the clinician implement for JS?

CASE EXEMPLAR: Patient With Acute Onset of Heart Failure With Fluid Retention

CC is a 60-year-old man who is seen in the clinic today with complaints of shortness of breath. He states he has been noticing that it is harder for him to do some activities, especially those that require additional exertion. He states this is new over the past 4 to 5 days.

Past Medical History
- Hypertension
- Angina
- Stent placement right coronary vessel
- Hypercholesteremia

Medications
- Lisinopril, 10 mg once daily
- Coumadin, 7.5 mg every other day; 5.0 mg on opposite days
- Simvastatin, 40 mg once daily

Physical Examination
- Height: 74″; weight: 220 lbs; blood pressure: 180/110; pulse: 122; respiration rate: 32
- 2+ pitting edema lower ankles
- Slight crackles throughout all lung fields
- S3 noted

Labs
- Total cholesterol: 210
- Liver function: normal
- Electrolytes: Sodium 138; Potassium 3.6 mEq

Discussion Questions
1. What is the likely diagnosis for CC and what is the appropriate medication treatment plan?
2. What clinical findings will indicate that the plan has been effective? What patient education does CC require?

KEY TAKEAWAYS

- AKI is an important clinical problem that is seen in upwards of 10% of hospitalized patients and up to 50% to 60% of ICU patients.
- Progression of CKD to ESRD necessitates dialysis or kidney transplantation; therefore, controlling the underlying etiology that led to CKD is paramount to slowing the progression.
- Types of diuretics include carbonic anhydrase inhibitors, loop, thiazide, potassium sparing, and osmotic.
- Types of acid–base disorders include metabolic acidosis, metabolic alkalosis, respiratory acidosis, and respiratory alkalosis. Calculation strategies are available to help define the disorder and determine if compensation is occurring.
- Electrolyte imbalances can occur with any electrolyte and manifest as electrolyte levels either too low or too high in the extracellular fluid. Treatment goals are implemented to restore balance throughout the systems.

REFERENCES

1. Kidney Disease Improving Global Outcomes. KDIGO clinical practice guideline for acute kidney in-jury. *Kidney Int Suppl.* 2012;2(1):1–132. https://kdigo.org/wp-content/uploads/2016/10/KDIGO-2012-AKI-Guideline-English.pdf
2. Hoste EA, Bagshaw S, Bellomo R, et al. Epidemiology of acute kidney injury in critically ill patients: the multinational AKI-EPI study. *Intensive Care Med.* 2015;41(8):1411–1423. doi:10.1007/s00134-015-3934-7
3. Paueksakon P, Fogo AB. Drug-induced nephropathies. *Histopathology.* 2017;70(1):94–108. doi:10.1111/his.13064
4. Mortensen LA, Bistrup C, Thiesson HC. Does mineralocorticoid receptor antagonism prevent calcineurin inhibitor-induced nephrotoxicity? *Front Med.* 2017;4:210. doi:10.3389/fmed.2017.00210
5. Viana SD, Reis F, Alves R. Therapeutic use of mTor inhibitors in renal diseases: Advances, drawbacks, and challenges. *Oxid Med Cell Longev.* 2018:3693625. doi:10.1155/2018/3693625
6. Diskin CJ, Stokes TJ, Dansby LM, et al. Toward the optimal clinical use of the fraction excretion of solutes in oliguric azotemia. *Ren Fail.* 2010;32(10):1245–1254. doi:10.3109/0886022X.2010.517353
7. Pepin MN, Bouchard J, Legault L, et al. Diagnostic performance of fractional excretion of urea and fractional excretion of sodium in the evaluations of patients with acute kidney injury with or without diuretic treatment. *Am J Kidney Dis.* 2007;50(4):566–573. doi:10.1053/j.ajkd.2007.07.001
8. Diskin CJ, Stokes TJ, Dansby LM, et al. The comparative benefits of the fractional excretion of urea and sodium in various azotemic oliguric states. *Nephron Clin Pract.* 2010;114(2):c145–c150. doi:10.1159/000254387
9. Baker RJ, Pusey CD. The changing profile of acute tubulointerstitial nephritis. *Nephrol Dial Transplant.* 2004;19(1):8–11. doi:10.1093/ndt/gfg464
10. Finfer S, Bellomo R, Boyce N, et al. A comparison of albumin and saline for fluid resuscitation in the intensive care unit. *N Engl J Med.* 2004;350(22):2247–2256. doi:10.1056/NEJMoa040232
11. Koyner JL, Davison DL, Brasha-Mitchell E, et al. Furosemide stress test and biomarkers for the prediction of

AKI severity. *J Am Soc Nephrol.* 2015. 26(8):2023–2031. doi:10.1681/ASN.2014060535

12. Kidney Disease Improving Global Outcomes. KDIGO clinical practice guideline for the evaluation and management of chronic kidney disease. *Kidney Int Suppl.* 2013;3(1):1–163. https://kdigo.org/wp-content/uploads/2017/02/KDIGO_2012_CKD_GL.pdf

13. Centers for Disease Control and Prevention. *Chronic kidney disease in the United States, 2019.* U.S. Department of Health and Human Services; 2019. https://www.cdc.gov/kidneydisease/pdf/2019_National-Chronic-Kidney-Disease-Fact-Sheet.pdf

14. Fried LF, Emanuele N, Zhang JH, et al. Combined angiotensin inhibition for the treatment of diabetic nephropathy. *N Engl J Med.* 2013;369(20):1892–1903. doi:10.1056/NEJMoa1303154

15. Kidney Disease Improving Global Outcomes. KDIGO clinical practice guidelines for anemia in chronic kidney disease. *Kidney Int Suppl.* 2012;2(4):1–335. https://kdigo.org/wp-content/uploads/2016/10/KDIGO-2012-Anemia-Guideline-English.pdf

16. Kidney Disease Improving Global Outcomes. KDIGO clinical practice guideline update for diagnosis, evaluation, prevention, and treatment of chronic kidney disease-mineral bone disorder (CKD-MBD). *Kidney Int Suppl.* 2017;7(1):1–59. doi:10.1016/j.kisu.2017.04.001

17. O'Malley CM, Frumento RJ, Hardy MA, et al. A randomized, double-blind comparison of lactated Ringer's solution and 0.9% NaCl during renal transplantation. *Anesth Analg.* 2005;100(5):1518–1524, table of contents. doi:10.1213/01.ANE.0000150939.28904.81

18. Semler MW, Self WH, Wanderer JP. Balanced crystalloids versus saline in critically ill adults. *N Engl J Med.* 2018;378(20):1951. doi:10.1056/NEJMc1804294

19. Finfer S, McEvoy S, Bellomo R, et al. Impact of albumin compared to saline on organ function and mortality of patients with severe sepsis. *Intensive Care Med.* 2011;37(1):86–96. doi:10.1007/s00134-010-2039-6

20. Myburgh JA, Finfer S, Bellomo R, et al. Hydroxyethyl starch or saline for fluid resuscitation in intensive care. *N Engl J Med.* 2012;367(20):1901–1911. doi:10.1056/NEJMoa1209759

21. Silversides JA, Major E, Ferguson AJ, et al. Conservative fluid management or deresuscitation for patients with sepsis or acute respiratory distress syndrome following the resuscitation phase of critical illness: a systematic review and meta-analysis. *Intensive Care Med.* 2017;43(2):155–170. doi:10.1007/s00134-016-4573-3

22. Felker GM, Lee KL, Bull DA, et al. Diuretic strategies in patients with acute decompensated heart failure. *N Engl J Med.* 2011;364:797–805. doi:10.1056/NEJMoa1005419

23. Salvador DR, Rey NR, Ramos GC, et al. Continuous infusion versus bolus injection of loop diuretics in congestive heart failure. *Cochrane Database Syst Rev.* 2005;(3):CD003178. doi:10.1002/14651858.CD003178.pub3

24. Bart BA, Goldsmith SR, Lee KL, et al. Ultrafiltration in decompensated heart failure with cardiorenal syndrome. *N Engl J Med.* 2012;367(24):2296–2304. doi:10.1056/NEJMoa1210357

25. Hamilton PK, Morgan NA, Connolly GM, Maxwell AP. Understanding acid-base disorders. *Ulster Med J.* 2017;86(3):161–166. https://www.ncbi.nlm.nih.gov/pmc/articles/PMC5849971

26. Rastegar M, Nagami GT. Non–anion gap metabolic acidosis: a clinical approach to evaluation. *Am J Kidney Dis.* 2017;69(2):296–301. doi:10.1053/j.ajkd.2016.09.013

27. Hopkins E, Sanvictores T, Sharma S. Physiology, acid base balance. [Updated September 14, 2020]. In: *StatsPearls* [Internet]. StatsPearls Publishing; 2020. https://www.ncbi.nlm.nih.gov/books/NBK507807

28. Duewall JL, Fenves AZ, Richey DS, et al. 5-Oxoproline (pyroglutamic) acidosis associated with chronic acetaminophen use. *Proc (Bayl Univ Med Cent).* 2010;23(1):19–20. doi:10.1080/08998280.2010.11928574

29. Martin RJ. Central pontine and extrapontine myelinolysis: the osmotic demyelination syndromes. *J Neurol Neurosurg Psychiatry.* 2004;75(suppl 3):iii22–iii28. doi:10.1136/jnnp.2004.045906

30. Greenberg A, Verbalis JG. Vasopressin receptor antagonists. *Kidney Int.* 2006;69(12):2124–2130. doi:10.1038/sj.ki.5000432

31. Zeltser D, Rosansky S, van Rensburg H, et al. Assessment of the efficacy and safety of intravenous conivaptan in euvolemic and hypervolemic hyponatremia. *Am J Nephrol.* 2007;27(5):447–457. doi:10.1159/000106456

32. Linder KE, Krawczynski MA, Laskey D. Sodium zirconium cyclosilicate (ZS-9): a novel agent for the treatment of hyperkalemia. *Pharmacotherapy.* 2016;36(8):923–933. doi: 10.1002/phar.1797

33. Kosiborod M, Rasmussen HS, Lavin P, et al. Effect of sodium zirconium cyclosilicate on potassium lowering for 28 days among outpatients with hyperkalemia: the HARMONIZE randomized clinical trial. *JAMA.* 2014;312(21):2223–2233. doi:10.1001/jama.2014.15688

34. Weir MR, Bakris GL, Bushinsky DA, et al. Patiromer in patients with kidney disease and hyperkalemia receiving RAAS inhibitors. *N Engl J Med.* 2015;372(3):211–221. doi:10.1056/NEJMoa1410853

35. Tertti R, Harmoinen A, Leskinen Y, et al. Comparison of calcium phosphate product values using measurement of plasma total calcium and serum ionized calcium. *Hemodial Int.* 2007;11:411–416. doi: 10.1111/j.1542-4758.2007.00210.x

Pharmacotherapy for Musculoskeletal and Rheumatologic Conditions

Rahnea Sunseri and Erica Barr

LEARNING OBJECTIVES

- Provide an overview of musculoskeletal and rheumatologic conditions, including epidemiological impact.
- Discuss the pathophysiology of musculoskeletal and rheumatologic disease states.
- Provide an overview of medications used to treat musculoskeletal and rheumatologic conditions.
- Compare and contrast pharmacotherapy for these conditions; understand the benefits and limitations of each drug.
- Select the most appropriate pharmacotherapeutic regimen to treat patients with musculoskeletal and rheumatologic conditions who may or may not have preexisting comorbidities and contraindications.

INTRODUCTION

Musculoskeletal (MSK) and rheumatologic disorders were second only to maintenance healthcare needs as the primary reason for ambulatory care visits in the United States in 2015.[1] Most were caused by mechanical trauma resulting in acute injuries and their sequelae. However, chronic disorders, chiefly osteoarthritis, were also common, accounting for 11% of the global burden of disease.[2] Immune-mediated rheumatologic diseases, such as rheumatoid arthritis (RA), occurred much less

frequently but were nonetheless important because of their significant morbidity and mortality.

The diagnosis of the majority of MSK and rheumatologic disorders is usually apparent, permitting empirical therapy. Additional factors to consider include whether the condition is due to a mechanical injury, is acute or chronic, or is of inflammatory or immune origin. These disorders affect all ages, sexes, and races so patient characteristics and comorbidities should also be considered when choosing treatments.

BACKGROUND

Therapeutic goals for MSK and rheumatologic disorders include controlling pain, reducing inflammation, repairing damaged tissue, and restoring function. Along with nonpharmacologic modalities, pharmacologic agents can achieve these goals. Specifically, opioid and nonopioid analgesics, including nonsteroidal anti-inflammatory drugs (NSAIDs) and adjunctive pain medications, are used for such therapy. However, disease-modifying antiarthritic drugs (DMARDs) are required in order to arrest or reverse tissue destruction.[3] Thus, drug selection is guided by underlying cause, pathophysiology, anticipated treatment duration, intended therapeutic goals, and patient factors. DMARDs are indicated for immune-mediated and autoimmune diseases, but analgesics and anti-inflammatories can provide temporary symptom control while awaiting the DMARD's effects, which may take several weeks to a few months depending upon the disorder and the DMARD. When the duration of pharmacotherapy is projected to be long-term, the potential for drug tolerance, adverse effects (AEs), and accumulative toxicity may preclude a drug's usefulness. Corticosteroids can control symptoms and modify disease but are rarely used long-term because of their deleterious effects.

PATHOPHYSIOLOGY OF INFLAMMATION

Understanding the pathophysiology of inflammation is fundamental for choosing an appropriate drug. The initial inflammatory process confines the injury, repairs the damage, and facilitates healing. The complex interactions between cellular components and chemical mediators defend against insults. Complement, clotting, and coagulation cascades are initiated at the site of injury and engage endothelial cells, neutrophils, and macrophages, followed by clot formation, vasodilatation, increased vascular permeability, and chemotactic signaling to other immune cells. Release of mediators—complement products, bradykinin, histamine, cyclooxygenase (COX) products (prostacyclins, prostaglandins, and thromboxane), leukotrienes, and cytokines—propagates these defenses. Cytokines include tumor-necrosis factors (TNFs), interleukins (ILs), colony-stimulating factors (CSFs), and chemokines. Resulting clinical manifestations of acute inflammation include pain, swelling, heat, redness, and dysfunction. In chronic inflammation, monocytes and macrophages phagocytize debris cause fibrosis and scarring, and release cytokines that produce systemic inflammatory responses (TNF-∝, IL-1 and IL6). To protect against future insults, lymphocytic humoral (B-cell) and cellular (T-cell) immunity are induced, sometimes resulting in autoimmune disease.

Preferred agents are those that control pain, resolve acute inflammation, abort tissue damage, and halt chronic immune processes, provided their benefits outweigh their risks. Selecting a drug with a mechanism of action (MOA) that acts on the intended target is key. Among the analgesics, opioids and acetaminophen only relieve pain. NSAIDs manage symptoms and signs in acute and chronic inflammation. Corticosteroids and other DMARDs restrain chronic inflammatory and immune changes and stop tissue-destroying metabolic processes. Adjuvant drugs for pain provide analgesic dose-sparing. Lastly, choice of drug formulations and routes of administration can ensure maximum efficacy with the least risk for side effects, such as the avoidance of systemic AEs with local therapy.

PHARMACOTHERAPY FOR MUSCULOSKELETAL AND RHEUMATOLOGIC CONDITIONS

The major categories of drugs that are effective for MSK and rheumatologic conditions include nonopioid analgesics, opioid analgesics, corticosteroids, skeletal muscle relaxants (SMRs), antidepressants, antiepileptic drugs (AEDs), specific topical agents, certain complementary and alternative medications (CAMs), and both traditional and biologic DMARDs. While evidence for efficacy in specific disorders is necessary, it is not always available for every drug and condition. In addition, it is important to keep in mind that different classes of drugs and even drugs within a class may have distinctive behaviors, which may change even further with the type of formulation and the route of administration.

Opioid analgesics, nonopioid analgesics such as acetaminophen and NSAIDs, and adjunctive pain medications provide relief of symptoms without disease modification. Drugs with anti-inflammatory activity are limited to NSAIDs, corticosteroids, DMARDS, and CAMs such as glucosamine and chondroitin. The effectiveness of adjunctive pain medications varies depending upon the MSK disorder. In general, topical NSAIDs are beneficial for localized pain. Despite their popularity, at this time there is limited evidence for the efficacy of various nutraceuticals.[4,5]

Although the following agents are described according to their individual uses, pain management often incorporates combinations of analgesics, anti-inflammatories, anesthetics, adjuvants, and other agents. Periprocedural and perioperative care may have pain "cocktail" protocols. Pain due to cancer and noncancer chronic pain are optimally controlled with drugs with different MOAs. It should be noted that pain management in general incorporates many nonpharmacologic therapies as well. A few examples of nonpharmacological therapies for pain management are hypnosis (e.g., distractions, relaxation, and guided imagery), comfort therapy (e.g., meditation, massage, hot/cold therapy, music, and visual arts), and neurostimulation (e.g., acupuncture, acupressure, and transcutaneous electrical nerve stimulation [TENS]). For further discussion of pain management, please refer to Chapter 33.

ANALGESICS

Acetaminophen

Acetaminophen or paracetamol (N-acetyl-p-aminophenol or APAP) exerts its analgesic and antipyretic effects via inhibition of prostaglandin synthesis (PGE2) in the brain at central cyclooxygenase one (COX-1). Its peripheral COX-1 and COX-2 inhibition is negligible; it has neither anti-inflammatory actions nor antiplatelet effects. APAP is a safe alternative to aspirin and other NSAIDs for patients with ASA or NSAID hypersensitivity, asthma, peptic acid disease, gastrointestinal (GI) bleeds, pregnancy, bleeding diatheses, and anticoagulation. However, its safety is limited by its risk of hepatotoxicity. Furthermore, recent evidence revealed that it was no better than placebo for pain relief in osteoarthritis (OA) of the knee and hip,[6] or for low back pain.[7] For these reasons, it is no longer the drug of choice for initial treatment of OA but may be tried nonetheless.

APAP has an ancillary use as a deterrent against opioid abuse as well as additive pain relief when combined with opioid medications.

Opioids

Opioids raise the pain threshold in spinal neurons and decrease pain perception in the brain, but do not prevent inflammation or tissue damage. Short-term (6 weeks) opioid use for analgesia is effective, but long-term use for chronic noncancer pain has questionable efficacy and is complicated by physical dependence and serious adverse effects.[8] For hip or knee OA and chronic back pain, opioids were no more effective for pain-related function than APAP or NSAIDs.[9] Opioids are now discouraged even for acute pain following injuries.[10] However, they can be useful for analgesia in patients who are pregnant or have contraindications to other analgesics, but their benefits must be weighed against their potential harms.

Tramadol, a synthetic opioid with serotonin–norepinephrine reuptake activity, has similar risk for physical dependence and adverse effects. Additionally, it lowers seizure thresholds, interacts with multiple drugs, and can cause serotonin syndrome. It is an alternative analgesic without clear benefits over harms. For further information about opioids and tramadol, please refer to Chapter 33.

Acetylsalicylic Acid and Other Nonsteroidal Anti-Inflammatory Drugs

NSAIDs are one of the most commonly used drug classes worldwide (**Table 22.1**).[11] Acetylsalicylic acid (ASA; aspirin), nonaspirin salicylates, and other NSAIDs prevent inflammation by blocking both cyclooxygenase enzymes (COX-1 & COX-2), which convert arachidonic acid (AA) to inflammatory mediators—prostacyclins (PGI_2), prostaglandins (PGF_2, PGE_2), and thromboxane (TXA; **Figure 22.1**).

COX-1 and COX-2 are present in most tissues, including the brain and spinal cord (i.e., the central nervous system [CNS]). COX-1 preferentially converts AA to TXA in platelets. In other tissues its constitutive activities (regulation of homeostatic processes) include temperature control, pain perception, platelet activity, renal function, and gastrointestinal mucosal protection. COX-2 acts constitutively but is inducible mostly by inflammatory mediators. ASA and salicylate salts irreversibly inhibit COX-1 and COX-2. Other NSAIDs have reversible and variable inhibition of COX-1 and COX-2, ranging from nonselective to COX-2-selective (coxib) inhibition. NSAID chemical classes predict their COX selectivity (**Exhibit 22.1**). As a group, NSAIDs have antipyretic, analgesic, antiplatelet, and anti-inflammatory effects, with the exception of nonacetyl salicylates and coxibs, which do not have antiplatelet activity.

NSAIDs are indicated for most MSK disorders, although ASA is not commonly used because of its irreversible antiplatelet effect and short analgesic duration. While NSAIDs have similar potencies, indomethacin and diclofenac are more potent, and their oral formulations are used infrequently to avoid their AEs. Nonacetyl salicylates are less potent and are used infrequently, except as topical preparations.[12] NSAIDs are contraindicated in persons with hypersensitivity to aspirin or who have aspirin-exacerbated respiratory disease (AERD), including asthma. Most NSAIDs are effective for acute MSK pain but are ineffective for fibromyalgia.[13]

The risk of AEs due to NSAIDs is greater with systemic therapy than with local therapy. In systemic treatment, except for hypersensitivity and idiosyncratic reactions, NSAID AEs are due to their COX inhibitory effects. Chief COX-related AEs include cardiovascular, gastrointestinal, renal, and asthma complications, as well as possible delayed bone healing. Extreme caution is advised for prescribing NSAIDs in patients with or at high risk for these AEs and for pediatric, pregnant, and elderly patients. In a Drug Safety Communication, the FDA has warned against the use of NSAIDs at around 20 weeks or later of pregnancy, because they may cause severe kidney problems in unborn babies.[14] During this period, the kidneys of the unborn baby produce primarily amniotic fluid. Consequently, the effects of NSAIDs may lead to a low level of amniotic fluid surrounding the baby, which provides a protective cushion and the development of the baby's lungs, digestive system, and muscles.

Nonaspirin NSAIDs increase risk for cardiovascular events, theoretically due to inhibition of COX-1 PGI_2 actions which negate TXA's thrombotic effects. ASA's cardioprotection is diminished by nonaspirin NSAIDs.[15] Even in patients without cardiovascular disease (CVD) or its risk factors, any use of nonaspirin NSAIDs can increase risks of myocardial infarction (MI), stroke, or heart failure. These risks increase with higher doses and longer durations of exposure.[16] In the first year after an MI, patient mortality increased with nonaspirin NSAID use.[16] Elevated CVD risk is similar for all nonaspirin NSAIDs,[16] except for oral diclofenac, which has greater CVD risk overall.[17]

NSAIDs' renal AEs are due to inhibition of renal prostaglandins in a dose-dependent manner, causing sodium and fluid retention, decreased renal blood flow, and elevated blood pressure. NSAIDs should be used with caution in the elderly and in persons with renal impairment, hypertension, and heart failure.

Hepatotoxicity is idiosyncratic and can range from transaminitis to fulminant liver failure and death.[18] As such, patients with preexisting transaminasemia from other causes would be difficult to monitor for idiosyncratic toxicity. NSAIDs should be used with caution in such patients. Hematopoietic toxicity is also idiosyn-

TABLE 22.1 Select Nonsteroidal Anti-Inflammatory Drugs for Musculoskeletal Disorders^a, b

Drug	Formulations	Dose (Adult)^c	Special Considerations^d
Nonselective COX Inhibitors—Salicylate Nonsteroidal Anti-Inflammatory Drugs			
Acetylated			
Aspirin (acetylsalicylic acid)	Tablets (immediate-release, enteric-coated, film-coated, chewable), caplets, rectal suppositories, chewing gum	Low dose: 81 mg once daily; Regular dose: 325–650 mg q4–6 h prn ≤4 g/24 h	MOA: COX-1 and COX-2 inhibition, irreversible PK/PD: good bioavailability, first pass hepatic metabolism, highly protein-bound, low volume of distribution, metabolism liver, both first order and zero-order kinetics; excreted in urine Use: low dose therapy for 2° CVD protection; regular doses for acute pain, fever, inflammation CI: bleeding disorders, anticoagulation, hypersensitivity, AERD, viral infections in persons ≤18 years old (Reyes syndrome), PUD, GI bleed, pregnancy (except low dose for preeclampsia prevention, antiphospholipid syndrome, anticoagulation in mechanical heart valves) Caution: asthma, AERD ADR: increased bleeding risk, asthma exacerbation risk Toxicity: CNS symptoms, tinnitus/hearing loss DDI: increased bleeding risk with anticoagulants and other antiplatelets Pro: inexpensive, available OTC Con: short duration of analgesic action, irreversible antiplatelet activity
Nonacetylated			
Diflunisal	Tablets	500 mg q8–12 h prn ≤1,500 mg/24 h	MOA: COX-1 and COX-2 inhibitor, irreversible; no antiplatelet activity PK/PD: Same as ASA, except no deacetylation necessary for activity Use: acute and chronic pain, fever, inflammation CI: hypersensitivity to other salicylates and NSAIDs ADR: similar to ASA, except no increased risk bleeding Toxicity: similar to ASA Pro: no antiplatelet activity, longer duration of action than ASA; some available OTC Con: weak COX-1 and COX-2 inhibitors, expensive
Choline magnesium trisalicylate	Tablets, liquid, caplets	1,500 mg bid or 3,000 mg qhs for inflammatory arthritis 2,000–3,000 mg daily in two or three divided doses prn pain or fever	
Salicylate	Tablets	500–750 mg q6 h, 1 g q12 h prn ≤3 g/24 h	
Trolamine salicylate	Cream, lotion	10% strength	

Drug	Formulations	Dose (Adult)^c	MOAs, Indications, CIs, ADRs, Cautions, BBWs, Toxicity, DDIs, Pros/Cons, Other Notes^d
Nonselective COX Inhibitors—Nonsalicylate Nonsteroidal Anti-Inflammatory Drugs			
Acetic Acid Derivatives			
Indomethacin	IV solution, capsules (immediate- and extended-release), oral suspension, rectal suppository	Oral: 25 mg bid–tid, 75 SR mg 2 bid ≤300 mg/24 h	MOA: COX-1 and COX-2 inhibitor, reversible at platelets PK/PD: bioavailability good, first pass hepatic metabolism, highly protein-bound, low volume of distribution, metabolism liver, t½ varies ∝ NSAID, COX selectivity varies Potency: generally equipotent; comparable to ASA and opioids; indomethacin, diclofenac, and ketorolac have greater potency Efficacy: usually equally effective, effective for acute and chronic pain with diminishing efficacy over time; except possibly for ankylosing spondylitis, NSAIDs do *not* modify disease in inflammatory and immune-mediated arthritides
Sulindac	Tablets	150–200 mg bid	
Etodolac	Tablets (immediate- and extended-release), capsules	200, 300, 400, 500, 600 mg; dose up to 1,200 mg/24 h; doses vary****	

Fenamates

Drug	Dosage forms	Dosing	Notes
			Use: fever, pain, acute and chronic pain, inflammatory arthritis and immune-mediated arthritides; IV indomethacin or oral ibuprofen (off-label) for ductus arteriosus closure in premature infants; etodolac approved for juvenile arthritis; mefenamic acid limited to pain, fever, gynecologic disorders; ketorolac intranasal formula used for migraine.
Mefenamic acid	Capsules	500 mg initially, followed by 250 mg q6 h depending upon the disorder	CI: bleeding disorders, anticoagulation, hypersensitivity to salicylates or other NSAIDs, AERD, PUD, UGI or LGI bleeding (COX-2 selective has less GI toxicity)
Meclofenamate	Tablets	50, 100 mg; doses vary^e ≤400 mg/24 h	Caution: asthma, AERD, poor renal and hepatic function, elderly and pediatric patients; Beers criteria recommend against use or minimal use of most NSAIDs; adjust doses for renal and hepatic insufficiencies
Diclofenac	IV and ophthalmic solutions, tablets (enteric-coated and extended-release), topical (solution, cream, gel)	Doses vary^e	ADR: increased bleeding risk, GI bleeding risk; increased CVD risk—MI, HF, Stroke; CVD risk with all NSAIDs except ASA; renal injury, fluid retention, worsening HF, HTN. ADR's greater with indomethacin, diclofenac, and ketorolac so their systemic use is limited to acute pain/inflammation; ketorolac use limited to 5 days duration; PPIs mitigate ASA mucosal damage at UGI, but not LGI tract; COX-2 inhibitor with PPI preferred for patients at high risk for UGI complications; all can be nephrotoxic (dose-dependent), hepatotoxic (idiosyncratic), toxic to bone marrow (idiopathic); avoid in pregnancy, especially last trimester due to premature closure of ductus arteriosus
Ketorolac	IV and IM solutions, intranasal spray, ophthalmic solution; tablets	10-mg tablet; IM and IV given in 15-, 30-, 60-mg doses; maximum dose varies with age and route, oral 40 mg/24 h	BBW: all NSAIDs (except ASA) carry a warning re: increased risk of CVD and GI bleeds and ulcerations
			Toxicity: CNS symptoms, tinnitus/hearing loss—stop if side effects occur

Propionic Acid Derivatives

Drug	Dosage forms	Dosing	Notes
Ibuprofen	IV solution, tablets (immediate-release and chewable), capsules (liquid-filled), suspensions	Oral tablets and capsules: 200, 400, 600 mg q4–6 h prn; 800 mg q6–8 h; ≤3,200 mg/24 h; Analgesic doses: 1,200–2,400 mg/24 h; Anti-inflammatory doses: 2,400–3,200 mg/24 h	Monitor: hematologic, renal, hepatic function at baseline and periodically, BP, fluid status
			Pro: relatively inexpensive, some are available OTC and in prescription-strengths, longer duration of analgesic action compared to ASA, reversible antiplatelet activity
Naproxen	Tablets (immediate-release and enteric-coated), suspensions	Oral tablets: 250, 375, 500 mg bid	Con: serious CVD, GI, renal toxicities; risk of bleeding and GI injury
Naproxen sodium	Tablets (immediate- and extended-release), capsules (liquid-filled)	220, 275, 375, 550 mg, doses vary^e	Pearl: Use the lowest effective dose for the shortest duration to avoid ADRs and toxicity
Fenoprofen	Tablets, capsules	200, 400, 600, doses vary^e; maximum dose 3,200 mg/24 h	
Ketoprofen	Capsules, topical cream	25, 50, 75, 200; 10%	
Flurbiprofen	Tablets (immediate-release)	50, 100 mg, maximum 100 mg/dose, 300 mg/24 h	

(continued)

TABLE 22.1 Select Nonsteroidal Anti-Inflammatory Drugs for Musculoskeletal Disorders[a]

Nonselective COX Inhibitors—Nonsalicylate Nonsteroidal Anti-Inflammatory Drugs

Enolic Acid Derivatives

Meloxicam	Tablets, suspensions, capsules	Tablet and suspension: 7.5, 15 mg, maximum dose 15 mg/24 h Capsule: 5 and 10 mg, maximum dose 10 mg/24 h	
Piroxicam	Capsules	10 mg bid or 20 mg once daily	
Nabumetone	Tablets	500 or 750 mg, range 1,000–2,000 mg/24 h	

Coxibs (COX-2 Selective Inhibitors)

Celecoxib	Capsules	50, 100, 200, 400, load with 400 mg × 1, then 200 mg q12 h, maximum 600 mg/24 h	See Nonselective NSAIDs Differences: COX-2 selective inhibitor has less GI ADRs. Combined with a PPI for GI mucosal protection; preferred in patients at high risk for upper and lower GI injury and bleeds, although PPI does not protect against LGI injury and bleeds
Rofecoxib	—		Withdrawn from market by manufacturer/developer in 2004 due to unacceptable increased risk of CVD events
Valdecoxib	—		Withdrawn from market by FDA in 2005 because of life-threatening skin reactions (SJS, TENS)

[a]Drugs available in United States.

[b]NSAIDs are contraindicated in pregnancy > or = 20 wks.

[c]Usual adult doses. Doses may require adjustment for diagnosis, age, sex, or renal or hepatic insufficiency.

[d]Notes include important drug characteristics applicable to patient care but are not all inclusive.

[e]Doses vary depending upon formulation, the condition to be treated, and the route of administration.

AERD, aspirin-exacerbated respiratory disease; ADR, adverse drug reaction; ASA, aspirin; BBW, "Black Box Warning"; bid, twice daily; BP, blood pressure; CI, contraindication; CNS, central nervous system; COX, cyclo-oxygenase; DDI, CV, cardiovascular; CVD, cardiovascular disease; drug–drug interaction; h, hour(s); HF, heart failure; HTN, hypertension; GI, gastrointestinal; H2Blkr, H2 Blockers; IM, intramuscularly; IV, intravenously; LGI, lower gastrointestinal; MOA, mechanism of action; NSAID, nonsteroidal anti-inflammatory drug; ns NSAID, nonselective NSAID; OTC, over-the-counter; PD, pharmacodynamics; PK, pharmacokinetics; PO, per oral/ by mouth; PPI, proton-pump inhibitor; PR, per rectum; prn, as needed; PUD, peptic ulcer disease; q, every; qd, daily; qid, four times daily; SJS, Stevens-Johnson syndrome; TENS, toxic epidermal necrolysis; tid, thrice daily; UGI, upper gastrointestinal.

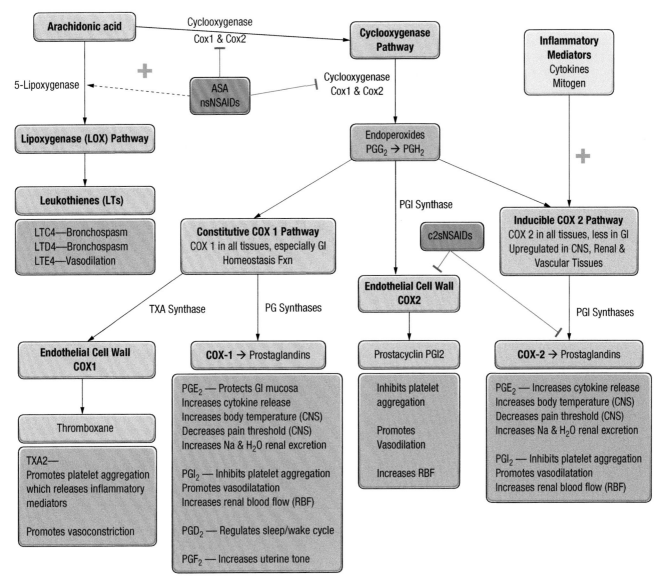

FIGURE 22.1 Arachidonic acid cascade with lipoxygenase pathway producing leukotrienes (LTs) and cyclooxygenase pathway producing prostacyclin (PGI$_2$), thromboxane (TXA), and prostaglandins (PGs). Different tissues have variable amounts of COX-1 and COX-2 activity. Aspirin (ASA) and nonselective NSAIDs (nsNSAIDs) inhibit both COX1 and COX2. COX2 selective NSAIDs (c2sNSAIDs) preferentially inhibit COX2, which is less prevalent in GI tissue. Inflammation is mediated via cytokines and platelet inflammatory mediators. nsNSAIDs inhibition of COX pathways indirectly pushes arachidonic acid toward the LOX pathway which increases LTs producing bronchospasm.

Source: Rahnea Sunseri, MD 2019.

cratic. Appropriate baseline and periodic laboratory monitoring are recommended.

ASA and NSAIDs interfere with COX-mediated gastrointestinal (GI) mucosal protection, increasing risks of ulceration, bleeding, and perforation. NSAIDs or ASA should not be given without a protective agent in patients at high risk for either upper- or lower-GI ulcerations and bleeds.[19] Proton-pump inhibitors (PPIs), H2-receptor blockers, and misoprostol may reduce upper gastrointestinal (UGI) bleeding risk of NSAIDs but do not protect against lower gastrointestinal (LGI) injury. Drugs such as rebamipide (not FDA -approved) may reduce the risks of UGI ulcers and small bowel in-

jury with NSAIDs, whereas misoprostol, irsogladine (not FDA-approved), and muscovite (not FDA-approved) may decrease small bowel mucosal injury due to diclofenac.[20] The combination of PPIs with celecoxib is preferred to prevent UGI AEs.[21] However, long-term therapy with protective agents such as PPIs may result in AEs due to these drugs.

Whether NSAIDs interfere with bone healing is controversial with conflicting results in the few available animal and human studies. Outcomes varied with NSAID type, dose, and anatomical location. While current evidence is insufficient to recommend against NSAID use in fractures or bone surgery, some

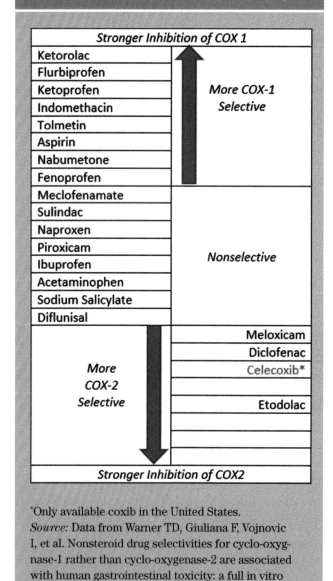

EXHIBIT 22.1: COX selectivity of NSAIDs. Relative COX selectivity of NSAIDs. (Nonselective or traditional NSAIDs in black. COX-2 selective NSAIDs in blue.)

*Only available coxib in the United States.
Source: Data from Warner TD, Giuliana F, Vojnovic I, et al. Nonsteroid drug selectivities for cyclo-oxygnase-1 rather than cyclo-oxygenase-2 are associated with human gastrointestinal toxicity: a full in vitro analysis. *Proc Natl Acad Sci USA.* 1999;96:7553–7568. doi:10.1073/pnas.96.13.7563.

orthopedic surgeons still avoid them in patients with more complex fractures and procedures.[11]

To avoid AEs from systemic NSAID therapy, the lowest effective dose for the shortest duration is advised. Alternatively, delivery of NSAIDs by topical application or local injection largely avoid AEs from systemic therapy. Topical NSAIDs are preferred in patients older than 75 years of age because they are relatively safe and have minimal potential to interact with drugs or exacerbate underlying diseases.

Topical NSAIDs—diclofenac, ibuprofen, ketoprofen, piroxicam, and indomethacin—have been used for pain relief in acute MSK pain. Only certain formulations of topical diclofenac and ketoprofen have good evidence for efficacy in acute MSK pain although they are not as effective for chronic pain.[5] Gastrointestinal AEs are significantly reduced with topical compared to oral NSAIDs. Whether risks of cardiovascular and renal AEs are diminished with chronic local therapy is unknown. Topical NSAID AEs are mainly mild transient rashes. Diclofenac is available by prescription in the United States as a solution (Pennsaid®), gel (Emulgel® or Voltaren®), or patch (Flector®); others must be compounded. Over-the-counter (OTC) rubefacient salicylates (salicylic acid and methyl salicylate) were shown to be ineffective for MSK pain.[22]

Local injections with ketorolac or indomethacin were shown to be equally or more effective than injected corticosteroids for pain relief and functional improvement.[23] Further research is necessary before concluding that injectable NSAIDs are superior.

ANTI-INFLAMMATORIES

Corticosteroids

Corticosteroids possess both anti-inflammatory and disease-modifying effects via inhibiting release of inflammatory products—prostaglandins, leukotrienes, nitric oxide, and cytokines (IL-1, 2, 3, 6, TNF-alpha).[12] Serious adverse effects of long-term therapy limit chronic glucocorticoid use,[24] but short-term use, low-dose systemic regimens, use in pregnancy, and intra-articular (IA) injections[25] provide safer alternatives for some patients.

The new extended-release triamcinolone formulation (Zilretta®),[26] triamcinolone acetonide, and methylprednisolone IA injections are effective for joint inflammation, pain, and function. Usually given with lidocaine, doses vary by anatomic locations.[27] Efficacy is modest overall but IA corticosteroids have been shown to decrease pain in adhesive capsulitis of the shoulder.[28] Improved pain and function in knee OA were limited and decreased over time.[25] The short-lived relief of symptoms necessitates repeat IA injections, commonly limited to 3-month or longer intervals to avoid glucocorticoid AEs. Decreased knee joint cartilage was observed even at this interval.[29] Systemic AEs are rare with IA glucocorticoids. Local AEs include pain, bleeding, infection, tissue atrophy and damage, osteonecrosis, and postinjection inflammatory flare. Contraindications include periarticular infection, septic arthritis, periarticular fracture, joint instability, juxta-articular osteoporosis.

Corticosteroid injections are also used for trigger points, tendonitis, bursitis, fasciitis, epicondylitis, and capsulitis. Overall volume of corticosteroid and anesthetic is small due to the limited space and tissue vulnerability at these sites. Evidence of efficacy varies with the site and typically lasts 6 to 8 weeks. AEs and complications are similar to IA corticosteroids. Contraindications include infection or weakness of the targeted soft tissue structures.

SKELETAL MUSCLE RELAXANTS

Antispasmodics and Antispasticity Agents

Skeletal muscle relaxants (SMRs) have a limited role in MSK disorders, restricted to pain relief for acute low back pain (LBP). SMRs are divided into antispasmodics and antispasticity agents, which have different indications and MOAs. Antispasmodics are used for MSK spasm, while antispasticity drugs are used for spastic upper motor neuron disorders (**Table 22.2**). Most antispasmodic agents interfere with CNS gamma aminobutyric acid (GABA).[30] Antispasticity drugs act on peripheral sites, spinal cord (baclofen), or skeletal muscle (dantrolene). Dantrolene is not approved for LBP.

TABLE 22.2 Skeletal Muscle Relaxants

Type[a]	Drug	Dose[b]	Notes[c]
Antispasticity agents	Baclofen	5 mg po tid, titrate to effect at 3-day intervals, maximum 80 mg/24 h	MOA-GABA$_B$ receptor agonist inhibits neuronal transmission at spinal cord. Elimination t½ 2–5 hours. BBW—abrupt withdrawal intrathecal drug. ADRs—hypotension, weakness, nausea, constipation, respiratory depression; withdrawal syndrome; transaminitis. Not indicated for MSK spasm. ODD.
	Dantrolene sodium	25 mg → 50 mg → 100 mg po tid at 7-day intervals	MOA-blocks calcium channel at muscle sarcoplasmic reticulum. BBW—potentially fatal hepatitis. ADRs—flushing, nausea, diarrhea. Not indicated for MSK spasm. Used to treat upper-motor neuron disorders, malignant hypothermia, and neuroleptic malignant syndrome. ODD.
Antispasmodic-antispasticity agents	Diazepam	2–10 mg po tid–qid	MOA-activates central neuronal GABA$_A$ receptors + spinal cord GABA activity. Abuse potential/physical dependence. Elimination t½ 20–50 hours. Active metabolites t½ up to 100 hours. ADRs—confusion. Beers criteria—avoid in elderly. Caution in renal or hepatic impairment.
	Tizanidine	4 mg po q6–8 h, titrate by 2–4 mg to effect, maximum 36 mg/24 hours	MOA-central alpha$_2$-adrenoreceptor agonist blocking presynaptic neurotransmission to motor neurons by ill-defined mechanism. Half-life 2.5 hours. ADRs—dry mouth, hypotension, asthenia. Hepatotoxicity. Contraindicated—concomitant potent CYP1A2 inhibitors. Monitor LFTs. ODD.
Antispasmodic agents	Cyclobenzaprine	5–10 mg po TID or 10–30 mg po at bedtime	MOA-centrally acting at brainstem; reduces tonic somatic motor activity by affecting alpha and gamma motor neurons. Elimination t½ 18–50 hours. ADRs—anticholinergic effects, QT prolongation. Avoid in patients with CVD, especially rhythm/conduction disorders and patients with glaucoma. Beers criteria—avoid in elderly. Indicated for MSK spasm.
	Carisoprodol	350 mg po qid	MOA-blocks reticular formation neurotransmission to spinal cord. Prodrug metabolized to meprobamate. Potential physical and psychologic dependence. Schedule IV. Withdrawal syndrome. Metabolism (CYP2C19). ADRs—headache. Indicated for MSK spasm. Beers criteria—avoid in elderly and children. Caution in patients with CYP2C19 polymorphism (high in Asians).
	Metaxalone	800 mg po tid–qid	MOA possibly due to CNS depression. Hepatic metabolism. Renal excretion. Half-life 8–9 hours. ADRs—GI upset, N&V, headache, irritability, hemolytic anemia, leukopenia, CNS depression, serotonin syndrome. Indicated for MSK spasm. Avoid in children, current or history of anemia. Beers criteria—avoid in elderly.
	Methocarbamol	Initial: 1,500 mg po qid × 2–3 days, then 4 g/day in divided doses	MOA possibly due to CNS depression. Hepatic metabolism. Renal excretion. ADRs—headache, lightheadedness, seizure, anaphylaxis. Beers criteria—avoid in elderly.
	Orphenadrine	100 mg po bid	MOA unknown; analgesic and anticholinergic activity. ADRs—fainting, lightheadedness, N&V, xerostomia, blurred vision. Half-life 13–20 hours. Avoid in glaucoma, myasthenia gravis, esophagospasm. Beers criteria—avoid in elderly.

[a]Antispasmodics treat musculoskeletal conditions; antispasticity agents treat upper motor neuron disorders.

[b]Doses for immediate-release oral formulations in adults. Dose adjustments may be required for age and hepatic and renal impairments.

[c]All skeletal muscle relaxants have ADRs of drowsiness and dizziness, plus ADRs noted in Table 22.2. All are metabolized primarily in the liver and eliminated by kidneys, except baclofen and carisoprodol which are eliminated chiefly by kidneys. Caution in elderly and children, and in renal and/or hepatic impairment for all. Patient counseling on ADRs imperative—avoid activities that may be unsafe or considered driving under the influence (DUI) while taking these drugs. All may cause impaired mental alertness.

ADR, adverse drug reaction; bid, twice daily; CNS, central nervous system; GABA, gamma aminobutyric acid; LFT, liver function test; MOA, mechanism of action; MSK, musculoskeletal; N&V, nausea and vomiting; ODD, orphan drug designation; po, by mouth; qid, four times daily; tid, thrice daily.

Of the SMRs, carisoprodol, cyclobenzaprine, and tizanidine have evidence for efficacy up to 2 weeks in acute back pain, but not for chronic LBP; no SMR was shown to be more effective than another.[31] SMR use in RA was not beneficial.[30] Addition of an SMR to NSAID analgesics did not provide further benefit and was associated with high rates of AEs, primarily dizziness and sedation.[32,33] Combining SMRs with opioids has not been shown to improve pain control. Due to AEs of sedation, anticholinergic effects, and increased falls and fractures, SMRs are inappropriate for persons older than 65 years of age per Beers criteria.[34]

ADJUNCTIVE PAIN MEDICATIONS

Antiepileptic Drugs and Antidepressants

AEDs gabapentin and pregabalin are not effective for acute, subacute, or chronic LBP with or without radiculopathy.[35] Pregabalin has evidence for pain relief in hand OA.[36] Possible sedation from both drugs and the abuse potential of pregabalin argue against their use for chronic MSK pain.

Duloxetine, a serotonin and norepinephrine reuptake inhibitor, has evidence for reducing pain and increasing function in LBP[7] and OA of the hand, knee, and hip.[7,37,38] Tricyclic antidepressants are not effective for chronic LBP.[7] Evidence is insufficient for MSK pain control with other antidepressants.

COMPLEMENTARY AND ALTERNATIVE MEDICATIONS AND MISCELLANEOUS AGENTS

Pharmaceutical grades of oral glucosamine sulfate and chondroitin sulfate each reduce pain in knee OA; no added benefit was evident with their combination.[39] Glucosamine is a precursor for glycosaminoglycan found in cartilage and synovial fluid and has good oral bioavailability, while chondroitin is a structural component of cartilage and has poor GI absorption. The nonpharmaceutical grade preparations of these agents vary widely, causing discrepancies in research results. Data on topical formulations are insufficient. Reduction of pain and inflammation and theoretical disease<space>modification are attributed to their inhibition of inflammatory cytokines, cartilage catabolism, and oxidative damages. The only AE of significance is that glucosamine increases blood glucose in diabetics. The relative safety, low cost, and potential efficacy of these agents suggest that they may be suitable alternatives for treating chronic MSK pain.

There is insufficient evidence for the efficacy of topical glyceryl trinitrate (nitroglycerin patch) in chronic rotator cuff pain; only one study using a dose of 5 mg daily found it to be effective for short-term treatment.[40] The most common side effect reported was headache.

Capsaicin, derived from chili peppers, binds to pain nociceptors when used topically, impeding transmission of painful stimuli. The high-concentration (8%) topical formulation is available only by prescription, is FDA-approved only for postherpetic neuralgia, and must be applied in a medical setting under a strict protocol, no more than every 3 months. Low-concentration OTC products (0.025%, 0.075%, 0.125%, and 0.25%) were not efficacious for MSK pain[5]; however, the 0.025% cream used in the United Kingdom is shown to be an equally effective topical NSAID for OA pain.[41] An isomer of capsaicin, civamide 0.075% cream was effective for knee OA.

Lidocaine, an amide local anesthetic—available in various topical formulations and strengths OTC (typically 4% for MSK pain) and as a 5% patch by prescription—does not relieve MSK pain, although it relieves postherpetic neuralgia.[5]

Nutraceuticals, both oral and topical, are not uniform in composition, hindering their clinical usefulness. Topical preparations for OA pain include[5]:

- **Arnica gel** (*Arnica montana*): as effective as topical ibuprofen but with same or worse AEs
- **Comfrey extract gel:** better than placebo
- **Capsaicin:** not effective in the doses studied

Other oral nutraceuticals lacked sufficient evidence for efficacy in OA pain.[4] For RA pain, only oral gamma-linolenic (GLA) oils—primrose, borage seed, blackcurrant seed—were effective; evidence for efficacy of other nutraceuticals was insufficient.[5]

Caution should be exercised with the use of any topical preparation. Hands should be washed after application, particularly with capsaicin, in order to avoid spreading the agent to sensitive mucosal areas and eyes where it can be irritating or cause local anesthesia. Heating pads and occlusive dressings (unless advised) should not be applied over topical medications because they may increase the systemic absorption and may result in skin irritation and injury.

DISEASE-MODIFYING ANTIRHEUMATIC DRUGS

DMARDs are commonly used to treat rheumatoid arthritis (RA) and other chronic immune-modulated arthritides, including ankylosing spondylitis, psoriatic arthritis, inflammatory bowel disease (IBD)-associated arthritis, and reactive arthritis. In addition, many DMARDs are also used in the treatment of other disease states, such as the treatment of certain cancers, GI disorders, systemic lupus erythematosus, and other connective tissue disorders. DMARDs slow disease progression and prevent further damage to the inflamed joints by suppressing the body's overactive immune systems/inflammatory pathways. The goal of therapy when using DMARDs is remission of the disease.

DMARDs are characterized as either traditional (nonbiologic) or biologic DMARDs. Some options require screening for exposure to infection (e.g., tuberculin skin test and hepatitis testing) prior to use. DMARDs can be utilized either as monotherapy or as combination therapy; however, two biologic options should never be used in combination due to the increased risk of severe infection. The most common DMARDs are methotrexate (MTX), hydroxychloroquine, sulfasalazine, and leflunomide. A summary of these as well as other DMARD options can be found in **Table 22.3**.

Methotrexate

Methotrexate is a folate antimetabolite which works by irreversibly binding and inhibiting dihydrofolate reductase, inhibiting the formation of reduced folates and purine, which interferes with DNA synthesis, cellular replication, and cellular repair during the S phase of the cell cycle.[42] It was originally used in the field of oncology, but has shown benefit in RA treatment at lower, weekly doses and is the preferred initial option for most patients.[42]

Methotrexate is available in a variety of formulations with side effects that vary by route and dosage. The most common side effects include GI upset, alopecia, and stomatitis. Some of these side effects can be offset with concurrent administration of folate. MTX also comes with a list of black box warnings due to its potential for serious hematological and hepatotoxic effects (see Table 22.3).

Hydroxychloroquine

Hydroxychloroquine is an immune modulator that is given daily as monotherapy or in combination with MTX and/or other DMARDs. It was originally developed as a treatment for malaria but has been found to have benefit in the treatment of inflammatory arthritis. It should be taken with food or milk.

Side effects include dose-related vision changes with a warning of possible irreversible retinopathy or loss of visual acuity. An eye exam, as well as muscle strength testing, should be performed at baseline and every 3 months during therapy. Other side effects include GI upset, rash, and rare pigmentation changes of the hair/skin.

Sulfasalazine

Sulfasalazine is an immune modulator. Patients with sensitivities to sulfa or salicylate allergies should avoid using sulfasalazine if possible. Sulfasalazine is also used in the treatment of inflammatory bowel disease. Common side effects include headache and rash. Sulfasalazine should be taken with food and at least 8 ounces of water to prevent crystalluria.

Leflunomide

Leflunomide is a prodrug that works by inhibiting pyrimidine synthesis, resulting in anti-inflammatory and antiproliferative effects. Because leflunomide carries a warning for embryo-fetal toxicity, a negative pregnancy test and agreement to use two forms of birth control are required prior to initiation of therapy, and patients must wait 2 years after discontinuation prior to becoming pregnant.[43] Leflunomide also carries a risk of hepatotoxicity and severe infections. Liver function tests and pregnancy screenings should be performed at baseline and regularly during treatment.

Biologic Agents and Disease-Modifying Antirheumatic Drugs

Biologic DMARDs target specific channels among the inflammation pathway. Though these drugs have some limitations, clinical studies suggest they are equally efficacious when compared to methotrexate,[44] and their use in combination with methotrexate may be more efficacious than use of methotrexate alone.[45] These biologic agents should not be combined with one another or given with live vaccines. They require testing for infections prior to initiation and carry an increased risk for developing infections and malignancies. For more information on the individual products, including the pathways they target (tumor necrosis factor-alpha inhibition/interleukin inhibition; see Table 22.3).

CONCLUSION

For acute and chronic pain with inflammation, NSAIDs and opioids are effective, but opioids are not considered first-line therapy. Corticosteroids may be used temporarily or intermittently. Because of their lessor AEs, topical NSAIDs and IA glucocorticoids are preferable to systemic formulations. Short-term SMRs may benefit acute LBP. Duloxetine is useful for chronic pain in LBP and OA. Pregabalin may benefit OA pain but has habit-forming potential. Except for systemic corticosteroids, and the use of NSAIDs for ankylosing spondylitis, none of these agents have disease-modifying activity.

DMARDs are commonly used to treat rheumatoid arthritis and other inflammatory arthritides. These drugs decrease inflammation and pain in affected joints as well as prevent or reverse damages and preserve function. The chief goal of therapy is disease remission. Selection of a DMARD regimen depends on several factors, including disease progress/severity, side-effect potential, and patient characteristics/preference. DMARDs can be given as mono- or combination therapy. The most commonly used initial DMARD is methotrexate. In more severe cases methotrexate can be combined with other traditional and/or biologic DMARDs to improve disease control.

Whether topical NSAIDs cause CVD or other systemic AEs needs to be determined to confirm their long-term safety. Additional exploration of the efficacy of glucosamine is warranted in view of its theoretical benefits, positive results in some trials, and relative safety. Nutraceutical therapy is hampered by inconsistent product composition and small or suboptimal studies, precluding reliable results and strong recommendations. DMARD therapy exploration continues and with further research disease targets may become more specific, thus decreasing potential AEs.

TABLE 22.3 Disease-Modifying Antirheumatic Drugs

Drug	Form/Strength	Typical Maintenance Dose*	Side Effects	Contraindications and Warnings	Monitoring and Notes
Methotrexate	Low weekly doses (for RA use) Subcutaneous autoinjectors, various doses Tablet: 5, 7.5, 10, 15 mg Pediatric oral solution: 2.5 mg/mL Injections available for oncology use	7.5, 15, 20 mg once weekly	N&V, diarrhea, mouth ulcers, increased LFTs, photosensitivity, alopecia, stomatitis, formulation-dependent side effects	Black Box Warning: bone marrow suppression and aplastic anemia, GI toxicity, hepatotoxicity, infections, pneumonitis, secondary malignancies, tumor lysis syndrome, renal impairment Pregnancy: category X	Monitor: LFTs (baseline and regularly throughout treatment), CBC, SCr Concurrent folate used to decrease side effects: give 5 mg po weekly on the day following MTX therapy
Hydroxychloroquine	Tablet: 200 mg	400 mg daily	Nausea and vomiting, diarrhea, rash, pruritus, headache, vision changes, rare pigmentation changes of the skin/hair	Irreversible retinopathy may occur; use with caution in patients with G6PD deficiency Pregnancy: caution	Monitor: eye exam, muscle strength, CBC, LFTs Take with food or milk
Sulfasalazine	Tablet and enteric-coated tablet: 500 mg	500, 1,000, 1,500 mg bid; enteric-coated tablets: 1,000, 2,000, 3,000 mg daily	Headache, skin rash, GI upset, oligospermia; can cause discoloration (yellow/orange) of urine and skin	May have cross-reactivity in those allergic to sulfonamide or salicylate medications; caution in patients with G6PD deficiency Pregnancy: caution	Monitor: CBC, LFTs, renal function Impairs folate absorption; can supplement with folate (1 mg/day)
Leflunomide	Tablet: 10, 20 mg	10, 20 mg daily	GI upset, respiratory infections, headache	Hepatotoxicity: avoid use in liver dysfunction/ALT above two times the upper limit of normal Pregnancy: embryo-fetal toxicity, do not use in pregnancy; must have negative pregnancy test and agree to two forms of birth control prior to use; must wait 2 years after discontinuation or use elimination product prior to becoming pregnant	Monitor: LFTs and CBC; screen for pregnancy and TB prior to initiation Cholestyramine or activated charcoal may be used as accelerated drug elimination products in event of toxicity or pregnancy
Azathioprine	Tablet: 50, 75, 100 mg Generic available as reconstituted solution for injection, 100 mg	Weight-based dosing titrated to lowest effective dose	Malaise, GI upset, leukopenia	Boxed warning: malignancy Pregnancy: category D	Monitor: CBC with differential and platelets Drug interactions with warfarin (decreases warfarin effect), allopurinol (increases azathioprine concentration)
Cyclosporine	Capsule, oral solution, IV solution	Weight-based dosing	Increased blood pressure, edema, GI upset, headache	Do not use in patients with abnormal renal function, uncontrolled hypertension, or malignancies Pregnancy: limited data suggests no link to birth defects, but possible increased incidence of premature birth and low birth weight	Monitor: plasma concentrations, renal function, blood pressure Avoid concurrent use with MTX (raise in levels of both drugs observed)

Drug	Formulation	Dosing	Adverse effects	Warnings/Contraindications	Monitoring
Penicillamine (not included in current clinical guidelines for treatment of RA)	Capsule: 250 mg Gluten-free tablet: 125 mg Tablet: 250 mg	Traditionally increased from 250 mg daily–tid prior to meals	Rash, GI upset, taste disorders, myelosuppression (rare)	Contraindicated with renal insufficiency; pregnancy/breastfeeding	Monitor: CBC, SCr, urinary protein Take without food (will decrease levels)
Auranofin (gold compound)	Capsule: 3 mg	9 mg/day in three divided doses	Rash, proteinuria, GI upset, myelosuppression (rare)	Contraindicated with a history of gold-induced disorders Boxed warnings: gold toxicity, including rash, persistent diarrhea hematologic depression Pregnancy: category C	Monitor: CBC with differential and platelets, renal and liver function tests, urinalysis Use with aspirin may increase risk of hepatotoxicity
Tofacitinib	Tablet: 5, 10 mg Extended-release tablet: 11 mg	5 mg po bid; XR: 11 mg po daily	Infections (upper respiratory, urinary), GI upset, headaches, increased blood pressure/lipids	Avoid live vaccines Risk of serious infections, increased risk of malignancies Pregnancy: limited data on use in pregnancy	Monitor: CBC, LFTs, signs of infection Do not use with biologics Increased frequency of side effects in patients of Asian decent
Baricitinib	Tablet: 2 mg (contains soy)	2 mg po daily	Upper respiratory tract infection, GI upset, hepatic issues, herpes zoster infection	Boxed warnings: malignancies, infections, and thrombosis Avoid live vaccines Pregnancy: Limited data available; adverse events observed in animal studies	Monitor: CBC, LFTs, signs of infection, lipids Do not use with biologics
Adalimumab	Pen injector: 40, 80 mg Prefilled syringe: 10, 20, 40, 80 mg	40 mg subcutaneously every other week; can give weekly if given in absence of MTX	Infections, injection site reactions, demyelinating disease, headache, increased CPK	Boxed warnings: serious infections and malignancies Contraindicated with active infection Pregnancy: limited data available; small studies have shown no increased risk of birth defects	Monitor: TB and HBV test prior to initiation, signs of infection, CBC, LFTs Do not use with other biologics or live vaccines Rotate injection sites
Etanercept	Prefilled syringe/auto-injector: 25, 50 mg	50 mg subcutaneously weekly	Infections, injection site reactions, demyelinating disease, headache	Boxed warnings: serious infections and malignancies Contraindicated with active infection, sepsis Pregnancy: limited data; adverse effects not observed in animal studies	Monitor: TB and HBV test prior to initiation, signs of infection, CBC, LFTs Do not use with other biologics or live vaccines Rotate injection sites
Certolizumab pegol	200 mg subcutaneous kits	200 mg subcutaneously every other week	Infections, injection site reactions, demyelinating disease, headache	Boxed warnings: serious infections and malignancies Contraindicated with active infection, sepsis Pregnancy: Avoid use in pregnancy, particularly after week 30	Monitor: TB and HBV test prior to initiation, signs of infection, CBC, LFTs Do not use with other biologics or live vaccines Rotate injection sites

(continued)

TABLE 22.3 Disease-Modifying Antirheumatic Drugs (continued)

Drug	Form/Strength	Typical Maintenance Dose*	Side Effects	Contraindications and Warnings	Monitoring and Notes
Golimumab	Solution: 50 mg Auto-injector: 50 mg, 100 mg Prefilled syringe: 50, 100 mg	Subcutaneously once a month (usually in combo with MTX) IV: 2mg/kg at 0, 4, and then every 8 weeks	Infections, injection site reactions, demyelinating disease, headache	Boxed warnings: serious infections and malignancies Contraindicated with active infection, sepsis Pregnancy: limited data; adverse effects not observed in animal studies	Monitor: TB and HBV test prior to initiation, signs of infection, CBC, LFTs Do not use with other biologics or live vaccines Rotate injection sites
Infliximab	IV infusion	3 mg/kg at weeks 0, 2, 6, and then every 8 weeks	Infusion reactions, delayed hypersensitivity reaction (3–12 days after receiving dose), infections, demyelinating disease, headache	Boxed warnings: serious infections and malignancies Contraindicated with doses >5mg/kg in moderate to severe heart failure, active infection, sepsis Pregnancy: category B	Monitor: vitals during infusion, TB and HBV test prior to initiation, signs of infection, CBC, LFTs Do not use with other biologics or live vaccines
Anakinra (give only after failure of other options)	Prefilled syringe: 100 mg	100 mg once daily at same time each day; give every other day if SCr <30 mL/min	Injection site reactions, headaches, GI upset, upper respiratory tract infections	Malignancies/ serious infection Pregnancy: Use during pregnancy not advised until more data becomes available	Monitor: TB test prior to therapy, CBC, SCr, signs of infection Do not use with other biologics or live vaccines
Abatacept (Orencia®)	Auto-injector: 125 mg/mL Prefilled syringe: 50, 87.5, 125 mg IV solution: 250 mg	IV: 500–1,000 mg based on weight at 0, 2, 4, and then every 4 weeks Subcutaneous:125 mg weekly	Injection site reactions/ infusion reactions, infections, headache, nausea	Malignancies/ serious infection; caution in patients with COPD Pregnancy: Use during pregnancy not advised until more data becomes available	Monitor: TB test prior to therapy; signs of infection/ hypersensitivity Do not use with other biologics or live vaccines
Rituximab	IV solution: 10 mg/mL	1,000-mg IV on day 1 and day 15	Infusion reactions, infections, GI upset, weight gain	Boxed warnings: infusion-related reactions, HBV reactivation Pregnancy: category C	Monitor: screen for HBV, HCV prior to therapy; infusion reaction symptoms, ECG, vitals during infusion, CBC, SCr, electrolytes Do not use with other biologics or live vaccines
Tocilizumab	Solution for infusion Auto-injector and pre-filled syringe: 162 mg	IV: weight based (4–8 mg/kg) Subcutaneous: 162 mg every other week; 162 mg every week if >100 kg	Infections, injection-site reactions, headache, increased lipids	Boxed warnings: serious infection, screen for TB prior to use Pregnancy: limited data available	Monitor: LFTs, CBC, lipids, signs of infection Do not use with other biologics or live vaccines
Sarilumab	Auto-injector and pre-filled syringe: 150 mg, 200 mg	200 mg every other week	Infections, injection-site reactions, headache, increased lipids	Boxed warnings: serious infection, screen for TB prior to use Pregnancy: limited data available	Monitor: LFTs, CBC, lipids, signs of infection Do not use with other biologics or live vaccines

*Note: Some therapies have an increased initial dosing regimen.

bid: twice daily; CBC: complete blood count; CPK, creatine phosphokinase; GI, gastrointestinal; HBV, hepatitis B virus; IV, intravenous; LFT, liver function test; MTX, methotrexate; po, by mouth; qd: once daily; SCr: serum creatinine; TB, tuberculosis; tid, thrice daily; XR, extended-release

KEY TAKEAWAYS

- APAP has negligible anti-inflammatory activity and limited analgesic effectiveness.
- NSAID selection should be based on patient risks of developing either GI or cardiovascular AEs; CVD risk assessment prior to prescribing is required.
- NSAID GI complications include both upper and lower GI. PPIs only protect against the UGI AEs.

- COX-2 selective coxibs have less upper and lower GI adverse effects than nonselective NSAIDs but have the same risks for cardiovascular, renal, and hepatic adverse reactions.
- SMRs, duloxetine, and pregabalin may be beneficial in some patients for MSK pain.
- Methotrexate should be given with folate to decrease adverse events.
- All DMARDs require negative TB and hepatitis screenings prior to initiation.
- Biologic DMARDs should not be given concomitantly with other biologics or with any live vaccine.

CASE EXEMPLAR: Patient With Rheumatoid Arthritis

GB, a 37-year-old female, presents with newly diagnosed rheumatoid arthritis involving her joints without extra-articular manifestations.

Past Medical History
- Painful, swollen, warm joints at third and fourth proximal interphalangeal (PIP) joints in both hands and at second and first metatarsophalangeal (MTP) joints
- Morning joint stiffness lasts 3 to 4 hours
- Otherwise healthy with no known drug allergies

Medications
- Ibuprofen as needed
- Oral contraceptives

Physical Examination
- Consistent with inflammatory arthritis

Labs and Imaging
- Hand and foot films: do not show joint narrowing, bony erosions, or periarticular osteopenia

Discussion Questions
1. What class of drugs must be given to prevent joint destruction?
2. When should it be initiated? What medications can GB take to control symptoms while her initial drug is taking effect?
3. What adverse effects are likely to occur with these drugs?

CASE EXEMPLAR: Patient With Joint Stiffness

PK is a 63-year-old male presenting for follow-up of chronic intermittent pains in his knees and ankles. He has worked as a carpenter for most of his adult life, although he has been more of a supervisor over the past few years. He has been using a variety of creams and lotions as well as hot baths to help with the pain. He does not like pills in general, but he might consider medications as long as he will not get addicted.

Past Medical History
- Actinic keratoses

Medications
- Acetaminophen, 500 mg once per day as needed for pain

Physical Examination
- Well-developed, well-nourished male in no distress
- Lungs: few scattered wheezes

- Heart: regular rate and rhythm
- Bony hypertrophy surrounding the joints of the hands; knees with palpable osteophytes and no effusion

Labs and Imaging
- Complete blood count: normal
- Sedimentation rate: normal
- X-rays: mild-to-moderate degenerative changes in both hands, knees, and ankles, with significant joint space narrowing in left knee

Discussion Questions
1. What class of drugs is considered the first drug of choice for PK's symptoms?
2. Are there nonprescription options available as adjuncts?
3. What role would corticosteroids play in the treatment of PK's osteoarthritis?

REFERENCES

1. Rui P, Okeyode T. *National Ambulatory Medical Care survey: 2015 state and national summary tables.* Published 2017. https://www.cdc.gov/nchs/data/ahcd/namcs_summary/2015_namcs_web_tables.pdf.

2. Global Health Data Exchange. GBD results tool. Accessed January 9, 2019. http://ghdx.healthdata.org/gbd-results-tool

3. Aletaha D, Smolen JS. Diagnosis and management of rheumatoid arthritis: a review. *JAMA.* 2018;320(13):1360–1372. doi:10.1001/jama.2018.13103

4. Wang A, Leong DJ, Cardoso L, et al. Nutraceuticals and osteoarthritis pain. *Pharmacol Ther.* 2018;*187*:167–179. doi:10.1016/j.pharmthera.2018.02.015

5. Derry S, Wiffen PJ, Kalso EA, et al. Topical analgesics for acute and chronic pain in adults—An overview of Cochrane reviews. *Cochrane Database Syst Rev.* 2017;(5):CD008609. doi:10.1002/14651858.CD008609.pub2

6. da Costa BR, Reichenbach S, Keller N, et al. Effectiveness of non-steroidal anti-inflammatory drugs for the treatment of pain in the knee and hip osteoarthritis: a network meta-analysis. *Lancet.* 2017;390:e21–e33. doi:10.1016/S0140-6736(17)31744-0

7. Chou R, Deyo R, Friedly J, et al. Systemic pharmacologic therapies for low back pain: a systematic review for an American College of Physicians clinical practice guideline. *Ann Intern Med.* 2017;*166*:480–492. doi:10.7326/M16-2458

8. Busse JW, Wang L, Kamaleldin M, et al. Opioids for chronic noncancer pain: a systematic review and meta-analysis. *JAMA.* 2018;320(23):2448–2460. doi:10.1001/jama.2018.18472

9. Krebs EE, Gravely A, Nugent S, et al. Effect of opioid vs nonopioid medications on pain-related function in patients with chronic back pain or hip or knee osteoarthritis pain, the SPACE randomized clinical trial. *JAMA.* 2018;319(9):872–882. doi:10.1001/jama.2018.0899

10. Oyler D, Bernard AC, VanHoose JD, et al. Minimizing opioid use after acute major trauma. *Am J Health Syst Pharm.* 2018;75(3):105–110. doi:10.2146/ajhp161021

11. Bryant B. ed. Do NSAIDs affect bone healing? *Prescriber's Letter.* February 2017. Resource #330205.

12. Brunton LL, Hilal-Dandan R, Knollmann BC, eds. *Goodman & Gilman's: The Pharmacological Basis of Therapeutics.* 13th ed. McGraw-Hill Education; 2018.

13. Derry S, Wiffen PJ, Häuser W, et al. Oral nonsteroidal anti-inflammatory drugs for fibromyalgia in adults. *Cochrane Database Syst Rev.* 2017;(3):CD012332. doi:10.1002/14651858.CD012332.pub2

14. U.S. Food and Drug Administration. *FDA drug safety communication: FDA recommends avoiding use of NSAIDs in pregnancy at 20 weeks or later because they can result in low amniotic fluid.* Published October 15, 2020. https://www.fda.gov/media/142967/download

15. Reed GW, Abdallah MS, Shao M, et al. Effect of aspirin coadministration on the safety of celecoxib, naproxen, or ibuprofen. *J Am Coll Cardiol.* 2018;71(16):1741–1751. doi:10.1016/j.jacc.2018.02.036

16. U.S. Food and Drug Administration. *FDA drug safety communication. FDA strengthens warning that non-aspirin nonsteroidal anti-inflammatory drugs (NSAIDs) can cause heart attacks and strokes.* Published July 9, 2015. https://www.fda.gov/drugs/drugsafety/ucm451800.htm

17. Schmidt M, Sørensen HT, Pedersen L. Diclofenac use and cardiovascular risks: series of nationwide Cohort studies. *BMJ.* 2018;362:K3426. doi:10.1136/bmj.k3426

18. Liver Tox. Drug Record. Nonsteroidal antiinflamatory drugs (NSAIDs). Accessed January 14, 2019. https://livertox.nlm.nih.gov//NonsteroidalAntiinflammatoryDrugs.htm

19. Ho KY, Gwee KA, Cheng YK, et al. Nonsteroidal anti-inflammatory drugs in chronic pain: implications of new data for clinical practice. *J Pain Res.* 2018;11:1937–1948. doi:10.2147/JPR.S168188

20. DynaMed. Prevention of NSAID-induced gastrointestinal toxicity. Accessed October 1, 2018. http://www.dynamed.com/topics/dmp~AN-T115775/Prevention-of-NSAID-induced-gastrointestinal-toxicity#References

21. Chan FKL, Ching YL, Tse YK, et al. Gastrointestinal safety of celecoxib versus naproxen in patients with cardiothrombotic diseases and arthritis after upper gastrointestinal bleeding (CONCERN): an industry-independent, double-blind, double-dummy, randomized trial. *Lancet.* 2017;389:2375–2382. doi:10.1016/S0140-6736(17)30981-9

22. Meng A, Huang R. Topical treatment of degenerative knee osteoarthritis. *Am J Med Sci.* 2018;355(1):6–12. doi:10.1016/j.amjms.2017.06.006

23. Sardana V, Burzynski J, Hasan, K, et al. Are non-steroidal antiinflammatory drug injections an alternative to steroid injections for musculoskeletal pain? A systematic review. *J Orthop.* 2018;15:812–816. doi:10.1016/j.jor.2018.08.022

24. Drugs for rheumatoid arthritis. *Med Lett Drugs Ther.* 2018;60(1552):123–128. https://secure.medicalletter.org/article-share?a=1552a&p=tml&title=Drugs%20for%20Rheumatoid%20Arthritis&cannotaccesstitle=125

25. Juni P, Hari R, Rutjes AWS, et al. Intra-articular corticosteroid for knee osteoarthritis. *Cochrane Database Syst Rev.* 2015;(10):CD005328. doi:10.1002/14651858.CD005328.pub3

26. Two new intra-articular injections for knee osteoarthritis. *Med Lett Drugs Ther.* 2018;60(1554):142–144. https://secure.medicalletter.org/article-share?a=1554b&p=tml&title=Two%20New%20Intra-Articular%20Injections%20for%20Knee%20Osteoarthritis&cannotaccesstitle=127.

27. Roberts WN. Intraarticular and soft tissue injections: What agent(s) to inject and how frequently? In Furst DE, Ramirez Curtis M, eds. *UpToDate.* Updated May 11, 2020. https://www.uptodate.com/contents/intraarticular-and-soft-tissue-injections-what-agents-to-inject-and-how-frequently

28. Wang W, Shi M, Zhou C, et al. Effectiveness of corticosteroid injections in adhesive capsulitis of shoulder: A meta-analysis. *Medicine (Baltimore).* 2017;96(28):e7529. doi:10.1097/MD.0000000000007529

29. McAlindon TE, LaValley MP, Harvey WF, et al. Effect of intra-articular triamcinolone vs saline on knee cartilage volume and pain in patients with knee osteoarthritis: a randomized clinical trial. *JAMA.* 2017;317(19):1967–1975. doi:10.1001/jama.2017.5283

30. Richards BL, Whittle SL, Buchbinder R. Muscle relaxants for pain management in rheumatoid arthritis. *Cochrane Database Syst Rev.* 2012;(1):CD008922. doi:10.1002/14651858.CD008922.pub2

31. Hardek B, Pruskowski J. Skeletal muscle relaxants #340. *J Palliat Med.* 2017;20(11):1293–1294. doi:10.1089/jpm.2017.0492

32. Friedman BW, Cisewski D, Irizarry E, et al. A randomized, double-blind, placebo-controlled trial of naproxen with or without orphenadrine or methocarbamol for acute low back pain. *Ann Emerg Med.* 2018;71(3):348–356. doi:10.1016/j.annemergmed.2017.09.031

33. Friedman BW, Irizarry E, Davitt M, et al. Diazepam is no better than placebo when added to naproxen for acute low back pain. *Ann Emerg Med.* 2017;70(2):169–176. doi:10.1016/j.annemergmed.2016.10.002

34. Derner MM, Linhart CA, Pederson LM, et al. Injuries in adults 65 years of age and older prescribed muscle relaxants. *Consult Pharm.* 2016;31(9):511–517. doi:10.4140/TCP.n.2016.511

35. Evidence staking up against gabapentin and pregabalin for low back pain. *BackLetter.* 2018;33(9):102–103. doi:10.1097/01.BACK.0000544944.44062.ee

36. Sofat N, Harrison A, Russell MD, et al. The effect of pregabalin or duloxetine in arthritis pain: a clinical and mechanistic study in people with hand osteoarthritis. *J Pain Res.* 2017;10:2437–2449. doi:10.2147/JPR.S147640

37. Wang G, Bi I, Li X, et al. Efficacy and safety of duloxetine in Chinese patients with chronic pain due to osteoarthritis: a randomized, double-blind, placebo-controlled study. *Osteoarthritis Cartilage.* 2017;25:832–838. doi:10.1016/j.joca.2016.12.025

38. Uchio Y, Enomoto H, Ishida M, et al. Safety and efficacy of duloxetine in Japanese patients with chronic knee pain due to osteoarthritis: an open-label, long-term, Phase III extension study. *J Pain Res.* 2018;11:1391–1403. doi:10.2147/JPR.S171395

39. Simental-Mendia M, Sánchez-Garcia A, Vilchez-Cavazos F, et al. Effect of glucosamine and chondroitin sulfate in symptomatic knee osteoarthritis: a systematic review and meta-analysis of randomized placebo-controlled trials. *Rheumatol Int.* 2018;38:1413–1428. doi:10.1007/s00296-018-4077-2

40. Cumpston M, Johnston RV, Wengier L, et al. Topical glyceryl trinitrate for rotator cuff disease. *Cochrane Database Syst Rev.* 2009;(3):CD006355. doi:10.1002/14651858.CD006355.pub2

41. Persson MSM, Stocks J, Walsh DA, et al. The relative efficacy of topical non-steroidal anti-inflammatory drugs and capsaicin in osteoarthritis: a network meta-analysis of randomized controlled trials. *Osteoarthritis Cartilage.* 2018;26:1575–1582. doi:10.1016/j.joca.2018.08.008

42. Steiman AJ, Pope JE, Thiessen-Philbrook H, et al. Non-biologic disease-modifying antirheumatic drugs (DMARDs) improve pain in inflammatory arthritis (IA): a systematic literature review of randomized controlled trials. *Rheumatol Int.* 2013;33(5):1105–1120. doi:10.1007/s00296-012-2619-6

43. Bérard A, Zhao J, Shui I, et al. Leflunomide use during pregnancy and the risk of adverse pregnancy outcomes. *Ann Rheum Dis.* 2017;77(4):500–509. doi:10.1136/annrheumdis-2017-212078

44. Donahue KE, Gartlehner G, Jonas DE, et al. Systematic review: Comparative effectiveness and harms of disease-modifying medications for rheumatoid arthritis. *Ann Intern Med.* 148(2):124. doi:10.7326/0003-4819-148-2-200801150-00192

45. Aaltonen KJ, Virkki LM, Malmivaara A, et al. Systematic review and meta-analysis of the efficacy and safety of existing TNF blocking agents in treatment of rheumatoid arthritis. *PLoS ONE.* 2012;7(1). doi:10.1371/journal.pone.0030275

23

Therapeutic Applications of Immunology and Vaccines

Sumathi Sankaran-Walters and Sara Boullt

LEARNING OBJECTIVES

- Describe the process of T-cell development, the role of each cell type in the immune process and response, and how T cells in combination with antibody-producing B cells target and kill cancer cells.
- Define when and how the role of T cells should be suppressed.
- Differentiate between T and B cells and define the role B cells play in immunity.
- Define the role of macrophages and natural killer cells in disease and cancer treatment.
- Outline the vaccines available to prevent disease in the United States.

INTRODUCTION

Immunology is a vast and developing field, which is due partly to the continuous emergence of new pathogens in various settings. For example, under the current pandemic, a new virus (i.e., COVID19) was identified, which has affected almost 7 million and killed more than 200,000 Americans at the time of this writing. Unfortunately, these numbers are expected to be further escalated as researchers are still looking for a new effective vaccine and treatment. A clear understanding of the immunologic pathways within our bodies is a crucial step in developing a preventive or curative treatment of an infection. In this chapter we discuss two aspects of immunology: Immunotherapy and vaccination.

MODIFYING THE IMMUNE RESPONSE, ONE CELL AT A TIME

T LYMPHOCYTES

T-Cell Development

The T cell is one of the two important lymphocytes that make up the adaptive immune system (**Figure 23.1**). T cells are derived from multipotent hematopoietic stem cells present in the bone marrow and go on to mature in the thymus. A mature T cell will express receptors as well as their associated coreceptor, either CD4 or CD8,[1] which are required epitopes for T-cell functions. However, there are T cells that are identified to have both the CD4 and CD8 receptors, termed "double positive" T cells.[2,3] As T cells mature in the thymus, the genes encoding the receptors will undergo rearrangement, leading to different T cells expressing different receptors, depending on how their genes are arranged. Sometimes this rearrangement can lead to the expression of T cell receptors that recognize the body's own cells, leading to autoimmune diseases.[4,5] Once rearrangement is completed and the receptors are expressed, maturing T cells need to undergo both positive and negative selection before they can finish maturation.[6] Undergoing positive and negative selection will ultimately decrease the likelihood of T cells attacking the body's own cells.

The goal of maturation is to produce T cells that express a variety of receptors that bind only to foreign antigens that are presented by the self-major histocompatibility complexes I and II (MHC I and MHC II). These antigens presenting MHC are found on the surface of other immune cells such as dendritic cells, macrophages, and B cells. If the maturing T cells bind to molecules other than the MHC-presenting molecules,

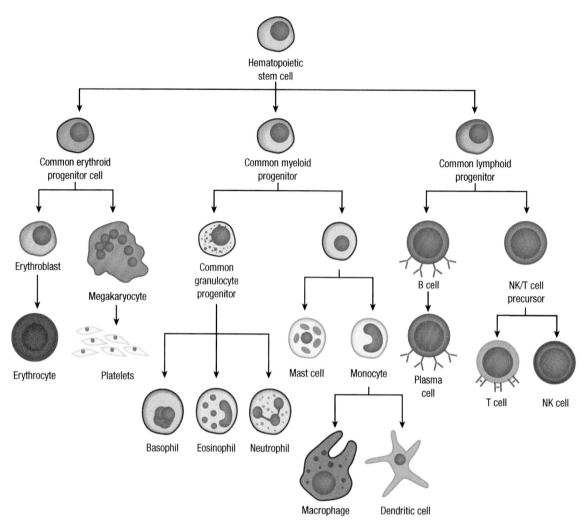

FIGURE 23.1 Cells of the immune system arise from a common hematopoietic stem cell. NK, natural killer.

then they do not pass the positive selection test and apoptosis is initiated to eliminate these malfunctioning T cells.[7–9] However, once they pass the positive selection they are then put through a negative selection test.[10] If the T cell binds strongly to a self-MHC molecule that is presenting a self-antigen or a self-MHC molecule that has no antigen bound, then it fails the negative selection test and apoptosis is initiated to eliminate the cell.[10] When T cells pass both positive and negative selections, they are able to complete maturation and become the various subsets of T cells, some of which include helper T cells, cytotoxic T cells, and regulatory T cells.

Types of T Lymphocytes

T cells may be classified into many different subtypes according to their surface molecules, how they function, and how they interact with the MHC. The most accepted classification is grouping T cells into three main subcategories: (a) T-helper (T_h) cells, (b) T-regulatory (T_{reg}) cells, and (c) T-cytotoxic (T_c) cells. Both T_h and T_{reg} cells have CD4 glycoprotein on their surfaces,

although T_{reg} cells have very different functions from T_h cells. Meanwhile, T_c cells have CD8 glycoprotein on their surface and are responsible for destroying the pathogens when they become activated.[11]

Helper T cells serve several purposes. They are needed to help activate B cells, macrophages, and cytotoxic T cells to attack and eliminate infected host cells.[1] Prior to activating these various other immune system cells, the helper T cells themselves must first be activated. This process involves a number of steps:

1. The dendritic cells ingest a pathogen and resynthesize the antigen that was presented by the pathogen.
2. The dendritic cells along with an associated MHC II molecule[12] now present a part of this antigen on their own cell surfaces.
3. The inactive helper T cells with the receptors that can specifically bind this antigen will bind to the MHC II molecule and the bound antigen on the surface of the dendritic cell and become activated.[12]

An activated helper T cell will begin to divide rapidly and differentiate into memory T cells and effector T cells.

Memory T cells will express the same receptors as the Helper T cell from which they are derived, to ultimately recognize the same antigen that activated the original Helper T cell. Should the body become infected with the same pathogen again, it will be able to mount a faster immune response as it will have more helper T cells—in the form of memory T cells—that are available to recognize the pathogen, bind to the antigen, and initiate an immune response.[13,14]

Effector T cells, on the other hand, can release cytokines that activate macrophages and cytotoxic T cells to begin fighting off an infection. These cytokines can also stimulate B lymphocytes to secrete specific types of antibodies.[15] One of the most important roles of effector T cells is to activate B cells that are already bound to an antigen that the original helper T cells have previously recognized. When a B cell ingests a pathogen, it breaks down the pathogen and presents a piece of the antigen on its cell surface by attaching to an MHC II molecule. The effector T cell subsequently recognizes this same antigen presented on the surface of the B cell. The binding of the effector T cell to the antigen, presented on the B cell surface, will activate the B cell allowing it to proliferate and differentiate into its own type of memory and effector B cells. Taken together, the response is specific to the antigen that has been presented.

Cytotoxic T cells are a special type of T cells that can recognize and mount an immune response toward host cells that have been infected by a virus or bacteria.[16] These cells typically express the CD8 marker and are otherwise known as CD8+ T cells. Like helper T cells, cytotoxic T cells must first be activated. This is done by the infected host cell breaking down the pathogen that has infiltrated the cell and presenting an antigen on its cell surface. The antigen is associated with an MHC I molecule on the host cell surface, which is expressed on all nucleated cells in the body. A cytotoxic T cell with a receptor that recognizes the antigen will bind to the host, present a pathologic antigen, and become activated.[16] An activated cytotoxic T cell will proliferate and differentiate into memory and effector T cells. The effector T cells will be able to bind these infected host cells by recognizing the same antigen present on the cell surface and secrete perforins and granzymes to kill the infected cell.[16]

Cytotoxic T cells can also recognize and mount a response to cancer cells. Cancer cells produce abnormal proteins.[17,18] A cancer cell can therefore also break down these proteins, attach them to the MHC I molecules, and express a piece of these proteins on their cell surfaces. Cytotoxic T cells with receptors that are able to recognize these proteins can bind them and carry out the same response as they do when binding to an infected host cell.

Regulatory T cells also play an important role in the body's immune response. These types of T cells work to modify and control the body's overall immune response, as well as maintain the immune system's tolerance to self-antigens that are presented on cells throughout the body.[19] Most importantly, because of their ability to promote tolerance to self-antigens, they can play a role in preventing the development of many autoimmune diseases. Regulatory T cells that have been altered and function abnormally, however, could therefore contribute to various autoimmune diseases.[19] Recent studies show that should regulatory T cell function be impaired, the consequences may include not only the development of autoimmune diseases but infectious and allergic diseases as well.[19] While this would suggest that regulatory T cells play a role in disease prevention, studies on various forms of cancer and several infectious diseases have also shown that regulatory T cells can impair necessary immune responses to cancer cells and invading pathogens, playing a role in promoting disease.[19]

There are two overarching categories of regulatory T cells that have been identified, the first being the thymus-derived naturally occurring CD4+ CD25+ T cells, and the second being inducible antigen-specific Regulatory T cells that secrete inhibitory cytokines.[19] Patients with multiple sclerosis were found to have CD4+ CD25+ regulatory T cells that could not downregulate the rapid expansion of T cells and their interferon production.[20,21] Inability to downregulate T-cell proliferation and interferon production could essentially contribute to the increased inflammation and T cell–mediated demyelination seen in patients with multiple sclerosis. The CD4+ CD25+ regulatory T cells cannot suppress the rapid T-cell expansion found in patients with type 1 and type 2 diabetes, as well as in patients with psoriasis and polyglandular syndrome.[22] Therefore, in the case of these autoimmune diseases, regulatory T cells appear to have a disease-preventing role, with their altered function consequently leading to the progression of the disease state.

Unlike observations in autoimmune diseases, it is not the alteration in function, but the decrease in number of CD4+ CD25+ regulatory T cells that contributes to several allergic diseases.[23,24] For example, researchers found that individuals with lower CD4+ CD25+ regulatory T-cell numbers there demonstrated an increase in allergen-specific T-helper type 2 cell proliferation and cytokine production in the presence of common allergens such as grass, milk, and nickel.[25] Because of uninhibited allergen-specific T-helper type 2 cell proliferation and cytokine production, these individuals experienced significant allergic reactions to these common allergens. These results therefore support the notion that in healthy individuals CD4+ CD25+ regulatory T cells can play a role in preventing the development of allergic diseases.[25]

As opposed to the results observed in various autoimmune and allergic diseases, regulatory T cells have been found to play a disease-promoting role in a multitude of cancers. Recent studies have shown that increased activity of regulatory T cells in cancer patients has been linked to an insufficient immune response to tumor antigens, resulting in decreased tumor cell killing.[26] More specifically, increased numbers of CD4+ CD25+ T regulatory cells that can inhibit other subsets of T cells and natural killer (NK) cells have been found in patients with lung, pancreatic, breast, and skin cancer.[27,28] These regulatory T cells potentially prevent tumor cell killing, by downregulating the number of T cells and NK cells that can infiltrate tumors and rid the body of cancerous cells.

Regarding infectious diseases, regulatory T cells seem to be playing the same disease-promoting role. For example, researchers found that in individuals infected with *Helicobacter pylori*, CD4+ CD25+ regulatory T cells appear to contribute to chronic infection by downregulating memory T cells' response to the infection.[29]

T-Cell–Derived Cancer Immunotherapy

T cells have long been a prime subject for cancer immunotherapy research as they are able to target and eliminate cancer cells. However, most research has focused on genetically engineering T cells to target specific types of cancer cells and eliminate them from the body.[30] Recently, new research has focused on using T cells in combination with antibody-producing B cells to target and kill cancer cells. A recent study explored the potential to use both T cells and B cells to target tumors.

First, B cells expressing tumor antigens on their cell surface were stimulated by binding the CD40 receptor on its cell surface with its designated ligand.[31] This resulted in the recruitment of T cells that specifically targeted the antigen expressed on the B cell surface. B cells were then stimulated using IL-21, IL-4, anti-CD40, and the tumor antigen of interest allowing them to proliferate and differentiate into Effector B cells that produce antibodies targeting the specific tumor cells of interest.[30]

T-Cell–Directed Immunosuppressive Therapy

While T cells can serve an invaluable purpose for cancer immunotherapy, there are also instances where T-cell suppression instead of expansion would be necessary. Such would be the case for transplant and cancer patients, as well as those with a variety of autoimmune diseases. Therefore, researchers have developed a multitude of drugs used for T-cell–directed immunosuppressive therapy. T-cell–directed immu-

nosuppressive therapeutic agents fall into two major categories: those that target signal one, and those that target signal two.[32] Signal one involves the T cell and its associated T-cell receptor binding with an antigen-presenting cell. For transplant patients, T cells would recognize the cells of the transplanted organ or tissue as the antigen themselves. On the other hand, signal two involves additional binding of various receptors on the T-cell surface with their associated ligands on an antigen-presenting cell, as binding with these receptors is necessary for the T cell to become fully activated.[32]

Agents that target signal one include cyclosporine and tacrolimus (**Table 23.1**). These therapeutic agents are calcineurin inhibitors.[32] Calcineurin plays a significant role in aiding the progression of full T-cell activation, specifically after T-cell receptor binding to associated antigens on an antigen-presenting cell. After binding, calcineurin is needed in a pathway that leads to the initiation of T-cell gene transcription, which is required for a T cell to become fully activated.[32] Therefore, these agents (e.g., cyclosporine and tacrolimus) can prevent T cells from being fully activated and mounting an immune response.

Therapeutic agents that specifically target signal two by blocking the interaction between CD80/86 on antigen-presenting cells with CD28 on T cells include abatacept and belatacept (Table 23.1). The binding of CD80/86 with CD28 on a T-cell surface is required for a T cell to become fully activated. These therapeutic agents compete for the binding with CD80/86 in order to downregulate T-cell activation, ultimately reducing the T-cell immune response.[32] Abatacept specifically has been approved for use in treatment of rheumatoid arthritis and is currently under investigation for potential use in treating a variety of autoimmune diseases.

ASKP1240 is another therapeutic agent currently in phase 2 clinical trials that targets signal two as well. This agent specifically blocks the interaction of CD154 on the activated T-cell surface with CD40 on antigen-presenting cells.[33] Should binding occur, antigen-presenting cells will experience an upregulation of the expression of CD80/86 on their cell surfaces. With increased expression of CD80/86 on the surfaces of antigen-presenting cells, T cells can more frequently bind CD80/86 and become fully activated. Therefore, ASKP1240 has the potential to downregulate T-cell activation and the overall T-cell immune response.

B Lymphocytes

The B lymphocyte is the second of the two important lymphocytes that make up the adaptive immune system (Figure 23.1). Like T cells, B cells are formed from multipotent hematopoietic stem cells present in the bone marrow. Following their development in the bone marrow, B cells move into the lymphatic system where they

TABLE 23.1 T-Cell–Directed Immunosuppressive Therapy Medications

Medication	Target	Functional in Signaling	Side Effects
Drugs That Target Signal One			
Cyclosporine (two formulations) **(a) nonmodified: Sandimmune** *organ transplant rejection prophylaxis: **PO:** 15mg/kg/dose PO x1 (give postop or 4–12hrs prior to procedure), then 10–15mg/kg/day PO x 1–2wk, then tapper 5% per wk to a maintenance dose of 5–10mg/kg/day. (Capsules and solution contain 12.5% alcohol; Sandimmune package insert) **IV:** 5–6mg/kg/day IV, give first dose 4–12hrs prior to procedure or postop. Daily single IV dose is given until patient can tolerate PO capsules. (IV dose is 1/3 of PO). IV formulation contains 32.9% alcohol by volume. (Sandimmune package insert) **(b) modified (for better absorption): Neoral** *organ transplant rejection prophylaxis: **PO:** 7–9mg/kg/day PO divided into BID. Give first dose 4–12hrs prior to procedure or postop. (Capsules and solution contain 11.9% alcohol)	Calcineurin	Involved in a pathway that leads to the activation of T-cell gene transcription, which is needed to continue with T-cell activation	Nephrotoxicity, posttransplantation diabetes mellitus, immunosuppression
Tacrolimus (Prograf) **organ transplant rejection prophylaxis: **PO:** 0.075–0.2 mg/kg/day PO divided Q12hrs. Start >6hrs and within 24hrs postop. Adjust dose based on trough levels. **IV:** Continuous IV infusion may be started for patient who cannot tolerate capsules. Switch to PO as soon as patient can tolerate PO. First PO dose should be given 8–12hrs after discontinuing IV infusion. (Tacrolimus package insert)			
Drugs That Target Signal Two			
Abatacept (Orencia) Moderate-severe Rheumatoid Arthritis **Intravenous infusion:** <60Kg: 500mg IV week 0, 2, 4, then Q4wks thereafter 60–100Kg: 750mg IV week, 0, 2, 4, then Q4wks thereafter >100Kg: 1,000mg IV week 0, 2, 4, then Q4wks thereafter **Subcutaneous Injection:** <60Kg: 500mg **IV** x 1, then 125mg SC x 1 in 24hrs, then 125mg SC Qwk 60–100Kg: 750mg **IV** x1, then 125mg SC x 1 in 24hrs, then 125mg SC Qwk >100Kg: 1,000mg **IV** x1, then 125mg SC x 1 in 24hrs, then 125mg SC Qwk	CD80/86	Binds with CD28 on a T cell to allow for optimal T-cell activation	Nausea, headache, nasopharyngitis, dyspepsia, immunosuppression
Belatacept (Nulojix) Restricted distribution in the U.S. (see manufacture's full prescribing information for further details)			

*Note: These formulations are not bio-equivalent; therefore, they are not interchangeable. Individualized dosing regimen is required.

will go on to circulate throughout the body and continue to mature. A mature B cell that has not yet been bound to an antigen will express thousands of a specific type of antibody on its cell surface. These are commonly known as "membrane-bound antibodies." All antibodies on the surface of a B cell will have the same unique antigen-binding site.[34,35] During development, rearrangement of the genes that encode the antibodies produced by the B cell will determine which type of antibody, and therefore which type of antigen-binding site, will be presented on the cell's surface. Rearrangement allows for a wide array of antibodies and antigen-binding sites to be pro-

duced, ultimately leading the immune system to respond to a variety of invading pathogens. Activation is accomplished by the binding of the antigen that the specific type of antibodies on the B cell surface can recognize.[36]

After having bound an antigen, engulfing the associated pathogen, and presenting a part of the antigen on its cell surface for an effector T cell to bind to, the B cell can now officially begin to divide and differentiate into effector B cells and memory B cells. Each of these types of cells plays a unique and crucial role in mounting an immune response toward an invading pathogen. Memory B cells produced by activated B cells will have longer life spans than the average B cell and express the same membrane-bound antibodies as the B cell from which it originates.[37] These two qualities will ensure that should this same pathogen invade the body in the future, there are plenty of B cells available—that are made to recognize this specific pathogen—to mount an even quicker immune response.

The effector B cells will essentially become antbody-producing factories (plasma cells).[38] An effector B cell will produce the same antibodies as the B cell from which it is derived, but instead of inserting these antibodies in the membrane, it will instead secrete these antibodies so that they can enter circulation.[38] These circulating antibodies can then bind the same antigen as the original B cell and mark the associated pathogen for elimination by other immune cells.[39]

B Lymphocyte Roles in Different Diseases

B cells can also play a role in the development of various diseases. Primarily, research has focused on abnormalities in B-cell maturation and regulation, and how abnormalities in either of these processes can lead to the development of immune deficiency disorders, autoimmune disorders, and even a variety of cancers. In these instances, B cells appear to have a more disease-promoting role, but overall, normally developing and properly regulated B cells do provide invaluable immune defense.

Aside from contributing to the development of immune-deficiency disorders, improper B-cell development also seems to be leading to the progression of certain cancers. More specifically, researchers have found that for every stage of B-cell development, there is a "malignant counterpart," where a cancerous B cell will emerge should there be an alteration in normal development, as in leukemias and lymphomas.

Abnormal regulation of B-cell growth and expansion plays a role in the development of several autoimmune diseases.[40,41] One theory for this dysfunction is based on the BCL2 dysregulation resulting in the lack of elimination of self-reactive B cells.

B-Cell–Derived Cancer Immunotherapy

B cells, along with various other immune cells, have the unique ability to infiltrate tumors, making them a prime target for use in cancer immunotherapy.[31] Multiple studies have shown that tumor-infiltrating B cells have contributed to a better overall prognosis for patients with various forms of cancer, including gastric cancer, breast cancer, ovarian cancer, and cutaneous melanoma. The exact mechanism by which B cells contribute to a better prognosis is not yet fully understood, but researchers believe there could be two possible explanations for this result. First, tumor-infiltrating B cells could be expressing antigens on their cell surfaces that recruit T cells to the site of the tumor for tumor cell "killing." Second, B

cells themselves could be activated in the tumor microenvironment to produce effector B cells to produce antibodies that specifically target the tumor cells. B cells have also been found to recruit and stimulate other immune cells.[31] One study found that when CD40-activated B cells were presented with a melanoma antigen in vitro, these B cells could promote the activation and expansion of T cells that specifically targeted melanoma.[31]

The mechanism by which B cells can activate T cells that have specific cancer cell targets has led to the recent development of a new cancer immunotherapy technique. Researchers have developed a new cytokine given the name GIFT4, which can turn naïve B cells into effector B cells.[42,43] These effector cells express CD40, as well as produce unique cytokines that can stimulate other immune cells. Based on these two properties, GIFT4-activated B cells could promote the production of cytotoxic T cells that selectively target human melanoma cells in vitro and in vivo.

B-Cell–Directed Immunosuppressive Therapy

While B cells can certainly make a significant contribution to cancer immunotherapy, there may also be times when B-cell maturation and proliferation would need to be suppressed instead of enhanced. This type of immunotherapy is termed "B-cell–directed immunosuppressive therapy." Researchers have developed a multitude of drugs that essentially inhibit B cells at various points during maturation and differentiation to decrease B cell numbers and downregulate their immune response. These drugs do so by targeting proteins on the B-cell surface, pathways involved in B-cell differentiation, and specific B-cell organelles (**Table 23.2**).

The first target of mention is CD20, a protein found on the cell surface of developing and mature B cells, but not specifically on the surface of effector B cells. CD20 plays a role in regulating activation of a B cell, prior to the cell's ability to proliferate and differentiate. By inhibiting CD20's ability to aid in B-cell activation, one can reduce B-cell expansion and differentiation into memory and effector B cells, lowering the number of immune cells available to mount an immune response.[44] Drugs that target the CD20 protein, termed "Anti-CD20 drugs," include rituximab, ocrelizumab, ofatumumab, and veltuzumab. Specifically, rituximab can lower B-cell numbers by inducing apoptosis or stopping further development of B cells after targeting CD20.

Another target of B-cell–directed immunosuppressive drugs is CD22. CD22 is a transmembrane protein found on the surface of B cells currently going through maturation. Like CD20, CD22 also regulates B-cell activation, and by inhibiting the phosphorylation of CD22, immunosuppressive drugs that target this protein can inhibit further B-cell proliferation and differentiation. However, researchers have noted that targeting CD22 appears to have much less impact on the suppression

TABLE 23.2 B-Cell–Directed Immunosuppressive Therapy Medications

Target	Target's Function	Drugs That Inhibit at This Target	Side Effects
CD20	Regulation of B-cell activation	Anti-CD20 drugs: Rituximab (used in chemotherapy) Ocrelizumab (used to treat multiple sclerosis) Ofatumumab (used to treat chronic lymphocytic leukemia) Veltuzumab (being developed to treat non-Hodgkin's lymphoma)	GI symptoms such as nausea and heartburn, muscle pain, night sweats, flu like symptoms
CD22	Regulation of B-cell activation	Epratuzumab (potential use in oncology and to treat SLE)	Not available
Pathways involved in B-cell differentiation	Promote B-cell differentiation and prevent apoptosis	Belimumab (used to treat SLE) Atacicept (under investigation for potential to treat SLE)	Nausea, diarrhea; fever, sore throat, runny or stuffy nose, cough; pain, itching, redness, or swelling at injection site; pain in the arms or legs; headache, depressed mood; sleep problems
Effector B-cell proteasome	Protein degradation	Bortezomib (used to treat multiple myeloma)	Fatigue, generalized weakness, peripheral neuropathy

GI, gastrointestinal; SLE, systemic lupus erythematosus.

of B-cell differentiation and expansion than does targeting CD20. Drugs that target CD22 are termed "anti-CD22 drugs," one of which is epratuzumab.[45]

Instead of targeting specific membrane proteins, some B-cell–directed immunosuppressive drugs also target pathways involved in B-cell differentiation. One specific pathway of importance involves the binding of the cytokine B-cell–activating factor and the cytokine proliferation-inducing ligand to their receptors on the B-cell surface. Binding of these molecules to their receptors initiates a chain of events that lead to the eventual advancement of B-cell differentiation, while preventing initiation of apoptosis as well. Drugs that inhibit the binding of the cytokine B-cell–activating factor and the cytokine proliferation-inducing ligand include telimomab and atacicept[46,47] (see Table 23.2).

Lastly, B-cell–directed immunosuppressive drugs exist to target B-cell organelles, in effector B cells specifically. One drug that targets an effector B cell organelle is bortezomib.[48] Bortezomib inhibits proper functioning of the proteasome, essentially preventing the effector B cell from degrading unneeded proteins. As a result of proteasome inhibition, the cell is not able to carry out normal cell cycling, eventually leading to apoptosis and cell death (see Table 23.2).

MACROPHAGES

Macrophages are members of the innate immune system and are derived from blood monocytes, which are white blood cells that can go on to differentiate into various immune cells (Figure 23.1). These monocytes will leave the general circulation and migrate to specific tissues in the body where they can proceed to differentiate into macrophages. The macrophage population is therefore highly diversified as macrophages will specialize based on the tissues in which they are found. A few types of common macrophages found in tissues throughout the body include alveolar macrophages found in lung alveoli, Kupffer cells found in the liver, and microglia found in the central nervous system. Each of these macrophages ultimately plays a different and highly specialized role.

The main roles of macrophages are to detect invading pathogens, phagocytose them, and destroy them by producing reactive oxygen species, one of which is nitric oxide.[49–51] Macrophages can also activate other immune cells by presenting antigens on their cell surfaces that other immune cells, such as T cells, can recognize. Lastly, macrophages can promote inflammation by producing cytokines that can activate other immune cells. Macrophages play an invaluable role in defending the body against invading pathogens and promoting an effective immune response.

Macrophage-Based Immunotherapy

A significant challenge in cancer immunotherapy research has been finding tumor-specific antigens presented by human tumor cells that can be recognized by the immune system and to which the immune system can mount a response.[52] Evidence has shown that very few human tumors in fact present tumor-specific antigens, making it difficult to stimulate immune cells that can target tumor cells without attacking the body's own cells. Therefore, recent research has focused on

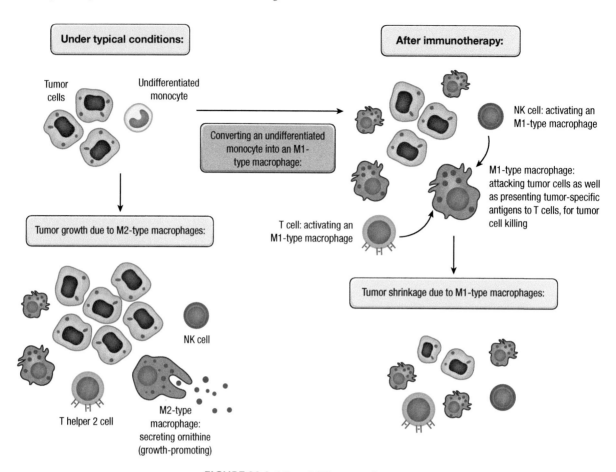

FIGURE 23.2 M1 and M2 macrophages.
NK, natural killer.

targeting macrophages for their potential use in cancer immunotherapy.

Evidence has shown that the tumor environment is essentially dominated by M2-type macrophages, which secrete ornithine, a growth-promoting molecule that promotes tumor-cell growth.[53] Therefore, macrophages appear to play a disease-promoting role when it comes to various forms of cancer. But, M2-type macrophages are just one of two types of macrophages into which a monocyte can differentiate. The second type of macrophage is an M1-type macrophage, which can inhibit cell growth by producing growth-inhibiting nitric oxide or "kill" target cells through phagocytosis. Researchers believe the tumor environment is dominated by the M2-type macrophages, however, due to tumor cells providing signals that essentially inhibit M1-type activation.[53] The absence of specific tumor antigens seems to also aid in inhibition of M1-type activation as well. There is even evidence that the lack of specific tumor antigens, as well as the nature of the tumor microenvironment itself, seem to be downregulating the activation of other immune cells like NK cells, which can attack tumor cells directly or activate nearby macrophages. Due to their ability to attack and eliminate tumor cells, researchers have therefore been attempting to develop a technique to essentially increase the number of M1-type macrophages in the tumor environment. They have described this technique as "macrophage-innate conversion (MIC) therapy" (**Figure 23.2**).

Macrophage-innate conversion therapy begins in the tumor environment, where an undifferentiated monocyte is present. Under typical conditions, this monocyte would differentiate into an M2-type macrophage that would secrete ornithine, promoting the growth of the tumor. Other immune cells, such as T-helper cells and NK cells, would be recruited to the site of the tumor, but would show little immune response as the lack of tumor-specific antigens, and the nature of the tumor microenvironment itself, would downregulate their activation.[52] The idea behind macrophage-innate conversion therapy is to instead modulate the differentiation of monocytes present in the tumor environment, essentially guiding them toward becoming M1-type macrophages instead. M1-type macrophages present in the environment would be available to become activated by nearby NK and T-helper cells, and eventually go on to initiate tumor cell "killing." Evidence to support this proposed therapeutic technique has shown that M2-type macrophages can indeed be converted to M1-type macrophages, and this conversion alone can cause the degradation of tumors.

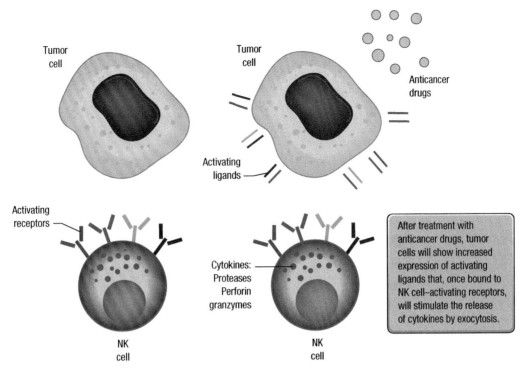

FIGURE 23.3 Natural killer (NK) cell therapy in cancer immunotherapy.

NATURAL KILLER CELL FUNCTION

NK cells are bone marrow–derived lymphocytes that, along with phagocytic leukocytes and dendritic cells, are members of the innate immune system (**Figure 23.3**). NK cells can be found in circulating blood as well as in the spleen, liver, lungs, lymph nodes, and even in the uterus during pregnancy. The primary role of NK cells is to patrol the body for both virally infected cells and tumor cells. When in contact with either type of cell, the NK cell, through a series of steps, releases cytokines to eventually "kill" its chosen target cell. NK cells therefore play a crucial role in the body's initial response to viral infection and the detection of early signs of cancer.[54]

Unlike T cells, NK cells do not require any priming to initiate a "killing" response when in contact with a tumor or virally infected cell. Instead, NK cells work through a system of activating and inhibitory receptors present on their cell surfaces. Depending on the type, ligands present on the surface of target cells will bind to either activating or inhibitory receptors and cause either the activation or suppression of the "killing" response of the NK cells. Specifically, if MHC class I ligands are present on the cell surface of a target cell, the ligand will bind to an NK cell inhibitory receptor and suppress the NK cell's release of cytokines, such as proteases, that would normally induce apoptosis of the target cell. In most cases, tumor and virally infected cells show a downregulation in the expression of MHC class I ligands, and therefore are more at risk for NK cell killing, as no inhibitory mechanism is in place. This system works to differentiate between host and virally infected or tumor cells, as host cells typically express MHC class I ligands that will suppress the NK cell "killing" response. Target cells can also express activating ligands such as MICA (MHC class 1 chain-related protein A), that will bind to NK cell–activating receptors and trigger the release of cytokines.[55]

Along with having the ability to induce apoptosis in tumor and virally infected cells, NK cells can also help enhance other immune responses. For example, NK cells found in lymphoid tissue can secrete cytokines that enhance the T-cell killing response. NK cells can also help initiate the inflammatory response in damaged tissue and further recruit other immune cells to the site of inflammation. Most notably, NK cells can exhibit significant variation in the types of inhibitory and activating receptors they express, leading to the ability to interact with a wide variety of ligands, and therefore increasing the range of stimuli to which they can respond.

ROLE OF NATURAL KILLER CELLS IN DISEASES

When it comes to the role of NK cells in various diseases, current research has shown conflicting results, as NK cells have been found to have both disease-controlling and disease-promoting effects. Whether attempting to control or promote a disease, NK cells in both the circulating blood and in various tissues have been shown to be significantly altered. For example, in patients with rheumatoid arthritis, researchers have found a decrease in the number of NK cells circulating in the bloodstream, as well as a suppression of their cytotoxic capability.[56] In contrast, there have been observed increases in the number of NK cells found in the synovial fluid for those with rheumatoid arthritis, and therefore researchers have labelled NK cells as having a disease-promoting role in this autoimmune disease. Similarly, in patients just recently diagnosed with Type I diabetes, NK cells have been found to be at abnormally high concentrations around the pancreatic islets, and are therefore believed to play a role in the destruction of beta cells prior to the time of diagnosis.[57]

Although NK cells appear to have disease-promoting roles in a multitude of diseases, they have nonetheless demonstrated proven disease-controlling capabilities. For example, in patients with asthma there is evidence that NK cells in circulating blood show increased cytotoxic activity and migrate to the lungs, and various lymphoid organs, to help combat the disease. Likewise, in systemic lupus erythematosus (SLE), another autoimmune disease, NK cells show a reduction in number and function. This is in an attempt to reduce an inflammatory response, and therefore NK cells appear to have a disease-controlling role in patients with SLE.[58] Although most research is focused on using adoptive NK cell therapy to treat various types of cancer, other forms of NKcell–derived immunotherapy are also being explored to treat diseases such as rheumatoid arthritis and diabetes, where NK cells are known to play a disease-enhancing role.

Natural Killer Cell–Derived Cancer Immunotherapy

Natural killer cells are known for their ability to recognize and destroy tumor cells in the body without any priming. Typically, tumor cells present a downregulation of the MHC class I ligands to avoid detection by T cells. Downregulation of the expression of these ligands results in tumor cells that no longer express the ligands that will bind to NK cell inhibitory receptors, thereby leaving the NK cell in a more active state and ready to release cytokines to either lyse or induce apoptosis in the tumor cells. Some tumor cells do not exhibit a downregulation of MHC class I ligands, and therefore can inhibit NK cell "killing," as the NK cells now recognize these tumor cells as "self." Patients with various types of cancer not only present with tumor cells that do not show downregulation of MHC class I ligands, but are also known to have a decrease in the number of NK cells circulating in the blood, as well as having NK cells with low activity.[59] Therefore, NK cells have become a focal point of cancer immunotherapy research, in hopes to increase their numbers, cytotoxic capabilities, and response to tumor cells that do express MHC class I ligands,[60,61]

Specifically, researchers are exploring the potential of adoptive NK cell therapy to treat various forms of cancer such as renal cell carcinoma, metastatic breast cancer, and malignant glioma. Adoptive NK cell therapy involves patients receiving NK cells either from sources within themselves or from a healthy donor. NK cells can be derived from bone marrow, umbilical cord blood, circulating blood, or embryonic stem cells. NK cells that are retrieved from these sources can be stimulated in vitro using IL-2 and IL-15 to expand them to greater numbers and increase their survivability once they are transplanted into a recipient.[62]

Using adoptive NK cell therapy in conjunction with anticancer drug treatments is currently a focus of cancer immunotherapy research (**Table 23.3**). The primary mechanism for how this form of NK cell-derived immunotherapy works first involves retrieving NK cells from a donor or from sources within the recipients themselves. Once retrieved, these NK cells are stimulated in vitro to increase their activity, and then later expanded to greater numbers before transplantation. After transplantation, the recipient is then treated with anticancer drugs that will increase expression of activating ligands on the surface of tumor cells, as tumor cells can also downregulate their activating ligands to avoid NK cell "killing." Once the tumor cells are stimulated by the anticancer drugs to increase their expression of activating ligands, they can bind NK cell–activating receptors when they encounter these innate immune cells that can initiate the release of cytokines that will eventually lyse or induce apoptosis in the tumor cells (Figure 23.3). Researchers have discovered a wide array of anticancer drugs that can increase the expression of activating ligands on the surface of tumor cells (some of which are listed in **Table 23.4** as well as many activating ligands that they can target for increased expression.[63] Therefore, using adoptive NK cell therapy in conjunction with anticancer drug treatments is a promising therapeutic approach to treatment of a wide array of cancers.

VACCINATION: PROTECTING THE WORLD, ONE PERSON AT A TIME

ADENOVIRUS

There are more than 50 distinct adenoviruses that cause infections in individuals. Adenoviruses typically cause various respiratory illnesses including, but not limited to, common cold, croup, and even pneumonia. Depending on the type of adenovirus, some have even been known to cause more severe illnesses such as gastroenteritis and cystitis.[64] Individuals with immunodeficiency are most at risk for developing these severe illnesses, and therefore special precaution should be taken. Adenovirus infections are spread from one individual to another typically through the air, by coughing

TABLE 23.3 Types of Anticancer Drugs That Can Induce Expression of NK-Activating Ligands

Antitumor Drug Type	Function	Drug Name
Antimetabolic agents	Interfere with activities involved in cell growth and replication	5-Fluorouracil (induces Fas) Gemcitabine (induces NKG2D) Cytarabine (induces ULBP2)
Plant alkaloids	Exhibit anticancer activity and have a range of effects on NK cells	Docetaxel (induces ULBPs and MICA) Vincristine (induces DNAM1-activating ligands) Docetaxel (induces ULBPs and MICA)
Antitumor antibiotics	Inhibit DNA replication and synthesis	Epirubicin (induces MICA) Radicicol (induces MICA and MICB) 17-Allylamino geldanamycin (induces MICA and MICB)
Alkylating agents	Attach an alkyl group to a guanine base in rapidly dividing cells, leading to damage of DNA and eventually to cell death	Cisplatin (induces expression of Fas) Oxaliplatin (induces MICA, MICB, and ULBP1) Melphalan (induces MICA)

DNAM1, DNAX accessory molecule 1; MICA, MHC class I polypeptide–related sequence A; MHC class I polypeptide–related sequence B; NK, natural killer; NKG2D, natural killer group 2D; ULBP, UL16-binding protein.

TABLE 23.4 Activating Ligands and Activating Receptors on Surface of NK Cells

Activating Ligands	Activating Receptors on NK Cells
MICA/MICB/ULBPs	NKG2D
PVR/Nectin2	DNAM1
TRAIL-R2	TRAIL
Fas	Fas-L

DNAM1, DNAX accessory molecule 1; MHC class I polypeptide–related sequence B; MICA, MHC class I polypeptide–related sequence A; NK, natural killer; NKG2D, natural killer group 2D; PVR, poliovirus receptor; TRAIL-R2, TNF-related apoptosis-inducing ligand receptor 2; ULBP, UL16-binding protein.

or sneezing, and through close personal contact. Due to the high transmissibility of the virus and severe outcomes from the infection, it is crucial to vaccinate approved personnel with the adenovirus vaccine.

In the United States, there is no adenovirus vaccine currently available for the general public. However, there is a vaccine that has been developed and approved for military personnel which provides protection against adenovirus types 4 and 7. While the original adenovirus vaccine was issued to military personnel from 1971 to 1999, a new live oral vaccine was approved in March 2011 for military personnel aged 17 to 50 years who are deemed at a higher risk for infection. This newly approved vaccination is currently administered orally in the form of two tablets to be taken simultaneously. The vaccine has demonstrated to be helpful in preventing the many illnesses that are caused by adenoviruses types 4 and 7 and is therefore critical for military personnel.[65]

The adenovirus vaccine works by inducing both a cell-mediated and antibody-mediated immune response. Essentially, the vaccine introduces a live, attenuated adenovirus to the immune system, which eventually allows for the activation of both T cells and B cells.[65] By stimulating both branches of the adaptive immune system, the vaccine is ultimately able to induce a long-lasting and highly effective immune response to adenovirus types 4 and 7.

HUMAN PAPILLOMAVIRUS

There are many types of human papillomaviruses (HPVs), with more than 30 distinct types infecting the genital tract alone. Teens and young adults are among the most likely to contract HPV, with transmission typically occurring via skin-to-skin contact. Those partaking in sexual intercourse specifically are considered at a higher risk of transmission. Unfortunately, infection with HPV can lead to the development of serious diseases such as cervical, vaginal, penile, and anal cancer.[66] Cutaneous types of HPV can even target the skin in areas such as the hands and feet, while mucosal types of the virus can infect the mucosal linings of the mouth, throat, and respiratory tract. Infection with HPV can lead to severe consequences; therefore, it is crucial for clinicians to provide patient education and follow HPV vaccination recommendations from the Centers for Disease Control and Prevention (CDC).

Gardasil-9 is an HPV vaccine approved for administration to the general public. The vaccine protects against nine different HPV strains, including types 6, 11, 16, 18, 31, 33, 45, 52, and 58. HPV types 6 and 11 cause primarily genital warts, while types 16 and 18 are associated mostly with cervical cancers. The vaccine is recommended for individuals between the ages of 11 and 12 years to protect against the various forms of cancer that are induced by HPV. Children who receive the vaccine at ages 11 or 12 are recommended to receive two doses of the vaccine, 6 to 12 months apart. Those who receive the first dose on or after their 15th birthday will need a total of three doses administered over 6 months. Gardasil® is a quadrivalent recombinant vaccine that includes types 6, 11, 16, and 18. Meanwhile, Cervarix™ is a bivalent recombinant vaccine that includes only types 16 and 18. These vaccines are prepared using purified virus-like particles.

Vaccines containing viral particles work by inducing an antibody-mediated immune response.[67] The viral particles, derived from the HPV, are antigens that B cells can recognize. Once the B cells bind these viral particles, they will become activated and continue with proliferating, differentiating, and completing maturation.

MEASLES

Infection with the measles virus, a paramyxovirus that is a member of the genus *Morbillivirus*, can lead to the development of measles. The measles virus enters the upper respiratory tract of an individual and goes on to infect the epithelium lining of the respiratory tract or the immune cells themselves.[68] Contracting the measles virus is particularly dangerous for young children, as they can develop pneumonia, brain damage, and deafness. In severe cases, measles can even cause encephalitis and death in children. Measles is spread primarily from person to person by coughing, sneezing, or even simply breathing on another individual. Therefore, the CDC recommends routine vaccination for the general public, specifically to prevent contracting the measles virus. The MMR vaccine protects against measles, mumps, and rubella.

MUMPS

Mumps, a disease caused by infection with an RNA virus, is a member of the genus *Rubulavirus*, within the family Paramyxoviridae. Mumps is a highly infectious disease in which the virus infects human peripheral leukocytes.[69] Mumps can easily be spread from person to person by one individual coughing or sneezing on another individual. Unfortunately, there is no current treatment for mumps, which is of great concern, considering mumps can lead to the development of many long-term health problems, including meningitis, deafness, mastitis in females, orchitis in males, and encephalitis. The most common symptoms of mumps though include fever, headache, tiredness, loss of appetite, and swollen glands near the ears and jaw. Due to the adverse consequences of contracting mumps, the CDC recommends routine vaccination, beginning in childhood.

RUBELLA

Rubella is a disease caused by the rubella virus and has been termed the "German measles." Contracting the rubella virus typically results in mild infection, where patients commonly present with a fever and rash. Contracting the rubella virus while pregnant can have significant consequences, as rubella can lead to miscarriage, early death of the child, or significant birth defects. Common symptoms of a rubella viral infection include a rash that starts on an individual's face and spreads to the rest of the body, a cough, runny nose, aching joints, and swollen glands. Rubella virus is spread from one person to another through respiratory secretions, often from one person coughing or sneezing on another.[70] Because of the dangers for pregnant women, and its easy transmission, the CDC highly recommends routine vaccination against the rubella virus.

MMR and MMRV are the two vaccines currently approved for protection against the measles, mumps, and rubella viruses. Both vaccines contain live, attenuated measles, mumps, and rubella viruses; MMRV contains a live, attenuated varicella-zoster virus as well. The CDC recommends children receive their first dose of either vaccine between 12 and 15 months old, while the second dose should be received between the ages of 4 and 6 years old.[71] Both vaccines are administered subcutaneously, the site of injection for children being the anterolateral side of the thigh, while for adults the vaccine is administered via the triceps muscles on the posterior side of the arm. Both vaccines have been shown to be highly effective in the prevention of measles, mumps, and rubella, with one dose of MMR being 93% effective in preventing measles, 78% effective in preventing mumps, and 97% effective in preventing rubella.[71]

The MMR and MMRV vaccines induce both a cell-mediated and antibody-mediated immune response. Because the vaccines introduce live, attenuated measles, mumps, and rubella viruses (as well as live attenuated varicella-zoster virus in the case of MMRV) to the immune system, immune cells will recognize antigens presented by these attenuated viruses and mount a response accordingly. T cells will become activated by antigen-presenting cells which have phagocytosed the attenuated viruses and are presenting pieces of the original antigens on their cells' surfaces.[72]

INFLUENZA

Influenza, more commonly known as "the flu," is an infection caused by the influenza virus. Influenza virus can infect the mucosa of the nose, throat, and lungs, and is easily spread from one individual to another. Symptoms of influenza include a fever, chills, runny or stuffy nose, tiredness, body aches, vomiting, and diarrhea. More severe complications of influenza can include the development of pneumonia, dehydration, and even the worsening of previously diagnosed medical conditions. The primary types of influenza viruses are types A and B. They differ based on the antigens present on cell surfaces. The transmission of influenza virus is often by talking, coughing, or sneezing, and therefore transferring droplets containing the virus to the mouths and/or noses of others.

The CDC recommends that individuals over 6 months of age receive a flu vaccine annually, prior to the start of flu season.[73] The vaccine is ultimately designed to protect people from three to four different strains of influenza virus that researchers have deemed to be the most common for that season. There are ultimately two overarching categories of flu vaccines available to the general public: trivalent and quadrivalent flu vaccines. Essentially, they differ by the number of strains against which they protect. The trivalent vaccines offer protection against three different strains (i.e., two influenza type A and one type B), and the quadrivalent provides protection against four strains (i.e., two influenza type A, and two type B). Because the composition of the vaccines varies from flu season to season, their effectiveness can vary and are dependent upon the accuracy of the predictions made as to which strains of influenza will likely be the most common of that flu season.

One of the formulations of the flu vaccines contains a live attenuated influenza virus, given as a nasal spray (FluMist Quadrivalent). The other injectable formulations of flu vaccine are acellular vaccines either egg-based or cell culture–based, which may be given intramuscularly (IM). The available formulations of influenza vaccines may be different each year in the United States. Examples of available influenza vaccines for the 2019 to 2020 flu season are shown in the summary table from the Advisory Committee on Immunization Practices (ACIP; **Table 23.5**). These vaccines ultimately will induce a cell-mediated response. The antigen of the virus first activates the innate immune system and is phagocytosed by dendritic and macrophage cells. These antigen-presenting cells will digest and present pieces of the original antigens on their own cell surfaces. T cells with the given receptors bind to these antigens and become activated,[72] thus providing immunity to the pathogens.

VARICELLA

Varicella is an infectious disease more commonly known as "chickenpox" and is caused by the varicella-zoster virus. A primary infection with the virus causes varicella, but after the initial infection, the virus may lay dormant in the dorsal root ganglia and reemerge at a later time causing a second infection, herpes zoster, or more commonly known as "shingles." Varicella-zoster virus is spread by exposure to an individual who is presenting with a varicella

or herpes zoster rash. The transmission may result from inhaling aerosols or direct contact of fluid from skin lesions on an infected individual. After infection, the incubation period for varicella can range from 10 to 21 days, while symptoms typically last from 4 to 7 days. In severe infection, it may lead to superimposed bacterial infections of the skin in children, and pneumonia in adults.[74] Due to these serious complications and the rapid transmission of the virus, vaccination is recommended for children and adults.

There are currently two approved varicella vaccines available to the general public in the United States, Varivax® and ProQuad® (which is also known as the "MMRV vaccine").[75] Both vaccines contain a live, attenuated varicella-zoster virus that is ultimately used to stimulate the immune system and induce long-term protection from the varicella-zoster virus. They induce both an antibody-mediated and cell-mediated immune response where both B cells and T cells will be able to recognize antigens presented by the virus and mount an immune response.

The CDC recommends individuals receive two doses of varicella vaccine, with the first dose delivered between 12 and 15 months of age, and the second dose delivered between 4 to 6 years of age.[76] Both vaccines have proved to be highly effective in protecting individuals from contracting the varicella-zoster virus, with one dose being 85% effective, and two doses being 98% effective in preventing infection.[77] The two approved varicella vaccines, with their high levels of effectiveness, have ultimately been instrumental in decreasing the amount of varicella and herpes-zoster cases seen in the United States each year. In the adult population, Zostavax® is the recommended vaccine to prevent herpes-zoster. The FDA has approved Zostavax for individuals at age 50 or older; however, according to the CDC recommendations, one dose of the vaccine is recommended for individuals aged 60 or older regardless of previous history with or without chickenpox (see CDC immunization schedule: www.cdc.gov/vaccines).

ROTAVIRUS

Rotavirus disease occurs in children especially under the age of 1 year. It is characterized by vomiting and watery diarrhea, which may be severe, for 3 to 8 days. It is also accompanied by fever and abdominal pain. Patients may also present with loss of appetite and dehydration. It is transmitted by the oral fecal route. In adults, the infection is self-limiting.

There are two available vaccines that are given within the first year of life. The vaccines provide 85% to 98% protection against severe rotavirus illness and against hospitalization from rotavirus illness. The RotaTeq® (RV5) is given in three doses at ages 2, 4, and 6

TABLE 23.5 Influenza Vaccines (United States, 2019–2020 Influenza Season)

Trade Name (Manufacturer)	Presentation	Age Indication	HA (IIVs and RIV4) or Virus Count (LAIV4) for Each Vaccine Virus (per Dose)	Route	Mercury (From Thimerosal; mcg/0.5 mL)
IIV4—Standard Dose—Egg-Based†					
Afluria® Quadrivalent (Seqirus)	0.25-mL PFS*	6–35 months	7.5 mcg/0.25 mL* 15 mcg/0.5 mL*	IM**	—
	0.5-mL PFS*	≥3 years			—
	5.0-mL MDV*	≥6 months (needle/syringe)18–64 years (jet injector)			24.5
Fluarix® Quadrivalent (GlaxoSmithKline)	0.5-mL PFS	≥6 months	15 mcg/0.5 mL	IM**	—
FluLaval® Quadrivalent (GlaxoSmithKline)	0.5-mL PFS	≥6 months	15 mcg/0.5 mL	IM**	—
	5.0-mL MDV	≥6 months			<25
Fluzone® Quadrivalent (Sanofi Pasteur)	0.25-mL PFS***	6–35 months	7.5 mcg/0.25 mL*** 15 mcg/0.5 mL***	IM**	—
	0.5-mL PFS***	≥6 months			—
	0.5-mL SDV***	≥6 months			—
	5.0-mL MDV***	≥6 months			25
IIV4—Standard Dose—Cell Culture–Based (ccIIV4)					
Flucelvax® Quadrivalent (Seqirus)	0.5-mL PFS	≥4 years	15 mcg/0.5 mL	IM**	—
	5.0-mL MDV	≥4 years			25
IIV3—High Dose—Egg-Based** (HD-IIV3)**					
Fluzone® High-Dose (Sanofi Pasteur)	0.5-mL PFS	≥65 years	60 mcg/0.5 mL	IM**	—
IIV3—Standard Dose—Egg-Based** With MF59 Adjuvant (aIIV3)**					
Fluad® (Seqirus)	0.5-mL PFS	≥65 years	15 mcg/0.5 mL	IM**	—
RIV4—Recombinant HA					
Flublok® Quadrivalent (Sanofi Pasteur)	0.5-mL PFS	≥18 years	45 mcg/0.5 mL	IM**	—
LAIV4—Egg-Based** **					
FluMist® Quadrivalent (AstraZeneca)	0.2-mL prefilled single-use intranasal sprayer	2–49 years	$10^{6.5–7.5}$ fluorescent focus units/0.2 mL	NAS	—

(continued)

TABLE 23.5 Influenza Vaccines (United States, 2019–2020 Influenza Season) (*continued*)

*The dose volume for Afluria Quadrivalent is 0.25 mL for children aged 6 to 35 months and 0.5 mL for persons aged ≥3 years.

**IM administered influenza vaccines should be given by needle and syringe only, with the exception of the MDV presentation of Afluria Quadrivalent, which may alternatively be given by the PharmaJet Stratis jet injector for persons aged 18 to 64 years only. For adults and older children, the recommended site for IM influenza vaccination is the deltoid muscle. The preferred site for infants and young children is the anterolateral aspect of the thigh. Additional guidance regarding site selection and needle length for IM administration is available in the ACIP General Best Practice Guidelines for Immunization (https://www.cdc.gov/vaccines/hcp/acip-recs/general-recs/downloads/general-recs.pdf).

***Fluzone Quadrivalent may be given to children aged 6 to 35 months as either 0.25 or 0.5 mL/dose. No preference is expressed for one or the other dose volume for this age group. Persons aged ≥3 years should receive the 0.5 mL/dose volume.

****Persons with a history of egg allergy may receive any licensed, recommended influenza vaccine that is otherwise appropriate for their age and health status. Those who report having had reactions to egg-involving symptoms other than urticaria (e.g., angioedema or swelling, respiratory distress, lightheadedness, or recurrent emesis) or who required epinephrine or another emergency medical intervention should be vaccinated in an inpatient or outpatient medical setting (including, but not limited to, hospitals, clinics, health departments, and physician offices). Vaccine administration should be supervised by a healthcare clinician who is able to recognize and manage severe allergic reactions.

ACIP, Advisory Committee on Immunization Practices; FDA, Food and Drug Administration; HA, hemagglutinin; IIV3, inactivated influenza vaccine, trivalent; IIV4, inactivated influenza vaccine, quadrivalent; IM, intramuscular; LAIV4, live attenuated influenza vaccine, quadrivalent; MDV, multidose vial; NAS, intranasal; PFS, prefilled syringe; RIV4, recombinant influenza vaccine, quadrivalent; SDV, single-dose vial.

Note: Clinicians should consult FDA-approved prescribing information for 2019 to 2020 influenza vaccines for the most complete and updated information, including (but not limited to) indications, contraindications, warnings, and precautions. Package inserts for U.S.-licensed vaccines are available at https://www.fda.gov/vaccines-blood-biologics/approved-products/vaccines-licensed-use-united-states. Availability of specific products and presentations might change and differ from what is described in this table and in the text of this report.

Source: From Centers for Disease Control and Prevention. Prevention and control of seasonal influenza with vaccines: Recommendations of the Advisory Committee on Immunization Practices—United States, 2019–20 influenza season (Table 2). U.S. Department of Health & Human Services; 2019. https://www.cdc.gov/mmwr/volumes/68/rr/rr6803a1.htm#T2_down

months, while Rotarix® (RV1) is given in two doses at ages 2 and 4 months.[78]

Rotarix is a live, attenuated rotavirus vaccine derived from the human 89-12 strain type. Rotarix replicates in the small intestine and induces immunity. The exact immunologic mechanism by which Rotarix protects against rotavirus gastroenteritis is unknown.

CHOLERA

While rare in the United States, there have been an increasing number of cholera cases seen around the world, mostly in Africa and Haiti. Cholera is ultimately an acute illness caused by the bacterium *Vibrio cholerae*, which infects the gastrointestinal tract and releases cholera toxin. Cholera is often contracted by ingesting contaminated food or water, often in areas with poor water sanitation systems. The infection is typically mild and can even be asymptomatic, but one in 10 people can develop severe cholera. A severe infection typically involves watery diarrhea (a consequence of cholera toxin release), vomiting, low blood pressure (due to the loss of fluids), thirst, and muscle cramps. If a severe infection is left untreated, patients can develop renal failure, electrolyte imbalance, and severe dehydration, which could even lead to shock and death.

Vaxchora® is the live oral cholera vaccine recommended by the CDC for adults 18 to 64 years old, who are traveling to an area with active cholera transmission.[79] An area with active cholera transmission is defined by the CDC as a "province, state, or other ad-

ministrative subdivision within a country where cholera infections may be reported regularly . . . or where cholera outbreak is occurring . . . and includes areas with cholera activity within the past year."[79] The vaccine is administered as a single oral dose, often in a suspension, to travelers prior to departure. The CDC reports that Vaxchora reduced the chance of people having severe diarrhea after infection by 90%, just 10 days after receiving the vaccination.[79] Unfortunately, Vaxchora does not provide protection from infection by *V. cholerae* serotype O139, the most common serotype seen in Southeast Asia; therefore travelers to these areas must take special precaution.[75]

The exact mechanism by which Vaxchora stimulates the immune system is not known, but researchers have hypothesized that the vaccine induces an antibody-mediated immune response.[80] Vaxchora contains live attenuated *V. cholerae* that will replicate in the gastrointestinal tract and release a nontoxic type of cholera toxin (PaxVax Connect).

DIPHTHERIA

Diphtheria is an acute, toxin-mediated disease caused by the bacterium *Corynebacterium diphtheria*. *C. diphtheria* can secrete toxins that inhibit protein synthesis in the cells that compose the infected area, cause tissue damage, and form pseudomembranes. The toxin secreted by *C. diphtheria* can even lead to severe complications that result from infection, including myocarditis, neuritis, and low platelet counts. Diphtheria is often transmitted via respiratory droplets, specifically spread by coughing or sneezing, and therefore can be easily transmitted. There are four available types of vaccines that may be used to prevent diphtheria, which are in combination with other vaccines:

1. Diphtheria plus tetanus (DT)
2. Diphtheria, tetanus, and pertussis (DTaP)
3. Tetanus plus diphtheria (Td)
4. Tetanus, diphtheria, and pertussis (Tdap)

PERTUSSIS

Pertussis is an acute disease caused by the bacterium *Bordetella pertussis*, seen primarily in children. Pertussis, more commonly known as "whooping cough," is a toxin-mediated disease similar to diphtheria and tetanus. *B. pertussis* attaches itself to the cilia of the respiratory epithelial cells and produces a toxin that ultimately paralyzes the cilia. Paralyzing the cilia can cause inflammation in the respiratory tract and disrupt the secretion of mucus. Transmission of pertussis is typically mediated by respiratory droplets, and causes symptoms to present primarily in three distinct stages. The first stage or catarrhal stage involves patients having a runny nose, low-grade fever, and mild cough. The second stage or paroxysmal stage is often the most severe and involves many outbursts of coughing that have the characteristic "whooping" sound. The coughing outbursts typically take place primarily at night, with the average patient having 15 attacks per day. The convalescent stage is the recovery stage which often takes 2 to 3 weeks for symptoms to fully disappear. Long-term complications that can result from having pertussis include difficulty sleeping, dehydration, neurological complications, and pneumonia, therefore making it imperative that individuals receive the recommended routine vaccinations.

TETANUS

Tetanus is an acute disease caused by the bacterium *Clostridium tetani*, which is often fatal. *C. tetani* produces two types of toxins, tetanolysin and tetanospasmin, which are a neurotoxin and cause the characteristic symptoms of a tetanus infection. Tetanus has been deemed to have three clinical forms: common, cephalic, and generalized. Generalized tetanus is the most common form of the disease and produces symptoms such as lockjaw, stiffness of the neck, and dysphagia. *C. tetani* typically enters the body through an open wound, in a low-oxygen environment, and often goes on to produce spores that survive in the body, germinate, and produce the two toxins. Tetanus can ultimately take months from infection to recovery and can even lead to long-term complications such as hy-

pertension, abnormal heart rhythms, and pulmonary embolisms. Therefore, it is imperative for individuals to receive routine vaccination against *C. tetani*.

The available vaccines to prevent diphtheria, tetanus, and pertussis infections may be separated into two groups. The first group is offered to pediatric patients and includes DTaP and DT. The CDC recommends infants and children receive five total doses of DTaP or DT, with the first dose occurring at 2 months old, again at 4 and 6 months old, while the last two doses should be administered from 15 to 18 months old, and lastly between 4 and 6 years old. The second group is offered to adults and adolescents, which includes Tdap and Td.[81] The CDC also recommends that individuals between the ages of 11 and 12 years old receive a dose of Tdap or Td, as a form of booster immunization, and should continue to do so every 10 years.[81] The DTaP and Tdap vaccines contain diphtheria and tetanus toxoids, as well as pertussis toxins, and the DT and Td vaccines contain only diphtheria and tetanus toxoids; however, all four vaccines still essentially induce an antibody-mediated immune response. Both groups of vaccines have been demonstrated to be highly effective in preventing the contraction of these three infectious diseases, with DTaP being 98% effective in protecting children within 1 year of their last dose. Tdap has also been shown to be 71% effective in protecting children from contracting these diseases within 5 years of receiving the last dose.[81]

MENINGOCOCCAL MENINGITIS

Meningococcal meningitis is a disease caused by the bacterium *Neisseria meningitides* that often affects infants, adolescents, and young adults. Individuals with medical conditions such as those that have had a splenectomy or are infected with human immunodeficiency virus (HIV), are at an even greater risk for contracting meningococcal disease. One in 10 people is a carrier of *N. meningitides*, present in the nasal cavity or pharynx, and does not lead to the development of meningococcal disease. If the bacterium does migrate and invade areas in the body that normally do not contain *N. meningitides*, one can develop meningococcal disease. In the disease case, *N. meningitides* invades primarily two distinct places in the body, the first being the meninges, which are membranous layers covering the brain and spinal cord. This form of meningococcal disease is termed "meningitis," and patients suffering from meningitis typically present with a fever, headache, stiff neck, vomiting, and even an altered mental status. The second type of meningococcal disease is termed "septicemia" and is an infection in the bloodstream that can cause patients to present with fever, chills, muscle and joint aches, and vomiting and diarrhea.[82] Both types of meningococcal diseases can be extremely dangerous diseases, making vaccination even more crucial.

There are currently four meningococcal vaccines available in the United States, which may be classified into two types: the meningococcal conjugate or MenACWY vaccines (e.g., Menactra® and Menveo®), and the serogroup B meningococcal or MenB vaccines (e.g., Bexsero® and Trumenba®). These vaccines provide protection from the five most common serotypes known to infect individuals today, which include serotypes A, B, C, W, and Y. The two recombinant vaccines, Trumenba and Bexsero, are monovalent vaccines that specifically provide protection against serotype B. Meanwhile, the two other conjugate vaccines, Menactra and Menveo, provide protection against serotypes A, C, W, and Y, making them quadrivalent vaccines. They are considered conjugate vaccines because they contain a protein that has been joined to an antigen and can go on to stimulate the immune system.[75] All four meningococcal vaccines ultimately induce an antibody-mediated immune response as their mechanism of action in providing immunity. The CDC recommends all 11- and 12-year-old children receive one of two conjugate vaccines with a booster recommended at age 16. Those between the ages of 16 and 18 are also recommended to receive one of two recombinant vaccines, to acquire protection from serotype B, as individuals within this age group have increased risk for contracting serotype B.[83]

POLIOMYELITIS

Poliomyelitis is a potentially life-threatening disease caused by the poliovirus. The poliovirus spreads from person to person by route of fecal–oral transmission, due to the contamination of food or water with fecal matter. Poliomyelitis is considered to be eradicated in the United States since 1979, due primarily to the effective vaccination programs of the inactivated polio vaccine (IPV). Nonetheless, the threat still exists in some countries.[84] IPOL® is the only current polio vaccine product offered in the United States since 2000; it is administered by intramuscular or subcutaneous injection. The vaccine protects against three types of poliovirus: type 1 (Mahoney), type 2 (MEF-1), and type 3 (Saukett).[85]

There are several products containing IPV together with other vaccines—for example, with the DTaP vaccine (Quadracel® and Kinrix®); with DTaP and *Haemophilus influenzae* type B (Pentacel®); and with DTaP, and hepatitis B vaccine (Pediarix®).[84]

The CDC currently recommends that children receive four doses of polio vaccine at 2 months, 4 months, and 6 to 18 months, and lastly at 4 to 6 years old. Adults deemed at a higher risk for infection, such as healthcare workers, laboratory workers, and those traveling internationally, should also receive one to three doses of inactivated polio vaccine.[86]

TYPHOID FEVER

Typhoid fever is characterized by a chronic fever that is caused by contracting the salmonella serotype typhi bacteria. Most U.S. citizens contract typhoid fever while traveling to other countries where typhoid fever is common. Therefore, the CDC recommends that individuals traveling to areas where typhoid fever is endemic should be vaccinated at least 1 to 2 weeks before traveling.[87] There are currently two types of typhoid fever vaccines available to the public in the United States, Vivotif® and Typhim Vi®.

Vivotif is delivered orally by capsule, and contains live attenuated *Salmonella serotype Typhi*. It can be administered to adults or children 6 years or older. The regimen consists of four capsules to be taken one capsule every other day 1 hour before meal with cold or lukewarm water. The last dose should be completed at least 1 week prior to potential exposure to the bacteria.[88] Typhim Vi is a polysaccharide conjugate vaccine that is injected intramuscularly. It may be given to individuals at age 2 years or older. The dose should be administered at least 2 weeks prior to traveling. The CDC currently recommends that individuals receive either four doses of the Vivotif vaccine or one dose or the Typhim Vi vaccine prior to their travels abroad.[89]

YELLOW FEVER

Yellow fever is caused by the yellow fever virus, an RNA virus that is a member of the genus *Flavivirus*. Yellow fever virus is transmitted to humans primarily through *Aedes* or *Haemagogus* species mosquitoes that have been infected by the virus after feeding on infected primates. The CDC recommends that individuals who are 9 months and older and traveling to areas where there is an increased risk for contracting yellow fever virus, such as South America and Africa, receive the yellow fever vaccine prior to traveling. The yellow fever vaccine is a live attenuated viral vaccine called "YF-Vax" and was made available again in the United States in 2019. Because there are several adverse effects to receiving the yellow fever vaccine, CDC recommends individuals be vaccinated only if they are traveling to an area where they are at an increased risk for exposure or to a country that requires proof of vaccination upon entry into the country.[90]

HAEMOPHILUS INFLUENZAE TYPE B

Haemophilus influenzae type b (Hib) is a serious illness caused by the *H. influenzae* bacteria. *H. influenzae* type b vaccines, which help to prevent Hib disease, include three different polysaccharide monovalent conjugate vaccines (ActHIB®, PedvaxHIB®, and Hiberix) and a fourth vaccine (Pentacel), where the Hib vaccine in combined with the DTaP vaccine and inactivated polio vaccine. The CDC recommends that all children under 2 years of age receive a Hib vaccine. The CDC recommends that four doses of Pentacel be given intramuscularly in a series beginning at 6 weeks old and concluding at 4 years of age. Three doses of ActHIB or Hiberix® are recommended to be given between 2 and 6 months of age, while two doses of PedvaxHIB are recommended to be given to children between 2 and 4 months of age.[91]

LYME DISEASE

Lyme disease, transmitted most commonly by ticks, is caused by the contraction of the *Borrelia burgdorferia* bacterium, and is characterized by the symptoms of fever, fatigue, headache, and a skin rash called "erythema migrans." Untreated patients with Lyme disease run the risk of the infection spreading to the heart and nervous system. In the United States, a Lyme disease vaccine is no longer offered to the general public; the vaccine manufacturer discontinued the production of the vaccine in 2002 after experiencing low demand for the vaccine. The CDC noted that protection offered from the vaccine diminishes over time, and therefore individuals immunized prior to 2002 are most likely no longer protected against Lyme disease.[92] Therefore, CDC also recommends taking preventative measures to reduce the risk of contracting Lyme disease, such as regularly examining clothing and pets for ticks.[93]

JAPANESE ENCEPHALITIS

Japanese encephalitis (JE) is an infectious disease caused by the JE virus, a *flavivirus* transmitted by mosquitoes that is the primary cause of encephalitis throughout Asia. JE is a serious life-threatening disease that has a fatality rate of 20% to 30%, and in 30% to 50% of survivors causes neurologic and psychiatric problems. According to the CDC, the risk of contracting JE by those traveling to Asia is very low, but risks could increase based on the exact destination, the season, and activities in which the traveler participates. Therefore, as a precaution, the CDC recommends those traveling to Asia receive two doses, 28 days apart, of the JE vaccine, Ixiaro®. This is an inactivated vaccine to be delivered intramuscularly to travelers ages 2 months and up.[75]

PLAGUE

Plague is an infectious disease caused by the bacterium *Yersinia pestis*, that commonly spreads to individuals after being bitten by a rodent flea carrying *Y. pestis*. Because today's antibiotics can effectively treat plague, human plague has become rare in most countries throughout the world. However, there are still cases of human plague infection in parts of the western United States, Africa, and Asia. The CDC ultimately recommends that only individuals considered to be at an increased risk for exposure to *Y. pestis* receive the plague vaccine, such as laboratory or field personnel who work with *Y. pestis*, and workers who are living in areas with epidemic plague (e.g., Peace Corps volunteers). The CDC also recommends these individuals receive a series of three injections of the inactivated plague vaccine intramuscularly, to aide in the prevention of contracting the disease.

RABIES

Rabies is a potentially fatal infectious disease caused by the rabies virus. Rabies can be transmitted to humans if one is scratched or bitten by an animal that has been infected with the rabies virus, most commonly by wild bats, raccoons, and skunks. The rabies virus attacks primarily the central nervous system, and if not treated in time, can spread to the brain and lead to death. There are two types of human rabies vaccines, Imovax Rabies® and RabAvert®, that can be administered before exposure, and most importantly, post-exposure. Both are inactivated vaccines to be delivered intramuscularly to adults and children before a known exposure, as well as after an exposure. Specifically, the CDC recommends that after one is exposed to the Rabies virus, a dose of human rabies immune globulin should be given together with the rabies vaccine on the same day as the exposure occurred. Following the first dose, three more doses of the vaccine should also be given at days 3, 7, and 14 after the initial exposure.[94]

PNEUMOCOCCAL DISEASE

Pneumococcal disease is caused by the gram-positive bacteria *Streptococcus pneumoniae*, which has more than 90 known serotypes. Only a small number of serotypes produce most pneumococcal infections. Anywhere from 5% to 90% of healthy individuals have *S. pneumoniae*, which commonly inhabits the nasopharynx and does not cause disease. When the bacteria migrate to formerly sterile parts of the body, however, disease can result. Transmission can occur via respiratory droplets being spread from an infected individual to another healthy individual. The CDC therefore recommends individuals receive the pneumococcal conjugate vaccine (PCV13 or Prevnar 13®) to receive protection from the 13 serotypes that most commonly cause serious illness. The CDC recommends children receive the PCV13 vaccine as a four-dose series at 2, 4, 6, and 12 to 15 months of age. The CDC also notes that all adults aged 65 years and older with conditions that cause increased risk for pneumococcal disease receive the PCV13. Lastly, the CDC recommends individuals receive a yearly influenza vaccine, as having the flu can increase one's chances for contracting pneumococcal disease.[75]

The vaccines discussed previously, as well as their mechanism of action, are summarized in **Table 23.6.**

TABLE 23.6 Vaccines for Viral and Bacterial Infectious Diseases

Viral Infectious Disease	Virus	Vaccine	Mechanism of Action
Adenovirus	Adenovirus	Adenovirus vaccine	Antibody-mediated and cell-mediated immune responses
HPV	HPV	HPV9 (Gardasil 9)	Antibody-mediated immune response
Measles	Measles virus	MMR, MMRV	Antibody-mediated and cell-mediated immune responses
Mumps	RNA Rubulavirus	MMR, MMRV	Antibody-mediated and cell-mediated immune responses
Rubella	Rubella virus	MMR, MMRV	Antibody-mediated and cell-mediated immune responses
Seasonal influenza	Influenza virus	Trivalent flu vaccine, Quadrivalent flu vaccine	Cell-mediated response
Varicella	Varicella-zoster virus	MMRV, Varivax, ProQuad	Antibody-mediated and cell-mediated immune responses

Bacterial Infectious Disease	Bacterium	Vaccine	Mechanism of Action
Cholera	*Vibrio cholerae*	Vaxchora	Antibody-mediated immune response
Diphtheria	*Corynebacterium diphtheria*	DTaP, DT, Tdap, Td	Antibody-mediated immune response
Pertussis	*Bordetella pertussis*	DTaP, DT, Tdap, Td	Antibody-mediated immune response
Tetanus	*Clostridium tetani*	DTaP, DT, Tdap, Td	Antibody-mediated immune response
Meningococcal	*Neisseria meningitides*	MenACWY (Menactra and Menveo), MenB (Bexsero and Trumenba)	Antibody-mediated immune response

DT, diphtheria; DTaP, diphtheria, tetanus, pertussis; HPV, human papillomavirus; MMR, measles, mumps, rubella; MMRV, measles, mumps, rubella, varicella; Tdap, tetanus, diphtheria, and pertussis.

CASE EXEMPLAR: Patient Requiring Updated Vaccinations

KB is a 65-year-old female presenting in the clinic for an annual review of her medications and recent lab work. All of her labs are normal. She asks about what new treatments or medications she might need. The clinician suggests several immunizations.

Past Medical History
- Breast cancer with mastectomy 10 years ago
- Chemotherapy 10 years ago
- Hypertension managed with medication

Medications
- Lisinopril, 5 mg once daily
- Furosemide, 10 mg once daily
- Ibuprofen for pain

Physical Examination
- Healthy female

Discussion Questions

1. KB says that she has heard about a shot for shingles. She has had shingles before and does not want to get it again. She asks how the vaccine works. How should the clinician respond?
2. KB says that one of her friends told her about the rise in whooping cough, and KB saw an ad on TV about how older people can spread it to their grandchildren. How should the clinician respond?
3. Based on her age, should KB receive any additional immunizations or vaccines?

CASE EXEMPLAR: Newborn Infant Requiring Vaccinations

RG delivered a healthy infant 23 hours ago. This is her first child and she has been very anxious throughout the entire pregnancy. She wants her baby to be safe and immunized. The clinician is scheduled to see RG and report on the baby's status. Following the initial exam, the clinician tells RG her baby requires several immunizations.

Past Medical History
- A healthy baby delivered 23 hours ago
- No respiratory distress
- Resolving acrocyanosis

Medications
- Scheduled immunizations
- Vitamin K

Family History
- Infant is awake and alert; APGARs 9 and 10

Physical Examination
- Infant stable with pulse: 120; respiration rate: 22; temperature: 97.6 °F

Discussion Questions

1. The clinician has completed the infant's initial assessment and is visiting with RG when RG asks what initial immunizations the baby will need. How should the clinician respond?
2. RG returns to see the clinician for a 6-month wellness check. What immunizations are required during this visit?
3. What immunizations should the infant receive by the age of 15 months?

KEY TAKEAWAYS

- The T cell is a lymphocyte of the adaptive immune system. The goal of maturation is to produce T cells that express a variety of receptors that bind only to foreign antigens and help fight disease. Interruptions can occur in the process and the T cell is altered and attacks the body's own cells, leading to autoimmune disorders.
- Helper T cells serve several purposes. They are needed to help activate B cells, macrophages, and cytotoxic T cells to attack and eliminate infected host cells.
- Should the body become infected with the same pathogen again, memory T cells are available to recognize the pathogen, bind to the antigen, and initiate an immune response.
- Cytotoxic T cells are a special type of T cell that can recognize and mount an immune response toward host cells that have been infected by a virus or bacteria. Cytotoxic T cells can also recognize and mount a response to cancer cells.

- Regulatory T cells modify and control the body's overall immune response, as well as maintain the immune system's tolerance to self-antigens that are present on cells throughout the body. Because of their ability to promote tolerance to self-antigens, regulatory T cells can play a role in preventing the development of many autoimmune diseases.
- In healthy individuals, certain regulatory T cells can play a role in preventing the development of allergic diseases.
- Normally developed and properly regulated B cells provide invaluable immune defense.
- The main roles of macrophages are to detect invading pathogens, phagocytose them, and destroy them.
- NK cells play a crucial role in the body's initial response to viral infection and the detection of early signs of cancer.
- Vaccines protect individuals of all ages from a variety of diseases. Because of vaccines, some diseases have been almost eradicated.

REFERENCES

1. O'Garra A, Robinson D. Development and function of T helper 1 cells. *Adv Immunol.* 2004;83:133–162. doi:10.1016/S0065-2776(04)83004-9
2. Parel Y, Aurrand-Lions M, Scheja A, et al. Presence of CD4+CD8+ double-positive T cells with very high interleukin-4 production potential in lesional skin of patients with systemic sclerosis. *Arthritis Rheum.* 2007;56:3459–3467. doi:10.1002/art.22927
3. Parel Y, Chizzolini C. CD4+ CD8+ double positive (DP) T cells in health and disease. *Autoimmun Rev.* 2004;3:215–220. doi:10.1016/j.autrev.2003.09.001
4. Ueno H. T follicular helper cells in human autoimmunity. *Curr Opin Immunol.* 2016;43:24–31. doi:10.1016/j.coi.2016.08.003

5. Zhu Y, Zou L, Liu YC. T follicular helper cells, T follicular regulatory cells and autoimmunity. *Int Immunol.* 2016;28:173–179. doi:10.1093/intimm/dxv079

6. Xu X, Zhang S, Li P, et al. Maturation and emigration of single-positive thymocytes. *Clin Dev Immunol.* 2013;*2013*:282870. doi:10.1155/2013/282870

7. Cohn M. Rationalizing thymic selection for functional T-cells: a commentary. *Cell Immunol.* 2015;298:83–87. doi:10.1016/j.cellimm.2015.09.008

8. Stritesky GL, Jameson SC, Hogquist KA. Selection of self-reactive T cells in the thymus. *Annu Rev Immunol.* 2012;30:95–114. doi:10.1146/annurev-immunol-020711-075035

9. Starr TK, Jameson SC, Hogquist KA. Positive and negative selection of T cells. *Annu Rev Immunol.* 2003;21:139–176. doi:10.1146/annurev.immunol.21.120601.141107

10. Guidos CJ. Positive selection of CD4+ and CD8+ T cells. *Curr Opin Immunol.* 1996;8:225–232. doi:10.1016/S0952-7915(96)80061-6

11. Tao X, Xu A. Basic knowledge of immunology. In: Xu A, ed. *Amphioxus Immunity: Tracing the Origins of Human Immunity.* China Science Publishing & Media / Elsevier; 2016:15–422.

12. Corthay A. A three-cell model for activation of naive T helper cells. *Scand J Immunol.* 2006;64:93–96. doi:10.1111/j.1365-3083.2006.01782.x

13. Burkett PR, Koka R, Chien M, et al. Generation, maintenance, and function of memory T cells. *Adv Immunol.* 2004;83:191–231. doi:10.1016/S0065-2776(04)83006-2

14. Metz DP, Bottomly K. Function and regulation of memory CD4 T cells. *Immunol Res.* 1999;19:127–141. doi:10.1007/BF02786482

15. Janeway CA Jr, Yagi J, Rojo J, et al. Immune recognition and effector function in subsets of CD4 T cells. *Princess Takamatsu Symp.* 1988;19:193–208. PubMed PMID: 2908353.

16. O'Rourke AM, Mescher MF. The roles of CD8 in cytotoxic T lymphocyte function. *Immunol Today.* 1993;14:183–188. doi:10.1016/0167-5699(93)90283-q

17. Sarkar S, Hewison M, Studzinski GP, et al. Role of vitamin D in cytotoxic T lymphocyte immunity to pathogens and cancer. *Crit Rev Clin Lab Sci.* 2016;53:132–145. doi:10.3109/10408363.2015.1094443

18. Melief CJ, Kast WM. Cytotoxic T lymphocyte therapy of cancer and tumor escape mechanisms. *Semin Cancer Biol.* 1991;2:347–354. PubMed PMID: 1773050.

19. Taams LS, Palmer DB, Akbar AN, et al. Regulatory T cells in human disease and their potential for therapeutic manipulation. *Immunology.* 2006;118:1–9. doi:10.1111/j.1365-2567.2006.02348.x

20. Danikowski KM, Jayaraman S, Prabhakar BS. Regulatory T cells in multiple sclerosis and myasthenia gravis. *J Neuroinflammation.* 2017;14:117. doi:10.1186/s12974-017-0892-8

21. Costantino CM, Baecher-Allan C, Hafler DA. Multiple sclerosis and regulatory T cells. *J Clin Immunol.* 2008;28:697–706. doi:10.1007/s10875-008-9236-x

22. Cools N, Ponsaerts P, Van Tendeloo VF, Berneman ZN. Regulatory T cells and human disease. *Clin Dev Immunol.* 2007;*2007*:89195. doi:10.1155/2007/89195

23. Akdis CA, Akdis M. Mechanisms and treatment of allergic disease in the big picture of regulatory T cells. *J Allergy Clin Immunol.* 2009;123:735–746; quiz 747–738. doi:10.1016/j.jaci.2009.02.030

24. Nouri-Aria KT, Durham SR. Regulatory T cells and allergic disease. *Inflamm Allergy Drug Targets.* 2008;7:237–252. doi:10.2174/187152808786848405

25. Xystrakis E, Boswell SE, Hawrylowicz CM. T regulatory cells and the control of allergic disease. *Expert Opin Biol Ther.* 2006;6:121–133. doi:10.1517/14712598.6.2.121

26. Najafi M, Farhood B, Mortezaee K. Contribution of regulatory T cells to cancer: a review. *J Cell Physiol.* 2019;234:7983–7993. doi:10.1002/jcp.27553

27. Zhang D, Chen Z, Wang DC, et al. Regulatory T cells and potential inmmunotherapeutic targets in lung cancer. *Cancer Metastasis Rev.* 2015;34:277–290. doi:10.1007/s10555-015-9566-0

28. Marshall EA, Ng KW, Kung SHY, et al. Emerging roles of T helper 17 and regulatory T cells in lung cancer progression and metastasis. *Mol Cancer.* 2016;15:67. doi:10.1186/s12943-016-0551-1

29. Kandulski A, Malfertheiner P, Wex T. Role of regulatory T-cells in *H. pylori*-induced gastritis and gastric cancer. *Anticancer Res.* 2010;30:1093–1103. http://ar.iiarjournals.org/content/30/4/1093.full.pdf+html.

30. Wennhold K, Thelen M, Schlößer HA, et al. Using antigen-specific B cells to combine antibody and T cell-based cancer immunotherapy. *Cancer Immunol Res.* 2017;5:730–743. doi:10.1158/2326-6066.CIR-16-0236

31. Wennhold K, Shimabukuro-Vornhagen A, Theurich S, et al. CD40-activated B cells as antigen-presenting cells: the final sprint toward clinical application. *Expert Rev Vaccines.* 2013;12:631–637. doi:10.1586/erv.13.39

32. Wiseman AC. Immunosuppressive medications. *Clin J Am Soc Nephrol.* 2016;11:332–343. doi:10.2215/CJN.08570814

33. Okimura K, Maeta K, Kobayashi N, et al. Characterization of ASKP1240, a fully human antibody targeting human CD40 with potent immunosuppressive effects. *Am J Transplant.* 2014;14:1290–1299. doi:10.1111/ajt.12678

34. Maggioni C, Carelli S, Cabibbo A, et al. Assembly and secretion of antibodies during B cell development. *Bratisl Lek Listy.* 1998;99:419–425. PubMed PMID: 9810765.

35. Tlaskalova-Hogenova H, Mandel L, Stěpánková R, et al. Autoimmunity: from physiology to pathology. Natural antibodies, mucosal immunity and development of B cell repertoire. *Folia Biol.* 1992;38:202–215. PubMed PMID: 1426416.

36. Reth M, Wienands J. The maintenance and the activation signal of the B-cell antigen receptor. *Cold Spring Harb Symp Quant Biol.* 1999;64:323–328. doi:10.1101/sqb.1999.64.323

37. Budeus B, de Reynoso SS, Przekopowitz M, et al. Complexity of the human memory B-cell compartment is determined by the versatility of clonal diversification in germinal centers. *Proc Natl Acad Sci USA.* 2015;112:E5281–E5289. doi:10.1073/pnas.1511270112

38. Calame KL, Lin KI, Tunyaplin C. Regulatory mechanisms that determine the development and function of plasma cells. *Annu Rev Immunol.* 2003;21:205–230. doi:10.1146/annurev.immunol.21.120601.141138

39. Frank MM, Joiner K, Hammer C. The function of antibody and complement in the lysis of bacteria. *Rev Infect*

Dis. 1987;9(suppl 5):S537–545. doi:10.1093/clinids/9.supplement_5.s537

40. Wu H, Deng Y, Feng Y, et al. Epigenetic regulation in B-cell maturation and its dysregulation in autoimmunity. *Cell Mol Immunol.* 2018;15:676–684. doi:10.1038/cmi.2017.133

41. Balomenos D, Martinez AC. Cell-cycle regulation in immunity, tolerance and autoimmunity. *Immunol Today.* 2000;21:551–555. doi:10.1016/s0167-5699(00)01748-5

42. Deng J, Pennati A, Cohen JB, et al. GIFT4 fusokine converts leukemic B cells into immune helper cells. *J Transl Med.* 2016;14:106. doi:10.1186/s12967-016-0865-1

43. Deng J, Yuan S, Pennati A, et al. Engineered fusokine GIFT4 licenses the ability of B cells to trigger a tumoricidal T-cell response. *Cancer Res.* 2014;74:4133–4144. doi:10.1158/0008-5472.CAN-14-0708

44. Kosmas C, Stamatopoulos K, Stavroyianni N, et al. Anti-CD20-based therapy of B cell lymphoma: state of the art. *Leukemia.* 2002;16:2004–2015. doi:10.1038/sj.leu.2402639

45. Origin and function of human plasma R-type vitamin B12 binding proteins. *Nutrition Rev.* 1976;34:148–150. doi:10.1111/j.1753-4887.1976.tb05741.x

46. Vilas-Boas A, Morais SA, Isenberg DA. Belimumab in systemic lupus erythematosus. *RMD Open.* 2015;1:e000011. doi:10.1136/rmdopen-2014-000011

47. Hartung HP, Kieseier BC. Atacicept: Targeting B cells in multiple sclerosis. *Ther Adv Neurol Disord.* 2010;3:205–216. doi:10.1177/1756285610371146

48. Adams J, Kauffman M. Development of the proteasome inhibitor Velcade (Bortezomib). *Cancer Invest.* 2004;22:304–311. doi:10.1081/cnv-120030218

49. Ganz T. Macrophage function. *New Horiz.* 1993;1:23–27. PubMed PMID: 7922389.

50. MacMicking J, Xie QW, Nathan C. Nitric oxide and macrophage function. *Annu Rev Immunol.* 1997;15:323–350. doi:10.1146/annurev.immunol.15.1.323

51. Rahat MA, Hemmerlein B. Macrophage-tumor cell interactions regulate the function of nitric oxide. *Front Physiol.* 2013;4:*144.* doi:10.3389/fphys.2013.00144

52. Mills CD, Lenz LL, Harris RA. A breakthrough: macrophage-directed cancer immunotherapy. *Cancer Res.* 2016;76:513–516. doi:10.1158/0008-5472.CAN-15-1737

53. Mills CD, Thomas AC, Lenz LL, et al. Macrophage: SHIP of immunity. *Front Immunol.* 2014;5:*620.* doi:10.3389/fimmu.2014.00620

54. Chung JW, Yoon SR, Choi I. The regulation of NK cell function and development. *Front Bioscie.* 2008;13:6432–6442. https://pdfs.semanticscholar.org/86e0/17e37f9a8342b95f34131747b39fd37ab1d3.pdf

55. Smyth MJ, Cretney E, Kelly JM, et al. Activation of NK cell cytotoxicity. *Mol Immunol.* 2005;42:501–510. doi:10.1016/j.molimm.2004.07.034

56. Lurati A, Marrazza MG, Re KA, Scarfpellini M. Relationship between NK cell activation and clinical response in rheumatoid arthritis treated with rituximab. *Int J Biomed Sci.* 2009;5:92–95. https://www.ncbi.nlm.nih.gov/pmc/articles/PMC3614777

57. Mehers KL, Long AE, van der Slik AR, et al. An increased frequency of NK cell receptor and HLA-C group 1 combinations in early-onset type 1 diabetes. *Diabetologia.* 2011;54:3062–3070. doi:10.1007/s00125-011-2299-x

58. Zippel D, Lackovic V, Kocisková D, et al. Abnormal macrophages and NK cell cytotoxicity in human systemic lupus erythematosus and the role of interferon and serum factors. *Acta Virol.* 1989;33:447–453. PubMed PMID: 2483602.

59. Waldhauer I, Steinle A. NK cells and cancer immunosurveillance. *Oncogene.* 2008;27:5932–5943. doi:10.1038/onc.2008.267

60. Chan CJ, Andrews DM, Smyth MJ. Can NK cells be a therapeutic target in human cancer? *Eur J Immunol.* 2008;38:2964–2968. doi:10.1002/eji.200838764

61. Di Vito C, Mikulak J, Zaghi E, et al. NK cells to cure cancer. *Semin Immunol.* 2019;41:101272. doi:10.1016/j.smim.2019.03.004

62. Mandal A, Viswanathan C. Natural killer cells: In health and disease. *Hematol Oncol Stem Cell Ther.* 2015;8:47–55. doi:10.1016/j.hemonc.2014.11.006

63. Cifaldi L, Locatelli F, Marasco E, et al. Boosting natural killer cell–based immunotherapy with anticancer drugs: a perspective. *Trends Mol Med.* 2017;23:1156–1175. doi:10.1016/j.molmed.2017.10.002

64. Lenaerts L, De Clercq E, Naesens L. Clinical features and treatment of adenovirus infections. *Rev Med Virol.* 2008;18:357–374. doi:10.1002/rmv.589

65. National Library of Medicine. Adenovirus type 4 and type 7 vaccine. In: *Drugs and lactation database (LactMed);* [Internet]. Updated June 15, 2020. https://www.ncbi.nlm.nih.gov/books/NBK501914

66. Hutchinson DJ, Klein KC. Human papillomavirus disease and vaccines. *Am J Health Syst Pharm.* 2008;65:2105–2112. doi:10.2146/ajhp070627

67. Stanley M. HPV—immune response to infection and vaccination. *Infect Agent Cancer.* 2010;5:*19.* doi:10.1186/1750-9378-5-19

68. Naim HY. Measles virus. *Hum Vaccin Immunother.* 2015;11:21–26. doi:10.4161/hv.34298

69. Duc-Nguyen H, Henle W. Replication of mumps virus in human leukocyte cultures. *J Bacteriol.* 1966;92:258–265. PubMed PMID: 5328751.

70. Leung AKC, Hon KL, Leong KF. Rubella (German measles) revisited. *Hong Kong Med J.* 2019;25:134–141. doi:10.12809/hkmj187785

71. Centers for Disease Control and Prevention. *Measles, mumps, and rubella (MMR) vaccination: what everyone should know.* https://www.cdc.gov/vaccines/vpd/mmr/public/index.html

72. Clem AS. Fundamentals of vaccine immunology. *J Glob Infect Dis.* 2011;3:73–78. doi:10.4103/0974-777X.77299

73. Centers for Disease Control and Prevention. *Influenza vaccination: a summary for clinicians.* https://www.cdc.gov/flu/professionals/vaccination/vax-summary.htm

74. Kennedy PGE, Gershon AA. Clinical features of Varicella-Zoster virus infection. *Viruses* 2018;10:609. doi:10.3390/v10110609

75. Vaccines for travelers. *Med Lett Drugs Ther.* 2018;60:185–192. https://pubmed.ncbi.nlm.nih.gov/30625125/

76. Centers for Disease Control and Prevention. *Varicella vaccine recommendations.* https://www.cdc.gov/vaccines/vpd/varicella/hcp/recommendations.html

77. Centers for Disease Control and Prevention. *Varicella vaccine effectiveness and duration of protection.* https://

www.cdc.gov/vaccines/vpd-vac/varicella/hcp-effective-duration.htm

78. Centers for Disease Control and Prevention. *About the vaccine.* https://www.cdc.gov/vaccines/vpd/rotavirus/hcp/about-vaccine.html

79. Centers for Disease Control and Prevention. *Cholera—Vibrio cholerae infection: vaccines.* https://www.cdc.gov/cholera/vaccines.html

80. Mosley JF II, Smith LL, Brantley P, et al. Vaxchora: The first FDA-approved cholera vaccination in the United States. *P T.* 2017;42:638–640. PubMed PMID: 29018300.

81. Centers for Disease Control and Prevention. *Diphtheria, tetanus, and whooping cough vaccination: what everyone should know.* https://www.cdc.gov/vaccines/vpd/dtap-tdap-td/public/index.html

82. Centers for disease control and prevention (CDC), 2017. https://www.cdc.gov/meningococcal/index.html

83. Centers for Disease Control and Prevention. *Meningococcal vaccination.* https://www.cdc.gov/vaccines/vpd/mening/index.html

84. O'Grady M, Bruner PJ. *Polio Vaccine.* StatPearls; 2019.

85. Sanofi Pasteur. Poliovirus vaccine inactivated: IPOL®. https://www.fda.gov/media/75695/download

86. Centers for Disease Control and Prevention. *Polio vaccination: what everyone should know.* https://www.cdc.gov/vaccines/vpd/polio/public/index.html

87. Centers for Disease Control and Prevention. *Typhoid fever and paratyphoid fever: vaccination.* https://www.cdc.gov/typhoid-fever/typhoid-vaccination.html

88. Crucell Vaccines. *Vivotif package insert.* Updated September 2013. https://www.fda.gov/media/75988/download

89. Van Camp RO, Shorman M. *Typhoid Vaccine.* StatPearls; 2019.

90. Centers for Disease Control and Prevention. *Yellow fever vaccine information for healthcare providers.* https://www.cdc.gov/yellowfever/healthcareproviders/vaccine-info.html

91. Centers for Disease Control and Prevention. *Table 1. Recommended Child and Adolescent Immunization Schedule for ages 18 years or younger, United States, 2020*: Haemophilus influenzae type b vaccination. https://www.cdc.gov/vaccines/schedules/hcp/imz/child-adolescent.html#note-hib

92. Centers for Disease Control and Prevention. *Lyme disease vaccine.* https://www.cdc.gov/lyme/prev/vaccine.html

93. Centers for Disease Control and Prevention. *Preventing tick bites.* https://www.cdc.gov/ticks/avoid/on_people.html

94. Centers for Disease Control and Prevention. *Rabies pPostexposure prophylaxis (PEP).* https://www.cdc.gov/rabies/medical_care/index.html

Pharmacotherapy for Endocrine Disorders

Prem Sahasranam, Michael Tran, Veronica T. Bandy, and Stanley Hsia

LEARNING OBJECTIVES

- Define the classes of pharmaceutical agents used in the treatment of diabetes, thyroid disorders, and osteoporosis.
- Explain the mechanism of action of pharmaceutical agents used in the treatment of the these selected endocrine disorders.
- Apply current treatment guidelines for these common endocrine diseases.
- Identify therapeutic options in the treatment of diabetes that would provide atherosclerotic cardiovascular disease (ASCVD) benefits.
- Develop alternative treatment plan for patients diagnosed with diabetes, thyroid disorders, and osteoporosis.

DIABETES MELLITUS

INTRODUCTION

Diabetes mellitus (DM) affects approximately 34 million individuals in the United States.[1] It is the most common cause of new cases of blindness among adults in developed countries,[2] the most common cause of end-stage renal failure and need for dialysis or transplantation in the United States.[2] Major cardiovascular diseases account for more than 20% of all hospital discharges among all patients with DM.[3] Among nonpregnant individuals, type 2 DM (T2DM) accounts for over 95% of all cases, with the remainder caused by type 1 DM (T1DM) or DM secondary to other factors (e.g., pancreatic destruction, glucocorticoid-induced).[1] Specific racial/ ethnic minority groups may be 50% to 200% more disproportionately affected as compared to non-Hispanic Whites.[1]

BACKGROUND

T1DM is caused by an autoimmune destruction of pancreatic islet cells, leading to a severe deficiency of insulin production. T2DM is a multifactorial condition caused by insufficient insulin production from cells to meet the body's increased insulin demands for maintaining normal carbohydrate and nutrient homeostasis (i.e., "insulin resistance," which in turn is typically associated with obesity, central adiposity, and/or aging). Insulin resistance interferes with total body glucose disposal and suppression of both endogenous hepatic glucose output and endogenous glucagon secretion, all of which predispose to hyperglycemia; thus, any degree of cell impairment relative to the severity of the insulin resistance will fail to compensate for these factors and result in hyperglycemia.[4]

DIAGNOSIS

In acute presentations, hyperglycemia causes polyuria and polydipsia, and in extreme cases, dehydration and hyperosmolarity, causing cognitive impairment or frank diabetic ketoacidosis (DKA). In milder cases of T2DM, patients are asymptomatic and the diagnosis is made biochemically (**Box 24.1**).[5] Routine screening of asymptomatic ambulatory adults is recommended (**Box 24.2**), since early detection and intervention at the "prediabetes" stage can slow the progression towards overt DM.[5,6]

TREATMENT: GENERAL CONSIDERATIONS

Nonpharmacological strategies (nutrition, lifestyle factors, weight control) are key, central components of optimal DM management, with pharmacological agents serving as important adjunctive therapies. However, such modifications can be complex and difficult for patients to properly implement and sustain long-term, so clinicians often rely on pharmacotherapies. Nonetheless, medical nutrition therapy and lifestyle counseling appropriate to each patient's needs should be reinforced regularly as a routine part of every patient encounter. Ideally, a specially trained Certified Diabetes Educator (CDE) should be closely involved with teaching Diabetes Self-Management Education and Support (DSMES) to all DM patients on an ongoing basis. Specific principles underlying these strategies are beyond the scope of this chapter.[7]

For T1DM, the overall aim is to achieve near-normoglycemia by replacing insulin in a manner that mimics as closely as possible normal endogenous insulin secretion profiles in response to usual daily glucose fluctuations. For T2DM, the overall aim is to achieve near-normoglycemia by overcoming each patient's defects of normal insulin action using additive and complementary treatments. Because T2DM usually coexists with a proatherogenic metabolic profile that contributes to atherosclerotic cardiovascular disease (ASCVD; the largest cause of mortality in T2DM), agents that reduce ASCVD risk and hyperglycemia should be used preferentially for T2DM patients with higher baseline ASCVD risk, and any concurrent ASCVD risk factors must be comanaged to their respective targets (**Table 24.1**; see Chapters 17 and 21).[2,8,9] For all DM patients, regular surveillance for end-organ complications should also take place at the recommended intervals, and any existing complications should be comanaged through appropriate referrals.

Targets of optimal glycemic control as recommended by the American Diabetes Association (ADA) are shown in **Table 24.2**. Hemoglobin A1c (HbA1c), a marker of integrated glycemic burden over the prior 2

TABLE 24.1 Recommended American Diabetes Association Treatment Guidelines

Guideline	Frequency	Treatment Goal
1. HbA1c	Minimum twice per year; quarterly if goal not attained	<7.0% (lower or higher goal may be reasonable for select patients)
2. Blood pressure	Every routine visit; home monitoring also recommended	Systolic <140 mmHg; diastolic <90 mmHg (lower goal of <130/80 mmHg may be reasonable for higher risk patients)
3. Dyslipidemia	Minimum every 5 years or more frequently if indicated (e.g., 1–2 years) and to monitor treatment	Use of a statin with LDL cholesterol–lowering intensity appropriate to the patient's risk profile; LDL cholesterol <70 mg/dL if prior ASCVD and very high risk (add adjunctive agents if necessary)
4. Aspirin	Prescribe if prior ASCVD, or high risk (e.g., age 50–70 years + one ASCVD risk factor)	Prescribe 75–162 mg once daily if no contraindications; clopidogrel 75 mg once daily if aspirin intolerant
5. Nephropathy	UACR and eGFR at least annually (twice yearly if abnormal)	Optimize blood pressure and glucose; use of an ACE inhibitor or ARB if coexisting hypertension with either albuminuria or eGFR <60 mL/min/1.73 m²
6. Retinopathy	Annual comprehensive dilated eye exam (or equivalent); may reduce to every 2 years if normal	Optimize blood pressure, glucose, dyslipidemia; ophthalmology referral for more intensive therapy (e.g., laser, anti-VEGF therapies)
7. Peripheral neuropathy	Sensory testing at least annually	Optimize glucose; analgesia for neuropathic pain if present
8. Foot care	Comprehensive foot exam at least annually (at each visit if sensory loss or prior ulcers)	Provide general preventive education; prevent ulceration or deformities; specialized therapeutic footwear or podiatry referral as needed
9. Smoking cessation/ prevention	Routinely counsel	Avoidance/cessation

ACE, angiotensin-converting enzyme; ADA, American Diabetes Association; ASCVD, atherosclerotic cardiovascular disease; eGFR, estimated glomerular filtration rate; HbA1c, hemoglobin A1c; LDL, low-density lipoprotein; UACR, urine albumin-creatinine ratio; VEGF, vascular endothelial growth factor.

Source: Adapted from American Diabetes Association. 11. Microvascular complications and foot care: *Standards of Medical Care in Diabetes—2020. Diabetes Care.* 2020;43(suppl 1):S135–S151. doi:10.2337/dc20-S011; American Diabetes Association. 10. Cardiovascular disease and risk management: *Standards of Medical Care in Diabetes—2020. Diabetes Care.* 2020;43(suppl 1):S111–S134. doi:10.2337/dc20-S010; Davidson MB, Hsia SH. *Meeting the American Diabetes Association standards of care: An algorithmic approach to clinical care of the diabetes patient;* 2017:13.

TABLE 24.2 American Diabetes Association Glycemic Recommendations

HbA1c	<7.0%*
Preprandial plasma glucose	80–130 mg/dL*
Peak postprandial plasma glucose	<180 mg/dL*

*More or less stringent glycemic goals may be appropriate for individual patients. Goals should be individualized based on duration of diabetes, age/life expectancy, comorbid conditions, known cardiovascular disease or advanced microvascular complications, hypoglycemia unawareness, and individual patient considerations.

HbA1c, hemoglobin A1c.

Source: Adapted from American Diabetes Association. 6. Glycemic targets: *Standards of Medical Care in Diabetes—2020. Diabetes Care.* 2020;43 (suppl 1):S66–S76. doi:10.2337/dc20-S006

to 3 months, is the best single marker of overall glucose control. A general HbA1c target of less than 7.0% is recommended for all DM patients, but actual targets should be individualized. More intensive control to below 7.0% can further reduce microvascular diabetes complications, but may also increase the risk of hypoglycemia.[11–13] If such risk places the patient at undue risk of harm, a less stringent HbA1c target may be considered. Older patients or those with longer duration of diabetes, multiple comorbidities, limited life expectancy, or other factors that complicate self-care may be less able to tolerate hypoglycemia; individual clinical judgment should be used to determine a patient's capacity to tolerate intensive control and thus the stringency of their HbA1c target.[10]

Self-monitoring of blood glucose (SMBG), using various devices to obtain capillary or interstitial glucose measurements, is another powerful tool for patients to monitor their own glucose fluctuations in real-time, if it is used in an informed and cost-effective manner. SMBG complements HbA1c by showing the variability of glucose control, and can be used to detect, anticipate, and/or prevent extreme excursions. SMBG can confirm a suspected hypoglycemic event and track its recovery as it is self-managed with oral carbohydrates. Depending on skill level, patients may also monitor on an as-needed (PRN) basis to improve self-management skills, such as better informing dietary choices by measuring postmeal glucose excursions, or anticipate, prevent, and/or manage potential hypoglycemia when engaging in physical activity. However, frequent SMBG also entails substantial costs related to consumable supplies (e.g., disposable test strips, lancets, sensors). Thus, while all insulin-treated patients are strongly encouraged to perform regular and frequent SMBG monitoring, for all other patients, it is prudent to use SMBG only if it will provide actionable information that can be properly interpreted to help improve the patient's control, either by the patient to improve their own DSMES, or by clinicians to educate the patient or inform treatment choices beyond the information provided by the HbA1c.[14]

TREATMENT: CHOOSING PHARMACOLOGICAL AGENTS

Many classes of pharmacological agents are available. Insulin is the only treatment option for T1DM. In contrast, several choices are available for T2DM, and the ADA has published a recommended treatment algorithm for choosing treatments for T2DM.[15] Effectively, these recommendations are based on a few general principles (**Table 24.3**):

1. Metformin is the best initial choice for all T2DM patients (unless contraindicated). Repeated reinforcement of dietary and lifestyle principles should occur frequently, irrespective of pharmacotherapy.
2. For T2DM patients with a prior history of ASCVD or significant ASCVD risk (including heart failure or chronic renal disease), the addition of either a GLP-1Ra or a SGLT-2i with proven ASCVD benefit should be considered, even if the patient's HbA1c is already at target, since they may still offer cardio-protective benefits independent of their glycemic effects.
3. If the maximum-tolerated dose of any T2DM agent fails to achieve the glycemia target, it is prudent to sequentially add an agent of a different class, each titrated up to their maximum-tolerated dose, until either the target is achieved or intolerance occurs.

TABLE 24.3 Summary of Major Available Classes of Agents for Type 2 Diabetes Mellitus

Agent	Macrovascular Benefits			Hypo	BW	Cost
	CV	HF	Renal			
Metformin	(+)	0	0	0	()[a]	$
Sulfonylurea/ meglitinide	0	0	0			$/$$
TZD	(+)[b]	X	0	0		$
AGi	0	0	0	0	0	$
DPP4i	0	(X)[c]	0	0	0	$$
SGLT2i	+[d]	+	+[e]	0		$$
GLP1Ra	+[f]	0	+[g]	0		$$
Insulin (NPH/Reg)	(+)[h]	0	0			$
Insulin (Analogue)						$$

+, beneficial; X, harmful; 0, neutral or no effect; ( ), possible or inconsistent effect; $ / $$, low versus high relative cost, respectively; AGi, a-glucosidase inhibitors; BW, body weight effects; CV, cardiovascular; DPP4i, dipeptidyl peptidase-4 inhibitor; GP1Ra, glucagon-like peptide-1 receptor agonist; HF, heart failure; Hypo, hypoglycemia risk; NPH, neutral protamine Hagedorn; Reg, regular (insulin); SGLT2i, sodium-glucose cotransporter-2 inhibitors; SU, sulfonylurea; TZD, thiazolidinedione.

[a]Usually weight neutral, but possible weight loss.

[b]Possible benefit with pioglitazone only.

[c]Possible harm with saxagliptin only.

[d]Benefit shown only with empagliflozin and canagliflozin, but not dapagliflozin.

[e]Benefit shown with empagliflozin, canagliflozin, dapagliflozin.

[f]Benefit shown with liraglutide, dulaglutide, and semaglutide, but not exenatide or lixisenatide.

[g]Benefit shown with liraglutide only.

[h]Possible benefit with long-term use of insulin in T1DM.

Source: Adapted from American Diabetes Association. 9. Pharmacologic approaches to glycemic treatment: *Standards of Medical Care in Diabetes—2020. Diabetes Care.* 2020;43(suppl 1):S98–S110. doi:10.2337/dc20-S009

4. At any stage, the choice of the next best agent for T2DM should be based on clinical judgment and discussion with the patient, accounting for: (a) the patient's ASCVD risk, (b) risk of hypoglycemia, (c) drug effects on body weight, (d) other medication side effects, (e) medication cost, and (f) other patient preferences (Table 24.3).[15]
5. Do not combine a GLP-1Ra with a DPP-4i, since both act through the same incretin system; evidence has shown no additive glucose lowering with this combination.[16] For the same reason, do not combine sulfonylureas (SUs) with meglitinides, since both these agents act through the same mechanism and confer no additive effect on glucose lowering.

TREATMENT: PHARMACOLOGICAL AGENT CLASSES

Oral Agents

Metformin
Long accepted as an inexpensive and ideal first-line agent for T2DM, metformin principally reduces hepatic glucose production, reduces intestinal glucose absorption, and improves insulin resistance (**Table 24.4**).[17]

Sulfonylureas
Also long accepted as a proven and inexpensive treatment, SUs potentiate B-cell insulin secretion is effective in any T2DM patient who does not have longstanding T2DM that has become insulin-requiring (**Table 24.5**). Older,

---

TABLE 24.4 Metformin

Medication	Dose/ Frequency	Advantages	Disadvantages
Metformin (Glucophage®, Riomet® [500 mg/5 mL])	500–1,000 mg bid daily (max: 2,550 mg/ day)	Reported to reduce ASCVD in overweight patients[18] No hypoglycemia (as monotherapy) No weight gain (or possible weight loss) Inexpensive	Potential dose-limiting GI side effects (diarrhea, nausea, cramping); may be modestly reduced if taken with meals or use of the XR formulation[17] Caution in renal insufficiency (discontinue if eGFR <30 mL/min/1.73 m²) and other states of lactic acidosis (but rarely ever the sole cause of lactic acidosis); hold for iodinated contrast if eGFR 30–60 mL/min/1.73 m² Potential vitamin B12 deficiency
Metformin XR (Glucophage XR®, Glumetza®, Fortamet®, Riomet ER® [500 mg/5 mL])	500–2,000 mg daily (max: 2,500 mg/ day)		

ASCVD, atherosclerotic cardiovascular disease; bid, twice daily; ER, extended-release; GI, gastrointestinal; max, maximum total dose; XR, extended-release.

TABLE 24.5 Sulfonylureas

Medication	Dose/Frequency	Advantages	Disadvantages
Glimepiride (Amaryl®)	1–4 mg daily (max: 8 mg/day)	Reduces microvascular complications[19]; does *not* increase ASCVD based on evidence from randomized trials (although controversy remains[20]) Inexpensive	Does not reduce ASCVD May cause hypoglycemia May cause weight gain Some caution is warranted in severe hepatic or renal insufficiency
Glipizide (Glucotrol®)	2.5–20 mg bid (max: 40 mg/day)		
Glipizide XL (Glucotrol XL®)	5–10 mg daily (max: 20 mg/day)		
Glyburide (DiaBeta®)	1.25–10 mg bid (max: 20 mg/day)		
Glyburide micronized (Glynase PresTab®)	0.75–6 mg bid (max: 12 mg/day)		

ASCVD, atherosclerotic cardiovascular disease; bid, twice daily; max, maximum total dose.

first-generation SUs (chlorpropamide, tolbutamide, tola-zamide) were associated with more side effects and are now best avoided. Glyburide possesses slightly faster kinetics than other available SUs, thus predisposing to slightly more hypoglycemia, and are best avoided in sensitive individuals (e.g., the elderly).

Meglitinides

Unlike SUs, meglitinides, or "glinides," are mealtime, short-acting insulin secretagogues (i.e., TID dosing, <30 minutes before each meal) that act only in the postprandial period to help lower postprandial glucose, thus predisposing to less risk of delayed hypoglycemia (**Table 24.6**).

Thiazolidinediones

Thiazolidinediones (TZDs), or "glitazones," are strong insulin sensitizers that act through activation of the nuclear receptor peroxisome proliferator-activated receptor-g (PPARg), which alters the expression of many genes relevant to glucose and lipid metabolism (**Table 24.7**).[22]

Glucosidase Inhibitors

Glucosidase inhibitors (AGi) inhibit intestinal a-glucoside hydrolase and pancreatic amylase, leading to delayed postprandial carbohydrate absorption and therefore reduced postprandial glucose excursions (i.e., TID dosing; **Table 24.8**).

TABLE 24.6 Meglitinides

Medication	Dose/Frequency	Advantages	Disadvantages
Repaglinide (Prandin®)	0.4–4 mg mg tid before meals (max: 4 mg/dose; 16 mg/day)	Less hypoglycemia than compared to SUs Flexible dosing (i.e., may skip dose if meal skipped)	Not studied for ASCVD May still cause hypoglycemia May still cause weight gain Less HbA1c-lowering than compared to SUs (particularly for nateglinide[21]) Caution in severe renal insufficiency (e.g., for repaglinide, creatinine clearance <40 mL/min) and severe hepatic insufficiency (for nateglinide) More expensive than SUs
Nateglinide (Starlix®)	60–120 mg tid before meals		

ASCVD, atherosclerotic cardiovascular disease; bid, twice daily; max, maximum dose; SU, sulfonylureas; tid, three times daily

TABLE 24.7 Thiazolidinediones

Medication	Dose/Frequency	Advantages	Disadvantages
Pioglitazone (Actos®)	15–45 mg daily	Pioglitazone reported to reduce ASCVD events[23] No hypoglycemia (as monotherapy, but potentiates hypoglycemic potential of SUs or insulin) Robust HbA1c-lowering	Rosiglitazone does not reduce ASCVD events (evidence that it may increase ASCVD events remains controversial) May cause weight gain (pro adipogenic) Potential fluid retention (use cautiously if severe peripheral edema; contraindicated if Class III–IV heart failure) Potential reduction in bone density
Rosiglitazone (Avandia®)	4–8 mg daily (max: 4 mg/day if combo with insulin)		

ASCVD, atherosclerotic cardiovascular disease; max, maximum total dose.

TABLE 24.8 Glucosidase Inhibitors

Medication	Dose/Frequency	Advantages	Disadvantages
Acarbose (Precose®)	25–100 mg tid at start of meals (max: 300 mg/day; 150 mg/day if wt <60 kg)	Favorable effects on ASCVD risk factors, although no clear reduction of ASCVD in T2DM (shown in pre diabetes only)[24] No hypoglycemia (as monotherapy) No weight gain	Possible dose-limiting increase in flatulence, loose stools, diarrhea; dose increases should be made gradually (q4–8 weeks); contraindicated in patients with luminal GI conditions[25] Modest HbA1c-lowering Caution in renal insufficiency (creatinine >2.0 mg/dL) or cirrhosis (i.e., luminal-acting, but absorbed metabolites) May attenuate effects of oral glucose in treating hypoglycemic reactions
Miglitol (Glyset®)	25–100 mg tid at start of meals (Max: 300 mg/day)		

ASCVD, atherosclerotic cardiovascular disease; GI, gastrointestinal; T2DM, type 2 diabetes mellitus; tid, three times daily

Dipeptidyl Peptidase-4 Inhibitors

Dipeptidyl peptidase-4 inhibitors (DPP4i), or "gliptins," facilitate specific inhibition of the degradation of endogenous incretins leads to enhanced incretin action (i.e., enhanced insulin secretion, reduced glucagon; **Table 24.9**).[26]

Sodium-Glucose Cotransporter-2 Inhibitors

Sodium-glucose cotransporter-2 inhibitors (SGLT2i), or "flozins," facilitate inhibition of renal tubular reabsorption of glomerular-filtered glucose, leading to reduced circulating glucose, albeit at the expense of increased glycosuria and a modest increase in the risk of urinary and genital infections.[29] This mechanism of action also represents a mild osmotic diuresis that can help to lower blood pressure and ameliorate heart failure, as well as contribute to a slight weight loss (**Table 24.10**).

Other Agents

Bromocriptine and colesevelam are approved by the U.S. Food and Drug Administration (FDA) for glucose lowering in T2DM, but their mechanisms of action remain unclear. Bromocriptine, a dopamine agonist, may benefit glucose homeostasis indirectly via effects on central neurotransmitters, independent of insulin action. A quick-release formulation of bromocriptine is approved for use in T2DM, although it may also predispose to nausea/vomiting, fatigue, headaches, rhinitis and dizziness/syncope, and needs to be taken with food; all other cautions and side effects associated with bromocriptine use also apply.[32] One small study also suggested a potential reduction in ASCVD events.[33] Colesevelam, a bile acid sequestrant used for lowering low-density lipoprotein (LDL) cholesterol, may improve hyperglycemia via indirect hepatic effects on reducing glucose production and/or pro incretin effects. The associated cautions and side effects of its use are those typical of bile acid sequestrants for lipid-lowering (e.g., constipation, adsorption of concomitant medications, higher triglycerides).[34] Neither agent causes hypoglycemia as monotherapy, but they are also not particularly potent glucose-lowering agents (**Table 24.11**).

Fixed-Combination Oral Agents

These agents simplify dosing regimens for patients but are generally more expensive and otherwise no different than prescribing the individual component agents separately (**Table 24.12**). All cautions and side-effect profiles remain those of the individual component agents.

TABLE 24.9 Dipeptidyl Peptidase-4 Inhibitors

Medication	Dose/Frequency	Advantages	Disadvantages
Sitagliptin (Januvia®)	100 mg daily	No hypoglycemia (as monotherapy) No weight gain Well tolerated	No reduction of ASCVD events; possible risk of heart failure with saxagliptin [27]
Saxagliptin (Onglyza®)	2.5–5 mg daily		Except for linagliptin, use progressively lower dosages in renal insufficiency (half-max dose if eGFR <45–60 mL/min/1.73 m²; ¼-max dose if eGFR <30 mL/min/1.73 m²)
Linagliptin (Tradjenta®)	5 mg daily		Contraindicated if history of pancreatitis (but only weak evidence as a cause of pancreatitis[28])
Alogliptin (Nesina®)	25 mg daily		More expensive

ASCVD, atherosclerotic cardiovascular disease; eGFR, estimated glomerular filtration rate.

TABLE 24.10 Sodium-Glucose Co-Transporter-2 Inhibitors

Medication	Dose/Frequency	Advantages	Disadvantages
Canagliflozin (Invokana®)	100–300 mg qAM	Canagliflozin[30] and empagliflozin[31] shown to reduce ASCVD events, particularly related to heart failure No hypoglycemia (as monotherapy) Possible weight loss Possible reduction of blood pressure; growing body of evidence of potential reno-protection	Increased risk of urinary/genital infections Canagliflozin may increase risk of lower limb amputations (particularly if pre-existing peripheral vascular disease or neuropathy) Possible increase in urinary frequency Caution if pre-existing volume depletion Contraindicated in advanced renal insufficiency (eGFR <30 mL/min/1.73 m²; if eGFR <45 mL/min/1.73 m² avoid empagliflozin, dapagliflozin; if eGFR <60 mL/min/1.73 m² avoid ertugliflozin, limit canagliflozin to 100 mg daily Rare complication of euglycemic diabetic ketoacidosis

ASCVD, atherosclerotic cardiovascular disease; qAM, once every morning.

TABLE 24.11 Bromocriptine and Colesevelam

Medication	Dose/Frequency
Bromocriptine-QR (Cycloset®)	0.8–4.8 mg qAM (with food within 2 hours of waking) max: 4.8 mg/day
Colesevelam (Welchol®)	3,750 mg daily or 1,875 mg bid

bid, twice daily; max, maximum total dose; qAM, once every morning.

Non-Insulin Injectable Agents

Glucagon-Like Peptide-1 Agonists

Glucagon-like peptide-1 (GLP-1) agonists (GLP1Ra), or "glutides," are subcutaneously injected analogues of the endogenous incretin GLP-1 potentiate glucose-stimulated insulin release, inhibition of glucagon, as well as slowing of gastric emptying and some central satiety, all of which improve glycemia without precipitating hypoglycemia (**Table 24.13**).[35] One oral

TABLE 24.12 Fixed-Combination Oral Agents for Diabetes Mellitus

Medication	Dose/Frequency
Glipizide/metformin (Metaglip®)	2.5/250–20/2000 mg/day
Glyburide/metformin (Glucovance®)	1.25/250–20/2000 mg/day
Repaglinide/metformin (PrandiMet®)	1/500–4/2000 mg/day
Pioglitazone/metformin (ACTOplus met®)	15/500–45/2550 mg/day
Pioglitazone/metformin XR (ACTOplus met XR®)	15/1000–45/2000 mg/day
Rosiglitazone/metformin (Avandamet®)	2/500–8/2000 mg/day
Sitagliptin/metformin (Janumet®)	50/500–100/2000 mg/day
Sitagliptin/metformin XR (Janumet XR®)	50/500–100/2000 mg/day
Saxagliptin/metformin XR (Kombiglyze XR®)	2.5/1000–5/2000 mg/day
Linagliptin/metformin (Jentadueto®)	5/1000–5/2000 mg/day
Linagliptin/metformin XR (Jentadueto XR®)	2.5/1000–5/2000 mg/day
Linagliptin/empagliflozin/metformin XR (Trijardy XR®)	2.5/5/1000–5/25/1000 mg/day
Alogliptin/metformin (Kazano®)	12.5/500–25/2000 mg/day
Canagliflozin/metformin (Invokamet®)	50/500–300/2000 mg/day
Canagliflozin/metformin XR (Invokamet XR)	50/500–300/2000 mg/day
Empagliflozin/metformin (Synjardy®)	5/500–25/2000 mg/day
Empagliflozin/metformin XR (Synjardy XR®)	5/1000–25/2000 mg/day
Dapagliflozin/metformin XR (Xigduo XR®)	5/500–10/2000 mg/day
Dapagliflozin/saxagliptin/metformin XR (Qternmet XR®)	2.5/2.5/1000–10/5/1000 mg/day
Ertugliflozin/metformin (Segluromet®)	2.5/500–15/2000 mg/day
Pioglitazone/glimepiride (Duetact®)	30/2–45/8 mg/day
Rosiglitazone/glimepiride (Avandaryl®)	4/1–8/4 mg/day
Alogliptin/pioglitazone (Oseni®)	12.5/15–25/45 mg/day
Ertugliflozin/sitagliptin (Steglujan®)	5/100–15/100 mg/day
Empagliflozin/linagliptin (Glyxambi®)	10/5–20/5 mg/day
Dapagliflozin/saxagliptin (Qtern®)	10/5 mg/day

TABLE 24.13 Glucagon-Like Peptide-1 Agonists

Medication	Dose/Frequency	Advantages	Disadvantages
Exenatide (Byetta®)	5–10 mg SC bid (1 hour before meals; increase monthly)	Liraglutide,[37] dulaglutide,[38] semaglutide[39] shown to reduce ASCVD events	Need for subcutaneous administration (except oral semaglutide)
Exenatide (Bydureon®, Bydureon BCise®)	2 mg SC weekly	No hypoglycemia (as monotherapy)	Transient nausea/vomiting/anorexia/diarrhea
Liraglutide (Victoza®)	0.6–1.8 mg SC daily (increase weekly)	Weight loss (may be sustained long-term)	Caution with exenatide in renal insufficiency (avoid if eGFR <45 mL/min/1.73 m²); caution with lixisenatide if eGFR <30 mL/min/1.73 m²; others safe in renal insufficiency
Dulaglutide (Trulicity®)	0.75–1.5 mg SC weekly	Generally favorable effects on ASCVD risk factors	Contraindicated if history of pancreatitis, pancreatic cancer, medullary thyroid carcinoma (but not well supported by the available evidence[40])
Lixisenatide (Adlyxin®)	10–20 mg SC daily (increase every 2 weeks)	Some formulations administered only once per week, although an oral formulation of semaglutide is also available	
Semaglutide (Ozempic®)	0.25–1 mg SC weekly (increase every 4 weeks)		
Semaglutide (oral; Rybelsus®)	3–14 mg po daily (before first meal; increase monthly)		

ASCVD, atherosclerotic cardiovascular disease; bid, twice daily; eGFR, estimated glomerular filtration rate; po, by mouth; SC, subcutaneously.

TABLE 24.14 Pramlintide

Medication	Dose/Frequency	Advantages	Disadvantages
Pramlintide (Symlin®)	T1DM: 15–60 mg SC qAc T2DM: 60–120 mg qAc (increase every 3 days)	Possible modest weight loss	Need for subcutaneous administration Indicated only as adjunct to concurrent prandial insulin (i.e., a separate injection); may potentiate hypoglycemia effects of the insulin (insulin dose reduction required) Transient nausea/vomiting Modest HbA1c-lowering Not recommended if creatinine clearance <15 mL/min More expensive

qAc, before every meal; T1DM, type 1 diabetes mellitus; T2DM, type 2 diabetes mellitus.

formulation of semaglutide is also now available, which provides HbA1c- and weight-lowering effects comparable to those of injected semaglutide, along with a comparable gastrointestinal (GI) side-effect profile if dose escalation is slow.[36]

Pramlintide

An injectable analogue of endogenous amylin, which suppresses glucagon, slows gastric emptying, and promotes central satiety, is indicated for use only as an adjunct to prandial (i.e., mealtime) insulin injections (i.e., TID dosing; **Table 24.14**).[41]

Insulins and Insulin Regimens

General Principles

Insulin is the only treatment option for T1DM. Insulin is also the most effective treatment for glucose control in T2DM. With longstanding T2DM, cumulative B-cell dysfunction renders many oral agents less effective, making insulin a more preferred choice later in the course of T2DM. However, insulin is less convenient

to use than other therapies; some patient subgroups harbor substantial misconceptions and fear of insulin; and many clinicians have limited experience managing complex insulin regimens.[42–44] The discussion that follows will help to guide the reader in the proper use of insulin (**Table 24.15**).

Rapid- or short-acting insulins are used as meal-associated ("prandial") insulins, while intermediate or long-acting insulins are used more for around-the-clock ("basal") coverage. Most insulin regimens include some combination of both. The ideal combination insulin regimen is one that is individualized to accommodate the patient's usual dietary pattern of carbohydrate peaks and nadirs, since most patients follow a relatively consistent day-to-day meal pattern (i.e., not vice versa: patients should not have to alter their usual dietary pattern simply to accommodate the insulin regimen). Alternatively, patients who must deal with fluctuating mealtimes or meal composition, either by choice or due to factors beyond their control, can learn how to rationally alter their own prandial insulin doses accordingly

TABLE 24.15 Available Insulin Formulations

Medication	Advantages	Disadvantages
Rapid-Acting Insulin	No maximum dose; will always be effective as long as dosing is guided by SMBG readings Reduces the progression of microvascular end-organ complications[19,45]; with long-term use, possibly also macrovascular events in T1DM[46] Native human insulin formulations are inexpensive Inhaled insulin helps to reduce the inconvenience of prandial injections Safe in renal and hepatic insufficiency as long as doses are reduced accordingly to avoid hypoglycemia	Need for subcutaneous injections, sometimes multiple times per day (except for inhaled insulin) Some combination insulin regimens can be complex Handling vials/syringes can be cumbersome (pen syringes may be easier) Frequent SMBG readings are *necessary* for dosage adjustments and safety monitoring May cause hypoglycemia May cause weight gain Inhaled insulin requires pulmonary function testing; contraindicated in smokers or history of pulmonary disease, or if FEV1 decreases >20% from baseline Synthetic insulin analogues can be expensive Insulin pumps can be expensive and complex to manage
Lispro (U-100, U-200) (Humalog®, Admelog®)		
Aspart (NovoLog®, Fiasp®)		
Glulisine (Apidra®)		
Inhaled (Afrezza®)		
Short-Acting Insulin		
Regular (Humulin R®, Novolin R®)		
Intermediate-Acting Insulin		
NPH (Humulin N®, Novolin N®)		
Regular U-500 (Humulin® R U-500)		
Long-Acting Insulin		
Glargine (U-100, U-300) (Lantus®, Toujeo®, Basaglar®)		
Detemir (Levemir®)		
Degludec (U-100, U-200) (Tresiba®)		
Premixed* Insulin		
70/30 (NPH/regular) (Humulin® 70/30, Novolin® 70/30)		
50/50 (NPH/regular) (Humulin® 50/50)		
Lispro Protamine/lispro 50/50 (Humalog® Mix 50/50)		
Lispro Protamine/lispro 75/25 (Humalog® Mix 75/25)		
Aspart Protamine/aspart 70/30 (NovoLog® Mix 70/30)		

*Premixed insulins are mixtures of an intermediate- and either a short- or a rapid-acting insulin in the proportions specified.

FEV1, forced expiratory volume in 1 second; NPH, neutral protamine Hagedorn. Standard insulin concentration is U-100 or 100 units/mL; U-200, U-300, and U-500 represent correspondingly higher concentrations. Regular and NPH are native human insulins; all others are synthetic insulin analogues.

("carbohydrate counting"). This is a more complex skill, usually learned by trial-and-error, that not all patients will be capable of; patients should ideally be referred to an endocrinologist for proper management of carbohydrate counting.

Before-meal ("preprandial") SMBG readings are generally preferred over "postprandial" readings because they are less labile. There are typically four SMBG-monitoring time points of interest: preprandial at each meal and at bedtime, as these time points typically coincide with the peak action of the insulin doses used in common regimens (**Table 24.16**). In general,

prandial insulins peak with a time course that disposes of a meal, thus controlling the preprandial reading by the time of the next meal (and in the case of a suppertime dose, controls the reading at bedtime). Intermediate-acting insulin, with its delayed peak, is best suited to control the predinner reading if injected at breakfast, and the prebreakfast (fasting) reading the next day if injected in the evening. Long-acting insulins, in contrast, being "peakless," provide largely constant profiles; when taken at bedtime, they effectively act through the night to control the prebreakfast reading the next morning.

TABLE 24.16 Monitoring Time Points of Different Insulin Doses

Injected at Breakfast	Injected at Lunch	Injected at Dinner	Injected at Bedtime
Rapid- or Short-Acting (Prandial) Insulin			
Monitor before lunch	Monitor before dinner	Monitor before bedtime	**
Intermediate-Acting Insulin			
Monitor before dinner	**	Monitor before breakfast	Monitor before breakfast
Long-Acting (Basal) Insulin			
Monitor before breakfast*	**	Monitor before breakfast	Monitor before breakfast

*Detemir or glargine injected in the morning may not last a full 24 hours; may consider monitoring before dinner or bedtime to better reflect its effect.
**injections that are not generally advised.

TABLE 24.17 Available Glucagon Formulations

Medication	Dose/Frequency	Advantages	Disadvantages
Crystalline (kit) (GlucaGen®)	1 mg SC/IM/IV (reconstitute in 1 mL sterile water in prefilled pen, makes 1 mg/mL solution) May repeat q15–20 min prn	Rapidly mobilizes glucose from hepatic glycogen stores, reversing hypoglycemia	May cause nausea/vomiting; precipitate tachycardia, hypertension, hyperglycemia Limited efficacy if prolonged fasting/starvation (depleted glycogen stores) Contraindicated if insulinoma or pheochromocytoma Caution if adrenal insufficiency is suspected
Liquid (Gvoke®)	0.5–1 mg SC (single-use prefilled injection syringe or auto-injector: 0.5 mg/0.1 mL; 1.0 mg/0.2 mL) May repeat × 1 after 15 min		
Intranasal device (Baqsimi®)	3 mg (1 actuation) intranasally × 1 May repeat × 1 after 15 min		

IM, intramuscularly; IV, intravenously; prn, as needed; q, every; SC, subcutaneously.

Common Insulin Regimens

T1DM patients need around-the-clock coverage, ideally with the MDI regimen. Insulin-requiring T2DM patients, in contrast, often prefer to start with the simplest regimen; as the natural history of T2DM progresses over time, other doses are progressively added and/or altered in a stepwise manner as needed, transforming eventually into the more complex regimens.

Bedtime Basal Insulin

Bedtime basal insulin is a single bedtime dose of intermediate or long-acting insulin, titrated to control next morning's prebreakfast reading; the patient otherwise continues on their prior daytime (noninsulin) agents. With only one insulin peak, SMBG monitoring is needed only prebreakfast. This regimen limits the associated weight gain, but also relies on the existing daytime (noninsulin) agents to control daytime excursions.

"Split-Mix" Insulin

"Split-Mix" insulin is an intermediate-acting neutral protamine Hagedorn (NPH), used largely as a basal insulin, plus short-acting regular insulin as a prandial insulin, typically given as a daily pre breakfast and pre dinner injection of a "mixture" of the two (i.e., combined into the same syringe each time), thus providing four independent insulin peaks that cover the 24-hour cycle but requiring only two injections per day (Table 24.16 shows peaks at all four time points using this regimen). Disadvantages include the need for relative consistency in day-to-day dietary and lifestyle patterns to avoid unexpected hypoglycemia—e.g., midday meal should not be missed, since NPH was delivered in the morning in anticipation of a midday meal. However, NPH and regular insulins are also substantially less expensive than the synthetic insulin analogues.

Premixed Insulins

Predetermined mixtures of a prandial plus an intermediate-acting insulin in a fixed ratio, administered twice daily, act as a split-mix-like regimen without the need to manually mix two insulins together (**Table 24.17**). However, the fixed ratio is also a major disadvantage since it prevents the two component insulins from being independently adjusted to individualize the regimen for a patient's unique daily pattern, thus limiting their utility in achieving tight control for many patients.

Multiple-Daily Injection

A "bolus" rapid-acting prandial insulin injection with each meal, plus the "peakless" long-acting basal insulin usually injected at bedtime (i.e., four daily injections), covers the 24-hour cycle while more closely mimicking the "basal-bolus" kinetics of endogenous insulin secretion. The multiple-daily injection (MDI), or "basal-bolus," regimen is the best choice for T1DM patients.

Inhaled insulin (Table 24.15) can be an alternative prandial insulin that eliminates the need for mealtime injections, but it does not replace the basal insulin and should not be used in patients with any pulmonary pathology (including smoking). A major advantage of MDI is that it allows the patient to vary the timing and dose of each prandial injection according to the timing and "carbohydrate counting" of each meal, respectively, which affords patients who must live with erratic or unpredictable dietary and lifestyle schedules greater flexibility and control.

Continuous Subcutaneous Insulin Infusion

Continuous subcutaneous insulin infusion (CSII), or "insulin pumps," are automated programmable devices that subcutaneously infuse a rapid-acting insulin, both continuously to mimic peakless basal action and as a manual prandial bolus at mealtimes—basically, a more convenient and discrete means of delivering MDI insulin. Users must be well-versed in the operation and programming of the device, as well as the insertion and care of the cutaneous infusion site. CSII pumps are *not* automated diabetes management systems; dose adjustments are still made manually by well-trained patients and clinicians based on SMBG readings. Patients on CSII are best managed by an endocrinologist.

Performing Frequent SMBG Readings

Insulin-treated patients must recognize the importance of obtaining frequent SMBG readings, although many patients dislike performing frequent daily fingerstick readings. Patients should avoid the sensitive tips of the fingers; but instead use the sides of each fingertip, and rotate sites across the fingers of both hands (avoiding thumbs). Patients may also stagger the time points measured across different days in an alternating manner (e.g., only two time points per day, but alternate time points across different days to accumulate over several days' readings that still cover all four time points); however, frequent daily readings should still be encouraged when possible. Direct download of the raw data from the device's digital memory avoids the potential transcribing errors of written logbook records and are thus more reliable and credible. All current devices can sync either directly to desktop software programs or via cloud-based storage networks. Alternatively, continuous glucose monitoring (CGM) systems, if available, can be worn discretely on the skin and can record interstitial glucose readings every few minutes around the clock, thus providing much greater ease and convenience of obtaining frequent daily readings, provided that patients can be taught to properly use and care for such devices. Recent innovations integrating both insulin pumps and CGM sensors ("closed-loop" systems) show promise in potentially automating dose-adjustment decision-making but are not yet widely available. Patients using CGM or closed-loop systems are best managed by an endocrinologist.

Adjusting Insulin Doses

Some general principles:

- Since dose requirements are dictated by the SMBG readings, there is effectively no upper limit to the allowable dose range for insulin, so long as there is no hypoglycemia. However, patients who require greater than 200 total units per day to achieve euglycemia are still best managed by an endocrinologist.

- The recommended target range for preprandial readings is 80 to 130 mg/dL as much as possible (i.e., day-to-day variability at any time point is to be expected).[10] A good rule of thumb is to aim for at least 50% of all readings at any given time point to be within this target range. It follows that dose changes should never be made because of a single outlier reading, but only if readings exceed the target range at a given time point in a recurring or sustained manner over at least several days. One exception to this principle would be a severe or significantly symptomatic hypoglycemia event that is otherwise unexplainable (and therefore not easily preventable with lifestyle modifications), especially if it endangers the patient.

- As demonstrated in Table 24.16, the SMBG reading obtained at a given time point does not inform the dose adjustment needed right then; instead it informs the dose adjustment that is needed starting the next day, for the insulin injection that normally peaks at that time point. This means that, for multi-dose regimens, the SMBG readings at each time point independently inform the adjustment needed for its corresponding insulin injection, although it is prudent not to make simultaneous adjustments to too many of the patient's insulin doses all at once.

- Whenever possible, always first explore if lifestyle/behavioral factors might explain the variation at that time point (e.g., a change in meal intake or physical activity in the hours prior) before any dose change is made. If identified, correcting such factors may obviate the need to make the dose change. This is particularly germane to readings that fluctuate wildly (i.e., extreme highs along with extreme lows) at any given time point, which would suggest erratic day-to-day variations in dietary, lifestyle, or other behavioral factors rather than a problem with the corresponding insulin dose.

- Since patients vary widely in their dose requirements, it is prudent to initially underestimate any dose increase, and then more gradually titrate further upward according to SMBG readings so as to avoid precipitating sudden hypoglycemia. Increments of two to four units at a time are usually safe, although larger dose increments are also safe if all readings are far above target. Note that T1DM patients are generally much more sensitive to small changes, so dose increments should be made more cautiously for them.
- Patients who are sophisticated enough to interpret their own SMBG reading patterns correctly and account for all of the preceding factors may be empowered to alter their own doses at home, but this is best avoided in patients who have not demonstrated the appropriate understanding and skills to do so effectively.

Insulin-Induced Hypoglycemia

Sporadic, mild hypoglycemia episodes may be unavoidable when patients are tightly controlled. All patients should be taught how to anticipate, recognize, and abort hypoglycemia episodes when early adrenergic symptoms and signs occur. Adrenergic symptoms of hypoglycemia can be nonspecific (e.g., nervousness, tachycardia, palpitations, tremors); patients should be encouraged to confirm the episode with a SMBG reading if possible. Alleviation of symptoms following the ingestion of carbohydrates usually secures the diagnosis as differentiated from other causes (e.g., arrhythmias, panic attacks). If it occurs only sporadically, before making dose reductions, attempts should first be made to identify possible causative lifestyle/behavioral factors (e.g., missed meals, unanticipated excess physical activity), and thus avoid them in the future. Severe hypoglycemia, defined as episodes that require the assistance of another person, suggests that adrenergic symptoms were missed or exceeded, leading to neuroglycopenic symptoms (impairment of CNS function—e.g., impaired judgment, confusion, obtundation) and thus the inability to self-manage the episode effectively. Severe hypoglycemia should be prevented from recurring. Patients who are prone to frequent or recurrent severe hypogly-cemia despite attempts to avoid potential causative factors are best managed by an endocrinologist, and may be advised to keep glucagon (Table 24.17) on hand for emergency use by caregivers or other bystanders.

Fixed-Combination Injectable Agents

For T2DM patients suboptimally controlled on basal insulin alone, an alternative to the addition of prandial insulin injections is the addition of a GLP1Ra instead, which would still improve glucose control but with fewer injections, precipitate less weight gain (or possibly greater weight loss), and incur less risk of hypoglycemia.[47,48] There are currently two such combination agents available (**Table 24.18**), although any basal insulin may be used together with any GLP-1Ra if prescribed separately; side effects and cautions related to the individual agents still apply.

THYROID DISORDERS

INTRODUCTION

Thyroid disorders are very common. More than 12% of the U.S. population will develop a thyroid condition during their lifetime. An estimated 20 million Americans have some form of thyroid disease and around 60% of those with thyroid disease are unaware of their condition. Women are five to eight times more likely than men to have thyroid problems.[49] The common thyroid disorders seen in clinical practice include hypothyroidism, hyperthyroidism, thyroid nodule, and thyroid cancer. Thyroid hormone is an important determinant in development and growth, and in adults plays a critical role in the regulation of the function and metabolism of virtually every organ system. Undiagnosed thyroid disease may put patients at risk for certain serious conditions, such as cardiovascular diseases, osteoporosis, and infertility. Most thyroid diseases are life-long conditions that can be managed with medical attention.[50,51]

The thyroid gland participates with the hypothalamus and pituitary gland in a classic feedback control

TABLE 24.18 Fixed-Combination Injectable Agents

Medication	Dose/Frequency	Advantages	Disadvantages
Glargine/lixisenatide (Soliqua® 100/33)	(Dosing based on glargine component): 15–60 units SC daily (titrate weekly by 2–4-units increments)	Provides additive glucose-lowering effects but offsets the weight gain of insulin Requires fewer injections than intensifying by adding a prandial insulin Decreased risk of hypoglycemia than intensifying with more insulin	GI side effects and all cautions related to the GLP1Ra agent still apply
Degludec/liraglutide (Xultophy® 100/3.6)	(Dosing based on degludec component): 10–50 units SC daily (titrate 2×/week by 2-unit increments)		

GI, gastrointestinal; SC, subcutaneously.

loop. The thyroid hormones thyroxine (T4) and triiodothyronine (T3) are secreted from the thyroid gland under the stimulatory influence of pituitary thyrotropin (thyroid-stimulating hormone [TSH]). The thyrotropin-releasing hormone (TRH), a hypothalamic peptide, stimulates the synthesis and release of TSH. The T4 and T3 directly inhibit pituitary TSH secretion. The thyroid hormone also exerts a feedback effect on hypothalamus. The hypothalamic-pituitary-thyroid axis auto regulation keeps the thyroid hormone levels regulated in the body.

HYPOTHYROIDISM

Causes of hypothyroidism include the following:

- Hypopituitarism or hypothalamic disorders
- Congenital hypothyroidism
- Hashimoto's thyroiditis
- Lymphocytic thyroiditis following transient hyperthyroidism
- Thyroid ablation, surgery, or following Radioactive I 131 therapy
- Drugs; antithyroid drugs, including propylthiouracil, methimazole, lithium

Although hypothalamic or pituitary disorders can affect thyroid function, localized disease of the thyroid gland that results in decreased thyroid hormone production is the most common cause of hypothyroidism. In the National Health and Nutrition Examination Survey (NHANES 1999–2002) of 4,392 individuals reflecting the U.S. population reported hypothyroidism (defined as TSH levels exceeding 4.5 mIU/L) in 3.7% of the population.[52] Diagnostic laboratory assay used in the diagnosis of thyroid disorders includes TSH, free T4, and free T3 levels. Primary hypothyroidism would show an elevated TSH, normal free T4 level in early and low free T4 level in later course of hypothyroidism. A hypothalamic pituitary etiology (central hypothyroidism) would show a normal/low TSH and low free T4 and free T3 levels. The thyroid peroxidase antibody (TPO antibody) is utilized if assessing for autoimmune thyroid disorders.

Subclinical hypothyroidism is an entity usually defined as asymptomatic state when serum-free T4 levels are normal but TSH is elevated in the range 5 to 10 mU/L. Hashimoto's is the leading cause of hypothyroidism. The typical symptoms of hypothyroidism include fatigue, loss of energy, lethargy, weight gain, decreased appetite, cold intolerance, dry skin, hair loss, sleepiness, muscle pain, joint pain, weakness in the extremities, depression, emotional lability, forgetfulness, impaired memory, inability to concentrate, constipation, menstrual disturbances, impaired fertility, decreased perspiration, paresthesia and nerve

entrapment syndromes, blurred vision, decreased hearing, fullness in the throat, and hoarseness.

PHARMACOTHERAPY FOR HYPOTHYROIDISM

Levothyroxine is the treatment of choice for hypothyroidism. The usual starting dose of levothyroxine is 50 to 75 mcg. The usual treatment dose is 1.6 mcg/kg/day and may be titrated up to correct metabolic derangements, as evidenced by normal TSH and free T4 levels. In the elderly and patients with heart disease, the starting dose should be half of the usual dose and slow increment titration should be made every 6 weeks. Clinical benefits begin in 3 to 5 days and level off after 4 to 6 weeks. Achieving a TSH level within the reference range may take several months because of delayed readaptation of the hypothalamic-pituitary axis. In patients receiving treatment with LT4, dosing changes should be made every 6 to 8 weeks until the patient's TSH is in target range. In patients with central hypothyroidism, T4 levels rather than TSH levels are used to guide treatment. In most cases, the free T4 level should be kept in the upper third of the reference range.

Most of the hypothyroidism could be treated with oral levothyroxine, except intravenous levothyroxine is indicated in cases of severe hypothyroidism (myxedema). Most of the patients could be treated with levothyroxine (T4), but a small subset of patients continue to be symptomatic in spite of having the TSH in the normal range and combination of T4/T3 could be considered. Liothyronine is the synthetic T3 medication and available in 5 and 25 mcg tablets.

The physiological way to replace hypothyroidism is to use the nature-thyroid combination of T4 to T3 in a ratio of 10 to 14:1. The desiccated thyroid preparations (Armour® and Nature-Throid® T3) are natural thyroid medications that have both T4 and T3. Desiccated thyroid is derived from extracts of bovine or porcine thyroid glands. Desiccated thyroid is referred to as "natural thyroid" and generally contains T3 and T4 in a 1:4 ratio. It is made in a range of strengths, with tablets including 1/8, 1/4, 1/2, 1, 2, 3, 4, or 5 grains. One grain (60 mg) contains about 38 mcg of T4 and 9 mcg of T3. Because these preparations contain variable quantities of T3, they should not be prescribed for patients with known or suspected cardiac disease and are generally avoided. They also are not preferred in pregnancy, because they lead to relatively lower T4 levels.

Levothyroxine is the drug of choice during pregnancy. Increased thyroid hormone dosage requirements should be anticipated during pregnancy, especially in the first and second trimesters. Studies have suggested that in pregnant women with hypothyroidism, the LT4 dose should be increased by 30% at the confirmation of pregnancy and subsequently adjusted in accordance

TABLE 24.19 Pharmacotherapy for Thyroid Disorders

Medication	Dose/Frequency	Half-Life	Adverse Reactions
Levothyroxine (Synthroid®, Levoxyl®, and Tirosint®)	25, 50, 75, 88, 100, 112, 125, 137, 150, 175, 200, 300 mcg	6–7 days	Palpitations, increased appetite, tachycardia, nervousness, tremor, weight loss, diarrhea, headache, heat intolerance, anxiety, rash, dyspnea, muscle spasm
Liothyronine (Cytomel®)	5, 25, 50 mcg	1 day	
Desiccated Thyroid (Armour®, Nature-Throid®)	Armour®: 15, 30, 60, 90, 120, 180, 240, 300 mg Nature-Throid®: 16.25, 32.5, 48.75, 65, 81.25, 97.5, 113.75, 130, 146.25, 195, 260, 325 mg	2–7 days	

For product conversion: 100 mcg of levothyroxine = 25 mcg liothyronine = 60–65 mg thyroid (porcine) = 1 grain.

with TSH levels.[53] The TSH levels should be checked every 4 weeks during the first trimester and then every 6 weeks during the second and third trimesters. The TSH goal is less than 2.0 mIU/mL during pregnancy.

Thyroid medication should be taken on an empty stomach for better absorption. Medications including calcium carbonate, aluminum-containing antacids, sucralfate, iron supplements, and cholestyramine decrease the absorption of thyroid medication. There is a need for dose adjustment and an increased requirement of thyroid medication dosage with concomitant therapy with estrogen-containing medications (**Table 24.19**).

HYPERTHYROIDISM

Hyperthyroidism is a condition that results from metabolism effects of excessive circulating concentrations of thyroid hormones. Subclinical hyperthyroidism refers to the combination of suppressed TSH with normal free T4 or free T3 levels, regardless of the presence or absence of symptoms. Hyperthyroidism could be secondary to increased thyroid hormone production as in Graves's disease (GD), toxic nodule, or toxic multinodular goiter. Hyperthyroidism could also result from release of thyroid hormone due to destruction of thyroid follicles (thyroiditis) as in subacute thyroiditis, Hashitoxicosis (as seen in autoimmune thyroid disorder), or postpartum thyroiditis. Subacute thyroiditis may be painful (mostly viral in origin) and other types of thyroiditis are painless. Certain drugs like interferon alpha, amiodarone, lithium, tyrosine kinase inhibitor, and interlukin-2 may also lead to thyroiditis. The natural course following thyroiditis is the development of temporary or permanent hypothyroidism, the pathogenesis being destruction of existing follicles and decreased new thyroid hormone production if there is no new development of thyroid follicles.

In the United States, the prevalence of hyperthyroidism is approximately 1.2% (0.5% overt and 0.7% subclinical); the most common causes include GD, toxic multinodular goiter (TMNG), and toxic adenoma (TA).[54,55] GD accounts for 60% to 80% of patients with hyperthyroidism. It is ten times more common in women and highest risk of onset is between 40 to 80 years of age. The diagnostic workup for hyperthyroidism shows low TSH levels and high free T4 and free T3 levels. The presence of positive thyroid peroxidase antibody levels suggests autoimmune thyroid disorder, and thyroid-stimulating immunoglobulin levels are often seen in GD. The positive thyroid-stimulating immunoglobulin corelates with development of GD. The radioactive iodine uptake (RAIU) test is performed by administering iodine-123 (^{123}I) orally and measuring the percent uptake anywhere from 4 hours to 24 hours. RAIU would differentiate GD (diffusely high uptake), TNMG (multiple area with high uptake), toxic adenoma (solitary area of increased uptake) from thyroiditis (low uptake). Evaluation with the help of thyroid ultrasound can complement the RAIU scan showing the presence of thyroid nodule in the areas of increased uptake as seen on the RAIU scan.

PHARMACOTHERAPY FOR HYPERTHYROIDISM

The common symptoms of hyperthyroidism include nervousness, anxiety, increased perspiration, heat intolerance, hyperactivity, palpitations, and weight loss. Treatment of hyperthyroidism includes symptom relief, as well as antithyroid pharmacotherapy, radioactive iodine-131 (^{131}I) therapy (the preferred treatment of hyperthyroidism among U.S. thyroid specialists), or thyroidectomy. However, antithyroid medications are not effective in thyrotoxicosis in which scintigraphy shows low uptake of ^{123}I, as in patients with subacute thyroiditis, because these cases result from release of preformed thyroid hormone. Many of the neurologic and cardiovascular symptoms of thyrotoxicosis are relieved by beta-blocker therapy. Propranolol 10 to 40 mg one to four times daily, atenolol 25 to 100 mg daily, or metoprolol succinate 25 to 100 mg daily may be used to control palpitation and tachycardia. Calcium channel blockers (e.g., verapamil and diltiazem) can be used for the same purposes when beta-blockers are contraindicated or poorly tolerated.

Antithyroid drugs (e.g., methimazole and propylthiouracil) have been used for hyperthyroidism since their introduction in the 1940s. In adult men and nonpregnant women, they are used to control hyperthyroidism before definitive therapy with radioactive iodine. Antithyroid medications inhibit the formation and coupling of iodotyrosines in thyroglobulin. Because these processes are necessary for thyroid hormone synthesis, this inhibition induces a gradual reduction in thyroid hormone levels over 2 to 8 weeks or longer. A second action of propylthiouracil (but not methimazole) is inhibition of conversion of thyroxine (T4) to triiodothyronine (T3). T3 is more biologically active than T4; thus, a quick reduction in T3 levels is associated with a clinically significant improvement in thyrotoxic symptoms.

The drug of choice for treating hyperthyroidism is methimazole. Propylthiouracil (PTU) is used during the first trimester of pregnancy and preferred in patients with thyroid storm as it could decrease the T4 to T3 conversion. Methimazole could cause cutis aplasia abnormalities if given during the first trimester of pregnancy. Generally, if a nonpregnant woman who is receiving methimazole desires pregnancy, she should be switched to propylthiouracil before conception. After 12 weeks of gestation, she can be switched back to methimazole, with frequent monitoring.

The antithyroid drug dose should be titrated every 4 weeks until thyroid functions normalize. Some patients with GD go into a remission after treatment for 12 to 18 months, and the drug can be discontinued. Notably, half of the patients who go into remission experience a recurrence of hyperthyroidism within the following year. Nodular forms of hyperthyroidism (i.e., toxic multinodular goiter and toxic adenoma) are permanent conditions and will not go into remission.[56]

Adverse reactions to antithyroid medications are uncommon (affecting only 1% to 3% of patients), but they do occur. PTU is available in dosages of 50 mg. The maximum allowed dose is 150 mg thrice daily. Methimazole is available in 5- and 10-mg tablets. The maximum recommended dose is 10 mg thrice daily, but up to 60 mg a day could be used. Side effects include rash, itching, abnormal hair loss, and fever. Less common side effects include nausea, swelling, heartburn, muscle and joint aches, numbness, and headache. In very rare instances, both drugs can cause liver injury. PTU has a higher risk of liver injury than methimazole. Methimazole could lead to cholestatic jaundice. Agranulocytosis is another serious side effect, occurring twice as often in patients taking PTU than methimazole.

Regardless of their dosage, patients taking PTU have the same risk of developing the condition. With methimazole, on the other hand, the risk is likely dependent on the dosage. The lower the dose, the lower the risk. A complete blood count analysis should be performed in response to signs of infection and symptoms of sore throat. Agranulocytosis and elevation of liver enzymes generally require prompt discontinuation of antithyroid drugs and definitive therapy like radioactive ablation or surgery should be considered.

OSTEOPOROSIS

INTRODUCTION

Osteoporosis affects both males and females but with a higher incidence in females in the United States. Osteoporosis affects the lumbar spine and femur neck in 24.5% of women 65 years of age and older, and 5.1% of men 65 years of age and older.[57] According to the International Osteoporosis Foundation (IOF), approximately 30% of postmenopausal women have osteoporosis, and 40% of these women experience one or more fractures within their lifetime.[58] As the U.S. population ages, it is estimated that the cost of treating osteoporosis-related fractures will exceed $25 billion by 2025. It has been estimated that 43.4 million Americans have low bone mass and 10.2 million Americans have osteoporosis.[59]

BACKGROUND

Diagnosis of osteoporosis or osteopenia can be made by T-score (bone mineral density [BMD] result) or by the occurrence of a low-trauma fracture without evidence of metabolic bone disease. **Table 24.20** summarizes the criteria set by the World Health Organization (WHO) for the classification of osteoporosis or osteopenia. A new update to the 2020 guidelines further clarifies diagnosis of osteoporosis in postmenopausal women by taking into account the fracture risk assessment tool (FRAX). See **Table 24.21** for the 2020 update to diagnosis in postmenopausal women.

A diagnosis of osteoporosis can now be made even if a BMD screening results in a T-score of better than –2.5.[59] The FRAX tool can be found at www.shef.ac.uk/FRAX; select the appropriate continent and country. The risk factors used to calculate the FRAX score include country of residence, ethnicity, age, sex, weight, height, previous fracture, parent fractured hip, current smoking tobacco, current oral glucocorticoid exposure, diagnosis of rheumatoid arthritis, secondary osteoporosis, alcohol consumption for three or more units per day, and BMD score.[60]

TABLE 24.20 Classification of Osteoporosis or Osteopenia

T-Score	Classification
–1.0 or above	Normal
–1.0 to –2.5	Osteopenia or low bone mass
–2.5 or below	Osteoporosis
–2.5 or below with fragility fracture	Established or Severe osteoporosis

TABLE 24.21 Diagnosis of Osteoporosis in Postmenopausal Women (2020 Update)

1	T-score –2.5 or below in total proximal femur, lumbar spine, femoral neck, or ⅓ radius
2	Low, trauma hip or spine fracture*
3	T-score between –1.0 and –2.5 *and* fragility fracture of distal forearm, pelvis, and proximal humerus
4	T-score between –1.0 and 2.52 *and* high FRAX score or trabecular bone score, adjusted FRAX

*Regardless of bone mineral density.

TREATMENT OF OSTEOPOROSIS

All postmenopausal women should follow lifestyle and nutritional recommendations to maintain bone health. Calcium and vitamin D levels should be assessed, and low levels should be treated. Postmenopausal women who are at least 50 years or older should be assessed for risk of osteoporosis. The 10-year risk of fracture should be determined to classify the patient as either high risk/no prior fractures or very high risk/prior fractures. The level of risk will determine treatment recommendation based on an algorithm for management of postmenopausal osteoporosis. Treatment classes for high risk/no prior fractures include alendronate, denosumab, risedronate, or zoledronate. If a patient is unable to tolerate these therapies, then ibandronate and raloxifene can be considered as alternative therapy. If a patient experiences a progression of bone loss or recurrent fractures, a clinician may switch to abaloparatide, romosozumab, teriparatide, or injectable antiresorptive if on previous oral agent. For patients classified as very high risk/prior fractures, abaloparatide, denosumab, romosozumab, teriparatide, and zoledronate are indicated. If a patient is unable to tolerate these therapies then alendronate and risedronate can be considered as alternative therapy.[59]

Pharmacological Treatment

Bisphosphonates

Bisphosphonates (**Table 24.22**) increase bone density by binding to hydroxyapatite in bone to inhibit osteoclast activity and bone resorption. It is important to test for and treat hypocalcemia prior to initiating therapy. Reassess fracture risk after 5 years of oral therapy and after 3 years for intravenous therapy. Calcium and other positive cation supplements should be spaced apart to prevent a decrease in absorption of bisphosphonates.[59,61]

Estrogen Agonists/Antagonists

Estrogen agonists/antagonists are selective estrogen receptor modulators (SERM) that cause bone resorption to reduce risk of vertebral fractures (**Table 24.23**). In patients over 60 years of age, consider raloxifene, bazedoxifene, hormone therapy, calcitonin, or calcium plus vitamin D.[59]

Receptor Activator of Nuclear Factor Kappa-B Ligand Inhibitor

Denosumab is a receptor activator of nuclear factor kappa-B ligand (RANKL) inhibitor that is the first biologic agent (human monoclonal antibody) for the treatment of osteoporosis (**Table 24.24**). It inhibits osteoclast formation, which then leads to decreased bone resorption and an increase in bone mass. If denosumab is discontinued, then bone loss can be rapid and indicates a need to consider alternative agent to maintain BMD.

Parathyroid Hormones

Parathyroid hormone agents are classified as recombinant parathyroid hormone (PTH) analogues. These agents mimic the physiological actions of PTH and stimulate new bone formation by stimulating osteoblastic activity (**Table 24.25**).

Sclerostin Inhibitors

Romosozumab is a sclerostin inhibitor that will inhibit the sclerostin protein from preventing bone formation, which then results in an increase in osteoblast activity (**Table 24.26**). Romosozumab injection should be kept under refrigeration while stored. The injection should be allowed to come to room temperature for 30 minutes prior to administration.

Calcitonin

Calcitonin is a treatment that directly inhibits bone resorption but it is less effective than other agents (**Table 24.27**).

TABLE 24.22 Bisphosphonates

Medication	Dose/Frequency	Advantages	Disadvantages
Alendronate (Fosamax®, Binosto®)	Prevention*: 5 mg po daily or 35 mg po weekly Treatment**: 10 mg po daily or 70 mg po weekly Not on estrogen: 10 mg po daily	Oral weekly and monthly formulations Parenteral quarterly and yearly formulations Alendronate, risedronate, zoledronic acid have shown evidence for reduction of vertebral, nonvertebral, hip fractures	Ibandronate indicated only to decrease vertebral hip fractures Alendronate and zoledronic acid should be avoided if CrCl <35 mL/min; risedronate and ibandronate should be avoided if CrCl <30 mg/min Contraindications: hypokalemia and drug hypersensitivity Oral formulations: patients should take with full glass of water and remain upright for 30 minutes; 60 minutes for monthly formulation (Boniva®) Common side effects: dyspepsia, heartburn, nausea, myalgia, diarrhea, nausea, back or joint pain; rare side effect of severe osteonecrosis of the jaw Zoledronic acid: associated with flulike symptoms (fever, achiness, headache, runny nose) Binosto®: an effervescent tablet that contains 91.37 mg of alendronate sodium equivalent to 70 mg of alendronic free acid. Each tablet also contains 650 mg of sodium; use with caution in heart failure, hypertension, cirrhosis, or sodium restricted patients Administer 2 hours apart for calcium, antacids, magnesium supplements
Risedronate (Actonel®, Atelvia®)	Prevention and treatment*: 5 mg po daily or 35 mg po weekly or 75 mg po on 2 consecutive days per month or 150 mg po monthly Treatment (males): 35 mg po weekly		
Ibandronate (Boniva®)	Prevention and treatment*: 150 mg po monthly Treatment*: 3 mg IV every 3 months (over 15–30 seconds)		
Zoledronic acid (Reclast®)	Prevention*: 5 mg IV every 2 years Treatment**: 5 mg IV once yearly		

*postmenopausal women.

**postmenopausal women and men.

IV, intravenously; PO, by mouth.

Sources: Merck & Co., Inc. Fosamax [package insert]. 2010. Accessed October 21, 2020. https://www.merck.com/product/usa/pi_circulars/f/fosamax/fosamax_pi.pdf; Procter & Gamble Pharmaceuticals, Inc. Actonel [package insert]. 2008. Accessed October 21, 2020; https://www.accessdata.fda.gov/drugsatfda_docs/label/2009/020835s035lbl.pdf; Genentech, Inc. Boniva [package insert]. 2016. Accessed October 21, 2020. https://www.gene.com/download/pdf/boniva_tablets_prescribing.pdf; Novartis. Reclast [package insert]. 2020. Accessed October 21, 2020. https://www.novartis.us/sites/www.novartis.us/files/reclast.pdf?campaign=xjffzswh

TABLE 24.23 Estrogen Agonists/Antagonists

Medication	Dose/Frequency	Advantages	Disadvantages
Raloxifene (Evista®)	Prevention and treatment®: 60 mg po daily	Raloxifene: associated with decreased incidence of invasive estrogen receptor+ breast cancer; shown evidence to prevent vertebral fractures	Raloxifene: boxed warning of increased risk of VTE (DVT/PE), increased risk of death due to stroke in women at risk for coronary events or coronary artery disease Duavee®: boxed warning of endometrial cancer, dementia in women >65 years, increased risk of VTE, stroke (postmenopausal aged 50–79); do not use with additional estrogen therapy Both agents contraindicated in pregnancy; raloxifene contraindicated in VTE; Duavee® contraindicated with history of breast cancer, hepatic impairment, undiagnosed uterine bleeding, active VTE, thromboembolic disease Raloxifene: should be discontinued if patients develop illness/condition that requires prolonged period of immobilization; common side effects include leg cramps, hot flashes, peripheral edema, arthralgia Duavee®: common side effects include dyspepsia, nausea, abdominal pain, muscle spasm, diarrhea
Conjugated estrogens/ bazedoxifene (Duavee®)	Prevention (females with uterus)®: 1 tab (0.45 mg/20 mg) po daily (An equine estrogen/ SERM combination product indicated for postmenopausal women with intact uterus to prevent osteoporosis and treat moderate/severe vasomotor symptoms)		

*postmenopausal women.

DVT, deep vein thrombosis; PE, pulmonary embolism; PO, by mouth; SERM, selective estrogen receptor modulator; VTE, venous thromboembolism.

Sources: Pfizer. Duavee [package insert]. 2019. Accessed October 21, 2020. https://www.accessdata.fda.gov/drugsatfda_docs/label/2015/022247s002lbl.pdf; Eli Lilly and Company. Evista [package insert]. 2018. https://www.accessdata.fda.gov/drugsatfda_docs/label/2007/022042lbl.pdf

TABLE 24.24 Receptor Activator of Nuclear Factor Kappa-B Ligand Inhibitor

Medication	Dose/ Frequency	Advantages	Disadvantages
Denosumab (Prolia®)	Treatment*: 60 mcg SC every 6 months; must be administered by a clinician	Evidence for reduction of vertebral, nonvertebral, and hip fractures	Indicated only for treatment of postmenopausal osteoporosis Drug holidays not recommended due to potential of increased risk of fracture Common side effects include fatigue, edema, dyspnea, hypertension, headache, nausea, vomiting, diarrhea Monitor for development of osteonecrosis of the jaw as side effect

*postmenopausal women and men

SC, subcutaneously.

Source: Amgen. Prolia [package insert]. 2019. Accessed October 21, 2020. https://www.accessdata.fda.gov/drugsatfda_docs/label/2017/125320s181lbl.pdf

TABLE 24.25 Parathyroid Hormone

Medication	Dose/ Frequency	Advantages	Disadvantages
Teriparatide (Forteo®)	Treatment*: 20 mcg SC daily	Abaloparatide and teriparatide have shown reduction of vertebral and nonvertebral fractures	No studies yet to show strong evidence for reduction of risk of hip fracture Teriparatide and abaloparatide: boxed warning of dose and therapy duration–dependent osteosarcoma in rats; not indicated in patients who have risk of development of osteosarcoma
Abaloparatide (Tymlos®)	Treatment**: 80 mcg SC daily		Common side effects of both agents include leg cramps, pain, nausea, orthostasis or dizziness, arthralgia; abaloparatide is also associated with increased uric acid levels, antibody development and injection site redness No more than 2 years of therapy in patient lifetime

*postmenopausal women and men

** postmenopausal women

SC, subcutaneously.

Sources: Eli Lilly and Company. Forteo [package insert]. 2020. Accessed October 21, 2020. https://www.accessdata.fda.gov/drugsatfda_docs/label/2009/021318s012lbl.pdf; Radius Health. Tymlos [package insert]. 2018. Accessed October 21, 2020. https://www.accessdata.fda.gov/drugsatfda_docs/label/2017/208743lbl.pdf

TABLE 24.26 Sclerostin Inhibitor

Medication	Dose/ Frequency	Advantages	Disadvantages
Romosozumab (Evenity®)	Treatment: 210 mg SC (administer via two separate injections) monthly; treat for up to 12 months	Shown evidence for reduction of hip fracture	Boxed warning: may increase the risk of myocardial infarction, stroke, or cardiovascular death. It should not be initiated with history of previous myocardial infarction or stroke within the previous year. If patient has a myocardial infarction or stroke while on therapy, it should be discontinued. Common side effects: injection site reaction, headache, arthralgia Contraindication: hypokalemia Duration of therapy is limited to 12 months

SC, subcutaneously.

Source: Amgen. Evenity [package insert]. 2019. Accessed October 21, 2020. https://www.accessdata.fda.gov/drugsatfda_docs/label/2019/761062s000lbl.pdf

TABLE 24.27 Calcitonin

Medication	Dose/Frequency	Advantages	Disadvantages
Calcitonin (Miacalcin®)	Treatment: One spray (200 IU) in one nostril daily or 100 IU SC/IM once daily	Shown evidence for reduction of vertebral fracture	Risk of cancer with long-term use Common side effects: myalgia, back pain, dizziness, nausea, nasal ulceration, epistaxis, rhinitis Contraindicated in individuals who are allergic to salmon calcitonin

IM, intramuscularly; SC, subcutaneously.

Source: Novartis. Miacalcin [package insert]. Accessed October 21, 2020. https://www.accessdata.fda.gov/drugsatfda_docs/label/2009/017808s030lbl.pdf

CASE EXEMPLAR: Patient With Polydipsia and Weight Gain

FM is a 52-year-old man complaining of excessive thirst. He was in his usual state of health until about 3 to 4 weeks ago when he experienced a significant weight gain that he blames on the stay-at-home order in response to the COVID-19 pandemic. He has been lonely and depressed and sitting at home "eating everything in sight." Over the past week he has noticed increasing thirst, urinary frequency, and blurred vision.

Past Medical History
- Hypertension
- Hyperlipidemia

Medications
- Lisinopril, 10 mg daily
- Hydrochlorothiazide, 25 mg daily
- Atorvastatin, 10 mg daily

Physical Examination
- Height: 68 inches; weight: 262 lbs.; BMI: 39.8; blood pressure: 158/96; pulse: 82; respiration rate: 16; temperature: 98.2 °F
- Well-developed obese Latino male in no distress
- Lungs: clear
- Heart: regular rate and rhythm
- Extremities: no edema
- Neurological: no deficits

Labs
- Hematocrit: 42%
- Random capillary blood glucose: 358 mg/dL
- Hemoglobin A1c: 11.4%
- Urinalysis: specific gravity 1.010, pH 7.4, 4+ glucose, zero acetone

Discussion Questions

1. What nonpharmacologic treatments should be recommended to FM?
2. What pharmacologic treatments should be recommended or avoided in FM?
3. What additional laboratory tests should be recommended to FM?

CASE EXEMPLAR: Patient With Constellation of Symptoms

YG is a 14-year-old female who presents to the office with complaints of polydipsia, polyuria, polyphagia, weight loss, and blurred vision. She noticed the onset of these symptoms about 1 week ago. She had been in excellent health up until this point and active in school sports. She denies fevers, chills, or sweats. She denies skin changes. Shortness of breath prompted today's visit.

Past Medical History
- Usual childhood illnesses
- Menarche about 6 months ago; last menstrual period 2 weeks ago
- Gravida 0

Physical Examination
- Height: 66 inches; weight: 112 lbs.; BMI: 18.1; blood pressure: 132/60; pulse: 110; respiration rate: 20; temperature: 97.2 °F
- Well-developed thin female with mild resting tachypnea; fruity odor to breath
- Lungs: clear
- Heart: regular rate and rhythm
- Abdomen: benign

Labs
- Hematocrit: 42%
- Random blood glucose: greater than 600 mg/dL
- Urinalysis: specific gravity 1.036; pH 5; glucose: 4+; ketones: 4+; protein: negative

Discussion Questions

1. Based on YG's physical examination and lab results, what is the likely diagnosis and what immediate action should the clinician take?
2. What immediate pharmacological treatments should be implemented, and what information about the diagnosis should be provided to YG at this time?
3. What additional information about monitoring and laboratory testing should be provided to YG?

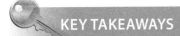

KEY TAKEAWAYS

- Nonpharmacological strategies (nutrition, lifestyle factors, weight control) are key, central components of optimal DM management, with pharmacological agents serving as important adjunctive therapies.
- For T1DM, the overall aim is to achieve near-normoglycemia by replacing insulin in a manner that mimics as closely as possible normal endogenous insulin secretion profiles in response to usual daily glucose fluctuations.
- For T2DM, the overall aim is to achieve near-normoglycemia by overcoming each patient's defects of normal insulin action using additive and complementary treatments.
- Metformin is the drug of choice as initial therapy for T2DM.
- Insulin is the only treatment option for T1DM and is also the most effective treatment for glucose control in T2DM.
- Levothyroxine is the drug of choice for hypothyroidism.
- The drug of choice for treating hyperthyroidism is methimazole.
- BMD together with FRAX score can be used to diagnose osteoporosis when T-scores are between –1 to –2.5.
- Lifestyle and adequate nutritional support are necessary to maintain bone health.
- Post menopausal women at 50 or older should be assessed for osteoporosis and 10-year risk of fractures.
- Patients with high risk of fracture should be treated with bisphosphonate such as alendronate or others.

REFERENCES

1. American Diabetes Association. *Statistics about diabetes.* Accessed March 1, 2020. https://www.diabetes.org/resources/statistics/statistics-about-diabetes
2. American Diabetes Association. 11. Microvascular complications and foot care: *Standards of Medical Care in Diabetes—2020. Diabetes Care.* 2020;43(suppl 1):S135–S151. doi:10.2337/dc20-S011.
3. Centers for Disease Control and Prevention. *National Diabetes Statistics Report, 2020.* https://www.cdc.gov/diabetes/data/statistics/statistics-report.html
4. Scheen AJ. Pathophysiology of type 2 diabetes. *Acta Clin Belg.* 2003;58(6):335–341. doi:10.1179/acb.2003.58.6.001
5. American Diabetes Association. 2. Classification and diagnosis of diabetes: *Standards of Medical Care in Diabetes—2020 Diabetes Care.* 2020;43(suppl 1):S14–S31. doi:10.2337/dc20-S002
6. The Diabetes Prevention Program Research Group. Reduction in the incidence of type 2 diabetes with lifestyle intervention or metformin. *N Eng J Med.* 2002;346(6):393–403. doi:10.1056/NEJMoa012512
7. American Diabetes Association. 5. Facilitating behavior change and well-being to improve health outcomes: *Standards of Medical Care in Diabetes—2020. Diabetes Care.* 2020;43(suppl 1):S48–S65. doi:10.2337/dc20-S005
8. Davidson MB, Hsia SH. *Meeting the American Diabetes Association standards of care: An algorithmic approach to clinical care of the diabetes patient.* American Diabetes Association; 2017:13.
9. American Diabetes Association. 10. Cardiovascular disease and risk management: *Standards of Medical Care in Diabetes—2020. Diabetes Care.* 2020;43(suppl 1):S111–S134. doi:10.2337/dc20-S010
10. American Diabetes Association. 6. Glycemic targets: *Standards of Medical Care in Diabetes—2020. Diabetes Care.* 2020;43(suppl 1):S66–S76. doi:10.2337/dc20-S006
11. The ADVANCE Collaborative Group. Intensive blood glucose control and vascular outcomes in patients with type 2 diabetes. *N Engl J Med.* 2008;358:2560–2572. doi:10.1056/NEJMoa0802987
12. The Action to Control Cardiovascular Risk in Diabetes Study Group. Effects of intensive glucose lowering in type 2 diabetes *N Engl J Med.* 2008;358:2545–2559. doi:10.1056/NEJMoa0802743
13. Ismail-Beigi F, Craven T, Banerji MA, et al. Effect of intensive treatment of hyperglycaemia on microvascular outcomes in type 2 diabetes: An analysis of the ACCORD randomised trial. *Lancet.* 2010;376:419–430. doi:10.1016/S0140-6736(10)60576-4
14. American Diabetes Association. 7. Diabetes technology: *Standards of Medical Care in Diabetes—2020. Diabetes Care.* 2020;43(suppl 1):S77–S88. doi:10.2337/dc20-S007
15. American Diabetes Association. 9. Pharmacologic approaches to glycemic treatment: *Standards of Medical Care in Diabetes—2020. Diabetes Care.* 2020;43(suppl 1):S98–S110. doi:10.2337/dc20-S009
16. Nauck MA, Kahle M, Baranov O, et al. Addition of a dipeptidyl peptidase-4 inhibitor, sitagliptin, to ongoing therapy with the glucagon-liker peptide-1 receptor agonist liraglutide: a randomized controlled trial in patients with type 2 diabetes. *Diab Obes Metab.* 2017;19(2):200–207. doi:10.1111/dom.12802
17. Rojas LBA, Gomes MB. Metformin: an old but still the best treatment for type 2 diabetes. *Diabetol Metab Syndr.* 2013;5:6. doi:10.1186/1758-5996-5-6
18. UK Prospective Diabetes Study (UKPDS) Group. Effect of intensive blood-glucose control with metformin on complication in overweight patients with type 2 diabetes (UKPDS 34). *Lancet.* 1998;352:854–865. doi:10.1016/S0140-6736(98)07037-8
19. UK Prospective Diabetes Study (UKPDS) Group. Intensive blood-glucose control with sulphonylureas or insulin compared with conventional treatment and risk of complications in patient with type 2 diabetes (UKPDS 33). *Lancet.* 1998;352:837–853. doi:10.1016/S0140-6736(98)07019-6

20. Riddle MC. A verdict for glimepiride: effsective and not guilty of cardiovascular harm. *Diabetes Care.* 2019;42(12):2161–2163. doi:10.2337/dci19-0034

21. Black C, Dennelly P, McIntyre L, et al. Meglitinide analogues for type 2 diabetes mellitus. *Cochrane Database Syst Rev.* 2007;18(2):CD004654. doi:10.1002/14651858.CD004654.pub2

22. Nanjan MJ, Mohammed M, Kumar BRP, et al. Thiazolidinediones as antidiabetic agents: a critical review. *Bioorganic Chem.* 2018;77:548–567. doi:10.1016/j.bioorg.2018.02.009

23. Dormandy JA, Charbonnel B, Eckland DJA, et al. Secondary prevention of macrovascular events in patients with type 2 diabetes in the PROactive Study (PROspective pioglitAzone Clinical Trial In macroVascular Events): a randomized trial. *Lancet.* 2005;366:1279–1289. doi:10.1016/S0140-6736(05)67528-9

24. Coleman RL, Scott CAB, Lang Z, et al. Meta-analysis of the impact of alpha-glucosidase inhibitors on incident diabetes and cardiovascular outcomes. *Cardiovasc Diabetol.* 2019;18:135. doi:10.1186/s12933-019-0933-y

25. Joshi SR, Standl E, Tong N, et al. Therapeutic potential of a-glucosidase inhibitors in type 2 diabetes mellitus: an evidence-based review. *Expert Opin Pharmacother.*2015;16(13):1959–1981. doi:10.1517/14656566.2015.1070827

26. Gallwitz B. Clinical use of DPP-4 inhibitors. *Front Endocrinol.* 2019;10:389. doi:10.3389/fendo.2019.00389

27. Santamaria M, Carlson CJ. Review of the cardiovascular safety of dipeptidyl peptidase-4 inhibitors and the clinical relevance of the CAROLINA trial. *BMC Cardiovasc Dis.* 2019;19:60. doi:10.1186/s12872-019-1036-0

28. Pinto L, Rados DV, Barkan SS, et al. Dipeptidyl peptidase-4 inhibitors, pancreatic cancer and acute pancreatitis: a meta-analysis with trial sequential analysis. *Sci Rep.* 2018;8:782. doi:10.1038/s41598-017-19055-6

29. Tentolouris A, Vlachakis P, Tzeravini E, et al. SGLT2 inhibitors: a review of their antidiabetic and cardioprotective effects. *Int J Environ Res Public Health.* 2019;16(16):E2925. doi:10.3390/ijerph16162965

30. Neal B, Perkovic V, Mahaffey KW, et al. Canagliflozin and cardiovascular and renal events in type 2 diabetes. *N Engl J Med.* 2017;377:644–657. doi:10.1056/NEJMoa1611925

31. Zinman B, Wanner C, Lachin JM, et al. Empagliflozin, cardiovascular outcomes, and mortality in type 2 diabetes. *N Engl J Med.* 2015;373:2117–2128. doi:10.1056/NEJMoa1504720

32. DeFronzo RA. Bromocriptine: a sympatholytic, D2-dopamineagonist for the treatment of type 2 diabetes. *Diabetes Care.* 2011;34(4):789–794. doi:10.2337/dc11-0064

33. Gaziano JM, Cincotta AH, O'Connor CM, et al. Randomized clinical trial of quick-release bromocriptine among patients with type 2 diabetes on overall safety and cardiovascular outcomes. *Diabetes Care.* 2010;33:1503–1508. doi:10.2337/dc09-2009

34. Handelsman Y. Role of bile acid sequestrants in the treatment of type 2 diabetes. *Diabetes Care.* 2011;34(suppl 2):S244–S250. doi:10.2337/dc11-s237

35. Romera I, Cebrian-Cuenca A, Alvarez-Guisasola F, et al. A review of practical issues on the use of glucagon-like peptide-1 receptor agonists for the management of type 2 diabetes. *Diabetes Ther.* 2019;10(1):5–19. doi:10.1007/s13300-018-0535-9

36. Davies M, Pieber TR, Hartoft-Nielsen ML, et al. Effect of oral semaglutide compared with placebo and subcutaneous semaglutide on glycemic control in patients with type 2 diabetes. A randomized clinical trial. *JAMA.* 2017;318(15):1460–1470. doi:10.1001/jama.2017.14752

37. Marso SP, Daniels GH, Brown-Frandsen K, et al. Liraglutide and cardiovascular outcomes in type 2 diabetes. *N Engl J Med.* 2016;375:311–322. doi:10.1056/NEJMoa1603827

38. Gerstein HC, Colhoun HM, Dagenais GR, et al. Dulaglutide and cardiovascular outcomes in type 2 diabetes (REWIND): a double-blind, randomized placebo-controlled trial. *Lancet.* 2019;394(10193):121–130. doi:10.1016/S0140-6736(19)31149-3

39. Marso SP, Bain SC, Consoli A, et al. Semaglutide and cardiovascular outcomes in patients with type 2 diabetes. *N Engl J Med.* 2016;375:1834–1844. doi:10.1056/NEJMoa1607141

40. Nauck MA, Friedrich N. Do GLP-1-based therapies increase cancer risk? *Diabetes Care.* 2013;36(suppl 2):S245–S252. doi:10.2337/dcS13-2004

41. Ryna G, Briscoe TA, Jobe L. Review of pramlintide as adjunctive therapy in treatment of type 1 and type 2 diabetes. *Drug Des Devel Ther.* 2008;2:203–214. doi:10.2147/DDDT.S3225

42. Machinani S, Bazargan-Hejazi S, Hsia SH. Psychological insulin resistance among low-income, U.S. racial minority patients with type 2 diabetes. *Prim Care Diabetes* 2013;7:51–55. doi:10.1016/j.pcd.2012.11.003

43. Hayes RP, Fitzgerald JT, Jacober SJ. Primary care physician beliefs about insulin initiation in patients with type 2 diabetes. *Int J Clin Pract.* 2008;62(6):860–868. doi:10.1111/j.1742-1241.2008.01742.x

44. Ellis K, Mulnier H, Forbes A. Perceptions of insulin use in type 2 diabetes in primary care: a thematic synthesis. *BMC Fam Pract.* 2018;19(1):70. doi:10.1186/s12875-018-0753-2

45. The Diabetes Control and Complications Trial Research Group. The effect of intensive treatment of diabetes on the development and progression of long-term complications in insulin-dependent diabetes mellitus. *N Engl J Med.* 1993;329:977–986. doi:10.1056/NEJM199309303291401

46. The Diabetes Control and Complications Trial/Epidemiology of Diabetes Interventions and Complications (DCCT/EDIC) Study Research Group. Intensive diabetes treatment and cardiovascular disease in patients with type 1 diabetes. *N Engl J Med.* 2005;353:2643–2653. doi:10.1056/NEJMoa052187

47. Eng C, Kramer CK, Zinman B, et al. Glucagon-like peptide-1 receptor agonist and basal insulin combination treatment for the management of type 2 diabetes: a systematic review and meta-analysis. *Lancet.* 2014;384:2228–2234. doi:10.1016/S0140-6736(14)61335-0

48. Maiorino MI, Chiodini P, Bellastella G, et al. Insulin and glucagon-like peptide 1 receptor agonist combination therapy in type 2 diabetes: a systematic review and meta-analysis of randomized controlled trials. *Diabetes Care.* 2017;40:614–624. doi:10.2337/dc16-1957

49. General Information/Press Room–American Thyroid Association. Accessed December 1, 2019. https://www.thyroid.org/media-main/press-room

50. Yen PM. Physiological and molecular basis of thyroid hormone action. *Physiol Rev.* 2001;81:1097–1142. doi:10.1152/physrev.2001.81.3.1097

51. Brent GA. Mechanisms of thyroid hormone action. *J Clin Invest.* 2012;122:3035–3043. doi:10.1172/JCI60047

52. Aoki Y, Belin RM, Clickner R, et al. Serum TSH and total T4 in the United States population and their association with participant characteristics: National Health and Nutrition Examination Survey (NHANES 1999–2002) *Thyroid.* 2007;17(12):1211–1223. doi:10.1089/thy.2006.0235

53. Alexander EK, Pearce EN, Brent GA, et al. 2017 Guidelines of the American Thyroid Association for the diagnosis and management of thyroid disease during pregnancy and the postpartum. *Thyroid.* 2017;27(3):315–389. doi:10.1089/thy.2016.0457

54. Ross DS, Burch HB, Cooper DS, et al. 2016 American Thyroid Association Guidelines for diagnosis and management of hyperthyroidism and other causes of thyrotoxicosis. *Thyroid.* 2016;26(10):1343–1421. doi:10.1089/thy.2016.0229

55. Girgis CM, Champion BL, Wall JR. Current concepts in graves. *Ther Adv Endocrinol Metabol.* 2011;2(3):135–144. doi:10.1177/2042018811408488

56. Porterfield JR Jr, Thompson GB, Farley DR, et al. Evidence-based management of toxic multinodular goiter (Plummer's disease). *World J Surg.* 2008;32(7):1278–1284. doi:10.1007/s00268-008-9566-0

57. Centers for Disease Control and Prevention. Percentage of adults aged 65 and over with osteoporosis or low bone mass at the femur neck or lumbar spine: United States, 2005–2010. Accessed November 6, 2015. https://www.cdc.gov/nchs/data/hestat/osteoporsis/osteoporosis2005_2010.htm

58. International Osteoporosis Foundation. Osteoporosis & musculoskeletal disorders—Osteoporosis—What is osteoporosis? https://www.iofbonehealth.org/epidemiology

59. Camacho PM, Petak SM, Binkley N, et al. American Association of Clinical Endocrinologists/American College of Endocrinology clinical practice guidelines for the diagnosis and treatment of postmenopausal osteoporosis—2020 Update. *Endocr Pract.* 2020;26(5):564–570. doi:10.4158/GL-2020-0524

60. Centre for Metabolic Bone Diseases. Welcome to FRAX®. http:// www.shef.ac.uk/FRAX

61. Rizzoli R, Reginster JY, Boonen S, et al. Adverse reactions and drug-drug interactions in the management of women with postmenopausal osteoporosis. *Calcif Tissue Int.* 2011;89(2):91–104. doi:10.1007/s00223-011-9499-8

Pharmacotherapy for Hematologic Disorders

Thamer Khasawneh and Matthew Horton

IRON-DEFICIENCY ANEMIA

In 1681 Sydenham first identified the importance of iron replacement in chlorosis; however, it was not until the 19th century that French physician Pierre Blaud would report cures after introducing pills that contained ferrous sulfate.[1] Approximately 30% of the world is estimated to be anemic with the most common nutritional deficiency and anemia being iron-deficiency anemia (IDA). Globally IDA affects females up to seven times more than males. In 2010 roughly 20,000 out of 100,000 or one in five females were affected by anemia globally.[2] Overall incidence of IDA has been down trending when comparing data from 1990 to 2010.[2]

BACKGROUND

There are two forms of iron: heme iron, and nonheme iron. Heme iron, which can be found in meat, poultry, and fish, is better absorbed by the body due to the presence of enzymes known as "heme-transporting ATPases," which catalyze transmembrane movement of iron into the bloodstream.

Sources of nonheme iron include plants, dairy, legumes, cereals, breads, and in elemental form as found in fortified foods.[3] Absorption of nonheme iron is enhanced by an acidic gastric environment, ascorbic acid, and meat or fish. Absorption is inhibited by phytates (e.g., legumes, whole grains, bran, oats, and rye fibers), tannins/polyphenols (e.g., tea, cereals, and select vegetables), calcium, and soy protein.

Calcium inhibits the absorption of both forms of iron; however, the effect of calcium on absorption rates for heme iron is less significant than on nonheme iron. So while heme iron may constitute only 10% to 15% of dietary iron intake, it represents 40% or more of total absorbed iron, indicating that this source of dietary iron may be more important to iron levels than the total amount of ingested iron. [4]

The protein hepcidin controls systemic iron hemostasis and is driven by erythropoietic needs of hemoglobin synthesis.[5] **Table 25.1** summarizes the recommended dietary reference intake (DRI) expressed as elemental iron.

RISK FACTORS FOR IRON-DEFICIENCY ANEMIA

Causes of IDA include insufficient intake of iron, provoked iron loss, decreased iron absorption, iron depletion due to increased demand, and redistribution of iron stores.[6] Insufficient intake of iron is commonly seen in individuals who consume meatless diets (e.g., vegans and vegetarians), those with malnutrition (more common in resource-scarce countries), and individuals with psychological conditions such as dementia.[7]

Iron loss can be provoked by hemorrhage (acute/traumatic and chronic) caused by a range of conditions.[6,8] Related gastrointestinal (GI) conditions include hematemesis (vomiting of blood); melena, the passage of black, tarry stools associated with bleeding in the upper GI tract or colon; ulcer; colonic vascular ectasia, dilated, tortuous vessels in the cecum and ascending colon that cause GI bleeding; hiatal hernia with linear erosions; colonic polyps; and Crohn's disease. It can also be caused by cancer (e.g., colon and gastric cancer) and occult bleeding from GI inflammation, malignancy, exercise, or parasites like hookworm and whipworm. Frequent blood removal via donation or blood draws for diagnostic testing can lead to iron loss, as well as menorrhagia, which can be mitigated by prescribing oral contraceptives.

Medications that reduce acid production, such as antacids (e.g., calcium carbonate), H2 receptor antagonists (H2RA), or proton pump inhibitors (PPIs), may reduce iron absorption. Celiac disease, autoimmune atrophic gastritis, *Helicobacter pylori*, and inflammatory bowel disease (IBD; e.g., Crohn's disease and ulcerative colitis) can impair iron absorption.[8-12] Patients with celiac disease, autoimmune atrophic gastritis, and *H. pylori* infection typically do not respond well to oral iron therapy.[5,9] This is true also of patients with IBD; however, several studies have shown ferric maltol to be a safe and effective alternative to intravenous therapy, which still remains first line.[5,13-15]

Iron depletion due to increased demand can be found in infants, toddlers, young children, and adolescents as a result of expanding erythropoiesis during phases of rapid growth. Pregnant, lactating, and postpartum women are susceptible to iron depletion and require oral iron therapy. Redistribution of iron stores is medication induced, primarily from erythropoiesis-stimulating agents (ESA) for hemodialysis (HD) patients.

Risk factors also include rare genetic causes, namely iron refractory iron deficiency anemia (IRIDA) and SLC11A2 mutation. IRIDA is a recessive anemia caused by mutations in the TMPRSS6 gene. It inhibits hepcidin transcription, leading to high serum hepcidin levels, which limits iron release from absorption sites and stores. This results in a microcytic anemia that is refractory to oral therapy. IRIDA is more prevalent in Caucasian and Asian populations. The most common variant is the rs855791, A736V, which influences hepcidin levels.[5] The SLC11A2 mutation encodes the divalent metal transporter 1 (DMT1), which is a transmembrane protein that is important for duodenal iron absorption and erythroid iron transport.[16]

SIGNS AND SYMPTOMS OF IRON-DEFICIENCY ANEMIA

Anemic patients may present with pallor, decreased palpation of the tongue, cheilosis (i.e., cracking at the corners of the mouth), and defects in the nail beds (e.g., spooning, Mees lines, and koilonychia). Symptoms are generally vague but those that may indicate

TABLE 25.1 Recommended Dietary Intake for Iron

Patient Age	Recommended Iron Intake	
	Males	Females
14–18 years	11 mg daily	15 mg daily Pregnancy: 30–60 mg daily Lactation: 10 mg daily
19–50 years	8 mg daily	18 mg daily Pregnancy: 30–60 mg daily Lactation: 9 mg daily
≥50 years	Recommended dietary allowance: 8 mg daily	Recommended dietary allowance: 8 mg daily

Source: Food and Nutrition Board Institute of Medicine. *Dietary Reference Intakes for Vitamin A, Vitamin K, Arsenic, Boron, Chromium, Copper, Iodine, Iron, Manganese, Molybdenum, Nickel, Silicon, Vanadium, and Zinc.* National Academies Press; 2001. doi:10.17226/10026

IDA include generalized fatigue, pica or the ingestion of non-nutrition materials (e.g., clay, dirt, paper), brittle nails, hair loss, and restless leg syndrome. Additionally, pagophagia, which is a craving for ice, is strongly associated with IDA and can lead to gingival disease. It is important to note that no symptoms may be apparent with mild cases of anemia.[1]

DIAGNOSIS OF IRON-DEFICIENCY ANEMIA

The "mean corpuscular volume" (MCV) is a measure of the average volume of a red blood cell (RBC). MCV measurement drives the classification of anemia—microcytic anemia, normocytic anemia, or macrocytic anemia. The measure is attained by multiplying a volume of blood by the proportion of blood that is cellular (the hematocrit) and dividing it by the number of erythrocytes (RBCs) in that volume. It is expressed as femtoliters (fL) or 10^{-15} L/cell.

The normal value for adult males and females is 80 to 100 fL. If anemia is present in this range, it is known as *normocytic anemia*; it could indicate blood loss (undiagnosed occult bleed, trauma, or surgery), bone marrow suppression (aplastic anemia), or anemia of chronic disease. An MCV of less than 80 fL indicates small RBC size or *microcytic anemia*, which is likely caused by IDA. Microcytic, *hypochromic anemia*, as the name suggests, is the type of anemia in which the circulating RBCs are smaller than the usual size of RBCs (microcytic) and have decreased red color (hypochromic). It is defined by a mean corpuscular hemoglobin (MCH) of less than 28 pg.[1,17] An MCV of greater than 100 fL indicates a large RBC size or *macrocytic anemia*, which is likely caused by drugs like hydroxyurea and zidovudine, alcohol consumption, and vitamin 12 or folate deficiency.[6,18] *Anisocytosis* is a condition in which the RBCs are unequal in size; greater red cell distribution width (RDW) is greater than 15 mcM.

Ferritin, or apoferritin, is protein in plasma that represents the body's iron stores that can be used for hemoglobin synthesis. It is labile and may increase with inflammation or hepatocellular injury. If inflammation and hepatic injury can be ruled out, then ferritin is the best indicator of ID and IDA. Normal serum ferritin levels are 30 to 300 ng/mL. A level of less than 30 ng/mL is indicative of ID with or without anemia (sensitivity: 92%; specificity: 98%), although it is usually seen only in IDA.[1,17]

Total iron-binding capacity (TIBC) and *transferrin saturation* (TSAT) measure the level of transferrin, a transport protein, which delivers iron to the bone marrow where it is incorporated into hemoglobin in circulation.[1,17] The measure is calculated as follows:

$$\text{TIBC (ug/dL)} = \text{transferrin (mg/dL)} \times 1.389$$
$$\text{TSAT \%} = (\text{serum iron level} \times 100)/\text{TIBC}$$

A TSAT of less than 16% to 20% indicates a very low iron supply that cannot sustain hemoglobin synthesis and red cell production; however, by itself it is not diagnostic of IDA.

Serum iron is the level of iron bound to transferrin. It is highly affected by inflammation, and the value can change daily due to iron demand from supporting the production of new RBCs. No value is indicative of IDA.[1] The *reticulocyte count*, often overlooked, is expressed as a percentage of all RBC or in absolute numbers per microliter of whole blood. If adjusted for premature release of cells from the bone marrow, it can be used to estimate the rate of effective marrow production compared to normal. Normal is a production index of 1. IDA is likely with a production index of greater than 2.[1]

In patients with inflammation, ferritin levels of 30 to 100 ng/mL are strong indicators of absolute iron deficiency.[17] If available, check MCH for hypochromic cells less than 28 pg and low hemoglobin density (LHD) of greater than 4%.

GUIDELINE-DIRECTED THERAPY FOR IRON-DEFICIENCY ANEMIA

There are no set guidelines specifically for IDA. Rather, treatment options for IDA are located in various guidelines for specific disease states.

Patients With Chronic Kidney Disease

Anemia in Chronic Kidney Disease (CKD) Guidelines (Kidney Disease: Improving Global Outcomes [KDIGO])[19]:

Recommend iron therapy (oral or parenteral) when TSAT less than or equal to 30%, serum ferritin less than or equal to 500 ng/mL, and Hbg less than 13 g/dL in males and 12 g/dL in females who desire an increase in Hgb level, to avoid blood transfusions, to reduce anemia-related symptoms, and/or to reduce erythropoiesis-stimulating agent (ESA) dose.

- Iron therapy is not recommended when TSAT is greater than 30% or serum ferritin is greater than 500 ng/mL due to lack of evidence.
- Also refer to National Institute for Health and Care Excellence (NICE) guidelines.[20]

Patients With Inflammatory Bowel Disease

The European Consensus on the Diagnosis and Management of Iron Deficiency and Anemia in Inflammatory Bowel Disease Guidelines (ECCO Guidelines)[17,21]:

- Recommend iron therapy (preferably parenteral) for patients with ferritin levels less than 30 ng/mL or ferritin less than 100 ng/mL and TSAT less than 20%

Patients With Symptomatic Chronic Heart Failure

European Society of Cardiology Heart Failure Guidelines[1,22,23]:

- Recommend starting parenteral iron therapy (e.g., ferric carboxymaltose) in patients with IDA defined by serum ferritin less than 100 ng/mL or ferritin between 100 to 299 ng/mL and TSAT less than 20% to help alleviate symptoms and improve exercise capacity and quality of life.
- Also refer to the American College of Physicians (ACP) Treatment of Anemia in Patients with Heart Disease guideline.[24]

Patients With Cancer

National Comprehensive Cancer Network (NCCN) guidelines[17,25–27]:

- Recommend iron therapy (oral or parenteral) for patients with absolute ID: ferritin less than 30 ng/mL and TSAT less than 20%.
- Recommend parenteral iron therapy for functional ID: ESA plus ferritin levels 30 to 800 ng/mL and TSAT less than 50%.
- Recommend no iron therapy for possible functional iron deficiency: ferritin greater than 500 to 800 ng/mL and TSAT less than 50%.
  - Recommend no iron therapy: ferritin greater than 800 ng/mL or TSAT greater than or equal to 50%.

Patients With Irritable Bowel Disease

Refer to the guidelines published by Gasche et al.[28]

PHARMACOTHERAPY FOR IRON-DEFICIENCY ANEMIA

Oral iron therapy in the form of ferrous sulfate is the common initial therapy for most patients with IDA. Patients with renal failure undergoing hemodialysis require parenteral iron repletion.[5] See **Table 25.2** for guidance on selection of appropriate iron therapy. For initial therapy options, it is important to avoid enteric-coated, controlled-, or slow-release formulations of ferrous sulfate as they release iron beyond the duodenum, which is the site of maximal absorption.[5,29,30]

Oral Iron Therapy

Oral therapy is the most cost-effective and direct approach to treating IDA. No formulation of oral iron has been found to be superior. While there is no consensus on the goal of therapy, current recommendations are to reduce reticulocytosis within a few days and increase hemoglobin by 1 to 2 g/dL every 2 weeks, replenishing iron stores in 3 to 6 months.[6,31] Oral therapy prevents the need for parenteral compounding, nursing administration, and monitoring for anaphylaxis.

The mechanism of action (MOA) is the same for all formulations except ferric maltol.[32] Oral iron formulations replenish iron stores found in hemoglobin, myoglobin, and other enzymes and are necessary for oxygen transport in hemoglobin. See **Table 25.3** for percentage of elemental iron in oral iron formulations.

Ferrous sulfate is the most common and cheapest option. The typical dose is 325 mg one to three times daily. This formulation is notorious for constipation and GI upset. Recent studies have shown that one tablet every other day results in greater absorption and possibly less adverse effects, although the latter did not reach statistical significance. One drawback is the duration of therapy must be doubled.[33,34] Two publications describe how there was a paradoxical effect of lower iron absorption when giving more frequent and higher doses of iron to iron-depleted women without anemia.[35,36] The mechanism appears to be due to increased hepcidin levels, which regulates iron metabolism. An increase in hepcidin due to an increase in iron intake or inflammation due to infection decreases iron absorption, recycling, and storage.[37] This supports giving lower less frequent doses might improve iron repletion and patient compliance. See **Table 25.4** for additional formulations and dosages.

Iron Absorption and Drug–Drug Interactions

Oral iron therapy is best taken on an empty stomach 1 or 2 hours before or after meals as absorption is reduced when taken with food; however, taking with meals may mitigate an adverse effect of GI upset and thus increase medication adherence. Medications that reduce acid production such as antacids (e.g., calcium carbonate),

H_2 blockers, or proton pump inhibitors (PPIs), may also reduce iron absorption; patients should take iron 2 hours before or 4 hours after taking these.

TABLE 25.2 Selection of Iron Agents

Consider Oral Iron Replacement	Consider IV Iron Replacement
Urgent replacement is not indicated (i.e., patient is not at risk of transfusion)	Urgent replacement is indicated (i.e., symptomatic, Hgb not at goal and at risk of requiring transfusion)
Patient is asymptomatic	
Patient has history of tolerating oral iron	Patient cannot tolerate oral iron replacement
Patient previously required IV iron replacement, but iron stores have stabilized and are at goal	Patient has history of GI ulceration, Crohn's disease, or ulcerative colitis. Black stool as side effect of iron may mask GI bleed
Patient has chronic infection	

GI, gastrointestinal; Hgb, hemoglobin.

TABLE 25.3 Elemental Iron in Oral Iron Formulations

Iron Salt	Percentage of Elemental Iron
Ferric maltol	100%
Carbonyl iron	>98%–100%
Iron polysaccharide complex	46%–100% (depends on formulation)
Ferrous fumarate	33%
Ferrous sulfate exsiccated (dried)	32%
Ferrous sulfate	20%
Ferrous gluconate	12%

Sources: Gasche C, Ahmad T, Tulassay Z, et al. Ferric maltol is effective in correcting iron deficiency anemia in patients with inflammatory bowel disease: results from a phase-3 clinical trial program. *Inflamm Bowel Dis.* 2015;21(3):579–588. doi:10.1097/MIB.0000000000000314; Gensavis Pharmaceuticals. NovaFerrum (polysaccharide-iron complex) [prescribing information]. Updated November 18, 2014. https://rxdruglabels.com/lib/rx/rx-meds/novaferrum-1; Gensavis Pharmaceuticals. NovaFerrum 50 (polysaccharide-iron complex) [prescribing information]. Updated October 31, 2013. https://dailymed.nlm.nih.gov/dailymed/lookup.cfm?setid=46abb133-711c-4219-ba6e-42cb64abf451; Manoguerra AS, Erdman AR, Booze LL, et al. Iron ingestion: an evidence-based consensus guideline for out-of-hospital management. *Clin Toxicol (Phila).* 2005;43(6):553–570. doi:10.1081/CLT-200068842; Martin Ekwealor Pharmaceuticals. Myferon 150 (polysaccharide-iron complex) [prescribing information]. Updated February 20, 2014. https://dailymed.nlm.nih.gov/dailymed/drugInfo.cfm?setid=c672cb8e-05a2-4ff5-b3bb-47acd955c2d9; McDonagh M, Cantor A, Bougatsos C, et al. Routine Iron Supplementation and Screening for Iron Deficiency Anemia in Pregnant Women: A Systematic Review to Update the U.S. Preventive Services Task Force Recommendation [Evidence Synthesis No. 123, AHRQ Publication No. 13-05187-EF-2; Table 1]. Agency for Healthcare Research and Quality; 2015. https://www.ncbi.nlm.nih.gov/books/NBK285987/table/ch1.t1; Schmidt C, Ahmad T, Tulassay Z, et al. Ferric maltol therapy for iron deficiency anaemia in patients with inflammatory bowel disease: long-term extension data from a Phase 3 study. *Aliment Pharmacol Ther.* 2016;44(3):259–270. doi:10.1111/apt.13665; Stallmach A, Büning C. Ferric maltol (St10): a novel oral iron supplement for the treatment of iron deficiency anemia in inflammatory bowel disease. *Expert Opin Pharmacother.* 2015;16(18):2859–2867. doi:10.1517/14656566.2015.1096929

TABLE 25.4 Pharmacotherapy for Iron-Deficiency Anemia

Medication	Dosage (Adult)/Frequency[a]	Side Effects
Ferrous sulfate	325 mg one to three times daily	Nausea, vomiting, constipation, abdominal pain or cramping, flatulence, dyspepsia, upset stomach, metallic taste, darkening of stools
Ferrous gluconate	324 mg one to three times daily	
Ferrous fumarate	324 mg one to three times daily	
Ferrous sulfate exsiccated (dried)	Varies based on formulation FeoSol® original: 200 mg one to three times daily	
Iron polysaccharide complex	Varies based on formulation 50–200 mg daily	
Ferric maltol (Accrufer®)	30 mg bid	
Carbonyl iron	Varies based on formulation Feosol® natural release: 45 mg once daily	
Ferrous sulfate slow release	Varies based on formulation Slow Fe®: 142 mg once daily	
Iron dextran (Infed®)	25-mg test dose, followed by 60 minutes of observation, then up to 1,000 mg total given once	Hypotension, dyspnea, pruritis, headache, muscle cramps, anaphylaxis (rare)
Iron sucrose (Venofer®)	HD-dependent CKD: 100 mg/dialysis session, up to 1,000 mg Peritoneal-dialysis CKD: 2,300-mg infusions 14 days apart, followed by 400-mg dose 14 days later (total: 1,000 mg) Nondialysis CKD: 200 mg once daily × 5 doses given anytime within 14 days or 500 mg on days 1 and 14[b]	
Ferric gluconate (Ferrlecit®)	IDA in HD patients: 125 mg to 250 mg (off label)/dialysis session, up to 1,000 mg or approximately eight dialysis sessions	
Ferumoxytol (Feraheme®)	Dose expressed as elemental iron: 510 mg × two doses 3–8 days apart; monitor for 30 minutes afterward	
Ferric carboxymaltose (Injectafer®)	Dose expressed as elemental iron: <50 kg: 15 mg/kg on day 1; repeat dose after at least 7 days ≥50 kg: 750 mg on day 1; repeat dose after at least 7 days Maximum: 750 mg/single dose; 1500 mg per course	

bid, twice daily; CKD, chronic kidney disease; HD, hemodialysis; IDA, iron-deficiency anemia.

[a]Expressed as formulation strength unless otherwise noted.

[b]Less data exists to support this dosing strategy.

Antibiotics such as cefdinir, fluoroquinolones, and tetracyclines—and, to a lesser extent, doxycycline and minocycline—can chelate iron and decrease absorption of both the iron and the antibiotic. Exceptions include ferric carboxymaltose, ferric gluconate, ferumoxytol, iron dextran complex, and iron sucrose. Cefdinir interacts with iron to form an insoluble complex, which results in red nonbloody stool. When taken with oral iron, tetracycline and quinolones should be taken 2 hours before (except moxifloxacin, which should be taken 4 hours before) and 4 hours after. Levofloxacin should be taken 2 hours after, ciprofloxacin should be taken 6 hours after, and moxifloxacin should be taken 8 hours after. With the exception of pamidronate and zoledronic acid, bisphosphonate derivatives (e.g., tiludronate, clodronate, and etidronate) should be taken

2 hours before and 2 hours after. Alendronate and risedronate should be taken 30 minutes after. Ibandronate should be taken 60 minutes after.

Antiviral medications like dolutegravir and raltegravir serum concentrations may be decreased and should be taken 2 hours before or 6 hours after. Oral iron should be avoided for patients taking baloxavir marboxil. For patients with Parkinson's disease, serum levels of entacapone and levodopa may be decreased and administration with oral iron should be separated by 2 hours. Serum levels of levothyroxine, used to treat hypothyroidism, may be decreased by oral iron and administration should be separated by 4 hours. Higher doses of vitamin C (≥200 mg) may increase acidity and thereby increase transportation of iron across cell membranes into the body and enhance absorption of iron.

Adverse Effects

Accidental iron overdose in children under 6 may be fatal. In cases of overdose, contact Poison Control or present to the nearest emergency department. The antidote for iron overdose is deferoxamine, which is not to be confused with deferiprone. Deferiprone is used for transfusion-related iron overload that is not responsive to deferoxamine.[38]

Approximately 70% of patients report significant GI side effects, making adherence difficult. Common side effects include nausea, constipation, upset stomach, and dark and tarry stool. Strategies to mitigate constipation include lower dose or frequency or switching to a formulation that contains a lower percent of elemental iron.[39] Adding fiber or docusate may help alleviate symptoms, but no published data is available supporting this.

Monitoring Parameters

For all types of IDA (e.g., cancer, chemotherapy or CKD with or without hemodialysis), serum ferritin and transferrin saturation (TSAT) testing will be the gold standard. Routine testing for hemoglobin and hematocrit, red blood cell (RBC) count, RBC indices, total iron binding capacity (TIBC), and serum iron are also encouraged.[19,40,41]

Parenteral Iron Therapy

Parenteral iron therapy is reserved for patients who do not respond to oral therapy or for patients with the inability to absorb oral iron due to GI diseases such as Crohn's. Currently, most literature supports a single loading with 1 g as there is no evidence to support use for more than 1 g.[19,42] Capacity for macrophage iron is approximately 600 mg. Parenteral iron therapy has a circulatory half life of approximately 2 weeks, where transferrin is regularly supplied with elemental iron for erythropoiesis.[42]

Patients with CKD stage 5 on hemodialysis are the most common patient population to receive parenteral iron. Randomized trials have shown that, compared to oral iron therapy, parenteral therapy is superior and has a greater increase in Hgb concentrations, requires a lower erythropoiesis-stimulating agent (ESA) dose, or both. Existing intravenous (IV) access allows for easy administration during dialysis sessions.[19] Parenteral iron therapy presents an increased risk for severe acute infusion-related reactions like hypotension, dyspnea, and rarely anaphylaxis.[19]

The etiology for anaphylaxis is unknown but may be immune related or release of free and reactive iron into the circulation.[19] Anaphylaxis occurs in approximately 0.6% to 0.7% of treated patients. There is a black box warning for iron dextran requiring a test dose—usually 25 mg and then observe patient for at least 1 hour. It was more common in the past with higher molecular-weight iron dextran formulations compared to the current lower molecular-weight iron dextran. Anaphylaxis may occur with any formulation but has not been well established in the literature.[19] When administering any IV formulation, emergent resuscitative medications are highly recommended with trained personnel present and close observation of the patient for 60 minutes afterward. Hypotension may be mitigated by infusing more slowly or giving a lower dose.

It is recommended to avoid and delay therapy in patients with active systemic infections as iron is essential for the growth and proliferation of various pathogens like bacteria, viruses, fungi, parasites, and helminths. There may also be minor effects on immune function, which might impair response to pathogens.[19] No IV formulation has been found to be superior regarding safety of efficacy.[17] Treatment may be repeated if necessary, for all patient populations. See Table 25.4 for available formulations and dosage information.

SICKLE CELL ANEMIA

Sickle cell anemia (SCA) affects millions of people worldwide; however, it is most common in people with ancestry from Sub-Saharan Africa. It is also prevalent in Spanish-speaking areas of the western hemisphere (e.g., South America, Caribbean, and Central America), Saudi Arabia, India, and Mediterranean countries such as Turkey, Greece, and Italy.[43,44] SCA, also called "sickle cell disease" (SCD), occurs in approximately 100,000 Americans, one out of 365 Black or African American births, and one out of every 16,300 Hispanic American births. One in 13 Black or African American births will carry the sickle cell trait (SCT).

From 1999 to 2002 deaths among Black or African American children decreased by 42%, which coincide with the introduction of a pneumococcal vaccine. Compared to data from 1983 to 1986, mortality rates decreased by 68% in children aged 0 to 3 years, 39% in children aged 4 to 9 years, and 24% in children aged 10 to 14 years.[43]

In 2005, the total annual medical expenditures for children with SCD averaged $11,702 for Medicaid and $14,772 for private insurance. Forty percent of patients from both groups had at least one hospital admission.[43] From 1989 to 1993, there were approximately 75,000 hospital admissions in the United States costing approximately $475 million.[43]

BACKGROUND

SCD is a genetic disorder that presents at birth when patients are homozygous for the sickle hemoglobin trait (HbSS), or if they have one sickle cell gene plus one abnormal hemoglobin trait (like beta thalassemia).[44]

Genetically a child has a 50% chance of carrying SCT if both parents have SCT and 25% chance of SCD if both parents have SCT.[45] Almost all SCD patients have chronic anemia.[46]

Complications of SCD include acute anemia, which may be caused by splenic sequestration, and is defined as a Hgb decrease by 2 g/dL lower than baseline. Splenic sequestration crisis is an acute drop in Hgb and sudden enlargement of the spleen caused by vaso-occlusion and pooling of RBCs in the spleen. Patients are treated with blood transfusions to partially correct anemia; excessive transfusions should be avoided with Hgb values greater than 8 g/dL as they may cause hyperviscosity.[46]

In SCD, RBCs are sickle or crescent shaped and are inflexible, deoxygenated, greater in blood viscosity, and are easily able to form blockages, which limits blood flow throughout the body.[44] This increases the risk of vascular complications, particularly stroke, vaso-occlusive crisis (VOC), and acute chest syndrome (ACS).[44] VOC is a hallmark acute complication that manifests as acute, excruciating pain. Nearly all SCD patients will experience VOC in their lifetime.[46] Subjective assessment by the patient is the only means of assessing severity of pain as there are no biomarkers to quantitatively validate the degree of pain. Pain management with long- and short-acting opioids for breakthrough pain is recommended. ACS is a frequent cause of acute lung disease in children with sickle cell disease.[44,46] It is defined as having new lung infiltrates with acute lower respiratory symptoms like cough or shortness of breath. ACS is less common than vaso-occlusive crisis, but potentially life threatening; it requires prompt diagnosis, antibiotics, and hospitalization.

A serious complication of SCD is aplastic crisis. This is caused by infection with Parvovirus B-19 (B19V), which infects RBC progenitors in bone marrow, resulting in impaired cell division and a rapid drop in Hgb (typically 3–6 g/dL lower than baseline). An aplastic crisis presents as gradual onset fatigue, shortness of breath, and syncope. The condition is self-limited, with bone marrow recovery occurring in 7 to 10 days, followed by brisk reticulocytosis.[46]

DIAGNOSIS OF SICKLE CELL ANEMIA

If a child is not diagnosed at birth, they may present later in life with anemia, severe or recurrent musculoskeletal or abdominal pain, aplastic crisis, ACS, splenomegaly or splenic sequestration, cholelithiasis, or vaso-occlusive pain.[47]

Infants in the United States are identified by routine neonatal screening using high-performance liquid chromatography (HPLC) or isoelectric focusing. HPLC is the gold standard test as it is fully automated, highly precise, sensitive, and specific.[48] It separates proteins based on differing interaction times and provides both quantitative and qualitative interpretations. One major disadvantage is cost. Isoelectric focusing is another gold standard test. It is highly accurate and cost effective. It separates proteins on a pH-gradient gel based on differences of isoelectric points.

High-risk infants not screened at birth should be screened with hemoglobin electrophoresis as soon as possible. If positive, a confirmatory test is required, which requires Hgb separation via either HPLC, electrophoresis (cellulose acetate and citrate agar), or isoelectric focusing.[48]

Point-of-care diagnostics are used in developing countries with few resources. These diagnostics have high sensitivity (93%) and specificity (94%) and are typically paper based so that they can be read by minimally trained medical staff. They can use either liquid or dry blood samples.[48]

TREATMENT OF SICKLE CELL ANEMIA

Treatment typically entails screening for preventable diseases, blood transfusion therapy, vaccine administration and antibiotic prophylaxis to prevent invasive pneumonia, hydroxyurea to promote blood flow, decrease symptoms that affect daily life, and manage acute pain crisis.[43,44,46]

Nonpharmacological Treatment

Screening for Preventable Diseases
Patients with SCD should be screened for ischemic retinopathy, renal disease, pulmonary hypertension, hypertension, pulmonary disease, vascular disease, and stroke.[44,46] Annual screening with transcranial doppler ultrasonography (TCD) should be used to assess stroke risk.[44] TCD measures average velocity of blood flow through the internal carotid and proximal middle cerebral arteries:

- TCD greater than or equal to 200 cm/s = 10% annual increase in stroke risk.
- TCD greater than or equal to 179 cm/s = candidate for blood transfusion therapy to prevent stroke and should be referred to a specialist for management.

Blood Transfusion Therapy
Blood transfusion therapy as primary stroke prevention in children was proven successful by the Stroke Prevention Trial in Sickle Cell Anemia (STOP).[44,46] It showed that incidence of stroke increase after transfusions stopped, resulting in the potential need for indefinite blood transfusions. Transfusions may be given to patients who have acute splenic sequestration and severe anemia, symptomatic severe ACS (oxygen saturation <90% despite supplemental oxygen),

symptomatic ACS and decreased Hgb of 1.0 g/dL below baseline, aplastic crisis, hepatic sequestration, intrahepatic cholestasis, multisystem organ failure, or symptomatic anemia. Blood transfusions should be avoided in patients with symptomatic anemia, priapism, or uncomplicated painful crisis.

Vaccine Administration

Pediatric patients with SCD should receive all recommended childhood vaccinations including hepatitis A and B; measles, mumps, rubella (MMR); measles, mumps, rubella, varicella (MMRV); rotavirus; *Haemophilus influenzae*; tetanus, diphtheria, and pertussis (Tdap); and poliovirus (only in countries where it is still endemic). Patients with SCD are at increased risk of illness and death from invasive pneumococcal disease; as a result, all children, as early as possible, should receive pneumococcal vaccines.[46,49] Refer to the latest recommendations on the CDC immunization schedule website and summary that follows.[49]

- **Influenza vaccine**: First dose at 6 months of age at the beginning of the annual influenza vaccine season.[50]
- **Meningococcal vaccines**[46,49]: Quadrivalent meningococcal conjugate vaccine (Menveo® [MenACWY-CRM] or Menactra® [MenACWY-D])
  ○ Menveo®:
    ■ First dose given at age 8 weeks: four dose series at 2, 4, 6, and 12 months
    ■ First dose given between ages 7 and 23 months: two doses at least 12 weeks after the first dose and after the first birthday
    ■ First dose given greater than or equal to 24 months: two dose series at least 8 weeks apart
  ○ Menactra®: Must be administered at least 8 weeks after completion of the PCV13 series
    ■ Ages 9 to 23 months: not recommended
    ■ Greater than or equal to 24 months: two doses at least 8 weeks apart
- **Meningococcal serogroup B vaccination (MenB-4C—Bexsero®; MenB-FHbp—Trumenba®)**[49]: Recommended for children aged greater than or equal to 10 years
  ○ Bexsero: two-dose series at least 1 month apart
  ○ Trumenba: three-dose series at 0, 1 to 2, 6 months
- **13-valent pneumococcal conjugate vaccine (PCV 13; Prevnar 13®)**: Four doses before 23 months of age; usually given to all children and on the same recommended schedule. If the child has been inoculated with the 7-valent conjugate vaccine (PCV7) they should still receive a supplemental dose of PCV13.
  ○ First three doses are given at 2, 4, and 6 months of age.
    ○ First dose can be given as early as 6 weeks of age.
    ○ Minimum of 4 weeks between the three doses is recommended.
    ○ Fourth dose can be administered between 12 and 15 months of age; give at least 2 months after the third dose.
- **23-valent pneumococcal polysaccharide vaccine (PPSV23; Pneumovax®)**: Two doses.
  ○ First dose is given at 24 months of age, at least 8 weeks after the completion of PCV13.
  ○ Second dose is given 3 to 5 years after the first dose.

Pharmacological Treatment

Invasive Pneumococcal Disease Prophylaxis

Invasive pneumococcal disease prophylaxis should be given to all children with SCD until they are 5 years of age. They may continue receiving prophylaxis if they have invasive pneumococcal disease, splenectomy, or have not completed their pneumococcal vaccine series. Penicillin VK is the preferred drug. It works by inhibiting cell wall synthesis by binding to penicillin-binding proteins and inhibiting peptidoglycan synthesis. Amoxicillin may be used as an alternative to penicillin and erythromycin may be used in those with allergies to penicillin (**Table 25.5**).[51] In consideration of local antibiotic resistance rates, the following drugs may also be used:

- For children and adults: cephalexin or other cephalosporins; azithromycin
- For adults only: fluoroquinolones (levofloxacin)

Hydroxyurea

Hydroxyurea can be used to promote blood flow and decrease symptoms that affect daily life. It is recommended for patients who have had three or more sickle cell–associated moderate-to-severe pain crisis in 12 months, severe or recurrent ACS, severe symptomatic chronic anemia that interferes with activities or quality of daily life, and children 9 months and older regardless of clinical severity to reduce complications.[44,46,52] Consult an expert in patients with beta-thalassemia, patients who have recurrent sickle-cell associated pain that interferes with activities or quality of daily life, or those with no clinical response to hydroxyurea therapy.

Hydroxyurea is a ribonuclease reductase inhibitor that increases RBC fetal hemoglobin levels (HbF), which is present in the fetus and in young infants that blocks the sickling of RBCs. Infants do not develop SCD symptoms until their HbF levels diminish after birth. Hydroxyurea increases MCV by increasing RBC water content, which improves cellular deformability and increases blood flow; lowers the number of circulating leukocytes and reticulocytes; and alters adhesion of RBCs to endothelium, all of which contribute

TABLE 25.5 Pharmacotherapy for Sickle Cell Anemia

Medication	Starting Dosage/Frequency	Side Effects
Hydroxyurea (pregnancy category: D)	Adult: 15 mg/kg/day (round up to the nearest 500 mg) Adult with CKD: 5–10 mg/kg/day Pediatric: 20 mg mg/kg/day	Bone marrow suppression: May cause severe myelosuppression; monitor blood counts at baseline and throughout treatment; interrupt treatment and reduce dose as necessary Secondary malignancy: Carcinogenic; advise sun protection and monitor patients for malignancies
Penicillin VK[a,b]	Pediatric (<3 years of age): 125 mg bid Pediatric (≥3 years of age): 250 mg bid	Nausea, vomiting, and diarrhea
Amoxicillin 20 mg/kg/day		

[a]Amoxicillin 20 mg/kg/day is an alternative to penicillin.

[b]Allergies to penicillin: children <5 years of age—erythromycin 125 mg twice daily; children ≥5 years of age—erythromycin 250 mg.

bid, twice daily; CKD, chronic kidney disease.

Sources: Cober MP, Phelps SJ. Penicillin prophylaxis in children with sickle cell disease. *J Pediatr Pharmacol Ther.* 2010;15(3):152–159. https://www.ncbi.nlm.nih.gov/pmc/articles/PMC3018247; National Heart, Lung, and Blood Institute. Evidence-based management of sickle cell disease. Expert Panel Report, 2014. Published September 2014. https://www.nhlbi.nih.gov/health-pro/guidelines/sickle-cell-disease-guidelines; Section on Hematology/Oncology and Committee on Genetics. Health supervision for children with sickle cell disease. *Pediatrics.* 2002;109(3):526–535. doi:10.1542/peds.109.3.526; Yawn BP, John-Sowah J. Management of sickle cell disease: Recommendations from the 2014 expert panel report. *Am Family Phys.* 2015;92(12):1069–1076A. https://www.aafp.org/afp/2015/1215/p1069.html

to vaso-occlusion. It should be used with caution in patients receiving other medications known to cause neutropenia like clozapine.

Hydroxyurea has a U.S. boxed warning for bone marrow suppression and secondary malignancy. Blood counts and comprehensive metabolic panel must be monitored at baseline and throughout treatment. Interrupt treatment and reduce dose as necessary. Advise sun protection and monitor patients for malignancies. When adjusting dosing monitor CBC with differential at a minimum every 4 weeks.

Clinical response takes 3 to 6 months, and the maximum tolerated dose must be tried for 6 months prior to discontinuation. The starting dosage for infants and children is 20 mg/kg/day, and the starting dosage for adults is 15 mg/kg/day (round up to the nearest 500 mg) and 5 to 10 mg/kg/day in patients with CKD (see Table 25.5). If dose increase is required and patient has stable blood levels, increase by 5 mg/kg/day increments every 8 weeks. It may be given until mild myelosuppression (ANC 2,000–4,000/uL) is achieved, up to a maximum of 35 mg/kg/day.

Once a stable dose is found, monitor CBC with differential, reticulocyte count, and platelet count every 2 to 3 months. The goal is an absolute neutrophil count (ANC) of greater than or equal to 2,000/uL and platelet count of greater than or equal to 80,000/uL; younger patients may safely tolerate ANC down to 1,250/uL. In the event of neutropenia or thrombocytopenia, hold hydroxyurea and monitor CBC with differential weekly. When the patient's blood counts have recovered, restart hydroxyurea at a dose of 5 mg/kg/day lower than the dose given before onset of abnormal blood readings. For further information, see current guidelines and the support evidences:

- American Academy of Pediatrics (AAP) Guidelines.[47,53]
- National Heart, Lung, and Blood Institute: Evidence-Based Management of Sickle Cell Disease: Expert Panel Report.[46]
- Advisory Committee on Immunization Practices (ACIP).[49]
- U.S. Preventive Services Task Force (USPSTF).[54]
- PROPS and PROPS II Trial.[51]

CHEMOTHERAPY-INDUCED NEUTROPENIA

INTRODUCTION

Chemotherapy-induced neutropenia is a complex and high-risk anemia that requires a hematology/oncology specialist and is unlikely to be treated by other specialists. The latest National Comprehensive Cancer Network Guidelines outline various strategies and recommendations. Neutropenia is typically treated based on the type of cancer and chemotherapy a patient receives as some therapies have a higher incidence of febrile neutropenia than others (**Table 25.6**). This section outlines general principles but, as noted, this type of neutropenia is generally treated by a specialist.[55]

"Febrile neutropenia" is defined as a single temperature of greater than or equal to 38.3°C orally or greater than or equal to 38°C over 1 hour plus either less than 500 or less than 1,000 neutrophils/mcL and predicted to decline to less than or equal to 500 neutrophils/mcL over the next 48 hours. For intermedia risk (10%–20%), assess patient risk factors, including prior chemotherapy or radiation therapy, persistent neutropenia; bone marrow involvement by tumor, recent surgery and/or

TABLE 25.6 Evaluation of Neutropenia

Evaluation Prior to First Chemotherapy Cycle	Risk Assessment for Febrile Neutropenia	Overall Neutropenia Risk	Recommendation
Evaluate risk for febrile neutropenia following chemotherapy in adults with solid tumors and non myeloid malignancies	Disease	High: >20%	G-CSF
	Chemotherapy regimen: high-dose therapy, dose-dense therapy, or standard-dose therapy	Intermediate: 10%–20%	Consider G-CSF based on patient risk factors
	Patient risk factors		
	Treatment intent (curative vs palliative)	Low: <10%	No G-CSF

G-CSF, granulocyte colony-stimulating factor.

Source: Smock KJ, Perkins SL. Thrombocytopenia: An update. *Int J Lab Hematol.* 2014;36(3):269–278. doi:10.1111/ijlh.12214

open wounds, liver dysfunction (bilirubin >2), renal dysfunction (creatinine clearance <50 mL/min), age greater than 65 and receiving full chemotherapy dose.

TREATMENT FOR CHEMOTHERAPY-INDUCED NEUTROPENIA

If the patient has no risk factors, then observation is warranted. But if the patient has one or more risk factors, consider using a G-CSF. If the patient is undergoing their second or subsequent chemotherapy sessions, then evaluate:

- Presence of febrile neutropenia or dose-limiting neutropenic event that could be either a nadir count or any count that may affect dose of chemotherapy the patient receives.
  - If the patient has received G-CSF in the past, consider reducing the chemotherapy dose or changing the drug regimen.
  - If the patient has not used G-CSF in the past, then consider using one.
- If the patient does not present with febrile neutropenia, then reassess at each visit.

Some drug regimens are associated with a high risk (>20%) for febrile neutropenia versus others that may be associated only with intermediate risk (10%–20%). There are a wide range of high-risk chemotherapy regimens based on type of cancer being treated.

G-CSFs work by stimulating the production, maturation, and activation of neutrophils, increasing their migration and cytotoxicity. These are typically used in patients with solid tumors receiving therapy that might cause myelosuppression. Febrile neutropenia is a major dose-limiting toxicity that has been associated with decreased quality of life, longer hospital stays, broad spectrum antibiotic use, and may result in a delay or dose reduction of chemotherapy. Currently the FDA-approved G-CSFs are filgrastim, (including

biosimilars such as filgrastim-aafi, filgrastim-sndz, tbo-filgrastim) and pegfilgrastim, (including biosimilars such as pegfilgrastim-jmdb and pegfilgrastim-cbqv). These have a longer half-life since they are pegylated allowing for less frequent dosing schedules.

The only granulocyte-macrophage colony stimulating factor (GM-CSF) that is FDA approved currently is sargramostim. It is used for patients with acute myeloid leukemia and various stem cell–transplant patients. Both G-CSFs and GM-CSF may be used for patients exposed to acute myelosuppressive doses of radiation.

Cheaper biosimilars have been appearing on the market since the Biologics Price Competition and Innovation Act was passed in 2009. A "biosimilar" is defined as a product that is almost identical in terms of efficacy, safety, and purity to its brand name. But it may different in methods of production and clinically inactive ingredients. They will contain the same amino acid sequence but due to the high complexity of protein folding the overall protein structure may differ between biosimilar products.

G-CSFs are notorious for causing mild-to-moderate bone pain affecting approximately 10% to 30% of patients. Thankfully, these are easily controlled with nonopioid analgesics. With GM-CSFs, 65% of patients reported adverse events that were typically mild to moderate and reversible. They include mild myalgias, facial flushing, low-grade fever, headache, bone discomfort, nausea, and dyspnea.

Dosing for filgrastim (including biosimilars: filgrastim-aafi, filgrastim-sndz, and tbo- filgrastim) is 5 mcg/kg subcutaneously daily until ANC returns to baseline. It is administered the day following or up to 3 to 4 days after completing chemotherapy. Dosing for pegfilgrastim (including biosimilars: pegfilgrastim-jmdb and pegfilgrastim-cbqv) is 6 mg (one syringe) subcutaneously as a single dose. It is administered the day after chemotherapy to prevent exacerbating neutropenia. There must be 12 days between doses of pegfilgrastim and the next cycle of chemotherapy. Sargramostim dosing is based on body surface area: 250 mcg/m^2 subcutaneously daily until ANC reverts back to baseline.

HEMOLYTIC ANEMIA

Hemolytic anemia (HA) is defined when RBCs are prematurely destroyed before their normal 120-day life span.[56] There are many potential causes for hemolytic anemia (**Table 25.7**). HA may range from chronic to life threatening and treatments greatly differ depending on underlying cause.[56]

AUTOIMMUNE HEMOLYTIC ANEMIA

Autoimmune hemolytic anemia (AIHA) results from antibody-mediated destruction and is confirmed by a positive direct antiglobulin test (DAT), or Coombs test.[56] Depending on the antibody-binding temperatures, it can be classified as either warm (more common) or cold agglutinins. Warm AIHA is treated with glucocorticoids, treatment of the underlying condition, blood transfusions, and supportive care. Cold AIHA usually develops with infections or malignancy. Treatment usually involves supportive care, avoiding triggers, and management of the underlying disease process.

DRUG-INDUCED HEMOLYTIC ANEMIA

The first suspected case of drug-induced hemolytic anemia occurred in 1953 and since then approximately 125 drugs have been identified that may cause immune-mediated hemolytic anemia.[56,57] The DAT is used to determine if RBCs have been coated in antibodies. Medications may affect this test and result in false G6PD positives. Medications that can cause a positive DAT/Coombs Test[58–61] include beta-lactam antibiotics like (e.g., cephalosporins and penicillins), beta-lactamase inhibitors, fluoroquinolones, isoniazid, levodopa, methyldopa, nitrofurantoin, quinine and quinidine, rifampin, and sulfonamides.

GLUCOSE-6-PHOSPHATE DEHYDROGENASE DEFICIENCY

G6P6 deficiency is an X-linked disorder usually affecting people with ancestry from the Mediterranean, Asia, or Africa.[56,62] Infants with jaundice or patients with a family history of G6PD should be tested for this deficiency. Oxidative stress can cause hemolysis by preventing the conversion methemoglobin or ferric (3+) iron to ferrous (2+) iron which carries oxygen. This results in methemoglobinemia, which is where the ferric hemoglobin denatures into multimers called "Heinz bodies," and the premature destruction of RBCs via phagocytosis. G6P6 deficiency is usually asymptomatic and hemolysis is short-lived, but some symptoms include back pain (caused by mild-to-severe anemia), abdominal pain (reticulocyte count increase 4 to 7 days after hemolysis), jaundice (Heinz bodies), transient splenomegaly (decreased haptoglobin), hemoglobinuria (increased bilirubin), and scleral icterus (DAT/Coombs test typically negative).[56,62]

TABLE 25.7 Hemolytic Anemia

Cause or Type	Classification or Disease	Mechanism	Diagnostic Lab Test	Treatment
Alloimmune	Transfusion-related reactions and fetal/newborn hemolytic disease	Phagocytosis	DAT	Stop transfusion and supportive care
Autoimmune HA	Warm or cold	Phagocytosis	DAT	Steroids, avoid any causative agents, treat underlying disease
Drug-induced	Oxidative and drug-induced HA	Direct-acting, toxin-induced phagocytosis	Schistocytes, DAT, Hienz bodies	Stop offending agent
Venom-induced	Insect, cobra, brown recluse	Direct-acting	—	—
Enzyme-induced	G6PD deficiency or pyruvate	Oxidative lysis	Enzyme-activity measurements	Avoid exacerbating agents, splenectomy
Hemoglobinopathy	SCD, thalassemias, or other Hgb defects	Blockages	HPLC or electrophoresis	Treat underlying disease

DAT, direct antiglobulin test; G6PD, glucose-6-phosphate-dehydrogenase; HA, hemolytic anemia; Hgb, hemoglobin; HPLC, high-performance liquid chromatography; SCD, sickle cell disease

Source: Phillips J, Henderson AC. Hemolytic anemia: Evaluation and differential diagnosis. *Am Family Phys*. 2018;98(6):354–361. https://www.aafp.org/afp/2018/0915/p354.html

Treatment for G6PD deficiency is avoidance of these oxidative stressors.[56,62] If anemia is severe, blood transfusions, folic acid, and iron supplementation may be considered. Splenectomy, vitamin E, and selenium are not recommended. There is a large number of medications that are contraindicated medications in G6PD deficiency. Chemicals and food that are unsafe include fava beans, henna compounds (black and red Egyptian), naphthalene, phenylhydrazine, and isobutyl and amyl nitrite.[56,62]

ANEMIA OF CHRONIC DISEASE

Anemia of chronic disease (ACD) is the most common hematological disorder and is usually observed in chronic disease states such as nonspecific anemia, which has multiple contributing etiologies. It is diagnosed with an MCV between 80 to 100 fL. Specific affected populations include patients with CKD, cancer, chronic infections, autoimmune diseases, and chronic rejection after solid organ transplantation.[63]

BACKGROUND

The erythropoiesis pathway is shown in **Figure 25.1**. Red blood cells carry oxygen to distribute to tissues. When pO_2 decreases, hypoxia-inducible factors (HIFs), a group of transcription factors, act as "masters of oxygen homeostasis." HIF-1, a transcription factor controls the expression of erythropoietin (EPO). EPO is a hormone that stimulates proliferation of erythroid precursors in bone marrow. Erythroblasts are generated as a result of this pathway in order to carry oxygen.

There are multiple distinct etiologies ACD. The immune system deprives invading cells, such as malignancies or pathogens, of iron, an important nutrient for proliferation of cancer cells and pathogens. Alterations of iron metabolism and diversion of body iron, hemophagocytosis, reduction in erythropoiesis, and diminished response to EPO stimulation all lead to the development of anemia.[63] For diminished response to EPO, known commonly as "EPO hypo-responsiveness," causes of inadequate response include iron deficiency, infection, noninfectious inflammatory states, chronic blood loss, hyperparathyroidism, inadequate dialysis (uremia), folic acid or vitamin B12 deficiency, vitamin C deficiency, malignancy, hemolysis, and bone marrow disorders.[64]

TREATMENT OF ANEMIA OF CHRONIC DISEASE

A diligent effort should be made to identify the underlying cause of anemia in all patients as well as to rule out iron deficiency. Treatment is reliant on making a correct diagnosis as well as targeting other inflammatory pathways.[63] The role of pharmacologic therapy is mainly to prevent the need for blood transfusions and to improve signs and symptoms of anemia.[65] Current guidelines used for management of anemia include the 2019 Guidelines on Hematopoietic Growth Factors by the National Comprehensive Cancer Network[65] and the 2012 Anemia in Chronic Kidney Disease Guideline by the Kidney Disease Improving Global Outcomes workgroup.[66] Landmark trials, CHOIR (2006) and TREAT (2009), showed targeting Hgb greater than 13 with ESAs was associated with a higher risk of death and

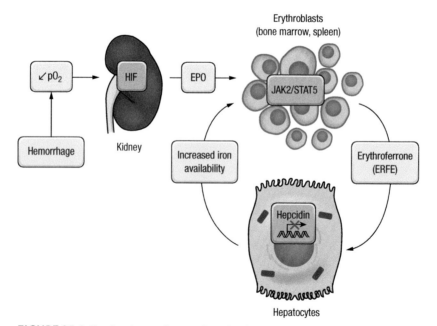

FIGURE 25.1 Production pathway of erythroblasts.
EPO, expression of erythropoietin; HIF, hypoxia-inducible factors; JAK2 = Janus kinase 2; pO_2 = partial pressure of O_2; STAT5 = Signal transducer and activator of transcription 5

hospitalizations for congestive heart failure (CHF) among patients with nondialysis-dependent CKD and anemia, and did not confer a survival benefit in diabetes mellitus type II with CKD, but did increase the risk of stroke, respectively.[67,68]

To treat ACD in FDA-approved indications such as adjuncts to chemotherapy and for chronic kidney disease, ESAs are used to augment endogenous erythropoietin hormone by stimulating iron uptake and heme biosynthesis in erythroid precursors. Increased hemoglobin concentration resulting from ESA use decreases

the risk of blood transfusion–associated adverse events and can improve signs and symptoms of anemia.[63,65] For dosing, it is dependent on indication and response of Hgb and is not generally observed until 2 to 6 weeks after initiation of therapy. For treatment of chemotherapy-induced anemia (Table 25.8), initiate ESAs only if Hgb is less than 10 g/dL, and if there is a minimum of 2 additional months of planned chemotherapy and use lowest dose necessary to avoid RBC transfusion. For treatment of anemia secondary to chronic kidney disease (Table 25.9), consider starting when Hgb is less

TABLE 25.8 Chemotherapy-Induced Anemia: ESA Dosing and Dose Adjustment

Erythropoiesis-Stimulating Agents	Dosing Options	Dose Increase	Dose Decrease
Epoetin alfa or epoetin alfa-epbx	Option 1: 150 units/kg SC 3 ×/week	Increase to 300 units/kg SC 3×/ week[a]	Reduce by 25% if Hgb increases >1 g/dL in any 2-week period or Hgb reaches a level needed to avoid RBC transfusion. Discontinue if no response in Hgb level or if RBC transfusion still required after 8 weeks of ESA
	Option 2: 40,000 units SC every week	Increase to 60,000 units SC every week[a]	
Darbepoetin alfa	Option 1: 2.25 mcg/kg SC every week	Increase up to 4.5 mcg/kg SC every week[b]	Reduce by 40% if Hgb increases >1 g/dL in any 2-week period or Hgb reaches a level needed to avoid RBC transfusion. Discontinue if no response in Hgb level or if RBC transfusion still required after 8 weeks of ESA
	Option 2: 500 mcg SC every 3 weeks	No dose increase recommended per manufacturer	

[a]Dose increase if after 4 weeks of ESA therapy, Hgb increases by <1 g/dL and Hgb remains <10 g/dL.
[b]Dose increase if after 6 weeks of ESA therapy, Hgb increases by <1 g/dL and Hgb remains <10 g/dL.
ESA, erythropoiesis-stimulating agents; Hgb, hemoglobin; SC, subcutaneously; RBC, red blood cells.

TABLE 25.9 Anemia Secondary to Chronic Kidney Disease: ESA Dosing and Dose Adjustment

Patient on Dialysis?	ESA	Starting Dose	Titration
On dialysis	Epoetin alfa or epoetin alfa-epbx	50–100 units/kg SC or IV 3×/week; patients may initially respond to 50–100 units/kg SC/IV every week. Maximum: 10,000 units 3×/week	Increase by 25% if Hgb does not increase by >1 g/dL after 4 weeks. Reduce by 25% if Hgb increased by >1 g/dL in any 2-week period
	Darbepoetin alfa	0.45 mcg/kg SC or IVP every week or 0.75 mcg/kg SC every 2 weeks	
	Methoxy polyethylene glycol-epoetin beta	0.6 mcg/kg SC or IVP every 2 weeks until stabilized, then may adjust to double dose every 4 weeks	
Not on dialysis	Epoetin alfa or epoetin alfa-epbx	50–100 units/kg SC every week	Increase by 25% if Hgb does not increase by >1 g/dL after 4 weeks. Reduce by 25% if Hgb increased by >1 g/dL in any 2-week period
	Darbepoetin alfa	0.45 mcg/kg SC every 4 weeks	
	Methoxy polyethylene glycol-epoetin beta	0.6 mcg/kg SC every 2 weeks until stabilized, then may adjust to double dose every 4 weeks	

ESA, erythropoiesis-stimulating agents; Hgb, hemoglobin; IV, intravenously; IVP, intravenous pyelogram; RBC, red blood cells; SC, subcutaneously

TABLE 25.10 Clinical Pearls for Erythropoiesis-Stimulating Agents

Erythropoiesis-Stimulating Agent	Clinical Pearl
Epoetin alfa or Epoetin alfa-epbx (Epogen®, Procrit®, Retacrit®)	• SC injection more effective than IV route of administration as patients have required 25% larger IV dose to achieve equivalent Hgb responses • Not as ideal for nondialysis treatment of anemia compared to darbepoetin in terms of frequency of injection • Easiest ESA to titrate as dose can be given multiple times per week
Darbepoetin alfa (Aranesp®)	• Half-life three times longer than epoetin alfa when given IV • Can be given monthly in outpatient, nondialysis-dependent CKD with monthly monitoring for efficacy/safety
Methoxy polyethylene glycol-epoetin beta (Mircera®)	• ESA with longest half-life (~120 hours) • Can be given monthly in outpatient, nondialysis-dependent CKD with monthly monitoring for efficacy/safety

CKD, chronic kidney disease; ESA, erythropoiesis-stimulating agent; IV, intravenous; SC, subcutaneously.

than 9 to 10 or dropping precipitously. It is important to consider black box warnings for ESA use, including[69–73]:

• Increased risk of death, MI, stroke, venous thromboembolism, thrombosis of vascular access.
• In patients with CKD, greater risk for death, serious adverse cardiovascular reactions, and stroke when ESAs are administered to target Hgb level greater than 11g/dL. No trial has identified a hemoglobin target level, ESA dose, or dosing strategy that does not increase these risks. Use the lowest ESA dose sufficient to reduce the need for RBC transfusions
• ESAs shortened the overall survival and/or increased the risk of tumor progression or recurrence in clinical studies of patients with breast, non-small cell lung, head and neck, lymphoid, and cervical cancers. To decrease these risks, as well as the risk of serious cardiovascular and thromboembolic reactions, use the lowest dose needed to avoid RBC transfusions. Use ESAs only for anemia from myelosuppressive chemotherapy. ESAs are not indicated for patients receiving myelosuppressive chemotherapy when the anticipated outcome is cure. Discontinue following the completion of a chemotherapy course. Do not use Mircera (methoxy polyethylene glycol-epoetin beta) for patients with cancer. A dose-ranging study was terminated early because of more deaths among patients receiving Mircera than another ESA.
• There is also a well-known adverse effect of increased blood pressure; consider aggressive management of hypertension if blood pressure is above 160/100 prior to ESA initiation.

Monitoring

It is important to check iron stores prior to initiating ESAs as iron deficiency leads to EPO hypo-responsiveness. Consider starting ESAs conservatively in patients not at risk of requiring blood transfusions to minimize risk of cardiovascular events or exacerbation of underlying cancers. If patients require RBC transfusions during initiation of ESAs for acute management, each unit of packed RBCs delivers 200 to 250 mg of iron.[73] For specific ESAs, clinical pearls are outlined in **Table 25.10**.

MACROCYTIC ANEMIA

Macrocytic anemia describes an anemic state characterized by the presence of abnormally large RBCs in the peripheral blood and is defined as MCV greater than or equal to 100 fL.[74] Historically, pernicious anemia, or lack of intrinsic factor, a cofactor necessary for B12 absorption, was first described in 1822 by Dr. James Scarth Combe.[75] In 1934, George Hoyt Whipple, George Richards Minot, and William Parry Murphy were awarded the Nobel Prize in Physiology or Medicine "for their discoveries concerning liver therapy in cases of anaemia." Whipple's diet, which included a rich intake of liver, changed the prognosis from a few months to years to management of a chronic disease.[76] Folate deficiency was first discovered by Lucy Wills in 1930 where she was studying macrocytic anemia in pregnancy, prevalent in female textile workers. She noticed that anemia was most frequent in populations with diets deficient in protein, fruit, and vegetables. She studied the effects of changes in diet on the macrocytic anemia of albino rats produced by a deficient diet and Bartonella infection. She added a yeast extract, "marmite," to the diets of these pregnant patients, and watched their hemoglobin recover.[77]

BACKGROUND

Dietary folic acid is absorbed by enterocytes and is converted to methyltetrahydrofolate by dihydrofolate reductase. Then, methyltetrahydrofolate (methyl THF) exits the enterocyte via the basolateral membrane and either enters the systemic circulation or undergoes enterohepatic circulation. Through the conversion of homocysteine and methyl THF, using Vitamin B12 as a cofactor for methionine synthase, methionine is produced for DNA synthesis (**Figure 25.2**). In addition, the demethylated THF then becomes methylene THF and is used by thymidylate synthase to convert dUMP to dTMP for purine synthesis.[78] Vitamin B12 has a distinct mechanism of absorption. B12 first binds to R protein, which is secreted by the salivary gland in order to protect from gastric acid degradation. In the duodenum and jejunum, R protein is degraded by pancreatic peptides and B12 is bound by intrinsic factor (IF). In the ileum, cubulin,[79] a cell receptor that recognizes the B12-IF complex, endocytoses the B12-IF complex and B12 binds to transcobalamin II in portal blood transport for liver storage or systemic circulation for tissue use.[80] B12 plays two separate roles. First, it is a cofactor to turn methyl-malonic-CoA into succinyl-CoA for use in the citric acid cycle. It also acts as a cofactor in the conversion of homocysteine to methionine. When there is insufficient dTMP necessary for DNA synthesis, uracil replaces these positions on the DNA strand. When uracil is incorporated into a purely DNA strand, repair enzymes unsuccessfully correct the error. As a result, the DNA strand is destroyed by p53-mediated cellular apoptosis of hematopoietic precursor cells and leads to ineffective erythropoiesis.[78]

RISK FACTORS FOR MACROCYTIC ANEMIA

For Vitamin B12 deficiency, risk factors include inadequate intake in strict vegans, chronic alcoholics, or low-solute diet due to financial limitations or poor dentition or decreased B12 absorption via loss of intrinsic factor by autoimmune mechanisms, chronic atrophic gastritis, or gastric-bypass surgery. Less common risk factors include overgrowth of bacteria that use B12, injury or surgery of ileum as in Crohns disease or small bowel surgery, blind loop syndrome, Whipple disease, Zollinger-Ellison syndrome, tapeworm infestations, pancreatic insufficiency, inflammatory bowel disease, advanced liver disease, metformin use, PPI and H2RA use for greater than 2 years.[81]

For folate deficiency, risk factors include inadequate nutritional intake in vegans, chronic alcoholics or low-solute diet,[82] increased folate demands as in pregnancy, infancy or diseases associated with rapid

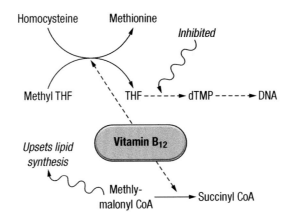

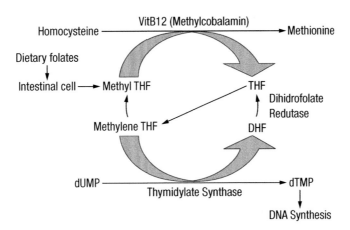

FIGURE 25.2 Folate and vitamin B12 and erythropoiesis.

CoA, co-enzyme A; DNA, deoxyribonucleic acid; dUMP, deoxyuridine monophosphate; dTMP, deoxythymidine triphosphate; THF, tetrahydrofolate; DHF, dihydrofolate.

cellular proliferation (i.e., hemolysis, leukemia), jejunal diseases, short bowel syndrome, bacterial overgrowth in GI tract leading to biologic competition, or drug-induced causes (anticonvulsants, oral contraceptives, sulfasalazine, methotrexate, triamterene).[83] Patients can mitigate these potential risk factors by eating a diet rich in vitamin B12 and/or folate depending on deficiency (**Table 25.11**).

DIAGNOSIS OF MACROCYTIC ANEMIA

After macrocytic anemia is diagnosed, it is important to determine the exact cause. Vitamin B12 deficiency is associated with nervous system demyelination and can additionally cause the following signs and symptoms[12,13]: paresthesias, numbness, ataxia, diminished vibratory sensation and proprioception in lower extremities, diminished or hyperactive reflexes, psychosis, mood disturbances, muscle spasticity, vision loss, and orthostatic hypotension.

In patients with macrocytic anemia, it is important to identify the underlying cause via laboratory diagnostic tests. A clinician should obtain B12 and folate levels directly for any person with an elevated MCV in order to determine deficiencies in either vitamin. If patients are borderline low on either B12/folate, then a clinician can order methyl-malonic acid (elevated in B12 deficiency), and homocysteine levels (elevated in either B12 or folate deficiency). Other causes of macrocytic anemia include alcohol use, medications, hypothyroidism, bone marrow dysplasias, nonalcoholic fatty liver disease, and reticulocytosis. In these cases, B12 and folate deficiencies may still be contributing factors, yet the underlying pathology is specific to the cause. Medications include reverse transcriptase inhibitors like zidovudine, phenytoin, valproic acid, carbamazepine, methotrexate, sulfamethoxazole–trimethoprim (SMX–TMP), purine, and pyrimidine inhibitors such as mycophenolate mofetil, and alkylating agents (e.g., cyclophosphamide, metformin, cholestyramine, hydroxyurea, 5-fluorouracil, pyrimethamine).[82] The available diagnostic tests will help differentiate potential causes (**Table 25.12**). Depending on the results of the diagnostic tests, a clinician should be able to ascertain the origin of the patient's macrocytic anemia. A diagnosis flowchart is provided in **Figure 25.3**.

TABLE 25.11 Foods High in Vitamin B12 and Folate

Foods High in Vitamin B12	Foods High in Folate
Lamb	Fortified cereal
Yogurt	Beans
Tuna	Spinach
Salmon	Turkey giblets
Beef	White rice
Milk	Beef liver

TABLE 25.12 Diagnostic Tests for Vitamin B12 or Folate Deficiencies

Test	Description
MCV for B12 deficiency	Sensitivity: 10.14% Specificity: 92.82%
RBC folate	Sensitivity (RBC folate levels <150 ng/mL): 20%–30% Specificity (RBC folate levels <150 ng/mL): 70%
RBC smear	Can indicate megaloblastic anemia (demonstrated by macroovalocytes and hypersegmented neutrophils); vitamin B12 or folate deficiency is the most likely cause
Reticulocyte count	Increased RBC production secondary to destruction or loss leads to reticulocytosis; reticulocytes are incompletely processed RBCs and are slightly larger than the average RBC
Schilling test	The Schilling test is not widely available anymore, but was used to test patients for B12 deficiency using radioactive cobalt given orally, then the subsequent percentage of radiolabeled B12 excreted during a 24-hour urine collection was measured.
Serum folate	Serum levels are variable, can decrease within a few days of dietary folate restriction Specificity: Folate levels can be normal or slightly low in patients; nonspecific as serum folate does not reflect tissue storage of folate
Serum homocysteine	Sensitivity (B12 deficiency): 86%–96% Sensitivity (folate deficiency): 91% Specificity difficult to determine as many factors cause alterations in serum levels, including B12 deficiency, pyridoxine deficiency, renal insufficiency, hypovolemia, hypothyroidism, and psoriasis
Serum methyl-malonic acid	Sensitivity (B12 deficiency): 86%–98% Specificity difficult to determine as many factors cause alterations in serum levels, including renal insufficiency, hypovolemia, and changes in bowel flora (e.g., antibiotic use)
Serum vitamin B12	Sensitivity (B12 levels <200 pg/mL): 50%–95% Sensitivity (B12 levels <100 pg/mL): 90% Lack of a consistently defined gold standard for B12 levels and their sensitivity and specificity to be considered deficient

MCV, mean corpuscular volume; RBC, red blood cell.

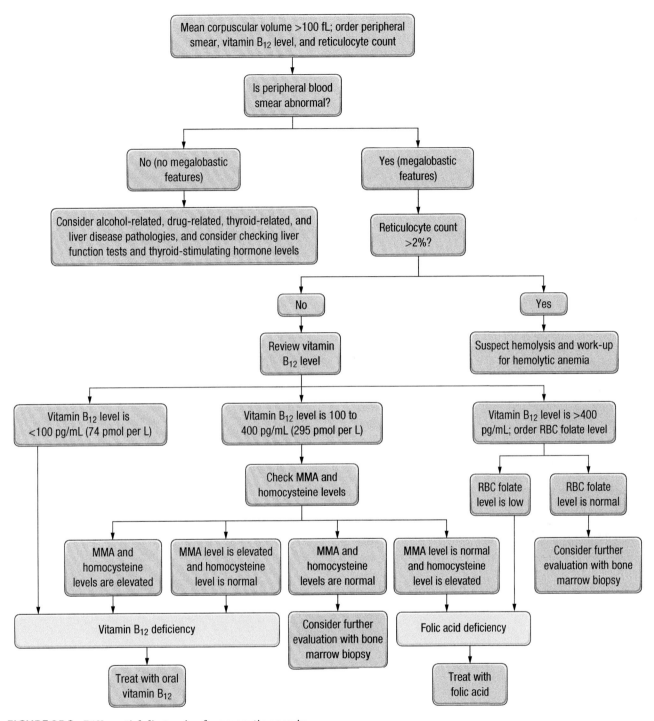

FIGURE 25.3 Differential diagnosis of macrocytic anemia.
Source: Kaferle J, Strzoda CE. Evaluation of macrocytosis. *Am Fam Physician.* 2009;79(3):203–208. https://www.aafp.org/afp/2009/0201/p203.html

For monitoring, there is no consensus for follow-up for macrocytic anemia. One may consider checking Hgb and other appropriate, patient-specific labs that originally diagnosed the deficiency every 3 months in accordance with RBC lifespan for chronic, asymptomatic management. For pregnant patients, follow-up should occur more frequently such as every few days to avoid birth defects as changes in serum levels can be identified. For neurologic/neuropsychiatric findings or anemia requiring hospitalization, consider monitoring B12/folate levels daily to every other day to ensure effectiveness. Monitoring should continue at least until a complete response has been documented and then rechecking 3 to 12 months after stopping therapy.

TABLE 25.13 Pharmacotherapy for Macrocytic Anemia

Drug	Dosage/Frequency
Folic acid	1–5 mg PO daily or 0.4–1 mg IM/IV daily
Vitamin B12	PO: 1,000–2,000 mcg daily × 1–2 weeks; then 1,000 mcg daily IM: 1,000 mcg every week × 8 weeks, then 1,000 mcg every month

IM, intramuscularly; IV, intravenously; PO, by mouth.

TREATMENT FOR MACROCYTIC ANEMIA

Nonpharmacologic treatment involves increasing dietary intake of vitamin B12 and/or folate. Pharmacologic treatment will replace the vitamin deficiency (**Table 25.13**). Treatment guidelines include the Evaluation of Macrocytosis (2009) by American Family Physician[82] and Diagnosis and Treatment of Macrocytic Anemias in Adults (2017) by the Journal of General and Family Medicine.[86] Clinicians should ensure proper repletion as neither B vitamin will replace a deficiency in the other vitamin.

THROMBOCYTOPENIA

Thrombocytopenia is a common clinical problem with numerous potential causes, including decreased bone marrow platelet production, increased peripheral platelet destruction, increased splenic sequestration, and hemodilution. A platelet count of less than 150×10^9/L is the typical laboratory lower limit of normal yet there is controversy over which level of platelet would contribute significant thrombocytopenia, as some clinicians prefer less than 100×10^9/L to be considered clinically significant. When approaching the workup of thrombocytopenia, it is important to utilize the clinical history and laboratory features.[87] **Table 25.14** displays acquired causes of thrombocytopenia and appropriate management.

TREATMENT FOR THROMBOCYTOPENIA

The offending drug should be discontinued. First-line treatment for immune thrombocytopenia caused by increased platelet destruction via formation of antibodies is steroids (prednisone, 0.5–2 mg/kg/day for 3–4 weeks, or dexamethasone, 40 mg daily for 4 days every 2–4 weeks for one to four cycles) or intravenous immunoglobulin (IVIG). IVIG dose depends on formulation. Options to consider include immune globulin (Gammagard®) 1 g/kg/day for 1 to 2 days or anti-D immune globulin, 50 to 75 mcg/kg/day.

If a patient presents with a sudden, severe decrease in platelets with possible complications of bleeding, drug-induced thrombocytopenia (DITP) should be considered.[88] Consider the following four questions to help determine the likelihood of a suspected DITP:

1. Did drug administration precede thrombocytopenia? Did complete, sustained recovery from thrombocytopenia occur after discontinuation of the suspected drug?
2. Were other drugs administered prior to the onset of thrombocytopenia continued or reintroduced after discontinuation of the suspected drug without a resulting decrease in platelet count?
3. Do other possible etiologies exist?
4. Was the patient re-exposed to the suspect drug that resulted in recurrent thrombocytopenia?

If all four criteria are met, then drug is considered a definite cause of DITP. If criteria 1 to 3 are met, then drug is considered a probable cause of DITP. If criterion 1 is met, then drug is considered a possible cause of DITP. If criterion 1 is not met, then drug is considered an unlikely cause of DITP. Be sure to add the drug to the patient's list of allergies/adverse drug reactions.

TABLE 25.14 Acquired Causes of Thrombocytopenia

Drug/Disease Process	Management/Clinical Pearls
Carbamazepine	Consider optimization of other AEDs. Induces own metabolism; may take 3–5 weeks to reach steady state. Adult half-life at steady state 12–17 hours; adult half-life 3.1–20.8 hours; initial half-life variable 25–65 hours Rapid withdrawal of AEDs precipitates seizures; consider up-titrating or starting alternative therapy as appropriate.
Chlorothiazide and hydrochlorothiazide	Consider alternative agents that are also first-line for hypertension. Thiazides contain a sulfur group; caution in patients allergic to sulfonamides. Cross-reactivity not well understood between antibiotics and nonantibiotics.
Ethanol	Advise patients to abstain from alcohol. Encourage social support to aid abstinence. Rebound thrombocytosis may occur with platelets increasing to 600–900 × 10^9/L and returning to normal levels within 7–10 days; this is a transient response that does not require intervention.

(continued)

Drug/Disease Process	Management/Clinical Pearls
Estrogens	Consider re-evaluation of need for estrogen therapy for chronic thrombocytopenia. Thrombosis is more clinically relevant and much more well documented.
Folate deficiency	Replete folate via supplementation. Folic acid: 1–5 mg PO daily or 0.4–1 mg IM/IV daily Monitor vitamin B12, folate, homocysteine, and methyl-malonic acid levels. Best considered if there are other findings suggestive of folate deficiency.
Interferon-alpha	IVIG or steroids Prednisone requires dose tapering and initial response of 4–14 days. Dexamethasone has faster onset of action than prednisone, 2–14 days. IVIG is first-line if steroids are contraindicated or produce suboptimal response. Anti-D immune globulin is used only for D-positive patients.
Isoniazid	IVIG given as 250 mg × 2 days may result in platelet recovery. If patient is taking rifampin and isoniazid, consider stopping rifampin first as thrombocytopenia due to rifampin use is more common than isoniazid.
Linezolid	Consider alternatives to linezolid for antibiotic therapy depending on the clinical scenario. Monitor patients with lower body weight or higher serum creatinine as these populations are at higher risk. Use >14 days increases risk.
Malaria	Evaluate patient for malaria treatment. Common complication of *Plasmodium vivax* and *Plasmodium falciparum;* no clear recommendation for management after initiating efficacious antimalarial treatment
Oxaliplatin	Consider alternative chemotherapeutic regimens and discontinue oxaliplatin. While 70% of patients receiving oxaliplatin can experience thrombocytopenia, only 3%–4% have grade 3–4 thrombocytopenia causing life-threatening bleeding.
Vitamin B12 deficiency	Vitamin B12: 1,000–2,000 mcg PO daily × 1–2 weeks; maintenance dose: 1,000 mcg IM daily or 1,000 mcg IM weekly × 8 weeks, then 1,000 mcg IM monthly Monitor vitamin B12, folate, homocysteine, and methyl-malonic acid levels. Best considered if there are other findings suggestive of vitamin B12 deficiency.
Viral infections	Consider investigating viral infections in unexplained thrombocytopenic patients. Identify and treat the underlying infection. HIV, HCV, CMV are more well-known causes. In self-limiting viral infections, platelet counts usually recover spontaneously.
Beta-lactams	Consider alternative antibiotic therapy depending on the clinical scenario. Penicillin, nafcillin, ampicillin piperacillin-tazobactam, cefazolin, cefotetan, ceftriaxone, and cefuroxime have all been implicated.
Calcineurin inhibitors	Consider alternative CNI and maintain goal trough targets. Patients have been converted between CNIs without the same recurrence of thrombocytopenia. Important to cross-titrate to preserve immunosuppressive actions for graft survival.
Daptomycin	Consider alternative antibiotic therapy depending on the clinical scenario. Case studies show successful conversion of vancomycin to daptomycin. In critically ill patients, rule out other potential causes of thrombocytopenia (e.g., heparin use and sepsis).
Mirtazapine	Consider alternatives for management of depression, such as bupropion. Medications that affect serotonin are more likely to affect platelets due to the 5-HT2A receptor and 5-HT transporter.
Quinine drugs	Consider changing therapy atovaquone/proguanil (250mg/100mg) tab. To take 4 tabs (1000mg/400mg) PO daily if not pregnant. IV quinidine has been discontinued by the manufacturer since April 2019; artesunate is now considered first-line treatment by WHO which is available via INF protocol from the FDA.
Sulfamethoxazole/ trimethoprim	Consider alternative agents depending on the clinical scenario for treatment of infection. Sulfonamide allergy and cross-reactivity is not well understood between antibiotics and non antibiotics.

(continued)

TABLE 25.14 Acquired Causes of Thrombocytopenia (*continued*)

Drug/Disease Process	Management/Clinical Pearls
Heparin-induced thrombocytopenia	Use the 4Ts clinical scoring system as a risk assessment tool. Recommend alternative anticoagulation. Therapeutic anticoagulation x 4 weeks with isolated HIT and 3 months for HIT patients with thrombosis. Fondaparinux is SC injection. It can be monitored for efficacy yet is not required by the ASH 2018 guidelines. Accumulates in renal failure. The largest bodies of evidence are for argatroban, bivalirudin, and fondaparinux. DOACs are a possible option, but evidence is not as robust as other agents and is limited to observational studies. Warfarin use requires overlap with parenteral agent and should be initiated only after recovery to stable platelet counts of >150 x109/L. If patients were being treated with warfarin at time of HIT onset or warfarin initiated before platelet recovery, this is contraindicated because of increased risk for venous limb gangrene and warfarin-induced skin necrosis.
GPIIb/IIIa inhibitors (abciximab, eptifibatide, tirofiban)	Consider alternatives such as P2Y12 receptor antagonist oral-loading dose prior to PCI: clopidogrel 600 mg, prasugrel 60 mg, ticagrelor 180 mg; or IV: cangrelor 30 mcg/kg bolus prior to PCI, then start 4 mcg/kg/min infusion for 2+ hours or duration of PCI, then give oral loading dose of P2Y12 antagonist after surgery. Abciximab has reported more cases because it is a modified monoclonal antibody to the GPIIb/IIIa receptor. Monitor platelets 2–4 hours after initiation and at 24 hours. Small-molecule eptifibatide and tirofiban are small molecules that have quicker recovery (<4 hours) of platelet aggregation than abciximab (14 days).
NSAIDs	Consider alternatives for pain management. Diclofenac, Ibuprofen, meloxicam, and naproxen have been shown to cause thrombocytopenia.
Rifampin	Consider alternatives in treatment of TB and other infectious cases depending on clinical presentation. Drug acts as a strong CYP3A4 and CYP2C19 inducer and moderate CYP2C8/9 inducer. If stopping medication, re-evaluate a patient's current medication list for therapeutic medication adjustments.
Valproic acid	Consider alternatives for management of epileptic and bipolar disorders. Persons of advanced age, female gender, and doses greater than 1 g/day are risk factors for development of thrombocytopenia.
Vancomycin	Consider alternative antibiotic therapy based on clinical presentation. Case studies show successful conversion of vancomycin to daptomycin. In critically ill patients, rule out other potential causes of thrombocytopenia (e.g. heparin use and sepsis).

AED, antiepileptic drug; aPTT, activated partial thromboplastin time; bid, twice daily; CMV, cytomegalovirus; CNI, calcineurin inhibitor; DOAC, direct oral anticoagulant; FDA, U.S. Food and Drug Administration; GPIIb, glycoprotein IIb; HCV, hepatitis C virus; HIT, heparin-induced thrombocytopenia; HIV, human immunodeficiency virus; IM, intramuscularly; INF, interferon; IV, intravenously; IVIG, intravenous immunoglobulin; NSAID, nonsteroidal anti-inflammatory drug; PCI, percutaneous coronary intervention; PO, orally; TB, tuberculosis; WHO, World Health Organization.

CASE EXEMPLAR: Patient With Fatigue

EM is a 74-year-old male with a history of rheumatoid arthritis (RA) who presents in the clinic with a complaint of fatigue. EM is ambulatory with a walker and recently has had intermittent flare-ups of his rheumatoid arthritis (RA) disease activity, with increasing pain and swelling in his affected joints. His energy has been declining over the past few months, so he thought it was a good time to come in for follow-up laboratory testing and reassessment of his medications. Most troublesome, he has fainted twice in the past 2 weeks, which resulted in falls onto his carpeted floor. He is afraid to go out into public and even more afraid to drive his car. He has also had some chest pains with exertion. He is eating and sleeping okay, although he does sleep better if his head is elevated on a few extra pillows. He lives alone and gets meals delivered by a local organization.

Past Medical History

- RA for 35 years, affecting hands, feet, knees, hips, and cervical spine
- Systolic hypertension
- Presbycusis

Medications

- Ibuprofen, 600 mg three to four times per day as needed
- Methotrexate, 7.5 mg weekly
- Atenolol, 25 mg daily
- Hydrocodone/acetaminophen, 5 mg/500 mg every 6 hours as needed for pain

Physical Examination

- Height: 71 inches; weight: 160 lbs.; BMI: 22.3; blood pressure: 162/60; pulse: 84; respiration rate: 16; temperature: 98.6 °F
- Well-developed, well-nourished elderly male in no distress; pale
- Lungs: bibasilar rales
- Heart: regular rate and rhythm, grade 3/6 systolic murmur, audible S3; positive carotid bruit on the left
- Abdomen: no masses, nontender
- Rectal: prostate 3+ enlarged, hemoccult negative brown stool
- Extremities: marked ulnar deviation of MCP and IP joints in both hands

Labs and Imaging

- Hemoglobin: 8.9 g/dL
- Mean corpuscular volume (MCV): 80 fL
- White blood cell count: 10.7×10^9/L
- Platelets: 250,000/L
- Reticulocyte count: 0.8%
- Ferritin: 415 mcg/L
- Electrocardiogram: no acute findings; some evidence of left ventricular hypertrophy

Discussion Questions

1. What is EM's diagnosis?
2. What is the underlying pathophysiology of EM's condition?
3. What is the best therapeutic approach to the treatment of EM's condition?

CASE EXEMPLAR: Patient With Muscle Pain

TS is a 22-year-old male from out of town who is visiting family. He presents with severe pain in his legs, back, and shoulders. He denies injury. He has been in excellent overall health and has not experienced anything like this before. The pain started while he was flying across the country. When the airplane landed, he could barely walk and asked for an ambulance. He remembers getting some mild leg cramps in the past when he was sick, but nothing like this.

Past Medical History
- Noncontributory

Social History
- Nonsmoker

Medications
- None

Physical Examination
- Height: 72 inches; weight: 182 lbs.; BMI: 24.4; blood pressure: 160/92; pulse: 110; respiration rate: 20; temperature 100.2 °F
- Well-developed, well-nourished, African American male in moderate distress

- Lungs: clear
- Heart: regular rate and rhythm
- Extremities: marked tenderness to palpation of major muscle groups of calves, thighs, and shoulders

Labs
- Hemoglobin: 10.4 g/dL
- White blood cell count: 11×10^9/L
- Mean corpuscular volume (MCV): 79 fL
- Peripheral smear: shows sickle cells
- Reticulocyte count: 4.9%
- Hemoglobin electrophoresis: hemoglobin A 60%, hemoglobin S 40%
- Creatine phosphokinase (CPK): 2500 U/L

Discussion Questions

1. What is the diagnosis for TS's muscle pains?
2. What is the underlying pathophysiology for TS's muscle pains?
3. What pharmacologic and nonpharmacologic interventions are appropriate to manage TS's condition?

KEY TAKEAWAYS

- Approximately 30% of the world is estimated to be anemic. IDA is the most common nutritional deficiency and anemia. Females are up to seven times more likely to be affected than males.
- Treatment of SCD consists of screening for co-morbid diseases, vaccination to prevent pneumonia, antibiotics to prevent complications, hydroxyurea to promote blood flow and improve quality of life, and pain control.
- Neutropenia is typically treated based on the type of cancer and the chemotherapeutic agent used as some therapies have a higher incidence of febrile neutropenia than others.
- "Hemolytic anemia" is defined as the premature destruction of RBCs before their normal 120-day lifespan; severity may range from chronic

and mild to life-threatening. Treatments vary widely based on the underlying etiology.
- "Anemia of chronic disease" is defined as a microcytic or normocytic anemia related to alterations of iron metabolism and diversion of body iron, hemophagocytosis, reduction in erythropoiesis, and diminished response to EPO.
- "Macrocytic anemia" describes an anemic state characterized by the presence of abnormally large RBCs in the peripheral blood. It is defined as MCV greater than 100 fL and is generally related to a lack of vitamin B12, deficiency of folic acid, or abuse of alcohol.
- Thrombocytopenia is a common clinical problem with numerous potential causes, including decreased bone marrow platelet production, increased peripheral platelet destruction, increased splenic sequestration, and hemodilution.

REFERENCES

1. Auerbach M, Adamson JW. How we diagnose and treat iron deficiency anemia. *Am J Hematol.* 2016;91(1):31–38. doi:10.1002/ajh.24201

2. Kassebaum NJ, Jasrasaria R, Naghavi M, et al. A systematic analysis of global anemia burden from 1990 to 2010. *Blood.* 2014;123(5):615–624. doi:10.1182/blood-2013-06-508325

3. Young I, Parker H, Rangan A, et al. Association between haem and non-haem iron intake and serum ferritin in healthy young women. *Nutrients.* 2018;10(1):81. doi:10.3390/nu10010081

4. West A-R, Oates P-S. Mechanisms of heme iron absorption: Current questions and controversies. *World J Gastroenterol.* 2008;14(26):4101–4110. doi:10.3748/wjg.14.4101

5. Camaschella C. Iron deficiency: new insights into diagnosis and treatment. *Hematology.* 2015;2015(1):8–13. doi:10.1182/asheducation-2015.1.8

6. Zhu A, Kaneshiro M, Kaunitz JD. Evaluation and treatment of iron deficiency anemia: a gastroenterological perspective. *Dig Dis Sci.* 2010;55(3):548–559. doi:10.1007/s10620-009-1108-6

7. MedlinePlus. Medical encyclopedia: iron deficiency anemia. Accessed August 31, 2019. https://medlineplus.gov/ency/article/000584.htm

8. Annibale B, Capurso G, Chistolini A, et al. Gastrointestinal causes of refractory iron deficiency anemia in patients without gastrointestinal symptoms. *Am J Med.* 2001;111(6):439–445. doi:10.1016/S0002-9343(01)00883-X

9. Hershko C, Hoffbrand AV, Keret D, et al. Role of autoimmune gastritis, Helicobacter pylori and celiac disease in refractory or unexplained iron deficiency anemia. *Haematologica.* 2005;90(5):585–595. Pubmed PMID: 15921373.

10. Kulnigg-Dabsch S, Resch M, Oberhuber G, et al. Iron deficiency workup reveals high incidence of autoimmune gastritis with parietal cell antibody as reliable screening test. *Semin Hematol.* 2018;55(4):256–261. doi:10.1053/j.seminhematol.2018.07.003

11. Hershko C, Lahad A, Kereth D. Gastropathic sideropenia. *Best Pract Res Clin Haematol.* 2005;18(2):363–380. doi:10.1016/j.beha.2004.10.002

12. Short MW, Domagalski JE. Iron deficiency anemia: evaluation and management. *Am Family Phys.* 2013;87(2):98–104. https://www.aafp.org/afp/2013/0115/p98.html

13. Stallmach A, Büning C. Ferric maltol (St10): A novel oral iron supplement for the treatment of iron deficiency anemia in inflammatory bowel disease. *Expert Opin Pharmacother.* 2015;16(18):2859–2867. doi:10.1517/14656566.2015.1096929

14. Schmidt C, Ahmad T, Tulassay Z, et al. Ferric maltol therapy for iron deficiency anaemia in patients with inflammatory bowel disease: long-term extension data from a Phase 3 study. *Aliment Pharmacol Ther.* 2016;44(3):259–270. doi:10.1111/apt.13665

15. Gasche C, Ahmad T, Tulassay Z, et al. Ferric maltol is effective in correcting iron deficiency anemia in patients with inflammatory bowel disease: results from a phase-3 clinical trial program. *Inflamm Bowel Dis.* 2015;21(3):579–588. doi:10.1097/MIB.0000000000000314

16. Iolascon A, d'Apolito M, Servedio V, et al. Microcytic anemia and hepatic iron overload in a child with compound heterozygous mutations in DMT1 (Scl11a2). *Blood.* 2006;107(1):349–354. doi:10.1182/blood-2005-06-2477

17. Muñoz M, Gómez-Ramírez S, Besser M, et al. Current misconceptions in diagnosis and management of iron deficiency. *Blood Transfus.* 2017. doi:10.2450/2017.0113-17

18. Tefferi A, Hanson CA, Inwards DJ. How to interpret and pursue an abnormal complete blood cell count in adults. *Mayo Clin Proc.* 2005;80(7):923–936. doi:10.4065/80.7.923

19. Chapter 2: use of iron to treat anemia in CKD. *Kidney Int Suppl.* 2012;2(4):292–298. doi:10.1038/kisup.2012.34

20. National Institute for Health and Care Excellence. Chronic kidney disease: managing anaemia. [NICE guideline NG8]. Published June 3, 2015. https://www.nice.org.uk/guidance/ng8

21. Dignass AU, Gasche C, Bettenworth D, et al. European consensus on the diagnosis and management of iron deficiency and anaemia in inflammatory bowel diseases. *J Crohns Colitis.* 2015;9(3):211–222. doi:10.1093/ecco-jcc/jju009

22. Ponikowski P, Voors AA, Anker SD, et al. 2016 ESC Guidelines for the diagnosis and treatment of acute and chronic heart failure: the Task Force for the diagnosis and treatment of acute and chronic heart failure of the European Society of Cardiology (ESC). Developed with the special contribution of the Heart Failure Association (HFA) of the ESC. *Eur J Heart Fail.* 2016;18(8):891–975. doi:10.1002/ejhf.592

23. Tim GL, Comin-Colet J, Leal-Noval S, et al. Management of anemia in patients with congestive heart failure. *Am J Hematol.* 2017;92(1):88–93. doi:10.1002/ajh.24595

24. Qaseem A, Humphrey LL, Fitterman N, et al. Treatment of anemia in patients with heart disease: a clinical practice guideline from the American College of Physicians. *Ann Intern Med.* 2013;159(11):770. doi:10.7326/0003-4819-159-11-201312030-00009

25. Lichtin AE. Clinical practice guidelines for the use of erythroid-stimulating agents: ASCO, EORTC, NCCN. *Cancer Treat Res.* 2011;157:239–248. doi:10.1007/978-1-4419-7073-2_14

26. National Comprehensive Cancer Network. Bone cancer. Accessed August 31, 2019. https://www.nccn.org/professionals/physician_gls/pdf/growthfactors.pdf

27. Schrijvers D, De Samblanx H, Roila F, et al. Erythropoiesis-stimulating agents in the treatment of anaemia in cancer patients: ESMO clinical practice guidelines for use. *Ann Oncol.* 2010;21(suppl 5):v244–v247. doi:10.1093/annonc/mdq202

28. Gasche C, Berstad A, Befrits R, et al. Guidelines on the diagnosis and management of iron deficiency and anemia in inflammatory bowel diseases. *Inflamm Bowel Dis.* 2007;13(12):1545–1553. doi:10.1002/ibd.20285

29. Feosol. Accessed August 31, 2019. https://www.feosol.com/

30. Slow Fe®. Slow release iron supplement. Accessed August 31, 2019. http://www.slowfe.com

31. Brittenham G. Disorders of iron metabolism: iron deficiency and iron overload. In: Hoffman R, Benz EJ, Shattil SJ, et al., eds. *Hematology: Basic principles and practice.* 5th ed. Elsevier Churchill Livingstone; 2009:453–468.

32. Shield Therapeutics Ltd. Accrufer (Ferric Maltol) [prescribing information]. Revised July 2019. https://www.accessdata.fda.gov/drugsatfda_docs/label/2019/212320Orig1s000lbl.pdf

33. Schrier SL. So you know how to treat iron deficiency anemia. *Blood.* 2015;126(17):1971. doi:10.1182/blood-2015-09-666511

34. Auerbach M, Schrier S. Treatment of iron deficiency is getting trendy. *Lancet Haematol.* 2017;4(11):e500–e501. doi:10.1016/S2352-3026(17)30194-1

35. Moretti D, Goede JS, Zeder C, et al. Oral iron supplements increase hepcidin and decrease iron absorption from daily or twice-daily doses in iron-depleted young women. *Blood.* 2015;126(17):1981–1989. doi:10.1182/blood-2015-05-642223

36. Stoffel NU, Cercamondi CI, Brittenham G, et al. Iron absorption from oral iron supplements given on consecutive versus alternate days and as single morning doses versus twice-daily split dosing in iron-depleted women: two open-label, randomised controlled trials. *Lancet Haematol.* 2017;4(11):e524–e533. doi:10.1016/S2352-3026(17)30182-5

37. Rossi E. Hepcidin—the iron regulatory hormone. *Clin Biochem Rev.* 2005;26(3):47–49. Pubmed PMID: 16450011.

38. Remacha Á, Sanz C, Contreras E, et al. Guidelines on haemovigilance of post-transfusional iron overload. *Blood Transfus.* 2013;11(1):128–139. doi:10.2450/2012.0114-11

39. Tolkien Z, Stecher L, Mander AP, et al. Ferrous sulfate supplementation causes significant gastrointestinal side-effects in adults: a systematic review and meta-analysis. *PLoS One.* 2015;10(2):e0117383. doi:10.1371/journal.pone.0117383

40. Centers for Disease Control and Prevention. Recommendations to prevent and control iron deficiency in the United States. *MMWR Recomm Rep.* 1998;47(RR-3):1–29. Pubmed PMID: 9563847.

41. Rizzo JD, Brouwers M, Hurley P, et al. American Society of Clinical Oncology/American Society of Hematology clinical practice guideline update on the use of epoetin and darbepoetin in adult patients with cancer. *J Clin Oncol.* 2010;28(33):4996–5010. doi:10.1200/JCO.2010.29.2201

42. Auerbach M, Deloughery T. Single-dose intravenous iron for iron deficiency: a new paradigm. *Hematology.* 2016;2016(1):57–66. doi:10.1182/asheducation-2016.1.57

43. Centers for Disease Control and Prevention. Data & statistics on sickle cell disease. Accessed October 5, 2019. https://www.cdc.gov/ncbddd/sicklecell/data.html

44. Yawn BP, John-Sowah J. Management of sickle cell disease: recommendations from the 2014 expert panel report. *Am Family Phys.* 2015;92(12):1069–1076. Pubmed PMID: 26760593.

45. Centers for Disease Control and Prevention. What is sickle cell trait? Accessed November 18, 2020. https://www.cdc.gov/ncbddd/sicklecell/traits.html

46. National Heart, Lung, and Blood Institute. Evidence-based management of sickle cell disease. Expert Panel Report, 2014. Published September 2014. http://www.nhlbi.nih.gov/health-pro/guidelines/sickle-cell-disease-guidelines

47. Section on Hematology/Oncology and Committee on Genetics. Health supervision for children with sickle cell disease. *Pediatrics.* 2002;109(3):526–535. doi:10.1542/peds.109.3.526

48. Bond M, Hunt B, Flynn B, et al. Towards a point-of-care strip test to diagnose sickle cell anemia. *Plos One.* 2017;12(5):e0177732. doi:10.1371/journal.pone.0177732

49. Centers for Disease Control and Prevention. Table 1: recommended child and adolescent immunization schedule for ages 18 years or younger, United States, 2020. https://www.cdc.gov/vaccines/schedules/hcp/imz/child-adolescent.html

50. Grohskopf LA, Alyanak E, Broder KR, et al. Prevention and control of seasonal influenza with vaccines: recommendations of the Advisory Committee on Immunization Practices—United States, 2019–20 influenza season. *MMWR Recomm Rep.* 2019;68(3):1–21. doi:10.15585/mmwr.rr6803a1

51. Cober MP, Phelps SJ. Penicillin prophylaxis in children with sickle cell disease. *J Pediatr Pharmacol Ther.* 2010;15(3):152–159. https://www.ncbi.nlm.nih.gov/pmc/articles/PMC3018247

52. Lederman HM, Connolly MA, Kalpatthi R, et al. Immunologic effects of hydroxyurea in sickle cell anemia. *Pediatrics.* 2014;134(4):686–695. doi:10.1542/peds.2014-0571

53. Kimberlin DW, Brady MT, Jackson MA, et al., eds. Pneumococcal infections. *Red Book: 2018–2021 report of the Committee on Infectious Diseases.* 31st ed. American Academy of Pediatrics; 2018:639–651.

54. Health Resources and Services Administration. Advisory committee on heritable disorders in newborns and children. Published June 2, 2017. https://www.hrsa.gov/advisory-committees/heritable-disorders/index.html

55. National Comprehensive Cancer Network. Hematopoietic growth factors. Published March 27, 2019. https://www.nccn.org/professionals/physician_gls/default.aspx#growthfactors

56. Phillips J, Henderson AC. Hemolytic anemia: evaluation and differential diagnosis. *Am Family Phys.* 2018;98(6):354–361. https://www.aafp.org/afp/2018/0915/p354.html

57. Garratty G. Immune hemolytic anemia associated with drug therapy. *Blood Rev.* 2010;24(4–5):143–150. doi:10.1016/j.blre.2010.06.004

58. Sarkar RS, Philip J, Mallhi RS, et al. Drug-induced immune hemolytic anemia (Direct antiglobulin test positive). *Med J Armed Forces India.* 2013;69(2):190–192. doi:10.1016/j.mjafi.2012.04.017

59. Arndt PA. Drug-induced immune hemolytic anemia: the last 30 years of changes. *Immunohematology: J Blood Group Serology Mol Genet.* 2014;30:44–54. https://www.redcrossblood.org/content/dam/redcrossblood/immunohematology-journal/Immuno%202014%20No.%202.pdf

60. Curtis BR. Drug-induced immune thrombocytopenia: incidence, clinical features, laboratory testing, and pathogenic mechanisms. *Immunohematology: J Blood Group Serology Mol Genet.* 2014;30:55–65. https://www.redcrossblood.org/content/dam/redcrossblood/immunohematology-journal/Immuno%202014%20No.%202.pdf

61. Garratty G, Arndt PA. Drugs that have been shown to cause drug-induced immune hemolytic anemia or positive direct antiglobulin tests: some interesting findings since 2007. *Immunohematology: J Blood Group Serology Mol Genet.* 2014;30:66–79. https://www.redcrossblood.org/content/dam/redcrossblood/immunohematology-journal/Immuno%202014%20No.%202.pdf

62. Frank JE. Diagnosis and management of G6PD deficiency. *Am Family Phys.* 2005;72(7):1277–1282. https://www.aafp.org/afp/2005/1001/p1277.html

63. Madu AJ, Ughasoro MD. Anaemia of chronic disease: an in-depth review. *Med Princ Pract.* 2016;26(1):1–9. doi:10.1159/000452104

64. Drüeke T. Hyporesponsiveness to recombinant human erythropoietin. *Nephrol Dial Transplant.* 2001;16(suppl 7):25–28. doi:10.1093/ndt/16.suppl_7.25

65. Becker PS. NCCN guidelines: Hematopoietic growth factors (Version 2.2019). Published March 27, 2019. https://www.nccn.org/professionals/physician_gls/pdf/growth-factors.pdf

66. KDIGO Anemia Work Group. KDIGO clinical practice guideline for anemia in chronic kidney disease. *Kidney Int Suppl.* 2012;2:279–335. https://kdigo.org/wp-content/uploads/2016/10/KDIGO-2012-Anemia-Guideline-English.pdf

67. Singh AK, Szczech L, Tang KL, et al. Correction of anemia with epoetin alfa in chronic kidney disease. *N Engl J Med.* 2006;355(20):2085–2098. doi:10.1056/NEJMoa065485

68. Pfeffer MA, Burdmann EA, Chen C-Y, et al. A trial of darbepoetin alfa in type 2 diabetes and chronic kidney disease. *N Engl J Med.* 2009;361(21):2019–2032. doi:10.1056/NEJMoa0907845

69. Amgen. Aranesp [package insert]. Revised June 2011. https://www.pi.amgen.com/~/media/amgen/repository-sites/pi-amgen-com/epogen/epogen_pi_hcp_english.pdf

70. Amgen. Epogen [package insert]. Revised July 2018. https://www.pi.amgen.com/~/media/amgen/repositorysites/pi-amgen-com/epogen/epogen_pi_hcp_english.pdf

71. Janssen Products. Procrit [package insert]. Revised August 2008. https://www.accessdata.fda.gov/drugsatfda_docs/label/2008/103234s5196pi.pdf

72. Pfizer. Retacrit [package insert]. Revised May 2018. https://www.accessdata.fda.gov/drugsatfda_docs/label/2018/125545s000lbl.pdf

73. Vifor Pharma. Mircera [package insert]. Revised April 2016. https://www.accessdata.fda.gov/drugsatfda_docs/label/2016/125164s071s072s073lbl.pdf

74. Aslinia F, Mazza JJ, Yale SH. Megaloblastic anemia and other causes of macrocytosis [published correction appears in *Clin Med Res.* 2006 Dec;4(4):342]. Clin Med Res. 2006;4(3):236–241. doi:10.3121/cmr.4.3.236

75. History of Leith, Edinburgh James Scarth Combe. Accessed October 10, 2019. http://www.leithhistory.co.uk/

76. Holmgren I. Award ceremony speech. December 10, 1934. https://www.nobelprize.org/prizes/medicine/1934/ceremony-speech

77. Hoffbrand AV, Weir DG. The history of folic acid. *Br J Haematol.* 2001;113(3):579–589. doi:10.1046/j.1365-2141.2001.02822.x

78. Castellanos-Sinco HB, Ramos-Peñafiel CO, Santoyo-Sánchez A, et al. Megaloblastic anaemia: folic acid and vitamin B12 metabolism. *Revista Médica Del Hospital General De México.* 2015;78(3):135–143. doi:10.1016/j.hgmx.2015.07.001

79. Fyfe JC, Madsen M, Højrup P, et al. The functional cobalamin (vitamin B12)-intrinsic factor receptor is a novel complex of cubilin and amnionless. *Blood.* 2004;103(5):1573–1579. doi:10.1182/blood-2003-08-2852

80. Schjønsby H. Vitamin B12 absorption and malabsorption. *Gut.* 1989;30(12):1686–1691. doi:10.1136/gut.30.12.1686

81. DiPiro, JT, Talbert RL, Yee, GC, et al., eds. *Pharmacotherapy: A Pathophysiologic Approach.* 10th ed. McGraw-Hill Education; 2017.

82. Kaferle J, Strzoda CE. Evaluation of macrocytosis. *Am Fam Physician.* 2009;79(3):203–208. https://www.aafp.org/afp/2009/0201/p203.html

83. Snow CF. Laboratory diagnosis of vitamin B12 and folate deficiency: a guide for the primary care physician. *Arch Intern Med.* 1999;159(12):1289–1298. doi:10.1001/archinte.159.12.1289

84. Healton EB, Savage DG, Brust JC, et al. Neurologic aspects of cobalamin deficiency. *Medicine.* 1991;70(4):229–245. doi:10.1097/00005792-199107000-00001

85. Lindenbaum J, Healton EB, Savage DG, et al. Neuropsychiatric disorders caused by cobalamin deficiency in the absence of anemia or macrocytosis. *N Eng J Med.* 1988;318(26):1720–1728. doi:10.1056/NEJM198806303182604

86. Nagao T, Hirokawa M. Diagnosis and treatment of macrocytic anemias in adults. *J Gen Fam Med.* 2017;18(5):200–204. doi:10.1002/jgf2.31

87. Smock KJ, Perkins SL. Thrombocytopenia: An update. *Int J Lab Hematol.* 2014;36(3):269–278. doi:10.1111/ijlh.12214.

88. James NG. Platelets on the web. University of Oklahoma Health Sciences Center. Updated April 16, 2015. https://ouhsc.edu/platelets/index.html

Hematology/Oncology and Supportive Care for the Nononcologist

Tianhong Li, Weijie Ma, and Xiaodong Feng

INTRODUCTION

Cancer causes significant disease burden worldwide. Each year, tens of millions of people are diagnosed with cancer around the world, and more than half of the patients eventually die from it. Globally, about one in six deaths is due to cancer. In many countries, cancer ranks the second most common cause of death following cardiovascular diseases, and accounts for an estimated 9.6 million deaths in 2018.[1] The economic impact of cancer is significant and has been increasing. The total annual economic cost of cancer in 2010 was estimated at approximately $1.16 trillion.

Cancer epidemiology defines the distribution, determinants, and frequency of cancer in specific populations.[2] Epidemiologic assessment provides clinicians and policy stakeholders with a quantification of cancer risk, formulates preventive strategies, outlines the basis for screening modalities for high-risk populations, and determines the efficacy of any preventive intervention. There is significant variation of cancer epidemiology worldwide. Approximately 70% of deaths from cancer occur in low- and middle-income countries. Knowledge of regional cancer trends helps to understand local cancer burden and develop individualized cancer control strategies; however, only one in five low- and middle-income countries have the necessary data to drive cancer policy.[3] Late-stage presentation and inaccessible diagnosis and treatment are common. In 2017, only 26% of low-income countries reported having pathology services generally available in the public sector. More than 90% of high-income countries reported treatment services are available compared to less than 30% of low-income countries. In this chapter, we focus on the cancer disease in the United States.

Cancer is the cause of 25% of deaths in the United States, second only to heart disease as a leading cause of death.[4] Each year, the American Cancer Society (ACS) compiles the most recent data on cancer incidence, mortality, and survival and publishes estimated numbers of new cancer cases and deaths that will occur in the United States nationally and for each state. In 2019, 1,762,450 new cancer cases and 606,880 cancer deaths were projected to occur in the United States. The cancer incidence rate (2006–2015) was stable in women and declined by approximately 2% per year in men, whereas the cancer death rate (2007–2016) declined annually by 1.4% and 1.8%, respectively. The overall cancer death rate dropped continuously from 1991 to 2016 by a total of 27%, translating into approximately 2,629,200 fewer cancer deaths than would have been expected if death rates had remained at their peak.[4] **Figure 26.1** summarizes the data for 10 leading cancer types for the estimated new cancer cases and deaths by sex in 2019 in the United States.

In addition to sex, factors that influence cancer incidence and mortality in the United States include age, race/ethnicity, geography, and socioeconomic status (SES). Cancer incidence and mortality rates are higher among males than females.[4] In addition, Americans over 65 years old have a tenfold greater risk of developing cancer than younger individuals. Despite an increase in the overall cancer mortality rate between 1950 and 1990, the mortality rates for all cancers combined have declined substantially for

individuals under 45 years of age but increased for individuals over 55 years of age. Most of the increase is attributable to deaths from lung cancer. African Americans have a higher cancer mortality rate than Whites.[5] Although the racial gap in cancer mortality is slowly narrowing, socioeconomic inequalities are widening, with the most notable gaps for the most preventable cancers. For example, compared with the most affluent counties, mortality rates in the poorest counties were twofold higher for cervical cancer and 40% higher for male lung and liver cancers during 2012 to 2016 in the United State. Some states are home to both the wealthiest and the poorest counties, suggesting the opportunity for more equitable dissemination of effective cancer prevention, early detection, and treatment strategies. A broader application of existing cancer control knowledge with an emphasis on disadvantaged groups would undoubtedly accelerate progress against cancer. Additional factors, such as timely

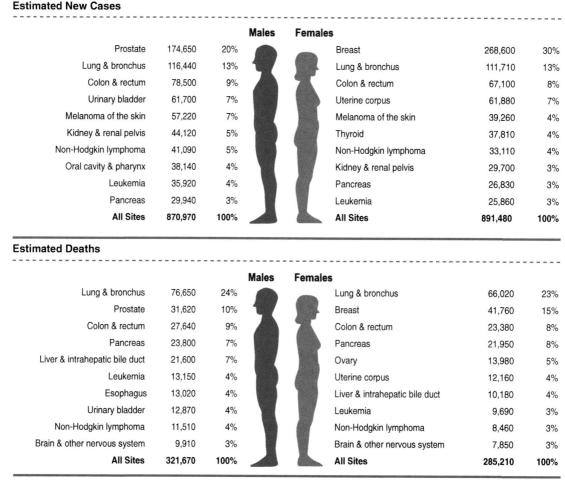

FIGURE 26.1 Most common new cancer rates and death in the United States. Ten leading cancer types for the estimated new cancer cases and deaths by sex, United States, 2019. Estimates are rounded to the nearest 10 and exclude basal cell and squamous cell skin cancers and in situ carcinoma, excluding urinary bladder. Ranking is based on modeled projections and may differ from the most recent observed data.

Source: With permission from Siegel RL, Miller KD, Jemal A. Cancer statistics. 2019. *CA Cancer J Clin.* 2019;69(1):7–34: Figure 1. doi:10.3322/caac.21551

access to healthcare, area of residence, immigration status, and even biologic differences, can also contribute to differential incidence and mortality by race.[6]

According to a report by the ACS, the cancer rates and death by cancer in the United States have been falling for more than 25 years due to the initiatives of smoking cessation, discouragement of hormone replacement therapy (HRT), frequent cancer screening, treatment of cancer at early stage, and availability of new technology and pharmacotherapy for cancers. The smoking cessation movement has contributed to almost 50% decline in lung cancer cases since 1960. Furthermore, screening high-risk patients (55–74 years old, 30 pack–years of cigarette smoking, quit less than 15 years prior) using low-dose computed tomography (LDCT) was shown to identify lung cancer at early stage and decrease lung cancer mortality by 20% in a randomized clinical trial in 2012.[7]

With the discontinuation of hormonal replacement therapy (HRT, estrogen-plus-progestin) since 2002, the cases of breast cancer in postmenopausal women have dropped significantly, which was not significantly related to the use of mammography.[8] Meanwhile, the routine screening of breast cancer by mammograms, early diagnosis, and early treatment of breast cancer have significantly decreased the death rate of breast cancer and increased the odds of survival for breast cancer patients.[9] According to a recent report, the 2018 mortality rate of breast cancer has dropped by 45.3% to 58.3% compared to the mortality rate of breast cancer

reported in 1989. Unfortunately, the new cancer cases and death of cancer related to obesity have been increasing.[10]

BACKGROUND

Cancer is a collection of more than 100 different diseases characterized by uncontrolled cellular growth and proliferation, high risk of invasion into surrounding tissue, and spreading or metastasizing to distance sites.[11] Metastases are a major cause of cancer-related death. Although almost any type of abnormal cell or tissues can develop into cancer anywhere, there are several main types of cancer categorized by the cell origins (**Table 26.1**). Carcinoma originates in the epithelial cells of skin, lungs, breasts, colon and rectum, pancreas, prostate, and other organs and glands. It remains as the most commonly diagnosed cancer type.[4]

Not all tumors are malignant or cancerous. The cells of benign tumor are generally well developed and have noncancerous, indolent growth. The benign tumor is usually encapsulated by the fibrous connective tissue, noninvasive to the surrounding normal tissues, and confined to the original site. Thus, the benign tumor, such as a common skin wart, is surgery curative. On the other hand, the cells of malignant tumors are poorly differentiated and genetically unstable. The malignant tumor generally loses the structure and function of the original tissue. The

---

TABLE 26.1 Cancer Types by the Cell Origins

Origin	Tissue Type	Cancer Type	Prevalence
Epithelial	Surface epithelium	Carcinoma	90% of human tumors
	Glandular tissue	Adenocarcinoma	
Connective	Fibrous	Fibrosarcoma	Sarcomas are rare in humans. They are solid tumors of connective tissues, including cartilage and fat.
	Bone	Osteosarcoma	
	Smooth or striated muscle	Leiomyosarcoma or rhabdomyosarcoma	
	Fat	Liposarcoma	
Hematological	Bone marrow	Leukemia	These tumors arise from blood-forming cells and immune cells. They count for about 8% of human malignancies.
	Lymphoid	Hodgkin and non-Hodgkin lymphoma	
	Plasma cell	Multiple myeloma	
Neural	Glial	Glioblastoma and astrocytoma	
	Nerve sheath	Neurofibrosarcoma	
	Melanocytes	Malignant melanoma	
Mixed	Gonadal tissue	Teratocarcinoma	

malignant tumor seldom has capsule and it is invasive to the surrounding normal tissue and can become metastatic by spreading to the distant sites. Malignant tumors of advanced stage are usually not curative by surgery.

Cancer development is a multiple-stage process including initiation, promotion, transformation, and progression (**Table 26.2**). "Cancer" is defined as a genetic disease that is caused by gene mutations in a few cells of the body. The somatic mutations usually derive from DNA damage or natural increase in age. These acquired mutations are present only in some of the cells and not passed between generations. A single mutation rarely causes cancer as the body will correct most mutations through apoptosis or programmed cell death. However,

cancer will occur as a result of multiple mutations over a lifetime, hence the higher chance for developing cancer in geriatric populations. Tumor suppressor genes are protective genes that repair mismatched DNA, slow down cell division, or start programmed cell death.

Oncogenes can cause cancer cells designated for apoptosis to survive and proliferate instead. When tumor suppressor genes do not work properly or oncogenes consistently activate, cells can grow out of control, which can lead to cancer. The arising tumor cells then acquire and accumulate some other abnormal characteristics at different stages and in different locations and patients become symptomatic for cancer disease (**Figure 26.2**). Substantial advances have been made in

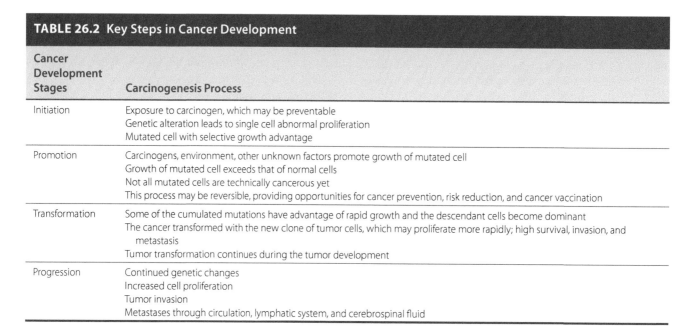

TABLE 26.2 Key Steps in Cancer Development	
Cancer Development Stages	**Carcinogenesis Process**
Initiation	Exposure to carcinogen, which may be preventable Genetic alteration leads to single cell abnormal proliferation Mutated cell with selective growth advantage
Promotion	Carcinogens, environment, other unknown factors promote growth of mutated cell Growth of mutated cell exceeds that of normal cells Not all mutated cells are technically cancerous yet This process may be reversible, providing opportunities for cancer prevention, risk reduction, and cancer vaccination
Transformation	Some of the cumulated mutations have advantage of rapid growth and the descendant cells become dominant The cancer transformed with the new clone of tumor cells, which may proliferate more rapidly; high survival, invasion, and metastasis Tumor transformation continues during the tumor development
Progression	Continued genetic changes Increased cell proliferation Tumor invasion Metastases through circulation, lymphatic system, and cerebrospinal fluid

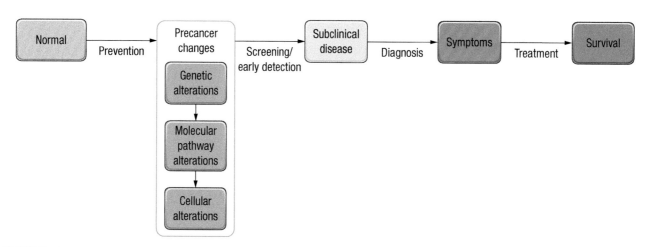

FIGURE 26.2 Cancer disease process and intervention. Cancer development is a complex process. Changes at the genetic level lead to modified intracellular signaling, which causes changes in cellular behavior and gives rise to cancerous tissue. Eventually, organs and the entire organism are affected. Asymptomatic patients have subclinical disease. Patients become symptomatic due to cancer and eventually die from cancer. Primary prevention, screening, early detection, diagnosis, and treatment are effective cancer management measures.

understanding the critical molecular and cellular mechanisms driving cancer development and progression that are summarized as "hallmarks of cancer," first described by Hanahan and Weinberg in 2000 and then revised in 2011.[12] Almost all these pathways have become drug targets over the past two decades. **Figure 26.3** illustrates the drug targets using lung cancer as an example.

The complex and heterogenous interplays of these critical molecular and cellular pathways contribute to different phenotypes of tumor progression. For instance, the rapid proliferation and expansion of solid tumors will slow down when the cells in the center of the tumor tissue cannot be reached by the existing vasculature, thus limiting the oxygen diffusion and nutrition supply. Hypoxia in the tumor tissues will stimulate tumor transformation. Hypoxia can potentially lead to high frequency of DNA mutations and less efficiency of DNA repairs. Hypoxia stimulates several intracellular signal transduction pathways, including hypoxia

inducible factor (HIF) pathway, PI3/AKT/mTOR pathway, and MAPK pathway, which play an essential role in regulating proliferation, survival, apoptosis, metabolism, migration, invasion, inflammation, and angiogenesis.[10] Angiogenesis, the growth of new blood vessels from preexisting vessels, is essential for tumor development. Angiogenesis is a complicated multistep process involving the activation, invasion, migration, proliferation, sprout formation, and tube and capillary network formation of vascular endothelial cells. All these steps are essential for the success of angiogenesis and controlled directly or indirectly by the dynamic balance between angiogenic stimulators and inhibitors. Hypoxia can induce the imbalance of angiogenesis regulations by upregulating the angiogenic stimulators, such as VEGF, SDF-1, Ang-2, and MMPs. Thus, investigating the cellular and molecular regulatory mechanism of angiogenesis provides potential drug targets to block angiogenesis and stop the tumor progression.

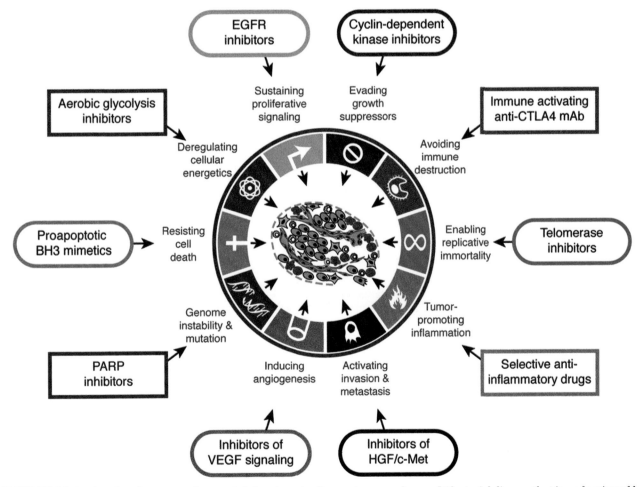

FIGURE 26.3 Hallmarks of cancer and potential drug targets. Cancer is a complex, multifactorial disease that is underpinned by the hallmarks of cancer that comprise several biological capabilities and two enabling characteristics (hypoxia and angiogenesis) that facilitate tumor growth and metastatic dissemination. Using lung cancer as an example, almost all these pathways have become drug targets over the past two decades.

c-met, mesenchymal-epidermal transition factor; EGFR, epidermal growth factor receptor; HGF, Hepatocyte growth factor; VEGF, vascular endothelial growth factor.

Source: With permission from Hanahan D, Weinberg RA. Hallmarks of cancer: The next generation. *Cell.* 2011;114(5):646–674: Figure 6. doi:10.1016/j.cell.2011.02.013

RISK FACTORS FOR CANCER

During the multistage process of cancer development, especially the early stages of initiation, promotion, and transformation, there are known interactions between a person's genetic factors and three categories of external agents, including: (i) physical carcinogens, such as ultraviolet and ionizing radiation; (ii) chemical carcinogens, such as asbestos, components of tobacco smoke, aflatoxin (a food contaminant), and arsenic (a drinking water contaminant); and (iii) biological carcinogens, such as infections from certain viruses, bacteria, or parasites. The World Health Organization (WHO), through its cancer research agency, International Agency for Research on Cancer (IARC), maintains a classification of cancer-causing agents.[13]

The cancer risk factors are classified as nonmodifiable and modifiable factors. Aging and inheritable genetic defects are nonmodifiable fundamental factors for the development of cancer. The incidence of cancer rises dramatically with age, most likely due to a build-up of risks for specific cancers that increase with age. The overall risk accumulation is combined with the tendency for cellular repair mechanisms to be less effective as a person grows older. Germline or hereditary mutations contribute to a small percentage of cancer patients. Because hereditary mutations are present in the DNA of sperm and egg cells, they can be passed down in families. An inherited gene means it is passed from parent to child within a family. These mutations are usually inherited from one or both parents and are present in nearly every cell of the body (**Table 26.3**).

About one-third of deaths from cancer are due to the leading behavioral and dietary risks, which are outlined in **Box 26.1**. Among these modifiable factors, tobacco use is the single most important risk factor for cancer and is responsible for approximately 22% of cancer-related deaths globally. Cancer-causing infections, such as hepatitis and human papillomavirus (HPV) are responsible for up to 25% of cancer cases in low- and middle-income countries.[14]

PREVENTION STRATEGIES

Primary Prevention Measures

Primary prevention measures are taken to prevent the onset of cancer or cancerous alterations and include avoidance of the known cancer risk factors. Reduced exposure to ultraviolet radiation and ionization radiation, immunization against HPV and hepatitis B virus, eating a healthy diet, and exercising regularly are all primary prevention measures. Vaccination against these HPV and hepatitis B viruses alone may prevent 1 million cancer cases each year.[15]

TABLE 26.3 Genetic Mutations Associated With Cancers

Oncogene	Associated Cancer
ALK	Lung cancer
BCL-2	Lymphoma
BCR-ABL	Chronic myelogenous leukemia
c-MYC	Burkitt lymphoma
HER2	Breast cancer
EGFR	Lung cancer
JAK2	Chronic myeloproliferative disorders
KRAS	Colon cancer, lung cancer
N-myc	Neuroblastoma
RET	Papillary thyroid carcinoma, lung cancer
Tumor Suppressor Gene	**Associated Cancer**
APC	Colorectal cancer
BRCA	Breast cancer, ovarian cancer
CDKN2A	Pancreatic cancer
DCC	Colon cancer
SMAD4	Pancreatic cancer
MEN1	Multiple endocrine neoplasia 1
NF1/2	Neurofibromatosis type 1/2
PTEN	Breast cancer, prostate cancer
RB	Retinoblastoma
TP53	Li-Fraumeni syndrome
VHL	Renal cell carcinoma
WT1	Wilms tumor
Gene Name	**Related Family Cancer**
MLHL, MSH2, MSH6, PMS2	Lynch syndrome
MEN	Multiple Endocrine Neoplasia
TP53	Li Fraumeni syndrome
STK11	Peutz-Jeghers syndrome

Secondary Prevention Measures

Screening is an important secondary prevention measure. Screening aims to identify presymptomatic individuals with abnormalities suggestive of a specific cancer or precancer and refer them promptly for diagnosis and treatment. Screening programs can be effective for select cancer types when appropriate tests are used, implemented effectively, linked to other steps

BOX 26.1
KNOWN CANCER RISK FACTORS FOR HUMAN MALIGNANCY

Nonmodifiable Risk Factors

Age
Race
Family history
Genetic susceptibility
- BRCA1/BRCA2

Inherited syndromes
- Down syndrome, Klinefelter syndrome, Fanconi's anemia

Geography

Modifiable Risk Factors

Tobacco
- Smokeless tobacco, environmental tobacco smoke, E-cigarettes

Alcohol
Diet
- High animal-fat intake; deficiencies in vitamins A and C and beta-carotenes

Environmental and occupational exposures
- Aromatic amines, arsenic, asbestos, nickel, pesticides, polycyclic hydrocarbons, vinyl chloride, lead, benzene, and others

Radiation
- Ionizing and ultraviolet radiation, radon

Medications
- See **Table 26.4**

Infection
- Bacterial (*Helicobacter pylori*)
- Parasites (*Schistosoma haematobium, Clonorchis sinensis*)

Viral
- Epstein-Barr virus
- Hepatitis B and C viruses
- Human immunodeficiency virus (HIV)
- Human papillomavirus (HPV)
- Human T-lymphotropic virus type 1

TABLE 26.4 Common Drugs That May Induce Human Cancers

Drug	Cancer Type
Antineoplastic Agents	
Alkylating agents	Leukemia
Cyclophosphamide	Urinary bladder
Androgen-anabolic steroids	Liver
Immunosuppressants	
Azathioprine, cyclosporine	Non-Hodgkin's lymphoma
Phenacetin-containing analgesics	Renal pelvis
Estrogens	
Steroid contraceptives	Liver
Conjugated	Endometrium
Synthetic (diethylstilbestrol)	Vagina, cervix (adenocarcinoma)

Pap test done every 3 years. HPV testing should not be used in this age group unless warranted after an abnormal Pap test result. Women between the ages of 30 and 65 should have a Pap test plus an HPV test (i.e., "cotesting") done every 5 years. Visual inspection with acetic acid (VIA) for cervical cancer is used in low-income settings. HPV testing and PAP cytology test for cervical cancer are used in middle- and high-income settings.[16]

Lung Cancer Screening
Lung cancer screening in high-risk patients (55–80 years old, 30 pack–years, quit less than 15 years prior) using LDCT was shown to identify lung cancer at an early stage and decrease lung cancer mortality by 20%.[17] However, only 4% of the 6.8 million eligible Americans reported being screened for lung cancer with LDCT in 2015.[18] In February 2015, the Centers for Medicare and Medicaid Services (CMS) first expanded coverage for LDCT.[19] Effective strategies are needed to improve lung cancer screening.

Breast Cancer Screening
Mammography (X-rays of the breast) is the most common screening test for breast cancer, recommended biannually for women aged 50 to 74 years. Screening should continue as long as a woman is in good health and is expected to live 10 or more years. Annual breast cancer screening with mammography is a choice for women aged 40 to 49.[20]

Colon Cancer Screening
For people at average risk for colorectal cancer, the ACS recommends regular screening beginning at age 50.

in the screening process, and when quality is assured. In general, a screening program is a far more complex public health intervention compared to early diagnosis. Currently, the U.S. Preventive Services Task Force (USPSTF) recommends screening for breast, cervical, lung, and colon cancer.

Cervical Cancer Screening
Cervical cancer screening should start at age 21. Women between the ages of 21 and 29 should have a

Screening for colorectal cancer is done either by a stool-based test that identifies signs of cancer in a patient's stool, or by a visual exam of the colon and rectum. Colonoscopy should begin at age 40 or 10 years before the youngest diagnosed relative for a patient with multiple first-degree relatives with colon cancer at any age or a first-degree relative diagnosed with colorectal cancer before age 60. In patients of families known to carry a Lynch syndrome gene mutation, screening should initiate during their early 20s, or 2 to 5 years younger than the youngest person in the family with a diagnosis. For people who have familial adenomatous polyposis (FAP) or test positive for the gene change linked to FAP, colonoscopy screening should start at 11 to 12 years old.[21]

Prostate Cancer Screening

Until recently, the blood prostate-specific antigen (PSA) test was used routinely to screen men for prostate cancer. However, research has not yet proven that the potential benefits of testing outweigh the harms of testing and treatment. Thus, the ACS recommends that men make an informed decision with a clinician about whether to be tested for prostate cancer before 55. Men should not be tested without first being educated on the risks and possible benefits of testing and treatment. For men aged 55 to 69 years, the decision to undergo periodic PSA-based screening for prostate cancer should be an individual one. Currently, Medicare provides coverage for an annual PSA test for all Medicare-eligible men aged 50 and older. Many private insurers cover PSA screening as well.[22]

Personalized Medicine

The advent of personalized genomic medicine offers an opportunity to maintain a healthier population by preventing disease. Studying a patient's genomic profile predicts the risk of disease, particularly if there is a family history of disease; for example, variants in the breast cancer genes (*BRCA*) increase the risk of breast and ovarian cancer. Patients with *BRCA* variants have the opportunity to pursue preventative treatment—such as elective surgery or close monitoring—to mitigate their high risk of disease or adopt changes in lifestyle to minimize the risk. Gene sequencing to evaluate the risk of transferring an inherited disease may become part of reproductive decisions.

DIAGNOSIS OF CANCER

The signs and symptoms of cancer vary significantly depending on the origin of the disease and tumor burden. Cancer can present with many signs and symptoms that are nonspecific, such as weight loss, hemoptysis, abdominal pain, severe fatigue, and others. Thus, it is important to evaluate the extent of tumor (i.e., stage) and to establish histological diagnosis when a cancer is suspected.

BIOMARKER-DRIVEN CANCER DIAGNOSIS

Tailoring therapy to an individual cancer patient by state-of-the-art technology has become a standard of care for selecting the most appropriate therapeutic regimen to maximize efficacy and minimize unwanted toxicity.

Taking lung cancer as an example, **Figure 26.4** illustrates a schema for biomarker-driven cancer diagnosis at multiscale levels. The extent of tumor at the organ and whole-body levels can be evaluated by imaging (e.g., positron emission tomography/computed tomography [PET/CT], CT scan with bone scans, or magnetic resonance imaging [MRI] of the brain). Histology, as well as molecular and immune biomarkers, are important to select the first-line systemic therapies for patients with nonoperable or metastatic lung cancer.[23] First, pathology assessment of tumor by biopsy is essential to establish a histological diagnosis of lung cancer based on a hematoxylin and eosin (H&E) stain and IHC stains. For example, PD-L1 IHC 22C3 pharmDx is the first companion diagnostic approved by the U.S. Food and Drug Administration (FDA) in patients with nonsmall cell lung cancer (NSCLC) for treatment with pembrolizumab.[24] It can be performed successfully on a variety of tumor specimens—formalin-fixed paraffin-embedded (FFPE) tissue blocks, fluid, and fine-needle aspiration cytology cell blocks or smears. Several studies have confirmed that the specimen should be considered to have positive membrane PD-L1 expression if total proportion score (TPS) ≥50% for first line monotherapy.

The different types of cancer are also described histologically under the microscope. For example, major histological subtypes of NSCLC include adenocarcinoma (LUAD), squamous cell carcinoma (LUSC), and large cell neuroendocrine tumor (LCNET). IHC with one LUAD marker (e.g., TTF1 and napsin A) and one LUSC marker (e.g., p40 and p63) will suffice.[25] Thyroid transcription factor-1 (TTF1) is expressed in 70% to 90% of primary LUAD and not expressed in LUSC, while p40 and p63 is highly expressed in LUSC and is not expressed in LUAD.[25,26]

The clinical application of multiplexed molecular biomarker assays has revolutionized cancer diagnosis and treatment, enabling the current era of precision cancer medicine.[27] Recent technology advances in genotyping and next-generation sequencing (NGS) now allow the possibility of rapidly and comprehensively interrogating the cancer genome of individual patients from small tumor biopsies.

Companion diagnostics have been developed for detecting a drug target by an FDA-approved test, such as real-time polymerase chain reaction (RT-PCR), flu-

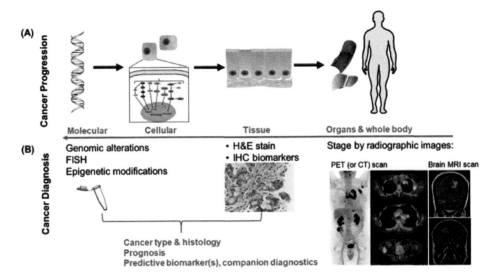

FIGURE 26.4 A schema for biomarker-driven cancer diagnosis at multiscale levels. Cancer development is a complex process. **(A)** Changes at the genetic level lead to modified intracellular signaling, which causes changes in cellular behavior and gives rise to cancerous tissue. Eventually, organs and the entire organism are affected. **(B)** Conversely, biomarker-driven cancer diagnosis also occurs at multiscale levels. Clinical staging includes radiographic images with PET/CT or CT with bone scans and possibly brain MRI scans to evaluate the extent of tumor at the organ and whole-body levels. An example from a patient with a primary left upper lobe squamous cell lung cancer with metastasis to regional lymph nodes, bones, and brain is shown. Histology evaluation at the tissue level and molecular and cellular biomarkers are all important to determine the cancer type and histology, prognosis, and predictive biomarkers important for treatment selection.

IHC: immunohistochemistry

orescence in situ hybridization (FISH), or multiplexed targeted NGS. For example, for newly diagnosed nonsquamous NSCLC patients, testing for epidermal growth factor receptor (*EGFR*; by a polymerase chain reaction method that takes <2 weeks, on either tissue or blood or fluorescence in-situ testing [FISH]) and c-ROS oncogene 1 (*ROS1*; by FISH) are all applied in clinic. NGS can be performed in parallel with these tests or reflexed if these tests are all negative.

Increasingly, these molecular biomarker assays have been used for selecting initial and subsequent therapy based on the tumor genomic makeups and clonal evolution of drug-sensitive or resistant mutations for either molecularly targeted therapy or ICI therapy.[28,29] Current NCCN guideline (Version 1 2020, accessed on February 8, 2020) recommends molecular testing for eight actionable molecular alterations in *EGFR, ALK, ROS1, BRAF, MET, RET, ERBB2,* and *NTRK1/2/3* genes, in patients with nonsquamous NSCLC.[23] The majority of these diagnostics improve their sensitivity by probing targeted genes with novel technologies using archival tumor specimens obtained by an invasive and expensive biopsy or surgical procedure. At diagnosis, these molecular assays can fail in up to 30% of reported cases due to insufficient tumor specimens procured.[29] Liquid biopsy, performed by a noninvasive blood draw for plasma circulating tumor DNA (ctDNA), has become a valuable alternative tumor resource for molecular

biomarker testing and has been recommended and increasingly used in the clinic when tumor tissue is limited and/or insufficient for molecular testing.[30-33] The sensitivity of the current FDA-approved companion diagnostics using plasma ctDNA for *EGFR* T790M is 70% to 82% with a specificity of ≥95%.[30-32] There is an unmet need to develop noninvasive or minimally invasive, low-cost, integrated blood biomarker assays that can improve the successful testing of molecular and immune biomarkers in those NSCLC patients who do not have sufficient tumor cells, ctDNA, or activated immune cells, with the goal of enabling precision oncology in every patient.

Given the importance of laboratory tests in cancer care, all laboratory testing that is performed on humans in the United States (except testing done in clinical trials and other types of human research) is regulated through the Clinical Laboratory Improvement Amendments (CLIA), which were passed by Congress in 1988. The CLIA laboratory certification program is administered by the CMS in conjunction with the FDA and the Centers for Disease Control and Prevention (CDC). CLIA ensures that laboratory staff are appropriately trained and supervised and that testing laboratories have quality-control programs in place so that test results are accurate and reliable. The FDA regulates the development and marketing of all laboratory tests that use test kits and equipment that are commercially manufactured in the United States. After the FDA approves a laboratory test, other federal and state agencies make sure that the test materials and equipment meet strict standards while they are being manufactured and then used in a medical or clinical laboratory.

CANCER STAGING

Cancer staging is the process of evaluating the size, location, and extent of the cancer. Knowing the stage of cancer helps clinicians know details about the tumor location, the seriousness of the cancer, and how to choose the best treatment options (e.g., surgery for an early-stage cancer, systemic therapies for an advanced-stage cancer). Clinicians may also identify clinical trials that may be treatment options for patients. **Table 26.5** summarizes the two most commonly used staging systems.

EARLY DETECTION AND EARLY DIAGNOSIS

Early detection identifies cancer at early stage, increasing effectiveness of treatment and resulting in a greater probability of survival, lower morbidity, and less-expensive treatment. Early diagnosis consists of three factors that must be integrated and provided in a timely manner: patient awareness and access to care; clinical evaluation, diagnosis, and staging; and access to treatment. Early diagnosis is relevant in all settings and the majority of cancers.

TREATMENT OF CANCER

Traditionally, pathologic diagnosis and clinical staging are essential for understanding the history, estimating the prognosis, and selecting the treatment options for each individual cancer patient. Modern cancer treatment regimens encompass one or more of the five treatment modalities: surgery, radiotherapy, chemotherapy, molecularly targeted therapy, and immunotherapy. When detected early and treated according to best practices, surgery offers high cure rates in most common cancer types, such as breast cancer, cervical cancer, NSCLC, oral cancer, and colorectal cancer. Radiation is an alternative local therapy option if patients are not candidates for the invasive surgical procedures. Chemotherapy and radiation are indicated for locally advanced cancer, and systemic chemotherapy is the mainstay treatment for nonoperable locally advanced and metastatic cancer.

It is important to recognize that certain cancer types—such as testicular seminoma, leukemias and lymphomas in children, and thyroid cancer in young adults—can have high cure rates if appropriate treatment is provided, even when cancerous cells have metastasized to other areas of the body. At the initial consultation, oncologists should provide cancer patients and their family members information related to cancer diagnosis and prognosis, evaluate the patient's fitness for therapy, and discuss the goal of care and

---

TABLE 26.5 Cancer Staging to Record the Anatomical Extent of Disease

AJCC TNM Stage*		Five-Category Stage	
Stage	Description	Stage	Description
Description			More often used by cancer registries than by doctors.
0	Abnormal cells are present but have not spread to nearby tissue. CIS is not cancer, but it may become cancer.	In situ	Abnormal cells are present but have not spread to nearby tissue.
1	T1-2N0M0	Localized (T1-2)	Cancer is limited to the place where it started, with no sign that it has spread
2	T3N0, or T1-2N1	Regional	Cancer has spread to nearby lymph nodes, tissues, or organs.
3	T4N0-3M0	Distant	Cancer has spread to distant parts of the body
4	anyT anyN M1	Unknown	No data available

Common users

AJCC TNM: Clinicians. The TNM classification comprises the clinical/pathological record algorithms for almost all cancers, with the primary exception of pediatric cancers.

Five category stage: cancer registries

*T, primary tumor size; N, regional lymph nodes involvement; M, presence or otherwise of distant metastatic spread.

AJCC, American Joint Committee on Cancer; CIS, carcinoma in situ; TNM, TNM Classification of Malignant Tumors.

Source: National Cancer Institute. *Cancer staging.* Published March 9, 2015. https://www.cancer.gov/about-cancer/diagnosis-staging/staging

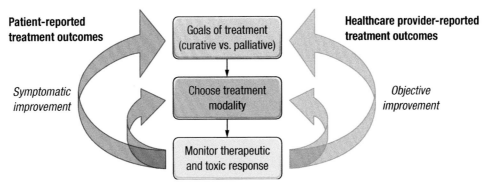

FIGURE 26.5   Initiation and management of cancer therapy.

treatment options (**Figure 26.5**). For those patients who are not curable or treatable for their cancer, it is important to inform the patients and family members the goal of palliative treatment and supportive care to reduce cancer-related symptoms, improve the patient's quality of life, and prolong life at the expense of potential treatment-related toxicities and even mortality. It is also important to provide integrated and patient-centered health services to support the patient's psychosocial distress and financial burden when possible.

P4 MEDICINE

Recent advances in new sequencing technologies and novel diagnostic techniques have allowed clinicians to use genomic data to both diagnose disease and predict how each patient will react to a particular medication.[34] P4 (predictive, preventive, personalized, and participatory) medicine,[35] uses the patient's genomic profile (e.g., FoundationOne CDx) to stratify patients into groups based on their subtype of mutations and response to drug therapies. Precise treatment, personalized to the genomic profile of the group, can then be offered. P4 medicine describes how personalized genomic medicine not only predicts a patient's response to treatment but also predicts their disease risk so they may pursue preventative treatment to reduce the risk.[36] Genomic personalized medicine enables clinicians to prescribe the most effective drug in the right combination with other medications to improve healthcare outcomes. As the population ages, there is a strain on healthcare systems to treat the increasing number of patients suffering from multiple medical conditions requiring polypharmacy. Personalized genomic medicine improves the prescribing patterns of drug treatments to help meet the challenge of delivering a more efficient and modern healthcare system, especially for those patients suffering with multimorbidities.[36]

CHEMOTHERAPY

All chemotherapy drugs work by attacking cells that are dividing rapidly by interfering with the division of these cells (**Figure 26.6**). Normal cells divide at a rate that is tightly controlled (cell growth) and die with a controlled program (apoptosis). Cancer cells have dysregulated the cell division, leading to uncontrolled production of new cells, and dysregulated cell death, leading to accumulation of cancer cells.[37] There are challenges to chemotherapy, including:

1. Cancer cells usurp normal cell replication and signal transduction pathways during their evolution for growth and survival.
2. There are no predictive surrogate markers for either response or toxicity of individual patients.
3. There has been limited success in controlling the toxicities from chemotherapy.

Before initiating chemotherapy, it is important to consider the goal of treatment (curative vs. palliative), duration of treatment (limited cycles vs. indefinite cycles), patient's factors such as performance status (commonly used ECOG or Karnofsky score), organ function and comorbidities, toxicities, and potential drug interaction. Depending on the goal of treatment, chemotherapy is classified by the terminology outlined in **Table 26.6**. Common side effects of chemotherapy include infusion reactions, hair loss, mucositis, nausea/vomiting, constipation or diarrhea, low blood counts (neutropenia, anemia, low platelet counts), peripheral neuropathy, cardiac toxicity, infertility, and rare complications from chemotherapy could cause death and second malignancies. Additionally, the treatment setting (inpatient vs. outpatient), intravenous access, family commitment, employment status, financial impact, and psychosocial support are also important in cancer-care planning. **Table 26.7** summarizes drugs approved for chemotherapy.

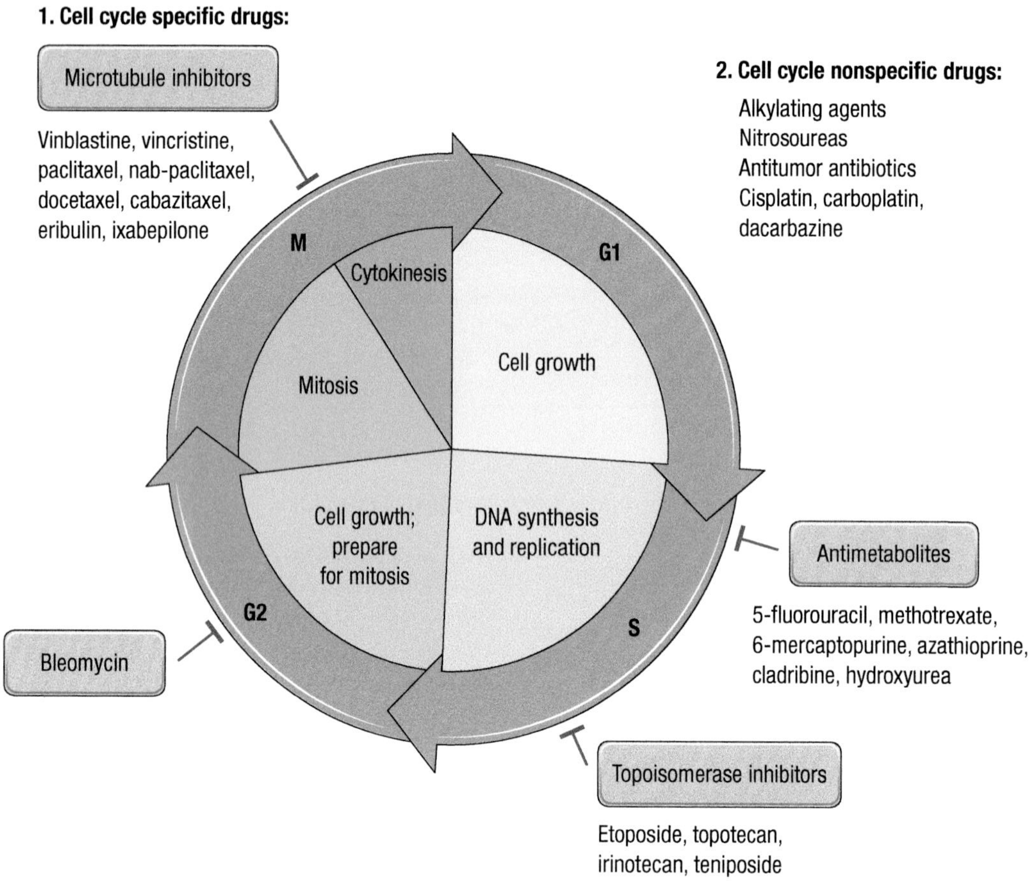

1. Cell cycle specific drugs:

Microtubule inhibitors

Vinblastine, vincristine, paclitaxel, nab-paclitaxel, docetaxel, cabazitaxel, eribulin, ixabepilone

2. Cell cycle nonspecific drugs:

Alkylating agents
Nitrosoureas
Antitumor antibiotics
Cisplatin, carboplatin, dacarbazine

M
Cytokinesis
Mitosis
G1
Cell growth

G2
Cell growth; prepare for mitosis
DNA synthesis and replication
S

Bleomycin

Antimetabolites

5-fluorouracil, methotrexate, 6-mercaptopurine, azathioprine, cladribine, hydroxyurea

Topoisomerase inhibitors

Etoposide, topotecan, irinotecan, teniposide

FIGURE 26.6 Principle of cytotoxic chemotherapy.

TABLE 26.6 Chemotherapy Classification Terminology

Classification Terminology	Description
Induction	Initial, high-dose regimen, usually combination, with intent of CR in a curative intent
Consolidation	Repetition of induction regimen for patients in CR, with intent of increasing cure rate or CR duration
Intensification	Treatment after achieving CR, using higher doses of induction regimen (or high doses of other regimen), with intent of increasing cure rate or CR duration
Maintenance	Long-term, low-dose regimen for patients in CR, with intent of delaying the regrowth of tumor cells
Adjuvant	Following successful eradication of measurable tumor by surgery or RT, a short course of high-dose chemo, with intent of destroying a small number of residual tumor cells in order to prolong either survival or disease-free survival
Neoadjuvant	Chemotherapy given in the pre- or perioperative period, with the intent of down-staging tumor, allowing for resection, or allowing for less disfiguring surgery
Primary chemotherapy	Sometimes used as a synonym for neoadjuvant, but also describes chemotherapy given in the absence of intended surgery or RT
Chemoradiation	Treatment that combines chemotherapy with radiation therapy for locally advanced cancer, such as head and neck, non-small cell lung cancer, small cell lung cancer, or rectal cancer. The chemotherapy acts as radiosensitizer to improve local control of cancer. The major limitation of combining two modalities has been cumulative normal-tissue toxicity.

CR, complete remission; RT, radiation therapy.

TABLE 26.7 Drugs Approved for Chemotherapy

Target	Medication	Indication	Side Effects
Purine (thiol) analogs	Azathioprine (Imuran®)	Preventing organ rejection, rheumatoid arthritis, IBD, SLE	Myelosuppression; GI, liver toxicity
Purine analog	Cladribine (Mavenclad®)	Hairy cell leukemia	Myelosuppression, nephrotoxicity, neurotoxicity
Pyrimidine analog	Cytarabine (arabinofuranosyl cytidine; Cytosar®)	Leukemias (AML), lymphomas	Myelosuppression with megaloblastic anemia
	5-fluorouracil (Adrucil®)	Colon cancer, pancreatic cancer, actinic keratosis, basal cell carcinoma (topical); effects enhanced with addition of leucovorin	Myelosuppression, palmar–plantar erythrodysesthesia (hand–foot syndrome)
Folic acid analog	Methotrexate (Trexall®)	Cancers: leukemias (ALL), lymphomas, choriocarcinoma, sarcomas / Nonneoplastic: ectopic pregnancy, medical abortion (with misoprostol), rheumatoid arthritis, psoriasis, IBD, vasculitis	Myelosuppression, hepatotoxicity, mucositis (e.g., mouth ulcers), pulmonary fibrosis, teratogenic (neural tube defects)
Breaks in DNA strands	Bleomycin (Blenoxane®)	Testicular cancer, Hodgkin lymphoma	Pulmonary fibrosis, skin hyperpigmentation, minimal myelosuppression
Intercalates into DNA	Dactinomycin (actinomycin D; Cosmegen®)	Wilms tumor, Ewing sarcoma, rhabdomyosarcoma; used for childhood tumors	Myelosuppression
	Doxorubicin (Adriamycin®)	Solid tumors, leukemias, lymphomas	Cardiotoxicity, myelosuppression, alopecia
Cross-link DNA at guanine	Cyclophosphamide, ifosfamide (Neosar®)	Solid tumors, leukemia, lymphomas	Myelosuppression, hemorrhagic cystitis
Cross-link DNA	Nitrosoureas (Lomustine®)	Brain tumors (including glioblastoma multiforme)	CNS toxicity (convulsions, dizziness, ataxia)
	Cisplatin, carboplatin (Platinol®)	Testicular, bladder, ovary, lung carcinomas	Nephrotoxicity, peripheral neuropathy, ototoxicity
Cell cycle phase–nonspecific alkylating agent	Procarbazine (Matulane®)	Hodgkin lymphoma, brain tumors	Bone marrow suppression, pulmonary toxicity, leukemia
Microtubule inhibitor	Paclitaxel, other taxanes (Taxol®)	Ovarian and breast carcinomas	Myelosuppression, neuropathy, hypersensitivity
	Vincristine, vinblastine (Leurocristine®)	Solid tumors, leukemias, Hodgkin (vinblastine) and non-Hodgkin (vincristine) lymphomas	Neurotoxicity; bone marrow suppression
Inhibits ribonucleotide reductase	Hydroxyurea (Droxia®)	CML, polycythemia vera	Severe myelosuppression
Inhibit topoisomerase II	Etoposide, teniposide (Etopophos®)	Solid tumors (particularly testicular and small cell lung cancer), leukemias, lymphomas	Myelosuppression, alopecia
Inhibit topoisomerase I	Irinotecan, topotecan (Camptosar®)	Colon cancer (irinotecan), ovarian and small cell lung cancers (topotecan)	Severe myelosuppression, diarrhea

ALL, acute lymphocytic leukemia; AML, acute myeloid leukemia; CML, chronic myeloid leukemia; GI, gastrointestinal; IBD, inflammatory bowel disease; SLE, systemic lupus erythematosus.

To improve the efficacy of chemotherapy, treatment including two or more chemotherapy drugs used simultaneously (i.e., "combination chemotherapy") and chemotherapy in combination with radiation—and most recently in combination with immune therapy—have been tested and applied in cancer treatment.

Therapeutic Drug Monitoring

Therapeutic drug monitoring (TDM) is an efficient tool for controlling the toxicity of therapeutic drugs, and trials have even demonstrated that it can improve efficacy. The therapeutic index is a quantitative measurement of the relative safety of a drug. Cancer therapeutics has the narrowest therapeutic index. Thus, clinicians need to assess and reassess the benefits and the risks of treatment constantly. The administered dose of anticancer drugs is sometimes adjusted individually using either a priori or a posteriori methods. The most frequent clinical application of a priori formulae concerns carboplatin and allows the computation of the first dose based on biometrical and biological data such as weight, age, gender, creatinine clearance, and glomerular filtration rate. A posteriori methods use drug plasma concentrations to adjust the subsequent dose(s). Thus, nomograms allowing dose adjustment on the basis of blood concentration are routinely used for 5-fluorouracil given as long continuous infusions. Multilinear regression models have been developed (e.g., for etoposide, doxorubicin, carboplatin, cyclophosphamide, and irinotecan) to predict a single exposure variable, such as area under concentration-time curve (AUC) from a small number of plasma concentrations obtained at predetermined times after a standard dose. These models can be applied only by using the same dose and schedule as the original study. Bayesian estimation offers more flexibility in blood-sampling times and, owing to its precision and to the amount of information provided, is the method of choice for ensuring that a given patient benefits from the desired systemic exposure.

Unlike the other a posteriori methods, Bayesian estimation is based on population pharmacokinetic studies and can take into account the effects of different individual factors on the pharmacokinetics of the drug. Bayesian estimators have been used to determine maximum tolerated systemic exposure thresholds (e.g., for topotecan or teniposide) as well as for the routine monitoring of drugs characterized by a very high interindividual pharmacokinetic variability such as methotrexate or carboplatin. The development of these methods has contributed to improving cancer chemotherapy in terms of patient outcome and survival.

Drug Resistance

The development of drug resistance during the course of chemotherapy is a formidable problem. While much has been learned about the cellular and molecular mechanisms of drug resistance, approaches to circumvent this problem have yet to be identified. Drug resistance in tumor cells might effectively decrease the dose of drugs available for radiosensitization. Several studies have shown that drug-resistant cells are not radioresistant.[38] However, no information exists as to whether drug-resistant cells can be radiosensitized by the drug(s) to which they are resistant. Stated differently, it is not known if a cell's mechanism for detoxication of cytotoxicity results in loss of radiosensitization.

TARGETED MOLECULAR THERAPY

Since 2001, there has been tremendous progress in the drug development against almost all drug targets contributing to cancer development (see Figure 26.3). As of January 2020, the U.S. FDA has approved a total of 52 small molecule kinase inhibitors, 40 of which are tyrosine kinase inhibitors, 10 are serine/threonine kinase inhibitors, and two are lipid kinase inhibitors.[39] Among these 52 drugs, 46 were approved for solid and hematological cancer types. **Table 26.8** summarizes the drugs currently approved for hematological cancers, and **Table 26.9** summarizes the drugs currently approved for solid cancers. Recent meta-analysis performed on more than 30,000 patients suggests that matched personalized therapy improves the outcome across cancer types and studies.[40,41] Mechanisms of resistance to drugs targeting kinase fusions have two categories. The first category is on-target alterations, in which mutation or amplification of the fusion happens itself. Acquired resistance mutations that cluster around the adenosine triphosphate (ATP) binding site of the kinase domain are emerging as common mechanisms of on-target resistance. These mutations may hinder drug binding by increasing the affinity for ATP, by altering the hydrogen bonds necessary for stabilization of the drug in the binding pocket, or by causing steric interference. The second category is off-target alterations, meaning activation of parallel bypass pathways. Different inhibitors have variable levels of activity against specific resistance mutations, which must be taken into account when making treatment-related decisions.[42] Ongoing studies are evaluating the strategies and drugs to overcome mechanism-based resistance mechanisms.

TABLE 26.8 Drugs Approved for Hematological Malignancies

Target	Medication	Indication	Side Effects
BCR-ABL	Imatinib (Gleevec®)	Chronic myelogenous leukemia	Vomiting, diarrhea, muscle pain, headache, rash
PML-RARα	ATRA (Vesanoid®)	Acute promyelocytic leukemia	Headache, fever, dry skin
FLT3 mutation	Midostaurin (Rydapt®)	Initial AML	Low blood counts; nausea and vomiting; diarrhea; swelling in hands, feet, ankles (edema); headache
IDH2 mutant	Enasidenib (Idhifa®)	Recurrent or refractory AML	Nausea and vomiting, diarrhea, decreased appetite
	Dual-drug liposomal encapsulation to deliver daunorubicin and cytarabine at a fixed molar ratio over a prolonged period of time (Vyxeos®)	tAML, AML-MRC	Bleeding, febrile neutropenia, rash, swelling, nausea
CD33+	Gemtuzumab ozogamicin (Mylotarg®)	AML, initial elderly	Fever, diarrhea, nausea, vomiting
IDH1 mutant	Ivosidenib (Tibosovo®)	Recurrent or refractory AML	Nausea, diarrhea, constipation, fever, tiredness, join paint, cough
Hypomethylation	Venetoclax (Venclexta®)	Chronic lymphocytic leukemia, small lymphocytic lymphoma	Neutropenia, diarrhea, nausea, upper respiratory tract infection
	Glasdegib (Daurismo®)	Chronic lymphocytic leukemia	Tiredness, bleeding, febrile neutropenia, muscle pain, nausea
FLT3 mutant	Gilteritinib (Xospata®)	Recurrent AML	Swelling, fatigue, fever, joint or muscle pain
BTK	Acalabrutinib (Calquence®)	Chronic lymphocytic leukemia	Headache, nausea, vomiting, abdominal pain, diarrhea
Bcl-2 blocker	Venetoclax (Venclexta®)	Chronic lymphocytic leukemia	Neutropenia, diarrhea, nausea, anemia
XPO1 antagonist	Selinexor (Xpovio®)	Multiple myeloma	Tiredness, infections, nausea, vomiting, loss of appetite, diarrhea, constipation

AML, acute myeloid leukemia; BTK, Bruton's tyrosine kinas; IDH, isocitrate dehydrogenase; MRC, myelodysplasia-related changes.

CANCER IMMUNOTHERAPY

Cancer immunotherapy refers to a diverse range of therapeutic approaches that attempt to harness the immune system to establish a targeted antitumor immune response.[43,44] Cancer cells have cumulative somatic mutations, which make them potentially recognizable by the immune system. However, cancer cells can evade the immune surveillance by several mechanisms such as defective antigen presentation, checkpoint pathways, immunosuppressive cell infiltration, upregulation, and secretion of immunosuppressive cytokines.[45] The field of cancer immunotherapy has undergone a renaissance due to a greater understanding of the complex pathways that regulate tumor-induced immuno-suppression. In particular, the knowledge of the ability of "cancer cells to up-regulate programmed cell death 1 ligand 1 (PD-L1) expression in order to 'turn off' effector CD8+ T cells that might destroy them" has provided a rationale for the development of novel immunotherapies that target immune checkpoints for reestablishing and augmenting effector CD8+ T cell function against cancer.[46]

Figure 26.7 illustrates the seven key events for generating an effective antitumor immune response in the cancer-immunity cycle. First-generation immune checkpoint inhibitors (ICIs) targeting programed cell death protein 1 (PD-1) or its ligand PD-L1 and cytotoxic T-lymphocyte-associated protein 4 (CTLA4) pathways have become the most potent

TABLE 26.9 Drugs Approved for Solid Malignancies

Target	Medication	Indications	Side Effects
VEGF	Bevacizumab (Avastin®)	Colorectal cancer, lung cancer, breast cancer, kidney cancer	Hypertension, bleeding, necrotizing fasciitis
VEGFR2	Ramucirumab (Cyramza®)	Stomach cancer, colorectal cancer, NSCLC	Diarrhea, hyponatremia, headache, high blood pressure
EGFR	Cetuximab (Erbitux®)	Colon cancer, head and neck cancer	Rash, allergy
EGFR	Panitumumab (Vectibix®)	Metastatic colorectal cancer	Skin rash, fatigue, nausea, diarrhea, fever, and decreased magnesium levels
EGFR	Erlotinib (Tarceva®)	NSCLC, pancreatic cancer	Rash, diarrhea, fatigue
EGFR L858R	Afatinib (Gilotrif®)	NSCLC	Diarrhea, rash, stomatitis, nosebleed
EGFR L858R/ T790M	Osimertinib (Tagrisso®)	First line NSCLC	Diarrhea, stomatitis, rashes
EGFR	Dacomitinib (Vizimpro®)	NSCLC	Skin rash, diarrhea, bacterial nail infection
EGFR	Necitumumab (Portrazza®)	NSCLC	Vomiting, diarrhea, low potassium in the blood
ALK/ ROS1/Met	Crizotinib (Xalkori®)	NSCLC	Edema (swelling), constipation, fatigue
ALK	Alectinib (Alecensa®)	NSCLC	Gastrointestinal, constipation, nausea, swelling, myalgia (muscle pain, anemia)
ALK/ROS1	Ceritinib (Zykadia®)	NSCLC	Diarrhea, nausea, elevated liver enzymes, vomiting, abdominal pain, fatigue, decreased appetite, and constipation
ALK/ROS1/ EGFR	Brigatinib (Alunbrig®)	NSCLC	Nausea, vomiting, diarrhea
ALK/ROS1	Lorlatinib (Lorbrena®)	NSCLC	High blood cholesterol, high blood triglycerides, edema, peripheral neuropathy, cognitive effects
ALK/MET	Cabozantinib (Cabometyx®)	Renal cell carcinoma, hepatocellular carcinoma	Low phosphorous, abdominal pain, constipation
HR	SERM: Tamoxifen Fulvestrant (Faslodex®)	Breast cancer	Hot flashes, nausea, endometrial carcinoma
	Aromatase Inhibitors (post-menopausal women) Nonsteroidal: Anastrozole, letrozole, exemestane (Arimidex®, Femara®, Aromasin®)	Breast cancer	Diarrhea, vomiting, dry mouth, headache, breast swelling
	Megestrol acetate	Advanced breast cancer and endometrial cancer	Nausea, vomiting, dizziness, weakness, blurred vision
HER2	Trastuzumab (Herceptin®)	Breast cancer, stomach cancer	Nausea, diarrhea, cardiac toxicity
	Pertuzumab (Perjeta®)	HER2-positive breast cancer	Diarrhea, hair loss, and loss of neutrophils
	Lapatinib (Tykerb®)	HER2-positive breast cancer	Diarrhea, hand-foot syndrome
BRCA	Olaparib (Lynparza®)	Ovarian cancer, metastatic breast cancer	Nausea, vomiting, loss of appetite, fatigue
	Niraparib (Nerlynx®)	Ovarian cancer	Thrombocytopenia, nausea, fatigue, and constipation

(continued)

TABLE 26.9 Drugs Approved for Solid Malignancies (*continued*)

Target	Medication	Indications	Side Effects
NTRK	Entrectinib (Rozlytrek®)	NTRK fusion-positive solid tumors	Fatigue, constipation, dysgeusia, edema,
	Larotrectinib (Vitrakvi®)	NTRK fusion-positive solid tumors	Stomach pain, vomiting, diarrhea, severe dizziness
Multi-target	Imatinib (Gleevec®)	Chronic myelogenous leukemia, rare gastrointestinal cancer	Vomiting, diarrhea, muscle pain, headache, and rash
	Pazopanib (Votrient®)	Renal cell carcinoma, soft tissue sarcoma	Headache, loss of appetite, weight loss, nausea and vomiting
CDK4/6	Palbociclib (Ibrance®)	Breast cancer	Neutropenia, weakness, anemia
	Ribociclib (Kisqali®)	Breast cancer	Shortness of breath, dizziness, low white blood cell counts
	Abemaciclib (Verzenio®)	Breast cancer	Diarrhea, nausea and vomiting, abdominal pain
PIK3CA	Alpelisib (Piqray®)	HR+/HER2-, PIK3CA-mutated, advanced, or metastatic breast cancer as detected by an FDA-approved test following progression on or after an endocrine-based regimen	Skin rash or dry skin, diarrhea, dyspepsia

CDK4, cyclin-dependent kinase 4; *EGFR*, epidermal growth factor receptor; HR, hormone receptor; NSCLC, nonsmall cell lung cancer; NTRK, neurotrophic tyrosine receptor kinase; VEGF, vascular endothelial growth factor.

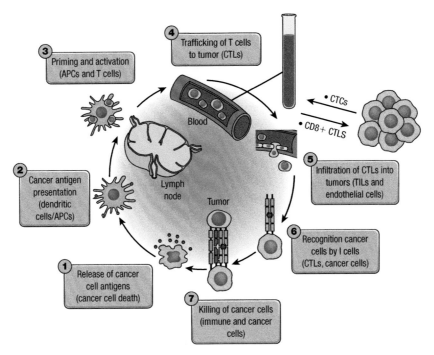

FIGURE 26.7 The cancer-immunity cycle. Generation of an effective antitumor immune response involves a series of seven stepwise events that ultimately form a cyclical response that increases the depth and breadth of the immune response against CSAs. Step 1: CSAs are released from cancer cells and captured by dendritic cells (DCs; a type of APC). This step must be accompanied by immunogenic signals such as proinflammatory cytokines. Step 2: The DCs present the captured CSAs to the immune effector cells—cytotoxic CD8+ T cells. Step 3: This activates and primes the cytotoxic CD8+ T cells to generate a specific immune response against the CSAs. Activated CD8+ T cells then migrate in blood (Step 4), infiltrate the tumor (Step 5), and recognize cancer cells by their expression of the specific CSAs. They then bind the specific antigen to their T-cell receptor (Step 6). The cytotoxic CD8+ T cell kills the cancer cells (Step 7), which results in the release of additional CSAs, thereby starting the whole process over again. APC, antigen-presenting cell; CSAs, cancer-specific antigens.

Source: Adapted from Chen DS, Mellman I. Oncology meets immunology: the cancer-immunity cycle. *Immunity.* 2013;39(1):1–10. doi:10.1016/j.immuni.2013.07.012

and durable cancer immunotherapy for patients with many cancer types.[47] Currently, FDA-approved ICIs include the anti-PD-1 monoclonal antibodies (mAbs) nivolumab and pembrolizumab; the anti-PD-L1 mAbs atezolizumab, durvalumab and avelumab; and the anti-CTLA-4 mAb ipilimumab.[24,48–52] These ICIs have improved overall survival in patients with advanced cancers and have been approved as first-line, second-line, or consolidation treatment for patients with NSCLC, first-line therapy for patients with metastatic small cell lung cancer (SCLC), melanoma,[53,54] and is promising for mesothelioma.[55,56] **Table 26.10**

TABLE 26.10 Summary of Immune Checkpoint Inhibitors

Target	Drug	Class	Company	Clinical Indication and Ongoing Evaluation
CTLA-4	Ipilimumab (Yervoy®, MDX-010, MDX-101)	Human IgG1/kappa	Bristol-Myers Squibb	*Metastatic melanoma* (U.S. FDA approved on March 28, 2011); *advanced (metastatic) renal cell carcinoma* (U.S. FDA approved on April 16, 2018, combo with Nivolumab); *advanced (metastatic) colon cancer* (U.S. FDA approved on July 11, 2018, combo with Nivolumab);
PD-1	Nivolumab (Opdivo®, ONO-4538, MDX-1106, BMS-936558)	Human IgG4/kappa	Bristol-Myers Squibb; Ono pharmaceuticals	*Metastatic melanoma* (U.S. FDA accelerated approval on December 22, 2014; U.S. FDA approval of nivolumab in combination with ipilimumab for *BRAF* V600 wild-type tumor on September 30, 2015); *Squamous NSCLC* (U.S. FDA approval on March 4, 2015; European Commission on July 20, 2015); expands to *nonsquamous NSCLC* (U.S. FDA approval on October 9, 2015); *advanced (metastatic) renal cell carcinoma* (U.S. FDA approval on November 23, 2015); *Hodgkin lymphoma* (U.S. FDA approval on May 17, 2016); *Head and neck carcinoma* (U.S. FDA approval on November 10, 2016); *Metastatic Urothelial Carcinoma* (U.S. FDA approval on February 2, 2017); *Hepatocellular carcinoma* (U.S. FDA approval on September 2, 2017 with previous treated by Sorafenib);
	Pembrolizumab (Keytruda®, MK-3475)	Humanized IgG4	Merck & Co.	*Metastatic melanoma* (United States accelerated approval on September 4, 2014); *metastatic NSCLC* (U.S. FDA approval on October 2, 2015; October 24, 2016; May 10, 2017; October 30, 2018, combo with Chemotherapy); *Head and neck carcinoma* (U.S. FDA approval on August 5, 2016; June 11, 2019); *Hodgkin lymphoma* (U.S. FDA approval on May 17, 2017); *Urothelial Carcinoma* (U.S. FDA approval on May 18, 2017); *Gastric Carcinoma* (U.S. FDA approval on September 22, 2017); *B-cell lymphoma* (U.S. FDA approval on June 13, 2018); *Merkel Cell Carcinoma* (U.S. FDA approval on December 19, 2018); *Advanced renal cell carcinoma* (U.S. FDA approved on April 22, 2019); *Esophagus cancer* (U.S. FDA approved on July 31 2019); *Endometrial Carcinoma* (U.S. FDA September 17, 2019)
	Cemiplimab (Libtayo®)	Humanized IgG4	Sanofi	*Advanced cutaneous squamous cell carcinoma* (U.S. FDA September 28, 2018)
PD-L1	Atezolizumab (Tecentriq™, MPDL3280A, RG7446)	Human IgG1	Roche & Genentech	*Metastatic bladder cancer* (U.S. FDA accelerated approval on May 18, 2016); *metastatic NSCLC* (U.S. FDA approval on December 6, 2018, combo with Avastin and Chemotherapy); *metastatic triple negative breast cancer* (U.S. FDA approval on March 8, 2019); *metastatic small cell lung cancer* (U.S. FDA approval on March 18, 2019)
	Durvalumab (MEDI4736)	Humanized IgG1	AstraZeneca	*Metastatic bladder cancer* (U.S. FDA approval on May 1, 2017); *metastatic NSCLC* (U.S. FDA approval on February 16, 2018); *Advanced renal cell carcinoma* (U.S. FDA approval on April 22, 2019)
	Avelumab (MSB0010718C)	Fully humanized IgG1	Merck KGaA, EMD Serono, Pfizer	*Merkel Cell Carcinoma* (U.S. FDA approval on March 23, 2017); *Urothelial cancer* (U.S. FDA approval on May 14, 2019)

CTLA-4, cytotoxic T-lymphocyte-associated protein 4; *NSCLC*, nonsmall-cell lung cancer; *PD-1*, programed cell-death protein 1; *PD-L1*, programed cell-death ligand 1.

summarizes the current available ICIs. The clinical benefit of ICIs is quite variable among different solid tumor types. However, objective tumor responses and durable long-term disease control are seen in only 10% to 40% of unselected patients with these solid tumor types. Currently, high PD-L1 expression on the membrane of tumor cells detected by immunohistochemistry for NSCLC and gastric cancer, and defective mismatch DNA repair (dMMR) or microsatellite instability high (MSI-H) for pan-tumor types have been approved as companion diagnostics for PD-1 inhibitor pembrolizumab. High tumor mutational burden (TMB) in tissue or plasma circulating tumor DNA has been shown to predict response in multiple tumor types to nivolumab plus ipilimumab or atezolizumab either alone or in combination. Additional biomarkers, such as the presence of CD8+ tumor infiltrating lymphocytes at tumor microenvironment and the T-cell inflamed gene expression profile, are promising for predicting responses to ICIs given either alone or in combination. Compared to molecular biomarkers, such as gain-of-function *EGFR* mutations and *ALK* gene rearrangements—which predict 60% to 80% of clinical responses to molecularly targeted therapy in NSCLC—immune biomarkers predict up to 50% with significant variations among different ICIs and tumor types. Further research is needed to optimize the use of these immune biomarkers either alone or in combination for patient selection.

These ICIs are not myelosuppressive and are usually well tolerated in geriatric patients and patients with performance status of 2. However, patients receiving ICIs may develop unique (and in rare cases, fatal) immune-related adverse events (irAEs) due to inflammatory infiltration of activated immune cells attacking normal organs.[57,58] These irAEs can affect any organ, including but not limited to skin, gastrointestinal tracts, lung, liver, heart, and bone marrow, giving them unique features that require new management strategies distinct from those of chemotherapy and molecularly targeted therapy.[59] A systematic review of 5,744 NSCLC patients from 23 studies treated with PD-1 or PD-L1 ICIs reported a global incidence of AEs of 64% (14% grade ≥3) with anti-PD-1 and 66% (21% grade ≥3) with anti-PD-L1 mAbs.[58] The incidence of grade 3 or 4 toxicity with the combination was increased compared with either single agent (59% vs. 21% and 28%, respectively, for nivolumab and ipilimumab) in cancer patients,[57,60] leading to early treatment discontinuation in approximately 18% of patients.[41] Of note, those patients who develop severe irAEs might benefit the most from ICIs.[61,62] Current National Comprehensive Cancer Network (NCCN) and American Society of Clinical Oncology (ASCO) guidelines recommend withholding immunotherapy after most irAEs reach grade 2 or higher (except macular rash, puritis, fatigue), and to consider resuming with caution when symptoms revert to grade 1.[63] For many patients this could cause a delay, and, potentially, discontinuation, of life-prolonging treatment. Standard of care for the treatment of irAEs at this time is limited to high-dose steroids, and infliximab for refractory disease.[64] Additionally, little is known regarding the safety and efficacy of retreatment with immunotherapy after an irAE. Much of the information available is based on retrospective studies.[65–67] Clinicians should be aware of these irAEs especially in cancer survivors who have long-term morbidities from irAEs.

The detection of both PD-1-positive tumor-infiltrating lymphocytes (TIL) and PD-L1-positive tumor cells at tumor microenvironment by IHC is a favorable prognostic factor and the best predictive factor of clinical response to ICI therapy. The combination of a T cell–inflamed gene expression profile (GEP) alone[68] or with PD-L1 IHC[69] or tumor mutation burden (TMB) might improve the prediction of favorable clinical response to pembrolizumab in combination with various agents. However, the assessment of *adaptive* expression of these markers requires post-treatment tumor biopsy, which is an invasive and expensive procedure that may be too risky to perform or be performed prematurely.[70] In addition, patients can develop unique immune-related adverse events, which include rare but severe autoimmune diseases due to inflammatory infiltration of activated immune cells attacking normal organs.[57,58] Together with the high cost and the availability of other emerging novel cancer therapeutics, there remains an unmet need to develop and validate minimally invasive immune-oncology biomarker assays that select the appropriate patients for cancer immunotherapy and monitor treatment response.

CLINICAL TRIALS

By monitoring effects on large groups of people, clinical research trials are vital to evaluating the effectiveness and safety of cancer drugs, diagnostic tests, or devices. **Table 26.11** summarizes the phases of clinical trials. Clinical research trials may be conducted by government health agencies such as the National Cancer Institute (NCI), researchers affiliated with a hospital or university medical program, independent researchers, or private industry. In fitted cancer patients who progressed to standard therapies, clinical research trials are sometimes life-saving. Whenever possible, cancer patients should be encouraged to participate in clinical trials; however, patient participation is voluntary, and it is important to emphasize four possible outcomes from a clinical trial:

TABLE 26.11 Summary of Clinical Trials

Phase	Purpose	Comment
0	Determines how a drug is processed in the body and how it affects the body	The first clinical trials done among people. In these trials, a very small dose of a drug is given to about 10–15 people
I	Determines maximum tolerated dose and describes pharmacology and pharmacokinetics	Dosing starts at 10% of the LD10 in mice Determine safe dose and schedule for phase II
II	Determines drug activity in specific tumors	Also determines administration schedule, toxicity, supportive care
III	New drug or drug combinations are compared against the standard therapy	Objective criteria: response rate, duration of response, survival, toxicity, and quality
IV	Role of drug in adjuvant/curative setting	Determines other uses, doses, schedules, and combination regimens

1. **Positive trial:** the clinical trial shows that the new treatment has a large beneficial effect and is superior to standard treatment.
2. **Noninferior trial:** the clinical trial shows that that the new treatment is equivalent to standard treatment.
3. **Inconclusive trial:** the clinical trial shows that the new treatment is neither clearly superior nor clearly inferior to standard treatment.
4. **Negative trial:** the clinical trial shows that a new treatment is inferior to standard treatment.

SPECIAL ISSUES

ONCOLOGIC EMERGENCIES

Oncologic emergencies are dangerous complications resulting from cancer. Common oncologic emergencies include neutropenia fever (sepsis), tumor lysis syndrome, metabolic disturbances and renal failure from tumor lysis syndrome, neurological compromise from symptomatic brain metastasis and spinal cord compression, cardiac arrest from malignant pericardial effusion/tamponade, respiratory failure from acute pulmonary embolism or malignant pleural effusion or superior vena cava (SVC) symptom, pain control, and coagulation emergencies, such as disseminated intravascular coagulation. The pathophysiology, etiology, and clinical presentation are described elsewhere.[71] It is important to recognize oncologic emergencies,

which often require multidisciplinary in-patient care for favorable clinical outcomes.

PALLIATIVE CARE

Palliative care is the treatment to relieve, rather than cure, symptoms caused by cancer and improve the quality of life of patients and their families. It is an urgent humanitarian need for people worldwide with cancer and other chronic fatal diseases and particularly needed in places with a high proportion of patients in advanced stages of cancer where there is little chance of cure. Palliative care can relieve the physical, psychosocial, and spiritual problems in over 90% of advanced cancer patients. For instance, more than 80% of cancer patients in terminal phase suffer from moderate to severe cancer pain, which can be effectively relieved by oral morphine. Effective public health strategies, comprising community- and home-based care, are essential to provide pain relief and palliative care for patients and their families in low-resource settings.

CARE FOR CANCER SURVIVORS

With the advances of cancer treatment, the number of cancer survivors has steadily increased in the recent years.[72] The majority of cancer survivors (64%) were diagnosed 5 or more years ago and 15% of cancer survivors were diagnosed 20 or more years ago. Nearly half (46%) of cancer survivors are 70 years of age or older.[72] It is essential to develop guidelines for posttreatment cancer survivorship care and to improve the quality of life of cancer survivors.

CHEMOTHERAPY-INDUCED ANEMIA

Anemia in cancer patients is a common side effect of myelosuppressive chemotherapy and may warrant treatment with erythropoiesis-stimulating agents.

Erythropoiesis-Stimulating Agents

Epoetin alfa (Epogen/Procrit), epoetin alfa-epbx (Retacrit), and darbepoetin alfa (Aranesp) are FDA-approved erythropoiesis-stimulating agents (ESA). Similar to endogenous erythropoietin, ESAs stimulate erythropoiesis by binding to progenitor stem cells, which leads to production and differentiation of red blood cells (RBC).[73–76] Epoetin alfa-epbx is an approved biosimilar to epoetin alfa.[76] These drugs carry a black box warning that use can increase the risk of death, myocardial infarction, stroke, venous thromboembolism, thrombosis of vascular access, and tumor progression or recurrence.[76]

Epoetin alfa (Epogen/Procrit) and epoetin alfa-epbx (Retacrit) increase the reticulocyte count within 10 days of initiation. This is followed by increases in the RBC count, hemoglobin, and hematocrit, usually within 2 to 6 weeks.[74–76] Hemoglobin levels are observed 2 to 6 weeks following the initiation of darbepoetin alfa (Aranesp).[73]

One of the FDA-approved indications of ESAs is for patients with nonmyeloid malignancies who have anemia due to myelosuppressive chemotherapy and have at least a minimum of 2 additional months of planned chemotherapy. Selected ESA is to be discontinued following the completion of a chemotherapy course.[73–76]

ESAs have not been shown to improve quality of life, fatigue, and patient well-being.[73–76] In addition, per manufacturer recommendations, ESAs are not indicated for use if the expected outcome is to cure with myelosuppressive chemotherapy, if anemia can be corrected by transfusion, or if the patient is receiving hormonal agents, biologics, or radiotherapy. However, administration of ESAs is indicated if patient is also on myelosuppressive chemotherapy in combination with hormonal agents, biologics, or radiotherapy.

Dosage for Chemotherapy Patients

Use of ESAs in chemotherapy patients should be initiated only if hemoglobin is <10 g/dL, and if a minimum of 2 additional months remain in the patient's planned chemotherapy course. The lowest necessary dose should be prescribed to avoid RBC transfusion. Typical adult ESA dosing and adjustment is outlined in **Table 26.12**.

CHEMOTHERAPY-INDUCED NEUTROPENIA

Anemia in cancer patients is a common side effect of myelosuppressive chemotherapy and may warrant treatment with erythropoiesis-stimulating agents.

Granulocyte Colony-Stimulating Factors

Granulocyte colony-stimulating factors (G-CSF) act on hematopoietic regulating production of neutrophils, progenitor proliferation, and differentiation and selected end-cell functional activation.[77–83]

They decrease the incidence of infection, as manifested by febrile neutropenia in patients with nonmyeloid malignancies receiving myelosuppressive chemotherapy.[78,80,81,83] Fulphila (pegfilgrastim-jmdb) and Udenyca (pegfilgrastim-cbqv) are approved as biosimilars to Neulasta (pegfilgrastim).

G-CSF are used to reduce the duration of neutropenia and neutropenia-related clinical sequelae in patients undergoing myelosuppressive chemotherapy or myeloablative chemotherapy followed by bone marrow transplantation. Filgrastim (Neupogen), filgrastim-sndz (Zarxio), or filgrastim-aafi (Nivestym) are FDA approved for patients undergoing bone marrow transplantation and those with acute myeloid leukemia receiving induction or consolidation chemotherapy.[80,81,83] Fulphila (pegfilgrastim-jmdb) and Udenyca (pegfilgrastim-cbqv) are approved as biosimilars to Neulasta (pegfilgrastim). These three agents are pegylated version of filgrastim and have a longer half-life.

Dosage for Chemotherapy Patients

Complete blood count (CBC) should be monitored twice weekly and it is recommended to consider increasing the dose in increments of 5 mcg/kg for each chemotherapy cycle according to the duration and severity of the absolute neutrophil count (ANC) nadir. G-CSF should be administered for up to 2 weeks or

TABLE 26.12 Adult Erythropoiesis-Stimulating Agent Dosing and Dose Adjustment

Erythropoiesis-Stimulating Agent	Dosing Options	Dose Increase*	Dose Decrease
Epoetin alfa or epoetin alfa-epbx	Option 1: 150 units/kg SC 3 × week or see below for Option 2	Increase to 300 units/kg SC 3 × week	Reduce by 25% Hgb increases greater than 1 g/dL in any 2-week period *or* Hgb reaches a level needed to avoid RBC transfusion Discontinue if no Hgb level response or if RBC transfusion still required after 8 weeks of ESA
	Option 2: 40,000 units SC every week	Increase to 60,000 units SC every week	
Darbepoetin alfa	Option 1: 2.25 mcg/kg SC every week or see below for Option 2	Increase up to 4.5 mcg/kg SC every week†	Reduce by 40% Hg increases greater than 1 g/dL in any 2-week period or Hb reaches a level needed to avoid RBC transfusion Discontinue if no Hgb level response or if RBC transfusion still required after 8 weeks of ESA
	Option 2: 500 mcg SC every 3 weeks	No dose increase recommended per manufacturer	

*Dose increase if after 4 weeks of ESA therapy, Hgb increases by less than 1 g/dL and the Hgb remains below 10 g/dL.[2–4]

†Dose increase if after 6 weeks of ESA therapy, Hgb increases by less than 1 g/dL and the Hgb remains below 10 g/dL.[1]

ESA, erythropoiesis-stimulating agents; Hgb, hemoglobin; RBC, red blood count; SC, subcutaneously.

until ANC increases beyond 10,000/mm³ after the expected chemotherapy-induced neutrophil nadir. Administer at least 24 hours after chemotherapy and do not administer within the 24-hour period prior to chemotherapy.[78,80,81,83] Typical adult G-CSF dosing and adjustment is outlined in **Table 26.13**.

TABLE 26.13 Granulocyte Colony-Stimulating Factor Dosage			
G-CSF	**Dosage**	**Start Time**	**Dose Adjustment**
Patients With Nonmyeloid Malignancies Receiving Myelosuppressive Chemotherapy			
Filgrastim, filgrastim-sndz, or filgrastim-aafi	5 mcg/kg/day SC or IV infusion	At least 24 hours after chemotherapy and do not administer within the 24-hour period prior to chemotherapy	Increase dose in increments of 5 mcg/kg for each chemotherapy cycle according to the duration and severity of the ANC nadir
tbo-filgrastim	5 mcg/kg/day SC		
Pegfilgrastim, pegfilgrastim-jmdb, or pegfilgrastim-cbqv	6 mg SC once/ chemotherapy cycle	Do not administer between 14 days prior to and 24 hours after the administration of chemotherapy	
Patients With Acute Myeloid Leukemia Receiving Induction or Consolidation Chemotherapy			
Filgrastim, filgrastim-sndz, or filgrastim-aafi	10 mcg/kg/day IV infusion no longer than 24 hours	At least 24 hours after chemotherapy and do not administer within the 24-hour period prior to chemotherapy	Increase dose in increments of 5 mcg/kg for each chemotherapy cycle according to the duration and severity of the ANC nadir
Patients With Cancer Undergoing Chemotherapy Followed by Bone Marrow Transplantation			
Filgrastim, filgrastim-sndz, or filgrastim-aafi	10 mcg/kg/day SC or IV infusion	Following bone marrow transplantation	Titrate daily dosage against neutrophil response. See package insert for dose adjustment.

ANC, absolute neutrophil count; G-CSF, Granulocyte colony-stimulating factor; IV, intravenously; SC, subcutaneously.

CASE EXEMPLAR: Patient With Chronic Cough and Weight Loss

TT is a 72-year-old male who presents in the clinic with complaints of a dry, hacking, nonproductive cough. He has experienced weight loss without intentionally working to slim down. He is fearful he might have lung cancer.

Past Medical History
- Cardiovascular disease, myocardial infarction (MI) 5 years ago
- Emphysema

Medications
- Phenobarbital, 10 mg once daily

Family History
- Parents deceased; father died of lung cancer

Social History
- Smoking history: half a pack/day, quit 4 years ago
- Sedentary lifestyle
- Active in community groups

Physical Examination
- Lungs: bilateral infiltrates, consolidation lower left lobe
- Clubbing of fingers bilaterally
- Vital signs within normal limits

Labs and Imaging
- Polycythemia
- Chest X-ray: mass 2 cm lower left lung

Discussion Questions
1. What diagnostic tests should the clinician perform to help determine the source of TT's cough?
2. A diagnosis of carcinoma is confirmed. TT says he has heard of cancer therapy with immune therapy. How should the clinician respond?
3. TT's lung cancer is nonoperable. What will the next steps be?

CASE EXEMPLAR: Chemotherapy Patient With Fatigue

JW is a 45-year-old male in the fourth round of chemotherapy for adenocarcinoma of the colon. He presents with complaints of tiredness, fatigue, and general malaise.

Past Medical History
- Colectomy 6 weeks ago
- Implanted port
- Receives chemotherapy every other week
- Wears a small pump that delivers 5 F U (Tuesday–Thursday)

Medications
- Phenergan, 12.5-mg tablet every 6 hours
- Zofran
- Vitamin C

Social History
- Continues to work
- Nonsmoker
- Active in the community

Physical Examination
- Weight loss of 5 pounds in 1 week
- Pale conjunctiva
- Tachycardia (Pulse 120) due to anemia

Labs and Imaging
- Hemoglobin (Hgb): 8
- Hematocrit (Hct): 23
- Red blood cell (RBC): 2.4
- White blood cell (WBC): 3,100
- Liver function: normal
- Carcinoembryonic antigen (CEA): 12
- Chest X-ray: lungs clear across all fields; heart not enlarged

Discussion Questions

1. The clinician has prescribed Epogen. How will the medication be administered? What initial results are expected?
2. What side effects can JW expect from the Epogen?
3. The clinician will prescribe Neupogen for the lowered white count. With a count this low, the risk of infection is great. What process is involved in administration of Neupogen and what does the patient need to know?

KEY TAKEAWAYS

- Cancer causes significant disease burden worldwide; it causes 25% of the deaths in the United States annually.
- Cancer is characterized by the cell of origin. Cancer cells can aggressively invade surrounding cells and generate their own blood supply through angiogenesis.
- Carcinogens occur in three categories: physical, chemical, and biological. Cancer risk factors are classified as nonmodifiable and modifiable.
- Primary prevention measures prevent the onset of cancer or cancerous alterations and secondary prevention includes all screening measures. Diagnosis is a cumulative process of lab, imaging, biopsy, and cellular detection that leads to staging of the cancer based on its aggressiveness.
- Modern cancer treatment regimens encompass one or more modalities of the five treatment modalities, including surgery, radiotherapy, chemotherapy, molecularly targeted therapy, and immunotherapy. All chemotherapy drugs work by attacking cells that are dividing rapidly by interfering with the division of these cells. Cancer immunotherapy aims to harness the immune system to establish a targeted antitumor immune response.

REFERENCES

1. Bray F, Ferlay J, Soerjomataram I, et al. Global cancer statistics 2018: GLOBOCAN estimates of incidence and mortality worldwide for 36 cancers in 185 countries. *CA Cancer J Clin.* 2018;68(6):394–424. doi:10.3322/caac.21492
2. Torre LA, Siegel RL, Ward EM, et al. Global cancer incidence and mortality rates and trends—An update. *Cancer Epidemiol Biomarkers Prev.* 2016;25(1):16–27. doi:10.1158/1055-9965
3. Tangka FK, Subramanian S, Edwards P, et al. Resource requirements for cancer registration in areas with limited resources: analysis of cost data from four low- and middle-income countries. *Cancer Epidemiol.* 2016;45(suppl 1):S50–S58. doi:10.1016/j.canep.2016.10.009
4. Siegel RL, Miller KD, Jemal A. Cancer statistics, 2019. *CA Cancer J Clin.* 2019;69(1):7–34. doi:10.3322/caac.21551

5. DeSantis CE, Miller KD, Goding SA, et al. Cancer statistics for African Americans, 2019. *CA Cancer J Clin.* 2019;69(3):211–233. doi:10.3322/caac.21555

6. Centers for Disease Control and Prevention. Cancer death rates—Appalachia, 1994–1998. *MMWR Morb Mortal Wkly Rep.* 2002;51(24):527–529. https://www.cdc.gov/mmwr/preview/mmwrhtml/mm5124a3.htm.

7. Chiles C. Lung cancer screening with low-dose computed tomography. *Radiol Clin North Am.* 2014;52(1):27–46. doi:10.1016/j.rcl.2013.08.006

8. Chlebowski RT, Kuller LH, Prentice RL, et al. Breast cancer after use of estrogen plus progestin in postmenopausal women. *N Engl J Med.* 2009;360(6):573–587. doi:10.1056/NEJMoa0807684

9. Tabar L, Dean PB, Chen TH, et al. The incidence of fatal breast cancer measures the increased effectiveness of therapy in women participating in mammography screening. *Cancer.* 2019;125(4):515–523. doi:10.1002/cncr.31840

10. De Pergola G, Silvestris F. Obesity as a major risk factor for cancer. *J Obes.* 2013;2013:291546. doi:10.1155/2013/291546

11. Gupta GP, Massague J. Cancer metastasis: building a framework. *Cell.* 2006;127(4):679–695. doi:10.1016/j.cell.2006.11.001

12. Hanahan D, Weinberg RA. Hallmarks of cancer: the next generation. *Cell.* 2011;144(5):646–674. doi:10.1016/j.cell.2011.02.013

13. World Health Organization. Cancer. Published September 12, 2018. https://www.who.int/news-room/fact-sheets/detail/cancer

14. Wild CP, Stewart BW, Wild C. *World Cancer Report 2014.* World Health Organization; 2014.

15. Plummer M, de Martel C, Vignat J, et al. Global burden of cancers attributable to infections in 2012: a synthetic analysis. *Lancet Glob Health.* 2016;4(9):e609–e616. doi:10.1016/S2214-109X(16)30143-7

16. Curry SJ, Krist AH, Owens DK, et al. Screening for cervical cancer: US Preventive Services Task Force recommendation statement. *JAMA.* 2018;320(7):674–686. doi:10.1001/jama.2018.10897

17. Jemal A, Fedewa SA. Lung cancer screening with low-dose computed tomography in the United States—2010 to 2015. *JAMA Oncol.* 2017;3(9):1278–1281. doi:10.1001/jamaoncol.2016.6416

18. Masters GA, Temin S, Azzoli CG, et al. Systemic therapy for stage IV non-small-cell lung cancer: American Society of Clinical Oncology clinical practice guideline update. *J Clin Oncol.* 2015;33(30):3488–3515. doi:10.1200/JCO.2017.74.6065

19. Ederer F, Axtell LM, Cutler SJ. The relative survival rate: a statistical methodology. *Natl Cancer Inst Monogr.* 1961;6:101–121. PubMed PMID: 13889176.

20. Siu AL. Screening for breast cancer: US Preventive Services Task Force recommendation statement. *Ann Intern Med.* 2016;164(4):279–296. doi:10.7326/M15-2886

21. Bibbins-Domingo K, Grossman DC, Curry SJ, et al. Screening for colorectal cancer: US Preventive Services Task Force recommendation statement. *JAMA.* 2016;315(23):2564–2575. doi:10.1001/jama.2016.5989

22. Grossman DC, Curry SJ, Owens DK, et al. Screening for prostate cancer: US Preventive Services Task Force recommendation statement. *JAMA.* 2018;319(18):1901–1913. doi:10.1001/jama.2018.3710

23. Ettinger DS, Wood DE, Aggarwal C, et al. Non-small cell lung cancer, version 1.2020: featured updates to the NCCN guidelines. *J Natl Compr Cancer Netw.* 2019;17(12):1464–1472. doi:10.6004/jnccn.2019.00592.

24. Reck M, Rodriguez-Abreu D, Robinson AG, et al. Pembrolizumab versus chemotherapy for PD-L1-positive non-small-cell lung cancer. *N Engl J Med.* 2016;375(19):1823–1833. doi:10.1056/NEJMoa1606774

25. Ao MH, Zhang H, Sakowski L, et al. The utility of a novel triple marker (combination of TTF1, napsin A, and p40) in the subclassification of non-small cell lung cancer. *Hum Pathol.* 2014;45(5):926–934. doi:10.1016/j.humpath.2014.01.005

26. Schilsky JB, Ni A, Ahn L, et al. Prognostic impact of TTF-1 expression in patients with stage IV lung adenocarcinomas. *Lung Cancer.* 2017;108:205–211. doi:10.1016/j.lungcan.2017.03.015

27. Li T, Kung HJ, Mack PC, et al. Genotyping and genomic profiling of non-small-cell lung cancer: Implications for current and future therapies. *J Clin Oncol.* 2013;31(8):1039–1049. doi:10.1200/JCO.2012.45.3753

28. Hugo W, Zaretsky JM, Sun L, et al. Genomic and transcriptomic features of response to anti-PD-1 therapy in metastatic melanoma. *Cell.* 2016;165(1):35–44. doi:10.1016/j.cell.2016.02.065

29. Zaretsky JM, Garcia-Diaz A, Shin DS, et al. Mutations associated with acquired resistance to PD-1 blockade in melanoma. *N Engl J Med.* 2016;375(9):819–829. doi:10.1056/NEJMoa1604958

30. Wan JCM, Massie C, Garcia-Corbacho J, et al. Liquid biopsies come of age: Towards implementation of circulating tumour DNA. *Nat Rev Cancer.* 2017;17(4):223–238. doi:10.1038/nrc.2017.7

31. Chung JH, Pavlick D, Hartmaier R, et al. Hybrid capture-based genomic profiling of circulating tumor DNA from patients with estrogen receptor-positive metastatic breast cancer. *Ann Oncol.* 2017;28(11):2866–2873. doi:10.1093/annonc/mdx490

32. California Cancer Registry. http://ccr.ca.gov

33. Lindeman NI, Cagle PT, Aisner DL, et al. Updated molecular testing guideline for the selection of lung cancer patients for treatment with targeted tyrosine kinase inhibitors: guideline from the College of American Pathologists, the International Association for the Study of Lung Cancer, and the Association for Molecular Pathology. *Arch Pathol Lab Med.* 2018;142(3):321–346. doi:10.5858/arpa.2017-0388-CP

34. Parkes M. Personalised medicine and genetic prediction—Are we there yet? *Clin Med (Lond).* 2013;13(suppl 6):s62–s64. doi:10.7861/clinmedicine.13-6-s62

35. Hood L, Friend SH. Predictive, personalized, preventive, participatory (P4) cancer medicine. *Nat Rev Clin Oncol.* 2011;8(3):184–187. doi:10.1038/nrclinonc.2010.227

36. Ginsburg GS, Willard HF. Genomic and personalized medicine: foundations and applications. *Transl Res.* 2009;154(6):277–287. doi:10.1016/j.trsl.2009.09.005

37. Wiman KG, Zhivotovsky B. Understanding cell cycle and cell death regulation provides novel weapons against human diseases. *J Intern Med.* 2017;281(5):483–495. doi:10.1111/joim.12609

38. Herscher LL, Cook JA, Pacelli R, et al. Principles of chemoradiation: theoretical and practical considerations. *Oncology (Williston Park)*. 1999;13(10 suppl 5):11–22. PubMed PMID: 10550823.

39. Roskoski R Jr. Properties of FDA-approved small molecule protein kinase inhibitors: a 2020 update. *Pharmacol Res*. 2020;152:104609. doi:10.1016/j.phrs.2019.104609

40. Kim C, Prasad V. Cancer drugs approved on the basis of a surrogate end point and subsequent overall survival: An analysis of 5 years of US Food and Drug Administration Approvals. *JAMA Intern Med*. 2015;175(12):1992–1994. doi:10.1001/jamainternmed.2015.5868

41. Schwaederle M, Zhao M, Lee JJ, et al. Impact of precision medicine in diverse cancers: a meta-analysis of phase II clinical trials. *J Clin Oncol*. 2015;33(32):3817–3825. doi:10.1200/JCO.2015.61.5997

42. Schram AM, Chang MT, Jonsson P, et al. Fusions in solid tumours: diagnostic strategies, targeted therapy, and acquired resistance. *Nat Rev Clin Oncol*. 2017;14(12):735–748. doi:10.1038/nrclinonc.2017.127

43. Chen DS, Irving BA, Hodi FS. Molecular pathways: next-generation immunotherapy—Inhibiting programmed death-ligand 1 and programmed death-1. *Clin Cancer Res*. 2012;18(24):6580–6587. doi:10.1158/1078-0432.CCR-12-1362

44. Topalian SL, Weiner GJ, Pardoll DM. Cancer immunotherapy comes of age. *J Clin Oncol*. 2011;29(36):4828–4836. doi:10.1200/JCO.2011.38.0899

45. Jager E, Jager D, Knuth A. Antigen-specific immunotherapy and cancer vaccines. *Int J Cancer*. 2003;106(6):817–820. doi:10.1002/ijc.11292

46. Vanneman M, Dranoff G. Combining immunotherapy and targeted therapies in cancer treatment. *Nat Rev Cancer*. 2012;12(4):237–251. doi:10.1038/nrc3237

47. Chen DS, Mellman I. Oncology meets immunology: the cancer-immunity cycle. *Immunity*. 2013;39(1):1–10. doi:10.1016/j.immuni.2013.07.012

48. Carbone DP, Reck M, Paz-Ares L, et al. First-line nivolumab in stage IV or recurrent non–small-cell lung cancer. *N Engl J Med*. 2017;376(25):2415–2426. doi:10.1056/NEJMoa1613493

49. Peters S, Gettinger S, Johnson ML, et al. Phase II trial of atezolizumab as first-line or subsequent therapy for patients with programmed death-ligand 1-selected advanced non–small-cell lung cancer (BIRCH). *J Clin Oncol*. 2017;35(24):2781–2789. doi:10.1200/JCO.2016.71.9476

50. Dirix LY, Takacs I, Jerusalem G, et al. Avelumab, an anti-PD-L1 antibody, in patients with locally advanced or metastatic breast cancer: a phase 1b JAVELIN Solid Tumor Study. *Breast Cancer Res Treat*. 2018;167(3):671–686. doi:10.1007/s10549-017-4537-5

51. Antonia SJ, Villegas A, Daniel D, et al. Durvalumab after chemoradiotherapy in Stage III non–small-cell lung cancer. *N Engl J Med*. 2017;377(20):1919–1929. doi:10.1056/NEJMoa1709937

52. Govindan R, Szczesna A, Ahn MJ, et al. Phase III trial of ipilimumab combined with paclitaxel and carboplatin in advanced squamous non-small-cell lung cancer. *J Clin Oncol*. 2017;35(30):3449–3457. doi:10.1200/JCO.2016.71.7629

53. Larkin J, Chiarion-Sileni V, Gonzalez R, et al. Five-year survival with combined nivolumab and ipilimumab in advanced melanoma. *N Engl J Med*. 2019;381(16):1535–1546. doi:10.1056/NEJMoa1910836

54. Hodi FS, Chesney J, Pavlick AC, et al. Combined nivolumab and ipilimumab versus ipilimumab alone in patients with advanced melanoma: 2-year overall survival outcomes in a multicentre, randomised, controlled, phase 2 trial. *Lancet Oncol*. 2016;17(11):1558–1568. doi:10.1016/S1470-2045(16)30366-7

55. Ott PA, Elez E, Hiret S, et al. Pembrolizumab in patients with extensive-stage small-cell lung cancer: results from the Phase Ib KEYNOTE-028 Study. *J Clin Oncol*. 2017;35(34):3823–3829. doi:10.1200/JCO.2017.72.5069

56. Alley EW, Lopez J, Santoro A, et al. Clinical safety and activity of pembrolizumab in patients with malignant pleural mesothelioma (KEYNOTE-028): preliminary results from a non-randomised, open-label, phase 1b trial. *Lancet Oncol*. 2017;18(5):623–630. doi:10.1016/S1470-2045(17)30169-9

57. Hellmann MD, Rizvi NA, Goldman JW, et al. Nivolumab plus ipilimumab as first-line treatment for advanced non-small-cell lung cancer (CheckMate 012): results of an open-label, phase 1, multicohort study. *Lancet Oncol*. 2017;18(1):31–41. doi:10.1016/S1470-2045(16)30624-6

58. Pillai RN, Behera M, Owonikoko TK, et al. Comparison of the toxicity profile of PD-1 versus PD-L1 inhibitors in non-small cell lung cancer: a systematic analysis of the literature. *Cancer*. 2018;124(2):271–277. doi:10.1002/cncr.31043

59. Remon J, Mezquita L, Corral J, et al. Immune-related adverse events with immune checkpoint inhibitors in thoracic malignancies: focusing on non-small cell lung cancer patients. *J Thorac Dis*. 2018;10(suppl 13):S1516–S1533. doi:10.21037/jtd.2017.12.52

60. Wolchok JD, Chiarion-Sileni V, Gonzalez R, et al. Overall survival with combined nivolumab and ipilimumab in advanced melanoma. *N Engl J Med*. 2017;377(14):1345–1356. doi:10.1056/NEJMoa1709684

61. Toi Y, Sugawara S, Kawashima Y, et al. Association of immune-related adverse events with clinical benefit in patients with advanced non-small-cell lung cancer treated with nivolumab. *Oncologist*. 2018;23(11):1358–1365. doi:10.1634/theoncologist.2017-0384

62. Haratani K, Hayashi H, Chiba Y, et al. Association of immune-related adverse events with nivolumab efficacy in non-small-cell lung cancer. *JAMA Oncol*. 2018;4(3):374–378. doi:10.1001/jamaoncol.2017.2925

63. Brahmer JR, Lacchetti C, Schneider BJ, et al. Management of immune-related adverse events in patients treated with immune checkpoint inhibitor therapy: American Society of Clinical Oncology Clinical Practice Guideline. *J Clin Oncol*. 2018;36(17):1714–1768. doi:10.1200/JCO.2017.77.6385

64. Puzanov I, Diab A, Abdallah K, et al. Managing toxicities associated with immune checkpoint inhibitors: consensus recommendations from the Society for Immunotherapy of Cancer (SITC) Toxicity Management Working Group. *J Immunother Cancer*. 2017;5(1):95. doi:10.1186/s40425-017-0300-z

65. Santini FC, Rizvi H, Plodkowski AJ, et al. Safety and efficacy of re-treating with immunotherapy after immune-related adverse events in patients with NSCLC. *Cancer Immunol Res.* 2018;6(9):1093–1099. doi:10.1158/2326-6066.CIR-17-0755

66. Schadendorf D, Wolchok JD, Hodi FS, et al. Efficacy and safety outcomes in patients with advanced melanoma who discontinued treatment with nivolumab and ipilimumab because of adverse events: a pooled analysis of randomized phase II and III trials. *J Clin Oncol.* 2017;35(34):3807–3814. doi:10.1200/JCO.2017.73.2289

67. Mouri A, Kaira K, Yamaguchi O, et al. Clinical difference between discontinuation and retreatment with nivolumab after immune-related adverse events in patients with lung cancer. *Cancer Chemother Pharmacol.* 2019;84(4):873–880. doi:10.1007/s00280-019-03926-y

68. Ayers M, Lunceford J, Nebozhyn M, et al. IFN-gamma-related mRNA profile predicts clinical response to PD-1 blockade. *J Clin Invest.* 2017;127(8):2930–2940. doi:10.1172/JCI91190

69. Ott PA, Bang Y-J, Razak ARA, et al. Relationship of PD-L1 and a T-cell inflamed gene expression profile (GEP) to clinical response in a multicohort trial of solid tumors (KEYNOTE [KN]028). *Ann Oncol.* 2017;28(suppl 5): v22. doi:10.1093/annonc/mdx363

70. Li H, Ma W, Yoneda KY, et al. Severe nivolumab-induced pneumonitis preceding durable clinical remission in a patient with refractory, metastatic lung squamous cell cancer: a case report. *J Hematol Oncol.* 2017;10(1):64. doi:10.1186/s13045-017-0433-z

71. Klemencic S, Perkins J. Diagnosis and management of oncologic emergencies. *West J Emerg Med.* 2019;20(2): 316–322. doi:10.5811/westjem.2018.12.37335

72. de Moor JS, Mariotto AB, Parry C, et al. Cancer survivors in the United States: prevalence across the survivorship trajectory and implications for care. *Cancer Epidemiol Biomarkers Prev.* 2013;22(4):561–570. doi:10.1158/1055-9965.EPI-12-1356

73. Amgen. Aranesp package insert. Updated January 2019. https://www.accessdata.fda.gov/drugsatfda_docs/label/2019/103951s5378lbl.pdf.

74. Ortho Biotech Products. Epogen package insert. Updated January 2019. https://www.pi.amgen.com/~/media/amgen/repositorysites/pi-amgen-com/aranesp/ckd/aranesp_pi_hcp_english.pdf.

75. Janssen Products. Procrit package insert. Updated July 2018. http://www.janssenlabels.com/package-insert/product-monograph/prescribing-information/PROCRIT-pi.pdf.

76. Pfizer. Retacrit package insert. Updated May 2018. https://www.accessdata.fda.gov/drugsatfda_docs/label/2018/125545s000lbl.pdf

77. Mylan. Fulphila package insert. Updated June 2018. https://www.accessdata.fda.gov/drugsatfda_docs/label/2018/761075s000lbl.pdf

78. Teva Pharmaceuticals USA. Granix package insert. Updated December 2014. https://www.accessdata.fda.gov/drugsatfda_docs/label/2014/125294s035lbl.pdf.

79. Amgen. Neulasta package insert. Updated November 2015. https://www.accessdata.fda.gov/drugsatfda_docs/label/2015/125031s180lbl.pdf

80. Amgen. Neupogen package insert. Updated September 2013. https://www.accessdata.fda.gov/drugsatfda_docs/label/2013/103353s5157lbl.pdf

81. Pfizer Labs. Nivestym package insert. Updated July 2018. https://www.accessdata.fda.gov/drugsatfda_docs/label/2018/761080s000lbl.pdf

82. Coherus BioSciences. Udenyca package insert. Updated April 2019. https://www.accessdata.fda.gov/drugsatfda_docs/label/2019/761039s001lbl.pdf

83. Sandoz. Zarxio package insert. Updated March 2015. https://www.accessdata.fda.gov/drugsatfda_docs/label/2015/125553lbl.pdf

ADDITIONAL RESOURCES

- Fact Sheets on Cancer From IARC
  - http://globocan.iarc.fr/Pages/fact_sheets_cancer.aspx
- World Cancer Report 2014
  - www.iarc.fr/en/publications/books/wcr/wcr-order.php
- International Agency for Research on Cancer (IARC)
  - www.iarc.fr
- Cancer Control: Knowledge Into Action
  - www.who.int/entity/cancer/modules/en/index.html
- WHO's Work on Cancer
  - www.who.int/entity/cancer/en/index.html
- Global Status Report on Noncommunicable Diseases 2014
  - www.who.int/entity/nmh/publications/ncd-status-report-2014/en/index.html
- WHO Report on the Global Tobacco Epidemic, 2008—The MPOWER Package
  - www.who.int/entity/tobacco/mpower/2008/en/index.html
- WHO Global Strategy on Diet and Physical Activity
  - www.who.int/entity/dietphysicalactivity/goals/en/index.html
- UN Interagency Task Force on the Prevention and Control of Noncommunicable Diseases
  - www.who.int/entity/nmh/ncd-task-force/en/index.html
- WHO: More on Cancer
  - www.who.int/topics/cancer/en/index.html

Pharmacotherapy Related to Women's Health Conditions

Elyse Watkins and Virginia McCoy Hass

- Differentiate the various treatment options for common infectious and noninfectious conditions commonly encountered in women's health.
- Create a management plan that includes evidence-based and approved pharmacologic products for common infectious and noninfectious conditions in women's health.
- Assess the risks, benefits, and alternatives of various pharmacologic options for treating common women's health issues.
- Compare and contrast each pharmacologic option for a given condition commonly seen in women's health.
- Discuss current relevant guidelines and best practices while managing conditions related to women's health.

INTRODUCTION

The continued escalation of healthcare costs in the United States has significantly impacted the female population. According to a 2018 Centers for Disease Control and Prevention (CDC) report, approximately 13.4% of women age 18 or older claimed fair or poor health. Consequently, the national demand for women's health services was estimated to increase. In fact, the forecast of demands was estimated to increase by 6% by 2020.[1] Due to this shift in demand of healthcare services, women's health is one of the important elements of any healthcare system. Furthermore, women's biological gestation and lactation are complex and subject to complications; therefore, it is prudent for clinicians to provide sufficient attention to maintain the well-being of this population. This chapter focuses on the commonly encountered conditions that relate to women's health and discusses the relevant therapeutic treatments according to the current guidelines and evidence. Generally, women's health-related conditions may be organized into two broad categories: those that are caused by infections and those that have noninfectious sources.

INFECTIOUS CONDITIONS AND GENERAL APPROACH

Vaginal discharge and sexually transmitted infections (STIs) are common presentations in women's health, primary care, urgent care, and emergency medicine. Recognition of the risk factors, presentation, diagnosis, and treatment options are important for treating an STI appropriately. Understanding can also help prevent the spread of infection to others and minimize complications related to delayed or inappropriate treatment. It is also important to recognize that some untreated or undertreated STIs can have deleterious effects on future reproductive potential.

All patients who are sexually active are at risk of contracting an STI and it should never be assumed that a patient is fully protected, even if they are using male or female condoms. Hence, the clinician should consider the possibility of STI in all patients who are sexually active. This section discusses yeast infections, bacterial vaginosis, genital condyloma, trichomoniasis, pelvic inflammatory disease, and cervical dysplasia/cancer.

VAGINAL YEAST INFECTION

The risk factors for yeast infection include exogenous estrogen use, diabetes mellitus, immunosuppression, recent antibiotic use, pregnancy, and possibly dietary ingestion of sugars.

Diagnosis of Vaginal Yeast Infection

Diagnosis of a vaginal yeast infection is fairly straightforward. Classic signs and symptoms include vaginal pruritus, burning, and vaginal discharge. Some patients may complain of dysuria and dyspareunia. Physical examination will reveal thick white cottage cheese-appearing vaginal discharge that adheres to the vaginal mucosa but is easily displaced. However, the yeast can sometimes appear slightly yellow or green. The vulva and vaginal mucosa may be erythematous. There may be small posterior fourchette fissures that cause itching and pain, especially with urination or sexual intercourse. The pH of the discharge is <4.5, and wet mount with potassium hydroxide (KOH) will reveal pseudohyphae and budding yeast.

Treatment of Vaginal Yeast Infection

The treatment of a vaginal yeast infection aims to eradicate the yeast and offer symptomatic relief of the pruritus. Antifungals are the mainstay of pharmacologic treatment. Other nonprescription remedies not approved by the United States Food and Drug Administration (FDA) have been purported to be helpful, such as gentian violet, boric acid, lactobacillus supplements for treatment and prevention, oral and vaginal yogurt, garlic, and vinegar. However, the evidence is weak or lacking so caution is advised in advocating for these options.

Most vaginal products for candidiasis are used at bedtime (hs) to avoid leakage from the vagina while sitting, standing, or ambulating. Oral fluconazole (Diflucan®) is a drug of choice for systemic therapy. There are six active ingredients that are approved for the treatment of yeast infection (see **Table 27.1**):

- **Miconazole:** Vaginal cream, suppository, and vulvar cream
- **Tioconazole:** Vaginal ointment
- **Clotrimazole:** Vaginal cream
- **Terconazole:** Vaginal cream, vaginal suppository
- **Butoconazole:** Vaginal cream
- **Fluconazole:** Oral antifungal

TABLE 27.1 Pharmacotherapy for Vaginal Yeast Infection

Medication	Dose/Frequency	Indications	Contraindications	Side Effects	Other Considerations
Miconazole	Use hs 2% cream: use for 7 days 4% cream: use for 3 days 100 mg suppository: use for 7 days 200 mg suppository: use for 3 days 1,200 mg suppository: use for 1 day Combination pack includes 2% cream for vulvar application	Vulvovaginal candidiasis; other dermatologic fungal infections	Hypersensitivity to the main ingredient	Erythema, burning, pruritus, edema	Available OTC
Tioconazole	Use hs	Vulvovaginal candidiasis	Hypersensitivity to the main ingredient	Erythema, burning, pruritus, edema	Available OTC; Ointment may stain clothes.
Clotrimazole	Use hs 1% cream: use for 7 days 2% cream: use for 3 days	Vulvovaginal candidiasis; other dermatologic fungal infections	Hypersensitivity to the main ingredient	Erythema, burning, pruritus, edema	Available OTC
Terconazole	Use hs 0.4% vaginal cream: use for 7 days 0.8% vaginal cream or suppository: use for 3 days	Vulvovaginal candidiasis	Hypersensitivity to the main ingredient	Erythema, burning, pruritus, edema	Rx only
Butoconazole	Use hs × one dose	Vulvovaginal candidiasis	Hypersensitivity to the main ingredient	Erythema, burning, pruritus, edema	Available OTC; Pre-filled applicator
Fluconazole	One 150 mg tablet PO × one; may repeat dose in 3 days if symptoms are still present	Vulvovaginal candidiasis Dosing different for systemic or severe fungal infections	Hypersensitivity to the main ingredient; concomitant use of other drugs that can cause Q-T prolongation and metabolized via CYTP3A4	Headache, nausea, abdominal pain	Rx only Not advised for use in pregnancy

hs, at bedtime; OTC, over-the-counter; PO, orally; Rx, prescription.

BACTERIAL VAGINOSIS

Risk factors for bacterial vaginosis (BV) include sexual activity, douching, and any other activity that reduces vaginal lactobacilli. Some patients will develop a bacterial vaginosis postcoitally when exposed to semen. BV is a common condition in females in general; lesbian women are also at risk of developing BV. According to one study, lesbians are shown to have 2.5-fold increase in risk of BV compared to heterosexual women.[2]

Diagnosis of Bacterial Vaginosis

Most patients with BV experience malodorous vaginal discharge but some patients may be asymptomatic. The diagnosis can be made with physical examination, pH testing, and wet mount findings. BV usually presents as a malodorous "milky" vaginal discharge. A fish odor (amine odor) will be apparent in the presence of potassium hydroxide. The vaginal pH is >4.5, and the pathognomonic wet prep finding is clue cells. Clue cells are vaginal epithelial cells stippled with clusters of bacteria. Nucleic-acid amplification (NAAT) testing is also approved.

Treatment of Bacterial Vaginosis

The treatment of BV requires antimicrobials. Due to the various organisms implicated in BV, treatment is with broad-spectrum antimicrobials aimed at eliminating the anaerobic bacteria most commonly isolated. Generally, pharmacotherapies for BV may be summarized as follows:

- **Clindamycin:** Vaginal cream, ovules, and oral tablets
- **Metronidazole:** Vaginal gel and oral tablets
- **Tinidazole:** Oral tablets

The CDC has outlined evidence-based treatment options for BV and STIs.[3] The 2015 guideline recommendations are listed in **Box 27.1. Table 27.2** provides a summary of pharmacotherapy for bacterial vaginosis.

TRICHOMONIASIS

Trichomoniasis is a sexually transmitted infection, so sexual activity is the primary risk factor. In addition, trichomoniasis infection is a risk factor for preterm labor, human immunodeficiency virus (HIV) acquisition, and pelvic inflammatory disease.

Diagnosis of Trichomoniasis

Patients with trichomoniasis may be asymptomatic, but most will complain of vaginal pruritus and vaginal discharge. Dyspareunia and dysuria may be present. On physical examination, the cervix may appear erythematous with punctations (called a "strawberry cervix"), the cervix may be friable, and a yellowish/greenish/grayish bubbly vaginal discharge may be present. The vaginal pH will be >4.5. Wet mount with normal saline

---

BOX 27.1
2015 CENTERS FOR DISEASE CONTROL AND PREVENTION GUIDELINES FOR TREATMENT OF BACTERIAL VAGINOSIS

Recommended Regimens

Metronidazole 500 mg orally twice a day for 7 days
   OR
Metronidazole gel 0.75%, one full applicator (5 g) intravaginally, once a day for 5 days
   OR
Clindamycin cream 2%, one full applicator (5 g) intravaginally at bedtime for 7 days

Alternative Regimens

Tinidazole 2 g orally once daily for 2 days
   OR
Tinidazole 1 g orally once daily for 5 days
   OR
Clindamycin 300 mg orally twice daily for 7 days
   OR
Clindamycin ovules 100 mg intravaginally once at bedtime for 3 days*

*Clindamycin ovules use an oleaginous base that might weaken latex or rubber products (e.g., condoms and vaginal contraceptive diaphragms). Use of such products within 72 hours following treatment with clindamycin ovules is not recommended.

Source: Centers for Disease Control and Prevention. *Bacterial vaginosis.* https://www.cdc.gov/std/tg2015/bv.htm

---

can reveal motile trichomonads. Nucleic-acid amplification (NAAT) testing is also approved.

Treatment of Trichomoniasis

The treatment of trichomoniasis involves treating both the patient and the patient's sexual partners. However, it is not reportable in any state in the United States. Therapy should also be aimed to prevent future infections and screen for other STIs as appropriate. Pharmacotherapies for trichomoniasis include (**Table 27.3**):

- Metronidazole: oral
- Tinidazole: oral

GENITAL CONDYLOMA

Genital condyloma (also called "condyloma acuminata" or "genital warts") is a sexually transmitted infection caused by human papillomavirus (HPV). Risk factors are generally related to sexual activity, including unprotected intercourse, multiple partners, coinfection with another STI, compromised immunity, and pregnancy. HPV is the most common sexually transmitted infection,

TABLE 27.2 Pharmacotherapy for Bacterial Vaginosis

Medication	Dose/Frequency	Indications	Contraindications	Side Effects	Other Considerations (as Needed)
Clindamycin	2% cream: hs for 7 days. 300 mg oral: one capsule bid for 7 days 100 mg ovule: hs for 3 days	Bacterial vaginosis; also used to treat a multitude of other bacterial infections	Hypersensitivity to clindamycin or lincomycin History of pseudomembranous colitis or ulcerative colitis	Superinfection of other bacteria Vaginal candidiasis Topical use can cause erythema, burning, or irritation	2% cream is CDC recommended first-line Capsules and ovules are CDC alternative recommendations
Metronidazole	500 mg tabs: PO bid for 7 days. 0.75% vaginal gel: bid for 5 days.	Bacterial vaginosis; also used to treat other bacterial, protozoal, and amoebic infections	Hypersensitivity to metronidazole	Disulfiram effect if taken with alcohol Bitter or metallic taste, gastro-intestinal upset, vaginal candidiasis	Both oral and gel are CDC recommended first-line Patients must abstain from alcohol use during treatment
Tinidazole	500 mg tablets: 2 g (4 tablets) PO once a day for 2 days 500 mg tablets: 1 g (2 tablets) PO once a day for 5 days	Bacterial vaginosis; also used to treat other protozoal and amoebic infections	Hypersensitivity to tinidazole	Bitter or metallic taste, gastro-intestinal upset, vaginal candidiasis	CDC alternative recommendation. Not recommended for use in pregnancy

bid, twice daily; CDC, Centers for Disease Control and Prevention; hs, at bedtime; PO, orally.

Source: Data from Centers for Disease Control and Prevention. *Bacterial vaginosis.* https://www.cdc.gov/std/tg2015/bv.htm

TABLE 27.3 Pharmacotherapy for Trichomoniasis

Medication	Dose/Frequency	Indications	Contraindications	Side Effects	Other Considerations (as Needed)
Metronidazole	500-mg tabs: Take four tabs PO × 1 Alternate regimen: 500-mg tabs: Take one tab bid for 7 days	Trichomoniasis; also used to treat other bacterial and amoebic infections	Hypersensitivity to metronidazole	Disulfiram effect if taken with alcohol Bitter or metallic taste, gastro-intestinal upset, vaginal candidiasis	The 2-g dose is CDC preferred Must advise patient to abstain from alcohol during use
Tinidazole	500-mg tabs: Take four tabs PO × 1	Trichomoniasis; also used to treat other protozoal and amoebic infections.	Hypersensitivity to tinidazole.	Bitter or metallic taste, gastro-intestinal upset, vaginal candidiasis	Not recommended for use in pregnancy

bid, twice daily; CDC, Centers for Disease Control and Prevention; PO, orally.

Source: Data from Centers for Disease Control and Prevention. *Trichomoniasis.* https://www.cdc.gov/std/tg2015/trichomoniasis.htm

with the majority of new infections occurring in the adolescent and young adult populations. Approximately 90% of genital condyloma are caused by HPV types 6 and 11.[4] Prevention of infection by these and high-risk (oncogenic) HPV types is discussed in Chapter 23, "Therapeutic Applications of Immunology and Vaccines".

Diagnosis of Genital Condyloma

Genital condyloma is a clinical diagnosis based upon physical examination and visualization of the lesions on the vulva, perineum, and/or perianal area. Routine testing of condylomatous lesions for oncogenic types

of HPV is not recommended because the vast majority of these lesions are caused by low-risk HPV types. Screening guidelines for women at average-risk of cervical cancer recommend cotesting for high-risk (oncogenic) HPV types along with pap smear every 5 years between ages 30 and 65.[5,6]

Treatment for Genital Condyloma

There are several treatment strategies for genital condyloma, including both pharmacologic and nonpharmacologic modalities. Nonpharmacologic modalities may involve cryoablation, laser ablation, electrosurgery, and excision with scissors or a scalpel. Biopsy is indicated if the diagnosis is not clear, the patient is immunocompromised, or if the lesions are atypical or do not respond or worsen during therapy.[7] Follow-up of patients treated with any modality should ensure resolution as a small percentage of patients may develop malignancy, particularly squamous cell carcinoma, also called "verrucous carcinoma." Cryotherapy is not recommended for treatment of intravaginal warts due to risk of fistula formation.[7] Cervical and intra-anal warts should be managed in consultation with a specialist.[7]

Pharmacologic therapies are classified as patient-applied or clinician-administered. FDA-approved medications include trichloroacetic acid (TCA), bichloroacetic acid (BCA), imiquod cream, podophyllotoxin, podophyllin, and sinecatchins (see **Table 27.4**).[7]

TABLE 27.4 Pharmacotherapy for Genital Condyloma

Medication	Dose/Frequency	Indications	Contraindications	Side Effects	Other Considerations (as Needed)
Imiquimod	Imiquimod 5% cream. Apply every other night for 3 nights/week; wash off after 6–8 hours; repeat until lesions resolve or up to 16 weeks. Imiquimod 3.75% cream: Apply once daily, wash off after 8 hours; may use until lesions resolve or up to 8 weeks	External anogenital condyloma; also used for actinic keratosis	Hypersensitivity to Imiquimod	Pain, pruritus, erythema, local irritation	Patient applied. May weaken condoms and vaginal diaphrams
Podophyllin	25% podophyllin in benzoin tincture; use sparingly on affected lesions only, allow to air dry before contact with clothing, leave on for max of 4 hours. Limit application to <0.5 mL or <10 cm² of warts per session. First application should be left in contact for approximately 30–40 minutes	External anogenital condyloma	Diabetes mellitus, immunocompromised, poor circulation	Can cause paresthesias, neuropathy/neuritis, leukopenia, thrombocytopenia, coma	Clinician-applied. Not for use in pregnancy. Over-application or application to open lesions/friable tissue is associated with increased risk of systemic toxicity
Podophyllotoxin (Podofilox®)	Podophyllotoxin 0.5% gel or solution. Apply bid for 3 consecutive days/week, then discontinue for 4 days. May repeat four times. Limit application to <0.5 mL or <10 cm² of warts per day	External genital condyloma	Hypersensitivity to podophyllotoxin	Erythema, skin erosion, bleeding, pruritus	Patient-applied. Preferably, the first treatment should be clinician-applied to demonstrate technique and sites for application.
Trichloroactiec acid or bichloroacetic acid	80%–90% solution applied to lesions. Recommended to protect peripheral skin with a petrolatum product	External anogential condyloma. Vaginal, cervical, and intra-anal condyloma*	Malignant, premalignant, bleeding, ulcerated lesions	Burning, erythema, irritation	Clinician-applied
Sinecatechins	15% ointment applied tid for up to 16 weeks	External anogenital condyloma	Hypersensitivity to green tea	Erythema, burning, localized irritation	Patient-applied. Can stain clothes and sheets. Not recommended in pregnancy. May weaken condoms and vaginal diaphrams

bid, twice daily; tid, three times daily.
*Cervical and intra-anal condyloma should be managed in consultation with a specialist.
Source: Centers for Disease Control and Prevention. *Anogenital warts.* https://www.cdc.gov/std/tg2015/warts.htm

PELVIC INFLAMMATORY DISEASE

Pelvic inflammatory disease (PID) is a spectrum of inflammatory/infectious disorders of the upper female genital tract. Risk factors include multiple sexual partners, a non monogamous sexual partner, coinfection with chlamydia and gonorrhea, immunocompromise, and prior history of PID.[8] Routine screening and treatment of sexually active women for STIs reduce the risk of PID.

Diagnosis

Acute PID can present with a wide range of symptoms and signs, making diagnosis difficult. The classic findings for PID are uterine tenderness, cervical motion tenderness (also called "the Chandelier sign"), and adnexal tenderness. Other findings suggestive of PID include the presence of white blood cells in a vaginal smear and mucopurulent discharge from the cervix. Some patients may present with fever >101°F (>38.3°C) orally and positive gonorrhea and/or chlamydia isolates on an endocervical swab. A patient with fever, leukocytosis with a left shift, and an adnexal mass must be ruled out for tubo-ovarian abscess, a potential consequence of untreated PID. All women diagnosed with PID should be screened for HIV, gonorrhea, and chlamydia.[8]

Treatment

The pharmacologic treatment of PID involves antimicrobials aiming at the most common pathogens. Although gonorrhea and chlamydia are common, other organisms have been isolated, including *Gardnerella vaginalis*, *Haemophilus influenzae*, *Streptococcus agalactiae*, *Mycoplasma genitalium*, *Staphylococcus aureus*, *Proteus* species, *Bacteroides* species and gram negative enteric rods.[8] Patients who are unable to tolerate oral medications, pregnant, or may have a tubo-ovarian abscess should be hospitalized for intravenous therapy.

According to the 2015 CDC guidelines, the treatments of PID for the in-patient and out-patient settings follows (**Box 27.2**).[8] Medications used in various regimens involve ceftriaxone, doxycycline, metronidazole (combined with ceftriaxone and doxycycline when anaerobes are suspected), cefoxitin, probenecid (adjuvant with cefoxitin to prolong cefoxitin half-life), cefotetan, clindamycin, and gentamicin (combined with clindamycin intravenously for synergy; **Table 27.5**).

CERVICAL DYSPLASIA/CANCER

Over 90% of cervical cancer is caused by infection with oncogenic strains of human papilloma virus (HPV).[9] Risk factors that increase pathogenicity include tobacco use, multiple sexual partners, early age of first intercourse, history of other STIs, age <30 years for HPV infection but >35 years for cervical cancer, and an immunocompromised state.

BOX 27.2
2015 CENTERS FOR DISEASE CONTROL AND PREVENTION GUIDELINES FOR PELVIC INFLAMMATORY DISEASE

Recommended Intramuscular/Oral Regimens (Outpatient)

Ceftriaxone 250 mg IM in a single dose
+ Doxycycline 100 mg orally twice a day for 14 days
*with** or *without* Metronidazole 500 mg orally twice a day for 14 days

OR

Cefoxitin 2 g IM in a single dose
+ Probenecid, 1 g orally administered concurrently in a single dose
+ Doxycycline 100 mg orally twice a day for 14 days
*with** or *without* Metronidazole 500 mg orally twice a day for 14 days

OR

Other parenteral third-generation cephalosporin (e.g., ceftizoxime or cefotaxime)
Doxycycline 100 mg orally twice a day for 14 days
*with** or *without* Metronidazole 500 mg orally twice a day for 14 days

Recommended Parenteral Regimens (Inpatient)

Cefotetan 2 g IV every 12 hours
+ Doxycycline 100 mg orally or IV every 12 hours
OR

Cefoxitin 2 g IV every 6 hours
+ Doxycycline 100 mg orally or IV every 12 hours
OR

Clindamycin 900 mg IV every 8 hours
+ Gentamicin loading dose IV or IM (2 mg/kg), followed by a maintenance dose (1.5 mg/kg) every 8 hours. Single daily dosing (3–5 mg/kg) can be substituted.

Alternative Parenteral Regimen (Inpatient)

Ampicillin/Sulbactam 3 g IV every 6 hours
+ Doxycycline 100 mg orally or IV every 12 hours

IM, intramuscularly; IV, intravenously.

*Addition of Metronidazole for extended anaerobic organism coverage should be considered
Source: Centers for Disease Control and Prevention. *Pelvic inflammatory disease (PID).* https://www.cdc.gov/std/tg2015/pid.htm

---

Diagnosis of Cervical Dysplasia/Cancer

The diagnosis of cervical dysplasia and cancer is done with Pap smear, colposcopy, and biopsy. HPV infection may also be detected by polymerase chain reaction (PCR).

TABLE 27.5 Pharmacotherapy for Pelvic Inflammatory Disease

Medication	Dose/Frequency	Indications	Contraindications	Side Effects	Other Considerations (as Needed)
Ceftriaxone	250 mg IM	PID, gonorrhea, and a multitude of other bacterial infections	Hypersensitivity to ceftriaxone. Patients with a true penicillin allergy may experience hypersensitivity reactions	Injection site erythema, burning, pain, induration	CDC-preferred therapy *combined with* doxycycline for mild-to-moderately severe acute PID
Doxycycline	100 mg PO bid × 14 days	Chlamydia and gonorrhea; a multitude of other bacterial infections	Hypersensitivity to doxycycline or any tetracycline	GI upset, rashes (including Stevens-Johnson syndrome, toxic epidermal necrolysis), hypersensitivity reactions, intracranial hypertension (particularly with prolonged use)	CDC-preferred therapy *combined with* ceftriaxone for mild-to-moderately severe acute PID
Metronidazole	500 mg PO bid × 14 days	PID if anaerobic organisms are suspected; also used to treat other bacterial, protozoal, and amoebic infections	Hypersensitivity to metronidazole	Disulfiram effect if taken with alcohol. Bitter or metallic taste, gastro-intestinal upset, vaginal candidiasis	CDC-preferred adjuvant with ceftriaxone and doxycycline if anaerobic organisms are suspected
Cefoxitin	2 g IM or IV	PID; a multitude of other bacterial infections	Hypersensitivity to cefoxitin or other cephalosporins Hemolytic anemia associated with any cephalosporin use	Nausea and diarrhea, hematologic abnormalities, injection site reactions (phlebitis)	CDC-preferred alternate cephalosporin for outpatient therapy, must be given with Probenecid. Is also a CDC-preferred inpatient option
Probenecid	1 g PO × one	PID; used with beta lactam antimicrobials to increase serum plasma levels Also used for hyperuricemia associated with gout	Hypersensitivity to probenecid or any component of the formulation; small- or large-dose aspirin therapy; blood dyscrasias; uric acid kidney stones. Precaution when used if patient has G6PD deficiency	Hypersensitivity reactions, can exacerbate gout, dizziness, rash	Used with cefoxitin and doxycycline for CDC alternative outpatient option
Cefotetan	2 g IV	PID; a multitude of other bacterial infections	Hypersensitivity to cefotetan or other cephalosporins Hemolytic anemia associated with any cephalosporin use	Nausea and diarrhea, hematologic abnormalities, injection site reactions (phlebitis)	CDC-preferred inpatient option
Clindamycin	900 mg IV q8h	PID; a multitude of other bacterial infections	Hypersensitivity to clindamycin or lincomycin	Hypersensitivity, colitis, severe dermatologic reactions (including Stevens-Johnson syndrome and toxic epidermal necrolysis), injection site reactions	CDC alternative inpatient option to be used with gentamicin
Gentamicin	2 mg/kg loading dose followed by 1.5 mg/kg q8h. Can also use 3–5 mg/kg/day)	PID; a multitude of bacterial infections	Hypersensitivity to gentamicin or other aminoglycosides	Hypersensitivity, vertigo, ototoxicity, nephrotoxicity	CDC alternative inpatient option to be used with clindamycin

CDC, Centers for Disease Control and Prevention; GI, gastrointestinal; IM, intramuscularly; IV, intravenously; PID, pelvic inflammatory disease; PO, orally; q8h, every 8 hours.

Treatment of Cervical Dysplasia/Cancer

There is no pharmacologic treatment of cervical dysplasia. The pharmacologic options to treat cervical cancer are beyond the scope of this chapter. Prevention of HPV infection, which significantly reduces the risk of cervical dysplasia and cervical cancer,[10] can be accomplished through vaccination. There are three HPV vaccines available: 9-valent (Gardasil 9®), quadrivalent (Gardasil®), and bivalent (Cervarix®). The 9-valent vaccine is the only HPV vaccine available in the United States. Outside the United States, vaccine avaiability should be confirmed locally.[11] **Table 27.6** summarizes HPV vaccines.

NONINFECTIOUS CONDITIONS AND CONDITIONS RELATED TO PRE- AND POSTMENOPAUSE

A common chief complaint among patients who are premenopausal is abnormal uterine bleeding. Abnormal bleeding can present as oligomenorrhea, amenorrhea, irregular menses, or heavy menstrual bleeding. A comprehensive history and physical exam should be conducted for all patients presenting with these complaints to identify the cause and to determine which patients have a potentially life-threating condition.

ABNORMAL UTERINE BLEEDING

All patients with an intact uterus are potentially at risk of developing abnormal uterine bleeding. However, patients with leiomyoma, adenomyosis, endocervical or endometrial polyps, ovarian dysfunction, endometrial hyperplasia and cancer, a blood dyscrasia, and patients who are taking tamoxifen, antiplatelet medications, and anticoagulants are all at greater risk. Patients who present with amenorrhea or oligomenorrhea will often have polycystic ovarian syndrome (see section on PCOS which follows).

Diagnosis of Abnormal Uterine Bleeding

The diagnosis of abnormal uterine bleeding is clinically based upon history and physical examination. Patients may present with sparse bleeding, irregular bleeding, or heavy menstrual bleeding. Infrequent menses are often due to polycystic ovarian syndrome, but pregnancy should always be ruled out in any reproductive-age patient with an intact uterus. Heavy menstrual bleeding requires a careful history and physical examination to rule out other serious causes.[12] Identification of the underlying cause usually requires laboratory testing, including a complete blood count, follicle stimulating hormone (FSH), leutenizing hormone (LH), thyroid stimulating hormone (TSH), and any other tests as appropriate. For example, a patient with significant bleeding who may require transfusion should have a type and cross,

prothrombin time (PT), partial thromboplastin time (PTT), and fibrinogen. Adolescents with heavy menstrual bleeding may need a von Willebrand factor panel.[12] Imaging with ultrasound can reveal structural abnormalities and gross pathology of the uterus and adnexa. Tissue diagnosis with endometrial biopsy can be completed in the office setting, with the addition of saline-infusion ultrasound increasing the yield.[12]

Treatment of Abnormal Uterine Bleeding

The treatment of abnormal bleeding depends upon the underlying etiology. However, common pharmacotherapies are listed here and in **Table 27.7**:

- **Nonsteroidal anti-inflammatory drugs (NSAIDs)** such as **ibuprofen** or **naproxen** are often used as adjunct therapy during heavy menstrual bleeding.
- **Tranexamic acid**. An antifibrinolytic used extensively for bleeding, including postpartum hemorrhage and trauma-related bleeding.
- **Conjugated equine estrogens**. Intravenous and oral preparations can be given depending upon the patient's presentation and the presence or absence of contraindications.
- **Progestins** or **progesterone** may be given in several delivery options (see Table 27.7).
- **Gonadotropin releasing hormone agonist**.
- **Combined hormonal contraception**. Used in patients who do not desire pregnancy and without contraindications.

DYSMENORRHEA

Primary dysmenorrhea is painful menses within the first 6 months of menarche without known pathology. Secondary dysmenorrhea is painful menses due to underlying pathology. Risk factors for primary dysmenorrhea are largely unknown, but the pathophysiology is due to excess prostaglandin production.[19] The risk factors for secondary dysmenorrhea depend upon the underlying pathology.

Diagnosis of Dysmenorrhea

Diagnosis is based on history, physical examination, and other testing as appropriate. Diagnosis of primary dysmenorrhea rarely requires advanced testing or imaging. Secondary dysmenorrhea should be worked up with a physical examination, Pap and STI testing as appropriate, ultrasound, and diagnostic laparoscopy when indicated.

Treatment of Dysmenorrhea

The treatment of dysmenorrhea depends upon the underlying pathophysiology/pathology. Various pharmacologic options include (**Table 27.8**): nonsteroidal anti-inflammatory drugs (NSAIDs; see Table 27.7), combined hormonal contraception, progestin-only contraception, and gonadotropin-releasing hormone agonists/antagonists.[16,17,20–23]

TABLE 27.6 Human Papillomavirus Vaccines

Medications	Dose/Frequency	Indications	Contraindications	Side Effects	Other Considerations
9-valent HPV vaccine	0.5 ml IM per dose Approved for use in males & females Age 9–14 years: 2 doses at 0 and 6 to 12 months. Age 15–45 years: 3 doses at 0, 2, and 6 months Immunocompromised, any age: 3 doses at 0, 1 to 2, and 6 months	Prevention of cervical, vulvar, vaginal, anal, oropharyngeal, and other head and neck cancers; anogenital precancerous and dysplastic lesions; and genital warts in females Prevention of anal, oropharyngeal, and other head and neck cancers, anal precancerous and dysplastic lesions, and genital warts in males	Hypersensitivity to any component of the vaccine	Injection site reactions, HA, fever Post vaccination syncope	Targets HPV types as 6, 11, 16, 18, 31, 33, 45, 52, and 58 Routine vaccination at age 11–12 years, can be administered starting at age 9 years Catch-up vaccination recommended for patients aged 13 to 26 years who have not been vaccinated or who have not completed the vaccine series Vaccination based on shared decision-making for adults age 27–45
Quadrivalent HPV vaccine*	0.5 ml IM per dose Males and females age 9 to 26 years: 3 doses at 0, 1, and 6 months	Prevention of vaginal, vulvar, and cervical precancers and cancers and genital warts in females Prevention of genital warts in males	Hypersensitivity to any component of the vaccine	Common: injection site pain Severe (<0.1%): Bronchospasm, HA, GI symptoms, HTN, vaginal hemorrhage, post injection movement impairment Post vaccination syncope	Targets HPV types 6, 11, 16, 18 In females, routine vaccination at age 11–12 years, can be administered starting at age 9 years Catch-up vaccination recommended for patients aged 13 to 26 years who have not been vaccinated or who have not completed the vaccine series Routine vaccination for males not recommended
Bivalent HPV vaccine*	0.5 ml IM per dose Females age 9–25 years: 3 doses at 0, 1, and 6 months	Prevention of cervical cancer, cervical intraepithelial neoplasia (CIN) Grade 2 or worse, adenocarcinoma in situ, and cervical intraepithelial neoplasia (CIN) Grade 1 caused by oncogenic HPV types 16 and 18	Hypersensitivity to any component of the vaccine	Common local adverse reactions (≥20%): pain, redness, swelling at injection site Common general adverse events (≥20%) fatigue, HA, myalgia, GI symptoms, arthralgia Post vaccination syncope	Routine vaccination at age 11–12 years, can be administered starting at age 9 years Catch-up vaccination recommended for patients aged 13–25 years who have not been vaccinated or who have not completed the vaccine series.

CDC, Centers for Disease Control and Prevention; FDA, Food and Drug Administration; GI, gastrointestinal; HA, headache; HPV, human papillomavirus; IM, intramuscularly

*Not available in the United States

Sources: Centers for Disease Control and Prevention. FDA licensure of quadrivalent human papillomavirus vaccine (HPV4, Gardasil) for use in males and guidance from the Advisory Committee on Immunization Practices (ACIP). *MMWR Morb Mortal Wkly Rep.* 2010; 59(20):630–632. https://www.cdc.gov/mmwr/preview/mmwrhtml/mm5920a5.htm; Centers for Disease Control and Prevention. *HPV vaccine schedule and dosing.* https://www.cdc.gov/hpv/hcp/schedules-recommendations.html; Cox JT, Palefsky JM. Human papillomavirus vaccination. In: Hirsch MS, Bloom A, eds. *UpToDate* . Updated October 30, 2020. https://www.uptodate .com/contents/human-papillomavirus-vaccination; U.S. Food and Drug Administration. Package insert and patient information—Ceravix. https://www.fda.gov/media/78013/download

TABLE 27.7 Common Pharmacotherapy for Abnormal Uterine Bleeding

Medication	Dose/Frequency	Indications	Contraindications	Side Effects	Other Considerations
Nonsteroidal anti-inflammatories	Ibuprofen 200–800 mg PO 3 to 4 times daily, usual dose 400 mg; maximum dose 3200 mg/day Naproxen sodium 220, 250, 375, 500, 550 mg. One tablet, every 8 to 12 hours as needed; maximum dose (as naproxen sodium) of 1650 mg/day	Adjunct therapy for pain and cramping associated with heavy menstrual bleeding or dysmenorrhea	Hypersensitivity to NSAIDs, IgE-mediated allergic reactions after use of NSAIDs (including aspirin) asthma after use of NSAIDs	Hypersensitivity reactions, GI upset, gastric ulcers, GI perforation, edema, headache, dizziness, rash, hemolysis, tinnitus, renal dysfunction, elevated hepatic enzymes, myocardial infarction, stroke	Take with food or milk. Monitor for drug–drug interactions as well as liver and kidney function
Tranexamic acid[12-14]	1,300 mg (650 mg two tablets) PO tid for 5 days as needed for heavy bleeding 10 mg/kg IV (max 600 mg/dose)	Heavy menstrual bleeding, acute and chronic	Thromboembolic events, acquired color vision impairments	GI upset, headache, back pain, abdominal pain, myalgias, arthralgias, thromboembolic events (increased risk with concomitant combined hormone contraception)	Tablets are large and may be difficult for some to swallow IV administration not to exceed 100 mg/minute (generally over 10 to 30 minutes)
Conjugated equine estrogens[12]	25 mg IV every 4–6 hours for 24 hours Can use IM but IV is preferred due to rapid onset of action	Heavy menstrual bleeding	Undiagnosed vaginal bleeding, breast cancer, uterine cancer, thromboembolic events, active hepatic disease, pregnancy	Long-term use associated with uterine cancer, breast cancer, thromboembolic events, myocardial infarction, stroke, GI upset, gallbladder disease, melasma, breakthrough seizures, arthralgias, edema, injection site reactions	Intravenous or intramuscular use indicated for short-term management in the absence of contraindications
Progestins or progesterone[12,14]	Medroxyprogesterone acetate: 5–10 mg PO daily × 5–10 days or tid × 7 days for acute heavy menstrual bleeding Depo-medroxyprogesterone acetate injection: 150 mg IM once every 12 weeks Micronized progesterone: 100 or 200 mg PO bid × 10 days Norethindrone acetate: 5 mg PO once daily Levonorgestrel-secreting intrauterine system (LNG-IUS)	Heavy menstrual bleeding. To induce a withdrawal bleed in oligo- or amenorrhea when pregnancy has been ruled out	Undiagnosed vaginal bleeding, pregnancy, breast cancer, thromboembolic events, hepatic disease, hypersensitivity to any of the active ingredients Peanut allergy: micronized progesterone Sepsis or active pelvic inflammatory disease: LNG-IUS	Abnormal uterine bleeding, breast tenderness, thromboembolic events, GI upset, depression, somnolence, acne, rash	Micronized progesterone and progestins are chemically distinct Can use norethindrone once daily long term

Drug class	Dosing	Indications	Contraindications	Side effects	Notes
Gonadotropin releasing hormone (GnRH) agonist[15-17]	Dosing for AUB due to uterine leiomyoma Leuprolide acetate 3.75 mg IM (once monthly), maximum dose 7.5 mg once monthly Depo-leuprolide acetate suspension 11.25 mg IM (once every 3 months), maximum dose 22.5 mg once every 3 months Goserelin acetate 3.6 mg SQ once monthly for one or two doses	AUB due to uterine leiomyoma, as adjunct and preparation for surgery Also used in treatment of endometriosis; adjunct therapy in breast and prostate cancers	Hypersensitivity to GnRH agonists, undiagnosed vaginal bleeding, pregnancy, breastfeeding	Vasomotor symptoms, bone loss with long-term use, headache, myalgias, arthralgias, depression, vaginitis, dizziness, decreased libido, lipid elevations, injection site reactions	Often used with norethindrone 5 mg PO once daily for endometriosis (See Table 27.8) Can be used to induce amenorrhea in patients undergoing myelosuppressive chemotherapy or premenopausal patients with breast cancer who are not candidates for endometrial ablation or the LNG-IUS
Combined hormonal contraception[12,18]	Monophasic pill pack with 35 mcg ethinyl estradiol: tid for 7 days Can use combined hormonal contraception daily or weekly (depending on delivery system) for long-term use in patients without contraindications who do not desire pregnancy (See Table 27.10)	Heavy menstrual bleeding, oligomenorrhea, irregular bleeding patterns when malignancy and pregnancy have been ruled out	Undiagnosed vaginal bleeding, breast cancer, uterine cancer, thromboembolic events, active hepatic disease, pregnancy, cigarette use in patients ≥ 35 years, ischemic heart disease, migraine with aura, diabetes mellitus with micro or macrovascular complications, immobility	Long-term use associated with uterine cancer, breast cancer, thromboembolic events, myocardial infarction, headaches, stroke, GI upset, gallbladder disease, melasma, breakthrough seizures, arthralgias, edema	Available as daily tablets, a patch, and a vaginal ring for long-term use. Combined oral contraceptive tablets tid can cause significant GI upset.

bid, twice daily; GI, gastrointestinal; HTN, hypertension; IM, intramuscularly; inj, injection; IV, intravenously; NSAID, nonsteroidal anti-inflammatories; PO, orally; tid, three times daily.

TABLE 27.8 Pharmacotherapy for Dysmenorrhea

Medication	Dose/Frequency	Indications	Contraindications	Side Effects	Other Considerations
Combined hormonal contraception[18,19]	Oral formulations: One tablet orally every day per package instructions. Various phasic formulations (i.e., mono-, bi-, or tri-phasic) available, which contain different doses of estradiol and various types and doses of progestins Patch: apply one patch once/week for 3 weeks, then off x 1 week. Monthly vaginal ring: insert one ring x 3 weeks, remove x 1 week. Restart with a new ring. Alternate schedule for cycle management: one ring x 12 weeks, off x 1 week. Restart with a new ring.	Dysmenorrhea, contraception	Undiagnosed vaginal bleeding, breast cancer, uterine cancer, thromboembolic events, active hepatic disease, pregnancy, cigarette use in patients ≥35 years, ischemic heart disease, migraine with aura, diabetes mellitus with micro or macrovascular complications, immobility	Long-term use associated with uterine cancer, breast cancer, thromboembolic events, myocardial infarction, headaches, stroke, GI upset, gallbladder disease, melasma, breakthrough seizures, arthralgias, edema	Available as daily tablets, a patch, and a vaginal ring
Progestin-only contraception[18,19]	Norethindrone: 0.35 mg PO every day Depo-medroxyprogesterone acetate injection: 150 mg IM once every 12 weeks Etonogestrel: 68 mcg subdermal implant for 3 years. LNG-IUS for 3–5 years	Dysmenorrhea, contraception	Undiagnosed vaginal bleeding, pregnancy, breast cancer, thromboembolic events, hepatic disease, hypersensitivity to any of the active ingredients Peanut allergy: micronized progesterone. Sepsis or active pelvic inflammatory disease: LNG-IUS	Abnormal uterine bleeding, breast tenderness, thromboembolic events, GI upset, depression, somnolence, acne, rash	Long-term use (>5 years) is associated with decreased bone mineral density
Gonadotropin-releasing hormone agonists[16,17,20–22]	For dysmenorrhea due to endometriosis in women age 18 years or more: Nafarelin nasal spray. Initial dose: one spray (200 mcg) into 1 nostril each AM, and 1 spray into the other nostril each PM (400 mcg/day). Maximum dose 2 sprays (1 in each nostril) twice daily (800 mcg/day) Goserelin acetate; dosed as for AUB (see Table 27.7) Leuprolide acetate injection and Depo-leuprolide acetate suspension for injection; both dosed as for AUB (see Table 27.7)	Endometriosis (second-line therapy) Uterine leiimyoma (adjunct therapy and preparation for surgery)	Hypersensitivity to GnRH agonists, undiagnosed vaginal bleeding, pregnancy, breastfeeding	Vasomotor symptoms, bone loss with long-term use, headache, myalgias, arthralgias, depression, vaginitis, dizziness, decreased libido, lipid elevations, injection site reactions	Norethindrone 5 mg PO daily may be used as adjunct therapy with Leuprolide for treatment of endometriosis Ovulation may not be suppressed with use of GnRH agonists at recommended dosage; use of an effective nonhormonal contraceptive is essential Initial therapy with GnRH agonist should not exceed 6 months due to risk of decreased bone mineral density. Total duration of therapy should not exceed 12 months
Gonadotropin-releasing hormone antagonist[22,23]	Elagolix 150 mg tablet, one tablet PO once daily for endometriosis 200 mg tablet, one tablet PO once daily for endometriosis with dyspareunia	Endometriosis, with or without dyspareunia	Pregnancy (increased risk of early pregnancy loss) Hypersensitivity to elagolix or its components, undiagnosed vaginal bleeding, known osteoporosis, severe (Child-Pugh class C) hepatic disease, concomitant use of strong OATP 1B1 inhibitors (e.g., cyclosporine, gemfibrozil)	Common: amenorrhea, menstrual changes, hot flashes, night sweats, headache, nausea, insomnia, joint pain Severe: Jaundice, mood changes, depression, anxiety and behavior change, allergic reaction	Many drug-drug interactions; consult a drug interactions database for detailed information Start within 7 days of menses onset (or exclude pregnancy prior to starting). Maximum treatment duration for endometriosis: 24 months Take at approximately the same time each day Maximum treatment duration for endometriosis with dyspareunia: 6 months

POLYCYSTIC OVARIAN SYNDROME

Polycystic ovarian syndrome (PCOS) is a common endocrine disorder among women of reproductive age, and is the most common cause of anovulatory infertility. The etiology is multifactorial; however insulin resistence and hyperandrogenism are key factors.[23-24] Several comorbid conditions are commonly found in PCOS, such as insulin resistance and type 2 diabetes mellitus, dyslipidemia, oligo- and amenorrhea, high body mass index, ovarian cysts, and infertility. The classic triad in PCOS is hyperandrogenism, cystic ovaries, and ovulatory dysfunction.[24,25]

Diagnosis of Polycystic Ovarian Syndrome

The diagnosis of PCOS should be considered in women with any of the previous presentations. PCOS should also be considered in females who present with hirsutism, acanthosis nigricans, androgenic alopecia, central adiposity, and acne.[24,25] Pregnancy should be excluded in women of reproductive age with menstrual irregularities or amenorrhea. The three diagnostic guidelines for PCOS (NIH Criteria [1990], Rotterdam Criteria [2003], and Androgen Excess and PCOS Society criteria [2009]) all include hyperandrogenism as a key criterion. The Rotterdam Criteria require two of the following: hyperandrogenism, oligomenorrhea, and/or polycystic ovaries. The Endocrine Society recommends use of the Rotterdam Criteria for diagnosis of PCOS.[25] If the patient meets diagnostic criteria, the following lab tests should be considered: follicle stimulating hormone (FSH), luteinizing hormone (LH), sex hormone binding globulin (SHBG), testosterone (free and total), and dehydroepiandrosterone sulfate (DHEAS) levels.[24-27] The ratio between FSH and LH is usually elevated in patients with PCOS. Furthermore, testosterone and DHEA-S levels will also be elevated, but SHBG will be low. Of note, cystic ovaries do not need to be present for the diagnosis. Once the diagnosis is confirmed, patients should have regular glucose and lipid screening as well as blood pressure evaluations.

Treatment for Polycystic Ovarian Syndrome

The choice of treatment options for PCOS is based on shared decision-making that takes the patient's desire for contraception and/or pregnancy into account. Medication options include metformin, combined hormonal contraception, progestin/progesterone, spironolactone, finasteride, eflornithine hydrochloride, clomiphene citrate, and letrozole (see **Table 27.9** for details).[24-33] Pregnancy should be excluded in all women of reproductive age prior to starting therapy with any of these medications.

CONTRACEPTION

Over 61% of women ages 15 to 44 in the United States currently use a contraceptive method. Choice of method varies with age, race/ethnicity, and socioeconomic status. The most commonly used methods are oral contraceptive pills (OCPs; 25.3%), tubal ligation (21.8%), male condom (14.6%), and long-acting reversible contraceptives (LARC)—IUD and implant (14.3%). Of note, use of LARCs increased by almost 140% between 2008 and 2014, while OCP use remained relatively constant.[34]

Any patient who is sexually active who does not desire pregnancy should be offered contraception. Choice of contraceptive is based upon shared decision-making that incorporates patient preferences and risk factors. Health history, to include patient preferences, pregnancy history and family planning goals, current number of sexual partners, history of sexually transmitted infection, smoking status, history of thromboembolic events, chronic illnesses (i.e. hypertension, heart disease, diabetes mellitus, liver/jaundice problems, kidney/renal disease, cervical/breast cancer) and history of pelvic surgery should be completed. Physical exam is guided by the history. Blood pressure should be measured in patients for whom hormonal contraception will be prescribed. Abdominal and pelvic (speculum and bimanual) exams should be completed in patients who will receive an intrauterine contraceptive device.

Pharmacologic Options for Contraception

Pharmacotherapy for contraception includes combined hormonal contraception, progestin-only contraception, and emergency contraception (**Table 27.10**).[34-39] Other non pharmaceutical contraceptive options exist but are beyond the scope of this chapter.

CONDITIONS RELATED TO POSTMENOPAUSE

Age of natural menopause ranges from late 40s to early 50s worldwide, and the average age of natural menopause is increasing. Globally, the prevalence of premature menopause (age < 40 years or bilateral oophorectomy) is 1% to 8.6%; the prevalence of early menopause (age 40–44 years) is 4.9% to 9.4%.[40,41] Many women have mild or no symptoms associated with menopause, and will require only health education on the prevention or treatment of osteoporosis. However, as many as 80% of women consult a clinician at least once for bothersome symptoms.[42] The prevalence varies with race/ethnicity. Though the incidence of such symptoms is greatest in the first 2 years after the last menstrual period, bothersome symptoms may persist for 10 years or more after the last menstrual period.[43-45] As reported in the 2017 North American Menopause Society (NAMS) position statement, hormone therapy (HT) continues to be the most effective treatment to relieve vasomotor symptoms (VMS), genitourinary syndrome of menopause (GSM), and to prevent bone loss and fracture.[46]

TABLE 27.9 Pharmacotherapy for Polycystic Ovarian Syndrome

Medication	Dose/Frequency	Indications	Contraindications	Side Effects	Other Considerations
Metformin[24–28]	1,500–2,250 mg PO daily	Off-label use for treatment of PCOS in absence of comorbid type 2 diabetes. Used to treat insulin resistance, anovulation, irregular menses, hirsutism	Severe renal disease (eGFR <30 mL/minute/1.73 m²) Acute or chronic metabolic acidoses	GI upset, lactic acidosis	Can be used together with other medications in this table. May induce spontaneous ovulation. If patient does not desire pregnancy, contraception should be offered.
Combined hormonal contraception[18, 24–27]	Oral formulations: One tablet orally every day per package instructions. Various phasic formulations (i.e., mono-, bi-, or tri-phasic) available, which contain different doses of estradiol and various types and doses of progestins Patch: apply one patch once/week for 3 weeks, then off x 1 week. Monthly vaginal ring: insert one ring x 3 weeks, remove x 1 week. Restart with a new ring Alternate schedule for cycle management: one ring x 12 weeks, off x 1 week. Restart with a new ring.	PCOS, contraception	Undiagnosed vaginal bleeding, breast cancer, uterine cancer, thromboembolic events, active hepatic disease, pregnancy, cigarette use in patients ≥35 years, ischemic heart disease, migraine with aura, diabetes mellitus with micro or macrovascular complications, immobility	Long-term use associated with uterine cancer, breast cancer; thromboembolic events, myocardial infarction, headaches, stroke, GI upset, gallbladder disease, melasma, breakthrough seizures, arthralgias, edema	Available as daily tablets, a patch, and a vaginal ring All combined hormonal contraceptives (CHCs) reduce hirsutism. Oral CHCs with antiandrogenic properties (clormadinone acetate, cyproterone acetate, drospirenone, dienogest, and "third-generation" progestins [desogestrel, gestodene, norgestimate]) may be more effective in obese patients. Long-term use of drospirenone combined with ethinyl estradiol may be associated with higher risk of thromboembolic and cardiovascular events as compared to other progestins.
Progestin/progesterone[18, 24–27]	Norethindrone: 0.35 mg PO every day Depot medroxyprogesterone acetate: 150 mg IM once every 12 weeks Etonogestrel: 68 mcg subdermal implant for 3 years LNG-IUS for 3–5 years	PCOS, contraception	Undiagnosed vaginal bleeding, pregnancy, breast cancer, thromboembolic events, hepatic disease, hypersensitivity to any of the active ingredients Peanut allergy: micronized progesterone Sepsis or active pelvic inflammatory disease: LNG-IUS	Abnormal uterine bleeding, breast tenderness, thromboembolic events, GI upset, depression, somnolence, acne, rash	Long-term systemic use (>5 years) is associated with decreased bone mineral density Significant drug–drug interactions exist. Consult drug interactions database for details.
Spironolactone[24–27, 29]	50–200 mg PO daily	PCOS: Treatment of hirsutism and acne in women for whom CHC is ineffective or contraindicated (off-label use)	Hyperkalemia, chronic adrenal insufficiency, anuria, severe renal impairment, severe hepatic impairment, concomitant use with other potassium-sparing diuretics, pregnancy	Hyperkalemia, other electrolyte disturbances, bradycardia, hypersensitivity reactions, renal failure, hepatic failure	Many drug–drug interactions; consult drug interactions database for detailed information Monitor blood pressure, serum electrolytes (including potassium) within 1 week of initiation and regularly thereafter, uric acid, glucose, renal function, and volume status
Finasteride[24–27, 30]	5 mg PO daily	Androgenic alopecia in men PCOS: Treatment of hirsutism or acne in women for whom CHC is ineffective or contraindicated (off-label use)	Hypersensitivity to finasteride or other 5-alpha reductase inhibitors, pregnancy, breastfeeding	Angioedema, depression, decreased libido	Not FDA approved for this use

Drug	Indication	Dosing	Contraindications	Adverse effects	Comments
Eflornithine hydrochloride[25,31]	Hirsutism	13.9% cream applied as a thin film bid at least 8 hours apart	Hypersensitivity to eflornithine; avoid in pregnancy and breastfeeding	Local skin irritation	No drug interactions Laser Do not wash treated area for at least 4 hours after application Marked improvement may occur after 8 weeks of use; hair growth usually returns 8 weeks after discontinuation
Clomiphene citrate 24-27,32	Infertility	Initial dose: 50 mg PO once daily for 5 days Subsequent doses: If ovulation occurs, continue with initial dosage of 50 mg once daily for 5 days starting on the fifth day of the menstrual cycle in subsequent treatment cycles If pregnancy is not achieved within 3 ovulatory responses, further treatment not recommended If ovulation does *not* occur after initial course of therapy, increase to 100 mg daily for 5 days, starting ≥30 days after previous course of therapy If ovulation does not occur after 3 courses of therapy, further treatment not recommended ≥6 cycles of therapy (including 3 ovulatory cycles) not recommended	Pregnancy, undiagnosed vaginal bleeding, hepatic dysfunction, pituitary tumors, uncontrolled thyroid or adrenal dysfunction	Ovarian hyperstimulation and enlargemen[t], pelvic bloating, vasomotor symptoms, GI upset, mastalgia	Can be used alone or in combination with metformin for ovulation induction in women with POCS and anovulatory infertility with no other infertility factors Considered second-line therapy Risk of multiple pregnancy higher with clomiphene citrate vs. letrozole or metformin alone
Letrozole 24-27, 33	Treatment of anovulatory infertility in women with PCOS (off-label) Also used in postmenopausal female with estrogen positive breast cancer.	2.5–7.5 mg PO once daily × 5 days, begin on day 3 of menstrual cycle	Pregnancy, breastfeeding	Vasomotor symptoms, decreased bone mineral density, thromboembolic events, myocardial infarction, arthralgias, headache	First line therapy for ovulation induction in women with POCS and anovulatory infertility with no other infertility factors Do not combine with DHEA or estrogens

bid, twice daily; DHEA, dehydroepiandrosterone sulfate; FDA, United States Food and Drug Administration; GI, gastrointestinal; PCOS, polycystic ovarian syndrome; PO, orally.

TABLE 27.10 Treatment Options for Contraception

Medication	Dose/Frequency	Indications	Contraindications	Side Effects	Other Considerations
Combined hormonal contraception[34–37]	Oral formulations: One tablet orally every day per package instructions. Various phasic formulations (i.e., mono-, bi-, or tri-phasic) available, which contain different doses of estradiol and various types and doses of progestins Patch: one patch every week, off × 1 week Monthly vaginal ring: one ring x 3 weeks, off x 1 week. Restart with a new ring. Alternate schedule for cycle management: one ring x 12 weeks, off x 1 week. Restart with a new ring. Annual vaginal ring: one ring x 3 weeks, off x 1 week; ring reusable x 1 year. Alternate schedule for cycle management: one ring x 12 weeks, off x 1 week; ring reusable x 1 year.	Contraception	Undiagnosed vaginal bleeding; breast cancer; uterine cancer; thromboembolic events; protein C, protein S, or antithrombin deficiency, or other known thrombophilic disorders; active hepatic disease; pregnancy; cigarette use in patients ≥35 years; ischemic heart disease; migraine with aura; diabetes mellitus with micro or macrovascular complications; immobility	Long-term use associated with breast cancer, thromboembolic events, myocardial infarction, headaches, stroke, GI upset, gallbladder disease, melasma, breakthrough seizures, arthralgias, edema	Available as daily tablets, a patch, and a vaginal ring Significant drug–drug interactions exist. Consult drug interactions database for details.
Progestin-only contraception[34–37]	Norethindrone 0.35 mg PO every day Depo-medroxyprogesterone acetate 150 mg IM once every 12 weeks. Etonogestrel 68 mcg subdermal implant for 3 years. LNG-IUS for 3–5 years	Contraception	Undiagnosed vaginal bleeding, pregnancy, breast cancer, thromboembolic events, hepatic disease, hypersensitivity to any of the active ingredients. Peanut allergy: micronized progesterone. Sepsis or active pelvic inflammatory disease: LNG-IUS	Abnormal uterine bleeding, breast tenderness, thromboembolic events, GI upset, depression, somnolence, acne, rash	Long-term systemic use (>5 years) is associated with decreased bone mineral density Significant drug–drug interactions exist. Consult drug interactions database for details.
Emergency contraception[34–36, 38, 39]	Levonorgestrel: 1.5 mg one tablet PO: must use within 72 hours of unprotected sex Ulipristal: 30 mg one tablet PO; must be taken within 120 hours of unprotected sex Combined hormonal contraceptive tablet with levonorgestrel as the progestin: various regimens are recommended depending upon the progestin dose; may require up to 6 tablets at once; two doses taken 12 hours apart	Emergency contraception up to 120 hours after unprotected intercourse	Pregnancy, breastfeeding, premenarche, postmenopause, active porphyria (combined and progestin tablets), thromboembolic events, migraine at the time of taking the medication, severe hepatic disease. Also see contraindications for combined oral contraceptive use above	GI upset, menstrual irregularities, dysmenorrhea, abdominal pain, headache, fatigue	Combined hormonal contraceptive tablet can cause GI upset if needing to take more than one tablet at a time Significant drug–drug interactions exist. Consult drug interactions database for details.

GI, gastrointestinal; IM, intramuscularly; PO, orally.

DIAGNOSIS OF MENOPAUSE

The diagnosis of menopause is generally based on patient history. Natural menopause can be diagnosed without laboratory testing in healthy women age 45 and above with a) amenorrhea for at least 1 year who are not using hormonal contraception; or b) based upon symptoms in women without a uterus. Routine laboratory testing to confirm the diagnosis is not recommended in these patients.[47] Serum FSH can be used to diagnose women aged less than 40 years in whom premature ovarian failure is suspected; and in women aged 40 to 45 years with menopausal symptoms.[47] Elevated FSH confirms the diagnosis. For patients in this age group in whom the diagnosis is still unclear, additional testing may be considered; elevated FSH, low or absent inhibin B, and low or absent anti-Müellerian hormone will be present.

HORMONE THERAPY

Patients who experience menopause often develop VMS, which include hot flashes and night sweats. They are described as episodes of sweating and flushing predominantly at around the chest, upper back, neck, and the head areas. The risk factors for VMS involve multiple aspects including racial/ethnic group, genetic polymorphism, obesity, and smoking. In the Study of Women's Health Across the Nation (SWAN), African American women reported VMH at a higher prevalence than other ethnic groups.[42] The genetic polymorphisms that alter the activity of sex steroid hormones may be another contributing factor. Furthermore, women with an average body mass index (BMI) of 31 kg/m^2 also reported VMS more frequently and women who are current smokers are approximately 60% more likely to report VMS compared to nonsmokers.[42,43] Women with comorbidities of anxiety, depressive symptoms, and perceived stress as well as lower socioeconomic status are also at higher risk for VMS.

The FDA-approved pharmacologic treatment options for menopausal symptoms are summarized in **Table 27.11** and include estrogen, progestin, dehydroepiandrosterone (DHEA), selective estrogen receptor modulators (SERMs), and selective serotonin reuptake inhibitors (SSRIs).[41, 46, 48–56] Of note, compounded hormone therapy is not recommended due to lack of standardization of dosing. Alternative and complementary therapies include acupuncture and black cohosh, but evidence is weak regarding their efficacy. Prevention and treatment of osteoporosis is discussed in **Chapter 20**.

BREAST CANCER

The well-established risk factors of breast cancer include female gender, *BRCA* mutations, increasing age, family history, prior radiation to the chest wall, age >30 years at time of first pregnancy resulting in birth, and menarche before age 13 years. Furthermore, changes in histological category from the initial to the subsequent biopsy could also significantly impact the risk of breast cancer. In fact, patients with nonproliferative initial findings converted to proliferative findings during subsequent biopsy have approximately 1.77-fold increase in risk of cancer compared to those who have no change in findings.[57] While having a *BRCA* mutation places a patient at tremendous risk of developing a breast or ovarian malignancy, less than 15% of all breast cancers are due to *BRCA* mutations.[58]

DIAGNOSIS

Findings that trigger concerns for breast cancer include a palpable breast mass and abnormalities on breast imaging. Mammographic findings in breast cancer include spiculations, posterior acoustic shadows, irregular borders, microcalcifications along a duct or lobule, and anatomic distortion. Diagnosis of breast malignancy is confirmed through tissue biopsy. Histopathology will report on estrogen and progesterone receptor status, human epidermal growth factor receptor-2 (HER-2), and other histologic components that help guide treatment decisions.[59]

HORMONAL THERAPIES FOR BREAST CANCER

The type and stage of breast cancer directs treatment options, which are determined based upon shared decision-making and patient preferences. Surgical options include lumpectomy or partial mastectomy followed by radiation, and mastectomy. In addition to stage at diagnosis, the molecular subtype (as determined by the presence or absence of biologic markers) impacts prognosis. The primary biologic markers in current use are estrogen receptor (ER), progesterone receptor (PR), and human epidermal growth factor 2 (HER2). The most common breast cancer molecular subtype is ER+/HER2-.[59,60] Because this subtype is usually responsive to hormonal therapy, it is associated with the best prognosis.[59] Adjuvant endocrine therapy targets the reduction of circulating estrogen and/or inhibition of estrogen receptors. Bilateral oophorectomy and ovarian ablation are surgical options that permanently stop ovarian production of hormones. Pharmacologic suppression of ovarian hormone production is accomplished with several drug classes. Gonadotropin-releasing hormone agonists (e.g., goserelin, leuprolide) suppress ovarian estrogen production. Aromatase inhibitors (e.g., anastrozole, letrozole, exemestane) prevent the conversion of androgens to estrogen by aromatase. Anti estrogens prevent the binding of estrogen receptors. Selective estrogen receptor modulators (SERMs; e.g., tamoxifen, toremifene) block estrogen from binding to its receptors. A novel class of medications, selective estrogen receptor degraders (SERDs; e.g., fulvestrant), alter the estrogen receptor, and may be useful in overcoming endocrine therapy resistance (see **Table 27.12**).[59,60,61] Adjuvant chemotherapy for advanced or metastatic breast cancer, and pharmacotherapy of HER2-positive breast cancers are beyond the scope of this chapter.

TABLE 27.11 Treatment Options for Menopause

Medication	Dose/Frequency	Indications	Contraindications	Side Effects	Other Considerations
Estrogen[41,46,48-50]	Estradiol tablets: 0.45, 0.5, 0.9, 1, 1.5, 2 mg; taken once daily Estradiol patches: 0.025, 0.0375, 0.05, 0.06, 0.075, 0.1 mg; one patch once or twice weekly depending on the delivery system with application sites rotated Estradiol emulsion: 4.3 mg/1.74 g (0.25%) applied daily Estradiol gels: 0.06% and 0.1% Estradiol transdermal spray: 1.53 mg in each spray, use daily Estradiol vaginal inserts: 10 or 25 mcg intravaginally once daily for 2 weeks, then twice a week Estradiol vaginal cream: 0.01% apply 2–4 g daily for 1–2 weeks, then 1 g 1–3 times weekly Estradiol vaginal ring: 2 mg reservoir (delivers 7.5 mcg/24 hours) leave in for 3 months Conjugated equine estrogen tablet: 0.3, 0.45, 0.625, 0.9, and 1.25 mg Conjugated equine estrogen vaginal cream: 0.625 mg/g, usual starting dose 0.5 g twice weekly	Oral, transdermal: vasomotor symptoms. Vaginal: atrophic vaginitis/genitourinary syndrome of menopause	Undiagnosed vaginal bleeding, breast cancer, uterine cancer, thromboembolic events, active hepatic disease, pregnancy, cigarette use in patients ≥35 years, ischemic heart disease, protein C, protein S, or antithrombin deficiency, or other known thrombophilic disorders; active hepatic disease migraine with aura, diabetes mellitus with micro or macrovascular complications, immobility	Breast tenderness, breast cancer, uterine cancer, thromboembolic events, myocardial infarction, headaches, stroke, GI upset, gallbladder disease, melasma, breakthrough seizures, arthralgias, edema	Patients with an intact uterus who use systemic estrogen must also use a progestin to prevent endometrial hyperplasia and cancer Not to be used to prevent heart disease or dementia
Progestin[41,46,48,51,52]	Medroxyprogesterone acetate 1.5, 2.5, 5-mg tablets once daily; also available as combination tablets with conjugated equine estrogens Norethindrone acetate 0.1- or 0.5-mg tablets (combination with estradiol) once daily Norethindrone acetate 0.5- or 1-mg (combination patches with estradiol) twice weekly	Used to prevent endometrial hyperplasia and cancer in patients with a uterus who are receiving systemic estrogen	Undiagnosed vaginal bleeding, pregnancy, breast cancer, thromboembolic events, hepatic disease, hypersensitivity to any of the active ingredients Peanut allergy: micronized progesterone. Sepsis or active pelvic inflammatory disease: LNG-IUS.	Abnormal uterine bleeding, breast tenderness, thromboembolic events, GI upset, depression, somnolence, acne, rash	Long-term systemic use (>5 years) is associated with decreased bone mineral density
Bazedoxifene[41,46,53]	20-mg tablet PO once daily in fixed combination with conjugated estrogens 0.45 mg	Management of moderate to severe VMS of menopause in women with an intact uterus Prevention of osteoporosis in postmenopausal women (off-label use in US)	Undiagnosed vaginal bleeding, breast cancer, uterine cancer, thromboembolic events, active hepatic disease, pregnancy, cigarette use in patients ≥35 years, ischemic heart disease, migraine with aura, diabetes mellitus with micro or macrovascular complications, immobility	GI upset, abdominal pain, dizziness, neck pain, muscle spasms, oropharyngeal pain	A selective estrogen receptor modulator Patients who experience vaginal bleeding while taking the product should have ultrasound evaluation of the endometrium for evidence of hyperplasia Use not recommended in renal impairment

Selective serotonin reuptake inhibitor[41,54]	Paroxetine 7.5-mg tablet once daily is the only FDA-approved SSRI for the treatment of VMS of menopause	Vasomotor symptoms during menopause	Monoamine oxidase inhibitor use within 14 days. Do not use with thioridazine or pimozide. Hypersensitivity to paroxetine	Headache, fatigue, GI upset, suicidal thoughts, serotonin syndrome	Other SSRIs and SNRIs have been shown to be effective in reducing vasomotor symptoms.[41] Avoid use when taking products requiring CYP2D6 metabolism
Ospemifene[41,46,48,55]	60-mg tablet PO daily	Genitourinary syndrome of menopause	Undiagnosed vaginal or uterine bleeding, estrogen-dependent malignancy, active or recent thromboembolic event, stroke, myocardial infarction, pregnancy, hypersensitivity to ospemifene	Vasomotor symptoms and night sweats, vaginal discharge, uterine bleeding, headache, muscle spasms, hyperhidrosis	Selective-estrogen receptor modulator with agonist effects on the endometrium. Patients should be counseled to report any vaginal bleeding and need to be assessed for hyperplasia/cancer
Prasterone[41,46,48,56]	6.5-mg vaginal insert at bedtime	Dyspareunia due to the genitourinary syndrome of menopause (genital atrophy, dyspareunia)	Undiagnosed vaginal bleeding	Vaginal discharge (6%–14%) Abnormal pap smear (2%)	DHEA derivative. Has not been studied in patients with breast cancer
Vaginal Lubricants (over-the-counter)	Lubricating gels/jelly, water-based (many brands) Topical emollients (many brands)	Vaginal dryness	Allergy to any component of the product	Irritation of skin, mucous membranes Personal lubricants that contain glycerol may trigger yeast infections	Ingredients vary with brand; read label carefully Petroleum-based products may damage latex condoms, diaphragms, or sex toys

FDA, United States Food and Drug Administration; GI, gastrointestinal; PO, orally.

TABLE 27.12 Pharmacotherapy of Estrogen-Receptor Positive Breast Cancer

Drug Class	Medication, Dose, & Frequency	Indications	Contraindications	Side Effects	Other Considerations
Anti estrogens: SERMs[59-64]	Tamoxifen Adjuvant therapy: 20-mg tablets one PO daily Metastatic breast cancer: 20-mg tablets one PO once or twice per day Toremifene (FDA approved for metastatic breast cancer only): 60-mg tablets one PO daily	Treatment of estrogen receptor-positive early stage and metastatic breast cancer Reduction of invasive breast cancer risk Following breast surgery and radiation in women with ductal carcinoma in situ (DCIS) Breast cancer risk reduction in women who are at high-risk	Thromboembolic events, concurrent warfarin therapy, pregnancy	Vaginal discharge, abnormal uterine bleeding, hepatotoxicity, nausea, vasomotor symptoms, depression	Many drug–drug interactions; consult drug interactions database for detailed information Metabolism (Tamoxifen): Hepatic, via CYP2D6 and CYP3A4/5 Do not use with other CYP2D6 inhibitors Metabolism (Toremifene): Hepatic, primarily by CYP3A4 Some SSRIs (particularly fluoxetine and paroxetine) compete with hepatic metabolism and reduce the effect of tamoxifen. Citalopram and venlafaxine do not appear to effect tamoxifen metabolism Effective non hormonal contraception should be used. Once postmenopausal or within 5 years of starting therapy, patients can be switched to an aromatase inhibitor. Continued use recommended in postmenopausal patients who cannot tolerate or refuse an aromatase inhibitor (NCCN guideline) Annual gynecologic exam recommended if uterus intact (NCCN guideline)
Anti estrogens: SERDs[59-62,65]	Fulvestrant is only FDA-approved SERD at this time. Others are under investigation. Fulvestrant injection 250 mg/5 mL: Initial: 500 mg IM on days 1, 15, and 29; Maintenance: 500 mg IM once monthly	Monotherapy or combination therapy of advanced or metastatic breast CA in postmenopausal women: Initial therapy in HR+/HER2- breast CA Second-line therapy of disease progression following endocrine therapy Combination therapy in pre-/perimenopausal women with advanced or metastatic HR+/HER2- breast CA	Hypersensitivity to fulvestrant or its components Pregnancy or lactation	Common: Pain at injection site CNS: Fatigue, HA GI: Nausea, stomatitis, diarrhea, abdominal pain, anorexia, elevated LFTs Hematologic: Neutropenia, leukopenia, anemia, thrombocytopenia CV: Vasodilation and hot flushes, VTE, chest pain, edema MSK: Bone, muscle, and joint pain Respiratory: Pharyngitis, dyspnea, cough, epistaxis GU: Pelvic pain, UTI, vaginal hemorrhage Derm: Alopecia, rash, dry skin, pruritus Immunologic: Hypersensitivity reactions, infections, influenza syndrome Renal: increased SCr	Hepatic via CYP3A4 and other pathways Use with caution in patients with history of bleeding disorders or who are on anticoagulant therapy Dose adjustment recommended in patients with moderate hepatic impairment For women of reproductive age, contraception should be used during therapy and for 1 year after the last fulvestrant dose For IM injection only: Administer 500 mg dose as two 5 mL IM injections (one in each buttocks) slowly over 1 to 2 minutes per injection Monitoring: Liver function tests Pregnancy testing recommended within 7 days prior to initiation for women of reproductive age Monitor for signs/symptoms of bleeding

GnRH agonists[16,17,59-62]	Goserelin: 3.6 mg SQ every 28 days Leuprolide Depot IM injection: 3.75 mg every 28 days for up to 24 months *OR* 11.25 mg every 3 months for up to 24 months	Goserelin: Breast cancer, advanced (off-label use) Leuprolide: Breast cancer, premenopausal ovarian suppression (off-label use)	Hypersensitivity to GnRH agonists, undiagnosed vaginal bleeding, pregnancy, breast feeding	Vasomotor symptoms, bone loss with long-term use, headache, myalgia, arthralgia, depression, vaginitis, dizziness, decreased libido, lipid elevations, injection site reactions	Many drug–drug interactions; consult drug interactions database for detailed information
Nonsteroidal aromatase inhibitors[59-62,66,67]	Anastrozole Monotherapy: 1-mg tablets one daily until tumor progression Letrozole 2.5-mg tablets one PO daily Consider dosing QOD if hepatic impairment present	Anastrozole: First-line therapy of HR+ advanced or metastatic breast CA Adjuvant therapy of early HR+ breast CA Treatment of advanced breast CA in women with disease progression after tamoxifen therapy Breast cancer risk reduction (off-label use) Letrozole Treatment of postmenopausal HR+ early breast cancer Adjuvant treatment of postmenopausal women with early breast cancer who completed prior tamoxifen therapy	Hypersensitivity to anastrozole or its components, pregnancy, lactation Caution in hepatic impairment Caution in preexisting ICVD (increased risk for ischemic events) Hypersensitivity to letrozole or its components, pregnancy Caution in hepatic impairment	Anastrozole: CV: HTN, edema, ICVHD GI: Nausea, vomiting, abdominal pain, diarrhea, constipation, anorexia, xerostomia, elevated LFTs, MSK: arthralgia, joint pain and stiffness, back pain, bone pain, osteoporosis, fracture, myalgia CNS: Fatigue, HA, dizziness, paresthesia, CVA, somnolence, confusion, changes in taste or smell Psych: mood changes, depression, insomnia Immune: Infection, influenza syndrome, fever, allergic reaction Derm: rash, alopecia, pruritus, Stevens-Johnson syndrome (rare) Respiratory: Dyspnea, cough, pharyngitis, bronchitis GU: UTI, mastalgia, vaginal discharge, vaginitis, vaginal bleeding, vaginal dryness, pelvic pain Metabolic: weight gain/loss, hyperlipidemia, decreased bone mineral density Hematologic: anemia, leukopenia Eye: cataracts Oncologic: tumor flare, neoplasm Letrozole—see Table 27.9 for side effects	Significantly decrease estrone sulfate levels Metabolism: Both primarily hepatic Hepatic impairment: Anastrozole: clearance decreased approximately 30% in stable cirrhosis, no dose adjustment required Letrozole: Use with caution, dose adjustment recommended with severe hepatic dysfunction or cirrhosis Renal impairment: Anastrolzole: renal clearance decreases proportional with CrCl Many drug–drug interactions; consult drug interactions database for detailed information Use of contraception during therapy and for at least 3 weeks after last dose recommended Aromatase inhibitors should not be used as *monotherapy* in premenopausal women with breast cancer. These women should be offered ovarian suppression/ablation along with endocrine therapy Patients on an aromatase inhibitor should receive supplemental vitamin D and calcium Monitoring: Bone mineral density, lipids Test for pregnancy prior to initial dose Women of reproductive age should use non-hormonal contraception during therapy and for at least 3 weeks after the final dose

(continued)

TABLE 27.12 Pharmacotherapy of Estrogen-Receptor Positive Breast Cancer (continued)

Drug Class	Medication, Dose, & Frequency	Indications	Contraindications	Side Effects	Other Considerations
Steroidal aromatase inhibitors[59-62,68]	Exemestane 25-mg tablets Adjuvant therapy (early breast CA): one tablet PO daily (after 2–3 years tamoxifen therapy) for total duration of 5 years of endocrine therapy Advanced breast CA: one tablet PO once daily, continue until tumor progression	Adjuvant treatment of postmenopausal estrogen-receptor positive early breast cancer who have completed 2 to 3 years of tamoxifen Treatment of advanced breast cancer in postmenopausal patients who experience disease progression on tamoxifen	Hypersensitivity to exemestane or its components, pregnancy Not indicated for use in premenopausal women	CV: HTN, edema (CHD, chest pain, heart failure (<1%), VTE (<1%) Derm: Hyperhidrosis, alopecia, dermatitis, pruritus GI: increased LFTs, nausea, vomiting, abdominal pain, diarrhea, constipation, increased appetite, anorexia, gastric ulcer (<1%) GU: UTI, endometrial hyperplasia (<1%) Heme/Onc: lymphedema Immune: fever, infection, influenza syndrome, hypersensitivity (<1%), urticaria (<1%) Metabolic: Hot flush, weight gain MSK: arthralgia, arthritis, back pain, limb pain, myalgia, osteoporosis, pathological fracture, cramping Neurologic: Fatigue, insomnia, pain, HA, paresthesia, confusion, CTS, neuropathy Eye: visual changes Psych: depression, dizziness, anxiety Renal: increased SCr Respiratory: dyspnea, cough, pharyngitis, sinusitis, URI	Extensive hepatic metabolism (CYP3A4) Many drug–drug interactions (particularly with CYP3A4 inducer); consult drug interactions database for detailed information Exemestane should not be given concurrently with estrogen-containing drugs Hepatic impairment: Dosage adjustment is recommended in patients with moderate impairment. Safety and efficacy have not been established in severe impairment. Patients on an aromatase inhibitor should receive supplemental vitamin D and calcium Monitoring: Vitamin D level at base line Bone mineral density Test for pregnancy prior to therapy. Women of reproductive age should use non-hormonal contraception during therapy and for at least 4 weeks after the final dose

bid, twice daily; CA, cancer; CTS, carpal tunnel syndrome; CV, cardiovascular; Derm, dermatologic; HA, headache; Heme/Onc, hematology/oncology; HER2, human epidermal growth factor receptor negative; HR+, hormone receptor positive; HTN, hypertension; GI, gastrointestinal; GnRH, gonadotropin-releasing hormone; GU, genitourinary; LFTs, liver function tests; MSK, musculoskeletal; PO, orally; Psych, psychiatric; QOD, every other day; SCr, serum creatinine; URI, upper respiratory infection; UTI, urinary tract infection; VTE, venous thromboembolism.

CASE EXEMPLAR: Patient With Amenorrhea

HH, a 26-year-old G0P0 presents with a chief complaint of "missing periods." Her last normal menstrual period was over 3 months ago, and prior to that it was irregular and light in flow. The patient does not use any contraception and is currently not sexually active.

Past Medical History
- Asthma, well controlled
- Menarche at age 11 years
- Last Pap test 2 years ago, normal

Medication
- Albuterol inhaler 2 puffs every 4 hours PRN

Family History
- Mother: type 2 diabetes mellitus
- Father: coronary heart disease

Social History
- Medical assistant in an orthopedics practice
- Single
- Nonsmoker
- Denies illicit drug or alcohol use

Physical Examination
- BP, 138/94 mm/Hg; pulse, 86 bpm; temperature, 98.6 °F; BMI, 32
- Alert and oriented in no acute distress
- Head, eyes, ears, nose, and throat (HEENT): mild acne present on face, scattered dark hair present above upper lip
- Thyroid: smooth, no nodules or thyromegaly
- Cardiac: regular rate and rhythm, no murmurs auscultated
- Pulmonary: clear to auscultation bilaterally
- Abdomen: normoactive bowel sounds, soft, no masses palpated
- Pelvic: external genitalia without lesions, vagina pink and moist, cervix long and closed without friability or lesions. Bimanual exam: nontender, uterus mobile, normal size, shape and consistency, adnexa difficult to palpate due to patient's body habitus

Labs
- Urine β-HCG: negative

Next Steps
- Patient to have the following labs drawn: thyroid-stimulating hormone, follicle-stimulating hormone, luteinizing hormone, sex hormone binding globulin, dehydroepiandrosterone sulfate, free and total serum testosterone, lipid panel, and hemoglobin A1c.
- Patient to have a transvaginal ultrasound.
- Based upon the patient's history and body habitus, the diagnosis is likely polycystic ovarian syndrome (PCOS).
- Once the diagnosis is confirmed, the patient should receive periodic progestin or progesterone to induce a withdrawal bleed. If the patient desires contraception, a progestin intrauterine system or combined hormonal contraceptives could be used.
- Metformin is indicated to help increase insulin sensitivity, reduce androgens, and improve ovulatory function. Patients who begin metformin therapy may spontaneously ovulate, so if the patient does not desire pregnancy, contraception should be offered.
- The two most important issues to address are the patient's underlying metabolic dysfunction and risk for Type 2 DM and heart disease, and to protect the endometrium from chronic anovulation which could lead to hyperplasia and cancer.
- Healthy weight loss is key for patients who are overweight or obese.

Discussion Questions

1. Additional labs confirm the diagnosis of polycystic ovarian syndrome (PCOS) in HH. Which pharmacologic treatment should the clinician initiate to induce a withdrawal bleed?
2. In a patient with PCOS who does not wish to conceive, what pharmacologic intervention can help restore ovulatory function?

CASE EXEMPLAR: Patient With Abnormal Menstrual Bleeding

DM, a 47-year-old G3P3 presents with approximately 6 months of heavy menstrual bleeding. The patient states she is soaking through several pads and tampons every day and often bleeds through her clothing. Last menstrual period was 2 weeks ago and states the bleeding usually lasts 7 to 10 days, but gets a bit lighter during the last several days. Husband is s/p vasectomy. Urine β-HCG is negative.

Past Medical History
- Spontaneous vaginal deliveries × 3 with no complications
- Last Pap test 4 years ago; no history of abnormal Paps
- Depression
- Hypothyroidism

Medication(s)
- Sertraline, 50 mg PO once daily
- Levothyroxine, 0.25 mg PO every morning
- Multivitamin daily

Family History
- Coronary heart disease (mother and father)
- Malignant melanoma (father)
- No known gynecologic malignancies

Social History
- High school English teacher
- Married; mutually monogamous
- Denies tobacco or illicit drug use; admits to occasional glass of white wine

Physical Examination
- BP, 128/78 mm/Hg; pulse, 80; temperature, 98.7 °F; BMI, 27
- Alert and oriented in no acute distress
- Head, eyes, ears, nose, and throat (HEENT): thyroid smooth, no nodules or thyromegaly
- Cardiac: regular rate and rhythm, no murmurs auscultated
- Pulmonary: clear to auscultation bilaterally
- Abdomen: normoactive bowel sounds, soft, no masses palpated
- Pelvic: external genitalia without lesions, vagina pink and moist, cervix long and closed without friability or lesions. Bimanual exam: nontender, uterus smooth and mobile, enlarged to about 12 weeks, adnexa no masses palpated.

Labs and Imaging
- Pap test
- Complete blood count, thyroid stimulating hormone (last test was 6 months ago)
- Transvaginal ultrasound
- Saline infusion sonohysterogram with endometrial biopsy

Next Steps
- An enlarged uterus in a patient with heavy menstrual bleeding may be due to adenomyosis or fibroids. Fibroids can be diagnosed with ultrasound imaging, and while adenomyosis is often diagnosed post hysterectomy, expert radiologists can detect findings associated with adenomyosis.
- If anemic, can start iron therapy.
- If the thyroid-stimulating hormone is high or low, appropriate adjustment to the dose is warranted, but not being euthyroid will rarely cause heavy menstrual bleeding.
- If the patient has no contraindications, tranexamic acid 650-mg tablets 2 PO TID for 5 days can be used.
- If the patient's endometrial biopsy is negative and there are no fibroids present, the patient can use a progestin-secreting intrauterine system or combined hormonal oral contraception until age 50 years if no contraindications exist.
- If there are fibroids present and the patient is not ready for definitive surgical management with hysterectomy, a gonadotropin-releasing hormone agonist can be used for 3 months.

Discussion Questions
1. What is the most serious diagnosis to rule out for DM?
2. What are the contraindications to tranexamic acid?

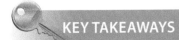

KEY TAKEAWAYS

- Accurate diagnosis and appropriate treatment of infectious diseases in women's health is imperative as all clinicians should strive for good antibiotic stewardship.
- Missed diagnosis and treatment of sexually transmitted infections can lead to pelvic inflammatory disease and tubo-ovarian abscess that may impair future fertility.
- Many issues in women's health have an underlying endocrine component. Thus, it is important to understand the physiology of the normal menstrual cycle, the myriad tissue effects of estrogen and progestin/progesterone, and the contraindications to using hormones to treat specific diseases.
- Polycystic ovarian syndrome is the most common underlying endocrinopathy in women's health, so a clear understanding of the different pharmacologic and non pharmacologic options for patients wishing to conceive or prevent pregnancy is essential.
- Multiple pharmacologic contraceptive options exist. Patients must receive the most up-to-date and evidence-based guidance on the risks, benefits, and alternatives of all options.
- Management of menopausal symptoms with approved pharmacologic medications requires a careful discussion regarding the risks, benefits, alternatives, contraindications, and current state of the evidence before making a decision of which option the patient may choose.
- Systemic hormone therapy for menopausal symptoms should never be used to prevent dementia or heart disease.

REFERENCES

1. Dall TM, Chakrabarti R, Storm MV, et al. Estimated demand for women's health services by 2020. *J Women Health.* 2013;22(7):643–648. doi:10.1089/jwh.2012.4119
2. Evans AL, Scally AJ, Wellard SJ, et al. Prevalence of bacterial vaginosis in lesbians and heterosexual women in a community setting. *Sex Transm Infect.* 2007;83(6): 470–475. doi:10.1136/sti.2006.022277
3. Centers for Disease Control and Prevention. Sexually transmitted disease treatment guidelines. Published 2015. Updated December 27, 2019. https://www.cdc.gov/std /tg2015/default.htm
4. Centers for Disease Control and Prevention. *Human papillomavirus (HPV) infection. Sexually transmitted diseases treatment guidelines.* 2015. Accessed November 10, 2020. http://www.cdc.gov/std/tg2015/hpv.htm
5. American College of Obstetricians and Gynecologists. Cervical cancer screening and prevention. Practice Bulletin No. 168. *Obstet Gynecol.* 2016;128:e111–e130. doi:10.1097/AOG.0000000000001708
6. Curry SJ, Krist AH, Owens DK, et al. Screening for cervical cancer: US Preventive Services Task Force Recommendation Statement. *JAMA.* 2018;320:674–686. doi:10.1001/jama.2018.10897
7. Centers for Disease Control and Prevention. Anogenital warts. 2015 STD treatment guidelines. https://www .cdc.gov/std/tg2015/warts.htm
8. Centers for Disease Control and Prevention. Pelvic inflammatory disease (PID). 2015 STD treatment guidelines. https://www.cdc.gov/std/tg2015/pid.htm
9. Centers for Disease Control and Prevention. HPV-associated cervical cancer rates by race and ethnicity. https://www.cdc.gov/cancer/hpv/statistics/cervical.htm
10. McClung NM, Gargano JW, Bennett NM, et al. Trends in human papillomavirus vaccine types 16 and 18 in cervical precancers, 2008–2014. *Cancer Epidemiol Biomarkers Prev.* 2019;28(3):602–609. doi:10.1158/1055-9965.EPI-18-0885
11. Cox JT, Palefsky JM. Human papillomavirus vaccination. In: Hirsch MS, Bloom A, eds. *UpToDate.* Updated October 30, 2020. https://www.uptodate.com/contents/ human-papillomavirus-vaccination
12. American College of Obstetricians and Gynecologists. ACOG Committee Opinion No. 557: management of acute abnormal uterine bleeding in nonpregnant reproductive-aged women. *Obstet Gynecol.* 2013;121(4):891–896. doi:10.1097/01.AOG.0000428646.67925.9a
13. Kost A, Pitney C. Tranexamic acid (Lysteda) for cyclic heavy menstrual bleeding. *Am Fam Physician.* 2011;84(8):883–886. https://www.aafp.org/afp/2011/1015/ p883.pdf
14. Sweet MG, Schmidt-Dalton TA, Weiss PM, et al. Evaluation and management of abnormal uterine bleeding in premenopausal women. *Am Fam Physician.* 2012;85(1):35–43. https://www.aafp.org/afp/2012/0101/ p35.pdf
15. Bradley LD, Gueye NA. The medical management of abnormal uterine bleeding in reproductive-aged women. *Am J Obstet Gynecol.* 2016;214(1):31–44. doi:10.1016/j .ajog.2015.07.044
16. Drugs.com. *Leuprolide.* Updated September 24, 2020. https://www.drugs.com/ppa/leuprolide.html
17. Drugs.com. *Goserelin acetate.* Updated October 6, 2020. https://www.drugs.com/ppa/goserelin.html
18. American College of Obstetricians and Gynecologists. ACOG Practice Bulletin No. 110: noncontraceptive uses of hormonal contraceptives. *Obstet Gynecol.* 2010;115(1):206–218. doi:10.1097/AOG .0b013e3181cb50b5
19. Bernardi M, Lazzeri L, Perelli F, et al. Dysmenorrhea and related disorders. *F1000Res.* 2017;6:1645. doi:10.12688/ f1000research.11682.1
20. Rafique S, Decherney AH. Medical management of endometriosis. *Clin Obstet Gynecol.* 2017;60(3):485–496. doi:10.1097/GRF.0000000000000292
21. Drugs.com. Nafarelin acetate. Updated October 6, 2020. https://www.drugs.com/ppa/nafarelin.html

22. Ferrero S, Barra F, Maggiore UL. Current and emerging therapeutics for the management of endometriosis. *Drugs.* 2018;78(10):995–1012. doi:10.1007/s40265-018-0928-0

23. Drugs.com. Elagolix. Updated October 6, 2020. https://www.drugs.com/ppa/elagolix.html

24. American College of Obstetricians and Gynecologists' Committee on Practice Bulletins—Gynecology. ACOG Practice Bulletin No. 194. Polycystic ovary syndrome. *Obstet Gynecol.* 2018;131(6):e157–e171. doi:10.1097/AOG.0000000000002656

25. Teede HJ, Misso ML, Costello MF, et al. Recommendations from the international evidence-based guideline for the assessment and management of polycystic ovary syndrome. *Hum Reprod.* 2018;33(9):1602–1618. doi:10.1093/humrep/dey256

26. Pasquali R. Contemporary approaches to the management of polycystic ovary syndrome. *Ther Adv Endocrinol Metab.* 2018;9(4):123–134. doi:10.1177/2042018818756790

27. Legro RS, Arslanian SA, Ehrmann DA, et al. Diagnosis and treatment of polycystic ovary syndrome. *J Clin Endocrinol Metab.* 2013;98(12):4565–4592. doi:10.1210/jc.2013-2350

28. Drugs.com. Metformin. Updated May 4, 2020. https://www.drugs.com/ppa/metformin.html

29. Drugs.com. Spironolactone. Updated March 25, 2020. https://www.drugs.com/ppa/spironolactone.html

30. Drugs.com. Finasteride. Updated April 21, 2020. https://www.drugs.com/ppa/finasteride.html

31. Drugs.com. Eflornithine. Updated June 22, 2020. https://www.drugs.com/monograph/eflornithine.html

32. Drugs.com. Clomiphene citrate. Updated October 22, 2020. https://www.drugs.com/monograph/clomiphene-citrate.html

33. Drugs.com. Letrozole. Updated May 14, 2020. https://www.drugs.com/mtm/letrozole.html

34. Kavanaugh ML, Jerman J. Contraceptive method use in the United States: Trends and characteristics between 2008, 2012 and 2014. *Contraception.* 2018;97(1):14–21. doi:10.1016/j.contraception.2017.10.003

35. American College of Obstetricians and Gynecologists' Committee on Practice Bulletins—Gynecology. ACOG Practice Bulletin No. 206: use of hormonal contraception in women with coexisting medical conditions. *Obstet Gynecol.* 2019;133(2):e128–e150. doi:10.1097/AOG.0000000000003072

36. World Health Organization. *Selected Practice Recommendations for Contraceptive Use.* 3rd ed. World Health Organization; 2016 https://www.who.int/reproductivehealth/publications/family_planning/SPR-3/en

37. Centers for Disease Control and Prevention. Summary of classifications for hormonal contraceptives methods and intrauterine devices. https://www.cdc.gov/reproductivehealth/contraception/mmwr/mec/appendixk.html

38. Centers for Disease Control and Prevention. Classifications for emergency contraception. https://www.cdc.gov/reproductivehealth/contraception/mmwr/mec/appendixj.html

39. American College of Obstetricians and Gynecologists' Committee on Practice Bulletins—Gynecology. ACOG Practice Bulletin No. 152: emergency contraception. *Obstet Gynecol.* 2015;126(3):e1–e11. doi:10.1097/AOG.0000000000001047

40. Choe SA, Sung J. Trends of premature and early menopause: a comparative study of the US National Health and Nutrition Examination Survey and the Korea National Health and Nutrition Examination Survey. *J Korean Med Sci.* 2020;35(14):e97. doi:10.3346/jkms.2020.35.e97

41. Shifren JL, Gass MLS. The North American Menopause Society recommendations for clinical care of midlife women. *Menopause.* 2014;21(10):1038–1062. doi:10.1097/gme.0000000000000319

42. Thurston RC, Joffe H. Vasomotor symptoms and menopause: Findings from the Study of Women's Health across the Nation. *Obstet Gynecol Clin.* 2011;38(3):489–501. doi:10.1016/j.ogc.2011.05.006

43. Politi MC, Schleinitz MD, Col NF. Revisiting the duration of vasomotor symptoms of menopause: a meta-analysis. *J Gen Intern Med.* 2008;23:1507–1513. doi:10.1007/s11606-008-0655-4

44. Gartoulla P, Worsley R, Bell RJ, et al. Moderate to severe vasomotor and sexual symptoms remain problematic for women aged 60 to 65 years. *Menopause.* 2015;22(7):694–701. doi:10.1097/GME.0000000000000383

45. Blümel JE, Chedraui P, Baron G, et al. A large multinational study of vasomotor symptom prevalence, duration, and impact on quality of life in middle-aged women. *Menopause.* 2011;18(7):778–785. doi:10.1097/gme.0b013e318207851d

46. North American Menopause Society. The 2017 hormone therapy position statement of the North American Menopause Society. *Menopause.* 2017;24(7):728–753. doi:10.1097/GME.0000000000000921

47. National Institute for Health and Care Excellence. *Menopause: Diagnosis and Management* (NICE Guideline, No. 23). National Institute for Health and Care Excellence (UK); 2019. https://www.ncbi.nlm.nih.gov/books/NBK552590

48. North American Menopause Society. The 2020 genitourinary syndrome of menopause position statement of the North American Menopause Society. *Menopause.* 2020;27(9):976–992. doi:10.1097/GME.0000000000001609

49. Drugs.com. Estradiol. Updated August 19, 2020. https://www.drugs.com/pro/estradiol.html

50. Drugs.com. Estradiol dosage. Updated August 19, 2020. https://www.drugs.com/dosage/estradiol.html

51. Drugs.com. Medroxyprogesterone acetate. Updated July 22, 2020. https://www.drugs.com/monograph/medroxyprogesterone-acetate.html

52. Drugs.com. Norethindrone. Updated September 11, 2020. https://www.drugs.com/ppa/norethindrone.html

53. Drugs.com. Bazedoxifene acetate. Updated February 10, 2020. https://www.drugs.com/monograph/bazedoxifene-acetate.html

54. Drugs.com. PARoxetine. Updated July 1, 2020. https://www.drugs.com/ppa/paroxetine.html

55. Drugs.com. Ospemifene. Updated July 1, 2020. https://www.drugs.com/ppa/ospemifene.html

56. Drugs.com. Prasterone. Updated July 1, 2020. https://www.drugs.com/ppa/prasterone.html

57. Visscher DW, Frank RD, Carter JM, et al. Breast cancer risk and progressive histology in serial benign biopsies.

J Natl Cancer Inst. 2017;109(10):djx035. doi:10.1093/jnci/djx035

58. Armstrong N, Ryder S, Forbes C, et al. A systematic review of the international prevalence of BRCA mutation in breast cancer. *Clin Epidemiol.* 2019;11:543–561. doi:10.2147/CLEP.S206949

59. American Cancer Society. *Breast Cancer Facts & Figures 2019–2020.* American Cancer Society; 2019. https://www.cancer.org/content/dam/cancer-org/research/cancer-facts-and-statistics/breast-cancer-facts-and-figures/breast-cancer-facts-and-figures-2019-2020.pdf

60. Gombos A. Selective oestrogen receptor degraders in breast cancer: a review and perspectives. *Curr Opin Oncol.* 2019;31(5):424–429. doi:10.1097/CCO.0000000000000567

61. Burstein HJ, Lacchetti C, Anderson H, et al. Adjuvant endocrine therapy for women with hormone receptor-positive breast cancer: ASCO clinical practice guideline focused update. *J Clin Oncol.* 2019;37(5):423–438. doi:10.1200/JCO.18.01160

62. National Comprehensive Cancer Network. Breast cancer (version 5.2020). 2020. https://www2.tri-kobe.org/nccn/guideline/breast/english/breast.pdf

63. Drugs.com. Tamoxifen. Updated May 24, 2020. https://www.drugs.com/ppa/tamoxifen.html

64. Drugs.com. Toremifene. Updated July 15, 2020. https://www.drugs.com/ppa/toremifene.html

65. Drugs.com. Fulvestrant. Updated August 23, 2020. https://www.drugs.com/ppa/fulvestrant.html

66. Drugs.com. Anastrozole. Updated August 29, 2020. https://www.drugs.com/ppa/anastrozole.html

67. Drugs.com. Letrozole. Updated April 10, 2020. https://www.drugs.com/ppa/letrozole.html

68. Drugs.com. Exemestane. Updated October 17, 2020. https://www.drugs.com/ppa/exemestane.html

Pharmacotherapy Related to Men's Health Conditions

Jon E. Siiteri

BENIGN PROSTATIC HYPERPLASIA

INTRODUCTION

Prostate disorders are common in the adult male population. The prevalence of histologic benign prostatic hyperplasia (BPH) is estimated to occur in 42% of men 51 to 60 years of age and in approximately 80% of men aged 71 to 80 years.[1,2] Lower urinary tract symptoms (LUTS) represent a cluster of chronic urinary disorders that occur in 15% to 60% of men older than 40 years of age. Specific symptoms include sense of incomplete bladder emptying, urinary hesitancy, weak urine stream, urinary frequency or urgency, and nocturia. The severity of symptoms increases with age as do associated adverse consequences, including risk of urinary tract infections (UTIs), bladder stones, urinary retention, and acute renal failure. Nonurologic adverse events that increase in older men with severe LUTS include risks of falling, associated debilitating morbidity, pain, and fractures. Adverse quality-of-life factors include increased risk of depression and impaired activities of daily living (ADLs).[3]

BACKGROUND

BPH is a result of the proliferation of prostatic epithelial and stromal cells that usually begins in men by age 40 and progresses in approximately two out of three men throughout the remainder of their lifetime. Hyperplasia of both cellular components, particularly in the transition zone through which the prostatic urethra passes, causes static obstruction of urine flow. Additionally, hypersensitivity to alpha adrenergic stimulation of fibromuscular elements in the prostate capsule, anterior portion of the prostate, and the detrusor sphincter smooth muscle results in increased muscle tone that contributes a dynamic component to the obstruction of urine flow. These dynamic and obstructive components of BPH provide two different pharmacotherapeutic approaches for the treatment of the symptoms of BPH, one to address the growth of the prostate and the other to relax detrusor sphincter and prostate smooth muscle tone. In a small subset of men, both obstructive and irritative urinary symptoms may be present which may respond to combined medical therapy.

DIAGNOSIS

The American Urological Association (AUA) established a validated symptom index score that is used to characterize the nature and severity of BPH symptoms (Table 28.1). A companion international survey (the International Prostate Symptom Score) assesses symptoms related to an enlarged prostate or bladder instability. Using the AUA symptom index score, symptoms are rated on a numerical scale ranging from 0 to 35 and are grouped into mild (0–8), moderate (9–18), and severe (19–35). In addition, a quality-of-life score on a scale

TABLE 28.1 American Urological Association Symptom Score

(Circle One Number on Each Line)	Not at All	<1 Time in 5	<Half the Time	About Half the Time	>Half the Time	Almost Always
Over the past month or so, how often have you had a sensation of not emptying your bladder completely after you finished urinating?	0	1	2	3	4	5
During the past month or so, how often have you had to urinate again less than 2 hours after you finished urinating?	0	1	2	3	4	5
During the past month or so, how often have you found you stopped and started again several times when you urinated?	0	1	2	3	4	5
During the past month or so, how often have you found it difficult to postpone urination?	0	1	2	3	4	5
During the past month or so, how often have you had a weak urinary stream?	0	1	2	3	4	5
During the past month or so, how often have you had to push or strain to begin urination?	0	1	2	3	4	5
Over the past month, how many times per night did you most typically get up to urinate from the time you went to bed at night until the time you got up in the morning?	0	1	2	3	4	5

Source: American Urological Association. *American Urological Association Guideline: Management of Benign Prostatic Hyperplasia.* American Urological Association; Revised 2010. http://www.24hmb.com/voimages/web_image/upload/file/20140627/65241403866150116.pdf

from 0 to 6 is completed by the patient. Providing patients with a bladder diary to record both volumes and types of fluid intake, voided urine volume, and times of voiding throughout a 24-hour period yields information that is helpful in characterizing the patient's symptoms and response to eventual medical therapy. Distinguishing between irritative and obstructive urinary symptoms utilizing the AUA symptom score may serve as a guideline for selecting initial medical therapy, which is generally most effective in men with moderate-to-severe symptoms. Men with severe symptoms, or any man with acute urinary retention or recurrent urinary tract infections, should be referred to a specialty clinic.

PHARMACOTHERAPY FOR BENIGN PROSTATIC HYPERPLASIA

5-alpha Reductase Inhibitors

The first medication to address the static symptoms due to BPH was the 5-alpha reductase inhibitor (5-ARI) finasteride approved by the U.S. Food and Drug Administration (FDA) in 1992.[4,5] This was followed by dutasteride in 2001. These medications inhibit the conversion of testosterone to the hormone dihydrotestosterone, which is directly responsible for the growth of acinar glands in the prostate. Both drugs inhibit further growth of the prostate and, in some men, can lead to a 25% reduction in the size of the prostate. These results are most effective in men who have a prostate gland larger than 40 cm³ or a serum prostate-specific antigen (PSA) greater than 1.5 ng/mL. Symptom relief is not apparent for 3 to 9 months; therefore 5-ARI can be used in combination with alpha adrenergic blockade to address any dynamic component resulting in obstructive urinary symptoms.[6] The advantage of this combination therapy is the adrenergic antagonists have a rapid onset, usually less than 48 hours. See **Table 28.2** for prescribing information.

Adverse Effects

The most common adverse reactions to 5-ARIs are erectile dysfunction (1.3%–8.1%), decreased libido (1.8%–6.4%), ejaculation disorders (0.8%–1.2%), and gynecomastia (0.5%–1.8%). Sexual dysfunction is the most common adverse effect. In 2012, the FDA required a revision to product labeling to state that decreased libido secondary to finasteride may persist after discontinuation of the drug. The FDA also required a change in the labeling to include a description of reports of male infertility and/or poor semen quality that normalized and/or were improved after drug discontinuation. Although finasteride and dutasteride have been studied for chemoprevention of prostate cancer, the FDA recommended against this use in 2010.

TABLE 28.2 Pharmacotherapy for Benign Prostatic Hyperplasia

Medication	Dose/Frequency	Side Effects	Contraindications
Alpha-Adrenergic Blockers			
Alfuzosin	10 mg once daily taken immediately after same meal each day	Dizziness, headache, orthostatic hypotension, fatigue, sinus congestion	Hypersensitivity to alfuzosin or any components of medication or quinazolines Moderate-to-severe liver impairment Concomitant use of potent CYP3A4 inhibitors or other alpha1-blocking agents Pregnancy/lactation Use with caution in patients with hypotension, liver disease, coronary artery disease, drugs that lower blood pressure
Doxazosin	**Immediate release:** Initial: 1 mg once daily at bedtime; titrate based on patient response and tolerability by doubling the daily dose (e.g., to 2 mg, then 4 mg, then 8 mg) at 1 to 2 week intervals up to 8 mg once daily (max: 8 mg/day) *Note:* If therapy is discontinued for several days, resume at 1 mg/day and titrate using initial dosing regimen. **Extended release:** 4 mg once daily; titrate based on response and tolerability every 3 to 4 weeks to 8 mg once daily (max: 8 mg/day) *Note:* If therapy is discontinued for several days, resume at 4 mg/day and titrate using initial dosing regimen. For conversion to extended release from immediate release: Omit final evening dose of immediate release prior to starting morning dosing with extended release product. Initiate extended release product using 4 mg once daily.	Dizziness, headache, fatigue	Hypersensitivity to doxazosin, any components of medication or quinazolines Pregnancy/lactation Use with caution in patients with hypotension, syncope, hepatic impairment
Silodosin	4–8 mg once daily CrCl 30–50 mL/min: 4 mg once daily with a meal	Orthostatic hypotension, dizziness, diarrhea, headache, sinus congestion, retrograde ejaculation	Hypersensitivity to silodosin or any components of medication Severe renal impairment (CrCl <30 mL/min) or severe hepatic impairment (Child–Pugh score >10) Concomitant use of potent CYP3A4 inhibitors or P-glycoprotein inhibitors
Terazosin	Initial: 1 mg daily at bedtime; titrate based on patient response and tolerability, over several weeks; most patients require 10 mg once daily; if no response after 4–6 weeks of 10 mg/day, may increase to 20 mg once daily (max: 20 mg/day) *Note:* If discontinued for several days or longer, consider beginning with initial dose and retitration as needed.	Dizziness, asthenia, hypotension, nasal congestion, somnolence	Use with caution in patients with angina, hypotension, syncope, hepatic impairment
Tamsulosin	Initial: 0.4 mg once daily May increase to 0.8 mg after 2–4 weeks (max: 0.8 mg/day)	Headache, dizziness, hypotension, rhinitis, abnormal ejaculation, arthralgia, infection	Hypersensitivity to tamsulosin Use with caution in patients with liver disease, coronary artery disease
5-alpha Reductase Inhibitors and Combination Product			
Dutasteride	0.5 mg once daily	Erectile dysfunction, decreased libido, ejaculation disorders, hypotension, rhinitis, gynecomastia; increased risk of prostate cancer	Hypersensitivity to dutasteride, tamsulosin, or any component to medications Use with caution in patients with liver disease, coronary artery disease
Dutasteride/ tamsulosin	Combination (0.5/0.4 mg) - 1 capsule daily 30 minutes after the same meal each day		
Finasteride	5 mg once daily	Erectile dysfunction, decreased libido, ejaculation disorders, gynecomastia	Hypersensitivity to finasteride or any component to medication Pregnant or potentially pregnant women should not handle crushed/broken tablets or semen of male partner Use with caution in patients with liver disease, obstructive uropathy

CrCl, creatinine clearance.

A well-known observed effect of 5-ARIs is a 50% decrease in PSA laboratory values.[7] As the clinical significance of this is currently unclear, PSA test results of all men who are taking 5ARI should be multiplied by two to ensure accuracy. Monitor side effects, especially in men older than 60 years of age.

Efficacy

5-ARIs have been available for more than 25 years and have been demonstrated to be very effective in relieving symptoms caused by prostatic obstruction.[4–6,8] Two large random-controlled clinical trials were conducted to evaluate the effectiveness of 5-ARIs alone or in combination with either doxazosin or alfuzosin. The Medical Therapy of Prostate Symptom Study (MTOPS) was conducted in select medical centers in the United States in over 3,000 men. It compared placebo versus finasteride versus doxazosin versus combination therapy.[9] Follow-up time was 5.5 years, and the endpoint was a composite progression of BPH symptoms. The second large study was the Combination of Avodart and Tamsulosin (CombAT) study that compared dutasteride versus tamsulosin versus combination therapy.[8] This enrolled more than 4,800 men for 4 years with the endpoint of change in a validated symptom score. The mean prostate size was 36.3 mL for the MTOPS and 55.0 mL for the CombAT trial. Both trials demonstrated that combination therapy with alpha blockers and 5-ARIs led to improvement in symptoms scores compared to either 5-ARIs or alpha blockers alone.

Alpha-Adrenergic Receptor Antagonists

Alpha-adrenergic receptor antagonists (alpha blockers) provide a second pharmacologic approach to the treatment of symptoms of an enlarged prostate. Alpha-blockers such as doxazosin and terazosin, developed over 25 years ago, were originally utilized for treatment of hypertension. Doxazosin mesylate extended release, was approved for treatment of BPH in 2005. Alpha-1a adrenoreceptors were identified upon further characterization of the specific adrenoreceptor subtype expressed by prostatic epithelial cells and fibromuscular elements within the prostate. This led to the development of antagonists specific for this receptor subtype, including tamsulosin, approved by the FDA in 1996, and alfuzosin in 2003, and silodosin in 2008. A product combining the 5-ARI dutasteride with tamsulosin (0.5/0.4 mg, respectively) was approved by the FDA in 2010.[8] See **Table 28.2** for prescribing information.

Adverse Effects

The adverse effect profile for alpha blockers includes dizziness, orthostatic hypotension, sinus congestion, and fatigue. Dizziness is the most common adverse event with incidence in 2% to 14% of patients. Elderly/frail patients should be carefully monitored for ortho-

static hypotension. Alpha blockers should be discontinued if correlation with onset of medication is identified.

Tamsulosin has been associated with ejaculatory disturbance in approximately 10% of patients due to relaxation of the detrusor sphincter at the time of orgasm. Additionally, tamsulosin has been correlated with intraoperative floppy iris syndrome. Patients who are planning cataract surgery should inform their ophthalmologists if they are taking tamsulosin prior to their surgery.[11]

Efficacy

The older alpha blockers such as doxazosin or terazosin must be titrated and monitored for hypotension. Dosing begins as low as 1 mg and increases up to 8 mg or 10 mg taken at night to decrease the risk of dizziness and falls. Tamsulosin is dosed at either 0.4 or 0.8 mg as needed for therapeutic effect.[10] Alfuzosin has a single dose of 10 mg daily. Silodosin is available in 4 mg and 8 mg doses. Though head-to-head trials have not been conducted, there appears to be no superiority of any one medication over the other in this class of medications.

A useful test for measuring the efficacy of alpha-adrenergic antagonists is a drug holiday.

Generally, men with symptoms due strictly to the dynamic component of BPH respond quickly to alpha-adrenergic antagonists and will notice an abrupt return and worsening of symptoms within 1 to 2 days after discontinuing medication.

Patient Evaluation

Assessment of treatment efficacy is measured by two office-based methods. *Uroflowmetry* measures urine flow rate, and results are interpreted based on a normal age and population-based values. Office-based *bladder or abdominal ultrasound* determines the postvoid residual urine volume. Abnormal findings with either measurement, in addition to evidence of urinary obstruction secondary to BPH, may indicate detrusor hypofunction, obstruction due to bladder neck contracture, or obstruction due to urethral structure.

Patients who fail to respond to medical therapy after dose adjustments, or who have worsening symptoms despite medical therapy, or have evidence of microscopic or gross hematuria, or cannot tolerate medical therapy should be referred for urologic evaluation.

ERECTILE DYSFUNCTION

INTRODUCTION

Erectile dysfunction (ED) is defined as the consistent or recurrent inability to obtain and maintain an erect penis that is satisfactory for sexual intercourse. Penile erection is a component of a series of psychophysiological steps, known as the "human sexual response cycle," which occurs in an orderly fashion. Originally defined by Masters and Johnson, the four-stage sequence begins with excitement, or initial arousal, sustained arousal, orgasm, and resolution.[12] ED is considered an impairment in the arousal phase.[12,13]

Estimates of the prevalence of ED in the United States range up to 30 million. Worldwide, 150 million men are estimated to be affected.[14,15] ED is significantly correlated with decreased quality of life in mental health, relationships, and overall well-being.[16]

BACKGROUND

According to the AUA 2018 Guideline on Erectile Dysfunction, independent risk factors for ED and cardiovascular disease (CVD) include age, smoking, obesity, diabetes mellitus, hypertension, dyslipidemia, depression, obesity, and sedentary lifestyle.[17] The preponderance of evidence suggests the underlying pathophysiology of both ED and CVD is vascular. Furthermore, the severity of ED is correlated with the degree of CVD. Recent studies suggest that ED may precede clinical signs and symptoms of CVD by 2 to 4 years.[18,19] Correlation of BPH and LUTS with ED is identified in a subset of men.[11] A significant percentage of men who had minimal or no symptoms of ED prior to radical prostatectomy or radiation therapy for prostate cancer will also acquire ED.[20,21]

PHARMACOTHERAPY FOR ERECTILE DYSFUNCTION

Phosphodiesterase-5 Inhibitors

Phosphodiesterase-five (PDE5) inhibitors inhibit the enzyme responsible for the cleavage of 5'-cyclic guanosine monophosphate (cGMP), leading to increased cGMP that is responsible for the relaxation of smooth muscle in the walls of the deep penile arteries and distal branches thereof that perfuse the corpus cavernosum. This allows engorgement of the erectile tissue, resulting in increased erection hardness and duration. Response in men with ED to PDE5 inhibitors requires adequate vascular compliance.

Sildenafil and other PDE5 inhibitors are metabolized by the liver via cytochrome P450:2C9 (CYP2C9) and cytochrome P450:3A4 (CYP3A4).

Contraindications and Adverse Effects

PDE5 inhibitors are contraindicated for patients with hypersensitivity, use of nitrates, or patients with a history of heart surgery within the past 6 months. Use of PDE5 inhibitors in combination with nitrates may lead to a precipitous decline in blood pressure that can be life-threatening. Men who take sublingual nitrate for ischemic heart disease should be instructed not to use the medication within 24 hours of taking a PDE5 inhibitor. Caution is advised for men with left ventricular outflow obstruction (e.g., aortic stenosis).

Drug–drug interactions occur with CYP2C9 and CYP3A4 substrates, including antidepressants, antifungals, antihypertensives, and HIV/AIDS drugs. Combined use of alpha blockers and PDE5 inhibitors may result in symptomatic hypotension. It is recommended that men take the two medications at least 4 hours apart. Men who perform penile self-injection therapy should be cautioned about the increased risk of priapism associated with combined use of PDE5 inhibitors.

Common side effects include facial flushing, nasal congestion, headache, dyspepsia, and blue-tinted vision.

Efficacy

Sildenafil, the first PDE5 inhibitor, was approved by the FDA for use in treatment of ED in 1988. Originally 25-, 50-, and 100-mg tablets were approved. Most patients respond to either 50 or 100 mg. Sildenafil must be taken 30 minutes to 1 hour prior to having sexual intercourse; it has a half-life of 4 hours. Taking sildenafil with alcohol or a heavy or high-fat meal decreases efficacy. Vardenafil, with a half-life of 4 to 5 hours, was approved by the FDA in 2003, followed by tadalafil, with a half-life 15 to 35 hours, in 2003. Avanafil is the latest PDE5 inhibitor released on the market. It was approved by the FDA in 2013 and has a half-life of 5 hours.

A comprehensive review of 191 individual trials plus pooled data across multiple trials and 15 reports of published systematic reviews published in the AUA 2018 ED guideline revealed the following[22]:

- Sildenafil, tadalafil, and vardenafil have equivalent efficacy.
- Data available for avanafil are limited; relative efficacy is unclear.
- Efficacy is comparable across all medications as measured by different assessments of erectile function.

There are differences in both onset of duration and duration of effectiveness among the different medications; see **Table 28.3**.

TABLE 28.3 Phosphodiesterase-5 Inhibitors

Medication	Onset of Action (Minutes)	Duration of Action (Hours)	Effect of Food Intake
Avanafil	15–30	Up to 6	Not affected
Sildenafil	30–60	Up to 12	High-fat meal decreases efficacy
Tadalafil	60–120	Up to 36	Not affected
Vardenafil	30–60	Up to 10	High-fat meal decreases efficacy

Intracavernosal Injection Therapy

Intracavernosal injection (ICI) increases vasodilaton in the erectile tissue of the penis by relaxing the smooth muscle in the walls of cavernosal arteries. ICI is a suitable alternative therapy for men who do not respond, or have contraindications, to PDE5 inhibitors.[23] Injected medications include papaverine, phentolamine, and alprostadil (a synthetic form of prostaglandin E1). Alprostadil is commercially available and may be used as a single agent. Papaverine and phentolamine are used in combination (papaverine + phentolamine) with or without alprostadil. These formulations must be mixed by a compounding pharmacy. Data directly comparing the efficacy of ICI drugs as single agents or in combination is insufficient.[23] Alprostadil is considered first-line due to its efficacy as a single agent, commercial availability, and lower rates of penile fibrosis and priapism compared to papaverine and phentolamine. Optimal dosing of these drug(s) varies widely from patient to patient. The ideal volume injected should be between 0.4 and 0.6 mL, regardless of the concentration required to elicit a satisfactory response. Dose titration of the selected drug(s) should occur in the office setting with patient education and observation by a clinician experienced in the procedure.[23]

Contraindications and Adverse Effects

ICI is contraindicated in men with a history of sickle cell anemia, Peyronie's disease, multiple myeloma, thrombocytopenia, or in those who receive heparin. Adverse reactions include penile or urethral pain, bleeding at the site of injection, hypotension, and dizziness. Serious reactions include priapism, which is a medical emergency, and syncope. Prolonged ICI use may lead to penile fibrosis at the injection sites. Efficacy and patient satisfaction rates are comparable to those of PDE5 inhibitors; however, dropout rates are high.

Transurethral Suppository

Alprostadil (MUSE®) is available in suppository formulation in dosages from 125 to 1,000 mcg. A unique applicator is used to deposit the suppository in the distal penile urethra. Dose adjustment is often needed to achieve a satisfactory erection, which usually occurs within 10 to 20 minutes after application.

Adverse effects are similar to ICI, although penile pain occurs more often (approximately 10%).

TESTOSTERONE DEFICIENCY

INTRODUCTION

There are wildly varying ranges of the estimated prevalence of testicular deficiency (TD) in American men. A recent review of studies conducted between 1966 and 2014 examining the clinical indication of low testosterone in combination with the measurement of serum testosterone indicated the prevalence in the United States ranged between 2% and 77%.[24] This review included 40 studies of more than 37,000 men aged 43 to 82 years old.

Testosterone levels are known to decline by an average of 3.1 to 3.5 ng/dL per year in men starting at age 30.[25] There are approximately 2.4 million men in the United States aged 40 to 69 years old who have TD, and this prevalence may increase to 6.5 million by 2025 in men 30 to 80 years of age.[26,27] Testosterone therapy prescribed for TD increased significantly between the time frame of 2000 to 2011 based on a multinational survey.[28]

Much of the uncertainty of identifying men who have low testosterone depends on which laboratory test was ordered—total serum testosterone, percent free testosterone, bioavailable testosterone, or a combination of one or the other—and what was considered as the lower limit of normal.[29] The AUA, the Endocrine Society, and the European Urology Association (EAU) define testosterone deficiency as a total serum testosterone less than 300 ng/dL in combination with symptoms of low testosterone, including fatigue, decreased libido, decreased motivation, and body mass changes (e.g., muscle mass loss and body fat weight gain).[30,31] Additional criteria include at least two serum total testosterone measurements obtained on different days early in the morning. Other considerations in screening men for TD include those who have unexplained anemia, bone-density loss, history of chronic corticosteroid use, history of male infertility, and a history of chronic opioid medication use.

BACKGROUND

The normal production of testosterone is under the influence of luteinizing hormone (LH), released from the anterior pituitary gland via stimulation of gonadotropin-releasing hormone (GNRH) from the hypothalamus. Systemic testosterone feeds back to the anterior pituitary to decrease the release of LH via a negative feedback loop. The normal production of testosterone is cyclical and episodic. Normal serum testosterone levels in men with typical sleep patterns between 10 p.m. and 6 a.m. are highest at 3 to 8 a.m. and decrease to a nadir by 4 p.m. with episodic serum level peaks and troughs occurring every 90 minutes.[32,33] This diurnal pattern is less prominent in men 70 years and older.[34]

Laboratory values of the normal range vary per lab and assay but generally are between 280 and 1,020 ng/dL in adult men. There is a normal age-related decrease in total testosterone beginning at age 40 with an approximate 1% decrease annually thereafter. Testosterone circulates in the blood tightly bound (44%) to a specific transport protein identified as sex hormone–binding globulin (SHBG) and in a nonspecific manner, loosely bound (50%) to serum albumin. A small amount of testosterone (4%) is also loosely bound to corticotropin-binding globulin. It is generally accepted that only loosely bound and free testosterone (2%), in sum called "bioavailable testosterone," is available for cellular uptake by cytoplasmic androgen receptor proteins. These hormone-bound receptors interact with hormone response elements associate with specific genes. The testosterone mediated cellular and tissue responses are eventually expressed. Examples of these responses include development and sperm production, masculine hair growth, skeletal muscle growth with development of lean body mass, as well as psychological effects such as libido, motivation, aggression, and general sense of well-being. Testosterone is also responsible for prostate growth and is considered a growth factor for prostate cancer.

Inadequate production of testosterone has many causes but is classified as either primary or secondary hypogonadism. *Primary hypogonadism* describes the failure of Leydig cells to respond to normal levels of LH. Causes of primary hypogonadism include acute testicular injury or infection such as mumps orchitis, vascular compromise to the testes, radiation treatment or chemotherapy to the pelvis, and prolonged or excessive exposure to heat as in hot baths or steam baths, all of which impair the response of Leydig cells to LH.

Secondary hypogonadism describes the failure of adequate production of either GnRH by the hypothalamus or LH by the anterior pituitary. Secondary hypogonadism, also known as "hypogonadotropic hypogonadism," occurs when there is inadequate LH production by the anterior pituitary due to traumatic brain injury, pituitary adenomas, and chronic opioid medication use, which has recently been correlated with testicular dysfunction by way of disruption of the hypothalamic-pituitary axis. Men who have a history of chronic corticosteroid use and those who have long-standing diabetes have been consistently found to have lower testosterone levels.

DIAGNOSIS

Signs and symptoms of TD include weight gain with loss of lean body mass and increased body fat, loss of bone density, fatigue, decreased cognition, loss of motivation, decreased libido, erectile dysfunction, and depressed mood. It is important to rule out other endocrine or medical disorders that have similar signs and symptoms, including hypothyroidism, diabetes mellitus, anemia, and metabolic syndrome. Current AUA guidelines recommend that patients be informed that TD may increase the risk for CVD. Men should be informed that evidence is inconclusive that testosterone therapy can improve cognition, measures of diabetes,

energy, fatigue, lipid profiles, or quality-of-life measures. Patients should also be informed that there is inconclusive evidence that testosterone supplementation increases the risk for prostate cancer.[35]

PHARMACOTHERAPY FOR TESTOSTERONE DEFICIENCY

Testosterone has been used in the treatment of hypogonadism since 1939. Because of testosterone and anabolic steroid abuse by athletes, testosterone was classified by the FDA as a schedule III drug in 1992. The FDA published a drug safety communication in March 2015 stating that testosterone products were approved only for men who have low testosterone levels caused by certain medical conditions and that the benefit and safety of testosterone medications has not been established for the treatment of low testosterone levels due to aging. The communication, also based on available evidence from published studies and expert input from an advisory committee meeting, concluded there was possible increased cardiovascular risk associate with testosterone use. Therefore, new label changes were required to reflect the possible increased risk of heart attacks and strokes associated with testosterone use.[36,37]

The effect of testosterone replacement therapy (TRT) on blood lipids and risks for cardiovascular disease (CVD) is controversial. Low testosterone is associated with increased low-density lipoprotein (LDL) and decreased high-density lipoprotein (HDL) in both cross-sectional and prospective observational studies. TRT is associated with decreased HDL coupled with beneficial decreases in LDL and total cholesterol. The overall impact of testosterone administration on CVD is still unclear, with mixed safety results from recent randomized controlled trials.[38]

Topical Therapy

Testosterone was the first synthesized anabolic steroid. Testosterone is available in the form of gels or liquids that are applied topically daily. Depending on the brand or generic name, they have three different sites of application that include the upper arm and shoulders, the thigh, and the axilla. Proprietary formulations of testosterone range in concentration from 1% to 2% gel with a dose range of 10 mg to a maximum of 120 mg. The starting dose is generally between 50 and 100 mg applied daily to the shoulders, upper arms, or thigh; it is important to note the specific manufacturer's instructions for application. A 2% solution is available as a pump with a dosing range of 30 to 120 mg and a starting dose of 60 mg applied to the axilla every morning. A transdermal patch is available in 2- or 4-mg strengths. The dose range for the patch is between 2 and 6 mg daily at bedtime.

An oral formulation available as a 30-mg testosterone buccal patch (tablet shaped patch, Striant@—not available in U.S.) is dosed every 12 hours. The buccal patch is applied to the upper gum above the incisor with instructions to rotate sides per application. An intranasal gel formulation, available as a pump, is delivered at a dose of 5.5 mg testosterone per pump with instructions to deliver one pump to each nostril for a total of 11 mg every 8 hours; max dose is 6 pumps/day.

The goal of testosterone therapy is to attain a steady-state serum testosterone level of between 450 and 600 ng/dL. This should be confirmed by a serum total testosterone lab test within 4 weeks of initiating therapy and every 6 to 12 months thereafter.[30] Topical testosterone preparations have the convenience of avoiding intramuscular injections, and in terms of pharmacodynamics, avoiding the wide ranges of serum testosterone levels associated with intramuscular injection.

Adverse Effects

There are specific adverse-effect profiles for the topical testosterone medications. Typical examples of serious reactions may include stimulation of prostate cancer and prostatic enlargement. PSA should be measured for all men over 40 years of age before starting testosterone. Those with elevated PSA require further evaluation to exclude prostate cancer prior to testosterone therapy. Periodic evaluation of PSA in patients taking testosterone should be decided upon using a shared decision-making approach in accordance the AUA guidelines.[30] Although there are conflicting clinical trial studies, the FDA requires warnings be given to patients regarding the potential risk for cardiovascular events, including myocardial infarction, stroke, and venous thromboembolism. TRT has been correlated with the development of polycythemia (hematocrit >50) in fewer than 10% of men treated. Common reactions to topical formulations include contact dermatitis, lability, mastodynia, worsening sleep apnea, and oligospermia.

Injectable Testosterone

There are three intramuscular injectable drugs with different half-lives, two that are short acting and one long acting.[30] Testosterone cypionate is a slow-acting, long-ester, oil-based injectable testosterone compound with a half-life of 8 to 9 days. It is commonly available at concentrations of 50 to 200 mg/mL for intramuscular injection into the gluteal muscle and lateral upper thigh. The starting dose generally begins at 100 mg per

week and is adjusted to 50 to 200 mg every 7 to 14 days. Testosterone enanthate is a another long-ester, oil-based injectable testosterone with comparable pharmacokinetics, available concentrations, and starting doses.

Testosterone undecanoate is available as a long-acting formulation of 750 mg/3 mL. The first dose is given intramuscularly, followed by a second dose 4 weeks later, and continued therapy every 10 weeks thereafter.

Following intramuscular injection, serum testosterone levels initially reach a supra-physiological level within 48 hours after intramuscular injection that can lead to overt increases in aggression, emotional lability, then sexual behavior. As the serum testosterone levels decline below 400 mg/dL, some men experience mild signs and symptoms of testosterone deficiency. Advantages of intramuscular injection include increased musculoskeletal benefits as blood levels are higher than transdermal-administrated testosterone.[30]

Adverse Effects

Adverse effects associated with injectable testosterone include injection site reaction, acne, edema, headache, elevated liver enzymes, promotion of male pattern baldness, and oligospermia. All men attempting to conceive a pregnancy should be informed of the risk of oligospermia and consult with a fertility specialist regarding alternative TRTs.[30]

Subcutaneous Pellets

Testosterone pellets that are implanted subcutaneously and slowly release the hormone were first approved by the FDA for testosterone therapy (TRT) in 1972 but were not marketed until 2008 as Testopel®, containing 75-mg crystalline testosterone.[39] The product insert recommends beginning with six pellets (450-mg testosterone) but peer-reviewed studies of Testopel and similar products licensed outside the United States suggest that higher doses up to 10 pellets (750-mg testosterone) are required to achieve the target blood levels of testosterone that are maintained for 3 to 6 months. The pellets are implanted in the subcutaneous fat in the medial aspect of the biceps muscle using a proprietary trocar. In addition to side effects associated with testosterone use, adverse effects include infection or hematoma at the site of pellet insertion, extrusion of pellets, and development of subcutaneous fibrosis associated with repeated insertions.

CASE EXEMPLAR: Patient With Benign Prostatic Hyperplasia

JK is a 63-year-old male who presents with complaints of difficulty starting his urine stream and that he has to get up to urinate at night at least three times. He states there are times when he does not think he will be able to go.

Past Medical History
- Controlled hypertension
- Hypercholesteremia
- Type 2 diabetes controlled by diet

Medications
- Zestril, 5 mg once daily
- Simvastatin, 40 mg
- Niacin, 1,000 mg
- Baby aspirin, daily

Social History
- A six-pack of beer on weekends
- Nonsmoker
- Active in Lions club

Physical Examination
- Well-developed male
- Chest: clear to auscultation
- Heart: regular rhythm; no gallops, thrills, or murmurs
- Digital rectal exam: enlarged prostate

Labs and Imaging
- Liver enzymes: normal
- Prostate specific antigen (PSA): 2.5 ng/mL
- Hemoglobin A1C: 6.9
- Office-based ultrasound: prostate enlargement approximately 41 cm^3
- Postvoid residual urine volume: 300 mL

Discussion Questions

1. The clinician prescribes dutasteride. What patient teaching should be included?
2. In addition to taking the prescribed medication, the clinician suggests JK keep a voiding diary. What information should JK track in this diary, and what value does this information provide?
3. JK fails to respond to the initial therapy. What second drug should the clinician add? What is the method of action of this drug and what advantage does this drug provide? What patient teaching should be included?

CASE EXEMPLAR: Patient With Testosterone Deficiency

YY is 52-year-old who presents with complaints of fatigue, decreased interest in sexual intercourse, difficulty maintaining an erection, and weight gain. He is wondering if he is experiencing testosterone deficiency.

Past Medical History
- Type 2 diabetes diagnosed 4 years ago
- Hypertension
- No surgeries or major illnesses

Medications
- Lisinopril, 10 mg daily
- Sitagliptin, 50 mg
- Baby aspirin, daily

Physical Examination
- Heart rate: normal rhythm; no gallops or murmurs
- Abdomen: soft; bowel sounds present throughout
- Liver: normal
- Mild prostatic enlargement, no difficulty with urination

Labs
- Liver function: normal
- Serum glucose: 180 mg/dL
- Serum testosterone: 200 ng/dL
- Serum cholesterol: 240 mg/dL
- Hemoglobin A1C: 6.9

Discussion Questions

1. What factors in YY's history would help confirm testosterone deficiency? What criteria would help confirm the diagnosis?
2. The clinician recommends topical testosterone as initial therapy. What diagnostic test should be performed prior to prescribing testosterone therapy? What does YY need to know about the drug and its application?
3. YY's testosterone levels have failed to elevate to the desired level. The clinician switches YY to an injectable form of testosterone. What does YY need to know about this drug? What side effects might he expect?

KEY TAKEAWAYS

- A validated symptom index score is useful to characterize the nature and severity of BPH symptoms. Medical therapy appears to be most effective in men with moderate to severe symptoms and consists of 5-ARI and alpha blockers.
- The underlying pathophysiology of both ED and CVD is vascular, and the severity of ED is correlated with the degree of CVD. Treatment options for ED include PDE5 inhibitors, intracavernosal injection therapy, and transurethral suppository.
- The PDE5 inhibitors are contraindicated in a variety of men, including those who take nitrates and those with recent cardiovascular surgery.
- Inadequate production of testosterone has many causes and is classified as either primary or secondary hypogonadism. Signs and symptoms of testosterone deficiency include weight gain with loss of lean body mass and increased body fat, loss of bone density, fatigue, decreased cognition, loss of motivation, decreased libido, erectile dysfunction, and depressed mood.
- Treatment of testosterone deficiency comes in several forms: gels or liquids that are applied topically daily, intramuscular drugs, and testosterone pellets that are implanted subcutaneously and slowly release the hormone. Each form comes with significant side effects that must be shared with the patient at the time of prescribing.

REFERENCES

1. Parsons JK. Benign prostatic hyperplasia and male lower urinary tract symptoms: Epidemiology and risk factors. *Curr Bladder Dysfunct Rep.* 2010 Dec; 5(4):212–218. https:// www.ncbi.nlm.nih.gov/pmc/articles/PMC3061630/#
2. Wei JT, Calhoun E, Jacobsen SJJ. Urologic diseases in America project: benign prostatic hyperplasia. *J Urol.* 2005 Apr;173(4):1256–1261. doi:10.1097/01.ju.0000155709.37840.fe
3. Parsons JK, Wilt TJ, Wang PY, Barrett-Connor E, Bauer DC, Marshall LM, & Osteoporotic Fractures in Men Research Group. Progression of lower urinary tract symptoms in older men: a community based study. *J Urol.* 2010 May;183(5): 1915–1920. doi:10.1016/j.juro.2010.01.026
4. Agency for Health Care Policy and Research. Benign prostatic hyperplasia: diagnosis and treatment. Guideline overview. *J Natl Med Assoc.* 1994;86(7):489, 548–549. https://www.ncbi.nlm.nih.gov/pmc/articles/PMC2607606
5. Nickel JC, Fradet Y, Boake RC, et al. Efficacy and safety of finasteride therapy for benign prostatic hyperplasia: results of a 2-year randomized controlled trial (the PROSPECT study). PROscar safety plus efficacy Canadian two year study. *CMAJ.* 1996;155(9):1251–1259. https://www.ncbi.nlm.nih.gov/pmc/articles/PMC1335066
6. McConnell J, Roehrborn C, Bautista O, et al. The long-term effect of doxazosin, finasteride, and combination therapy on the clinical progression of benign prostatic hyperplasia. *N Engl J Med.* 2003;349:2387. doi:10.1056/NEJMoa030656
7. Cote RJ, Skinner EC, Salem CE, et al. The effect of finasteride on the prostate gland in men with elevated serum prostate-specific antigen levels. *Br J Cancer.* 1998 Aug; 78(3):413–418. doi:10.1038/bjc.1998.508
8. Roehrborn C, Siami P, Barkin J, et al. The effects of dutasteride, tamsulosin and combination therapy on lower urinary tract symptoms in men with benign prostatic hyperplasia and prostatic enlargement: 2-year results from the CombAT study. *J Urol.* 2008;179:616–621. doi:10.1016/j.juro.2007.09.084
9. McConnell JD, Roehrborn CG, Bautista OM, et al. The long-term effect of doxazosin, finasteride, and combination therapy on the clinical progression of benign prostatic hyperplasia. *N Engl J Med.* 2003 Dec;349(25):2387–2398. doi:10.1056/NEJMoa030656
10. Barry M, Fowler F Jr, O'Leary M, et al. The American Urological Association symptom index for benign prostatic hyperplasia. *J Urol.* 1992;148:1549–1557. doi:10.1016/s0022-5347(17)36966-5
11. Chang D, Campbell J. Intraoperative floppy iris syndrome associated with tamsulosin. *J Cataract Refract Surg.* 2005;31(4):664–673. doi:10.1016/j.jcrs.2005.02.027
12. Masters WH, Johnson VE. *Human Sexual Response.* Bantam Books; 1966.
13. McCabe MP, Sharlip ID, Atalla E, et al. Definitions of sexual dysfunctions in women and men: a consensus statement from the Fourth International Consultation on Sexual Medicine 2015. *J Sex Med.* 2016;13:135–143. doi:10.1016/j.jsxm.2015.12.019
14. McKinlay JB. The worldwide prevalence and epidemiology of erectile dysfunction. *Int J Impot Res.* 2000;12(suppl 4):S6–S11. doi:10.1038/sj.ijir.3900567
15. Feldman HA, Goldstein I, Hatzichristou DG, et al. Impotence and its medical and psychosocial correlates: results of the Massachusetts Male Aging Study. *J Urol.* 1994;151:54–61. doi:10.1016/s0022-5347(17)34871-1
16. Corona G, Lee DM, Forti G, et al. Age-related changes in general and sexual health in middle-aged and older men: results from the European Male Ageing Study (EMAS). *J Sex Med.* 2010;7:1362–1380. doi:10.1111/j.1743-6109.2009.01601.x
17. American Urological Association Education and Research. *Erectile dysfunction: AUA guideline.* American Urological Association; 2018.
18. Montorsi P, Ravagnani PM, Galli S, et al. The triad of endothelial dysfunction, cardiovascular disease, and erectile dysfunction: clinical implications. *Eur Urol.* 2009;8:58–66. doi:10.1016/j.eursup.2008.10.010

19. Inman BA, Sauver JL, Jacobson DJ, et al. A population-based, longitudinal study of erectile dysfunction and future coronary artery disease. *Mayo Clin Proc.* 2009;84:108. doi:10.4065/84.2.108

20. De Nunzio C, Roehrborn CG, Andersson KE, et al. Erectile dysfunction and lower urinary tract symptoms. *Eur Urol Focus.* 2017 Oct;3(4–5):352–363. doi:10.1016/j.euf.2017.11.004

21. Walz J, Epstein JI, Ganzer R, et al. A critical analysis of the current knowledge of surgical anatomy of the prostate related to optimization of cancer control and preservation of continence and erection in candidates for radical prostatectomy: an update. *Eur Urol.* 2016;70:301–311. doi:10.1016/j.eururo.2016.01.026

22. Gaither TW, Awad MA, Osterberg EC, et al. The natural history of erectile dysfunction after prostatic radiotherapy: a systematic review and meta-analysis. *J Sex Med.* 2017 Sep;14(9):1071–1078. doi:10.1016/j.jsxm.2017.07.010

23. Belew D, Klassen Z, Lewis RW. Intracavernosal injection for the diagnosis, evaluation, and treatment of erectile dysfunction: a review. *Sex Med Rev.* 2015 Mar;3(1):11–23. doi:10.1002/smrj.35

24. Millar AC, Lau AN, Tomlinson G, et al. Predicting low testosterone in aging men: a systematic review. *CMAJ.* 2016;188: E321. doi:10.1503/cmaj.150262

25. Zmuda JM, Cauley JA, Kriska A, et al. Longitudinal relation between endogenous testosterone and cardiovascular disease risk factors in middle-aged men: a 13-year follow-up of former multiple risk factor intervention trial participants. *Am J Epidemiol.* 1997;146:609–617. doi:10.1093/oxfordjournals.aje.a009326

26. Harman SM, Metter EJ, Tobin JD, et al. Longitudinal effects of aging on serum total and free testosterone levels in healthy men. *J Clin Endocrinol Metab.* 2001;86:724–731. doi:10.1210/jcem.86.2.7219

27. Malik RD, Lapin B, Wang CE, et al. Are we testing appropriately for low testosterone? Characterization of tested men and compliance with current guidelines. *J Sex Med.* 2015;12(1):66–75. doi:10.1111/jsm.12730

28. Handelsman DJ. Global trends in testosterone prescribing, 2000–2011: expanding the spectrum of prescription drug misuse. *Med J Aust.* 2013;199(8):51. doi:10.5694/mja13.10111

29. Khera M. Controversies in testosterone supplementation therapy. *Asian J Androl.*2015;17:175–176. doi:10.4103/1008-682X.148728

30. Mulhall JP, Trost LW, Brannigan RE, et al. Evaluation and management of testosterone deficiency. *J Urol.* 2018;200(2):423–532. doi:10.1016/j.juro.2018.03.115

31. Bhasin S, Brito JP, Cunningham GR, et al. Testosterone therapy in men with hypogonadism: an Endocrine Society clinical practice guideline. *J Clin Endocrinol Metab.* May 2018;103(5):1–30. doi:10.1210/jc.2018-00229

32. Bremner WJ, Viriello MV, Prinz, PN. Loss of circadian rhythmicity in blood testosterone levels with aging in normal men. *J Clin Endocrinol Metab.* 1983;56:1278–1281. doi:10.1210/jcem-56-6-1278

33. Plymate SR, Tenover JS, Bremner WJ. Circadian variation in testosterone, sex hormone binding globulin, and calculated non-sex hormone binding globulin bound testosterone in healthy young and elderly men. *J. Androl.* 1989;10:366–371. doi:10.1002/j.1939-4640.1989.tb00120.x

34. Crawford ED, Barqawi AB, O'Donnell C, et al. The association of time of day and serum testosterone concentration in a large screening population. *BJU Int.* 2007 Sep;100(3):509–513. doi:10.1111/j.1464-410X.2007.07022.x

35. O'Rourke TK Jr, Wosnitzer MS. Opioid-Induced Androgen Deficiency (OPIAD): Diagnosis, management, and literature review. *Curr Urol Rep.* 2016;17(10):76. doi:10.1007/s11934-016-0634-y

36. Clavell-Hernández J, Wang R. Emerging evidences in the long standing controversy regarding testosterone replacement therapy and cardiovascular events. *World J Mens Health.* 2018;36(2):92–102. doi:10.5534/wjmh.17050

37. U.S. Food and Drug Administration. FDA drug safety announcement. Accessed March 3, 2015. http://www.fda.gov/Drugs/DrugSafety/ucm436259.htm

38. Monroe AK, Dobs AS. The effect of androgens on lipids. *Curr Opin Endocrinol Diabetes Obes.* 2013 Apr;20(2):132–139. doi:10.1097/MED.0b013e32835edb71

39. McCullough A. A review of testosterone pellets in the treatment of hypogonadism. *Curr Sex Health Rep.* 2014;269. doi:10.1007/s11930-014-0033-7

Pharmacotherapy Related to Transgender Care

Diane M. Bruessow and Joanne Rolls

LEARNING OBJECTIVES

- Define key terminology and concepts as they relate to gender-diverse patients.
- Discuss the overall therapeutic approach to gender transition.
- Support the selection of pharmacological therapies to eliminate gender incongruence.
- Develop an overall multidisciplinary plan for a person with gender incongruence.

INTRODUCTION

Gender diversity is a common, culturally diverse phenomenon that occurs across all cultures and is not inherently pathological or negative.[1-4] In this way, gender diversity is akin to left-handedness and homosexuality. Although gender diversity is not a new concept, transgender medicine is an emerging area in medicine. A 2016 systematic review of the literature notes the availability of data regarding the health risks and resilience for transgender people in terms of biological, behavioral, social, and structural factors.[5] In 2013 the American Psychiatric Association (APA) stated that "it is important to note that gender nonconformity is not in itself a mental disorder."[6] It is the distress associated with gender incongruence that pharmacological and nonpharmacological interventions seek to resolve.[4,7] The existing research demonstrates improved quality of life and functioning when gender identity and expression are affirmed.[3,8-15] Efforts to change a person's gender identity or expression are not considered ethical.[8,14]

Within the United States, 0.6% (0.3% to 0.8%, 2.77% in the District of Columbia) of adults—or 1.4 million total adults—and 1 out of every 137 adolescents at age 13 to 17 years is estimated to experience incongruence between their assigned sex at birth (ASAB) and gender identity.[16,17] U.S. prevalence is likely underreported. Prevalence among adolescents in New Zealand is almost 4% (1.2% report being transgender, 2.5% report being unsure) suggesting that the form taken by sex and gender are dependent upon whether the environment is permissive or restrictive.[18,19]

TERMINOLOGY AND CONCEPTS

Sex is documented in one of two ways: *ASAB* or *legal sex*. In the United States, ASAB is limited to male or female, and is determined primarily by a newborn's phenotype (physical characteristics) regardless of genotype or differences of sexual development (DSD).[20] ASAB is either assigned female at birth (AFAB) or assigned male at birth (AMAB). Legal sex, such as what is represented on a birth certificate and other official identification documents, may be changed but governmental requirements vary.

Gender identity refers to the deeply held self-identification of gender. By age four, most children have a stable sense of their gender identity; however, self-actualization can occur at any age. Gender identity and gender expression are different constructs and may be discordant, particularly in restrictive environments.[21] *Cisgender* is a descriptor for concordance between ASAB and gender identity.[20,22] *Transgender* is a descriptor for discordance between ASAB and gender identity. Some but not all who meet these criteria may self-identify as transgender when describing themselves.[3,23,24]

Nonbinary (NB) is a gender identity other than exclusively male or female.[25] Gender is understood differently in different cultures. There are many kinds of NB gender identities across cultures, including Hijra (South Asia), Nandi (Africa), Muxe (Mexico), and Two-Spirit (Native American).[26] Some countries (e.g., Australia, Austria, Argentina, Bangladesh, Canada, Denmark, Germany, Malta, Nepal, New Zealand) offer an alternative to M/F gender markers (e.g., X [unspecified], T [transgender], I [intersex], E [eunuch], O [other], or a blank) on official documents such as passports. In the United States, 15 states and the District of Columbia recognize NB genders for state-issued identification documents such as drivers' licenses.[27] All but two states (Tennessee, Ohio) permit amendments to birth certificates, with nine states allowing NB gender designation as of October 2019. [27]

Transition describes the period during which a person makes physical, social, and/or legal changes toward congruence with their gender identity. Transition is a temporary status. Best practices in transition-related care include providing individualized and nonlinear patient-centered care.[3,21]

BACKGROUND

Incongruence between ASAB and gender identity will present differently at different developmental stages, although dysphoria becomes reliably more debilitating with the onset of secondary sex characteristics during natal puberty when a spike in suicides and suicide attempts has been documented.[14,15]

Although awareness of gender identity may occur at any age, a retrospective study of transgender adults in the United States ($N = 27,715$) found that 60% of transgender adults were aware of their gender being different than their ASAB before puberty, while 81% knew before age 16.[24] In another survey of over 3,400 transgender adults, 82.6% were aware before the age of 12 that they "felt different" from the gender associated with their ASAB and of them, the majority reported having expressed their gender in hiding. The gap between when an individual knows and when an individual expresses their gender identity should be kept in mind when considering criteria for eligibility for medical interventions.[28]

RISK FACTORS

Children with incongruence between their ASAB and gender identity and whose gender identity is affirmed and supported in all social domains, appear psychologically indistinguishable from cisgender controls and have developmentally normative levels of depression.[15,29] In addition, family acceptance correlates with increased resilience and improved psychological health and well-being. A lack of family acceptance, however, results in up to eight times higher rates of suicidal behavior, substance use, and other unhealthy behaviors.[14,15,29,30] Emerging data suggests a lack of social support in key developmental areas during childhood results in long-term negative psychosocial outcomes in adulthood.[31]

In restrictive societies such as the United States, gender incongruence is associated with social stigma that may precipitate discrimination, abuse, and decreased access to both general and gender-affirming healthcare, as well as increased incidence of unhealthy behaviors (e.g., alcohol, smoking, substance abuse).[24,32] Populations that face discrimination are more vulnerable to internalized disorders such as depression and anxiety, which compound health disparities.[33-36] Adolescents and adults who lack affirmation of their gender identity consistently experience dramatically elevated rates of internalized disorders, including anxiety, depression, and suicidality.[24,37,38] Studies note a marked decrease in the prevalence of depression after the initiation of masculinizing hormone therapy/feminizing hormone therapy (MHT/FHT) of 24.9% to 2.4% and 13.9% to 1.4%, respectively.[39,40]

Risk factors can be reduced by implementing best and promising practices for creating a safe and welcoming healthcare environment for gender-diverse patients. This is based primarily upon avoiding assumptions that patients are cisgender. Ideal professional practices include using every patient's correct name and pronoun; having an awareness of gendered language; avoiding assumptions about sexual attraction, behavior, and identity; and having knowledge of transition-related care.[41] In addition, a welcoming environment will allow for a patient's disclosure of ASAB and gender identity at four critical opportunities within healthcare systems: patient registration, clinical encounter, measurements of patient satisfaction, and health outcomes.[42]

DIAGNOSIS

FROM DIAGNOSIS TO DIVERSITY

The APA, which produces the *Diagnostic and Statistical Manual of Mental Disorders, Fifth Edition (DSM-5)*, and the World Health Organization (WHO), which produces the *International Classification of Diseases for Mortality and Morbidity Statistics, Eleventh Revision (ICD-11)*, agree that gender diversity must be destigmatized, and both organizations have taken explicit actions to do so within their publications.[3,23]

"Gender incongruence" is the term utilized in the *ICD-11* to further depathologize gender dysphoria in a manner similar to how pregnancy is not considered an illness or pathology.[4,43] Gender incongruence is characterized by a marked and persistent incongruence between an individual's gender identity and ASAB, while gender dysphoria focuses on distress resulting from incongruence.[44] Both the *ICD-11* and *DSM-5* differentiate prepubertal patients (i.e., gender incongruence of childhood), from peri- or postpubertal (i.e., gender incongruence of adolescence and adulthood).[4,43]

ASSESSMENT OF READINESS

As the science of transgender care has evolved, the medical belief in an underlying pathology has been replaced by an understanding of gender incongruence as a person's characteristic, and the practice of making mental health diagnoses has been replaced by an understanding of gender diversity. Similarly, the framework of diagnostic criteria has been replaced with an assessment of readiness for transgender persons. Guidelines are consistent in their recommendation for the assessment of the adolescent and adult patient's readiness to initiate partially irreversible pharmacologic interventions.[3]

Any master's-level medical or mental health clinician with the ability to assess both a patient's capacity to provide informed consent and whether the patient's psychiatric comorbidities (if present) are reasonably well-controlled may recommend the initiation of pharmacologic interventions for gender incongruence without requiring additional assessment or referral.[3,45] When assessment is conducted by a therapist or other master's-level licensed mental health professional, patients will be referred to a prescriber for management with pharmacological agents.[3]

Because pubertal suppression is completely reversible—natal puberty will commence upon discontinuation of this intervention—a different approach is recommended. Delaying or withholding treatment at Tanner Stage 2 may result in irreversible harm. If time is of the essence and the patient is indeed at Tanner Stage 2, pharmacological agents to suppress puberty can be initiated for 6 to 12 months while the patient undergoes assessment. This approach has the added benefit of making psychotherapy more effective by reducing distress and is often "diagnostic" for parents.[3,23,46]

> *Refusing timely medical interventions for adolescents might prolong gender dysphoria and contribute to an appearance that could provoke abuse and stigmatization.* **Withholding puberty suppression and subsequent feminizing or masculinizing hormone therapy is not a neutral option for adolescents.**[3]
> —World Professional Association for Transgender Health (WPATH)

It is recommended that clinicians also assess readiness to begin MHT/FHT.[3] Psychotherapy is not an absolute requirement, nor is the absence of mental health or medical disorders.[3] It is possible for a patient experiencing gender incongruence to be living with a mental health disorder; however, mental health disorders need to be reasonably well controlled.[3]

Several questions about gender dysphoria and incongruence remain unanswered, starting with the need for its nature to be clarified. Gender incongruence does not imply that gender dysphoria is present or that treatment is needed, nor do all individuals experiencing gender dysphoria require treatment. When treatment is needed, appropriate diagnostic coding should be available. However, formal guidance is not available to address dysphoria or incongruence that resolves with treatment, or spontaneously is in remission, or shifts to a new diagnosis (e.g., gender incongruence of childhood shifts to gender incongruence of adolescence and adulthood). As gender dysphoria can be resolved, criteria for resolution should be explicit. Subject matter experts often employ endocrine disorder not otherwise specified (NOS) for patients who are no longer dysphoric or incongruent but require ongoing maintenance of their hormone therapy.[47]

GUIDELINES

The seminal work on transgender healthcare, *Standards of Care for the Health of Transsexual, Transgender, and Gender Nonconforming People (SOC)*, was published in 1979 by the WPATH and is now in its seventh version (2012).[3] It is notable for demonstrating a North American and western European bias, necessitating that some guidelines be reframed for cultural competence.[3]

The *SOC* is not the preferred resource at the point of care. Publications designed for point-of-care utilization include the University of California San Francisco Center of Excellence (CoE) for Transgender Health's *Guidelines for the Primary and Gender-Affirming Care of Transgender and Gender Nonbinary People, Second edition* (2016), which explores the topic from a primary care perspective, as well as the Endocrine Society's "Endocrine Treatment of Gender-Dysphoric/Gender-Incongruent Persons: An Endocrine Society Clinical Practice Guideline" (2017).[23,46] In a philosophical shift from the Endocrine Society's 2009 guideline, which recommended that the pharmacologic transition-related care be the exclusive domain of endocrinologists, the revised guideline (2017) supports the provision of hormone therapy by primary care providers.[23] Canada, Australia, New Zealand, the United Kingdom, the United Nations, and Pan American organizations have also developed guidelines for the care of transgender and gender-diverse persons.

TABLE 29.1 Common Gender-Affirming Medically Necessary and Effective Approaches

Approach	Examples	Ages	Reversibility	Medical
Social transition	Gender-affirming hairstyles, clothing, name, gender pronouns, restrooms	Any	Completely reversible	No
Pubertal suppression	Gonadotropin-releasing hormone/GnRH analogs (leuprolide/histrelin)	Tanner Stage G2/B2, not age	Completely reversible	Yes
Masculinizing /feminizing hormone therapy	Testosterone (for patients AFAB); estradiol ± an androgen inhibitor (for patients AMAB)	Adults, adolescents when appropriate	Partially reversible	Yes
Surgical interventions	"Top" surgeries (to create a male-typical chest shape or breast augmentation); "bottom" surgeries (genitals and/or reproductive organs); other: facial feminization, chondrolaryngoplasty	Adults (*adolescents when appropriate)	Irreversible	Yes
Other interventions	Chest binding, electrolysis/laser hair removal, voice therapy, prosthetics	Varies	Varies	Sometimes
Legal transition	Changing name and gender on birth certificate, school records, and other identity documents	Any	Reversible	Sometimes

AFAB, assigned female at birth; AMAB, assigned male at birth; GnRH, gonadotropin-releasing hormone.

Source: Adapted with permission from Murchison G, Adkins D, Conrad LA, et al. *Supporting & caring for transgender children.* Human Rights Campaign Foundation; September 2016.

These guidelines are peer-reviewed and utilize a ranking system of available evidence.[3,23,46] Common across all guidelines are the following[3,23,46]:

- A focus on improved quality of life and function
- A reiteration that gender diversity is not pathologic
- The incorporation of mental healthcare as individually indicated rather than as a requirement in adults
- The encouragement of a multidisciplinary team-based approach to care
- The utilization of adjunct, nonpharmacologic treatments to affirm a person's gender

The guidelines vary slightly on recommended starting doses and lab-monitoring intervals, as well as usability at the point-of-care versus utility as a reference.[3,23,46] There are also some agents, specifically antiandrogens, which are available only outside the United States.[3,23,46] At the time of this publication, there are no large, highly powered, prospective studies available to inform care. The first longitudinal study on patients prior to and serially after the initiation of MHT/FHT is underway in Sweden.[48]

INTERVENTIONS

GENERAL APPROACH

In patients with gender incongruence, the objective is to improve the quality of life by reducing distress and improving function.[49] Gender affirmation may involve interventions within the specialties of pharmacology,

mental healthcare, speech and communication therapy, surgery, social work, and legal realms, among others (**Table 29.1**). Pharmacologic interventions, including pubertal suppression and MHT/FHT, are considered primary care.[46,50]

PHARMACOLOGIC APPROACHES TO CARE

The three categories of drugs that are discussed in this chapter include gonadotropin-releasing hormone analogs, sex steroids, and antiandrogens. All of the drugs referenced in this chapter are used off-label.

There is consensus among guidelines and medical and mental health associations that pharmacologic interventions are considered medically necessary and effective. This includes the suppression of endogenous puberty in peripubertal adolescents, which halts the development of secondary sex characteristics associated with ASAB, as well as MHT/FHT in adolescents and adults, which initiates development of secondary sex characteristics consistent with the patient's gender identity.[3,23,46] Among AMAB patients who have experienced a natal puberty, an antiandrogen is commonly added to facilitate feminization with a lower dose of estradiol to mitigate estradiol's dose-dependent side effects.[3,23,46] Antiandrogens are no longer necessary after orchiectomy.[3,23,46]

Initiation of pharmacologic interventions are recommended at developmental maturation stage Tanner 2, regardless of age.[3,23,46,49] Prior to Tanner 2, no pharmacologic interventions are indicated. An individualized, patient-centered approach is taken for all patients, and is even more important for nonbinary patients who

TABLE 29.2 Desirable Effects of Masculinizing/Feminizing Hormone Therapy

Masculinizing	Feminizing
Growth of and increased coarseness of body and facial hair[b]	Gynecomastia[a]
Deepening of voice[b]	Enlarged areola and nipple[a]
Increased muscle mass[b]	Decreased spontaneous genital activity[d]
Clitoromegaly[c]	Softened skin[a]
Redistribution of body fat[c]	Redistribution of body fat[a]
Vaginal atrophy[b]	Reduced testicular volume[a]
Scalp hair loss (male-pattern baldness)	Decreased sperm production

[a]Desirable effects first noticeable at 3–6 months after hormonal therapy.
[b]Desirable effects first noticeable at 6–12 months after hormonal therapy.
[c]Desirable effects first noticeable at 1–6 months after hormonal therapy.
[d]Desirable effects first noticeable at 1–3 months after hormonal therapy.

may be seeking a modified level of masculinization or feminization.[3,46,49]

Mechanism of Action

Pubertal Suppression With Gonadotropin-Releasing Hormone Analogs

Regardless of ASAB, endogenous puberty may be suppressed in peripubertal adolescents with a gonadotropin-releasing hormone (GnRH) analog.[3,23,46,49] GnRH analogs desensitize the pituitary gland by GnRH receptor downregulation.[49] This results in the subsequent suppression of pituitary gonadotropin (luteinizing hormone [LH] and follicle-stimulating hormone [FSH]) secretion and suspension of germ cell maturation responsible for sex steroid production and, ultimately, puberty.[49] Pituitary desensitization occurs typically within 4 weeks of initiation.[49] The initial exposure to GnRH analogs leads to a spike in LH and FSH secretion, which triggers a spike in natal sex steroid production, described as a "puberty flare."[49] This flare effect can result in a temporary increase in secondary sex characteristics, exacerbating dysphoria, before desensitizing the pituitary and suppressing the hypothalamic-pituitary-gonadal axis. Techniques to mitigate the flare effect exist within the literature, such as employing a short- and long-acting GnRH analog simultaneously, or using anti-gonadotropins, antiandrogens, or androgen synthesis inhibitors.

Initiation of GnRH analogs during Tanner Stage 2 will completely prevent undesirable natal secondary sex characteristics. Initiation at Tanner Stage 3 will suspend further development.[3,23,46,49,51] Pubertal suppression has been shown to reduce the need for future medical and surgical interventions, reduce depression and risk-taking behavior, and allow for the establishment of early and strong social support.[12,49] GnRH analogs have the added benefit of being fully reversible and offer significantly more effective suppression than alternatives.

Sex Steroids

Sex steroids bind to their respective androgen and estrogen receptors within target cells. The presence or absence of various sex steroids influences physiological effects, ranging from composition of body mass to fat, renal function, immune reactivity, drug-metabolizing enzymes, circulating proteins that may bind to medications, gastric acid secretion, and gastric emptying time; however, these and other neuroendocrine, reproductive, and metabolic effects of sex steroids are not addressed in this chapter.[52,53] Sex steroids are utilized in gender-affirming transition for their physiological effects that are directly related to the development of secondary sex characteristics (**Table 29.2**).

For transition-related purposes, clinicians should focus on the suppression of natal sex steroids and development of secondary sex characteristics, as well as the risks associated with the absence of sex steroids. After gonadectomy, lifelong maintenance therapy is recommended.

Testosterone

Masculinizing effects of testosterone include development of coarser and more oily skin; growth and increased coarseness of body and facial hair; thickening of vocal cords and deepening of the voice; increased lean body mass; clitoromegaly; redistribution of fat from hips, thighs, buttocks, and breasts to abdomen; vaginal atrophy; and possibly male-pattern baldness.

Estradiol

Feminizing effects of estradiol include gynecomastia, enlargement of the areola and nipple, softened skin, and redistribution of body fat from abdomen to hips, thighs, buttocks, and breasts. Decrease in spontaneous genital activity, reduction in testicular volume, and decreased sperm production may be considered desirable among some patients, including those who are "bottom dysphoric," a term referring to a negative association with natal genitalia. Estradiol has no effect on the voice, laryngeal prominence, or facial features. However, speech therapists and surgical options are available.

Anti-Androgens

The addition of pharmacologic agents with anti-androgen effects has allowed for a reduction in the dose of estradiol necessary for feminization, thereby reducing dose-dependent risks. Spironolactone is a mineralocorticoid-receptor agonist with antiandrogenic properties. Compared to alternatives, it is clinically preferred for its effectiveness and the ability to directly monitor serum total testosterone levels.[3,46] Cyproterone acetate is an antiandrogen with progestational properties that inhibit secretion of LH.[3,46] It is included within guidelines; however, it is not available in the United States. Alternatives such as finasteride and dutasteride inhibit the conversion of testosterone to dihydrotestosterone.[3,46] They are neither effective nor allow for direct lab monitoring.[3,46]

Dosing, Side Effects, Contraindications, and Black Box Warnings

Pubertal Suppression With GnRH Analogs

Contraindications to GnRH analogs are limited to sensitivity to medication. Adverse effects, which should be reviewed during the informed consent process, are noted in **Table 29.3**. Though there are no black box warnings, there are rare case reports of pituitary apoplexy occurring within the first few hours to days after initial administration in patients with pituitary adenoma. Presentation includes headache, nausea or vomiting, and vision changes.

Dosing for pubertal suppression is noted in Table 29.3. For patients receiving injections every 4 to 12 weeks, emphasis is placed on weight-based dosing as well as the dosing interval, which may need to be shortened to maintain hypothalamic-pituitary-gonadal axis suppression. An insufficient interval is detrimental because patients will experience recurring puberty flares. Ultrasensitive pediatric FSH/LH and endogenous sex-steroid levels may be helpful to support clinical suspicion of insufficient axis suppression. Clinical monitoring occurs every 3 to 4 months, emphasizing the growth chart's trend line which should slow but not stall. Suppression of endogenous puberty is often followed by coadministration of MHT/FHT to initiate puberty congruent with gender identity.

Masculinizing and Feminizing Hormone Therapy

In adolescent patients who are concurrently on a GnRH analog for puberty suppression, consider starting with 25% of the lowest adult dose when initiating MHT/FHT.[23,46] Patches may be cut into quarters, and topical creams may be compounded.[23,46] In adolescent patients concurrently receiving exogenous estradiol while on a GnRH analog, in addition to lab monitoring for toxicity, it is important to keep in mind that estradiol

TABLE 29.3 Pubertal Suppression (GnRH analog) Dosing and Adverse Effects

Medication	Dose	Frequency
Leuprolide acetate	50 mcg/kg SC	Daily
Leuprolide acetate for depot suspension (1-month administration)	Patient weight <25 kg: 7.5 mg IM Patient weight <25–37.5 kg: 11.25 mg IM Patient weight >37.5 kg: 15 mg IM	Monthly
Leuprolide acetate for depot suspension (3-month administration) 3-month admin has 2 doses: 11.25 and 30 mg	11.25 mg IM or 30 mg IM	Every 3 months
Histrelin implant	50 mg	Every 12–36 months
Adverse Effects		
Injection site reactions, including sterile abscess		
Suboptimal bone-mineral density accrual		
Mood alterations or emotional lability		
Irregular vaginal bleeding		

GnRH, gonadotropin-releasing hormone; IM, intramuscular; SC, subcutaneous.

Source: Adapted with permission from Olson J, Garofalo R. The peripubertal gender-dysphoric child: Puberty suppression and treatment paradigms. *Pediatr Ann.* 2014;43(6):e132–e137.

has a dose-dependent effect of stimulating closure of epiphyseal plates while simultaneously enhancing the growth-curve's trend line upward over that of pubertal suppression alone.[23,46] Antiandrogens are unnecessary while on GnRH analogs.[23,46]

Although guidelines provide a target range of sex-steroid serum levels, experienced clinicians in transgender healthcare use the lowest dose of MHT/FHT that results in clinical feminization/masculinization and monitor levels only to identify toxicities. For optimum feminization, serum total testosterone levels below 55 are recommended. This should not be a requirement for prescribing FHT, however, as there are patients who prefer to maintain their testosterone level. For patients who wish to achieve maximum feminization while also maintaining erectile function, a phosphodiesterase type 5 (PDE5) inhibitor may be beneficial.

Major side effects from HT are uncommon. Findings from 15 gender centers globally saw virtually no side effects when the Endocrine Society guidelines were followed, noting a thrombus rate of 1%. To further optimize health outcomes, daily activity and a tobacco-free lifestyle are recommended in all MHT/FHT patients.

MHT/FHT dosing for adolescents and adults should be adjusted clinically every 3 months during the first year (**Tables 29.4 and 29.5**). Mode of delivery is determined by patient preference. In addition to the noted effects, additional clinical effects of spironolactone include inhibition of spontaneous genital activity (therapeutic in patients whose dysphoria is exacerbated by erections) followed by dry or almost dry orgasms.

There is a lack of consensus on how to best integrate clinical and lab monitoring (**Table 29.6**). MHT/FHT dose titration should be based on safety and the patient's clinical response at 3-month intervals during the first year. Keep in mind that early breast development—experienced by the patient as soreness behind the nipples—may be seen 3 to 6 months after initiating FHT. If not present and no breast growth is determined on physical examination, the estradiol dose should be increased if it can be done safely. Deepening of the voice and body/facial hair are usually seen 6 to 12 months after initiating MHT. Patients may describe an improved psychological sense of well-being from the first dose. It is common for sex-steroid lab levels to be low by cisgender standards.

Elevated prolactin levels of 40 to 60 ng/mL are common, which is consistent with female levels. On rare occasions, the levels can be as high as 80 to 100 ng/mL. As long as the prolactin level plateaus, and the patient does not report symptoms consistent with a prolactinoma (e.g., headache, vision disturbances, nausea, vomiting), prolactin can be monitored. Conversely, if a patient complains of headache, vision changes, nausea, or vomiting, a workup for a prolactinoma should be initiated regardless of prolactin level.

After orchiectomy and oophorectomy, exogenous HT doses are decreased by up to 40% and antiandrogens are discontinued.[3,46] After gonadectomy, HT must be maintained to ensure adequate bone density.[3,46]

In patients on spironolactone, monitoring serum potassium is recommended if potassium-sparing medications are taken concurrently.[46]

Contraindications to testosterone include pregnancy as well as androgen-sensitive cancers.[3,46] Relative contraindications and undesirable effects include erythrocytosis (hematocrit over 50%), and severe liver dysfunction (transaminases >3 × upper limits), as well as coronary artery disease (CAD), cardiovascular disease (CVD), hypertension (HTN), and breast or uterine cancer.[3,46]

Absolute contraindications to estradiol include thromboembolism while on therapeutic doses of anticoagulation therapy, severe thrombophlebitis while on anticoagulation therapy, estrogen-sensitive cancers, or end-stage chronic liver disease.[3,46] Decision trees are available to assist in the management of patients with known hypercoagulative states and increased thrombogenicity.[46] Relative contraindications and undesirable effects include hyperprolactinemia, prolactinoma, severe liver dysfunction (transaminases >3 × upper limits, applicable to oral dosing), severe migraine headaches, cholelithiasis, hypertriglyceridemia, CAD, CVD, and breast cancer.[3]

Notable Pharmacokinetics

The presence and absence of various sex steroids, as well as sex chromosomes, influence the absorption, distribution, metabolism, and elimination of other medications. This has the potential to result in adverse drug reactions.[53] Additional research is needed to further individualize therapeutic interventions across combinations of hormone status and sex chromosomes.[53]

HIV Antiretrovirals and Feminizing Hormone Therapy
Within the United States, 14% of transfeminine people are living with HIV, with a disproportionate burden among transwomen of color; specifically, 44% Black/African American, 26% Hispanic/Latina, and 7% White.[55] One area where published data on pharmacokinetics exists is antiretroviral medication used in the prevention and management of HIV.[56–58] HIV-prevention technologies including PrEP are effective at reducing seroconversion when taken as prescribed. However, transfeminine patients receiving feminizing hormone therapy have expressed concern that PrEP may have a negative effect on their feminizing hormone levels, though data reflects the inverse effect: various FHT regimens, including estrogen/cyproterone and ogestrogen/spironolactone, result in reduced concentrations of PrEP in plasma as well as rectal tissue.[56,58,59] These reductions were consistent with concentrations seen in patients on PrEP regimens of five to six doses per week, thus prescribers

TABLE 29.4 Feminizing Hormone Therapy Dosing and Side Effects

Medication	Start/Usual and Typical Max Dose	Frequency	Pros and Cons	Notes
Estrogens				
Estradiol IM or SQ[1] injection	**Valerate** *Start/usual:* 5–10 mg (0.25 mL–0.5 mL of 20-mg/mL solution or (0.125 mL–0.25 mL of 40-mg/mL solution) *Typical max:* 20 mg (1 mL of 20-mg/mL solution or 0.5 mL of 40-mg/mL solution) **Cypionate** *Start/usual:* 1.25–2.5 mg (0.25 mL–0.5 mL of 5-mg/mL solution) *Typical max:* 5 mg (1 mL of 5-mg/mL solution)	Weekly[2]	**Pros:** Less frequent administration; systemic effect, avoids first-pass effect on liver (when at peak circulating levels of estrogen, amount delivered to liver may be higher than other modes of delivery); peak of injectable may help better suppress endogenous hormone production **Cons:** Peak/trough fluctuation effect; self-injection or frequent in-office injections; needle use	**Valerate:** Formulated in castor oil (use if allergic to cottonseed) and typically used with weekly dosing; national shortages of injectable formulation, especially generic estradiol valerate, not applicable **Cypionate:** Formulated in cottonseed oil (use if allergic to castor oil) and is typically a quarter of the dose of valerate and can be given at every 2-week interval rather than weekly due to the longer half life
Estradiol patch	*Start/usual:* 0.1–0.2 mg (1–2 × 0.1-mg patch) *Typical max:* 0.4 mg (4 × 0.1-mg patch)	Bi-weekly or per manufacturer's recommendation	**Pros:** No needle use; less fluctuation in levels; no first-pass metabolism **Cons:** Adhesive irritation, can fall off with sweat*; daily application; may be expensive if not covered by insurance	Preferred method for those with increased risk of DVT/PE/CVD For those who have had DVT/PE/CVD, shared clinical decision-making to resume low-dose (0.05-mg) transdermal estrogen may be done, but should be administered with continuous anticoagulation For transdermal formulations, consider using higher doses for those with more adipose tissue
Estradiol oral	*Start/usual:* 2–6 mg (1–3 × 2-mg tablet) *Typical max:* 8 mg (4 × 2-mg tablets daily)	Daily	**Pros:** No needle use; less fluctuation in levels **Cons:** Daily dose; first-pass metabolism	Single or divided doses dependent on preference; if on higher dose of 6–8 mg, divide to decrease first-pass impact and hepatotoxicity Some providers recommend SL administration to attempt to bypass first-pass metabolism, but it is unclear how much is actually absorbed SL vs. oral; consider switch to injectable if not seeing results with oral DO NOT USE estradiol ethinyl or other conjugated equine estrogens as they are associated with higher thromboembolism risk and can interact with HIV medications
Premarin[*] oral	*Start/usual:* 1.25–2.5 mg (1–2 × of 1.25-mg tablet) *Typical max:* 5 mg (4 × 1.25-mg tablet)	Daily	**Pros:** No needle use; less fluctuation in levels **Cons:** Daily dose; rarely used and not preferred due to higher thrombogenic risk compared to estradiol; difficult to monitor estrogen level as it may not reflect true serum levels related to dose; may be expensive if not covered by insurance; first-pass metabolism	See estradiol

Aldosterone Antagonist

Spironolactone oral	*Start/usual:* 100–300 mg (1–3 × 100-mg tablet) *Typical max:* 400 mg (4 × 100-mg tablet)	Daily	**Pros:** Inexpensive; very effective to decrease endogenous testosterone levels **Cons:** Potential risk of hyperkalemia, especially if kidney function is compromised; diuretic effect can result in fatigue, dehydration side effects; erectile dysfunction**	Single or divided doses dependent on preference

GnRH Receptor Agonist

Leuprolide acetate IM	*Start/usual:* 11.25 mg (1 shot of 11.25-mg/1.5- mL dilutant) *Typical max:* 22.5mg (2 shot of 11.25-mg/1.5- mL dilutant)	Every 3 months	**Pros:** GnRH receptor agonist, very effective; for teens: best option for puberty suppression, can use either alone or with exogenous hormones; for adults: especially beneficial if can't use spironolactone, on a lower estrogen dose, and/or having difficulty suppressing endogenous hormone production **Cons:** May be expensive if not covered by insurance; not ideal for long-term use due to bone-density loss***	—
Histrelin pellet	*Start/usual:* 50 mg *Typical max:* 50 mg	Every 1 year	**Pros:** See leuprolide acetate **Cons:** More invasive, requires minor surgery to implant; may be expensive if not covered by insurance; not ideal for long-term use due to bone-density loss***	—

Progestins

Micronized progesterone oral	*Start/usual:* 100–200 mg (1 × 100-mg or 1 × 200-mg tablet) *Typical max:* 200 mg (1 × 200-mg tablet daily)	Daily	**Pros:** In addition to suppressing testosterone production, progesterone also has weak androgen receptor activation that can improve mood and sex drive; weak evidence shows areola size may increase, but no evidence that it increases breast size; it may increase weight gain with a side effect of fuller breasts **Cons:** May increase risk of breast cancer additionally over estrogen use alone; with personal history of breast cancer or known BRCA-mutation carrier, consider not prescribing; avoid using cyclically due to higher risk of breast cancer compared to daily use	Research is low quality to advise for or against; for those with a strong desire to try, a limited prescription is reasonable (e.g., 6 months) Engage in shared clinical decision-making about risks and benefits. Consider separate informed consent form or well-documented consent
Medroxyprogesterone oral	*Start/usual:* 2.5–10 mg (1 × 2.5-mg,1 × 5-mg, or 1 × 10-mg tablet) *Typical max:* 10 mg (1 × 10-mg tablet)	Daily	**Pros/Cons:** See micronized progesterone	Use only if micronized progesterone is cost-prohibitive

Anti-Androgens

(continued)

TABLE 29.4 Feminizing Hormone Therapy Dosing and Side Effects *(continued)*

Medication	Start/Usual and Typical Max Dose	Frequency	Pros and Cons	Notes
Cyproterone acetate oral	*Start/usual:* 50 mg (1 × 50-mg tablet) *Typical max:* 100 mg (2 × 50-mg tablet)	Daily	**Pros:** Steroidal androgen receptor antagonist, blocks T & DHT very effectively **Cons:** Risk of meningioma; however, adverse effects are unlikely if using 100 mg or less daily dose	Unavailable in the United States
Finasteride oral (as adjuvant anti-androgen)	*Start/usual:* 5 mg (1 × 5-mg tablet) *Typical max:* 5 mg (1 × 5-mg tablet)	Daily	**Pros:** Slows and prevents balding due to androgenic alopecia and decreases other secondary sexual hair growth in youth **Cons:** Not typically covered by insurance	Used as adjuvant as it decreases DHT but not testosterone Can use alone (without estrogen) if goal is only for partial feminization
Dutasteride oral (as adjuvant anti-androgen)	*Start/usual:* 5 mg (1 × 5-mg tablet) *Typical max:* 5 mg (1 × 5-mg tablet)	Every 3 days	**Pros:** Slows and prevents balding due to androgenic alopecia and decreases other secondary sexual hair growth in youth; can take every 3 days rather than every day with finasteride **Cons:** May be expensive and not typically covered by insurance	See finasteride
Less Commonly Used Anti-Androgens				
Bicalutamide oral	*Start/usual:* 50 mg (1 × 50-mg tablet) *Typical max:* 50 mg (1 × 50-mg tablet)	Daily	**Pros:** Nonsteroidal androgen receptor antagonist **Cons:** See flutamide; however, bicalutamide has less hepatotoxicity, so if choosing between nonsteroidal androgen antagonists, choose bicalutamide over flutamide	If utilized, must check LFT at baseline, 1 month, 2 months, then every 6 months for lifetime
Flutamide oral	*Start/usual:* 250 mg (2 × 125-mg tablet) *Typical max:* 250 mg (2 × 125-mg tablet)	Daily	**Pros:** Nonsteroidal androgen receptor antagonist **Cons:** Potential risk of rapid-onset, severe, life-threatening liver toxicity, use extreme caution and monitor closely; don't use if +G6PD or increased risk of methemoglobinemia (e.g, smokers); caution if other hepatotoxic drugs or alcohol	See bicalutamide
Combination therapy				
Esterified estrogen/ methyltestosterone oral	*Start/usual:* 0.625 mg/1.25 mg *Typical max:* 1.25 mg/2.5 mg	Daily	**Pros:** Alleviation of fatigue and low libido associated with lack of androgen **Cons:** Same risks as those associated with estrogen; controlled substance	Dose of main source of estrogen should be adjusted to accommodate the increase included in the combo tablet. Generally, this is not a concern as most use drug after orchiectomy so they're less likely to require higher doses of estrogen for feminization.

*To diminish irritation, apply 1% hydrocortisone to patch area for 1-hour duration before and then clean area prior to patch application. Tincture of benzoin applied to patch area will promote adhesion.

**If patient would like to experience erections with endogenous testosterone suppression and does not want to decrease anti-androgen dose, consider prescription of sildenafil, tadalafil, or, if postorchiectomy, consider low-dose testosterone or esterified estrogen/methyltestosterone.

***If using anastrozole or leuprolide acetate in the presence of other risk factors for osteoporosis, consider dual-energy X-ray absorptiometry (DEXA) scan after 2 years of use.

BRCA, breast cancer gene; CVD, cardiovascular disease; DHT, dihydrotestosterone; DVT, deep vein thrombosis; GnRH, gonadotropin-releasing hormone; HIV, human immunodeficiency virus; IM, intramuscular; LFT, liver function test; PE, pulmonary embolism; SQ, subcutaneous.

Source: With permission from Jaffe JM, Gorton RN, Menkin D, et al. Gender affirming hormone therapy prescriber guidelines. *TransLine.* Published April 4, 2019. https://transline.zendesk.com/hc/en-us/articles/229373288-TransLine-Hormone-Therapy-Prescriber-Guidelines

TABLE 29.5 Masculinizing Hormone Therapy Dosing and Side Effects

Medication	Start/Usual and Typical Max Dose	Frequency	Pros and Cons	Notes
Exogeneous Testosterone				
IM or SQ[1] injectable testosterone	*Start/usual:* 50–80 mg (0.25–0.4 mL of 200 mg/mL solution or 0.5–1.0mL of 100 mg/mL solution) *Typical max:* 100 mg (0.5 mL of 200 mg/mL solution)	Weekly[2]	**Pros:** Less frequent administration compared with transdermal; peak of injectable may better suppress endogenous hormone production **Cons:** Peak/trough fluctuation effect; self-injection or frequent in-office injections; needle use	Cypionate formulated in cottonseed oil (use if allergic to sesame) Enanthate formulated in sesame oil (use if allergic to cottonseed) Enanthate has slightly shorter halflife than cypionate
Transdermal testosterone topical gel	*Start/usual:* 20–62.5 mg (Androgel 1%, 12.5 mg/actuation, 2–5 pumps; Androgel 1.62%, 20.25 mg/actuation, 1–3 pumps; Axiron, 30 mg/actuation, 1–2 pumps; Testim, 50 mg/5 g, 2.5–5g) *Typical max:* 100 mg (Androgel 1%, 12.5 mg/actuation, 8 pumps; Androgel 1.62%, 20.25 mg/actuation, 5 pumps; Axiron, 30 mg/actuation, 3 pumps; Testim, 50 mg/5 g, 10 g)	Daily	**Pros:** No needle use; less fluctuation in levels; good for more gradual effects **Cons:** Slower to stop menses and may not fully stop at lower doses; risk of transferring to others/pets so must instruct how to apply per package insert; some products are scented and may not be appropriate for those with scent-sensitivities; daily application; may be expensive if not covered by insurance	Consider using higher doses for those with more adipose tissue
Transdermal testosterone patch	*Start/usual:* 2–6 mg (1–3 x 2-mg patches) *Typical max:* 8 mg (2 x 4-mg patches)	Daily	**Pros:** No needle use; less fluctuation in levels; good for more gradual effects; less risk of transfer to others **Cons:** Slower to stop menses and may not fully stop at lower doses; adhesive irritation, can fall off with sweat[3]; daily application; may be expensive if not covered by insurance	Consider using higher doses for those with more adipose tissue
Testosterone pellets	*Start/usual:* 450–600 mg (6–8 x 75-mg pellets) *Typical max:* 750 mg (10 x 75-mg pellets)	Every 3–4 months	**Pros:** No needle use; less frequent administration; less fluctuation in levels **Cons:** More invasive, requires minor surgery to implant; may be expensive if not covered by insurance	Lab draw frequency: Baseline draw prior to starting, once at 1 month, then at 3 months prior to next insertion Consider using higher doses for those with more adipose tissue
IM testosterone undecanoate	*Start/usual:* 750 mg (6–8 x 75-mg pellets) *Typical max:* N/A	Initial injection at 4 weeks, then every 10 weeks thereafter	**Pros:** Less frequent injection; less fluctuation in levels **Cons:** Pulmonary oil embolism risk; primary care provider and facility need registration; may be expensive and unlikely to be covered by insurance at present	Formulated in castor oil

(continued)

TABLE 29.5 Masculinizing Hormone Therapy Dosing and Side Effects *(continued)*

Medication	Start/Usual and Typical Max Dose	Frequency	Pros and Cons	Notes
Oral testosterone undecanoate	*Start/usual:* 316–474 mg (1 × 158-mg capsule BID; 1 × 198-mg capsule BID; 1 × 237-mg capsules BID) *Typical max:* 790mg (1 × 158-mg + 1 × 237-mg capsules BID)	Daily	**Pros:** No needle use; less fluctuation in levels **Cons:** First pass metabolism; daily dose	Recommend divided doses (BID) to decrease first pass effect and hepatotoxicity Starting dose 237 mg BID, then adjust dose to minimum of 158 mg BID with a max of 395 mg BID
Testosterone nasal gel	*Start/usual:* 33 mg (2 pump actuations, one 5.5-mg actuation per nostril = 11 mg TID) *Typical max:* N/A	Daily	**Pros:** No needle use; less fluctuation in levels **Cons:** Administration three times per day	Not recommended for use with other nasally administered drugs other than sympathomimetic decongestants
Medications to Supplement Testosterone				
Finasteride oral	*Start/usual:* 1 mg (1/4 of 5-mg or 1 × 1-mg tablet) *Typical max:* 5 mg (1 × 5-mg tablet)	Daily	**Pros:** Prevent or slow balding due to androgenic alopecia **Cons:** May slow other DHT-dependent changes like secondary hair growth and clitoral growth; discuss with patients, especially if considering using at the beginning of testosterone use, unless they are deliberately trying to prevent aforementioned changes	5 mg cheaper than 1 mg; can split 5 mg into quarters
Dutasteride oral	*Start/usual:* 0.5 mg (1 × 0.5- mg tablet) *Typical max:* 0.5 mg (1 × 0.5- mg tablet)	Every 3 days	**Pros:** Slows and prevents balding due to androgenic alopecia; can take every 3 days rather than every day with finasteride **Cons:** See finasteride	—
Compounded testosterone cream (applied to genitals)	*Start/usual:* 12.5–50 mg[a] (0.25–1 g of 5% cream) *Typical max:* 100 mg (2 g of 5% cream or 1 g of 10% cream)	Daily	**Pros:** Clitoral enlargement; can also be used as a cheaper transdermal alternative to AndroGel® **Cons:** May worsen balding due to androgenic alopecia	Some surgeons may suggest the topical application of testosterone to the clitoris as an adjunct to growth. There is no definitive evidence for this practice; if undertaken, the applied dose should be subtracted from the patient's total testosterone dosage (if it is used in addition to another formulation of testosterone). Contact compounding pharmacy to determine equivalent amount to be subtracted from total dose, as equivalency depends greatly on the chemicals it is compounded with. Long-term efficacy is not well established.
Compounded dihydrotestosterone cream (applied to genitals)	*Start/usual:* 6 mg over course of day (20 mg of 10% cream) *Typical max:* 6 mg over course of day (20 mg of 10% cream)	Apply 2mg 3x per day	**Pros:** Clitoral enlargement **Cons:** May worsen balding due to androgenic alopecia	See compounded testosterone cream Not sold or FDA approved in the US; very expensive and illegal to import due to being a schedule III drug Available as an alcohol-based gel overseas; when used on mucous membranes, can result in a burning sensation after topical application

Drug	Dose	Frequency	Pros/Cons	Notes
Leuprolide acetate IM	*Start/usual*: 11.25 mg (1 shot of 1.25-mg/1.5-mL dilutant) *Typical max*: 22.5 mg (2 shots of 11.25-mg/1.5-mL dilutant)	Every 3 months	**Pros**: GnRH receptor agonist, very effective at suppressing endogenous hormone production; typically used only for puberty suppression in teens; can use either alone or with exogenous hormones **Cons**: May be expensive if not covered by insurance; not ideal for long-term use due to bone-density loss[b]	—
Vaginal estradiol	Dosing same as postmenopausal ciswomen	N/A	**Pros**: Treats vaginal atrophy, pain with penetration, and unsatisfactory cytology result on pap smear **Cons**: N/A	If used in preparation for vaginal exam and/or pap smear, 2-week course prior can help with pain and obtaining satisfactory cytology Approach discussion with sensitivity as some may not feel comfortable using estrogen due to gender dysphoria
Medroxyprogesterone acetate IM	*Start/usual*: 150 mg (1 mL of 150-mg/mL solution) *Typical max*: 150 mg (1 mL of 150-mg/mL solution)	Every 3 months	**Pros**: Stops persistent vaginal bleeding on T[c]; contraception **Cons**: N/A	3-month course, then re-evaluate
Medroxyprogesterone oral	*Start/usual*: 5 mg (1 × 5-mg tablet) *Typical max*: 10 mg (1 × 10-mg tablet)	Daily	**Pros**: Stops persistent vaginal bleeding on T[c] **Cons**: N/A	7–10-day course to as long as a 3-month course
Anastrozole	*Start/usual*: 1 mg *Typical max*: 1 mg	Daily	**Pros**: Stops persistent vaginal bleeding on T[c] **Cons**: Not ideal for long-term use due to bone-density loss[b]	3-month course; may cause menopausal symptoms
Levonorgestrel IUD	*Start/usual*: 20 mcg/day (Mirena®); 14 mcg/day (Skyla®); 19.5 mg/day (Kyleena®) *Typical max*: N/A	N/A	**Pros**: Stops persistent vaginal bleeding on T[c]; contraception **Cons**: N/A	Mirena® lasts 5 years; Skyla® lasts 3 years; Kyleena® lasts 4 years

DHT, dihydrotestosterone; GnRH, gonadotropin-releasing hormone; IM, intramuscular; IUD, intrauterine device.

[a]Testosterone Cypionate/Enanthate and Estradiol Valerate/Cypionate are FDA approved for delivery only through intramuscular injections. However, for many patients, subcutaneous injection serves as a safe and effective alternative option due to decreased pain with injection. There are limited studies supporting subcutaneous delivery, but anecdotally, some patients and providers prefer this method. There is a caveat that hormone level may be more variable due to variable absorption, and, for those with more adipose tissue, it may take a longer time to achieve steady state.

[2]For injectable can alter dose to every 10- or 14-day regimen if preferred

[3]To diminish irritation, apply 1% hydrocortisone to patch area for 1-hour duration before, then clean area, prior to patch application. Tincture of benzoin applied to patch area will promote adhesion.

[a]Dosing depends on compounded formulation. Consult with pharmacy to determine usual cisgender-male replacement dose and start at approximately 25% to 50% of that dose.

[b]If using anastrozole or leuprolide acetate in the presence of other risk factors for osteoporosis, consider dual-energy X-ray absorptiometry (DEXA) scan after 2 years of use.

[c]First rule out if testosterone usage has been variable—testosterone level too high (and aromatizing into estrogen) or too low. Persistent vaginal bleeding while on testosterone requires work-up if >12 months amenorrhoeic

Source: With permission from. Jaffe JM, Gorton RN, Menkin D, et al. Gender affirming hormone therapy prescriber guidelines. *TransLine.* Published April 4, 2019. https://transline.zendesk.com/hc/en-us/articles/229373288-TransLine-Hormone-Therapy-Prescriber-Guidelines

TABLE 29.6 Monitoring for Feminizing/Masculinizing Hormone Therapy

Timing	Lab Monitoring	Clinical Monitoring
Transmasculine: Exogenous Testosterone		
Baseline	CBC, CMP	PCP exam, BP, UPT[c]
Once amenorrhoeic (or 2–3 months after start)	Testosterone (total)	PCP check-in, BP
After change in dose (1–3 months after change)	Testosterone (total)	PCP check-in, BP
6 months after first achieving maintenance dose[a]	CBC, testosterone (total)	PCP check-in, BP
12 months on stable maintenance dose[b]	CBC, testosterone (total), CMP[c], lipids[d]	PCP check-in, BP
Timing of testosterone draw	Injectable: 1 week after injection[e]; transdermal: trough (don't take/apply on the day of the draw); oral: 6 hours after morning dose at least 7 days after starting or adjusting dose	
Transfeminine: Exogenous Estrogen		
Baseline	BMP[f] Prolactin (only if on meds known to increase prolactin)	PCP exam, BP
6–8 weeks after initiation	Testosterone (total), Estrogen (total)	PCP exam, BP
After change in dose (6–8 weeks)	Testosterone (total), Estrogen (total)	PCP exam, BP
6 months after first achieving maintenance dose[a]	Testosterone (total), Estrogen (total), Prolactin[g]	PCP exam, BP
12 months on stable maintenance dose[b]	BMP[f], Testosterone (total), Estrogen (total), Prolactin	PCP exam, BP
Timing of estrogen/prolactin draw	Injectable: 1 week after injection[h]; oral and transdermal: trough (don't take/apply on the day of the draw)	

[a]Optional, especially if otherwise young and healthy.

[b]Unless other concerns.

[c]Only if at risk for pregnancy.

[d]In all patients, check lipids 12 months after starting and repeat every 12 months if there is a concern of fatty liver, chronic liver disease, high cholesterol.

[e]Level will be higher on every 10- or 14-day dosing than on every 7-day dosing. Timing of testosterone draw is not important; instead, it's important to know if it's trough, mid-level, or peak to determine if the results are as expected.

[f]Basic metabolic panel most important while using spironolactone. Check comprehensive metabolic panel, rather than basic panel, if using maximum or above-maximum estrogen dosages, Estrace⁻, flutamide, or bicalutamide, or if other medications or risks for hepatotoxicity present.

[g]If using maximum or above-maximum estrogen dosages or if using Premarin⁻, prolactin should be checked more rigorously. Otherwise, it's more important to screen for symptoms of prolactinoma than to check a level.

[h]Level will be higher on every 10- or 14-day dosing than on every 7-day dosing.

BMP, basic metabolic panel; BP, blood pressure; CBC, complete blood count; CMP, comprehensive metabolic panel; CP, primary care provider; UPT, urinary pregnancy test.

Source: With permission from Jaffe JM, Gorton RN, Menkin D, et al. Gender affirming hormone therapy prescriber guidelines. *TransLine.* Published April 4, 2019. https://transline.zendesk.com/hc/en-us/articles/229373288-TransLine-Hormone-Therapy-Prescriber-Guidelines

are discouraged from offering PrEP regimens with reduced dosing schedules to patients on FHT. Patients on FHT should be counseled in this regard.[56,60]

Sickle Cell Disease and Hormone Therapy

Sickle cell trait increases thromboembolic and cardiovascular risk, which can also be provoked by sex steroids. Exogenous testosterone contributes to dose-dependent increases in hemoglobin, thereby increasing viscosity. The thrombus risk of exogenous

estrogens is dependent upon preparation, dose, and route of administration.[53,61]

NONPHARMACOLOGIC APPROACHES TO TREATMENT

There are several nonpharmacologic approaches to support gender affirmation. While some are individual, others are socially implemented.

Social Transition

Social transition involves adopting a new nickname, pronouns, hair length, and/or clothing that reflects the person's gender identity. It is completely reversible and may be implemented by gender-incongruent patients of any age.[62] The benefits of social transition among children and adolescents include improved states of mental health, approaching similar rates of mental health conditions to cisgender control groups. Children who are supported with social transition and medical therapy achieve improved mental health outcomes as adults.[62]

Surgical Interventions

A variety of surgical interventions are available for adult patients and older adolescents and are not reversible. They are commonly referred to as "GCS," or gender confirmation surgeries, and grouped into the categories of "top surgery," "bottom surgery," and "other procedures," which can include facial feminization and tracheal shaves. GCS is effective in treating gender dysphoria and is considered medically necessary, not cosmetic or elective.[3,23] The authors recommend working with experienced surgical teams and following the criteria for surgery outlined within the *SOC7*.[3]

Top Surgeries

For the person AFAB who desires a more masculine chest wall, masculinizing chest procedures involve a subcutaneous mastectomy, the construction of a male chest wall, and nipple relocation and reduction.[3,63] There are several surgical approaches that are dictated by breast size and body habitus.[63] Chest binding results in changes that will limit some of the surgical approaches as well. Testosterone therapy is not required for any duration of time prior to masculinizing surgery.[63]

While testosterone therapy is not required for masculinizing top surgery, persons AMAB who desire a feminine chest are recommended to receive hormone therapy for at least 1 year prior to chest feminization.[3] This allows the person an opportunity to experience the effect of exogenous estrogen on the development of glandular breast tissue prior to surgery.[3,63] Chest feminization typically involves breast augmentation with or without fat grafting. Serial procedures may be required depending on body habitus and desired breast size.[63]

Bottom Surgeries

Masculinizing bottom surgery options include metoidioplasty or phalloplasty with optional vaginectomy, scrotoplasty, testicular implants/prostheses, and implantable erection devices. Surgical technique decisions are based on a person's clitoral growth in response to testosterone therapy, desire to maintain full sensation, and personal goals such as standing to urinate or engaging in penetrative intercourse. Other bottom surgical options include hysterectomy and salpingo-oophorectomy.[3,63] Continuous testosterone therapy is recommended for 12 months prior to these procedures.[3]

Feminizing bottom surgical options include bilateral orchiectomy, which in addition to treating dysphoria can also reduce the need for antiandrogen medication, vulvoplasty, and vaginoplasty. Vulvoplasty creates external female genitalia without the creation of a neovagina, such as that created by vaginoplasty. Vaginoplasty requires significant postoperative management to prevent stenosis and maintain vaginal depth. Surgical choice is dictated by patient preference, postoperative rehabilitation, and goals.[3,63] Continuous feminizing hormone therapy is recommended for 12 months prior to these surgical procedures.[3]

Other Surgical Procedures

Several facial feminization surgery (FFS) procedures are available for the person AMAB who would benefit from a more feminine facial mosaic. These include both structural facial procedures and soft-tissue procedures such as Adam's apple reduction (also called "tracheal shave"), chin reduction, jawline shaping, zygomatic arch or frontal bone reduction, rhinoplasty, cheekbone augmentation, brow lifts, hairline advancement or transplantation, blepharoplasty, lip lift, face lift, and fat grafting.[63]

Legal Transition

Legal transitioning is often dependent on the state in which a person was born and currently resides. This can involve updating name and gender markers on identification documents and legal records and may require a letter of support from a medical professional.[7,27]

Other Nonpharmacologic Gender-Affirming Interventions

There are several additional gender-affirming treatments and care options available for transgender and gender nonconforming persons. Voice and speech therapy is considered a fundamental aspect of transition-related care and allows a person to achieve a communication and vocal style that is congruent with their gender.[64] Hair-removal treatments, such as electrolysis or laser hair removal, are associated with decreased dysphoria and increased psychological well-being in transfeminine persons and should not be considered cosmetic or elective.[65] Breast, hip, or penile prostheses may be used to reduce dysphoria and assist with a gender expression that affirms a person's gender identity.[3] The use of penile prostheses is often referred to as "packing."[63] Persons wishing to reduce the appearance of breast tissue may engage in breast or chest binding. Commercial binding devices are preferred to the use of ace-wraps or other homemade options as these can lead to skin and musculoskeletal complications.[63]

CASE EXEMPLAR: Patient Initiating Masculinizing Hormone Therapy

MM is an 18-year-old male, assigned female at birth (AFAB), who presents with his parents to initiate masculinizing hormone therapy (MHT) for gender incongruence. MM's long-term goals for therapy include top surgery and changing his driver's license gender marker. He is unsure about bottom surgery at this point. He does not want to carry biological children and is currently not sexually active due to his dysphoria.

Past Medical History
- Depression
- Psychotherapy treatment (6 years)

Medications
- Fluoxetine, 20 mg; well-controlled

Family History
- Remarkable for diabetes and coronary artery disease

Social History
- No tobacco or alcohol use
- Infrequent use of marijuana
- Describes family support as "okay"; notes positive support of siblings and mother

Discussion Questions

1. Does MM meet the criteria for readiness to initiate MHT?
2. What organ systems should a clinician explore during MM's physical examination, and what lab studies should be ordered initially?
3. What are the clinician's next steps in clinical management for MM, including medication initiation?
4. What patient education should be provided to MM in regard to drug–drug interactions, drug–food interactions, and side effects?
5. MM returns to the clinic 3 months after starting testosterone. Overall, he is happy with starting MHT. He feels that his mood is improving, and he feels more confident. He is looking forward to facial hair and is hoping to attain greater upper body muscle mass. MM has started lifting weights at the gym 3 days a week. He denies depression or aggression. His periods have lightened and are more irregular, but have not completely stopped, which triggers dysphoria. He has developed some acne, particularly under his chest binder, which he wears daily. What are the clinician's next steps for management of MM?

CASE EXEMPLAR: Patient With Gender Dysphoria

VF is a 10.5-year-old male, assigned female at birth (AFAB), who presents with his parents to address recent breast budding. VF's medical record includes a referral letter from a child-trained therapist who has been working with him since he was a toddler. The referral letter recommends pubertal suppression at the appropriate developmental stage (Tanner 2). His parents have anticipated that VF may have entered puberty and are both present to initiate informed consent.

Past Medical History
- Remarkable for gender dysphoria/incongruence of childhood, which has mostly abated with social transition and gender affirmation in all domains (home, school, community).
- Up-to-date on all immunizations, well check-ups, and developmental milestones

Medications
- None

Discussion Questions

1. What organ systems would a clinician explore during VF's physical examination, and what lab studies should be initially ordered?
2. VF's physical examination and lab work are consistent with Tanner 2. Are there any contraindications to initiating pubertal suppression at this time? Are there any drug–drug or drug–food interactions to consider?
3. What are the clinician's next steps in the clinical management of VF?
4. If VF had not previously been assessed by a mental health professional, would it be appropriate to initiate pubertal suppression at this visit?

KEY TAKEAWAYS

- Sex is documented as assigned sex at birth (ASAB) or legal sex, and gender identity refers to the deeply held self-identification of gender.
- Incongruence between ASAB and gender identity will present differently at different developmental stages, although dysphoria becomes reliably more debilitating with the onset of secondary sex characteristics during puberty.
- Children with incongruence between their ASAB and gender identity, whose gender identity is affirmed and supported in all social domains, appear psychologically indistinguishable from cisgender controls and have developmentally normative levels of depression. Family acceptance correlates with increased resilience and improved psychological health and well-being.
- Gender incongruence is characterized by a marked and persistent incongruence between an individual's gender identity and ASAB, while gender dysphoria focuses on distress resulting from incongruence.
- The recommended therapeutic strategy at Tanner Stage 2 is to delay puberty using pharmacologic interventions.
- Gender affirmation may involve interventions within the specialties of pharmacology, mental health care, speech and communication therapy, surgery, social work, and legal realms. Pharmacological interventions, including pubertal suppression and MHT/FHT, are considered primary care.
- Suppression of endogenous puberty is often followed by coadministration of MHT/FHT to initiate puberty congruent with gender identity.

REFERENCES

1. Knudson G, De Cuypere G, Bockting W. Recommendations for revision of the DSM diagnoses of gender identity disorders: consensus statement of the World Professional Association for Transgender Health. *Int J Transgenderism.* 2010;12(2):115–118. doi:10.1080/15532739.2010.509215
2. Hidalgo MA, Hidalgo MA, Ehrensaft D, et al. The Gender affirmative model: what we know and what we aim to learn. *Hum Dev.* 2013;56(5):285–290. doi:10.1159/000355235
3. Coleman E, Bockting W, Botzer M, et al. Standards of care for the health of transsexual, transgender, and gender-nonconforming people, Version 7. *Int J Transgenderism.* 2012;13(4):165–232. doi:10.1080/15532739.2011.700873.
4. American Psychiatric Association. *Diagnostic and statistical manual of mental disorders.* 5th ed. American Psychiatric Association; 2013.
5. Reisner SL, Poteat T, Keatley J, et al. Global health burden and needs of transgender populations: A review. *Lancet.* 2016;388(10042):412–436. doi:10.1016/S0140-6736(16)00684-X
6. American Psychiatric Association. Gender dysphoria. Accessed 2013. https://www.psychiatry.org/File%20Library/Psychiatrists/Practice/DSM/APA_DSM-5-Gender-Dysphoria.pdf
7. Murchison G, Adkins D, Conrad LA, et al. Supporting & caring for transgender children. *Human Rights Campaign Foundation.* Published September 2016.
8. Substance Abuse and Mental Health Services Administration. *Ending conversion therapy: Supporting and affirming LGBTQ youth.* U.S. Department of Health and Human Services; 2015. HHS Publication No. (SMA) 15–4928.
9. Byne W, Bradley SJ, Coleman E, et al. Report of the American Psychiatric Association Task Force on treatment of gender identity disorder. *Arch Sex Behav.* 2012;41(4):759–796. doi:10.1007/s10508-012-9975-x
10. Minter SP. Supporting transgender children: new legal, social, and medical approaches. *J Homosex.* 2012;59(3):422–433. doi:10.1080/00918369.2012.653311
11. Wallace R, Russell H. Attachment and shame in gender-nonconforming children and their families: toward a theoretical framework for evaluating clinical interventions. *Int J Transgenderism.* 2013;14(3):113–126. doi:10.1080/15532739.2013.824845
12. de Vries ALC, Steensma TD, Doreleijers TAH, et al. Puberty suppression in adolescents with gender identity disorder: a prospective follow-up study. *J Sex Med.* 2011;8(8):2276–2283. doi:10.1111/j.1743-6109.2010.01943.x
13. Edwards-Leeper L, Spack NP. Psychological evaluation and medical treatment of transgender youth in an interdisciplinary "Gender Management Service" (GeMS) in a major pediatric center. *J Homosex.* 2012;59(3):321–336. doi:10.1080/00918369.2012.653302
14. Ryan C, Russell ST, Huebner D, et al. Family acceptance in adolescence and the health of LGBT young adults. *J Child Adolesc Psychiatr Nurs.* 2010;23(4):205–213. doi:10.1111/j.1744-6171.2010.00246.x
15. Olson KR, Durwood L, DeMeules M, et al. Mental health of transgender children who are supported in their identities. *Pediatrics.* 2016;137(3):e20153223. doi:10.1542/peds.2015-3223
16. Herman JL, Flores AR, Brown TNT, et al. *Age of individuals who identify as transgender in the United States.* The Williams Institute; 2017. https://williamsinstitute.law.ucla.edu/publications/age-trans-individuals-us/
17. Flores AR, Herman JL, Gates GJ, et al. *How many adults identify as transgender in the United States?* The Williams Institute; 2016. https://williamsinstitute.law.ucla.edu/publications/trans-adults-united-states/
18. Clark TC, Lucassen MF, Bullen P, et al. The health and well-being of transgender high school students: results from the New Zealand adolescent health survey (Youth'12). *J Adolesc Health.* 2014;55(1):93–99. doi:10.1016/j.jadohealth.2013.11.008

19. Bruessow D, Poteat T. Primary care providers' role in transgender healthcare. *JAAPA.* 2018;31(2):8–11. doi:10.1097/01.JAA.0000529780.62188.c0

20. American Psychological Association. Guidelines for psychological practice with transgender and gender nonconforming people. *Am Psychol.* 2015;70(9):832–864. doi:10.1037/a0039906

21. Guss C, Shumer D, Katz-Wise SL. Transgender and gender nonconforming adolescent care: psychosocial and medical considerations. *Curr Opin Pediatr.* 2015;27(4): 421–426. doi:10.1097/MOP.0000000000000240

22. Green ER. Debating trans inclusion in the feminist movement: a trans-positive analysis. *J Lesbian Stud.* 2006;10(1–2):231–248. doi:10.1300/J155v10n01_12

23. Hembree WC, Cohen-Kettenis PT, Gooren L, et al. endocrine treatment of gender-dysphoric/gender-incongruent persons: an Endocrine Society* clinical practice guideline. *J Clin Endocrinol Metabol.* 2017;102(11):3869–3903. doi:10.1210/jc.2017-01658

24. James SE, Herman, JL, Rankin S, et al. *The report of the 2015 U.S. transgender survey.* National Center for Transgender Equality; 2016. https://www.transequality .org/sites/default/files/docs/USTS-Full-Report-FINAL.PDF

25. National Center for Transgender Equality. *Understanding non-binary people: How to be respectful and supportive.* National Center for Transgender Equality; 2018. https://transequality.org/issues/resources/understanding -non-binary-people-how-to-be-respectful-and-supportive

26. Werft M, Sanchez E. Male, female, and muxes: places where a third gender is accepted. Published 2016. https:// www.globalcitizen.org/en/content/third-gender-gay -rights-equality/

27. National Center for Transgender Equality. ID documents center. *National Center for Transgender Equality.* https://transequality.org/issues/resources/understanding -non-binary-people-how-to-be-respectful-and-supportive

28. Beemyn G, Rankin S. Introduction to the special issue on "LGBTQ campus experiences." *J Homosex.* 2011;58(9):1159–1164. doi:10.1080/00918369.2011.605728

29. Olson KR, Key AC, Eaton NR. Gender cognition in transgender children. *Psychol Sci.* 2015;26(4):467–474. doi:10.1177/0956797614568156

30. Durwood L, McLaughlin KA, Olson KR. Mental health and self-worth in socially transitioned transgender youth. *J Am Acad Child Adolesc Psychiatr.* 2017;56(2): e116–e123, e112. doi:10.1016/j.jaac.2016.10.016

31. Newcomb ME, LaSala MC, Bouris A, et al. The influence of families on LGBTQ youth health: a call to action for innovation in research and intervention development. *LGBT Health.* 2019;6(4):139–145. doi:10.1089/ lgbt.2018.0157

32. Winter S, Diamond M, Green J, et al. Transgender people: health at the margins of society. *Lancet.* 2016;388(10042): 390–400. doi:10.1016/S0140-6736(16)00683-8

33. Bariola E, Lyons A, Leonard W, et al. Demographic and psychosocial factors associated with psychological distress and resilience among transgender individuals. *Am J Public Health.* 2015;105(10):2108–2116. doi:10.2105/ AJPH.2015.302763.

34. Nuttbrock L, Bockting W, Rosenblum A, et al. Gender abuse and major depression among transgender women:

a prospective study of vulnerability and resilience. *Am J Public Health.* 2013;104(11):2191–2198. doi:10.2105/ AJPH.2013.301545

35. Bockting WO, Miner MH, Swinburne Romine RE, et al. Stigma, mental health, and resilience in an online sample of the US transgender population. *Am J Public Health.* 2013;103(5):943–951. doi:10.2105/AJPH.2013.301241

36. Institute of Medicine. *The Health of Lesbian, Gay, Bisexual, and Transgender People: Building a Foundation for Better Understanding.* National Academies Press; 2011. https://www.ncbi.nlm.nih.gov/books/NBK64806

37. Grant JM, Mottet LA, Tanis J, et al. *Injustice at every turn: A report of the National Transgender Discrimination survey.* National Center for Transgender Equality and National Gay and Lesbian Task Force; 2011. https://www.transequality.org/sites/default/files/docs/ resources/NTDS_Report.pdf

38. Colizzi M, Costa R, Todarello O. Transsexual patients' psychiatric comorbidity and positive effect of cross-sex hormonal treatment on mental health: results from a longitudinal study. *Psychoneuroendocrinol.* 2014;39:65–73. doi:10.1016/j.psyneuen.2013.09.029

39. Asscheman H, T'Sjoen GG, Goren LJ. Morbidity in a multisite retrospective study of cross-sex hormone-treated transgender persons. *Joint Meeting of the International Society of Endocrinology and the Endocrine Society: ICE/ENDO 2014.* Published June 24, 2014.

40. Louden K. Largest study to date: transgender hormone treatment safe. Published July 2, 2014. https://www.medscape .com/viewarticle/827713#vp_1

41. Bruessow D, Wong H, Wilson-Stronk A. The welcoming environment. In: Schneider JS, Silenzio VMB, Erickson-Schroth L, eds. *The GLMA Handbook on LGBT Health. Vol. 2.* Praeger; 2019.

42. Bruessow D. Keeping up with LGBT health: Why it matters to your patients. *JAAPA.* 2011;24(3):14. Pubmed PMID: 21434493.

43. World Health Organization. *International Statistical Classification of Diseases and Related Health Problems.* 11th ed. World Health Organization; 2018.

44. Beek TF, Cohen-Kettenis PT, Bouman WP, et al. Gender incongruence of adolescence and adulthood: acceptability and clinical utility of the World Health Organization's proposed ICD-11 criteria. *PLoS One.* 2016;11(10):e0160066. doi:10.1371/journal.pone.0160066

45. Deutsch MB, Feldman JL. Updated recommendations from the World Professional Association for Transgender Health Standards of Care. *Am Fam Physician.* 2013;87(2):89–93. https://www.aafp.org/afp/2013/0115/ p89.html

46. Deutsch MB, ed. *Guidelines for the primary and gender-affirming care of transgender and gender nonbinary people.* 2nd ed. UCSF Transgender Care, Department of Family and Community Medicine, University of California; 2016. https://transcare.ucsf.edu/sites/transcare.ucsf .edu/files/Transgender-PGACG-6-17-16.pdf

47. Moser C. ICD-11 and gender incongruence: language is important. *Arch Sex Behav.* 2017;46(8):2515–2516. doi:10.1007/s10508-016-0936-7

48. Wiik A, Andersson DP, Brismar TB, et al. Metabolic and functional changes in transgender individuals follow-

ing cross-sex hormone treatment: design and methods of the Gender Dysphoria Treatment in Sweden (GETS) study. *Contemp Clin Trials Commun.* 2018;10:148–153. doi:10.1016/j.conctc.2018.04.005

49. Olson J. Hormonal therapy for transgender youth. *Society for Adolescent Health and Medicine.* Published 2010.

50. Olson J, Garofalo R. The peripubertal gender-dysphoric child: puberty suppression and treatment paradigms. *Pediatr Ann.* 2014;43(6):e132–e137. doi:10.3928/00904481-20140522-08

51. American College of Obstetricians and Gynecologists. Care for transgender adolescents. *American College of Obstetricians and Gynecologists.* Published 2017. https://www.acog.org/clinical/clinical-guidance/committee-opinion/articles/2017/01/care-for-transgender-adolescents

52. Soldin OP, Mattison DR. Sex differences in pharmacokinetics and pharmacodynamics. *Clin Pharmacokinet.* 2009;48(3):143–157. doi:10.2165/00003088-200948030-00001

53. Moyer AM, Matey ET, Miller VM. Individualized medicine: sex, hormones, genetics, and adverse drug reactions. *Pharmacol Res Perspect.* 2019;7(6):e00541. doi:10.1002/prp2.541

54. Jaffe JM, Gorton GN, Menkin D, et al. Gender affirming hormone therapy prescriber guidelines. *TransLine.* Published April 4, 2019. https://transline.zendesk.com/hc/enus/article_attachments/360047702053/TransLine_HRT_Guidelines_FINAL.pdf

55. Becasen JS, Denard CL, Mullins MM, et al. Estimating the prevalence of HIV and sexual behaviors among the US transgender population: a systematic review and meta-analysis, 2006–2017. *Am J Public Health.* 2018;109(1):e1–e8. doi:10.2105/AJPH.2018.304727

56. Shieh E, Marzinke MA, Fuchs EJ, et al. Transgender women on oral HIV pre-exposure prophylaxis have significantly lower tenofovir and emtricitabine concentrations when also taking oestrogen when compared to cisgender men. *J Int AIDS Soc.* 2019;22(11):e25405. doi:10.1002/jia2.25405

57. Radix A, Sevelius J, Deutsch MB. Transgender women, hormonal therapy and HIV treatment: a comprehensive review of the literature and recommendations for best practices. *J Int AIDS Soc.* 2016;19(3S2):20810. doi:10.7448/IAS.19.3.20810

58. Deutsch MB, Glidden DV, Sevelius J, et al. HIV pre-exposure prophylaxis in transgender women: a subgroup analysis of the iPrEx trial. *Lancet HIV.* 2015;2(12):e512–e519. doi:10.1016/S2352-3018(15)00206-4

59. Poteat T, Cooney E, Malik M, et al. Predictors of willingness to take PrEP among Black and Latina transgender women. *Conference on Retroviruses and Opportunistic Infections.* March 4–7, 2018.

60. Hiransuthikul A, Janamnuaysook R, Himmad K, et al. Drug-drug interactions between feminizing hormone therapy and pre-exposure prophylaxis among transgender women: the iFACT study. *J Int AIDS Soc.* 2019;22(7):e25338. doi:10.1002/jia2.25338

61. Ronda J, Nord A, Arrington-Sanders R, et al. Challenges in the management of the transgender patient with sickle cell disease. *Am J Hematol.* 2018;93(11):E360–E362. doi:10.1002/ajh.25242

62. Connolly MD, Zervos MJ, Barone CJ 2nd, et al. The mental health of transgender youth: advances in understanding. *J Adolesc Health.* 2016;59(5):489–495. doi:10.1016/j.jadohealth.2016.06.012

63. Narayan SK, Morrison T, Dugi DD 3rd, et al. Gender confirmation surgery for the endocrinologist. *Endocrinol Metab Clin North Am.* 2019;48(2):403–420. doi:10.1016/j.ecl.2019.02.002

64. Gray ML, Courey MS. Transgender voice and communication. *Otolaryngol Clin North Am.* 2019;52(4):713–722. doi:10.1016/j.otc.2019.03.007

65. Bradford NJ, Rider GN, Spencer KG. Hair removal and psychological well-being in transfeminine adults: associations with gender dysphoria and gender euphoria. *J Dermatol Treat.* 2019;1–8. doi:10.1080/09546634.2019.1687823

Antimicrobial Pharmacotherapy

Eric C. Nemec II and Kevin Michael O'Hara

LEARNING OBJECTIVES

- Describe the process for determining an infectious disease diagnosis, including the indications from findings related to antimicrobial susceptibility testing, minimum inhibitory concentration, and minimum bactericidal concentration.
- Define the importance of antibiotic stewardship.
- Differentiate between pharmacokinetics and pharmacodynamics and the impact of drug interactions and allergy as each relates to antimicrobial therapy.
- Identify the various methods for grouping antimicrobials, including the terms "bacteria cell wall activity," "generation," "bacteriostatic and bactericidal," and "classification."
- Describe the activity of antivirals, including their mechanisms of action and classifications.
- Describe the mechanisms of action of various antifungal agents that are currently available.

INTRODUCTION

Antimicrobial pharmacotherapy is a broad topic incorporating knowledge of microbiology, pharmacology, and medicine. This chapter intends to provide applied pharmacology knowledge, with clinical practice pearls as appropriate. Evidence-based practice guidelines from the Infectious Diseases Society of America (IDSA) can help direct appropriate therapy for specific infectious disease syndromes.

GENERAL APPROACH TO INFECTIOUS DISEASES

There are several important considerations for the clinician when prescribing antimicrobial therapy.[1] These include obtaining an accurate diagnosis of infection; understanding the difference between prophylactic, empiric, and definitive therapy; identifying opportunities to transition to narrower spectrum, and/or cost-effective oral agents for the shortest duration necessary; understanding drug characteristics of individual antimicrobial agents (e.g., pharmacodynamics and efficacy at the site of infection); and recognizing the adverse effects of antimicrobial agents.[1]

Generally, the treatment of infectious processes falls into one of three major categories: prophylactic, empiric, and definitive. Antimicrobial prophylaxis (AP) is the administration of a drug to prevent infection. Typically, prophylactic therapy should be limited to specific, well-accepted indications to avoid excess cost, toxicity, and antimicrobial resistance.[2] Antimicrobial prophylaxis is often recommended for surgical procedures; however, there are many other indications including herpes simplex infection, rheumatic fever, recurrent cellulitis, meningococcal disease, recurrent uncomplicated urinary tract infections in women, spontaneous bacterial peritonitis in patients with cirrhosis, influenza, infective endocarditis, and pertussis.[2]

An infectious disease diagnosis is reached by determining the site of infection, defining the host (e.g., immunocompromised, diabetic, of advanced age), and establishing, when possible, a microbiological diagnosis.[1] A microbiological diagnosis is important to ensure appropriate therapy. The timing of dosing versus microbiological sampling should be guided by individual patient acuity. Ideally, a clinician would collect a sample prior to—or at least concurrent with—the administration of an antimicrobial agent as it can suppress or inhibit culture growth. This microbiological diagnosis will typically take 48 to 72 hours; therefore, initial therapy is referred to as "empiric." The selection of empiric therapy is based on clinical presentation along with the best hypothesis of the causative pathogen. For example, most common bacterial causes of community-acquired pneumonia are *Streptococcus pneumoniae*, *Haemophilus influenzae*, *Chlamydia pneumoniae*, and *Mycoplasma pneumoniae*; thus, a regimen that would affect these organisms should be selected. The spectrum of empiric therapy is often broader than required.

When a pathogenic microorganism is identified in clinical cultures, the next typical step is antimicrobial susceptibility testing (AST). Using guidelines established by the Clinical and Laboratory Standards Institute (CLSI), a clinician can determine if a specific organism can grow in the presence of a given antimicrobial. Minimum inhibitory concentration (MIC) is defined as the concentration that inhibits visible bacterial growth at 24 hours of growth in specific media, at a specific temperature, and at a specific carbon dioxide concentration. The minimum bactericidal concentration (MBC) is the concentration of a drug that results in a 1,000-fold reduction in bacterial density at 24 hours of growth in the same specific conditions. An MIC result is clinically useful in terms of antimicrobial selection; however, these results are typically interpreted by the laboratory as "susceptible," "resistant," or "intermediate," according to CLSI criteria. A report of "susceptible" indicates that the isolate is likely to be inhibited by the usually achievable concentration of a particular antimicrobial agent when the recommended dosage is administrated for the particular site of infection. A result of "intermediate" would indicate a variable response based on site of infection and potential drug concentration. A "resistant" organism will not respond to that given drug and may impart resistance to the entire class of drugs. Once microbiology results have helped to identify the etiologic pathogen and/or antimicrobial susceptibility data are available, the clinician should attempt to narrow the antibiotic spectrum.

ANTIMICROBIAL STEWARDSHIP AND OVERPRESCRIBING

The rapid global emergence of resistant microorganisms presents a public health crisis, endangering the efficacy of antibiotics, which have already transformed medicine and saved countless lives.[3] Unfortunately, the overuse and inappropriate use of antibiotics clearly drives the evolution of resistance. This, coupled with the limited numbers of new drugs in the pharmaceutical industry pipeline, decreases the clinical

armamentarium. One of the largest contributors to overuse errors is prescribing antibiotics for viral infections. Patients may attempt to pressure clinicians into prescribing an antibiotic. In the outpatient setting, the cost and ability to obtain cultures in low-acuity infections may lead to unwarranted empiric treatment. In addition to a missing indication there are a few other errors common when using antimicrobials. First is the continued use of empiric treatment without evidence of infection. Second is the treatment of a positive culture in the absence of disease. Bacterial colonization of the urinary tract is relatively common occurrence in a geriatric female patient, so while one may find a "positive" urine culture, the treatment of asymptomatic bacteriuria has not been shown to improve patient outcomes. The last major pitfall of antimicrobial therapy is when a clinician fails to narrow antimicrobial therapy pursuant to identifying a causative agent. Once culture and susceptibility data are available, an antibiotic with the narrowest possible spectrum and most feasible dosing strategy should be selected for continuation of therapy. Antimicrobial stewardship refers to coordinated interventions designed to improve and measure the appropriate use of antimicrobial agents by promoting the selection of the optimal antimicrobial drug regimen including dosing, duration of therapy, and route of administration.[4] Simply put, clinicians should use the right drug for the right patient, for the right duration.

PHARMACOKINETICS AND PHARMACODYNAMICS

The pharmacodynamics and pharmacokinetics of any antimicrobial agent determine drug efficacy at the site of the infection. Knowledge of the drug's antimicrobial pharmacodynamic effects (e.g., rate and extent of bactericidal action and postantibiotic effect) provides a rational basis for determination of optimal dosing regimens. Suppression of bacterial growth that persists after short exposure of organisms to antimicrobial agents has been seen since early investigations with penicillin. The postantibiotic effect (PAE) is defined as persistent suppression of bacterial growth after a brief exposure (1 or 2 hours) to an antibiotic in the absence of host defenses.[5,6]

Pharmacokinetics describes the time course of drug levels in body fluids as a result of absorption, distribution, and elimination of a drug after administration. (Refer to Chapter 2, for further discussion.) Most antimicrobial drugs are administered either by the intravenous (IV) or oral administration (PO) routes. Absorption is important for antimicrobials as it will help determine the route of administration based upon available/appropriate drugs and care setting. A drug's bioavailability (abbreviated as F), is measured as the proportion of a drug's dose that reaches the systemic circulation. When administered intravenously, a drug is considered 100% bioavailable; however, when administered orally, the proportion of available drug may be less. A number of antimicrobial drugs have excellent oral bioavailability, meaning there is minimal difference in absorption when comparing IV to PO. For example, metronidazole, doxycycline, linezolid, trimethoprim–sulfamethoxazole, and the fluoroquinolones all have good oral bioavailability. Ciprofloxacin (a fluoroquinolone) has a bioavailability of approximately 80%; this pharmacokinetic property can be illustrated by comparing the typical oral and intravenous doses (400 mg IV = 500 mg PO).

Administration of an antimicrobial medication must achieve a concentration equal to or greater than the MIC at the site of infection in order to be effective. For this reason, it is important to note a drug's distribution prior to administration. Some anatomical sites such as the ocular fluid, cerebrospinal fluid, and bone often have much lower concentrations than serum levels.

Although there are many classes of antimicrobial agents, each with distinct mechanisms of action, they can be categorized as either "bacteriostatic" and "bactericidal" based on how they affect microbes. Bacteriostatic means that the agent prevents the growth of bacteria (i.e., it keeps them in the stationary phase of growth), and bactericidal means that it kills bacteria.[7] Bactericidal drugs include drugs that act primarily on the cell wall (e.g., beta-lactams) or cell membrane (e.g., daptomycin). Bacteriostatic agents inhibit bacterial replication without killing the organism. Bacteriostatic drugs require the aid of host defenses to clear tissues of the infecting microorganism. Most bacteriostatic drugs, including sulfonamides, tetracyclines, and macrolides, act by inhibiting protein synthesis.[1] There are a few clinical situations in which bactericidal activity is considered necessary: endocarditis, meningitis, osteomyelitis, and neutropenia.[7] However, virtually all available data from high-quality, randomized controlled trials demonstrate no intrinsic superiority of bactericidal compared to bacteriostatic agents.[8]

The last important pharmacodynamic characteristics are based upon concepts of time-dependent versus concentration-dependent effects. Drugs that exhibit time-dependent activity (beta-lactams and vancomycin) exhibit bactericidal activity based upon the time the serum concentration is above the organism MIC. In contrast, drugs that exhibit concentration-dependent effects (aminoglycosides, fluoroquinolones, metronidazole, and daptomycin) have enhanced bactericidal activity as the serum concentration is increased.[1]

DRUG–DRUG INTERACTIONS

As with all medications, there is the potential for drug–drug interactions, which may require closer monitoring or alteration of therapy. Antimicrobials are especially challenging because they are prescribed only for a limited course. Almost all antibiotics can potentiate the effects of warfarin by inhibiting intestinal flora that produce Vitamin K. Inhibition of the hepatic metabolism of warfarin is another possible mechanism for increased bleeding.[9] Divalent cations (calcium and magnesium) and trivalent cations (aluminum and ferrous sulfate) can form insoluble complexes in the gut if they are taken concurrently with fluoroquinolones; this can be avoided by separating the dose timing. The interaction between oral contraceptives and other antibiotics is controversial in that no definitive studies have demonstrated contraceptive failure from such combinations. One concern often reported is the potential of lower efficacy of oral contraceptives when taken concomitantly with antibiotics; however, rifampin is the only antibiotic proven to decrease serum ethinyl estradiol and progestin levels in women.[10]

DRUG ALLERGIES

Antibiotics are the most common cause of life-threatening immune-mediated drug reactions, so treatment of patients with identified allergies should be approached with care.[11] Antibiotics can result in adverse drug reactions (ADRs) and hypersensitivity reactions (HSRs) through a variety of mechanisms though rashes and hives are the most commonly reported HSRs. Often these documented allergies will require a clinician to change therapies to broader spectrum agents of a different class which may lead to antimicrobial resistance, prolonged hospitalizations, readmissions, and increased costs.[12] In most cases, a true drug allergy will preclude the use of drugs within the same class. For example, a patient with an anaphylactic reaction to ciprofloxacin should likely not receive levofloxacin.

Of significant concern are allergies to beta-lactam antibiotics as 5% to 15% of all people in developed countries report a penicillin allergy, which in theory could affect the selection of a cephalosporin, carbapenem, or monobactam drug.[11] Despite this reported prevalence, 80% to 90% of those reporting a penicillin allergy will have a negative response to penicillin skin testing.[13] A common myth is that about 10% of patients with a penicillin allergy history will experience an allergic reaction if administered a cephalosporin; however, more recent prospective studies have found this to be less than 1%.[14,15] This cross-reactivity theory postulated that the allergenicity was related to the beta-lactam ring itself; however, it appears that cross-reactivity between penicillins and cephalosporins is more likely associated with structurally similar side chains. It is important to determine whether the allergy represents an immunoglobulin (IgE)-mediated reaction, a delayed-onset reaction, an adverse effect, or simply an intolerance. For patients with a history of nonsevere, nonIgE–mediated reactions to penicillins, the use of cephalosporins and carbapenems may not be precluded; however, clinicians should attempt to employ agents with nonsimilar side-chains.[16] Of note, aztreonam is a monobactam that is less immunogenic and is associated with fewer allergic reactions compared with other beta-lactams. It can be used safely in most beta-lactam allergies (e.g., a patient with both a penicillin and cephalosporin allergy) unless a patient has a specific allergy to ceftazidime.

ANTIMICROBIAL DRUGS

The different ways to categorize antimicrobial medications are by class, indication, or mechanism of action. This chapter seeks to employ the latter organization as it allows readers to logically categorize drugs, understand side effects, spectrum of activity, and more easily recall the mechanism of action. Each section begins with the prototypical agent and expands upon the class as new drugs were approved that broaden the spectrum of activity, as well as decrease unwanted adverse effects.

DRUGS THAT TARGET THE CELL WALL

The discovery of penicillin is one of the greatest milestones in modern medicine.[17] It serves as the prototypical agent for the beta-lactam class of antimicrobial drugs. All penicillins are derivatives of 6-aminopenicillanic acid and possess the beta-lactam ring structure responsible for its antibacterial activity. High doses of beta-lactam drugs can cause seizures.

MECHANISM OF ACTION

Bacterial cell walls are created via a complex metabolic pathway that combines mucopeptides and peptidoglycans resulting in a cytoplasmic membrane.[18,19] The enzymatic targets for these antibiotics are absent from mammalian cells allowing for a selective toxicity to the bacteria. The beta-lactam class of drugs exerts its action in the final stage of bacterial cell wall synthesis by binding to species-specific proteins named "penicillin-binding proteins" (PBPs). Beta-lactams are analogues of the terminal D-Alanine-D-Alanine amino acid of the peptidoglycan chain. By binding to the PBP, these drugs inhibit the transpeptidase activities responsible for cross-linking of the peptidoglycan chain, which is important for cell wall integrity, especially in gram-positive bacteria. Inhibition of these enzymes by beta-lactam antibiotics results in decreased

cell wall synthesis and can also activate autolytic enzymes that destroy the cell wall. In susceptible organisms, these drugs are bactericidal. Beta-lactams share a similar mechanism of action; therefore, using two drugs from this class for the same infection may not be advantageous.

RESISTANCE

There are three major mechanisms of bacterial resistance that can limit the clinical utility of the beta-lactam drugs.[20] Beta-lactamases are hydrolytic enzymes that disrupt the amide bond of the beta-lactam ring rendering the drug ineffective. Beta-lactamases are most common in gram-negative organisms. There are beta-lactamases specific to each of the drugs in the class—for example, penicillinase is specific to penicillin, extended-spectrum beta-lactamase, and cephalosporinase which affect cephalosporins and monobactams, and carbapenemase will hydrolyze all beta-lactams. Alterations to the PBP may also impart resistance to a given antibiotic. Enterococci often have low-affinity PBPs. Last, efflux and modification or deletion of porin function can play a role in resistance to specific beta-lactam drugs. To counteract resistance, some drugs are manufactured in combination with a beta-lactamase inhibitor such as sulbactam, clavulanic acid, or tazobactam.

BETA-LACTAM DRUGS

Natural Penicillins

Natural penicillins include oral (Penicillin V Potassium) and parenteral (Penicillin G).[21,22] As one of the oldest antimicrobial agents available, bacteria has developed significant resistance; thus it is a poor choice for empiric therapy. The natural penicillins are most active against nonbeta-lactamase–producing gram-positive bacteria such as *Streptococcus pyogenes*, anaerobes, and select gram-negative cocci such as *Neisseria*. Penicillin remains the drug of choice in neurosyphilis (*Treponema pallidum*). See **Table 30.1** for adult and pediatric dosages.

Antistaphylococcal Penicillins

Antistaphylococcal penicillins include nafcillin, oxacillin, dicloxacillin, methicillin, and cloxacillin. These drugs were developed to be penicillinase-stable penicillins and were used primarily for staphylococcal infections until the emergence of methicillin-resistant *S. aureus* (MRSA). Methicillin is not used today because of the high risk of nephritis; however, it remains part of standard nomenclature when referring to resistant organisms. These drugs still are a good choice for infections caused by methicillin-sensitive *S. aureus* (MSSA) and streptococci. Both the natural and

TABLE 30.1 Penicillins

Medication	Typical Dosage Range
Natural Penicillins	
Penicillin G	Adult: 2–4 million units IV q4–6h Pediatric: 100,000–400,000 units/kg/d IV divided q4–6h
Penicillin G benzathine	Adult: 1.2–2.4 million units IM at specified intervals Pediatric: 300,000–2.4 million units IM at specified intervals
Penicillin G procaine	Adult: 600,000–4.8 million IM divided q12–24h Pediatric: 25,000–50,000 units/kg/d IM divided 1–2 times/d
Penicillin V potassium	Adult: 250–500 mg PO q6h Pediatric: 25–50 mg/kg/d PO divided q6–8h
Antistaphylococcal Penicillins	
Cloxacillin	Adult: 250–500 mg PO q6h Pediatric: 25–50 mg/kg/d PO divided q6h
Dicloxacillin	Adult: 250–500 mg PO q6h Pediatric: 12.5–100 mg/kg/d PO divided q6h
Nafcillin	Adult: 500 mg–1 g IV q4–6h Pediatric: 50 mg–200 mg/kg/d IV divided q4–6h
Oxacillin	Adult: 500 mg–2 g IV q4–6h Pediatric: 100–200 mg/kg/d IV divided q4–6h
Aminopenicillins	
Ampicillin	Adult: 1–2 g IV q4–6h Pediatric: 100–400 mg/kg/d IV divided q4–6h
Amoxicillin	Adult: 250–500 mg PO q8h *or* 875 mg–1,000 mg PO q12h Pediatric: 80–90 mg/kg/day po divided q8–12h mg/kg/d PO divided q8–12h
Antipseudomonal Penicillins and Beta-Lactamase Inhibitor Drugs	
Amoxicillin/clavulanate	Adult: 250–500 mg PO q8h *or* 500 mg–875 mg PO q12h *or* 2,000 mg PO q12h (Augmentin® extended-release) Pediatric: 20–40 mg/kg/d PO divided q8–12h
Ampicillin/sulbactam	Adult: 1.5–3 g IV q6h Pediatric: 100–400 mg/kg/d IV divided q6h
Piperacillin/tazobactam	Adult: 4.5 g IV q6–8h *or* 3.375 g IV q6h Pediatric: 240–300 mg/kg/d IV divided q8h

d, day; h, hour; IM, intramuscularly; IV, intravenously; PO, orally; q, every.

antistaphylococcal penicillins have short half-lives necessitating frequent dosing. See Table 30.1 for adult and pediatric dosages.

Aminopenicillins

Ampicillin and amoxicillin are aminopenicillins which were developed with improved activity against Gram-negative pathogens and have sufficient bioavailability to allow for oral administration.[23] Of the two, amoxicillin has better bioavailability, less incidence of diarrhea, and is administered less frequently and thus is often a better option for an oral agent. The antibacterial spectrum of aminopenicillins includes nonbeta-lactamase–producing gram-positive cocci, anaerobes, and gram-negative cocci, including *Neisseria* and *Enterobacteriaceae* that do not produce beta-lactamase. These agents are not active against *Pseudomonas* spp. and are hydrolyzed by beta-lactamases, making them ineffective against beta-lactamase-producing strains of bacteria. The major adverse effects associated with ampicillin use are rashes, which tend to occur more commonly than with other penicillins. These macular rashes usually appear 4 to 5 days after the initiation of therapy; these nonurticarial rashes are not indicative of a true hypersensitivity reaction. Amoxicillin can also cause a morbilliform rash if given to a patient acutely infected with Epstein–Barr virus. Conventional doses of amoxicillin (45 mg/kg/day) are effective against all susceptible strains of *S. pneumoniae*; however, high doses (80–90 mg/kg/day) are required for adequate concentrations in the middle ear for the treatment of acute otitis media. See Table 30.1 for adult and pediatric dosages.

Antipseudomonal Penicillin and Beta-Lactamase Inhibitor Drugs

Antipseudomonal penicillins which include piperacillin and ticarcillin are administered only parenterally and are important in the treatment of gram-negative infections; however, they remain susceptible to penicillinase. The antibacterial spectra of antipseudomonal penicillins and aminopenicillins can be broadened by combining them with beta-lactamase inhibitors; thus, these drugs are currently used only in combination with a beta-lactamase inhibitor. They are available in the following products: ampicillin/sulbactam (Unasyn), amoxicillin/clavulanate (Augmentin), and piperacillin/tazobactam (Zosyn). Clavulanic acid is a potent inhibitor of beta-lactamases produced by *Klebsiella pneumoniae*, *Proteus mirabilis*, *Proteus vulgaris*, *Bacteroides fragilis*, *S. aureus*, *H. influenzae*, and other anaerobes; however, it does not affect the pharmacokinetics of amoxicillin, nor does it enhance its activity; rather it protects the penicillin from a beta-lactamase. Of note within this group, only piperacillin/tazobactam has activity against *Pseudomonas aeruginosa*, which makes it especially important in healthcare-acquired infections. Amoxicillin/clavulanic acid is the only product available in an oral formulation. There is a fixed ratio of clavulanic acid within a preparation; this lower dose of clavulanic acid is associated with a lower incidence of diarrhea. Also of note regarding the beta-lactamase inhibitors is that sulbactam has useful activity against *Acinetobacter baumannii*, which is often resistant to many drugs. High-dose ampicillin/sulbactam can be an effective treatment against *A. baumannii* where the sulbactam is actually the active drug.

These drugs, especially piperacillin/tazobactam, have a very wide spectrum of activity and make them a good choice for empiric therapy; clinicians must remember to select a narrower spectrum agent once AST results are available. For example, if a patient is at risk for hospital-acquired (nosocomial) pneumonia, empiric therapy should include coverage for *Pseudomonas aeruginosa*; if AST identifies *Streptococcus pneumoniae* as the responsible pathogen, then a drug with a narrower spectrum should be selected. See Table 30.1 for adult and pediatric dosages.

Cephalosporins

Cephalosporins are generally grouped into generations based upon their spectrum of activity against aerobic and gram-negative bacilli and gram-positive bacteria. Cephalosporins are used very frequently because they cover a broad range of organisms, do not have many serious adverse effects, and are easy to administer. While in a different class than penicillin drugs, they employ the same mechanism as all beta-lactam drugs: inhibition of the peptidoglycan cross-linking of a bacterial cell wall, leading to cellular death. This text organizes cephalosporins by generation. See **Table 30.2** for adult and pediatric dosages.

First-Generation Cephalosporins

First-generation cephalosporins include:

- **Oral:** Cefadroxil and cephalexin
- **Parenteral:** Cefazolin

These drugs are often used as alternatives for antistaphylococcal penicillins as they have a similar spectrum of activity and require less frequent administration which helps to reduce incidence of infusion-related adverse effects such as phlebitis. The first-generation cephalosporins are good for skin and skin structure infections caused by Methicillin-sensitive *S. aureus* or streptococci. Cefazolin is the only parenteral first-generation cephalosporin available in the United States and is most commonly used for surgical prophylaxis, which should be limited to a total of 24 hours of therapy.

Second-Generation Cephalosporins

Second-generation cephalosporins include:

- **Oral:** cefaclor, cefprozil, and cefuroxime
- **Parenteral:** cefuroxime, cefoxitin, and cefotetan

Compared with first-generation agents, the second-generation cephalosporins are less active against gram-positive microbes such as staphylococci; however, they have greater gram-negative activity. There are two subgroups of the second-generation cephalosporins. First, the cephamycins, which include cefoxitin and cefotetan, are active against bacteroides in addition to *Escherichia coli*, *P. mirabilis*, and *Klebsiella*. The second subgroup, which includes cefuroxime and cefprozil, has greater activity against *H. influenzae*. Similar to first-generation cephalosporins, second-generation agents do not cross the blood–brain barrier in concentrations high enough to effectively treat central nervous system (CNS) infections.

Third-Generation Cephalosporins

Third-generation cephalosporins include:

- **Oral:** cefpodoxime, cefixime, cefdinir, ceftibuten, cefditoren
- **Parenteral:** ceftriaxone, ceftazidime, cefotaxime

TABLE 30.2 Cephalosporins

Medication	Typical Dosage Range
First-Generation Cephalosporins	
Cefadroxil	Adult: 500–1,000 mg PO q12h Pediatric: 30 mg/kg/d PO divided q12h
Cephalexin	Adult: 250–1,000 mg PO q6h Pediatric: 25–100 mg/kg/d PO divided q6h
Cefazolin	Adult: 500 mg–1 g IV q8h Pediatric: 50–100 mg/kg/d IV divided q8h
Second-Generation Cephalosporins	
Cefaclor	Adult: 250–500 mg PO q8h Pediatric: 20–40 mg/kg/d PO divided q8–12h
Cefotetan	Adult: 1–2 g IV q12h Pediatric: 40–80 mg/kg/d IV divided q12h
Cefoxitin	Adult: 1–2 g IV q6–8h Pediatric: 80–160 mg/kg/d IV divided q4–8h
Cefprozil	Adult: 250–500 mg PO q12h Pediatric: 15–30 mg/kg/d PO divided q12h
Cefuroxime axetil (oral)	Adult: 250–500 mg PO q12h Pediatric: 20–30 mg/kg/d PO divided q12h
Cefuroxime sodium (parenteral)	Adult: 750 mg–1.5 g IV q8h Pediatric: 50–240 mg/kg/d IV divided q8h mg/kg/d IV divided q8h
Third-Generation Cephalosporins	
Cefdinir	Adult: 300–600 mg PO q12–24h Pediatric: 7 mg/kg/d PO divided q12h
Cefditoren	Adult: 200–400 mg PO q12h Pediatric >12 years: 200–400 mg PO q12h
Cefixime	Adult: 400 mg/d PO q12–24h Pediatric: 8 mg/kg/d PO divided q12h
Cefotaxime	Adult: 1–2 g IV q8h Pediatric: 100–300 mg/kg/d IV divided q6–8h
Cefpodoxime	Adult: 100–400 mg PO q12h Pediatric: 10 mg/kg/d PO divided q12h
Ceftazidime	Adult: 1–2 g IV q8h Pediatric: 90–1,500 mg/kg/d IV divided q8h
Ceftibuten	Adult: 400 mg PO q24h Pediatric: 9 mg/kg/d PO divided q24h
Ceftriaxone	Adult: 1–2 g IV q12–24h Pediatric: 50–100 mg/kg/d IV divided q12–24h
Fourth-Generation Cephalosporins	
Cefepime	Adult: 1–2 g IV q8–12h Pediatric: 50 mg/kg/d IV divided q8h
Fifth-Generation or Anti-MRSA Cephalosporin	
Ceftaroline	Adult: 600 mg IV q8h
Fifth-Generation or Anti-MRSA Cephalosporin	
Ceftazidime/avibactam	Adult: 2.5 g IV q8h
Ceftolozane/tazobactam	Adult: 750 mg IV q8h

d, day; h, hour; IV, intravenously; MRSA, methicillin-resistant *Staphylococcus aureus*; PO, orally; q, every.

The third-generation cephalosporin class has more gram-negative activity compared to the first- and second-generation cephalosporins due to its stability to the common beta-lactamases of gram-negative bacilli. Third generation cephalosporins are highly active against Enterobacteriaceae; however, when compared to previous generations, have less staphylococcal activity. Additionally, they can cross the blood–brain barrier making them effective in many central nervous system infections. Similar to the second generation, the third generation of cephalosporins can also be subdivided. In one subgroup, cefotaxime and ceftriaxone have poor activity against *Pseudomonas aeruginosa*, whereas ceftazidime has activity against *Pseudomonas*, but has poor activity against gram-positive organisms. Ceftriaxone has the longest serum half-life of this class and can be administered typically once a day, with twice a day reserved for meningitis. Ceftriaxone has a few unique challenges in the neonatal population: first, it should never be administered in a line that contains a calcium-related product as it can crystallize in the kidneys and lungs. Second, it can precipitate biliary sludging. Cefotaxime is typically safer in this population as it does not exhibit these same adverse effects.

Fourth-Generation Cephalosporin

Cefepime is the only fourth-generation cephalosporin currently available in the United States. Like third-generation drugs, it is active against Enterobacteriaceae, *Neisseria*, and *H. influenzae*; however, it has greater activity against gram-negative enteric bacteria and *P. aeruginosa*. Due to its broad spectrum of activity, cefepime is a good choice for many nosocomial infections. Patients treated with cefepime are at an increased risk of seizures (specifically nonconvulsive status epilepticus); especially patients with renal dysfunction in whom the dose is not appropriately adjusted.

Fifth-Generation Cephalosporin or Anti-MRSA Cephalosporin

Ceftaroline can be considered a fifth-generation cephalosporin; however, the CLSI would classify it as an anti-MRSA cephalosporin. It is different in that it loses gram-negative activity in comparison to the fourth-generation cephalosporin cefepime and therefore does not follow the pattern of improved gram-negative coverage as the generations increase. Its mechanism of action is similar to all other cephalosporins except it has a higher affinity for penicillin-binding protein 2a, which is expressed by methicillin-resistant staphylococci; thus, it is unique as it is the only beta-lactam to have this activity. Also unique is that it has activity against *Enterococcus faecalis*.

Cephalosporin and Beta-Lactamase Inhibitor Drugs

Ceftolozane/tazobactam and Ceftazidime/avibactam are two newer agents that combine cephalosporins with a beta-lactamase inhibitor. Ceftolozane is a novel cephalosporin whose gram-negative activity is expanded by the addition of tazobactam. It has activity against most aerobic and gram-negative organisms, including *Pseudomonas aeruginosa* and most extended-spectrum beta-lactamase (ESBL) Enterobacteriaceae; however, it has limited gram-positive activity. Avibactam is a novel beta-lactamase inhibitor, similar to other beta-lactamase inhibitors; it has limited efficacy by itself. Avibactam helps preserve activity against ESBL-producing organisms, and some carbapenemase producing organisms.

Carbapenems

Carbapenems, to include imipenem/cilastatin, meropenem, ertapenem, and doripenem, have the broadest spectrum of activity against gram-negative organisms. They are structurally similar to the beta-lactams, and thus have a similar mechanism of action; however, they are resistant to effects by most beta-lactamases. Carbapenems cover gram-negative organisms (including the Enterobacteriaceae, *P. aeruginosa*, *H. influenzae*, and *N. gonorrhoeae*), anaerobes, and gram-positive organisms. They are not active against MRSA, *Stenotrophomonas maltophilia*, *Burkholderia cepacia*, or *E. faecium*. Imipenem/cilastatin, meropenem, and doripenem generally have the same spectrum of activity; however, ertapenem lacks activity against *P. aeruginosa* and *Acinetobacter*. This is an important consideration when attempting to narrow therapy; it also has a long half-life which allows for once daily dosing in contrast to the other carbapenems that are given multiple times per day. Imipenem is inactivated by renal enzymes which is why it is coformulated with cilastatin which prevents this breakdown. While most of the carbapenems are well tolerated, imipenem is associated with central nervous system toxicity and seizures. Meropenem is available as a combination with a beta-lactamase inhibitor vaborbactam. Vaborbactam is a novel broad-spectrum beta-lactamase inhibitor that potently inhibits carbapenemases, including *K. pneumoniae* carbapenemases, which have been particularly problematic as they are resistant to most antimicrobial therapy. However, it does not enhance activity against carbapenem-resistant *P. aeruginosa* or *Acinetobacter* spp. While the broad spectrum of activity appears appealing in terms of empiric therapy, if resistance develops to carbapenems, there are very limited options in treating carbapenem-resistant organisms. See **Table 30.3** for adult and pediatric dosages.

TABLE 30.3 Carbapenems

Medication	Typical Dosage Range
Doripenem[a]	Adult: 500 mg IV q8h
Ertapenem	Adult: 1 g IV/IM daily Pediatric: 30 mg/kg/d IV divided q12h
Imipenem/cilastatin	Adult: 250 mg–1 g IV q6h Pediatric: 25–100 mg/kg/d IV divided q6h
Meropenem	Adult: 500 mg–1 g IV q8h Pediatric: 30–120 mg/kg/d IV divided q8h

[a]The brand name Doribax® (Doripenem) is no longer available in the United States; no generic is available.

h, hour; IM, intramuscularly; IV, intravenously; q, every.

Monobactam

Aztreonam is the only available monobactam antibiotic available. These are similar to other beta-lactam drugs; however, its beta-lactam ring is not fused to another ring. It has activity similar to ceftazidime or the aminoglycosides. Aztreonam is clinically useful in patients who have both true penicillin and cephalosporin allergies as it does not appear to exhibit cross-allergenicity. Patients specifically allergic to ceftazidime may be allergic to aztreonam because they have a similar side-chain. Dosages vary based on severity of infection, from 500 mg to 2 g intravenously every 6 to 12 hours for adults, and 90 to 120 mg/kg/day intravenously divided every 6 to 8 hours for children.

Glycopeptides

There are currently two glycopeptides available for use in the United States: vancomycin and telavancin. Glycopeptides bind to terminal D-ala-D-ala chains on peptidoglycan in the cell wall, preventing cross links of peptidoglycan chains; telavancin has a secondary mechanism in that it also disrupts bacterial cell membrane barrier functions. Glycopeptides are clinically important because they possess activity against gram-positive bacteria, specifically MRSA. Telavancin is technically a synthetic lipoglycopeptide but is distinct from other lipoglycopeptides in that it still requires daily dosing (dalbavancin can be given as a single dose regimen, or a two-dose regimen with the second dose given a week later). Telavancin has activity against most gram-positive organisms such as methicillin-resistant *S. aureus* (MRSA), *E. faecalis* and *E. faecium*.

Vancomycin dosing requires careful consideration of pharmacokinetics and is based upon the severity of infection, patient weight, and renal function. Generally, vancomycin is dosed at 15 mg/kg of actual body weight every 12 hours, in 250-mg increments. Similar to the beta-lactam antibiotics, vancomycin exhibits time-dependent antimicrobial properties, meaning in order for the bactericidal activity to continue, the free concentration of these drugs should be maintained above the MIC. Traditionally, trough concentrations (lab level drawn immediately before the fourth dose or after reaching a steady state concentration) have been considered useful as a surrogate measurement for area under the time-concentration curve (AUC) and an indicator of the time where the concentration was greater than the MIC. There is no role for routine monitoring of peak vancomycin concentrations.

Vancomycin is associated with several adverse drug reactions. Red man syndrome is a histamine-mediated flushing that occurs during or after infusion; it is considered an infusion reaction and can typically be avoided by extending the infusion time. While less common, telavancin also exhibits a similar infusion-related reaction. Vancomycin also has the potential to cause nephrotoxicity and ototoxicity. Nephrotoxicity has been associated with steady-state vancomycin trough concentrations exceeding 15 mcg/mL; however, it is more likely to occur when coadministered with other nephrotoxic drugs such as aminoglycosides. Nephrotoxicity is usually reversible. Ototoxicity is more common in older patients and presents as tinnitus or ataxia. Vancomycin has very limited oral bioavailability; however, oral administration is the first line treatment for Clostridioides (formerly clostridium) difficile infection.

Lipoglycopeptides (Long-Acting Glycopeptides)

Dalbavancin and oritavancin are lipoglycopeptides that employ a glycopeptide structure, and slow their elimination allowing for one-time or two-time dosing for an entire treatment course. As glycopeptide derivatives, they still work by binding to the D-alanyl-D-alanine terminus of the cell wall peptidoglycan preventing cross-linking and cell wall synthesis. Both are approved for treatment of adults with acute bacterial skin and skin structure infections (ABSSSI) caused by susceptible gram-positive pathogens which include MRSA. These drugs are generally well tolerated; however, their convenient one- or two-time dosing (**Table 30.4**) come with the tradeoff of being extremely expensive.

TABLE 30.4 Lipoglycopeptides (long-acting glycopeptides)

Medication	Typical Dosage Range
Dalbavancin	Adult: 1 g IV followed by 500 mg IV 1 week later
Oritavancin	Adult: 1.2 g IV as a single injection

IV, intravenously.

DRUGS THAT BLOCK PROTEIN SYNTHESIS

AMINOGLYCOSIDES

Several aminoglycosides are available for clinical use in the United States.[24] These include gentamicin, tobramycin, amikacin, plazomicin, streptomycin, neomycin, and paromomycin. Of these, gentamicin, tobramycin, and amikacin are most commonly used for systemic treatment of infections caused by aerobic gram-negative bacilli. They are sometimes used in combination with other drugs such as beta-lactams for the treatment of select gram-positive infections. The combination of aminoglycosides and beta-lactam drugs exhibits synergism, meaning that when used together they produce an effect more potent than if they were used alone.[25] Beta-lactams can increase cellular penetration which allow the aminoglycosides to more readily exert their mechanism of action within the cell.

The aminoglycosides act primarily by binding to the aminoacyl site within the 30S ribosomal subunit, leading to misreading of the genetic code and premature termination. Aminoglycosides have a broad spectrum of activity against aerobic gram-negative organisms as well as mycobacteria. They have poor coverage against atypical and anaerobic bacteria. Compared to other antibiotic classes, aminoglycosides enjoy limited antimicrobial resistance; organisms that possess either ESBL or klebsiella pneumoniae carbapenemase (KPC) are often also resistant to aminoglycosides. Aminoglycosides exhibit concentration-dependent microbiologic activity, meaning higher concentrations of aminoglycosides (relative to the organism's MIC) to induce more rapid, and complete, killing of the pathogen.[26]

While aminoglycosides have limited resistance problems, their clinical utility is limited because there are lesser toxic agents available that have similar efficacy and no monitoring requirements.

Traditional parenteral aminoglycoside dosing in adults involves the administration of a weight-based dose divided two to three times daily in patients with normal renal function. In contrast, extended-interval aminoglycoside therapy (also known as "once-daily aminoglycosides," "single daily aminoglycoside dosing," "consolidated or high-dose aminoglycoside therapy") utilizes a higher weight-based dose administered at an extended interval (every 24 hours for those with normal renal function and longer for those with renal dysfunction). While both strategies have similar efficacy, extended-interval dosing takes advantage of two pharmacodynamic properties, the postantibiotic effect and concentration-dependent killing, to offer a number of potential advantages to traditional dosing. This includes simpler dosing and monitoring (which also has

a cost advantage) and potentially decreasing the risk of nephrotoxicity.

There are two main adverse effects that require caution for aminoglycosides: ototoxicity and nephrotoxicity. Aminoglycosides are associated with cochlear and vestibular toxicity in a substantial proportion of patients receiving the drug for prolonged periods.[27] Acute kidney injury (AKI) due to acute tubular necrosis is a relatively common complication of aminoglycoside therapy; up to 20% of patients will experience a 50% increase in serum creatinine concentration from baseline.[28] Gentamicin is considered the most nephrotoxic, followed in decreasing order of nephrotoxicity by tobramycin and amikacin. To prevent these toxicities, patients should have electrolytes repleted (potassium and magnesium), be appropriately hydrated, and undergo pharmacokinetic monitoring. For traditional dosing methods, a peak level should be drawn half an hour after the end of the infusion, while trough levels should be drawn within 30 minutes before the next dose. For extended-interval dosing, a published nomogram, such as the Hartford Nomogram, should guide monitoring.[29]

FLUOROQUINOLONES

Fluoroquinolones available for systemic use in the United States include ciprofloxacin, levofloxacin, moxifloxacin, ofloxacin, and delafloxacin.[30] Fluoroquinolones have a wide spectrum and accessible pharmacokinetic properties and are among the most commonly prescribed antibiotics. Their spectrum includes gram-positive, gram-negative, atypical organisms, and are particularly effective against Enterobacteriaceae and *Haemophilus* spp. The spectrum is generally the same; however there are some notable differences. Only levofloxacin and ciprofloxacin have activity against *Pseudomonas* and only moxifloxacin has activity against anaerobes.

Unfortunately, they are associated with a growing number of potentially serious adverse effects. The U.S. Food and Drug Administration (FDA) has issued warnings about the risk of delirium, memory impairment, disorientation, tendinopathy and tendon rupture, QT interval prolongation, liver failure, hypo and hyperglycemia, retinal detachment, aortic dissection, and rupture. In 2016, the FDA stated that these serious adverse effects outweigh the benefits for infections such as sinusitis, bronchitis, and uncomplicated urinary tract infections.

Fluoroquinolones are the only class of antimicrobial agents in clinical use that are direct inhibitors of bacterial DNA synthesis and are considered to be bactericidal. Fluoroquinolones inhibit two bacterial enzymes, DNA gyrase and topoisomerase IV, which have essential and distinct roles in DNA replication. Typically, gram-negative bacterial activity correlates with inhibition of DNA gyrase, and gram-positive bacterial activity corresponds with inhibition of DNA type IV topoisomerase.

Levofloxacin and moxifloxacin have near 100% bioavailability and therefore when transitioning from parenteral to oral therapy the clinician can administer the same dose. Ciprofloxacin has approximately 80% bioavailability and will require a proportionally higher oral dose; fortunately, the parenteral formulation typically is supplied as 400 mg and the oral is 500 mg, accounting for this (see **Table 30.5** for adult dosage ranges). A common problem with fluoroquinolones is that co-administration of divalent cations such as aluminum-, magnesium-, or, to a lesser extent, calcium-containing antacids will chelate the drug molecule and result in reduced oral bioavailability. Fluoroquinolones, with the exception of moxifloxacin, will require dose adjustment in patients with renal insufficiency.

LIPOPEPTIDES

Daptomycin, a cyclic lipopeptide, has rapid bactericidal activity against a wide range of gram-positive bacteria including methicillin-resistant *S. aureus*.[31] Daptomycin is approved for use in skin and skin-structure infections and *S. aureus* bacteremia (including endocarditis). While it has good penetration into the lungs, it cannot be used for pneumonia as daptomycin was shown to interact in vitro with pulmonary surfactant, resulting in inhibition of antibacterial activity.[32]

Daptomycin exerts its activity by binding to components of the cell membrane of susceptible organisms and causing rapid depolarization and cell lysis; it also inhibits intracellular synthesis of DNA, RNA, and protein. Daptomycin is bactericidal in a concentration-dependent manner. Although daptomycin resistance has been documented, it remains uncommon despite the increasing use of daptomycin.

Daptomycin is generally well tolerated; however, it has effects on skeletal muscle such that patients should be monitored for pain or weakness in distal extremi-

ties. To monitor for this, CPK should be monitored at least weekly during therapy, and more frequent monitoring if a patient in on current or prior statin therapy.

BACTERIOSTATIC ANTIBIOTICS

This section discusses how bacteriostatic antibiotics limit the growth of bacteria by interfering with bacterial protein synthesis, DNA replication, or other aspects of bacterial cellular metabolism.[33] After disrupting replication, these antibiotics require the host immune system and require phagocytic cells to definitively clear bacteria. Bacteriostatic antimicrobials include: tigecycline, linezolid, macrolides, sulfonamides, tetracyclines, and streptogramins.[33] There exists the potential for an antagonist effect when combining bacteriostatic and bactericidal antimicrobials.[34] Bactericidal antibiotics are most potent against actively dividing cells and require an organism to be actively dividing to be effective, whereas bacteriostatic agents prevent cellular division. Therefore, if a bacteriostatic antibiotic which prevents active division is used in combination with a bactericidal antibiotic, one could expect to see an antagonistic effect.

TETRACYCLINES

Commonly used tetracyclines include doxycycline, minocycline, and tetracycline. There are a number of tetracycline derivatives that include tigecycline, a glycylcycline, as well as newer agents such as eravacycline, sarecycline, and omadacycline. Tetracyclines work by reversibly binding to the 30S ribosomal subunit at a position that blocks the binding of the aminoacyl-tRNA to the acceptor site on the mRNA-ribosome complex. Protein synthesis is ultimately inhibited, leading to a bacteriostatic effect.

The antimicrobial activity of all the tetracyclines is essentially the same and can be used to treat infection caused by many aerobic gram-positive and gram-negative bacteria as well as many atypical pathogens. Tigecycline has a broader spectrum of activity when compared to the tetracyclines; however, it carries an FDA black box warning regarding an increased risk of all-cause mortality. Tigecycline should be reserved for situations where alternative treatments are not available.

Tetracyclines, with the exception of tigecycline, are generally safe drugs; however, they do cause a number of gastrointestinal-related side effects. Photosensitivity is also often seen in patients treated with tetracyclines; therefore, they should avoid the sun or use sunscreen during treatment. Tetracycline antibiotics have been associated with permanent tooth discoloration in children less than 8 years of age if used repeatedly or for prolonged

TABLE 30.5 Fluoroquinolones	
Medication	Typical Dosage Range
Ciprofloxacin	Adult: 200–400 mg IV q12h *or* 400 mg IV q8h (severe infections); 250–750 mg PO q12h
Delafloxacin	Adult: 300 mg IV q12h *or* 450 mg PO q12h
Levofloxacin	Adult: 250–750 mg PO/IV daily
Moxifloxacin	Adult: 400 mg PO/IV daily
Ofloxacin	Adult: 200–400 mg PO q12h

d, day; h, hour; PO, orally; IV, intravenously; q, every.

courses. However, doxycycline binds less readily to calcium than other tetracyclines, and the risk of dental staining with doxycycline is minimal if a short course (<21 days) is administered. Therefore, in these populations the benefits outweigh the risks of doxycycline for certain infections like Rocky Mountain spotted fever.

The newer tetracyclines, eravacycline, sarecycline, and omadacycline offer an expanded spectrum of activity. For example, eravacycline is a parenteral agent approved for complicated intra-abdominal infections, and appears to have similar efficacy to carbapenems; however, it appears to have activity against carbapenem resistant *Acinetobacter*.[35] Sarecycline is an oral agent used for the treatment of acne. Omadacycline is available in both oral and parenteral formulations and is used to treat acute bacterial skin and skin structure infections. See **Table 30.6** for adult dosing information.

MACROLIDES AND KETOLIDE

Erythromycin is the prototypical macrolide; however, it is associated with many adverse effects and drug interactions. It has limited clinical utility as an antimicrobial agent. Later agents such as azithromycin and clarithromycin are structural improvements over erythromycin which provide improved bioavailability and pharmacokinetic properties. Telithromycin is the only one of the ketolide class of antimicrobials that is structurally related to the macrolides; it is no longer available in the United States due to significant risk of hepatotoxicity and myasthenia gravis exacerbations.

The macrolides exert their antimicrobial activity by binding to the 50S subunit of bacterial ribosomes, leading to inhibition of transpeptidation, translocation, chain elongation, and, ultimately, bacterial protein synthesis.

Macrolide is active against pathogens of the respiratory tract such as *S. pneumoniae*, *Haemophilus spp.*, *Moraxella catarrhalis*, and the atypicals including *Mycoplasma pneumoniae*, *Chlamydia trachomatis*, *Chlamydia (Chlamydophila) pneumoniae*, *Bordetella pertussis*, and *Legionella* species.

Macrolide antibiotics are frequently used in the treatment of community-acquired respiratory tract infections, particularly pneumonia. In the 2007 IDSA/ATS guidelines, the macrolides were recommended for those without significant risk factors for macrolide-resistant *S. pneumoniae*; unfortunately, the overall rate of macrolide of *S. pneumoniae* is greater than 25% in almost all the United States and may not be appropriate for monotherapy.

Macrolides have significant gastrointestinal side effects, including nausea, vomiting, and diarrhea. As mentioned previously, erythromycin is rarely used as an antimicrobial agent; it is still employed as a prokinetic agent. The class also carries the risk of QT interval prolongation; caution should be taken when coadministering antiarrhythmic drugs. Azithromycin has a longer intracellular half-life when compared to the other macrolides; a "Z-Pak" or once-daily administration for 5-day regimen has similar efficacy to a 10-day course of other macrolides. See **Table 30.7** for dosing information.

LINCOSAMIDES

Clindamycin (Cleocin) and lincomycin (Lincocin), which, despite sharing a similar naming convention and a similar mechanism of action with the macrolides, are not chemically related and belong to the lincosamide class of antimicrobials (**Table 30.8**). Clindamycin is clinically useful in the treatment of gram-positive infections and has a spectrum of activity that covers anaerobic, streptococcal, and staphylococcal infections.

Lincosamides exert their antimicrobial activity by binding to the 50S ribosomal subunit of bacteria and disrupting protein synthesis by interfering with the transpeptidation reaction, which thereby inhibits early chain elongation. These drugs may compete for this binding site with macrolide antibiotics.

TABLE 30.6 Tetracyclines

Medication	Typical Dosage Range (Adult)
Doxycycline	100 mg IV/PO q6h
Eravacycline	1 mg/kg IV q12h (infuse over 60 minutes)
Minocycline	100–200 mg PO q12h
Omadacycline	Loading dose (day 1): 200 mg IV once *or* 100 mg IV × 2 doses; maintenance: 100 mg IV daily *or* Loading dose (days 1 and 2): 450 mg PO daily; maintenance: 300 mg PO daily
Sarecycline	60–150 mg PO daily
Tetracycline	250–500 mg PO q6h

d, day; h, hour; PO, orally; IV, intravenously; q, every.

TABLE 30.7 Macrolides

Medication	Typical Dosage Range
Azithromycin	Typical Z-pak adult dose = 500 mg PO × 1, then 250 mg PO daily × 4 days. Other dosing regimens for adults: 250–500 mg IV/PO daily or 2,000 mg PO single dose (extended-release) Pediatric: 5–12 mg/kg IV/PO daily *or* 30 mg/kg PO single dose (extended-release)
Clarithromycin	Adult: 250–500 mg PO q12h *or* 1,000 mg PO daily (extended-release) Pediatric: 15 mg/kg/d PO divided q12h
Erythromycin base	Adult: 250–1,000 mg PO q6h Pediatric: 30–50 mg/kg/d PO divided q6–8h

d, day; h, hour; PO, orally; IV, intravenously; q, every.

TABLE 30.8 Lincosamides

Medication	Typical Dosage Range
Clindamycin	Adult: 150–450 mg PO q6–8h *or* 600 mg IV q8h Pediatric: 10–30 mg/kg/d PO divided q6–8h *or* 25–40 mg/kg/d IV divided q6–8h
Lincomycin	Adult: 600 mg IM q12–24h *or* 600 mg–1 g IV q8–12h (max dose: 8 g/d) Pediatric: 10 mg/kg IM q12–24h *or* 10–20 mg/kg/d IV q12–24h

d, day; h, hour; PO, orally; IM, intramuscularly; IV, intravenously; q, every.

TABLE 30.9 Folate antagonists

Medication	Typical Dosage Range
Sulfadiazine	Adult: 4,000–8,000 mg PO divided q6–12h Pediatric: 100–150 mg/kg/d PO divided q6h
Sulfadoxine	Adult: 4,000–8,000 mg PO divided q4–6h Pediatric: 120–150 mg/kg/d PO divided q4–6h
Trimethoprim– sulfamethoxazole	Adult: 160/800 mg PO q12h *or* 10–200 mg/kg/d IV divided Pediatric: 6–20 mg/kg/d PO/IV divided q6–12h

d, day; h, hour; PO, orally; IV, intravenously; q, every.

Lincosamides are associated with a number of serious adverse effects. *Clostridioides* (formerly *Clostridium*) *difficile*-associated diarrhea (CDAD) has been reported with use of nearly all antibacterial agents, including clindamycin, and may range in severity from mild diarrhea to fatal colitis. Treatment with antibacterial agents alters the normal flora of the colon, leading to overgrowth of *C. difficile*. However, clindamycin has been associated with severe and even fatal colitis; it should be reserved for serious infections that do not have other treatment options. A maculopapular skin rash is also relatively common and has been noted in up to 10% of patients receiving clindamycin.

FOLATE ANTAGONISTS

Drugs such as dapsone, pyrimethamine, sulfadiazine, and sulfadoxine are all considered folate antagonists; however, trimethoprim–sulfamethoxazole (TMP–SMX), also known as "cotrimoxazole," is the most commonly used.[36] TMP–SMX is effective against a wide variety of aerobic gram-positive and gram-negative bacteria, *P. jirovecii*, and some protozoa; TMP–SMX can also be used to treat outpatient MRSA infections. Unfortunately, due to widespread use, significant resistance has developed.

The two components, TMP and SMX, work sequentially to inhibit enzyme systems involved in the bacterial synthesis of tetrahydrofolic acid (THF). Reduced availability of THF inhibits thymidine synthesis and subsequently DNA synthesis.

Dosing of TMP–SMX is based on the trimethoprim component and expressed as a mg/kg/day of TMP (**Table 30.9**). TMP–SMX dosing should be altered for patients with renal insufficiency. Side effects associated with TMP–SMX include gastrointestinal tract upset and dermatological issues such as rash. The TMP component can act like a potassium-sparing diuretic, leading to hyperkalemia. More serious side effects such as Stevens-Johnson syndrome and lactic acidosis have also been reported. TMP–SMX has also been shown to have significant drug–drug interactions (warfarin, cyclospo-rine, phenytoin, and oral hypoglycemics) that may require dose adjustment and additional monitoring.

OXAZOLIDINONES

Linezolid and tedizolid are oxazolidinones. Both exhibit bacteriostatic activity against MRSA and streptococci. The drugs are very similar and have been observed to have equivalent cure rates for MRSA; tedizolid is considered to be noninferior to linezolid for the treatment of skin and soft tissue infections.[37] Linezolid can be used for pneumonia, skin and skin structure infections, urinary tract infections, and others; tedizolid is currently indicated only for acute bacterial skin and skin structure infections but may be useful in others.

Oxazolidinones inhibit bacterial protein synthesis by binding to bacterial 23S ribosomal RNA of the 50S subunit. This prevents the formation of a functional 70S initiation complex that is essential for the bacterial translation process. Linezolid is bacteriostatic against enterococci and staphylococci and bactericidal against most strains of streptococci. Tedizolid is bacteriostatic against enterococci, staphylococci, and streptococci.

Both drugs are available in parenteral and oral formulations (**Table 30.10**). The oral formulation provides a convenient treatment option for patients who may in the past have required parenteral medications. The most common adverse effect associated with linezolid is gastrointestinal disturbance. Reversible myelosuppression including thrombocytopenia and anemia have been reported after prolonged therapy. Linezolid was originally discovered as a psychotropic agent that exhibited mild reversible nonselective inhibition of monoamine oxidase (MAO). Patients are at risk for developing serotonin syndrome when linezolid and selective serotonin reuptake inhibitors are simultaneously administered. Serotonin syndrome, also known as "serotonin toxicity," is caused by excessive levels of circulating serotonin in the central nervous system (CNS) and the periphery.[38]

TABLE 30.10 Oxazolidinones

Medication	Typical Dosage Range
Linezolid	Adult: 400–600 mg PO/IV q12h Pediatric: 20–30 mg/kg/d PO/IV divided q8–12h
Tedizolid	Adult: 200 mg PO/IV daily

d, day; h, hour; PO, orally; IV, intravenously; q, every.

TABLE 30.11 Nitrofurans and Fosfomycin

Medication	Typical Dosage Range
Nitrofurantoin	Adult: 50 mg PO q6h (crystalline) or 100 mg PO q12h (monohydrate) Pediatric: 5–7 mg/kg/d PO divided q6h (crystalline)
Fosfomycin	Adult: 3 g PO once (powder)

d, day; h, hour; PO, orally; IV, intravenously; q, every.

STREPTOGRAMINS

Quinupristin/dalfopristin (Synercid) is the only available streptogramin.[39] It was approved for the treatment of serious or life-threatening infections associated with vancomycin-resistant *Enterococcus faecium* bacteremia and complicated skin and skin structure infections caused by methicillin-susceptible *Staphylococcus aureus* and *Streptococcus pyogenes*. Quinupristin/dalfopristin is not active against *E. faecalis*. The use of quinupristin/dalfopristin has generally been supplanted by more tolerable drugs such as linezolid and daptomycin.

The combination of quinupristin and dalfopristin is synergistic and is generally bactericidal compared with either agent used alone or compared with similar antibiotics in the macrolide group. Quinupristin/dalfopristin inhibits bacterial protein synthesis by binding to different sites on the 50S bacterial ribosomal subunit thereby inhibiting protein synthesis.

The most common side effects of quinupristin/dalfopristin are arthralgias and myalgias. It also causes significant phlebitis and thus should be administered only through a central access catheter. Quinupristin/dalfopristin significantly inhibits CYP3A4 enzyme, and therefore has several significant drug–drug interactions.

NITROFURANS AND FOSFOMYCIN

Nitrofurantoin and fosfomycin are structurally unique and have different mechanisms of action; however, they share a similar clinical utility in the treatment of acute uncomplicated cystitis. While fosfomycin is included in clinical practice guidelines as a first-line agent for acute uncomplicated cystitis, it has been reported to have decreased efficacy when compared to other first-line agents.[40] However, fosfomycin may have additional clinical utility in the treatment of MRSA UTIs.[41]

Fosfomycin inhibits bacterial wall synthesis (bactericidal) by inactivating the enzyme, pyruvyl transferase, which is critical in the synthesis of cell walls by bacteria. Meanwhile, nitrofurantoin is reduced by bacterial flavoproteins to reactive intermediates that inactivate or alter bacterial ribosomal proteins leading to inhibition of protein synthesis, aerobic energy metabolism, DNA, RNA, and cell wall synthesis. Nitrofurantoin is bactericidal in urine at therapeutic doses.

Nitrofurantoin is generally well tolerated, though it can cause gastrointestinal upset. It can also cause a rare pulmonary toxicity that presents as either an acute onset approximately 9 days after starting therapy or a chronic onset developing after several months. Nitrofurantoin should be avoided if there is suspicion for early pyelonephritis or if the creatinine clearance is less than 30 mL/min. Observational studies have suggested that the agent is effective and safe with mild renal impairment, even in older women.[42] Nitrofurantoin is available in two dosage formulations, crystalline and monohydrate, dosed four times daily and twice daily respectively. Fosfomycin is available as a powder, which is administered as a one-time dose. See **Table 30.11** for additional dosing information.

FIDAXOMICIN

Fidaxomicin is the first macrocyclic lactone antibiotic agent that is classified as a macrolide by the FDA. It is selectively active against gram-positive anaerobes, including *Clostridioides*.[43] It exerts its action by inhibiting RNA polymerase, thereby preventing transcription. Current guidelines recommend fidaxomicin as a treatment option for the initial episode of *Clostridioides difficile* infection (CDI).[44]

When administered orally, fidaxomicin (similar to oral vancomycin) is minimally absorbed, being excreted almost entirely through the feces; thus, there are few side effects apart from gastrointestinal upset.

DRUGS THAT TARGET *MYCOBACTERIUM TUBERCULOSIS* (TB)

Tuberculosis (TB), caused by the organism *Mycobacterium tuberculosis*, is the leading cause of death worldwide from a bacterial infectious disease among adults.[45] In the majority of infected individuals, *Mycobacterium tuberculosis* establishes a latent TB infection (LTBI) in the lungs, where the individual is asymptomatic and noninfectious. However, the organism remains viable and if the host immune system were to be compromised, there is a possibility that this would progress to an active symptomatic infection.[46]

The overall goals of tuberculosis treatment focus on eradicating LTBI, curing the individual patient with active infection, and minimizing the transmission of *Mycobacterium tuberculosis* to other persons.[47] The overall disease state management from screening to diagnosis and treatment is highly complex; however, this section focuses on first-line treatment of a pansusceptible active tuberculosis infection in HIV-uninfected adults as the knowledge regarding these first line agents is transferrable to the treatment of LTBI and are other regimens. The preferred treatment regimen consists of four drugs (isoniazid, rifampicin, pyrazinamide, and ethambutol) given for a total of 2 months followed by two drugs (isoniazid and rifampicin) given for an additional 4 months.[47]

Isoniazid (commonly abbreviated INH) has a very complex mechanism of action; however, one of the more important aspects of this mechanism is that it selectively inhibits mycolic acid syntheses which are cellular wall components of *Mycobacterium tuberculosis* and *Mycobacterium kansaii* making INH selective to *Mycobacterium spp.*[48] INH, in combination with other antitubercular drugs, remains the drug of choice for the treatment of tuberculosis despite the fact that it can cause a number of significant adverse reactions.[49] Most notably, INH carries a FDA–boxed warning for severe and sometimes fatal hepatitis which may develop even after many months of treatment. The risk of hepatotoxicity increases with age and for persons 35 years and older, clinicians should conduct monthly symptom reviews as well as measure hepatic enzymes (ALT & AST) at baseline and periodically throughout treatment. Additionally, INH therapy also increases the risk of developing neuropathy. Therefore, Pyridoxine (vitamin B6), 25–50 mg/day, is given with INH to all persons at risk of neuropathy (e.g., pregnant women; breastfeeding infants; persons with HIV; patients with diabetes, alcoholism, malnutrition, or chronic renal failure; or patients with advanced age).[47] Last, while rare, INH can precipitate sideroblastic anemia especially in patients with a concomitant folate deficiency.[50]

Rifampin (RIF) is a member of the rifamycin class of drugs along with rifabutin, rifapentine, and rifaximin (this last medication is used for *Clostridioides* and other GI disorders, not tuberculosis).[51] The rifamycins work by binding specifically to the β subunit of bacterial RNA polymerases preventing the production of mRNA. One of the major side effects of rifampin is that it colors bodily secretions such as sweat, saliva, and tears an orange-red color. In regard to other adverse effects, rifamycins can contribute to hepatotoxicity as well as cause nausea, though typically not to an extent that would require discontinuation of treatment.[52]

Unlike other antimicrobials, Pyrazinamide (PZA) has no defined target of action, though it is active only against *Mycobacterium tuberculosis*.[53] It is used in combination with other antitubercular drugs for the first 2 months of tuberculosis therapy. In regard to adverse effects, most notably PZA contributes to an increased risk of hepatotoxicity; it also may cause hyperuricemia, overall malaise, and arthralgia.

The last of the multidrug tuberculosis cocktail is ethambutol (EMB) which works by interfering with the biosynthesis of arabinogalactan, a component of the *Mycobacterium* cell wall.[54] The most important adverse effect of EMB is optic neuropathy or neuritis which can present a loss of visual acuity, blurred vision, or color blindness (specifically red-green discrimination). Vision should be evaluated at baseline and monitored throughout therapy; in patients reporting changes in vision, therapy should be discontinued as irreversible blindness has been reported. Otherwise, EMB is generally well tolerated.

There are a number of mnemonic devices that can assist with remembering the components of tuberculosis treatment such as "RIPE" (Rifampin, Isoniazid, Pyrazinamide, Ethambutol).

The widespread occurrence of multidrug-resistant TB (MDR-TB) presents major challenges in the management and eradication of TB. Multidrug-resistant TB strains do not respond to the standard 6-month treatment with first-line anti-TB drugs discussed previously. Patients may require up to 2 years or more of treatment with drugs that are less potent, more toxic, and much more expensive.[55] Current guidelines from various international agencies, such as the Infectious Disease Society of America (IDSA), recommend that treatment should be tailored based on drug-susceptibility testing, and that individuals should not receive medicines to which the *Mycobacterium tuberculosis* strain is resistant.[56]

ANTIVIRAL AGENTS PRIMARILY USED TO TREAT HERPES SIMPLEX VIRUS AND VARICELLA ZOSTER VIRUS

Herpes simplex virus (HSV) 1 and 2 and varicella zoster virus (VZV) are part of the Herpesviridae family. There is no cure for either infection and only VZV has a successful vaccine. This vaccine has resulted in reduced prevalence of VZV, but HSV still infects the majority of the world. Most individuals infected with HSV and VZV are without signs or symptoms. When outbreaks occur from the latent form of these viral infections, cutaneous manifestations are the most common.

Herpes simplex virus (HSV) typically causes a cutaneous eruption of vesicular lesions that may recur throughout the life span. HSV-1 and HSV-2 result in similar disease, with the exception that HSV-2 is more implicated in genital infection and prone to more frequent recurrences. The virus transmits through skin-to-skin contact with other persons. As a result, it often appears in the genital region as a sexually transmitted infection. The clinical manifestations of HSV are diverse, especially in the immunocompromised host. This virus is implicated in aseptic meningitis/encephalitis. VZV is the pathogen behind the viral exanthem syndrome of chicken pox. Later in life when the virus reactivates it can cause the painful dermatomal vesicular lesions of shingles.

When HSV-1, HSV-2, and VZV result in cutaneous eruptions, the diagnosis is made through nucleic acid amplification technology (NAT) of a swabbed vesicular lesion. Other manifestations are typically diagnosed with NAT of the tissue/fluid suspected to be infected such as cerebrospinal fluid via lumbar puncture. First-line treatment for both these viral infections is acyclovir or its prodrug valacyclovir. While the treatment does not offer a cure, it has been shown to reduce severity and duration of symptoms.

ACYCLOVIR/VALACYCLOVIR

Acyclovir is used to treat and prevent recurrent outbreaks of HSV and VZV. When acyclovir, and its prodrug valacyclovir, are used for treatment the duration and severity of symptoms may be reduced. Thus, some individuals who have had a HSV/VZV cutaneous outbreak may take antiviral therapy in order to reduce the frequency of symptomatic recurrences and asymptomatic viral shedding.

Acyclovir has clinical activity against HSV-1, HSV-2, and VZV.[57] However, it is approximately 10 times more potent against HSV. Thus, higher doses are utilized to treat VZV disease. The oral bioavailability is low (15%); therefore multiple daily doses are required. As a result, the prodrug valacyclovir is commonly used. Additionally, IV acyclovir is used when high drug concentration is required in cases such as resistant or CNS infections. There is no IV formula for valacyclovir. The dose and duration of these drugs depends on which virus the clinician is treating and its clinical manifestation. For example, the dose and duration for an initial (primary) genital HSV-2 infection is different than a recurrent outbreak, and certainly different for HSV–induced hepatitis or meningitis.

Acyclovir is a guanosine analogue that is converted to a monophosphate derivative by viral thymidine kinase. This means the active drug accumulated in infected cells. Host cell kinases eventually convert to acyclovir triphosphate compounds. This triphosphate form of acyclovir inhibits viral DNA polymerase and incorporates into the developing viral DNA causing chain termination. Valacyclovir is rapidly converted to acyclovir by esterases. Acyclovir is cleared by glo-

merular filtration and tubular secretion and should be renally adjusted. Mechanisms of resistance include mutations to viral thymidine kinase or DNA polymerase. Fortunately, resistance is rare, especially in those with competent immune systems. When resistance occurs, Foscarnet is often the prescribed agent.

FAMCICLOVIR/PENCICLOVIR

Famciclovir is an oral drug that is deacetylated and oxidized through first pass metabolism to penciclovir. Penciclovir requires phosphorylation and activation by viral thymidine kinase. The activated form of the drug interferes competitively with DNA polymerase. Penciclovir exists in topical and intravenous form. Unfortunately, the commonly found HSV/VZV resistance patterns are cross resistant to famciclovir/penciclovir.

FOSCARNET

Foscarnet, which is available only intravenously, has clinical use against HSV, VZV, Human Herpes Virus-6 (HHV-6), and Cytomegalovirus (CMV) infection. This drug inhibits herpesvirus DNA and RNA polymerase through blockade of their pyrophosphate binding site and inhibits cleavage of pyrophosphate from deoxynucleotide triphosphates.[58] Resistance can occur and is often secondary to mutation in the DNA polymerase.

One of the more noteworthy adverse effects of foscarnet is nephrotoxicity, often presenting with renal tubular injury. Intravenous normal saline bolus preadministration reduces the risk of nephrotoxicity. Electrolyte dyscrasias are frequent and monitoring with repletion is essential. Common abnormalities include hypocalcemia, hypokalemia, hyperphosphatemia, and hypomagnesemia. Additionally, hallucination, headache, nausea, hepatitis, and genital ulceration are reported.

AGENTS PRIMARILY USED TO TREAT CYTOMEGALOVIRUS

Cytomegalovirus (CMV) is another member of the herpesvirus family. Following primary infection, which may or may not be symptomatic, the virus enters a latent stage and infects the human host for life. The most important risk factor for developing symptoms due to CMV, also known as CMV disease, is immune system compromise.

The most common presentation of CMV disease in those with a competent immune system is a mononucleosis-like syndrome. In addition to disseminated disease, like the mononucleosis syndrome, we see a wide range of tissue invasive disease in the compromised immune system. The most common tissue invasive CMV diseases include retinitis and colitis. The varied manifestations of CMV disease are, in part, related to its diverse cellular tropism. Disseminated disease can be diagnosed by CMV DNA PCR of the blood. The gold standard for diagnosis of tissue-invasive disease is histology that is aided by immunohistochemistry. Diagnosis of the varied manifestations of CMV is complex and beyond the scope of this review. There are several antiviral drugs used in the treatment and prevention of CMV. The dose and duration depend on the manifestation of disease and immune function.

GANCICLOVIR/VALGANCICLOVIR

Ganciclovir and its prodrug Valganciclovir are widely used for treatment and prevention of CMV disease.[59] Ganciclovir is available only in IV form due to its poor bioavailability. Ganciclovir is converted intracellularly by viral kinase encoded by the CMV gene UL97. This drug's active phosphorylated form is a nucleoside guanosine analog and competitively inhibits as it incorporates into the new DNA chain.[59] Resistance is possible and originates primarily from mutations in the UL97 gene.

Both agents have been used for the initial treatment of CMV disease, prophylaxis, and preemptive treatment in those at high risk. One example of a patient who may receive preemptive treatment is a recent transplant patient with rising CMV viremia and no evidence of disease. Depending on the location and severity of the disease, Ganciclovir is sometimes used as induction treatment and then the patient is transitioned to oral valganciclovir. The exact dose and duration depend on host and disease manifestation, and is beyond the scope of this chapter. For example, the drug must be renally dosed and has been associated with renal injury. Another noteworthy toxicity is myelosuppression.

CIDOFOVIR

Cidofovir, which is available only intravenously, has clinical use against HSV, CMV, VZV, HHV-6, BK polyomavirus, and Adenovirus. The half-life of this drug is long and typically dosed weekly based on current renal function. Its role in CNS infection is limited by poor penetration. Cidofovir is an inhibitor of viral DNA polymerase and incorporated into the developing viral DNA chain. Phosphorylation to the active form of Cidofovir is independent of viral enzymes; therefore it has activity against strains of HSV and CMV where these enzymes are altered.

One of the more noteworthy adverse effects is nephrotoxicity, often presenting as a proximal tubular ne-

phropathy. To reduce this risk, intravenous normal saline bolus is given prior to drug administration and probenecid. Renal monitoring is necessary as each dose is adjusted based on current GFR. Concurrent use of other nephrotoxic drugs should result in extreme caution.

LETERMOVIR

This drug is available orally and has activity against CMV. Letermovir is currently used in the prophylaxis of CMV disease in allogeneic stem cell–transplant patients and its role may expand as more data becomes available. This drug inhibits terminase complex which plays a significant role late in the CMVZ replication cycle.[60]

AGENTS PRIMARILY USED TO TREAT INFLUENZA

The influenza virus spreads person to person through respiratory droplets. Common manifestations are the influenza syndrome that include fever, rhinorrhea, myalgias, sore throat, headache, and cough. However, manifestations range from asymptomatic to fatal pneumonia. Influenza types A and B are the common human pathogens. Diagnosis is typically made through a nasopharyngeal swab that looks for influenza antigen, antibody, or RNA via nucleic acid amplification technology. Several rapid tests have been validated that allow for diagnosis in the context of a single clinic visit. Rapid diagnosis is important because treatment has been shown to be effective only if started within 48 hours of symptom onset. Early awareness of infection can also be important for prevention in high-risk settings such as a nursing home or immune-compromised person exposure. Those individuals exposed, and at greatest risk, may begin a course of antiviral therapy such as oseltamivir.

NEURAMINIDASE INHIBITORS

This drug class includes oseltamivir, zanamivir, and peramivir. These agents are typically active against influenza types A and B. Neuraminidase is a viral enzyme that cleaves sialic acid residues on the surface of host cells. This cleavage allows for release of new influenza virus from infected host cells. The neuraminidase inhibitors are analogs of sialic acid. They block the function or neuraminidase and prevent new virus from being released.

Zanamivir is administered as an inhaled powder due to poor oral bioavailability. This agent is not recommended for those with pulmonary disease such as COPD as the delivery system may cause exacerbation.

Oseltamivir is the only orally administered neuraminidase inhibitor. Peramivir is available only in IV formula. Generally speaking, these drugs are well tolerated.

Oseltamivir has been shows to reduce the duration of symptoms if started within 48 hours of symptom onset. In addition, Oseltamivir has been studied in the prevention of influenza for those with a high-risk exposure and is somewhat effective.

CAP-DEPENDENT ENDONUCLEASE INHIBITORS

The single drug in this class is baloxavir marboxil and it is orally administered. This is a newer drug and class without much data to guide practice. The likely mechanism of action is inhibition of cap-dependent endonuclease activity of the viral polymerase which reduced influenza A and B replication.[61] Currently recommended for initial treatment of influenza in those 12 years of age and older, it is not recommended for pregnant women, breastfeeding mothers, outpatients with complicated or progressive illness, or hospitalized patients. This recommendation stems from the current lack of data about use in these populations. Resistance to this drug is possible.

ADAMANTANES

Amantadine and rimantadine are two drugs of this class. Given significant influenza A resistance and lack of influenza B activity, this drug class is no longer recommended for typical influenza therapy. This drug class interferes with M2 viral proton channel which prevents acidification of the interior of the virion and as a result does not initiate viral replication. Through a different mechanism of action, Amantadine has been used to treat Parkinson's Disease.

AGENTS USED PRIMARILY TO TREAT HEPATITIS C

Hepatitis C infects over 100 million persons worldwide, including approximately 2.4 million in the United States.[62] The virus spreads through blood contact which makes intravenous drug abuse the biggest risk factor in the United States. Rarely do those infected have symptoms, unless liver failure has resulted. Fortunately, not everyone infected with hepatitis C will develop liver failure. Also, about one-fourth of those infected will resolve the infection without antiviral therapy. Individuals are typically screened with a hepatitis C antibody test. If this is positive, a NAT study is done through blood draw to confirm presence of current infection. If hepatitis C infection is confirmed, a liver elastography test is often performed to determine extent of fibrosis and a genotype blood test to deter-

mine the virus type. Those who do not clear the virus and have a life expectancy where further liver injury will reduce quality of life should be treated. The treatment is curative. Given the risk of resistance two or more drugs are typically utilized. The type and duration of the drugs depend primarily on the viral genotype and presence of cirrhosis.[63]

The main targets of these new direct-acting antiviral agents are the HCV-encoded proteins that enable viral replication. After hepatocyte entry, the viral RNA is translated through host cell machinery into a polyprotein which is cleaved into a number of proteins. The new drugs block several of these new proteins, including those that play a role in processing and replication.[63] Throughout these direct-acting antiviral drug classes are frequent drug to drug interactions.

Resistance is also an issue with varied degrees of risk. As a result, drugs are frequently paired together. Approximately 10% to 15% of genotype 1-infected patients without prior exposure to NS5A inhibitors have detectable NS5A RASs prior to treatment.

NS3/4A PROTEASE INHIBITORS

Drugs in this class inhibit a viral enzyme called NS3/4A serine protease. This enzyme helps process and replicate hepatitis C virus. Simeprevir, telaprevir, boceprevir, grazoprevir, and voxilaprevir are examples of drugs in this class.

NUCLEOSIDE NS5B POLYMERASE INHIBITORS AND NON-NUCLEOSIDE NS5B INHIBITORS

NS5B is an RNA polymerase involved in posttranslational processing of hepatitis C viral proteins. This enzyme function is essential for HCV replication. Nucleoside/tide drugs block the nucleoside binding site of the polymerase whereas nonnucleoside drugs bind to several nonnucleoside sites and result in allosteric alteration. Sofosbuvir is an example of a nucleoside drug and Dasabuvir is a nonnucleoside inhibitor.

NS5A INHIBITORS

Drugs in this class block NS5A protein which plays a role in replicating and packaging new virus. The exact mechanism is uncertain, but it is likely multifactor and includes hyperphosphorylation. As a class, these drugs are typically active against all hepatitis C genotype and include daclatasvir, elbasvir, ledipasvir, and velpatasvir.

RIBAVIRIN

This drug is used to treat several viral infections including hepatitis C, hepatitis E, respiratory syncytial virus, and some of the viral hemorrhagic fevers.

Nowadays this antiviral is rarely used for Hepatitis C given the development of aforementioned direct-acting antiviral drugs. Its mechanism of action is that of a nucleoside analogue that can resemble adenosine or guanosine. This causes mutations in RNA-dependent replication in RNA viruses. The mechanism for its activity against DNA virus is less understood. Noteworthy side effects include red blood cell breakdown and birth defects.

AGENTS USED PRIMARILY TO TREAT HEPATITIS B

Hepatitis B virus (HBV) is another prevalent viral hepatitis with a large global burden. It spreads not only through blood, but other body fluids including semen and saliva. Thanks to an effective vaccine, the incidence has decreased dramatically in resource-rich countries. Some infected with HBV will clear the infection without treatment. However, those who require treatment typically have a lifelong therapeutic course as the most common antiviral drug strategy is not curative.[64] HBV is diagnosed by NAT quantification and presence of hepatitis B surface antigen in the blood stream. Treatment is determined by virulence of the infection and degree of liver damage. The class of drugs often used are nucleoside/nucleotide reverse transcriptase inhibitors and are covered in the HIV section. Patients infected with both HBV and HIV often go on a drug regimen which addresses both infections. Drugs in this class, with activity against HBV, include entecavir, tenofovir, emtricitabine, lamivudine, and adefovir.[64]

ANTIFUNGAL AGENTS

Fungi are eukaryotic organisms with chitin in their cell wall. There are millions of fungal species, but only a few hundred are known human pathogens. Most of us have experienced fungal infections in the form of dermatologic disease such as tinea versicolor or onychomycosis. However, fungi have the possibility to cause infectious disease in all tissues including the blood, solid organs, and skin. Fungal infections are more common in persons with immune system compromise, especially those manifestations that are noncutaneous. Fungi do not always cause disease as some are part of our normal flora occupying areas such as the skin, intestinal tract, and vagina.

One group of fungi is molds which grow multicellular filaments called "hyphae." Aspergillus is a well-known pathogenic genus of mold. Yeasts, such as the Candida genus, are a different group of fungi that are single celled. Dimorphic fungi switch between the two depending on environmental factors. It is important for

a clinician to recognize that there are many antifungal agents, and each has a unique adverse effect profile and spectrum of activity.

The diagnosis of fungal infection depends on the location and type of infection. Fungal cultures can be obtained from urine, blood, and other tissue samples. Specific antigen, antibody, and NAT testing are available for a wide range of fungal organisms.

AZOLE ANTIFUNGAL AGENTS

There are two main groups of Azole antifungals: the triazoles and imidazoles. Both groups work primarily by inhibiting the cytochrome P450-dependent enzyme lanosterol 14-alpha-demthylase which is necessary to convert lanosterol to ergosterol. The substance ergosterol is an essential component of the fungal cell wall. Without an effective cell wall there is cell death. All azoles are metabolized by cytochrome P450 system which leads to frequent drug-to-drug interactions. Resistance to azoles occurs through several mechanisms.

The triazole drugs include fluconazole, itraconazole, voriconazole, posaconazole, and isavuconazole. Each drug has a different spectrum of activity and adverse effect profile. Triazole drugs are tolerated in PO or systemic fairly well. Clinical hepatitis can occur and is rare.

Fluconazole has good yeast and Cryptococcus coverage. It also covers many endemic U.S. mycotic infections such as histoplasmosis, coccidiomycosis, and blastomycosis. However, it lacks coverage of the yeasts *Candida glabrata* and *krusei*. It comes in both oral and IV formula.

Itraconazole offers a broader spectrum of activity but has inconsistent bioavailability. It covers a spectrum of fungi similar to fluconazole plus the dematiaceous brown-black molds. The CSF penetration is poor.

Voriconazole is a preferred initial agent for Aspergillus fusarium. It has broad coverage of antifungal, including activity against *C. glabrata and krusei*. The agent may cause changes in heart rate or rhythm, blurred vision, or visual color disturbances and hallucination. The steady state trough plasma level is generally achieved approximately 5 days after the oral or intravenous dosing without a loading dose regimen. However, when a loading dose is employed, the steady state may be achieved within 1 day.[65] Genetic polymorphisms of cytochrome P450 enzymes such as 2C9, 2C19, and 3A4 significantly impact the drug levels of voriconazole. Studies have shown that individuals who are poor metabolizers on average may have four-fold higher of drug exposure compare to their homozygous extensive metabolizers. Drug levels are routinely drawn when there are drug-drug interactions that may significantly impact the therapeutic level.[65]

Isavuconazole and posaconazole are newer agents with expanded spectrum of activity to include mucorales infection.[66,67] The drugs have wide range of coverage including aspergillosis and candida.

Common imidazole group drugs include ketoconazole miconazole and clotrimazole. The imidazole group is less selective for fungal cell cytochrome P 450 enzymes which render greater toxicity. As a result, these agents are primarily for topical use. Clotrimazole uniquely comes in a troche formula, which can be a nice alternative for oral candida infection when nystatin is not effective or poorly tolerated secondary to taste. This drug group is useful for cutaneous dermatophyte and Candida infections.

OTHER AGENTS USEFUL FOR MUCOCUTANEOUS FUNGAL INFECTION

In addition to imidazoles, there are numerous antifungal agents used to treat mucocutaneous infection. Many are topical, but some oral agents exist for more significant cutaneous infection or onychomycosis. This section reviews several of the most common agents.

Nystatin is similar to Amphotericin B as it is a polyene antifungal. It forms pores in the fungal cell wall by binding to ergosterol. It is too toxic for systemic use and is available only in topical and mouth wash formula. It is active against Candida species but resistance is possible. It is commonly used to treat oropharyngeal thrush.

The allylamines class includes drugs such as terbinafine and naftifine. This drug class has good activity against Dermatophyte and Candida cutaneous infections. Both mentioned drugs have topical formulas. The oral formula of terbinafine is used primarily to treat onychomycosis and not systemic fungal disease. This class interferes with an enzyme required for ergosterol synthesis and is fungicidal. Both agents are tolerated well and the oral formula of terbinafine has few drug interactions.

Griseofulvin is administered in an oral formula for treatment of several types of dermatophytosis. It is typically reserved for larger burden of disease. The drug binds to keratin which makes them resistant to fungal infections. As a result it would not have activity where this protein is not present such as blood stream and lungs. A therapeutic course is typically several weeks as it is fungistatic. It is well tolerated.

Ciclopirox olamine has activity against Dermatophyte and Candida cutaneous infections. In addition to typical topical vehicles, it comes as a lacquer that is often used to treat onychomycosis. The exact mechanism of action is not well understood but likely interferes with several enzymes important for fungal cell metabolism.

AMPHOTERICIN B

This drug is produced by Streptomyces nodosus and is classified as a polyene antifungal drug. Amphotericin B has broad fungicidal activity that is typically reserved for sicker patients without better options given the noteworthy adverse-effect profile. It is sometimes used as induction treatment given its rapid reduction of fungal burden. After the induction period a less toxic antifungal agent is continued. The drug covers Candida spp., Aspergillus spp., and hyaline and brown-black molds and also provides good coverage for Mucorales and many of the U.S. endemic mycoses.

Intravenous Lipid-based formulations of amphotericin B have been introduced in an attempt to reduce the toxicities associated with *amphotericin B deoxycholate* administration. The drug has poor oral bioavailability which makes PO not an option unless the infection is within the intestinal tract itself. Amphotericin B has formulas available for intraperitoneal, intravitreal, intrathecal, and direct bladder administration.

The drug binds to cell wall sterols, especially ergosterol, which leads to pore formation and ultimately destruction as contents leak out of the fungal cell. While amphotericin B has a higher affinity for the ergosterol component of the fungal cell membrane, it can also bind to the cholesterol component of the mammalian cell leading to cytotoxicity.

Nephrotoxicity is often the most concerning adverse effect of Amphotericin B.[68] Some evidence shows that renal injury can be prevented with sodium loading and typically a normal saline bolus is delivered intravenously with each dose. Electrolyte abnormalities such as hypokalemia and hypomagnesemia are common and should be monitored for.

In addition to normal saline fluid a patient is typically premedicated with acetaminophen and antihistamine. This is done to prevent common infusion reaction of nausea, chills, rigor, and nausea.

FLUCYTOSINE

This intravenous drug is typically used in synergy with another antifungal class, and has good bioavailability including into the CNS. It has activity against some Candida species, and the molds that cause chromoblastomycoses. This drug converts to fluorouracil and inhibits DNA and RNA synthesis. It is brought into fungal cells by the enzyme cytosine permease. Resistance is possible and drug levels are sometimes obtained as the therapeutic window is quite narrow. Primary toxicity is myelosuppression and nephrotoxicity. Caution should be had if the drug is being paired with another adverse effect–prone drug such as Amphotericin B.

ECHINOCANDINS

This antifungal class is available only intravenously and includes three drugs: micafungin, caspofungin, and anidulafungin. Classwide there is good fungicidal activ-ity against most Candida spp. and Aspergillus.[69] However, Candida Neoformans is not adequately covered. Echinocandins typically have modest or weak activity against non-*Aspergillus* molds. Drugs in this class are noncompetitive inhibitors of beta-D-glucan synthesis. Beta-D-glucans are branched polysaccharides that serve as essential linking components of the cell wall of many fungi. Compared with other antifungals this class has less toxicity especially with regards to liver and kidney.

CASE EXEMPLAR: Patient With Fever, Malaise, Systemic Myalgias

JF is a 22-year-old female who presents at the urgent care center with complaints of fever, malaise, systemic myalgias, and painful vesicular eruptions on her right labia.

Physical Examination
- Fever, malaise, systemic myalgias
- Painful vesicular lesions on right labia
- Right-sided inguinal adenopathy

Labs
- Nucleic acid amplification testing (NAAT) swab for HSV-1 and HSV-2: positive for HSV-1

Next Steps
- Given the high clinical suspicion for primary HSV infection, the clinician prescribes valacyclovir.

Discussion Questions

1. JF asks how she acquired the disease and when the lesions will be gone. How should the clinician respond?
2. What should the patient understand about how valacyclovir will affect the disease?
3. What side effects, if any, can JF expect?

CASE EXEMPLAR: Patient With Treatment-Resistant Herpes Simplex Virus

SS is a 48-year-old male who presents to the emergency department (ED) with painful perioral vesicular eruptions.

Past Medical History
- History of labial HSV-1 infection
- Acute myeloid leukemia (AML), no evidence of current disease
- 4 months postallogenic stem cell transplant

Medications
- Immunosuppressive medications to prevent graft versus host disease
- Antimicrobial prophylaxis that includes acyclovir

Physical Examination
- Painful perioral vesicular eruptions

Labs
- Herpes simplex virus/varicella zoster virus (HSV/VZV) polymerase chain reaction (PCR) swab with resistance testing: pending

Assessment
- Given the progression of these painful lesions and immunocompromised state, the clinician admits the patient for intravenous (IV) foscarnet therapy while awaiting test results.

Discussion Questions

1. What method of action makes foscarnet the drug of choice in the case of SS?
2. What major side effect may be life threatening from the use of foscarnet?
3. What lab monitoring is required while SS is receiving foscarnet?

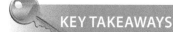

- The treatment of infectious processes falls into one of three major categories: prophylactic, empiric, and definitive. Clinicians must follow antibiotic stewardship while managing infections and be vigilant in prescribing antimicrobials.

- Diagnosis is reached by determining the site of infection, defining the host (e.g., immunocompromised, diabetic, of advanced age), and establishing, when possible, a microbiological diagnosis, which is important to ensure appropriate therapy.

- A drug's pharmacodynamics provides a rational basis for determination of optimal dosing regimens while pharmacokinetics describes the time course of drug levels in body fluids as a result of absorption, distribution, and elimination of a drug after administration. Administration of an antimicrobial must achieve a concentration equal to or greater than the MIC at the site of infection to be effective.

- The potential for drug–drug interactions requires closer monitoring. Antimicrobials are especially challenging because they are prescribed only for a limited course. Antibiotics are also the most common cause of life-threatening immune-mediated drug reactions.

- Antimicrobial medications are categorized by class, indication, or mechanism of action. Examples include drugs that inhibit the cell wall, drugs that block protein synthesis, and drugs that inhibit DNA synthesis.

- Antivirals include Ganciclovir and its prodrug valganciclovir, which are used for treatment and prevention of CMV disease, and neuraminidase inhibitors (oseltamivir, zanamivir, and peramivir), which are typically active against influenza type A and B.

REFERENCES

1. Leekha S, Terrell CL, Edson RS. General principles of antimicrobial therapy. *Mayo Clin Proc.* 2011;86(2):156–167. doi:10.4065/mcp.2010.0639

2. Enzler MJ, Berbari E, Osmon DR. Antimicrobial prophylaxis in adults. *Mayo Clin Proc.* 2011;86(7):686–701. doi:10.4065/mcp.2011.0012

3. Ventola CL. The antibiotic resistance crisis: part 1: Causes and threats. *P T.* 2015;40(4):277–283. https://www.ncbi.nlm.nih.gov/pmc/articles/PMC4378521

4. Dyar OJ, Huttner B, Schouten J, et al. What is antimicrobial stewardship? *Clin Microbiol Infect.* 2017;23(11):793–798. doi:10.1016/j.cmi.2017.08.026

5. Levison ME, Levison JH. Pharmacokinetics and pharmacodynamics of antibacterial agents. *Infect Dis Clin North Am.* 2009;23(4):791–815, vii. doi:10.1016/j.idc.2009.06.008

6. Craig WA, Vogelman B. The postantibiotic effect. *Ann Intern Med.* 1987;106(6):900–902. doi:10.7326/0003-4819-106-6-900.

7. Pankey GA, Sabath LD. Clinical relevance of bacteriostatic versus bactericidal mechanisms of action in the treatment of gram-positive bacterial infections. *Clin Infect Dis.* 2004;38(6):864–870. doi:10.1086/381972

8. Wald-Dickler N, Holtom P, Spellberg B. Busting the myth of "static vs cidal": a systemic literature review. *Clin Infect Dis.* 2019;66(9):1470–1474. doi:10.1093/cid/cix1127

9. Ament PW, Bertolino JG, Liszewski JL. Clinically significant drug interactions. *Am Fam Physician.* 2020;61(6):1745–1754. https://www.aafp.org/afp/2000/0315/p1745.html

10. Barditch-Crovo P, Trapnell CB, Ette E, et al. The effects of rifampin and rifabutin on the pharmacokinetics and pharmacodynamics of a combination oral contraceptive. *Clin Pharmacol Ther.* 1999;65(4):428–438. doi:10.1016/S0009-9236(99)70138-4

11. Blumenthal KG, Peter JG, Trubiano JA, et al. Antibiotic allergy. *Lancet.* 2019;393(10167):183–198. doi:10.1016/S0140-6736(18)32218-9

12. Har D, Solensky R. Penicillin and beta-lactam hypersensitivity. *Immunol Allergy Clin North Am.* 2017;37(4):643–662. doi:10.1016/j.iac.2017.07.001

13. Frumin J, Gallagher JC. Allergic cross-sensitivity between penicillin, carbapenem, and monobactam antibiotics: What are the chances? *Ann Pharmacother.* 2009;43(2):304–315. doi:10.1345/aph.1L486

14. Herbert ME, Brewster GS, Lanctot-Herbert M. Ten percent of patients who are allergic to penicillin will have serious reactions if exposed to cephalosporins. *West J Med.* 2000;172(5):341. doi:10.1136/ewjm.172.5.341

15. Daulat S, Solensky R, Earl HS, et al. Safety of cephalosporin administration to patients with histories of penicillin allergy. *J Allergy Clin Immunol.* 2004;113(6):1220–1222. doi:10.1016/j.jaci.2004.03.023

16. Joint Task Force on Practice Parameters; American Academy of Allergy, Asthma and Immunology; American College of Allergy, Asthma and Immunology; Joint Council of Allergy, Asthma and Immunology. Drug allergy: An updated practice parameter. *Ann Allergy Asthma Immunol.* 2010;105(4):259–273. doi:10.1016/j.anai.2010.08.002

17. Lobanovska M, Pilla G. Penicillin's discovery and antibiotic resistance: lessons for the future? *Yale J Biol Med.* 2017;90(1):135–145. https://www.ncbi.nlm.nih.gov/pmc/articles/PMC5369031

18. Bush K. Antimicrobial agents targeting bacterial cell walls and cell membranes. *Rev Sci Tech.* 2012;31(1):43–56. doi:10.20506/rst.31.1.2096

19. Waxman DJ, Strominger JL. Penicillin-binding proteins and the mechanism of action of beta-lactam antibiotics. *Ann Rev Biochem.* 1983;52:825–869. doi:10.1146/annurev.bi.52.070183.004141

20. Poole K. Resistance to beta-lactam antibiotics. *Cell Mol Life Sci*. 2004;61(17):2200–2223. doi:10.1007/s00018-004-4060-9

21. Bush K, Bradford PA. β-lactams and β-lactamase inhibitors: an overview. *Cold Spring Harb Perspect Med*. 2016;6(8):a025247. doi:10.1101/cshperspect.a025247

22. Malik ZA, Litman N. The penicillins. *Pediatr Rev*. 2006;27(12):471–473. doi:10.1542/pir.27-12-471

23. Malik ZA, Litman N. Ampicillin and amoxicillin. *Pediatr Rev*. 2006;27(11):434–436. doi:10.1542/pir.27-11-434

24. Mingeot-Leclercq MP, Glupczynski Y, Tulkens PM. Aminoglycosides: activity and resistance. *Antimicrob Agents Chemother*. 1999;43(4):727–737. doi:10.1128/AAC.43.4.727

25. Davis BD. Bactericidal synergism between beta-lactams and aminoglycosides: mechanism and possible therapeutic implications. *Rev Infect Dis*. 1982;4(2):237–245. doi:10.1093/clinids/4.2.237

26. McLean AJ, IoannidesDemos LL, Li SC, et al. Bactericidal effect of gentamicin peak concentration provides a rationale for administration of bolus doses. *J Antimicrob Chemother*. 1993;32(2):301–305. doi:10.1093/jac/32.2.301

27. Dobie RA, Black FO, Pezsnecker SC, et al. Hearing loss in patients with vestibulotoxic reactions to gentamicin therapy. *Arch Otolaryngol Head Neck Surg*. 2006;132(3):253–257. doi:10.1001/archotol.132.3.253

28. Humes HD. Aminoglycoside nephrotoxicity. *Kidney Int*. 1988;33(4):900–911. doi:10.1038/ki.1988.83

29. Nicolau DP, Freeman CD, Belliveau PP, et al. Experience with a once-daily aminoglycoside program administered to 2,184 adult patients. *Antimicrob Agents Chemother*. 1995;39(3):650–655. doi:10.1128/AAC.39.3.650

30. Oliphant CM, Green GM. Quinolones: a comprehensive review. *Am Fam Physician*. 2019;65(3):455. –465. https://www.aafp.org/afp/2002/0201/p455.html

31. Gonzalez-Ruiz A, Seaton RA, Hamed K. Daptomycin: an evidence-based review of its role in the treatment of Gram-positive infections. *Infect Drug Resist*. 2016;9:47–58. doi:10.2147/IDR.S99046

32. Silverman JA, Mortin LI, Vanpraagh AD, et al. Inhibition of daptomycin by pulmonary surfactant: in vitro modeling and clinical impact. *J Infect Dis*. 2005;191(12):2149–2152. doi:10.1086/430352

33. Nemeth J, Oesch G, Kuster SP. Bacteriostatic versus bactericidal antibiotics for patients with serious bacterial infections: systematic review and meta-analysis. *J Antimicrob Chemother*. 2019;70(2):382–395. doi:10.1093/jac/dku379

34. Ocampo PS, Viktória L, Balázs P, et al. Antagonism between bacteriostatic and bactericidal antibiotics is prevalent. *Antimicrob Agents Chemother*. 2014;58(8):4573–4582. doi:10.1128/AAC.02463-14

35. Koulenti D, Song A, Ellingboe A, et al. Infections by multidrug-resistant Gram-negative bacteria: What's new in our arsenal and what's in the pipeline? *Int J Antimicrob Agents*. 2018;53(3):211–224. doi:10.1016/j.ijantimicag.2018.10.011

36. Ho JM, Juurlink DN. Considerations when prescribing trimethoprim-sulfamethoxazole. *CMAJ*. 2011;183(16):1851–1858. doi:10.1503/cmaj.111152

37. Bozdogan B, Appelbaum PC. Oxazolidinones: activity, mode of action, and mechanism of resistance. *Int J Antimicrob Agents*. 2004;23(2):113–119. doi:10.1016/j.ijantimicag.2003.11.003

38. Quinn DK, Stern TA. Linezolid and serotonin syndrome. *Prim Care Companion J Clin Psychiatry*. 2009;11:353–356. doi:10.4088/PCC.09r00853

39. Manzella J. Quinupristin-dalfopristin: a new antibiotic for severe gram-positive infections. *Am Fam Physician*. 2001;64(11):1863–1867. https://www.aafp.org/afp/2001/1201/p1863.html

40. Huttner A, Kowalczyk A, Turjeman A, et al. Effect of 5-day nitrofurantoin vs single-dose fosfomycin on clinical resolution of uncomplicated lower urinary tract infection in women: a randomized clinical trial. *JAMA*. 2018;319(17):1781–1789. doi:10.1001/jama.2018.3627

41. Falagas ME, Roussos N, Gkegkes ID, et al. Fosfomycin for the treatment of infections caused by Gram-positive cocci with advanced antimicrobial drug resistance: a review of microbiological, animal and clinical studies. *Expert Opin Invest Drugs*. 2009;18(7):921–944. doi:10.1517/13543780902967624

42. Singh N, Gandhi S, McArthur E, et al. Kidney function and the use of nitrofurantoin to treat urinary tract infections in older women. *CMAJ*. 2015;187(9):648–656. doi:10.1503/cmaj.150067

43. Zhanel GG, Walkty AJ, Karlowsky JA. Fidaxomicin: A novel agent for the treatment of clostridium difficile infection. *Can J Infect Dis Med Microbiol*. 2015;26(6):305–312. doi:10.1155/2015/934594

44. McDonald LC, Gerding DN, Johnson S, et al. Clinical practice guidelines for clostridium difficile infection in adults and children: 2017 update by the Infectious Diseases Society of America (IDSA) and Society for Healthcare Epidemiology of America (SHEA). *Clin Infect Dis*. 2018;66(7):e1–e48. doi:10.1093/cid/cix1085

45. Furin J, Cox H, Pai M. Tuberculosis. *Lancet*. 2019;393:1642–1656. doi:10.1016/S0140-6736(19)30308-3

46. Tang P, Johnston J. Treatment of latent tuberculosis infection. *Curr Treat Options Infect Dis*. 2017;9(4):371–379. doi:10.1007/s40506-017-0135-7

47. Nahid P, Dorman SE, Alipanah N, et al. Official American Thoracic Society/Centers for Disease Control and Prevention/Infectious Diseases Society of America Clinical Practice Guidelines: Treatment of Drug-Susceptible Tuberculosis. *Clin Infect Dis*. 2016;63(7):e147–e195. doi:10.1093/cid/ciw376

48. Unissa AN, Subbian S, Hanna LE, Selvakumar N. Overview on mechanisms of isoniazid action and resistance in Mycobacterium tuberculosis. *Infect Genet Evol*. 2016;45:474–492. doi: 10.1016/j.meegid.2016.09.004

49. Metushi I, Uetrecht J, Phillips E. Mechanism of isoniazid-induced hepatotoxicity: then and now. *Br J Clin Pharmacol*. 2016;81(6):1030–1036. doi:10.1111/bcp.12885

50. Piso RJ, Kriz K, Desax M-C. Severe isoniazid related sideroblastic anemia. *Hematol Rep*. 2011;3(1):e2. doi:10.4081/hr.2011.e2

51. Rothstein DM. Rifamycins, alone and in combination. *Cold Spring Harb Perspect Med*. 2016;6(7):a027011. doi:10.1101/cshperspect.a027011

52. LiverTox: Clinical and research information on drug-induced liver injury. Rifampin. Bethesda, MD: National Institute of Diabetes and Digestive and Kidney Diseases. 2012. PMID: 31643176

53. Zhang Y, Mitchison D. The curious characteristics of pyrazinamide: A review. *Int J Tuberc Lung Dis.* 2003;7(1):6–21.

54. Lee N, Nguyen H. Ethambutol. *StatPearls.* Treasure Island, FL: StatPearls Publishing; 2020. PMID: 32644476.

55. World Health Organization. Multidrug and extensively drug-resistant TB (M/XDR-TB): 2010 report on global surveillance and response (No. WHO/HTM/TB/2010.3). Published 2010.

56. Nahid P, Mase SR, Migliori GB, et al. Treatment of drug-resistant tuberculosis. An official ATS/CDC/ERS/IDSA clinical practice guideline. *Am J Respir Crit Care Med.* 2019; 200(10):e93–e142. doi:10.1164/rccm.201909-1874ST

57. Whitley RJ, Gnann JW Jr. Acyclovir: A decade later. *N Engl J Med.* 1992;327(11):782–789. doi:10.1056/ NEJM199209103271108.

58. Wagstaff AJ, Bryson HM. Foscarnet. A reappraisal of its antiviral activity, pharmacokinetic properties and therapeutic use in immunocompromised patients with viral infections. *Drugs.* 1994;48(2):199–226. doi:10.2165/00003495-199448020-00007

59. Faulds D, Heel RC. Ganciclovir. A review of its antiviral activity, pharmacokinetic properties and therapeutic efficacy in cytomegalovirus infections. *Drugs.* 1990;39(4):597–638. doi:10.2165/00003495-199039040-00008

60. Marty F, Ljungman P, Chemaly R. Letermovir prophylaxis for cytomegalovirus in hematopoietic-cell transplantation. *N Engl J Med.* 2017;377:2433–2444. doi:10.1056/ NEJMoa1706640

61. Hayden, Sugaya N. Baloxavir marboxil for uncomplicated influenza in adults and adolescents. *N Engl J Med.* 2018;379:913–923. doi:10.1056/NEJMoa1716197

62. GBD 2015 Disease and Injury Incidence and Prevalence, Collaborators. Global, regional, and national incidence, prevalence, and years lived with disability for 310 diseases and injuries, 1990–2015: A systematic analysis for the Global Burden of Disease Study 2015. *Lancet.* 2016;388(10053):1545–1602. doi:10.1016/S0140-6736(16)31678-6

63. AASLD-IDSA HCV Guidance Panel. Hepatitis C guidance 2018 update: AASLD-IDSA recommendations for testing, managing, and treating hepatitis C virus infection. *Clin Infect Dis.* 2018;67(10):1477–1492. doi:10.1093/cid/ ciy585

64. Terrault N, Lok A, McMahon B, et al. AASLD guidelines for treatment of chronic hepatitis B. *Hepatology.* 2018;63(1):261–283. doi:10.1002/hep.28156

65. Pfizer, Inc. *VFEND® (voriconazole)* [package insert]. Published June 2010. https://www.accessdata.fda.gov/ drugsatfda_docs/label/2010/021266s032lbl.pdf

66. Thompson GR 3rd, Wiederhold NP. Isavuconazole: A comprehensive review of spectrum of activity of a new triazole. *Mycopathologia.* 2010;170(5):291–313. doi:10.1007/s11046-010-9324-3

67. Nagappan V, Deresinski S. Reviews of anti-infective agents: Posaconazole: A broad-spectrum triazole antifungal agent. *Clin Infect Dis.* 2007;45(12):1610–1617. doi:10.1086/523576

68. Sawaya BP, Briggs JP, Schnermann J. Amphotericin B nephrotoxicity: the adverse consequences of altered membrane properties. *J Am Soc Nephrol.* 1995;6(2):154–164. https:// jasn.asnjournals.org/content/jnephrol/6/2/154.full.pdf

69. Denning DW. Echinocandin antifungal drugs. *Lancet.* 2003;362(9390):1142–1151. doi:10.1016/S0140-6736(03)14472-8

Antiretroviral Pharmacotherapy

Sampath Wijesinghe, Andrew Nevins, Simon Paul, and Tegest Hailu

LEARNING OBJECTIVES

- Summarize the emergence of human immunodeficiency virus (HIV) as it relates to the development of drug therapy in the course of the disease.
- Outline the process of transmission of HIV and describe the risk factors that impact this process.
- Differentiate between the risks of HIV through sexual transmission, exposure to blood or blood products, and perinatal transmission and outline the various methods used for screening and diagnosis.
- Describe the basic principles of treatment of HIV, differentiate by class the various treatment options available to manage HIV, and describe the monitoring and patient education involved.
- Describe the nonpharmacological treatment that comprises the overall management of the patient with HIV. Review the factors involved in the prophylaxis and treatment of opportunistic infections and illustrate the challenges involved in the entire process of managing this population.

INTRODUCTION

More than 1.1 million individuals in the United States live with human immunodeficiency virus (HIV) today.[1] According to 2018 data, for every 100 people who were diagnosed with HIV, 65 received medical care and 56 had viral suppression. In the United States, those most at risk of contracting HIV infection include homosexual men and African Americans. Recently, a significant rise of newly diagnosed cases has been noted among Hispanic/Latino gay or bisexual men. A report from 2018 data showed that there were 15,820 deaths among adults and adolescents diagnosed with HIV in the United States.[1] Fortunately, there have been significant developments in antiretroviral therapy (ART) that allow HIV-positive patients an improved quality of life and increased life expectancy. As HIV/acquired immunodeficiency syndrome (AIDS) becomes a chronic disease, research recommends utilizing a chronic disease management model.[2] This involves a multidisciplinary team of HIV specialists, counselors, and primary care clinicians. This chapter addresses current approaches to antiretroviral pharmacotherapy and covers the treatment of opportunistic infections.

BACKGROUND

The development of antiretroviral pharmacotherapy can be traced as far back as the early 1980s when the retrovirus was identified as the causative agent of HIV/AIDS. Barré-Sinoussi and colleagues[3] identified the virus and Gallo et al.[4] demonstrated that the loss of T cells (CD4+ cells) is the primary cause of immunodeficiency. The other milestones were the ability to measure HIV ribonucleic acid (RNA) levels in clinical specimens,[5,6] and the development and approval of effective antiretroviral therapy (ART).[7,8]

The emergence of HIV drugs started with the identification of the HIV virus, specifically its structure, virulence, and pathogenesis. HIV is an RNA virus with a life cycle that allows many targets for ART (**Figure 31.1**). The HIV binds to a CD4 surface molecule and a chemokine receptor, both present on activated CD4-cells (also known as T cells or *helper cells*). After cell entry, the enzyme *reverse transcriptase* transcribes the viral RNA into a deoxyribonucleic acid (DNA) copy. Subsequently, this viral DNA fragment is integrated into the host's CD4 cell chromosomal DNA. The integrated viral DNA is now transcribed under the host's cell transcription process to produce messenger

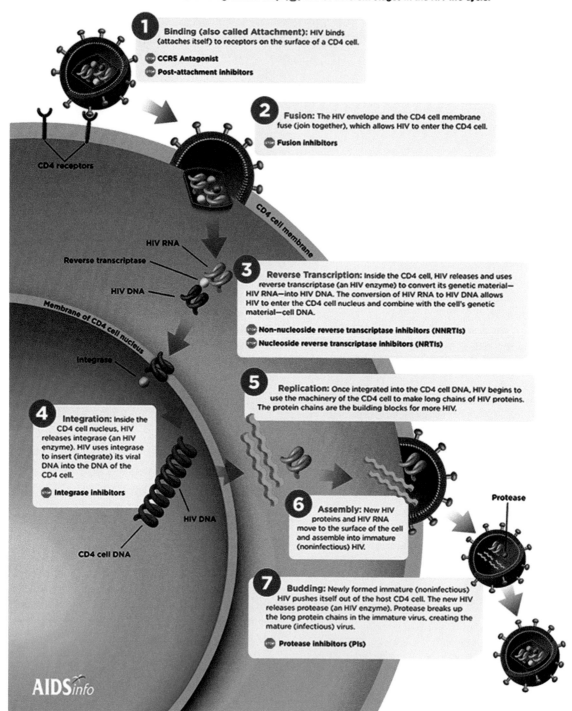

FIGURE 31.1 The HIV life cycle.

Source: U.S. National Library of Medicine. https://hivinfo.nih.gov/understanding-hiv/fact-sheets/hiv-life-cycle

RNA (mRNA), which is then translated into viral proteins. Eventually, the HIV protease cleaves the newly synthesized polypeptides into individual HIV proteins that allow the virus to assemble itself and buds from the host cells.[9] Over time, the HIV infection will deplete the host CD4 cells, leading to immunodeficiency.

In addition to the death of CD4 cells leading to long-term cell decline, chronic immune activation has also been proposed as an etiology leading to immune exhaustion.[10] It has been demonstrated that HIV infection leads to significant chronic systemic inflammation and opportunistic infections due to persistent exposure of viral antigens.[11] For example, loss of gut-associated lymphoid tissue has been shown to occur early in HIV infection, leading to chronic systemic exposure to highly inflammatory bacterial lipopolysaccharides (LPS).[11–14] Furthermore, chronic inflammation and a depletion of CD4 cells lead to stress on naive T cells, which subsequently create short-lived activated CD4 cells. In most patients, CD4 cells decline from a normal value of near 1,000 cells/µL to below 200 cells/µL over time.[15] The cell-mediated immunity of the host becomes considerably impaired when these CD4 cell counts fall below the threshold (i.e., 200 cells/µL, an AIDS-defining event). Because of the immunodeficiency, the host becomes more susceptible to opportunistic infections (OI). Examples of OI associated with AIDS include *Pneumocystis jirovecii* pneumonia, cryptococcal meningitis, disseminated *Mycobacterium avium*, and cancers such as Kaposi's sarcoma or non-Hodgkin's lymphoma.

While ART can stop viral replication and allow regeneration of CD4 cell counts, inflammation persists even after years of treatment.[16] This chronic inflammation may be the cause of a higher incidence of renal and cardiac diseases now seen in aging HIV patients who have been on ART for many years.[17] The inability to cure HIV infection with ART is partly due to the infection of long-lived memory T-cells. While the HIV does not infect these quiescent memory cells (not active CD4 cells) directly, it is believed that HIV by chance may infect active T-cells just at the time they become inactivated to remain as long-lived memory CD4 cells.[18,19] The integrated HIV DNA is not transcribed while these cells remain in quiescence. However, if these "latent" HIV-infected memory cells become activated, the HIV genes will be transcribed. It has been estimated that the reservoir of infected quiescent cells slowly decays with a half-life of approximately 40 to 44 months.[20,21] Investigations are still underway to target and eradicate these long-lived quiescent cells. However, even with maximum suppression of viral replication using the current ART, these memory cells will allow for reappearance of viremia if treatment is stopped.[22]

RISK FACTORS FOR HUMAN IMMUNODEFICIENCY VIRUS

HIV infection is acquired through sexual contact, through exposure to infected blood or blood products, or during childbirth. For all modes of transmission, a higher viral load in the HIV-infected person is associated with a higher risk of transmission to others. Although the incidence of HIV has decreased since the height of the epidemic, understanding risk factors for infection is important for individual patient assessment and screening. It is also the cornerstone of ongoing prevention strategies.

SEXUAL TRANSMISSION

The incidence of sexual transmission of HIV varies by behavior and extent of exposure. In general, sexual behavior that disrupts the mucosa and causes bleeding is associated with higher risk than behaviors that do not disrupt the mucosa. HIV transmission between men who have sex with men (MSM) is generally higher than transmission between heterosexual partners. Among heterosexual partners, male-to-female transmission is thought to be slightly more common than female-to-male. Interestingly, female-to-female sexual transmission of HIV has rarely been reported.[23]

Sexually transmitted infections (STI) may increase the risk of HIV infection. Although the risk is greatest with concomitant genital ulcer disease (e.g., herpes simplex virus, primary syphilis), other STIs that cause significant urethral irritation (e.g., gonococcal urethritis) are also associated with an increased risk of transmission. Studies have shown that HIV transmission rates tend to be higher in uncircumcised than circumcised males. Although circumcision has been shown to decrease the risk of female-to-male HIV transmission, it has not shown to decrease risk of transmission to a female partner.[24,25] Additionally, the risk of reduction in MSM has not been demonstrated.

BLOODBORNE TRANSMISSION

The risk of HIV transmission by exposure to blood or blood products varies based on a specific exposure. Prior to the development of effective screening methods in the 1980s, the greatest risk of transmission was via blood transfusion. Fortunately, the incidence of this type of transmission has markedly diminished in most industrialized countries.[26] Today, one of the greatest risks of bloodborne transmission is through needle sharing (particularly among intravenous [IV] drug users) and percutaneous needle-stick injuries in healthcare workers.[27,28] It is important to note that many individuals who inject illegal/street drugs also engage in high-risk sexual behaviors that increase risk of infection. The risk of HIV acquisition from a needle-stick injury depends upon the infection status of the source and characteristics of the injury.[23] Exposure to blood sources from an individual with a high viral load is associated with a higher risk of transmission. Deep injuries, injury with a hollow-bore needle, injury with a needle that had been in an artery or vein, and injuries with a visibly contaminated needle or other device also carry very high risk of transmission. Lastly, HIV infection may be acquired via large mucous membrane exposure (e.g., a splash of infected blood into the eye), although transmission through this route is relatively rare. Studies have shown the risk of HIV transmission related to percutaneous exposure of infected blood is approximately at 0.3%.[29]

PERINATAL TRANSMISSION

The risk of perinatal HIV transmission depends on maternal risk factors and whether the mother is breast-feeding.[30] The transmission of HIV may occur during pregnancy, at delivery, or following delivery. High viral loads of maternal plasma and breast milk are associated with increased risk of transmission.[31] Additionally, micro-transfusions of maternal blood across the placenta to a fetus are also thought to be a source of perinatal infection, since the majority of in utero exposures of HIV occur during the third trimester.[32] Placental inflammation (particularly chorioamnionitis) is also thought to increase in utero transmission.[33]

Intrapartum transmission occurs from contact of infant mucosal membranes with the HIV virus in blood and secretions in the vaginal canal. In addition, a prolonged duration of membrane rupture (longer than 4 hours) has been associated with an increased risk of transmission.[34] Although the exact mechanism of transmission during breastfeeding is unknown, HIV has been detected in both colostrum and breast milk.[35]

SCREENING AND DIAGNOSIS OF HUMAN IMMUNODEFICIENCY VIRUS

In 2006, the Centers for Disease Control (CDC) revised HIV testing guidelines recommending routine, opt-out testing for everyone between the ages of 13 and 64.[36,37] In addition, the United States Preventive Services Task Force[38] recommended routine HIV screening for all individuals between the ages 15 and 65. HIV screening no longer requires an individualized risk-factor assessment, special counseling, or signed consent.[37,39] Despite recommendations, HIV screening has been a challenge to implement and remains underused and inconsistently applied across the United States. Although universal HIV testing was established over a decade ago, as many as 14% of HIV-positive individuals are unaware of their status. In 2014, 23% of individuals newly diagnosed with HIV already had AIDS, underscoring the disparity of the screening process.[40] It has been clearly documented that individuals with HIV who are under consistent medical care and have viral suppression are less likely to transmit HIV.[1] These findings support the need to maximize early screening, testing, and treatment. Timely diagnosis is critical.

The period of acute HIV infection is the first 6 months of virus acquisition. During this period, individuals are highly infectious due to high viremia and lack of awareness of their HIV status.[41] The acute infection is marked by a high HIV RNA level and presence of P24 antigen along with a negative or indeterminate antibody testing. When an acute HIV infection is suspected, an HIV RNA and subsequent confirmatory HIV antibody test should be used for diagnosis.

HIV infection has four distinctive stages. The *eclipse* stage is the first 10 to 12 days postinfection. The eclipse stage is without consistently detectable laboratory markers making diagnosis unlikely. The next stage is the *seroconversion window*, the period between infection and the first antibody detection (IgG). This is followed by *acute HIV infection*, which is the stage of HIV acquisition and detectable HIV RNA or P24 antigen and an absent antibody. It is at this stage that a person is highly infectious. The final stage is *established HIV infection/seroconversion*, during which time there is a detectable IgG antibody test.[42]

During the acute stage of infection, an infected individual may develop an *acute retroviral syndrome*. The symptoms are frequently mistaken for a common viral infection due to a transient surge of viremia and a drop in CD4 count. They include fever, fatigue, myalgia, headache, pharyngitis, cervical lymphadenopathy, and a skin rash on the trunk, which commonly appear within 28 days of infection and may last for days to weeks.[42]

TYPES OF SCREENING FOR HUMAN IMMUNODEFICIENCY VIRUS

According to the CDC,[43] three types of HIV diagnostic tests are commonly utilized: nucleic acid tests (NAT), antibody tests, and antigen/antibody tests. NATs can detect HIV RNA within 10 to 33 days after infection. These tests are expensive and are generally reserved for acute infection or recent high-risk exposure. Antibody tests are reliable but do not detect early infection or effectively differentiate HIV-1 from HIV-2. Because they rely on antibody formation the diagnostic capacity varies from 23 to 90 days. Antigen/antibody tests were approved by the U.S. Food and Drug Administration (FDA) in 2010 and are the fourth generation of HIV immunoassay. These tests screen for both antigen P24 and the IgM and IgG antibodies. They have a diagnostic capacity from 18 to 45 days after infection.

The HIV fourth generation (antigen/antibody) assays also have greater than 99.7% sensitivity and 99.3% specificity.[44] Positive results from a fourth-generation screening test require a supplemental HIV-1/HIV-2 differentiation assay.[45] The differentiation between HIV-1 and HIV-2 is crucial as HIV-2 is genetically different; therefore, it is more prone to develop resistance to some of the recommended ARV agents.[46] To date, the HIV-1 Western blot is no longer recommended as a confirmatory test, since the HIV-1/HIV-2 antibody test has greater sensitivity for detecting early infection, can rapidly be performed, and accurately differentiate HIV-1 from HIV-2.[45]

TREATMENT FOR HUMAN IMMUNODEFICIENCY VIRUS

BASIC PRINCIPLES OF TREATMENT

The cornerstone for the management of HIV infection should involve a complete history, comprehensive

BOX 31.1
BASELINE EVALUATION IN NEW HUMAN IMMUNODEFICIENCY VIRUS INFECTION

- HIV antibody testing (if no documentation available or HIV RNA is below the assay's limit)

- CD4 lymphocyte cell count*

- Plasma HIV RNA (viral load)*

- Complete blood count

- Complete metabolic panel

- Fasting blood sugar

- Fasting lipids

- Urinalysis

- Pregnancy test (women of childbearing potential)

- Hepatitis A, B, and C serologies

- Genotypic resistance testing**

- Testing for gonorrhea, chlamydia, syphilis, and other sexually transmitted infections

- Viral tropism assay***

- HLA-B*5701****

*CD4 count and Plasma HIV RNA are two surrogate markers routinely used to monitor patients with HIV.
**If patient's viral load is <500 to 1,000 copies/mL, viral amplification for resistance may fail.
***Prior to initiation of CCR5 antagonist or if there is a virologic failure while patient is on CCR5 antagonist.
****Prior to initiation of abacavir (ABC). Baseline assessment allows rapid response if ABC is needed.
RNA, ribonucleic acid.

Source: Panel on Antiretroviral Guidelines for Adults and Adolescents. Guidelines for the use of antiretroviral agents in adults and adolescents with HIV. Department of Health and Human Services. Updated December 18, 2019. https://clinicalinfo.hiv.gov/sites/default/files/guidelines/documents/AdultandAdolescentGL.pdf

physical examination, pertinent laboratories, and counseling. With a newly diagnosed patient, it is important to find out if they were on any HIV pre-exposure prophylaxis (PrEP). For patients with established diagnosis, it is also vital to obtain history of prior ARV treatment and the results of resistance testing.

For a patient with a new HIV infection, the Guidelines for the Use of Antiretroviral Agents in Adults and Adolescents with HIV[42] recommend the baseline tests listed in **Box 31.1**.

The development of effective ART has changed HIV into a chronic disease that can be effectively managed. The goal of ART is to reduce HIV-related morbidity and mortality and prevent transmission. When managing HIV infection, ART should be initiated as soon as possible regardless of CD4 count.[42] Studies show early initiation of ART reduces risk of progression to AIDS, reduces T-cell activation, and increases host immune-response to vaccines.[47–49] The primary goal of ART is HIV viral load suppression. Changing the ART regimen is not indicated in patients with an undetectable viral load even if the CD4 count does not increase.

Up to 10% to 15% of patients may be infected with a virus that has developed drug resistance.[50] Cross resistance is more common with older drug classes such as the nucleoside/nucleotide reverse transcriptase inhibitors (NRTI); therefore, a drug resistance test (HIV genotype) should be completed to determine if the viral strain is resistant to any ARV agent prior to starting ART.

PHARMACOTHERAPY FOR HUMAN IMMUNODEFICIENCY VIRUS

Presently, there are more than 30 different ARV agents in seven drug classes used for treatment of HIV infection. Each ARV class generally targets a unique step in the life cycle of HIV.

- NRTIs
- Nonnucleoside/nucleotide reverse transcriptase inhibitors (NNRTIs)
- Protease inhibitors (PIs)
- Fusion inhibitors (FIs)
- CCR5 receptor antagonists
- Integrase strand transfer inhibitors (INSTIs)
- Postattachment inhibitors

In order to maximize the effectiveness of ART and reduce drug resistance, the initial regimen should include three medications from at least two drug classes that target different steps of the life cycle. Some formulations are available in combinations of active ingredients. According to the 2019 PAGAA recommendations, the first-line regimens for antiretroviral naïve patients typically include two NRTIs plus an INSTI. A combination of one NRTI plus an INSTI may be considered *except* for individuals with HIV RNA >500,000 copies/mL, HBV coinfection, or in whom ART is to be started before the results of HIV genotypic resistance testing for reverse transcriptase or HBV testing are available.[42] **Table 31.1** presents typical initial combination regimens for ARV-naïve HIV-positive patients. The combination of tenofovir disoproxil and emtricitabine (TDF/FTC) is commonly used as PrEP in HIV-negative persons. In the setting of a new HIV diagnosis in persons who are currently taking or have previously taken PrEP, drug-resistance results are particularly important. However, one of the regimens listed in **Table 31.2** may be initiated pending resistance testing results.[42,51] Additionally, clinicians should adjust drug regimens based on patient-specific factors such as age, pregnancy, and

TABLE 31.1 Recommended Initial Combination Regimens in the Antiretroviral-Naïve Patient

INSTI Plus Two NRTIs (in Alphabetical Order)

INSTI	NRTI Combinations	Level of Evidence
Bictegravir	TAF plus FTC	AI
Dolutegravir	ABC plus 3TC*	AI
Dolutegravir	TAF or TDF** plus (FTC or 3TC)	AI
Raltegravir	(TAF or TDF)** plus (FTC or 3TC)	BI for TDF/FTC or 3TC BII for TAF/FTC

INSTI Plus One NRTI***

INSTI	NRTI	Level of Evidence
Dolutegravir	3TC	AI

*Only for individuals who are HLA-B*5701 negative and without chronic hepatitis B virus coinfection.

**TAF and TDF are two forms of tenofovir that are approved by the FDA. TAF has fewer bone and kidney toxicities than TDF, while TDF is associated with lower lipid levels. Safety, cost, and access are among the factors to consider when choosing between these drugs.

***3TC is recommended for use with DTG in ART-naive persons, and with DRV/r if ABC, TDF, and TAF are not optimal. Otherwise, dual-NRTI backbones are recommended.

Note: **Rating of recommendations:** A, Strong; B, Moderate; C, Optional.

Rating of evidence: I, Data from randomized controlled trials; II, Data from well-designed nonrandomized trials, observational cohort studies with long-term clinical outcomes, relative bioavailability/bioequivalence studies, or regimen comparisons from randomized switch studies; III, Expert opinion.

3TC, lamivudine; ABC, abacavir; FTC, emtricitabine; INSTI, integrase strand transfer inhibitor; NRTI, nucleoside reverse transcriptase inhibitor; TAF or TDF, tenofovir alafenamide.

Source: Panel on Antiretroviral Guidelines for Adults and Adolescents. Guidelines for the use of antiretroviral agents in adults and adolescents with HIV. Department of Health and Human Services. Updated December 18, 2019. https://clinicalinfo.hiv.gov/sites/default/files/guidelines/documents/AdultandAdolescentGL.pdf

TABLE 31.2 Prophylaxis to Prevent Opportunistic Infections

Opportunistic Infection	Indication	Preferred	Alternative
Pneumocystis pneumonia	CD4 count <200 cells/ mm³ **(AI)**, *or* CD4 <14% **(BII)**, *or* CD4 count >200 but <250 cells/ mm³ if monitoring CD4 cell count every 3 months is not possible **(BII)**	TMP–SMX* one double-strength (DS) po daily **(AI)**, *or* TMP–SMX* one single-strength (SS) daily **(AI)**	TMP–SMX* one DS po three times weekly **(BI)**, *or* dapsone** 100 mg po daily or 50 mg po bid **(BI)**, *or* dapsone** 50 mg po daily + (pyrimethamine 50 mg + leucovorin 25 mg) po weekly **(BI)**, *or* (dapsone** 200 mg + pyrimethamine*** 75 mg + leucovorin 25 mg) po weekly **(BI)**; *or* aerosolized pentamidine 300 mg via Respirgard II™ nebulizer every month **(BI)**, *or* atovaquone 1,500 mg po daily **(BI)**, *or* (atovaquone 1,500 mg + pyrimethamine*** 25 mg + leucovorin 10 mg) po daily **(CIII)**
Toxoplasma gondii encephalitis	Toxoplasma IgG-positive patients with CD4 count <100 cells/µL **(AII)**	TMP–SMX* 1 DS po daily **(AII)**	TMP–SMX* one DS po three times weekly **(BIII)**, *or* TMP–SMX* one SS po daily **(BIII)**, *or* dapsone** 50 mg po daily + (pyrimethamine*** 50 mg + leucovorin 25 mg) po weekly **(BI)**, *or* (dapsone** 200 mg + pyrimethamine*** 75 mg + leucovorin 25 mg) po weekly **(BI)**; *or* atovaquone 1,500 mg po daily **(CIII)** ; *or* (atovaquone 1,500 mg + pyrimethamine*** 25 mg + leucovorin 10 mg) po daily **(CIII)**

(continued)

TABLE 31.2 Prophylaxis to Prevent Opportunistic Infections (*continued*)

Opportunistic Infection	Indication	Preferred	Alternative
Mycobacterium tuberculosis infection (i.e., treatment of latent TB infection)	(+) screening test for LTBI, with no evidence of active TB, and no prior treatment for active TB or LTBI (**AI**), or close contact with a person with infectious TB, with no evidence of active TB, regardless of screening test results (**AII**).	(INH 300 mg + pyridoxine 25–50 mg) po daily × 9 months (**AII**), or INH 900 mg po BIW (by DOT) + pyridoxine 25–50 mg po daily × 9 months (**BII**).	Rifampin 600 mg po daily × 4 months (**BIII**), or rifabutin (dose adjusted based on concomitant ART)***** × 4 months (**BIII**), or (rifapentine [see dose below] po + INH 900 mg po + pyridoxine 50 mg po) once weekly × 12 weeks Rifapentine dose: 32.1 to 49.9 kg: 750 mg 50 mg: 900 mg; rifapentine recommended only for patients receiving raltegravir- or efavirenz-based ART regimen For persons exposed to drug-resistant TB, select anti-TB drugs after consultation with experts or public health authorities (**AII**).
Disseminated *Mycobacterium avium* complex disease	CD4 count <50 cells/µL—after ruling out active disseminated MAC disease based on clinical assessment (**AI**).	Azithromycin 1,200 mg po once weekly (**AI**), or clarithromycin 500 mg po bid (**AI**), or azithromycin 600 mg po twice weekly (**BIII**)	Rifabutin (dose adjusted based on concomitant ART)***** (**BI**); rule out active TB before starting rifabutin
Histoplasma capsulatum infection	CD4 count ≤150 cells/µL and at high risk because of occupational exposure or live in a community with a hyperendemic rate of histoplasmosis (>10 cases/100 patient-years) (**BI**)	Itraconazole 200 mg po daily (**BI**)	
Coccidioidomycosis	A new positive IgM or IgG serologic test in patients who live in a disease-endemic area and with CD4 count <250 cells/µL (**BIII**)	Fluconazole 400 mg po daily (**BIII**)	
Penicilliosis	Patients with CD4 cell counts <100 cells/µL who live or stay for a long period in rural areas in northern Thailand, Vietnam, or Southern China (**BI**)	Itraconazole 200 mg once daily (**BI**)	Fluconazole 400 mg po once weekly (**BII**)

*TMP–SMX DS once daily also confers protection against toxoplasmosis and many respiratory bacterial infections; lower dose also likely confers protection.

**Patients should be tested for glucose-6-phosphate dehydrogenase (G6PD) before administration of dapsone or primaquine. Alternative agent should be used in patients found to have G6PD deficiency.

***Screening tests for LTBI include tuberculin skin test (TST) or interferon-gamma release assays (IGRA).

****Refer to "Drug Interactions" section in the Adult and Adolescent ARV Guidelines for dosing recommendation.

*****For more detailed guidelines on use of different ARV drugs, clinicians should refer to the Drug-Drug Interactions section of the Adult and Adolescent Antiretroviral Guidelines.

Note: Vaccinations not listed.

Evidence rating:

Strength of recommendation: A, strong recommendation for the statement; B, moderate recommendation for the statement; C, optional recommendation for the statement.**Quality of evidence for the recommendation:** I, one or more randomized trials with clinical outcomes and/or validated laboratory endpoints; II, one or more well-designed, nonrandomized trials or observational cohort studies with long-term clinical outcomes; III, expert opinion. In cases where there are no data for the prevention or treatment of an OI based on studies conducted in HIV-infected populations, but data derived from HIV-uninfected patients exist that can plausibly guide management decisions for patients with HIV/AIDS, the data will be rated as III but will be assigned recommendations of A, B, C depending on the strength of recommendation.

ART, antiretroviral therapy; bid, twice daily; BIW, twice a week; CD4, CD4 T lymphocyte cell; DOT, directly observed therapy; DS, double strength; IgG, immunoglobulin G; IgM, immunoglobulin M; INH, isoniazid; LTBI, latent tuberculosis infection; MAC, *Mycobacterium avium* complex; po, orally; SS, single strength; TB, tuberculosis; TMP–SMX, trimethoprim–sulfamethoxazole.

Source: Panel on Opportunistic Infections in Adults and Adolescents with HIV. *Guidelines for the Prevention and Treatment of Opportunistic Infections in Adults and Adolescents With HIV: Recommendations From the Centers for Disease Control and Prevention, the National Institutes of Health, and the HIV Medicine Association of the Infectious Diseases Society of America* [Table 1]. Updated November 21, 2019. https://clinicalinfo.hiv.gov/sites/default/files/guidelines/documents/Adult_OI.pdf

comorbidities. For further information, please also refer to population-specific guidelines available on the HIVinfo website (hivinfo.nih.gov).

While ART is recommended for all patients, the PAGAA advises urgent initiation of therapies in the following conditions: pregnancy, AIDS-defining conditions, CD4 count below <200 cells/μL, HIV-associated nephropathy, acute/early infection, HIV/hepatitis B virus coinfection, or HIV/hepatitis C virus coinfection. Currently, drugs used in ART can be combined for almost all patients. These drugs have long half-lives allowing once-daily dosing and a relatively low viral resistance rate. In addition, disease response can be monitored by clinicians with highly sensitive HIV RNA assays. Typically, viral suppression can be achieved in 12 to 24 weeks after initiating ART. Viral load rebound can also be monitored for HIV drug(s) resistance. If drug resistance develops, a different regimen without cross-resistant pattern should be implemented. In general, the predictors of virologic success are based on low baseline viremia, high potency of the ARV regimen, regimen tolerability, convenience, and patient adherence.[42]

Many of the currently available HIV medications are small molecules that target viral replication by binding to the active site of a viral protein or structure or enzyme. However, there are three notable exceptions. Maraviroc, a CCR5 antagonist, targets a human protein, the chemokine receptor on the surface of T-cells that the HIV uses for binding and entry to the host cells. The NRTIs are DNA nucleoside analogues that lack the hydroxyl group required to add the next base to the growing DNA chain. As the HIV reverse transcriptase transcribes the viral RNA into a DNA copy, NRTIs are incorporated to prevent the elongation of the DNA copy. NRTI is one of the original drug classes of ARV agents. Zidovudine or AZT was the first clinically effective drug available for HIV treatment.[52] Finally, the NNRTI drug class inhibits HIV reverse transcriptase by binding to the "NNRTI-binding pocket" of the enzyme, which then causes a conformational change of its active site.[53]

HIV resistance to ARV medications often results from a more traditional mechanism of viral mutations leading to amino acid changes at the drug binding site that reduce the ability of the drug to bind and effectively inhibit the enzymes. However, in the case of a drug that targets the human chemokine receptor CCR5 (e.g., maraviroc), resistance does not occur by changing the chemokine receptor; instead, the HIV virus develops the ability to bind an alternate chemokine receptor, CXCR4, on which this drug has no effect.[42,54]

The viral burden of HIV is commonly expressed as log viral load (VL). Using this method of reporting, clinicians can track the viral burden. With effective ART, the HIV VL may be suppressed to levels below detection by the currently available HIV RNA assays at 20 copies RNA/μL or less. The use of the log VL allows

comparison of drug effectiveness in patients with widely varying baseline VL. Most single ARV agents can lower the HIV log VL by 1 to 2 units; meanwhile, the baseline log VL is usually >4, and may be as high as 6 to 7. Therefore, monotherapy is **not** recommended to treat HIV; a three-drug regimen from two or more drug classes is usually required to lower the log VL to <1.[42]

The high mutation rate of the HIV virus also necessitates the use of combination ART. HIV reverse transcriptase has poor accuracy, which introduces multiple mutations with every transcript.[55] Based on the number of HIV virions present in an average person infected with the virus and the number of mutations introduced while generating this number of virions, it has been estimated that even prior to beginning ART every possible amino acid mutation already exists in the viral population.[56] Thus, if the HIV virus only requires a single amino acid mutation to become resistant to an ARV medication, that mutant virus already exists in a patient's viral population and will be selected immediately if that ARV agent is given as a single treatment. If multiple ARV medications are given, and especially if medications require more than two to three viral mutations for resistance, there will be adequate effectiveness to stop viral replication and prevent ongoing mutation. It should be noted that there is no pharmacological agent (i.e., ART) to date that is able to completely eradicate the virus from the host.[57]

Current trends in medication development focus on potency, longer durations of action, and intramuscular (IM) route of administration. One of the newer developments includes the use of broadly neutralizing antibodies that bind to the viral protein gp120, a CD4-binding molecule.[58,59] Antibodies that bind to almost all clinical isolates of HIV gp120 have been isolated. Infusion of these antibodies can prevent HIV virions from infecting T-cells and may have prolonged effectiveness.[58,59] Despite the various developments in the field of HIV treatment, most ART stops viral replication but has no direct effect on CD4 cell replication. A meta-analysis of interleukin 2 infusion as a strategy to increase CD4 count showed transient increases in CD4 cell count but no clinically significant benefits such as reductions in mortality, VL, or opportunistic infections.[60] While an international collaboration (the HIV Trials Network) is currently focused on the development of vaccines to prevent HIV/AIDS, there is no vaccine available that will prevent HIV infection as of this writing.[61]

NONPHARMACOLOGIC THERAPY FOR HUMAN IMMUNODEFICIENCY VIRUS

Many studies have found associations between disease progression, wasting, and one or more nutrient deficiencies in HIV-positive persons, associated with disease progression and poor outcomes.[62,63] To date, routine supplementation of multiple micronutrients has not shown consistent beneficial outcomes on disease progression or mortality. However, these observations should not exclude or deny supplementation of nutrients that have been shown to be deficient in specific cases. Therefore, daily multivitamin with minerals supplementation may still be beneficial and appropriate for HIV-positive patients with minimal risk.[64]

Studies have demonstrated 53% to 89.7% of persons with HIV use one or more nonpharmacologic therapies.[65,66] The most common indications for using nonpharmacologic therapies include improving general health, increasing overall sense of well-being and energy (61.4%), preventing or alleviating side effects of ART (50%), or relieving HIV-related conditions such as dermatological problems, nausea, depression, insomnia, and weakness.[67–69]

Despite various benefits reported such as improved quality of life (70%), improvement of general malaise (62%), and improvement in neuropathy (54.7%), nonpharmacologic therapies are not without risk.[68,70] This is particularly true when ART is taken together with St. John's wort or garlic supplements, which reduce the ART therapeutic drug levels. In addition, echinacea, milk thistle, ginseng, cat's claw, and grapefruit can reduce concentrations of indinavir and saquinavir.[71] It is important to note that interactions between herbal remedies and ARV drugs have not been subjected to robust controlled trials, though patients should be cautioned about combining herbal remedies with ART and their potential safety implications.[71]

PROPHYLAXIS AND TREATMENT OF OPPORTUNISTIC INFECTIONS

The compromised immune system of HIV-positive persons makes them susceptible to a wide spectrum of opportunistic infections (OIs). Fortunately, effective ART has reduced the risk of OIs in this population. When a CD4 count is lower than 200 cells/μL, various recommended prophylactic regimens should be implemented. The indications for prophylaxis and preferred treatments for OI are summarized in Tables 31.2 and **31.3**.

TABLE 31.3 Treatment for Common Opportunistic Infections

Opportunistic Infection	Preferred Therapy
Pneumocystis pneumonia	Patients who develop PCP despite TMP–SMX prophylaxis can usually be treated with standard doses of TMP–SMX **(BIII)**; duration of PCP treatment: 21 days **(AII)**. **For moderate-to-severe PCP:** TMP–SMX: (TMP 15–20 mg and SMX 75–100 mg)/kg/day IV given q6h or q8h **(AI)**; may switch to po after clinical improvement **(AI)** **For mild-to-moderate PCP:** TMP–SMX: (TMP 15–20 mg and SMX 75–100 mg)/kg/day, given po in three divided doses **(AI)**, *or* TMP–SMX: (160 mg/800 mg or DS) two tablets po tid **(AI)** **Secondary prophylaxis, after completion of PCP treatment:** TMP–SMX DS: one tablet po daily **(AI)**, *or* TMP–SMX (80 mg/400 mg or SS): one tablet po daily **(AI)**
Toxoplasma gondii encephalitis	**Treatment of acute infection:** Pyrimethamine* 200 mg po one time, followed by weight-based therapy: if <60 kg, pyrimethamine* 50 mg po once daily + sulfadiazine 1,000 mg po q6h + leucovorin 10–25 mg po once daily; if ≥60 kg, pyrimethamine* 75 mg po once daily + sulfadiazine 1,500 mg po q6h + leucovorin 10–25 mg po once daily; leucovorin dose can be increased to 50 mg daily or bid. **Duration for acute therapy:** At least 6 weeks **(BII)**; longer duration if clinical or radiologic disease is extensive or response is incomplete at 6 weeks. After completion of acute therapy, all patients should be initiated on chronic maintenance therapy. **Chronic maintenance therapy:** Pyrimethamine* 25–50 mg po daily + sulfadiazine 2,000–4,000 mg po daily (in two to four divided doses) + leucovorin 10–25 mg po daily **(AI)**
Cryptosporidiosis	Initiate or optimize ART for immune restoration to CD4 count >100 cells/μL **(AII)**, *and* aggressive oral or IV rehydration and replacement of electrolyte loss **(AIII)**, *and* symptomatic treatment of diarrhea with antimotility agents **(AIII)**.
Mycobacterium tuberculosis disease	After collecting specimen for culture and molecular diagnostic tests, empiric TB treatment should be started in individuals with clinical and radiographic presentation suggestive of TB **(AIII)**. Refer to AIDSInfo.gov for dosing recommendations. **Initial phase (2 months, given daily, 5–7 times/week by DOT) (AI):** INH + (RIF or RFB) + PZA + EMB **(AI)** **Continuation phase:** INH + (RIF or RFB) daily (5–7 times/week) **Total duration of therapy (for drug-susceptible TB):** Pulmonary, drug-susceptible TB: 6 months **(BII)**; pulmonary TB and culture-positive after 2 months of TB treatment: 9 months **(BII)**; extra-pulmonary TB w/CNS infection: 9–12 months **(BII)**; extra-pulmonary TB w/bone or joint involvement: 6–9 months **(BII)**; extra-pulmonary TB in other sites: 6 months **(BII)** Total duration of therapy should be based on number of doses received, not on calendar time.
Disseminated *Mycobacterium avium* complex disease	**At least two drugs as initial therapy with:** Clarithromycin 500 mg po bid **(AI)** + ethambutol 15 mg/kg po daily **(AI)**, *or* (azithromycin 500–600 mg + ethambutol 15 mg/kg) po daily **(AII)** if drug interaction or intolerance precludes the use of clarithromycin **Duration:** At least 12 months of therapy; can discontinue if no signs and symptoms of MAC disease and sustained (>6 months) CD4 count >100 cells/μL in response to ART.

(continued)

TABLE 31.3 Treatment for Common Opportunistic Infections *(continued)*

Opportunistic Infection	Preferred Therapy
Mucocutaneous candidiasis	**For oropharyngeal candidiasis; initial episodes (for 7–14 days):** Oral fluconazole 100 mg po daily **(AI)** **For esophageal candidiasis (for 14–21 days):** Fluconazole 100 mg (up to 400 mg) po or IV daily **(AI)**, *or* itraconazole oral solution 200 mg po daily **(AI)** **For uncomplicated vulvo-vaginal candidiasis:** Oral fluconazole 150 mg for one dose **(AII)**, *or* topical azoles (clotrimazole, butoconazole, miconazole, tioconazole, or terconazole) for 3–7 days **(AII)** **For severe or recurrent vulvo-vaginal candidiasis:** Fluconazole 100–200 mg po daily for ≥7 days **(AII)**, *or* topical antifungal ≥7 days **(AII)**
Cryptococcosis	**Cryptococcal meningitis** *Induction therapy (for at least 2 weeks, followed by consolidation therapy):* Liposomal amphotericin B 3–4 mg/kg IV daily + flucytosine 25 mg/kg po qid **(AI)** (Note: Flucytosine dose should be adjusted in patients with renal dysfunction.) *Consolidation therapy (for at least 8 weeks **(AI)**, followed by maintenance therapy):* Fluconazole 400 mg po (or IV) daily **(AI)** *Maintenance therapy:* Fluconazole 200 mg po daily for at least 12 months **(AI)** **For non CNS, extrapulmonary cryptococcosis and diffuse pulmonary disease:** Treatment same as for cryptococcal meningitis **(BIII)** **Non CNS cryptococcosis with mild-to-moderate symptoms and focal pulmonary infiltrates:** Fluconazole, 400 mg po daily for 12 months **(BIII)**
Coccidioidomycosis	**Clinically mild infections (e.g., focal pneumonia):** Fluconazole 400 mg* po daily **(AII)**, *or* itraconazole 200 mg* po bid **(BII)** **Bone or joint infections:** Itraconazole 200 mg* po bid **(AI)** **Severe, nonmeningeal infection (diffuse pulmonary infection or severely ill patients with extrathoracic, disseminated disease):** Lipid formulation amphotericin B 3–5 mg/kg IV daily **(AIII)**, *or* amphotericin B deoxycholate 0.7–1.0 mg/kg IV daily **(AII)** *Duration of therapy:* Continue until clinical improvement, then switch to a triazole **(BIII)** **Meningeal infections:** Fluconazole 400–800 mg* IV or po daily **(AII)**
Cytomegalovirus disease	**CMV Retinitis:** *Induction therapy (followed by chronic maintenance therapy):* For immediate sight-threatening lesions (within 1,500 μm of the fovea)—intravitreal injections of ganciclovir (2 mg) or foscarnet (2.4 mg) for 1–4 doses over a period of 7–10 days to achieve high intraocular concentration faster **(AIII)**; plus valganciclovir 900 mg po bid for 14–21 days, then 900 mg once daily **(AI)** *For peripheral lesions:* Valganciclovir 900 mg po bid for 14–21 days, then 900 mg once daily **(AI)** *Chronic maintenance:* Valganciclovir 900 mg po daily (AI) for 3–6 months until ART-induced immune recovery **CMV esophagitis or colitis:** Ganciclovir 5 mg/kg IV q12h; may switch to valganciclovir 900 mg po q12h once the patient can tolerate oral therapy **(BI)** *Duration:* 21–42 days or until symptoms have resolved **(CII)**; maintenance therapy is usually not necessary but should be considered after relapses **(BII)**. **Well-documented, histologically confirmed CMV pneumonia:** Experience for treating CMV pneumonitis in HIV patients is limited. Use of IV ganciclovir or IV foscarnet is reasonable (doses same as for CMV retinitis) **(CIII)**. The optimal duration of therapy and the role of oral valganciclovir have not been established. **CMV neurological disease (Note: Initiate treatment promptly):** Ganciclovir 5 mg/kg IV q12h + (foscarnet 90 mg/kg IV q12h or 60 mg/kg IV q8h) to stabilize disease and maximize response; continue until symptomatic improvement and resolution of neurologic symptoms **(CIII)**. The optimal duration of therapy and the role of oral valganciclovir have not been established. Optimize ART to achieve viral suppression and immune reconstitution **(BIII)**.
Herpes simplex virus disease	**Orolabial lesions (for 5–10 days):** Valacyclovir 1 g po bid **(AIII)**, *or* famciclovir 500 mg po bid **(AIII)**, *or* acyclovir 400 mg po tid **(AIII)** **Initial or recurrent genital HSV (for 5–14 days):** Valacyclovir 1 g po bid **(AI)**, *or* famciclovir 500 mg po bid **(AI)**, *or* acyclovir 400 mg po tid **(AI)** **Severe mucocutaneous HSV:** Initial therapy acyclovir 5 mg/kg IV q8h **(AIII)**; after lesions begin to regress, change to po therapy as previously noted; continue until lesions are completely healed. **Chronic suppressive therapy:** For patients with severe recurrences of genital herpes **(AI)** or patients who want to minimize frequency of recurrences **(AI)**—valacyclovir 500 mg po bid **(AI)**; famciclovir 500 mg po bid **(AI)**; acyclovir 400 mg po bid **(AI)**; continue indefinitely regardless of CD4 cell count.
HHV-8 diseases (Kaposi sarcoma, primary effusion lymphoma, multicentric Castleman's disease)	**Mild-to-moderate KS (localized involvement of skin and/or lymph nodes):** Initiate or optimize ART **(AII)** **Advanced KS (visceral [AI] or disseminated cutaneous KS [BIII]):** Chemotherapy (per oncology consult) + ART; liposomal doxorubicin first-line chemotherapy **(AI)** **Primary effusion lymphoma:** Chemotherapy (per oncology consult) + ART **(AIII)**; valganciclovir po or IV ganciclovir can be used as adjunctive therapy **(CIII)** **MCD therapy options (in consultation with specialist, depending on HIV/HHV-8 status, presence of organ failure, and refractory nature of disease):** ART **(AIII)** along with one of the following—valganciclovir 900 mg po bid for 3 weeks **(CII)**, *or* ganciclovir 5 mg/kg IV q12h for 3 weeks **(CII)**, *or* valganciclovir po or ganciclovir IV + zidovudine 600 mg po q6h for 7–21 days **(CII)**; rituximab ± prednisone **(CII)**; monoclonal antibody targeting IL-6 or IL-6 receptor **(BII)** **Concurrent KS and MCD:** Rituximab + liposomal doxorubicin **(BII)**

TABLE 31.3 Treatment for Common Opportunistic Infections *(continued)*

Opportunistic Infection	Preferred Therapy
Malaria	Because *Plasmodium falciparum* malaria can progress in hours from mild symptoms or low-grade fever to severe disease or death, all HIV-infected patients with confirmed or suspected *P. falciparum* infection should be hospitalized for evaluation, initiation of treatment, and observation **(AIII)**. Treatment recommendations for HIV-infected patients are the same as for HIV-uninfected patients **(AIII)**. Choice of therapy is guided by the degree of parasitemia, the species of *Plasmodium*, a patient's clinical status, region of infection, and the likely drug susceptibility of the infected species, and can be found at www.cdc.gov/malaria.

* Refer to www.daraprimdirect.com for information regarding how to access pyrimethamine.

Note: **Evidence rating**:

Strength of recommendation: A, strong recommendation for the statement; B, moderate recommendation for the statement; C, optional recommendation for the statement. **Quality of evidence for the recommendation:** I, one or more randomized trials with clinical outcomes and/or validated laboratory endpoints; II, one or more well-designed, nonrandomized trials or observational cohort studies with long-term clinical outcomes; III, expert opinion. In cases where there are no data for the prevention or treatment of an OI based on studies conducted in HIV-infected populations, but data derived from HIV-uninfected patients exist that can plausibly guide management decisions for patients with HIV/AIDS, the data will be rated as III but will be assigned recommendations of A, B, C, depending on the strength of recommendation.

ART, antiretroviral therapy; bid, twice a day; CD4, CD4 T lymphocyte cell; CDC, The Centers for Disease Control and Prevention; CMV, cytomegalovirus; CNS, central nervous system; DOT, directly-observed therapy; DS, double strength; EMB, ethambutol; g, gram; HHV-8, human herpes virus-8; HSV, herpes simplex virus; INH, isoniazid; IV, intravenous; mg, milligram; KS, Kaposi sarcoma; MAC, *Mycobacterium avium* complex; MCD, multicentric Castleman's disease; PCP, pneumocystis pneumonia; po, oral; PZA, pyrazinamide; q(n)h, every "n" hours; qid, four times a day; RFB, rifabutin; RIF, rifampin; SS, single strength; TB, tuberculosis; tid, three times daily; TMP–SMX, trimethoprim–sulfamethoxazole; TVR, telaprevir; ZDV, zidovudine.

Source: Patel P, Borkowf CB, Brooks JT, et al. Estimating per-act HIV transmission risk: a systematic review. *AIDS.* 2014;28(10):1509–1519. doi:10.1097/QAD .0000000000000298

CHALLENGES ASSOCIATED WITH TREATMENT

There are multiple medical, social, and psychiatric challenges associated with the management of HIV and AIDS. Issues such as stigma of the disease, side effects, adherence to medications, and opportunistic infections should be continuously addressed by clinicians. Prior to initiating ART, clinicians should assess the patient's readiness for ART. This assessment should include evaluation of high-risk behaviors such as substance use (e.g., illicit drugs, alcohol, and tobacco), high-risk sexual behavior, social support, mental illness, comorbidities, and economic factors (e.g., employment, housing, transportation, and health insurance). Additionally, patients should be provided with counseling on how to disclose HIV status to sexual or needle-sharing partners. Patients should also be educated on HIV risk behaviors and strategies to prevent transmission. In general, the management of HIV/AIDS should follow a chronic-disease model involving a multidisciplinary care team with HIV specialists, primary care clinicians, pharmacists, case/social workers, psychologists/psychiatrists, dentists, registered dietitians, dermatologists, and all other necessary medical and support clinicians.[72] The HIV/AIDS care team should focus on evidence-based practices and patient-centered care.

CASE EXEMPLAR: Patient With Respiratory Symptoms

WE is a 37-year-old female who presents with complaints of a sore throat, fever, cough, and shortness of breath that has "gotten worse" over the past 3 days. She tested positive for HIV 3 years ago. She had been prescribed medication, which she took for 1 year and then stopped taking because she "felt better." She has not seen a clinician since that time.

Past Medical History
- HIV positive
- No known drug allergies

Medications
- Pain medication, as needed
- Allergy medication, as needed

Social History
- Does not smoke or drink
- Occasional illicit drug use with cocaine
- Sexually active with men

Physical Examination
- Blood pressure: 98/62; pulse: 110; respiration rate: 28; temperature: 102.0 °F
- Regular sinus, no murmurs or gallops noted on auscultation
- Candida present on tongue
- Chest: Bilateral crackles with rales and rhonchi; decreased lung sounds in lower lobes bilaterally

(continued)

- Abdomen: Nontender, no splenomegaly or hepatomegaly

Labs and Imaging
- White blood count (WBC): 10,000 mm³
- Segmented neutrophils (segs): 38
- Lymphocytes: 45
- Monocytes: 9
- Eosinophils: 8
- Hemoglobin (Hgb): 9.6 g/dL
- Hematocrit (Hct): 28.8%
- Platelets: 221 mm³

- CD4 count: 225
- Viral load: 50,000
- X-ray: Confirms infiltrates

Discussion Questions
1. Given WE's history and physical findings, what is the likely diagnosis? What one additional test will help confirm this diagnosis?
2. How will WE's condition likely be managed?
3. What patient teaching and follow-up should WE receive?

CASE EXEMPLAR: Patient With Diarrhea

AD is a 26-year-old male who presents with complaints of diarrhea with watery stools, severe abdominal cramping, and an inability to eat or drink. He thinks he has lost weight. He has been taking lamivudine/zidovudine and nelfinavir. He has been faithful about taking his medications. He says he has had an undetectable viral load and his CD4 has been 420. He did some traveling outside the United States to Mexico.

Past Medical History
- Does not smoke or drink
- No known drug allergies

Medications
- Pain medication, as needed
- Allergy medication, as needed
- Lamivudine/zidovudine, 150 mg two times a day
- Nelfinavir, 250 mg three times a day

Social History
- Sexually active with men

Physical Examination
- Blood pressure: 98/62; pulse: 80; respiration rate: 13; temperature: 101.0 °F

- Regular sinus, no murmurs or gallops noted on auscultation
- Hyperactive bowel sounds all quadrants
- Abdomen: Tender to palpation, but no splenomegaly or hepatomegaly

Labs
- White blood count (WBC): 6,000 mm³
- Segmented neutrophils (segs): 38
- Lymphocytes: 45
- Monocytes: 10
- Eosinophils: 7
- Hemoglobin (Hgb): 13.8 g/dL
- Hematocrit (Hct): 41.8%
- Platelets: 180 mm³
- CD4 count: 200
- Viral load: Undetectable

Discussion Questions
1. Given AD's history and physical findings, what is the likely diagnosis? What additional test will help confirm the diagnosis?
2. How will AD's condition likely be managed?
3. What changes, if any, should be made to AD's ART therapy?

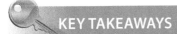

KEY TAKEAWAYS

- HIV is an RNA virus with a life cycle that allows many targets for ART.
- Research recommends utilizing a chronic disease management approach, involving a multidisciplinary team of HIV specialists, counselors, and primary care clinicians.
- HIV infection is acquired through sexual contact or exposure to infected blood or blood products or during childbirth. For all modes of transmission, a higher viral load in the HIV-infected person is associated with a higher risk of transmission to others.
- Sexual behavior that disrupts the mucosa and causes bleeding is associated with higher risk than behaviors that do not disrupt the mucosa.
- The risk of HIV transmission by exposure to blood or blood products varies based on a specific exposure.
- The transmission of HIV may occur during pregnancy, at delivery, or following delivery. High viral loads of maternal plasma and breast milk are associated with increased risk of transmission.
- Individuals with HIV who are under consistent medical care and have viral suppression are less likely to transmit HIV.
- Three types of HIV diagnostic tests are commonly utilized: NATs, antibody tests, and antigen/antibody tests. NATs can detect HIV RNA within 10 to 33 days after infection.
- Agents in seven drug classes are used for treatment of HIV infection, and each ARV class generally targets a unique step in the life cycle of HIV.
- Current trends in medication development focus on potency, longer durations of action, and intramuscular route of administration.
- The compromised immune system of HIV-positive persons makes them susceptible to a wide spectrum of OIs. Effective ART has reduced the risks.
- Patient compliance throughout the necessary course of treatment remains a hurdle.

REFERENCES

1. Centers for Disease Control and Prevention. *HIV in the United States and dependent areas*. 2020. https://www.cdc.gov/hiv/statistics/overview/ataglance.html
2. Gallant JE, Adimora AA, Carmichael JK, et al. Essential components of effective HIV care: a policy paper of the HIV medicine Association of the Infectious Diseases Society of America and the Ryan White Medical Providers Coalition. *Clin Infect Dis.* 2011;53:1043–1050. doi:10.1093/cid/cir689
3. Barré-Sinoussi F, Chermann JC, Rey F, et al. Isolation of a T-lymphotropic retrovirus from a patient at risk for acquired immune deficiency syndrome (AIDS). 1983. *Rev Invest Clin.* 2004;56(2):126–129. PMID: 15378805.
4. Gallo RC, Salahuddin SZ, Popovic M, et al. Frequent detection and isolation of cytopathic retroviruses (HTLVIII) from patients with AIDS and at risk for AIDS. *Science.*1984;224(4648):500–503. doi:10.1126/science.6200936
5. Pachl C, Todd JA, Kern DG, et al. Rapid and precise quantification of HIV-1 RNA in plasma using a branched DNA signal amplification assay. *J Acquir Immune Defic Syndr Hum Retrovirol.* 1995;8(5):446–454. doi:10.1097/00042560-199504120-00003
6. Dewar RL, Highbarger HC, Sarmiento MD, et al. Application of branched DNA signal amplification to monitor human immunodeficiency virus type 1 burden in human plasma. *J Infect Dis.* 1994;170(5):1172–1179. doi:10.1093/infdis/170.5.1172
7. Hammer SM, Squires KE, Hughes MD, et al. A controlled trial of two nucleoside analogues plus indinavir in persons with human immunodeficiency virus infection and CD4 cell counts of 200 per cubic millimeter or less. *N Engl J Med.* 1997;337(11):725–733. doi:10.1056/NEJM199709113371101
8. Ho DD, Moudgil T, Alam M. Quantitation of human immunodeficiency virus type 1 in the blood of infected persons. *N Engl J Med.* 1989;321(24):1621–1625. doi:10.1056/NEJM198912143212401
9. Potempa M, Lee SK, Wolfenden R, et al. The triple threat of HIV-1 protease inhibitors. *Curr Top Microbiol Immunol.* 2015;389:203–241. doi:10.1007/82_2015_438
10. Vidya Vijayan KK, Karthigeyan KP, Tripathi SP, Hanna LE. Pathophysiology of CD4+ T-cell depletion in HIV-1 and HIV-2 infections. *Front Immunol.* 2017;8:580. doi:10.3389/fimmu.2017.00580
11. Zicari S, Sessa L, Cotugno N, et al. Immune activation, inflammation, and non-AIDS co-morbidities in HIV-infected patients under long-term ART. *Viruses.* 2019;11(3):200. doi:10.3390/v11030200
12. Birx DL, Redfield RR, Tencer K, et al. Induction of interleukin-6 during human immunodeficiency virus infection. *Blood.* 1990;76(11):2303–2310. doi:10.1182/blood.V76.11.2303.2303
13. Février M, Dorgham K, Rebollo A. CD4+ T cell depletion in human immunodeficiency virus (HIV) infection: role of apoptosis. *Viruses.* 2011;3(5):586–612. doi:10.3390/v3050586
14. Sandler NG, Douek DC. Microbial translocation in HIV infection: causes, consequences and treatment opportunities. *Nat Rev Microbiol.* 2012;10(9):655–666. doi:10.1038/nrmicro2848
15. Melhuish A, Lewthwaite P. Natural history of HIV and AIDS. *Medicine.* 2018;46(6):356–361. doi:10.1016/j.mpmed.2013.05.009
16. Falasca F, Di Carlo D, De Vito C, et al. Evaluation of HIV-DNA and inflammatory markers in HIV-infected individuals with different viral load patterns. *BMC Infect Dis.* 2017;17(1):581. doi:10.1186/s12879-017-2676-2

17. Aberg JA. Aging, inflammation, and HIV infection. *Top Antivir Med.* 2012;20(3):101–105. https://www.ncbi.nlm.nih.gov/pmc/articles/PMC6148943

18. Finzi D, Blankson J, Siliciano JD, et al. Latent infection of CD4+ T cells provides a mechanism for lifelong persistence of HIV-1, even in patients on effective combination therapy. *Nat Med.* 1999;5(5):512–517. doi:10.1038/8394

19. Kulkosky J, Bray S. HAART-persistent HIV-1 latent reservoirs: their origin, mechanisms of stability and potential strategies for eradication. *Curr HIV Res.* 2006;4(2):199–208. doi:10.2174/157016206776055084

20. Margolis DM, Archin NM. Proviral latency, persistent human immunodeficiency virus infection, and the development of latency reversing agents. *J Infect Dis.* 2017;215(suppl 3):S111–S118. doi:10.1093/infdis/jiw618

21. Siliciano JD, Kajdas J, Finzi D, et al. Long-term follow-up studies confirm the stability of the latent reservoir for HIV-1 in resting CD4+ T cells. *Nat Med.* 2003;9(6):727–728. doi:10.1038/nm880

22. Jones RB, Walker BD. HIV-specific CD8+ T cells and HIV eradication. *J Clin Invest.* 2016;126(2):455–463. doi:10.1172/JCI80566

23. Patel P, Borkowf CB, Brooks JT, et al. Estimating per-act HIV transmission risk: a systematic review. *AIDS.* 2014;28(10):1509–1519. doi:10.1097/QAD.0000000000000298

24. Auvert B, Taljaard D, Lagarde E, et al. Randomized, controlled intervention trial of male circumcision for reduction of HIV infection risk: the ANRS 1265 Trial. *PLoS Med.* 2006;3(5):e226. doi:10.1371/journal.pmed.0020298

25. Gray R, Kigozi G, Kong X, et al. Male circumcision for HIV prevention and effects on risk behaviors in a posttrial follow-up study. *AIDS.* 2012;26(5):609–615. doi:10.1097/QAD.0b013e3283504a3f

26. Centers for Disease Control and Prevention. HIV transmission through transfusion—Missouri and Colorado, 2008. *MMWR Morb Mortal Wkly Rep.* 2010;59:1335–1339. https://www.cdc.gov/mmwr/pdf/wk/mm5941.pdf

27. Baggaley RF, Boily M-C, White RG, Alary M. Risk of HIV-1 transmission for parenteral exposure and blood transfusion: a systematic review and meta-analysis. *AIDS.* 2006;20(6):805–812. doi:10.1097/01.aids.0000218543.46963.6d

28. Smith DK, Grohskopf LA, Black RJ, et al. Antiretroviral post-exposure prophylaxis after sexual, injection drug use, or other non-occupational exposure to HIV in the United States: recommendations from the U.S. Department of Health and Human Services. *MMWR Recomm Rep.* 2005;54(RR-2):1–20. https://www.cdc.gov/mmwr/preview/mmwrhtml/rr5402a1.htm

29. Wyżgowski P, Rosiek A, Grzela T, Leksowski K. Occupational HIV risk for health care workers: risk factor and the risk of infection in the course of professional activities. *Ther Clin Risk Manag.* 2016;12:989–994. doi:10.2147/TCRM.S104942

30. Nesheim SR, FitzHarris LF, Mahle Gray K, Lampe, MA. Epidemiology of perinatal HIV transmission in the United States in the era of its elimination. *Pediatr Infect Dis J.* 2019;38(6):611–616. doi:10.1097/INF.0000000000002290

31. John GC, Kreiss J. Mother-to-child transmission of human immunodeficiency virus type 1. *Epidemiol Rev.* 1996;18(2):149–157. doi:10.1093/oxfordjournals.epirev.a017922

32. Lee T-H, Chafets DM, Biggar RJ, et al. The role of transplacental microtransfusions of maternal lymphocytes in in utero HIV transmission. *J Acquir Immune Defic Syndr.* 2010;55(2):143–147. doi:10.1097/QAI.0b013e3181eb301e

33. King CC, Ellington SR, Kourtis AP. The role of co-infections in mother-to-child transmission of HIV. *Curr HIV Res.* 2013;11(1):10–23. doi:10.2174/1570162x11311010003

34. Aagaard-Tillery KM, Lin MG, Lupo V, et al. Preterm premature rupture of membranes in human immuno-deficiency virus-infected women: a novel case series. *Infect Dis Obstet Gynecol.* 2006;2006:53234. doi:10.1155/IDOG/2006/53234

35. Buranasin P, Kunakorn M, Petchai B, et al. Detection of human immunodeficiency virus type 1 (HIV-1) proviral DNA in breast milk and colostrum of seropositive mothers. *J Med Assoc Thai.* 1993;76(1):41–45. https://www.ncbi.nlm.nih.gov/pubmed/8228693

36. Branson BM, Handsfield HH, Lampe MA, et al. Revised recommendations for HIV testing of adults, adolescents, and pregnant women in health-care settings. *MMWR Recomm Rep.* 2006;55(RR-14):1–17. https://www.cdc.gov/mmwr/preview/mmwrhtml/rr5514a1.htm

37. Rothman RE, Merchant RC. Update on emerging infections from the Centers for Disease Control and Prevention. Revised recommendations for HIV testing of adults, adolescents, and pregnant women in health-care settings. *Ann Emerg Med.* 2007;49(5):575–579. doi:10.1016/j.annemergmed.2007.03.002

38. U.S. Preventive Services Task Force. *Final recommendation statement human immunodeficiency virus (HIV) infection: screening.* Published June 11, 2019. https://www.uspreventiveservicestaskforce.org/uspstf/document/RecommendationStatementFinal/human-immunodeficiency-virus-hiv-infection-screening#bootstrap-panel–6

39. Bayer R, Philbin M, Remien RH. The end of written informed consent for HIV testing: not with a bang but a whimper. *Am J Public Health.* 2017;107(8):1259–1265. doi:10.2105/AJPH.2017.303819

40. Centers for Disease Control and Prevention. *Today's HIV/AIDS epidemic.* Published August 2016. https://www.cdc.gov/nchhstp/newsroom/docs/factsheets/todays epidemic-508.pdf

41. Pilcher CD, Tien HC, Eron JJ, Jr, et al. Brief but efficient: acute HIV infection and the sexual transmission of HIV. *J Infect Dis.* 2004;189(10):1785–1792. doi:10.1086/386333

42. Panel on Antiretroviral Guidelines for Adults and Adolescents. *Guidelines for the Use of Antiretroviral Agents in Adults and Adolescents With HIV.* Department of Health and Human Services. Updated December 18, 2019. https://clinicalinfo.hiv.gov/sites/default/files/guidelines/documents/AdultandAdolescentGL.pdf

43. Centers for Disease Control and Prevention. *HIV testing.* Accessed November 3, 2020. https://www.cdc.gov/hiv/testing/index.html

44. Daskalakis D. HIV diagnostic testing: evolving technology and testing strategies. *Top Antivir Med.* 2011;19(1):18–22. https://www.ncbi.nlm.nih.gov/pmc/articles/PMC6148855

45. Branson BM, Owen SM, Wesolowski LG, et al. *Laboratory testing for the diagnosis of HIV infection: updated recommendations.* Published June 27, 2014. doi:10.15620/cdc.23447

46. Charpentier C, Eholié S, Anglaret X, et al. Genotypic resistance profiles of HIV-2-treated patients in West Africa. *AIDS*. 2014;28(8):1161–1169. doi:10.1097/QAD.0000000000000244

47. Le T, Wright EJ, Smith DM, et al. Enhanced CD4+ T-cell recovery with earlier HIV-1 antiretroviral therapy. *N Engl J Med*. 2013;368(3):218–230. doi:10.1056/NEJMoa1110187

48. Okulicz JF, Le TD, Agan BK, et al. Influence of the timing of antiretroviral therapy on the potential for normalization of immune status in human immunodeficiency virus 1-infected individuals. *JAMA Intern Med*. 2015;175(1):88–99. doi:10.1001/jamainternmed.2014.4010

49. Kernéis S, Launay O, Turbelin C, et al. Long-term immune responses to vaccination in HIV-infected patients: a systematic review and meta-analysis. *Clin Infect Dis*. 2014;58(8):1130–1139. doi:10.1093/cid/cit937

50. Ross LL, Shortino D, Shaefer MS. Changes from 2000 to 2009 in the prevalence of HIV-1 containing drug resistance-associated mutations from antiretroviral therapy-naive, HIV-1-infected patients in the United States. *AIDS Res Hum Retroviruses*. 2018;34(8):672–679. doi:10.1089/AID.2017.0295

51. Panel on Opportunistic Infections in Adults and Adolescents with HIV. *Guidelines for the Prevention and Treatment of Opportunistic Infections in Adults and Adolescents With HIV: Recommendations From the Centers for Disease Control and Prevention, the National Institutes of Health, and the HIV Medicine Association of the Infectious Diseases Society of America.* Updated August 18, 2020. https://clinicalinfo.hiv.gov/sites/default/files/guidelines/documents/Adult_OI.pdf

52. Pau AK, George JM. Antiretroviral therapy: current drugs. *Infect Dis Clin North Am*. 2014;28(3):371–402. doi:10.1016/j.idc.2014.06.001

53. Sluis-Cremer N, Temiz NA, Bahar I. Conformational changes in HIV-1 reverse transcriptase induced by nonnucleoside reverse transcriptase inhibitor binding. *Curr HIV Res*. 2004;2(4):323–332. doi:10.2174/1570162043351093

54. Wagner TA, Frenkel LM. Potential limitation of CCR5 antagonists: drug resistance more often linked to CXCR4-utilizing than to CCR5-utilizing HIV-1. *AIDS*. 2008;22(17), 2393–2395. doi:10.1097/QAD.0b013e328312c72c

55. Abram ME, Ferris AL, Das K, et al. Mutations in HIV-1 reverse transcriptase affect the errors made in a single cycle of viral replication. *J Virol*. 2014;88(13):7589–7601. doi:10.1128/JVI.00302-14

56. Boltz VF, Shao W, Bale MJ, et al. Linked dual-class HIV resistance mutations are associated with treatment failure. *JCI Insight*. 2019;4(19):e130118. doi:10.1172/jci.insight.130118

57. Spivak AM, Planelles V. Novel latency reversal agents for HIV-1 cure. *Annu Rev Med*. 2018;69:421–436. doi:10.1146/annurev-med-052716-031710

58. Gruell H, Klein F. Antibody-mediated prevention and treatment of HIV-1 infection. *Retrovirology*. 2018;15(1):73. doi:10.1186/s12977-018-0455-9

59. Stephenson KE, Barouch DH. Broadly neutralizing antibodies for HIV eradication. *Curr HIV/AIDS Rep*. 2016;13(1):31–37. doi:10.1007/s11904-016-0299-7

60. Onwumeh J, Okwundu CI, Kredo T. Interleukin-2 as an adjunct to antiretroviral therapy for HIV-positive adults. *Cochrane Database Syst Rev*. 2017;(5):CD009818. doi:10.1002/14651858.CD009818.pub2

61. HIV Vaccine Trials Network. *Science.* Accessed April 3, 2020. http://www.hvtn.org/en/science.html

62. Koethe JR, Heimburger DC. Nutritional aspects of HIV-associated wasting in sub-Saharan Africa. *Am J Clin Nutr*. 2010;91(4):1138S–1142S. doi:10.3945/ajcn.2010.28608D

63. Pienaar M, van Rooyen FC, Walsh CM. Reported health, lifestyle and clinical manifestations associated with HIV status in people from rural and urban communities in the Free State Province, South Africa. *South Afr J HIV Med*. 2017;18(1):465. doi:10.4102/sajhivmed.v18i1.465

64. Visser ME, Durao S, Sinclair D, et al. Micronutrient supplementation in adults with HIV infection. *Cochrane Database Syst Rev*. 2017;(5):CD003650. doi:10.1002/14651858.CD003650.pub4

65. Chang BL, van Servellen G, Lombardi E. Factors associated with complementary therapy use in people living with HIV/AIDS receiving antiretroviral therapy. *J Altern Complement Med*. 2003;9(5):695–710. doi:10.1089/107555303322524544

66. Hsiao A-F, Wong MD, Kanouse DE, et al. Complementary and alternative medicine use and substitution for conventional therapy by HIV-infected patients. *J Acquir Immune Defic Syndr*. 2003;33(2):157–165. doi:10.1097/00126334-200306010-00007

67. Cho M, Ye X, Dobs A, Cofrancesco J. Jr. Prevalence of complementary and alternative medicine use among HIV patients for perceived lipodystrophy. *J Altern Complement Med*. 2006;12(5):475–482. doi:10.1089/acm.2006.12.475

68. Agnoletto V, Chiaffarino F, Nasta P, et al. Reasons for complementary therapies and characteristics of users among HIV-infected people. *Int J STD AIDS*. 2003;14(7):482–486. doi:10.1258/095646203322025803

69. Sparber A, Wootton JC, Bauer L, et al. Use of complementary medicine by adult patients participating in HIV/AIDS clinical trials. *J Altern Complement Med*. 2000;6(5):415–442. doi:10.1089/acm.2000.6.415

70. Duggan J, Peterson WS, Schutz M, et al. Use of complementary and alternative therapies in HIV-infected patients. *AIDS Patient Care STDS*. 2001;15(3):159–167. doi:10.1089/108729101750123661

71. Lorenc A, Robinson N. A review of the use of complementary and alternative medicine and HIV: issues for patient care. *AIDS Patient Care STDS*. 2013;27(9):503–510. doi:10.1089/apc.2013.0175

72. Hass V, Kayingo G. Chronic care perspectives. In: Ballweg R, Brown D, Vetrosky D, Ritsema TS, eds. *Physician Assistant: A Guide to Clinical Practice*. 6th ed. Elsevier; 2018:197–213.

ADDITIONAL RESOURCES

For additional information, please refer to the following sites:

- AIDS *info* (HIV Guidelines): www.aidsinfo.nih.gov/guidelines
- AIDSUnited: www.aidsunited.org
- amfAR: www.amfar.org
- Avert: www.avert.org
- Centers for Disease Control and Prevention: www.cdc.gov/hiv
- HIV.gov (Department of Health and Human Services): www.hiv.gov
- UNAIDS (United Nations): www.unaids.org/en
- University of California, San Francisco (UCSF) Clinician Consultation Center: https://nccc.ucsf.edu

Psychopharmacology and Integrative Health: Combined Treatment of Psychiatric and Neurocognitive Conditions

Simone T. Lew, Jeremy M. DeMartini, Emmanuel A. Zamora, and Amir Ramezani

LEARNING OBJECTIVES

- Briefly compare and contrast the signs and symptoms of the various affective, anxiety, obsessive-compulsive, trauma-related, and psychotic disorders.
- Outline the signs and symptoms of the neurocognitive and neurodevelopmental disorders.
- Discuss the method of action, expected and adverse reactions, and any lab monitoring required for antidepressants, mood stabilizers, sedative-hypnotics, and other anxiolytics. Include in the discussion the rationale for patient teaching regarding extended times to drug effectiveness.
- Describe the uses of antipsychotic agents and explain the management of side effects.
- Explain the rationale and indications for the use of stimulants throughout the life span.
- Delineate the relationship between integrative behavioral therapy and psychopharmacology.

INTRODUCTION

The World Health Organization (WHO) estimates that most countries experience an 18.1% to 36.1% prevalence rate for psychiatric illness.[1] Psychiatric conditions are highly comorbid in individuals living with chronic medical conditions, and these conditions can impact one another in a reciprocal manner.[2] For example, research has shown an increased risk of developing major depression in patients with chronic medical disorders. The rate of depression in primary care patients is estimated to be between 5% and 10%, while the rate of depression in patients with chronic diabetes is 12% to 18% and the rate in coronary artery disease is 15% to 23%.[2] Additionally, psychiatric illnesses (e.g., depression, bipolar disorder, and psychosis) have been shown to be risk factors for developing many chronic diseases, including diabetes, coronary artery disease, asthma, osteoarthritis, epilepsy, and hypertension.[2] Individuals with comorbid chronic medical and psychiatric conditions often have an increased frequency of suicidal ideation.[3]

The healthcare clinician's ability to prescribe and monitor psychopharmacological agents is an essential skill set, which also must be balanced with integrative behavioral interventions to fully address patient needs (Figure 32.1). The goals of this chapter are to: (a) increase knowledge of psychopharmacology for common psychiatric and neurocognitive conditions; (b) discuss practical applications of psychotropic medications; and (c) apply knowledge of clinical conditions and psychopharmacology to integrative behavioral treatments.

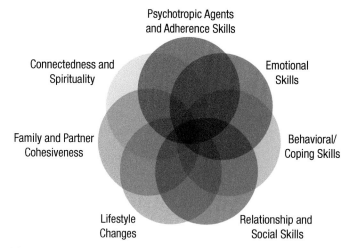

FIGURE 32.1 Diagram review.

PSYCHIATRIC AND NEUROCOGNITIVE DISORDERS

The clinician's ability to make a specific diagnosis is key in directing and monitoring the effects of treatment. The following text briefly describes symptoms associated with common psychiatric and neurocognitive conditions.[4]

AFFECTIVE DISORDERS

Depression is defined by the presence of dysphoric mood and/or loss of pleasure or interest, and is often associated with sleep disturbance, appetite changes, psychomotor changes, and suicidal ideation. Depression can be episodic (e.g., major depressive episode), low grade/nonepisodic (e.g., persistent depressive disorder/formerly known as dysthymia), and/or present with psychotic features (e.g., hallucinations or paranoia). In some patients, depression may be masked by the expression of somatic (e.g., functional neurological disorder) or cognitive (e.g., pseudodementia) symptoms rather than clear mood symptoms.[4]

Bipolar affective disorder exists on a spectrum and may present in different ways. Bipolar I disorder is characterized by the presence of at least one major manic episode. Symptoms of mania include elevated mood, increased energy, decreased need for sleep, irritability, racing thoughts, risky behaviors, and pressured speech. These symptoms occur for at least 7 days and/or lead to psychiatric hospitalization. People with bipolar I disorder may also experience one or more depressive episodes. Bipolar II disorder is characterized by at least one episode of hypomania and one episode of depression. The hypomanic episode must last at least 4 days. Hypomania is less severe than mania and usually does not cause functional impairment or lead to hospitalization. Patients are typically able to preserve normal

day-to-day functioning. Most patients with bipolar II disorder present with a depressive episode when they first seek treatment. In general, they will experience more depressive episodes compared to hypomanic episodes over the course of their illness. Cyclothymia is characterized by numerous periods of hypomania and depression over at least 2 years.[4]

ANXIETY AND OBSESSIVE-COMPULSIVE DISORDERS

Anxiety disorders can present with a wide range of somatic, cognitive, and behavioral symptoms. Anxiety can manifest in uncontrollable worrying as in generalized anxiety disorder (GAD), excessive fear of being judged as in social anxiety disorder (SAD), or specific phobias. Obsessive-compulsive disorder (OCD) is characterized by obsessions (recurrent intrusive thoughts—e.g., fear of contamination, doubt, and loss of control) and compulsions (repetitive behaviors the individual is compelled to act upon, including hand washing, rituals, or internal counting). Uncontrolled anxiety may escalate into panic. During a panic attack, patients may experience increased heart rate, shortness of breath, and sweating, among other symptoms. Patients may even feel as if they are dying during a severe panic attack. Related disorders include trichotillomania (hair-pulling disorder), hoarding disorder, skin-picking disorder, and body dysmorphia.[4]

TRAUMA-RELATED DISORDERS

A traumatic event is defined as an emotionally disturbing experience that may involve the threat of death, serious injury, sexual violence, or threat to physical integrity. Some individuals, though not all, present with posttraumatic stress disorder (PTSD). Symptoms related to the trauma include intrusive thoughts, nightmares, flashbacks, and avoidance. Heightened arousal states, in which the individual is irritable or easily startled, are also common. In some cases, dissociative symptoms occur. Repeated PTSD scales or psychological testing can help monitor the effects of treatment over time as well as distinguish trauma conditions from other psychiatric illness (e.g., personality disorders or psychosis). Persistent complex bereavement disorder (PCBD) can present with depression and anxiety symptoms that center around loss or grieving.[4]

PSYCHOTIC DISORDERS

Psychotic symptoms, including delusions and hallucinations, can accompany depressive or manic episodes and often occur independent of mood. Major stressors may precede a psychotic episode. Disordered thinking and speech are common in schizophrenia-spectrum disorders, as are negative symptoms such as flattened affect and avolition. Medications and recreational drugs may also cause hallucinations and/or delusions. For example, marijuana, lysergic acid diethylamide (LSD), spice, methamphetamine, benzodiazepines, smoking-cessation drugs, hypnotics, and opioids are among the most common drugs to cause psychotic symptoms.[4]

NEUROCOGNITIVE AND NEURODEVELOPMENTAL DISORDERS

Attention-deficit/hyperactivity disorder (ADHD) is a neurodevelopmental disorder that impairs functioning with symptoms of inattention, impulsivity, and/or excessive motor activity and restlessness. Rating scales and neuropsychological testing are the gold standards to make this diagnosis and to monitor effectiveness of treatment. Major or minor neurocognitive disorders are impairments in attention, executive function, learning and memory, language, perceptual-motor, or social cognition as a result of an organic brain change (e.g., Alzheimer's, Parkinson's, Lewy-Body, Huntington's, traumatic brain injury, stroke, HIV encephalopathy). Neuropsychological assessment is often necessary to rule out such neurocognitive conditions, create differential diagnosis, and monitor progression to determine suitability for driving, capacity for performing the activities of daily living, level of supervision needed, fitness for work/return to work, and the stage of disease.[4]

PSYCHOPHARMACOLOGICAL TREATMENTS

ANTIDEPRESSANTS

Antidepressants are the most commonly prescribed psychiatric medications. They are effective for moderate-to-severe major depressive disorder but may be less useful in milder forms of depression.[5] As seen in **Table 32.1**, antidepressants have a wide range of U.S. Food and Drug Administration (FDA) indications. These include depression, anxiety disorders, PTSD, eating disorders, chronic pain disorders, vasomotor symptoms in menopause, and smoking cessation.

Selective serotonin reuptake inhibitors (SSRIs) and serotonin–norepinephrine reuptake inhibitors (SNRIs) are considered first-line antidepressants. They are relatively well tolerated and have fewer drug–drug interactions and less toxicity than tricyclic antidepressants (TCAs) and monoamine oxidase inhibitors (MAOIs).[5] While SSRIs (fluoxetine, sertraline, paroxetine, fluvoxamine, citalopram, and escitalopram) quickly increase the postsynaptic activity of serotonin, the antidepressant effect may take 4 to 6 weeks to obtain the full effect of a certain dose. SNRIs (venlafaxine, desvenlafaxine, and duloxetine) have a similar mechanism of action to SSRIs, but with the additional postsynaptic activity of norepinephrine. The liver largely metabolizes SSRIs and SNRIs and several are associated with significant drug–drug interactions through cytochrome P450 enzyme inhibition, including fluoxetine (CYP2D6-potent, CYP2C19-moderate), fluvoxamine (CYP1A2-potent, CYP2C19-moderate), paroxetine (CYP2D6-potent), and duloxetine (CYP2D6-moderate). Citalopram and escitalopram have the fewest drug–drug interactions. However, they have dose-dependent risks of QT-interval prolongation with potential for serious arrhythmias such as torsades de pointes. This limits their dosage, especially in patients who are older adults, have hepatic impairment, and/or take other drugs that may increase SSRI levels. Sertraline tends to have fewer drug–drug interactions and less QT-interval prolongation and may be a good choice when both are concerns. Fluoxetine provides many patients with an increase in energy but tends to have more of a dose-dependent effect on sexual dysfunction.

SSRIs and SNRIs are best tolerated when started at low dosages, especially for anxiety disorders and those with prior antidepressant intolerance. In the first 1 to 2 weeks of therapy, the patient may complain of a jittery feeling, which almost always subsides by the third week. These antidepressants may be increased (in no sooner than weekly intervals) toward their maximum dosages for the most benefit. This may take as long as 6 to 8 weeks.[6] Patients should be counseled that the gut has a high concentration of serotonin receptors, and they may experience nausea or diarrhea initially, but this often improves after the first few days. Clinicians should also monitor for sexual dysfunction, increased bleeding, hyponatremia, switch into mania, and serotonin syndrome. There is a U.S. boxed warning that antidepressants increase the risk of suicidal thoughts and behavior in children and young adults in short-term

TABLE 32.1 Antidepressants				
Medication	Adult Dose/Frequency	Indications	Off-Label Uses	Common Adverse Effects and Other Considerations*
Selective Serotonin Reuptake Inhibitors				
Fluoxetine	20–80 mg daily Doses > 20 mg/day may be dosed bid; max dose 80 mg/day	Bipolar depression (combined with olanzapine), bulimia nervosa, MDD, OCD, panic disorder, PMDD	Binge eating disorder, body dysmorphic disorder, fibromyalgia, GAD, PTSD, premature ejaculation, SAD	Anxiety, weakness, tremor, pharyngitis Long half-life Inhibits CYP2D6 (potent) and CYP2C19 (moderate) Caution in hepatic impairment
Sertraline	50–200 mg daily Max dose 200 mg/day; taper dose gradually to D/C, especially high dose	MDD, OCD, panic disorder, PMDD, PTSD, SAD	Binge eating disorder, body dysmorphic disorder, bulimia nervosa, GAD, premature ejaculation	Fatigue Caution in hepatic impairment
Citalopram	10–40 mg daily Taper dose gradually to D/C, especially high dose	MDD	Binge eating disorder, dementia-associated agitation and aggression, GAD, OCD, panic disorder, PMDD, premature ejaculation, PTSD, SAD, vasomotor symptoms in menopause	Diaphoresis Maximum dose is 20 mg/d in poor CYP2C19 metabolizers and adults >60 years of age due to risk of QT prolongation Caution in hepatic impairment
Escitalopram	10–20 mg daily Taper dose gradually to D/C	GAD, MDD	Binge eating disorder, body dysmorphic disorder, bulimia nervosa, OCD, panic disorder, PTSD, PMDD, premature ejaculation, vasomotor symptoms in menopause	Ejaculatory disorder Maximum dose is 10 mg/d in adults >60 years of age due to risk of QT prolongation Caution in renal and hepatic impairment
Paroxetine	IR: 20–50 mg daily Max dose 50 mg/d ER: 25–62.5 mg ER daily max dose 62.5 mg/day ER Both formulations: Taper dose gradually to D/C, especially high dose	GAD, MDD, OCD, panic disorder, PTSD, PMDD, SAD, vasomotor symptoms in menopause	Body dysmorphic disorder, premature ejaculation	Diaphoresis, ejaculatory disorder, weakness, tremor Short half-life increases risk of discontinuation syndrome (nausea, dizziness, lightheadedness) Inhibits CYP2D6 (potent) Caution in renal and hepatic impairment
Fluvoxamine	IR: 50–150 mg bid; max dose 300 mg/d ER: 100–300 mg ER PO qhs; max dose 300 mg/d ER Both forms: Titrate slowly in older adult pts; taper dose gradually to D/C, especially high dose	OCD	Bulimia nervosa, MDD, panic disorder, PTSD, SAD	Weakness Inhibits CYP1A2 (potent) and CYP2C19 (moderate)
Serotonin–Norepinephrine Reuptake Inhibitors				
Desvenlafaxine	25–50 mg daily. There is no evidence that doses > 50 mg per day provide additional benefit.	MDD	Vasomotor symptoms in menopause	Hyperhidrosis Dose adjustment required in renal and hepatic impairment
Duloxetine	30–120 mg daily Max dose 120 mg/d	Fibromyalgia, GAD, MDD, musculoskeletal pain (chronic), neuropathic pain (diabetic)	Chemotherapy-induced peripheral neuropathy, stress urinary incontinence	Fatigue, weight loss, weakness Inhibits CYP2D6 (moderate) Caution in renal impairment and avoid use when CrCl <30 mL/minute and ESRD

(continued)

TABLE 32.1 Antidepressants (continued)

Medication	Adult Dose/Frequency	Indications	Off-Label Uses	Common Adverse Effects and Other Considerations*
Serotonin–Norepinephrine Reuptake Inhibitors				
Venlafaxine	IR: 75 mg daily divided bid or tid initially, increase by ≤ 75 mg/day not faster than every 4 days; max dose 375 mg/day divided q 8–12 hrs ER: 37.5–75 mg daily initially; may increase by 75 mg/day every 4 days; max dose 225 mg/day	GAD, MDD, panic disorder, SAD	Migraine prevention, narcolepsy with cataplexy, neuropathic pain (diabetic), OCD, PTSD, PMDD, vasomotor symptoms in menopause	Diaphoresis, weakness Caution in renal impairment: Reduce total daily dose by 25%–50% Caution in hepatic impairment: Reduce total daily dose by 50%
Tricyclic Antidepressants				
Amitriptyline	Typical effective dose: 50–150 mg daily; range 10–300 mg/day; max dose 300 mg/day Dose at HS; may be given in divided doses Taper gradually to D/C, especially at high dosage	MDD	Chronic fatigue syndrome, fibromyalgia, functional dyspepsia, interstitial cystitis, headaches (migraine and tension), neuropathic pain, postherpetic neuralgia, sialorrhea	TCA poisoning: Convulsions, coma, cardiotoxicity Start 10-25 mg qhs in older adult pts and titrate 10-25 mg every 2-3 days
Nortriptyline	10–150 mg daily	MDD	Chronic pain, myofascial pain, neuropathy (diabetic), orofacial pain, postherpetic neuralgia, smoking cessation	TCA poisoning: convulsions, coma, cardiotoxicity
Clomipramine	25–250 mg daily Taper dose gradually to D/C, especially at high dosage	OCD	MDD, panic disorder	Diaphoresis, difficulty in micturition, dyspepsia, ejaculation failure, impotence, myalgia, myoclonus, nervousness, pharyngitis, rhinitis, tremor, visual disturbance, weight gain TCA poisoning: Convulsions, coma, cardiotoxicity
Monoamine Oxidase Inhibitors				
Phenelzine	15–90 mg daily Divide doses > 15 mg/d into TID dosing; taper dose gradually to D/C, especially at high dosage	Depression	N/A	Contraindicated in severe renal failure and hepatic impairment Avoid tyramine-containing foods (e.g., cheese, alcohol); can result in MAOI-induced hypertensive crisis
Tranylcypromine	10–60 mg daily Start: 10 mg tid x 2wk; may increase by 10 mg/d q1–3 wk; max dose 60 mg/d; Taper dose gradually to D/C, especially at high dosage	MDD	N/A	Avoid tyramine-containing foods (e.g., cheese, alcohol)
Isocarboxazid	10–60 mg daily Start: 10 mg bid, may increase by 10 mg/d q2–4 days; max dose 60 mg/d; taper dose gradually to D/C, especially at high dosage	Depression	N/A	Dizziness, headache Avoid tyramine-containing foods (e.g., cheese, alcohol) Contraindicated in severe renal failure and hepatic impairment

(continued)

TABLE 32.1 Antidepressants (*continued*)

Medication	Adult Dose/Frequency	Indications	Off-Label Uses	Common Adverse Effects and Other Considerations*
Atypical/Other Antidepressants				
Bupropion	SR 100–400 mg daily; XL 150–450 mg daily	MDD, seasonal affective disorder, smoking cessation (SR formulation)	ADHD, bipolar depression, SSRI augmentation, SSRI-induced sexual dysfunction	Agitation, blurred vision, diaphoresis, tachycardia, tremor, weight loss, nasopharyngitis, pharyngitis, rhinitis Contraindicated in patients with anorexia/bulimia, seizure disorder Caution in mild/moderate renal impairment; avoid use in severe renal and hepatic impairment
Mirtazapine	15–45 mg qhs Taper dose gradually to D/C, especially at high dosage	MDD	Panic disorder, tension headache prophylaxis	Weight gain, sedation, increased serum cholesterol
Trazodone	Typical dose 50–100 mg bid-tid Start: 25–50 mg bid-tid, may increase by 50 mg/d q3–4 days; max dose 400 mg/d; taper dose gradually to D/C, especially at high dosage	MDD	Dementia-associated agitation and aggression, insomnia	Blurred vision, falls, fatigue, nervousness, orthostatic hypotension

*FDA Boxed Warning: Antidepressants increase risks of suicidal thoughts and behavior in children and young adults in short-term studies. Monitor all patients for these risks. Other concerns with many antidepressants include allergic events, akathisia, anticholinergic effects, bleeding risk, CNS depression, fractures, ocular effects (glaucoma), QT prolongation, serotonin syndrome, syndrome of inappropriate antidiuretic hormone secretion, hyponatremia, ventricular arrhythmia, and weight loss. Adverse effects common to many antidepressants include headache, insomnia, drowsiness, dizziness, xerostomia, abdominal pain, nausea, vomiting, diarrhea, constipation, anorexia, increased appetite, and sexual dysfunction.

ADHD, attention-deficit/hyperactivity disorder; CNS, central nervous system; CrCl, creatinine clearance; D/C, discontinue; ER, extended release; FDA, U.S. Food and Drug Administration; GAD, generalized anxiety disorder; IR, immediate release; MAOI, monoamine oxidase inhibitor; MDD, major depressive disorder; OCD, obsessive-compulsive disorder; PMDD, premenstrual dysphoric disorder; PTSD, posttraumatic stress disorder; SAD, social anxiety disorder; SR, sustained release; SNRI, serotonin-norepinephrine reuptake inhibitor; SSRI, selective serotonin reuptake inhibitor; TCA, tricyclic antidepressant; XL, extended release.

Source: Data from Lexicomp Online. *Lexi-Drugs.* Wolters Kluwer Clinical Drug Information; 2019.

studies. Other studies did not find increased suicide risk in these groups. While clinicians should not be deterred from treating younger patients, they may require more counseling, education, and monitoring.

Atypical antidepressants can also be used as first-line treatment for depression or as adjunctive therapy to SSRIs and SNRIs. Bupropion is structurally similar to amphetamines and is associated with the release and reuptake inhibition of dopamine and norepinephrine. Compared to other antidepressants, it tends to be activating; therefore, it can potentially worsen anxiety or irritability in some patients. It is not associated with weight gain or sexual dysfunction. In fact, it can improve sexual function and be used to treat SSRI-induced sexual dysfunction. Conversely, mirtazapine tends to be sedating and increases appetite, and therefore may cause weight gain. Its effect on sexual function is neutral. The mechanism of action

of mirtazapine is related to the antagonism of presynaptic alpha-2 adrenergic receptors and postsynaptic serotonin receptors. Drug–drug interactions are not a significant problem with mirtazapine. Historically, trazodone was used as an antidepressant at dosages from 200 to 400 mg/day; however, this was associated with more sedation and orthostatic hypotension than other antidepressants. Therefore, the contemporary use of trazodone is as a sleep aid, at dosages from 50 to 100 mg/day. Caution is advised in using trazodone in the older adults due to risk of sedation, confusion, and falls. In addition, a possible side effect of trazodone is priapism, and males should be advised to seek medical assistance for erections lasting more than 4 hours.

Tricyclic antidepressants (TCAs) and monoamine oxidase inhibitors (MAOIs) are older antidepressants that are now used less frequently due to their increased risk of serious side effects. MAOIs block the metabolism of tyramine in the gastrointestinal tract, which can lead to a hypertensive crisis after consumption of a meal rich in tyramine such as beer, wine, cheese, and cured foods. Selegiline is available in a transdermal patch for patients who cannot take other antidepressants by mouth; it tends to be more selective to monoamine oxidase-B (MAO-B) and, at lower doses, may not require a special diet. There are several significant drug–drug interactions associated with MAOIs. Patients should wait at least 2 weeks, for example, prior to switching between an SSRI and MAOI due to the risk of serotonin syndrome when combining these medications. Since fluoxetine has a longer half-life, it should be stopped at least 5 weeks before starting an MAOI. TCAs also work through serotonin and norepinephrine reuptake inhibition, but they have myriad other pharmacologic effects, including antihistaminic and anticholinergic properties, which lead to dizziness, drowsiness, dry mouth, and urinary hesitation. These medications also cause calcium and sodium channel inhibition, which may lead to life-threatening cardiac arrhythmias. They are useful in treating chronic pain disorders, including fibromyalgia, and for migraine prophylaxis. It is important to monitor suicidality in patients as TCAs are extremely toxic and often result in death upon overdose due to torsades de pointes.

MOOD STABILIZERS

Mood stabilizers (valproate, lithium, lamotrigine, carbamazepine, oxcarbazepine) are the treatment of choice for bipolar spectrum disorders (**Table 32.2**); antipyschotics, which are discussed on page 521, are also effective in treating bipolar disorder. With the exception of lithium, mood stabilizers are also used as antiepileptic drugs.

Lithium is indicated by the FDA for the manic phases and maintenance of bipolar disorder. Lithium is sometimes used off-label and in lower doses in the depressive phases of bipolar disorder and for the augmentation of antidepressants in major depressive disorder. Lithium is effective in decreasing the frequency and severity of bipolar episodes and is one of the only medications that have been shown to decrease suicidal ideation and behavior.[7] However, lithium has a very narrow therapeutic window and an overdose may be lethal. Therefore, candidate selection and monitoring are crucial. Therapeutic drug levels are from 0.5 to 1.2 mEq/L. Levels greater than 1.5 mEq/L are associated with toxicity. Lithium toxicity is based on clinical presentation and symptoms may include abdominal pain, diarrhea, tremors, muscle spasms, seizures, and coma. Electrocardiograms (EKGs) are necessary for patients over 40 years old and for those with underlying cardiac disease due to risk of heart block and arrhythmias. Kidney disease and hypothyroidism are associated with lithium and require periodic lab monitoring. Other common side effects include tremor, hair thinning, weight gain, polyuria, and acne.

Valproate is most useful in treating and preventing the manic phase of bipolar disorder. The mechanism of action is related to increasing gamma-aminobutyric acid (GABA) activity, as well as blocking voltage-dependent sodium channels. This has an overall inhibitory effect.[8] Valproate also helps treat irritability. Possible side effects include weight gain, hair loss, liver-enzyme elevation, and drowsiness, especially at the start of therapy. Drowsiness, if experienced, often resolves after 1 or 2 weeks of continued treatment. For rapid symptom control, valproate may be dosed by weight (20–30 mg/kg/day). Valproate levels are typically checked 4 days after initiating therapy or changing the dose with the goal level between 50 and 125 mcg/mL. The valproate level should be in the lower range for older adult patients and higher range for patients with severe mania. Valproate carries an FDA boxed warning for hepatotoxicity, teratogenicity, and pancreatitis. Despite these warnings, valproate is commonly used as first-line treatment for acute and maintenance phases of bipolar disorder.

Lamotrigine is primarily indicated for the maintenance phase of bipolar disorder to prevent depression but is often used off-label for the depressive phase itself.[8] Clinicians should counsel patients on the rare but serious side effect of Stevens-Johnson syndrome, which starts with flu-like symptoms and then evolves into widespread red or purple blistering rash of the skin and mucous membranes. Patients should be advised to stop the medication and seek medical advice or emergency care for a severe rash (e.g., mouth or genital rash). The risk of Stevens–Johnson syndrome is minimized by slowly titrating the medication to a therapeutic dosage over a period of 6 to 8 weeks when initiating treatment. The initial dose is 25 mg daily, and the dose should not be increased sooner than every 2 weeks. Valproate increases lamotrigine levels; therefore, the lamotrigine dose should be decreased when valproate is taken concurrently.

Carbamazepine is used as an alternative to first-line agents (lithium, valproate, and second-generation antipsychotics) for manic and depressive phases of bipolar disorder.[8] It is chemically related to tricyclic antidepressants and limits sodium ion influx. Carbamazepine may help with irritability and violence in some patients. Carbamazepine may be associated with serious side effects such as aplastic anemia and agranulocytosis. It is also associated with fatal skin reactions in patients with the HLA-B*1502 allele, which should be screened for in those with Asian ancestry. Carbamazepine is associated with significant drug–drug interactions as it is an inducer of CYP2B6 (moderate) and CYP3A4 (strong). Oxcarbazepine is chemically similar to carbamazepine and is associated with less risk of blood dyscrasias and drug–drug interactions. However, it has not been as extensively

TABLE 32.2 Mood Stabilizers

Medication	Dose/Frequency	Indications	Off-Label Uses	Common Adverse Effects and Other Considerations*
Lithium	IR: 300–1,800 mg/day divided bid-tid Adjust dose q 3 days based on treatment response and serum levels Dose adjustment may be needed during pregnancy and/or postpartum ER: 1,800 mg/d ER divided bid-tid Adjust dose q3 days based on treatment response and serum levels Do not cut/crush/chew ER tab	Bipolar maintenance and mania	Bipolar depression, MDD, headache (cluster)	Acne vulgaris, cognitive impairment, dry or thinning hair, hypothyroidism, polydipsia, polyuria, tremor, weight gain Administer with meals to decrease GI upset Caution in renal impairment and hypothyroidism **Therapeutic level: 0.5–1.2 mEq/L**
Valproic acid	Typical dose: 250–500 mg tid Max dose: 2,500 mg/d Decrease start dose and titrate slowly in older adults patients Adjust dose based on treatment response and serum levels Taper dose gradually to D/C	Bipolar mania, focal and generalized onset seizures, migraine prophylaxis	Bipolar depression and maintenance, status epilepticus	Abdominal pain, diarrhea, infection, thrombocytopenia, tremor, visual disturbance Risk of hyperammonemic encephalopathy Fetal risk of neural tube defects in pregnancy Contraindicated in severe hepatic impairment **See Chapter 11 for therapeutic level.**
Lamotrigine	Monotherapy: 200 mg daily Start: Orange starter pack (25 mg once daily x 2 wk, then 50 mg once daily x 2 wk, then 100 mg once daily x 1 wk); max: 200 mg/day Valproate adjunct: 100 mg daily Start: Blue starter pack (25 mg once daily x 2 wk, then 25 mg once daily x 2 wk, then 50 mg once daily x 1 wk); max: 100 mg/day Applies to any regimen containing a valproic acid derivative Enzyme-inducing AED adjunct: 200 mg bid Start: Green starter pack (50 mg once daily x 2 wk, then 50 mg bid x 2 wk, then 100 mg bid x 1 wk), then 150 mg bid x1 wk; max: 400 mg/day Enzyme-inducing AEDs include carbamazepine, phenytoin, phenobarbital, primidone Dose adjustment may be needed during pregnancy and/or postpartum Taper dose over 2 wk to D/C	Bipolar maintenance, focal and generalized onset seizures	Bipolar depression, unilateral neuralgiform headache attacks/prophylaxis	Serious skin reactions (e.g., Stevens-Johnson syndrome) Caution in renal and hepatic impairment
Carbamazepine	800–1,200 mg/d divided bid-qid Start: 200 mg bid, may increase by 200 mg/day Max dose: 1,600 mg/d Adjust dose based on treatment response and serum levels Give with food; divide dose qid for susp Taper dose gradually to D/C	Bipolar mania and depression, focal and generalized onset seizures, neuropathic pain	Bipolar maintenance	Ataxia, vomiting Monitor for hyponatremia, aplastic anemia, and agranulocytosis HLA-B*1502 allele is associated with fatal skin reactions (screen patients with Asian ancestry) Induces CYP2B6 (moderate) and CYP3A4 (strong) Caution in renal impairment **See Chapter 11 for therapeutic level**

(continued)

TABLE 32.2 Mood Stabilizers (*continued*)

Medication	Dose/Frequency	Indications	Off-Label Uses	Common Adverse Effects and Other Considerations*
Oxcarbazepine	600–1,200 mg bid Start: 300 mg bid, increase by 300 mg/day q3 days or by 600 mg/d qwk Dose adjustment may be needed during pregnancy and/or postpartum Taper dose gradually to D/C	Focal onset seizures	Bipolar disorder, neuropathic pain	Abdominal pain, abnormal gait, ataxia, fatigue, hyponatremia, hypothyroidism, tremor, vertigo, visual disturbance, vomiting Induces 3A4/3A5 (strong) and inhibits CYP2C19 (strong) Caution in renal and hepatic impairment

*Adverse effects and other concerns common to many mood stabilizers include dizziness, drowsiness, headache, nausea, anticholinergic sensitivity, hypersensitivity, CNS depression, blood dyscrasias, hyponatremia, hepatic and renal impairment, suicidal ideation, and serious dermatologic reaction.

CNS, central nervous system; ER, extended release; FDA, U.S. Food and Drug Administration; GI, gastrointestinal; IR, immediate release; MDD, major depressive disorder.

Source: Data from Lexicomp Online. *Lexi-Drugs.* Wolters Kluwer Clinical Drug Information; 2019.

studied as a mood stabilizer and is only used off-label to treat bipolar disorder. Carbamazepine and oxcarbazepine can lower levels of oral steroid contraceptives and reduce their efficacy. Therefore, the patient should be advised to use an alternative or additional form of contraception to prevent an unplanned pregnancy. Carbamazepine has a narrow therapeutic window. Blood/serum trough levels should be drawn immediately prior to the next dose, and levels maintained at 4–12 mg/L. Oxcarbazepine levels are not measured.

SEDATIVE-HYPNOTIC DRUGS AND OTHER ANXIOLYTICS

Many adult and older adult patients in the United States are prescribed benzodiazepines[9] (**Table 32.3**). While they are useful in procedural sedation and in treating the acute phases of anxiety, insomnia, mania, and alcohol withdrawal, there are many disadvantages associated with long-term use of benzodiazepines. The primary mechanism of action of benzodiazepines is binding to GABAa, potentiating the inhibitory effect of GABA.[10] Most benzodiazepines require hepatic oxidation for metabolism and have active metabolites, which can lead to accumulation. The exceptions are oxazepam, lorazepam, and temazepam, which tend to be safer in patients with liver disease and older adult patients.

Benzodiazepine dependence is common in those who use these drugs for longer than 1 month. Chronic benzodiazepine users should be tapered slowly due to rebound anxiety and insomnia, as well as the risk of serious withdrawal symptoms (e.g., seizures and delirium).[10] While the risk of fatal overdose with monotherapy is low, deaths from patients who are concurrently taking other sedating substances (e.g., opiates, alcohol)

with benzodiazepines have increased substantially. Other side effects include drowsiness, amnesia, impaired cognition, behavioral disinhibition, impaired driving, falls, and respiratory insufficiency. Benzodiazepine receptor antagonists, commonly referred to as Z-drugs, including zolpidem, zaleplon, and eszopiclone, are primarily used to treat insomnia and share many similarities and risks with benzodiazepines.

Some patients taking benzodiazepines or Z-drugs may experience side effects such as sleepwalking, nighttime eating, unusual sexual appetite, and other types of behavioral disinhibition. Care should be used when prescribing these medications to patients who have other psychiatric diagnoses as they may be worsened.

Cognitive-behavioral therapy (CBT), sleep-hygiene techniques, and mindfulness therapies for insomnia are favored over chronic Z-drug and benzodiazepine use, especially in older adults.[11]

Other anxiolytics are often used to avoid benzodiazepine use and dependence although they may not be as effective for acute anxiety.[6] Buspirone is FDA indicated for GAD and used off-label for unipolar depression augmentation. It can be associated with dizziness. Buspirone is often effective but is dosed as a scheduled medication, not an as-needed medication. Anxiolytic effects may not be observed for 2 to 4 weeks after initiation of medication. Hydroxyzine is a first-generation antihistamine. The hydrochloride salt form is often used for allergic conditions and as an antiemetic while the pamoate salt is used to treat anxiety. Patients should be counseled on the risks of drowsiness, confusion, dry mouth, constipation, and other anticholinergic effects. Hydroxyzine should be avoided in older adults. Gabapentin is FDA indicated for postherpetic neuralgia and focal seizures but is used off-label for many conditions, including other chronic pain disorders, alcohol

TABLE 32.3 Sedative-Hypnotic Drugs and Other Anxiolytics

Medication	Dose/Frequency	Indications	Off-Label Uses	Common Side Effects and Other Considerations*
Benzodiazepines				
Alprazolam	**Anxiety disorders:** IR: 0.25–0.5 mg tid; max dose 4 mg/day in divided doses **Panic disorders:** IR: Starting dose 0.5 mg tid; max dose 10 mg/day in divided doses ER: Starting dose 0.5–1 mg once daily Maintenance dose 3–6 mg once daily; max dose 10 mg/day	Anxiety disorders, panic disorder	N/A	Increased/decreased appetite, ataxia, cognitive dysfunction, constipation, depression, dizziness, drowsiness, dysarthria, fatigue, irritability, decreased libido, memory impairment, difficulty in micturition, paradoxical reaction, sedation, skin rash, weight gain/loss, xerostomia Avoid concomitant use of benzodiazepines with opioids given risk for sedation, respiratory depression, coma, and death
Lorazepam	0.5–10 mg daily PO; 1–8 mg daily IV/IM	Anxiety, anesthesia premedication, status epilepticus	Alcohol delirium and withdrawal, chemotherapy-associated nausea and vomiting, psychogenic catatonia, sedation, tranquilization	Risk of dependence, tolerance, and abuse
Clonazepam	**Anxiety disorder:** 0.25–0.5 mg bid-tid; start 0.25 mg bid, may increase by 0.25 mg/day q1-2 days; max dose 4 mg/day **Panic disorder:** 0.5–2 mg po bid; start 0.25 mg bid, increase by 0.25–0.5 mg/day q3 days; max dose 4 mg/day			Use lowest possible effective dose; frequently reassess need for continued treatment When D/C or decreasing daily dose, reduce by no more than 0.5 mg every 3 days Use in renal impairment: IV/IM forms not recommended. Caution advised with diazepam
Diazepam	2–10 mg bid-qid po; Alt: 2–10 mg IM/IV q3–4h prn; max dose 40 mg/day in divided doses	Panic disorder, seizure disorders Anxiety, ethanol withdrawal, muscle spasm, preoperative, seizures, status epilepticus	Bipolar mania, burning mouth syndrome, essential tremor, REM sleep disorder, RLS, TD, tic disorders Sedation in ICU patient	Use in hepatic impairment: Caution advised in mild-moderate impairment; contraindicated in severe disease
Z-Drugs				
Zolpidem	IR 5–10 mg daily; ER 6.25–12.5 mg daily	Insomnia	N/A	Dizziness, drowsiness, dysgeusia (eszopiclone only), headache FDA boxed warning: Complex sleep behaviors (e.g., sleep-walking, driving) may occur and can result in serious injury and/or death Dose ≥7 hrs before planned awakening Avoid taking with a high-fat meal Lower dosage in older adults For women, max dose of zolpidem IR and ER: 5 and 6.25 mg/day, respectively Caution in hepatic impairment
Zaleplon	5–20 mg daily	Note: Zaleplon is FDA indicated for short-term treatment up to 30 days		
Eszopiclone	1–3 mg daily			
Other Anxiolytics				
Buspirone	20–30 mg/day divided bid-tid Start 7.5 mg bid, then increase 5 mg/day q2–3 days Max dose 60 mg/day	GAD	Unipolar depression, augmentation	Dizziness Not recommended in severe renal and hepatic impairment

(continued)

TABLE 32.3 Sedative-Hypnotic Drugs and Other Anxiolytics (continued)

Medication	Dose/Frequency	Indications	Off-Label Uses	Common Side Effects and Other Considerations*
Other Anxiolytics				
Hydroxyzine	50–100 mg q6h prn po Alt: 50–100 mg q4–6h prn IM Max dose 400 mg/day in divided doses	Allergic conditions, anxiety, pruritus, perioperative sedation, peripartum antiemetic	N/A	GFR ≤50 mL/minute: administer 50% of normal dose Risk of generalized exanthematous pustulosis
Gabapentin	Start: 300 mg once daily x 1 day, then 300 mg bid x 1 day, then 300 mg tid; may continue to increase by 300 mg/day maintaining divided doses, to max dose of 3,600 mg/day In older adult patients, start at 100 mg/day and titrate up by 100 mg/day as previously noted to max dose 1,800 mg/day Taper dose over >7 days to D/C	Postherpetic neuralgia, focal onset seizures	Alcohol use disorder, alcohol withdrawal, cough, fibromyalgia, hiccups, pruritis, pain (neuropathic, postoperative), RLS, SAD, menopause-associated vasomotor symptoms	Ataxia, dizziness, drowsiness, edema, fatigue, viral infection Dose adjustment needed for renal impairment [adjust dose amount, frequency]: CrCl 30–59: 200–700 mg bid CrCl 16–29: 200–700 mg once daily CrCl 15: 100–300 mg once daily CrCl <15: decrease dose proportionately from CrCl 15 HD: decrease dose proportionately from CrCl 15; give 125–350 mg as supplement after dialysis PD: 300 mg q48h; supplement not defined

*Adverse effects and other concerns common to many sedative-hypnotic medications include abnormal thinking, anterograde amnesia, behavioral changes, complex sleep behaviors, CNS depression, hypersensitivity reaction, paradoxical reactions, akathisia, serotonin syndrome, QTc prolongation/torsades de pointes, anaphylaxis, angioedema, multiorgan hypersensitivity, neuropsychiatric effects, and suicidal ideation.

CNS, central nervous system; ER, extended release; FDA, U.S. Food and Drug Administration; GAD, generalized anxiety disorder; GFR, glomerular filtration rate; ICU, intensive care unit; IM, intramuscular; IR, immediate release; IV, intravenous; PO, by mouth; REM, rapid eye movement; RLS, restless leg syndrome; SAD, social anxiety disorder; TD, tardive dyskinesia.

Source: From Lexicomp Online. Lexi-Drugs. Wolters Kluwer Clinical Drug Information; 2019.

use disorder, and anxiety. Sedation is common, especially in patients with renal impairment.

ANTIPSYCHOTICS

There are approximately 20 antipsychotic medications available in the United States.[12] Several of the more commonly used medications in this class are listed in **Table 32.4**. Antipsychotics share D2 receptor blockade or mitigation as a common mechanism; however, they have varying activity at many other receptors including serotonin. They are indicated for the treatment of psychotic disorders (schizophrenia, schizoaffective, other psychosis), bipolar disorders, and antidepressant augmentation. Antipsychotics are more effective in relieving the positive symptoms of psychosis (hallucinations, delusions, disorganized speech and behavior), and are less effective at treating negative symptoms (flat affect, social withdrawal, low motivation, and decreased speech).[13]

The first-generation antipsychotics have long been implicated in causing extrapyramidal symptoms (EPS), including akathisia, dystonia, parkinsonism, and tardive dyskinesia. They can also cause neuroleptic malignant syndrome (NMS), which requires urgent and/

or emergent psychiatric care. Clinicians must monitor for these side effects carefully, and, depending on their severity, consider whether the medication should be decreased or discontinued. Beta-blockers (propranolol), anticholinergics (benztropine, trihexyphenidyl, and diphenhydramine), and benzodiazepines (lorazepam and clonazepam) are helpful in treating many of the mild-to-moderate EPS symptoms. The exception is tardive dyskinesia. Tardive dyskinesia can be treated with vesicular monoamine transporter 2 inhibitors (tetrabenazine and deutetrabenazine) or, rarely, clozapine. The second-generation antipsychotics, especially olanzapine, quetiapine, and clozapine, have more recently been associated with metabolic disorders, including weight gain, hyperlipidemia, hypertension, and diabetes. Metabolic side effects are often not dose dependent. Clinicians should recommend behavioral modifications (e.g., proper diet and exercise) and pharmacotherapy for metabolic disorders. Clinicians should be aware that the metabolic side effects may happen with any antipsychotics, although there are exceptions. Haloperidol, chlorpromazine, and all other first-generation antipsychotics may cause moderate weight gain, while aripiprazole, risperidone, lurasidone, asenapine,

TABLE 32.4 Antipsychotics

Medication	Typical Dose	FDA Indications	Off-Label Uses	Common Adverse Effects and Other Considerations*
First-Generation (Typical) Antipsychotics				
Chlorpromazine	30–800 mg daily PO; 25–800 mg daily IV/IM	Severe behavioral problems, bipolar mania, hiccups, nausea/vomiting, porphyria, SZP, other psychotic disorders, tetanus	Nausea and vomiting of pregnancy, dementia-associated psychosis and agitation	TD and akathisia less common than other first-generation antipsychotics
Fluphenazine	2.5–40 mg daily PO; 12.5–100 mg IM	Psychotic disorders	Huntington chorea, chronic tic disorders, dementia-associated psychosis and agitation	Contraindicated in hepatic impairment Long-acting injectable available
Haloperidol	0.5–20 mg daily PO; 2–20 mg daily IV/IM	Behavioral disorder, hyperactivity, SZP, Tourette disorder	Chemotherapy-associated nausea and vomiting; Huntington chorea; ICU delirium and agitation; nausea and vomiting treatment and prevention; OCD; dementia-associated psychosis and agitation; rapid tranquilization of agitation, aggression, violent behavior	Extrapyramidal reaction, parkinsonism Contraindicated in Parkinson's disease Risk of QT prolongation, especially with IV formulation Long-acting injectables available
Second-Generation (Atypical) Antipsychotics				
Aripiprazole	2–30 mg daily	Aggression associated with conduct disorder, bipolar mania, irritability associated with autism, MDD augmentation, SZP, Tourette disorder	Dementia-associated psychosis and agitation	Increased total serum cholesterol, LDL cholesterol and triglycerides, decreased HDL cholesterol Caution in patients with seizure disorder Long-acting injectables available
Clozapine	12.5–900 mg daily	SZP, suicidal behavior in SZP or schizoaffective disorder	Bipolar disorder (treatment-resistant), dementia-associated psychosis and agitation, Parkinson disease psychosis	Dyspepsia, fever, HTN, orthostatic hypotension, sialorrhea, tachycardia, vertigo FDA boxed warnings: Severe neutropenia (requires periodic ANC monitoring by clozapine REMS); orthostatic hypotension, bradycardia, syncope; seizures; myocarditis
Lurasidone	20–160 mg daily	Bipolar depression, SZP	MDD with mixed features, dementia-associated psychosis and agitation	Increased serum glucose and triglycerides, viral infection Caution in renal and hepatic impairment
Olanzapine	5–30 mg daily PO; 2.5–10 mg IM	Bipolar mania and depression (combination with fluoxetine), SZP	Prevention of chemotherapy-associated nausea and vomiting, ICU delirium and agitation, delusional infestation, dementia-associated psychosis and agitation, PTSD, Tourette syndrome	Accidental injury, dyspepsia, orthostatic hypotension, increased serum AST/ALT, increased serum prolactin, decreased serum bilirubin, weakness, weight gain (common) Long-acting injectables available
Paliperidone	3–12 mg daily	Schizoaffective disorder, SZP	Delusional infestation, dementia-associated psychosis and agitation	Dystonia, hyperglycemia, hyperkinesia, parkinsonian-like syndrome, increased serum cholesterol and triglycerides, increased serum prolactin, tachycardia, tremor Associated with intraoperative floppy iris syndrome and priapism Caution in renal and hepatic impairment Long-acting injectables available

(continued)

TABLE 32.4 Antipsychotics *(continued)*

Medication	Typical Dose	FDA Indications	Off-Label Uses	Common Adverse Effects and Other Considerations*
Second-Generation (Atypical) Antipsychotics				
Quetiapine	12.5–800 mg daily	Bipolar mania and depression, MDD, SZP	Bipolar maintenance, ICU agitation and delirium, delusional infestation, GAD, MDD, OCD, PTSD, dementia-associated psychosis and agitation, Parkinson disease psychosis	Agitation, hyperglycemia, HTN, increased serum cholesterol and triglycerides, tachycardia Caution in patients with hypothyroidism or QT prolongation
Risperidone	0.5–8 mg daily	Bipolar mania and maintenance, irritability associated with autistic disorder, SZP	Delusional infestation, MDD augmentation, PTSD, dementia-associated psychosis and agitation, Tourette syndrome	Anxiety, cough, drooling, fever, hyperprolactinemia, rhinorrhea, tremor, urinary incontinence, nasopharyngitis Associated with intraoperative floppy iris syndrome and priapism
Ziprasidone	20–160 mg daily PO; 10–40 mg daily IM	Bipolar disorder (acute and maintenance), SZP	ICU delirium and agitation, delusional infestation, MDD, dementia-associated psychosis and agitation	Risk of QT prolongation Risk of priapism

*FDA Boxed Warning: Older adult patients with dementia-related psychosis are at an increased risk of death when treated with antipsychotics. Other serious antipsychotic concerns include altered cardiac conduction, anticholinergic effects, aspiration, blood dyscrasias, cerebrovascular effects, CNS depression, insomnia, suicidal ideation, EPS, TD, tremors, NMS, falls, hyperprolactinemia, orthostatic hypotension, ocular effects, photosensitivity, temperature dysregulation, weight gain, abdominal pain, esophageal dysmotility, aspiration, and severe constipation.

ANC, absolute neutrophil count; CNS, central nervous system; EPS, extrapyramidal symptoms; GAD, generalized anxiety disorder; HDL, high-density lipoproteins; HTN, hypertension; ICU, intensive care unit; IM, intramuscular; IV, intravenous; LDL, low-density lipoproteins; MDD, major depressive disorder; NMS, neuroleptic malignant syndrome; OCD, obsessive-compulsive disorder; PO, by mouth; PTSD, posttraumatic stress disorder; REMS, risk evaluation and mitigation strategy; SZP, schizophrenia; TD, tardive dyskinesia.

Source: Data from Lexicomp Online. *Lexi-Drugs.* Wolters Kluwer Clinical Drug Information; 2019.

brexpiprazole, cariprazine, and ziprasidone (all second-generation) often cause little to no weight gain. Risperidone has a moderate risk of EPS, especially at high dosages, and may also increase prolactin levels, resulting in gynecomastia in men or women or lactation in non-pregnant females.

When treating patients with dementia-associated agitation or psychosis, clinicians should be aware that there is an FDA boxed warning that antipsychotics are associated with an increased risk of death in older adult patients with dementia-related psychosis. Therefore, using an antipsychotic requires careful risk–benefit discussions with patients and their families and strong consideration of optimal behavioral management options. Furthermore, antipsychotics with potent D2 blockade (e.g., haloperidol) should be avoided when treating patients with Lewy body dementia, as this may lead to severe parkinsonism. Low-dose clozapine or quetiapine is less likely to cause parkinsonism in these patients. Antipsychotic-associated QT prolongation is a concern for many patients who are older adults, especially those with polypharmacy, critical illness, or those who are prescribed ziprasidone or IV haloperidol. In these cases, frequent EKG monitoring is needed, and alternative medications or behavioral therapies should be considered.

Clozapine, the original second-generation antipsychotic, may be the most effective antipsychotic. Initially it was withdrawn from the European market after multiple reports of agranulocytosis.[14] However, it was later approved in the United States after a large randomized controlled trial showed superiority over chlorpromazine in patients that were refractory to multiple antipsychotics. Since that time, it has been reserved for patients with treatment-refractory schizophrenia but has also been approved for use for suicidal behavior in patients with psychotic disorders. In addition to the risk of death in patients with dementia, clozapine includes four unique FDA boxed warnings:

1. Severe neutropenia
2. Orthostatic hypotension, bradycardia, and syncope
3. Seizures
4. Myocarditis, cardiomyopathy, and mitral valve incompetence

While these side effects are more likely with clozapine, they may also be associated with other antipsychotics. The risk of severe neutropenia is rare (1%–2%) and is managed through the clozapine Risk Evaluation and Mitigation Strategy (REMS) system, which requires periodic absolute neutrophil count (ANC) monitoring. This risk decreases over time the longer the patient remains on the medication. Prescribers and pharmacies using clozapine must be nationally certified. The risks related to the second and third boxed warnings are dose dependent, and therefore it is recommended to titrate the drug slowly from 12.5 mg/day to the target dose of 300 to 450 mg/day. Myocarditis typically occurs early in the course of clozapine initiation; therefore, clinicians should consider baseline EKG and troponin/c-reactive protein (CRP) levels to rule out underlying cardiovascular disease, followed by 1 month of weekly troponin-/CRP-level monitoring. Any patients with concerning symptoms require a cardiac workup prior to initiating treatment. It should be noted that clozapine can also cause severe constipation; therefore, patients require a good bowel regimen. Clozapine also causes sialorrhea,

which may be lessened with the use of anticholinergic liquids in the mouth such as ipratropium bromide.

When nonadherence is a concern, as it is when treating many patients with psychosis, clinicians should consider a long-acting injectable, also known as "depot," formulations of aripiprazole, fluphenazine, haloperidol, olanzapine, and paliperidone.

STIMULANTS AND OTHER AGENTS FOR ATTENTION DEFICIT HYPERACTIVITY DISORDER

The most efficacious treatments for ADHD are stimulants (**Table 32.5**), which have clinical response rates of 65% to 75%.[15] While the ability of these drugs to improve focus is notable, all stimulant drugs for ADHD are controlled substances and may cause drug dependence. Stimulants may be divided into subclasses of

TABLE 32.5 Stimulants and Other Agents for Attention-Deficit/Hyperactivity Disorder

Medication	Dose/Frequency	Indications	Off-Label Uses	Common Side Effects and Other Considerations*
Stimulants				
Amphetamine/Dextroamphetamine	5–60 mg daily	ADHD, narcolepsy	N/A	Short-acting stimulant dosed one to two times daily
Lisdexamfetamine	20–70 mg daily	ADHD, binge eating disorder	N/A	Upper abdominal pain Caution in renal impairment
Methylphenidate	IR 5–60 mg daily; ER 25–100 mg daily	ADHD, narcolepsy	Fatigue, MDD	Irritability, nausea
Dexmethylphenidate	IR 2.5–20 mg daily; ER 10–40 mg daily	ADHD	N/A	Anxiety, jitteriness
Other (Nonstimulant) Agents				
Atomoxetine	40–100 mg daily	ADHD	N/A	Drowsiness, constipation, erectile dysfunction, hyperhidrosis, nausea, vomiting Reduce dose by 25%–50% in moderate-to-severe liver impairment
Clonidine (Available in transdermal patch)	IR and ER 0.1–0.4 mg daily	ADHD (ER formulation), HTN	ADHD (IR formulation), ICU sedation, opioid withdrawal	Dizziness, drowsiness, transient skin rash
Guanfacine	IR 0.5–4 mg daily; ER 1–7 mg daily	ADHD (ER formulation), HTN (IR formulation)	ADHD (IR formulation)	Dizziness, drowsiness, fatigue

*Adverse effects and other concerns common to many ADHD medications include headache, insomnia, xerostomia, abdominal pain, decreased appetite, weight loss, cardiovascular events/altered cardiac conduction, peripheral vasculopathy, serotonin syndrome, visual disturbance, hypersensitivity, priapism, and psychiatric effects.

ADHD, attention deficit/hyperactivity disorder; ER, extended release; HTN, hypertension; ICU, intensive care unit; IR, immediate release; MDD, major depressive disorder.

Source: Data from Lexicomp Online. *Lexi-Drugs.* Wolters Kluwer Clinical Drug Information; 2019.

amphetamine (amphetamine/dextroamphetamine, lisdexamfetamine) and methylphenidate (methylphenidate, dexmethylphenidate) preparations. Both subclasses are equally efficacious, and clinicians should consider switching to another subclass if a patient fails one type of stimulant prior to changing to a nonstimulant agent. The mechanism of action for stimulants is primarily through norepinephrine and dopamine reuptake blockade.[16] The patient's response to methylphenidate is often more subtle and is usually prescribed before the straight amphetamine derivatives. If the response to methylphenidate is not adequate at the target dose, amphetamine salts and dextroamphetamine can be prescribed.

Long-acting stimulants tend to be better tolerated and have better adherence than immediate-release formulations. Possible side effects of stimulants include headaches, insomnia, nausea, anorexia, growth restriction, and anxiety. If a patient has a history of cardiovascular disease or a family history of sudden cardiac death, an EKG and cardiology consultation should be obtained prior to initiating treatment.[15] Caution should be taken when considering stimulants for patients with a history of a substance use disorder, and psychiatric consultation is recommended.

Several other (nonstimulant) agents may be effective in treating ADHD. These medications are not controlled substances and do not cause dependence. Clonidine extended release (ER) and guanfacine ER are FDA approved only for children and adolescents, while atomoxetine is also approved for adults. Clonidine and guanfacine are alpha-2 agonists with an overall inhibitory effect. These medications may also lessen irritability and improve insomnia. Both drugs are well tolerated at low dosages but have risks of bradycardia, hypotension, and sedation. Atomoxetine selectively inhibits norepinephrine reuptake and has a similar side effect profile to antidepressants. Sedation is the most common adverse effect. Atomoxetine also carries an FDA boxed warning of increased risk of suicidal behavior and thoughts in children and adolescents because it is an antidepressant by class.

INTEGRATIVE BEHAVIORAL TREATMENTS

The clinician's ability to educate and implement behavioral treatment when initiating pharmacotherapy will often yield more successful outcomes. Behavioral treatments may be effective as independent or integrative treatments for psychiatric and some neurocognitive conditions. See **Table 32.6** for a list of behavioral interventions. Motivational Interviewing (MI) has been shown to be effective for improving treatment adherence and can help patients make fundamental changes in their emotional and physical health.[17] Studies show

that Cognitive Behavioral Therapy (CBT), as well as third-generation/third-wave therapies (e.g., Dialectical Behavior Therapy [DBT], Acceptance and Commitment Therapy [ACT], Mindfulness-Based Cognitive Therapy [MBCT], compassion therapies), have been found to effectively treat a wide range of disorders including affective, anxiety, trauma-related, obsessive-compulsive, somatic, and sleep disorders.[18,19] Psychodynamic therapies also show efficacious results in treating trauma, anxiety, depression, eating disorders, and mood dysregulation.[20] Clinicians may wish to learn a conceptual framework to implement such therapeutic modalities (e.g., Behavioral Medicine Y-Model).[21] The American Psychological Association's Division 12 has an up-to-date database of evidence-based behavioral practices that can be found online (www.div12.org/psychological-treatments). **Figure 32.2** provides a general frame of comprehensive behavioral care services in a multidisciplinary setting.

CONCLUSION

A clinician's knowledge of common symptoms associated with psychiatric and neurocognitive disorders is important to make an accurate diagnosis and select appropriate psychotropic medications and integrative behavioral treatments.

SSRIs and SNRIs are helpful to treat affective disorders, PMDD, SAD, GAD, panic disorder, eating disorders, PTSD, OCD, and ADHD. TCAs and SNRIs can treat some chronic pain conditions; however, TCAs need to be closely monitored as they can lead to life-threatening cardiac arrhythmias and are extremely toxic in overdose situations. Counseling patients on potential side effects helps foster realistic expectations and improve medication adherence, particularly during the first month of treatment. A wide range of behavioral treatments have been validated for affective and anxiety conditions. Integrating exercise, CBT, MBCT, ACT, psychodynamic, and compassion therapies (e.g., mindful self-compassion) often leads to successful treatment outcomes. It is also important for patients to remain socially active when depressed. Depressed and anxious individuals often isolate themselves from others and their symptoms worsen. For those who have good mental resiliency, stamina, and ego strength, Eye Movement Desensitization and Reprocessing (EMDR), mindfulness-based therapies, and/or prolonged exposure therapy may be good options for patients who have a history of trauma or who are diagnosed with PTSD.

Mood stabilizers, especially lithium carbonate and valproic acid derivatives, are effective for bipolar spectrum disorders. Lithium can also augment antidepressants when treating depression. Prescribers need to monitor symptoms and the levels of certain mood

TABLE 32.6 Integrative Behavioral Interventions

Intervention	Affective and Anxiety Disorders	Trauma	OCD	ADHD	Psychosis
Mindfulness therapies* (e.g., mindfulness-based cognitive therapy)	✓	✓	✓	✓	✓
Nutritional counseling**	✓	✓	✓	✓	✓
Behavioral weight and sleep management	✓	✓	✓	✓	✓
Integration of family, couples, and spiritual therapy or professionals	✓	✓	✓	✓	✓
Motivational interviewing	✓	✓	✓	✓	✓
Cognitive-behavioral therapy	✓	✓	✓	✓	✓
Psychodynamic therapy	✓	✓	✓		
Acceptance and commitment therapy	✓	✓	✓		✓
Exposure and response prevention and prolonged exposure	✓	✓	✓		
Compassion therapies (e.g., mindful self-compassion, compassion-focused therapy)	✓	✓			
Dialectical behavioral therapy	✓	✓			
Eye movement desensitization and reprocessing	✓	✓			
Cognitive processing therapy	✓	✓			
Executive functioning training				✓	
Neurofeedback	✓	✓		✓	
Cognitive remediation/rehabilitation				✓	

*Mindfulness therapies include a wide range of evidence-based interventions specifically studied for particular conditions (e.g., mindfulness for attention deficit/hyperactivity disorder, mindfulness for relapse prevention and depression, mindful eating).

**Delivered by dietitian and/or education by clinicians about importance of dietary interventions and lifestyle changes.

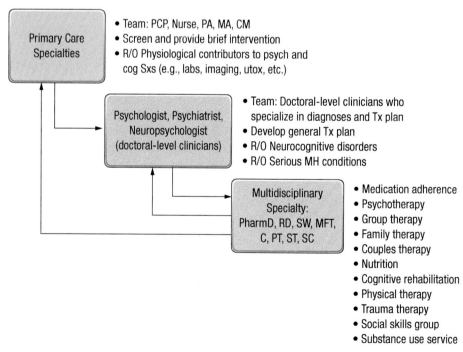

FIGURE 32.2 Multidisciplinary clinician and referral process.
C, counselor; CM, case manager; MA, medical assistant; MFT, marriage and family counselor; MH, mental health; NP, nurse practitioner; PA, physician assistant; PCP, primary care provider; PharmD, pharmacist; PT, physical therapy; RD, registered dietitian; R/O, rule out; SC, substance use counselor; ST, speech therapy; SW, social worker; Sxs, symptoms; Tx, treatment.

stabilizers (lithium, sodium valproate, and carbamazepine) to avoid toxicity or elevations above their therapeutic ranges. Prescribers should consider obtaining and EKG prior to starting therapy and regularly during treatment in patients who are over 40 years old or who have underlying cardiac disease. Continuous monitoring should be performed for anemia, agranulocytosis, and skin reactions in patients with Asian ancestry taking carbamazepine. Utilization of MI, CBT, and mindfulness therapies are helpful in optimizing medication adherence, symptom awareness, impulse control, and self-management strategies.

Short-term use of benzodiazepines or Z-drugs may help with initial treatment of anxiety while waiting for buspirone or other antidepressant medications to take effect. Benzodiazepines should only be used short-term for initial treatment of anxiety disorders. Treatment with SSRIs or SNRIs, when paired with CBT, sleep hygiene techniques, and mindfulness therapies, are help patients experience long-term success. Clinicians need to assess psychological dependency and use slow and stepwise tapering of medications to avoid serious withdrawal symptoms. Gabapentin can be used for alcohol use disorder, anxiety, and some chronic pain conditions, but should be avoided in patients with major neurocognitive disorders (e.g., Alzheimer's disease, delirium, and cognitive impairment).

Antipsychotic medications are effective for psychotic disorders, bipolar disorder, suicidal behaviors, aggressive behaviors, and depression. Prescribers should counsel and monitor for potential side effects including but not limited to EPS, tardive dyskinesia, neutropenia, orthostatic changes, weight gain, and cardiovascular disease.

Stimulant and nonstimulant medications often improve the functioning of individuals with ADHD. Prior to starting stimulant medications, an EKG and/or cardiology consultation should be considered for those with a history of cardiac disease or family history of sudden cardiac death. Prescribers may consult a psychiatrist when working with complex cases (e.g., substance use history, personality disorders) and consult a neuropsychologist with complex cognitive cases (e.g., history of neurodevelopmental disorders, mild TBI, dyslexia, stroke/TIA conditions). Executive functioning training, CBT, neurofeedback, and mindfulness therapies should also be considered to manage behavioral, cognitive, and emotional regulation issues in ADHD.

CASE EXEMPLAR: Patient With Depression and Generalized Anxiety Disorder

OV, a 51-year-old perimenopausal woman with major depressive disorder (MDD) and generalized anxiety disorder (GAD), presents with severe hot flashes, worsening lower extremity pain, and blurry vision. Her lab results show she has poorly controlled diabetes, which is likely causing diabetic neuropathy and retinopathy. Which medication is the best choice to treat many of her symptoms? What nonpharmacological treatments should be considered?

CASE EXEMPLAR: Patient With Bipolar Disorder

SW is a 28-year-old woman being treated for bipolar disorder. Valproate had to be discontinued due to worsening confusion thought to be secondary to hyperammonemia. Her clinician decides to start lamotrigine. What potentially fatal side effect should the SW be warned about? What behavioral treatment should be considered for a patient with bipolar disorder?

KEY TAKEAWAYS

- The World Health Organization (WHO) estimates that most countries experience an 18.1% to 36.1% prevalence rate of psychiatric illness.
- Healthcare professionals' ability to prescribe and monitor psychopharmacological agents needs to be balanced with integrative behavioral interventions to address patient needs.

- The clinician's ability to make a specific diagnosis is key in directing and monitoring the effects of treatment.
- Depression is defined by the presence of dysphoric mood and/or loss of pleasure or interest and is often associated with sleep disturbance, appetite changes, psychomotor changes, and suicidal ideation. These symptoms may be masked by other somatic or cognitive conditions.

- Bipolar I disorder is characterized by the presence of at least one major manic episode. Bipolar II disorder is characterized by at least one episode of hypomania and one episode of depression.
- Anxiety can manifest in uncontrollable worrying as in generalized anxiety disorder (GAD), excessive fear of being judged as in social anxiety disorder (SAD), or specific phobias. Obsessive-compulsive disorder (OCD) is characterized by obsessions and compulsions.
- A traumatic event is an emotionally disturbing experience that may involve the threat of death, serious injury, sexual violence, or threat to physical integrity. Some individuals present with posttraumatic stress disorder (PTSD).
- Psychotic symptoms can accompany depressive or manic episodes and often occur independent of mood disturbance. Disordered thinking and speech are common in schizophrenia spectrum disorders, as are negative symptoms such as flattened affect and avolition.
- Attention deficit/hyperactivity disorder (ADHD) is a neurodevelopmental disorder that impairs functioning with symptoms of inattention, impulsivity, and/or excessive motor activity and restlessness.
- Selective serotonin reuptake inhibitors (SSRIs) and serotonin-norepinephrine reuptake inhibitors (SNRIs) as first-line antidepressants. These agents are best tolerated when started at low dosage. Atypical antidepressants (e.g., bupropion) can also be used as first-line treatment or as adjunctive therapy to SSRIs and SNRIs. Tricyclic antidepressants (TCAs) and monoamine oxidase inhibitors (MAOIs) are older antidepressants that are used less frequently due to their increased risk of serious side effects.
- Mood stabilizers (valproate, lithium, lamotrigine, carbamazepine, and oxcarbazepine) are the treatment of choice for bipolar spectrum disorders. With the exception of lithium, mood stabilizers are also used as antiepileptic drugs.
- The benzodiazepines are used for sedative-hypnotic therapy. Benzodiazepine dependence is common in those who use these drugs for longer than 1 month.
- There are approximately 20 antipsychotic medications in use today. They are indicated for the treatment of psychotic disorders (schizophrenia, schizoaffective, other psychosis), bipolar disorders, and antidepressant augmentation. The first-generation antipsychotics can result in extrapyramidal symptoms (EPS) including akathisia, dystonia, parkinsonism, and tardive dyskinesia. They can also cause neuroleptic malignant syndrome (NMS).
- The most efficacious treatments for ADHD are stimulants, all of which have an amphetamine base.
- The clinician's ability to educate and implement behavioral treatment when initiating pharmacotherapy will often result in more successful outcomes.

REFERENCES

1. Kessler RC, Aguilar-Gaxiola S, Alonso J, et al. *The global burden of mental disorders: an update from the WHO World Mental Health (WMH) surveys. Epidemiologia e psichiatria sociale. 2009;*18(1):23. doi:10.1017/s1121189x00001421
2. Katon WJ. Epidemiology and treatment of depression in patients with chronic medical illness. *Dialogues Clin Neurosci.* 2011;13(1):7–23. doi:10.31887/DCNS.2011.13.1/wkaton
3. Ilgen MA, Zivin K, McCammon RJ, et al. Pain and suicidal thoughts, plans and attempts in the United States. *Gen Hosp Psychiatry.* 2008;30(6), 521–527. doi:10.1016/j.genhosppsych.2008.09.003
4. American Psychiatric Association. *Diagnostic and Statistical Manual of Mental Disorders.* 5th ed. American Psychiatric Association; 2013.
5. Park LT, Zarate CA. Depression in the primary care setting. *N Engl J Med.* 2019;380(6):559–568. doi:10.1056/NEJMcp1712493
6. DeMartini J, Patel G, Fancher TL. Generalized anxiety disorder. *Ann Intern Med.* 2019;170(7):ITC49–ITC64. doi:10.7326/AITC201904020
7. Lewitzka U, Severus E, Bauer R, et al. The suicide prevention effect of lithium: More than 20 years of evidence—a narrative review. *Int J Bipolar Disord.* 2015;3(1):15. doi:10.1186/s40345-015-0032-2
8. López-Muñoz F, Shen WW, D'ocon P, et al. A history of the pharmacological treatment of bipolar disorder. *Int J Mol Sci.* 2018;19:2143. doi:10.3390/ijms19072143
9. Olfson M, King M, Schoenbaum M. Benzodiazepine use in the United States. *JAMA Psychiatry.* 2015;72(2):136–142. doi:10.1001/jamapsychiatry.2014.1763
10. Soyka M. Treatment of benzodiazepine dependence. *N Engl J Med,* 2017;376(12):1147–1157. doi:10.1056/NEJMra1611832
11. Richards K, Demartini J, Xiong G. Understanding sleep disorders in older adults. *Psychiatric Times.* 2018;35(2):17-20. Accessed October 24, 2020. https://ucdavis.pure.elsevier.com/en/publications/understanding-sleep-disorders-in-older-adults

12. Lieberman JA, First MB. Psychotic disorders. *N Engl J Med*.2018;379(3):270–280. doi:10.1056/NEJMra1801490

13. Owen MJ, Sawa A, Mortensen PB. Schizophrenia. *Lancet*. 2016;388(10039):86–97. doi:10.1016/S0140-6736(15)01121-6

14. Warnez S, Alessi-Severini S. Clozapine: a review of clinical practice guidelines and prescribing trends. *BMC Psychiatry*. 2014;14(1):102. doi:10.1186/1471-244X-14-102

15. Pliszka S, AACAP Work Group on Quality Issues. Practice parameter for the assessment and treatment of children and adolescents with attention-deficit/hyperactivity disorder. *J Am Acad Child Adolesc Psychiatry*. 2007;46(7):894–921. doi:10.1097/chi.0b013e318054e724

16. Mattingly GW, Wilson J, Rostain AL. A clinician's guide to ADHD treatment options. *Postgraduate Medicine*. 2017;129:657–666. doi:10.1080/00325481.2017.1354648

17. Miller WR, Rollnick S. *Motivational Interviewing: Preparing People for Change*. 2nd ed. Guilford Press; 2002.

18. Butler AC, Chapman JE, Forman EM, et al. The empirical status of cognitive-behavioral therapy: a review of meta-analyses. *Clin Psychol Rev*. 2006;26(1):17–31. doi:10.1016/j.cpr.2005.07.003

19. Hofmann SG, Asmundson GJG. *The Science of Cognitive Behavioral Therapy*. Academic Press; 2017.

20. Levy RA, Ablon JS, Kächele H. (Eds.). *Psychodynamic Psychotherapy Research: Evidence-Based Practice and Practice-Based Evidence*. Humana Press–Springer; 2012.

21. Ramezani A, Rockers DM, Wanlass RL, et al. Teaching behavioral medicine professionals and trainees an elaborated version of the Y-Model: implications for the integration of cognitive-behavioral therapy (CBT), psychodynamic therapy, and motivational interviewing. *J Psychother Integr*. 2016;26(4):407–424. doi:10.1037/int0000048

Pharmacotherapy for Pain Management

Theresa Mallick-Searle, Joy Vongspanich, Aliyah Ali, Paramjit Kaur,
Erielle Anne P. Espina, Phil Emond, and Brent Luu

LEARNING OBJECTIVES

- Identify the classes of pharmacological agents used in the treatment of pain.
- Distinguish between pain syndromes that require opioids and those that do not.
- Apply guidelines from national pain societies in the assessment of patients in pain.
- Select the appropriate class of pain medication for a given type of pain syndrome.
- Compare therapeutic alternatives that can be used in the treatment of pain.
- Design an evidence-based treatment protocol for a patient in pain.

INTRODUCTION

The International Association for the Study of Pain (IASP) defines pain as "[a]n unpleasant sensory and emotional experience associated with, or resembling that associated with, actual or potential tissue damage."[1] This definition enables clinicians to recognize the connection between the objective, physiological, subjective, and emotional aspects of pain. Pain can be classified by pathophysiology into categories of nociceptive pain and neuropathic pain. Pain is a normal symptom and serves a protective function. Once nociceptors are stimulated by injury or tissue damage, nerve impulses are generated and interpreted by the brain.[2] The unpleasant nature of pain is what contributes to the emotional aspect, and this can lead to a patient becoming depressed as well as anxious as they anticipate the oncoming dysphoria associated with pain.[3,4] The American Academy of Pain Medicine (AAPM) describes pain as a temporal continuum "beginning with an acute stage, which may progress to a chronic state of variable duration."[5]

The field of pain management has changed significantly over the last several decades; and continues to evolve based upon emerging evidence-based practice. The 2011 Institute of Medicine (IOM) report, *Relieving Pain in America*, called for comprehensive population-health strategies to address pain management, education, and research.[6] Based upon this IOM report, the Interagency Pain Research Coordinating Committee of the National Institutes of Health created a National Pain Strategy (NPS) to address the social, environmental, political, and economic factors that contribute to the causes, recognition, and treatment of pain in the United States.[7] The NPS outlines strategic plans aimed at reducing the burden of chronic pain in the United States. These programs and implementation activities fall into six major areas:

- **Professional education and training:** focus on the skills and training that clinicians require for better management of pain.
- **Public education and communication:** responsibility for the development of high quality, evidence-based education programs for patients and the public.
- **Disparities**: need for identification of the under-treatment and inappropriate treatment of pain among racial and ethnic minorities.
- **Prevention and care:** creation of programs that substantially increase the accessibility and quality of pain care.
- **Services and payments:** engagement with public health entities in pain care and prevention.
- **Population research:** focus on improvements in state and national data on pain and treatment.

TABLE 33.1 Acute versus Chronic Pain

Characteristic	Acute Pain	Chronic Pain
Pathophysiology	Commonly results from noxious stimuli	Natural cause may be absent
Typical sources	Results from injury, tissue damage, or inflammatory response (e.g., surgery, fractures, acute injury)	Typically results from chronic disease or untreated conditions (e.g., neuropathy, cancer, arthritis, headaches)
Duration	Can resolve over days to weeks	Persistent pain lasting longer than 3–6 months (potentially years)
Dependence/tolerance to medication	Less likely	Common

Source: Adapted from Yam MF, Loh YC, Tan CS, et al. General pathways of pain sensation and the major neurotransmitters involved in pain regulation. *Int J Mol Sci*. 2018;19(8):2164. doi:10.3390/ijms19082164.

This chapter will focus primarily on the available pharmacological treatments for acute and chronic pain, with a brief overview of nonpharmacological considerations. The major categories of pharmacologic agents for pain management include nonopioid analgesic medications and opioids. For many patients, an approach using combinations of drugs that target different mechanistic pathways may result in improved analgesia and fewer side effects because lower doses of each drug can be used. As the practice of pain management is best done through a multimodal approach, the use of pharmaceuticals is one of the aspects that clinicians should consider in relationship to psychological, behavioral, and mind–body therapies and procedural interventions.

CHARACTERIZING PAIN

Pain can be classified by several means, such as duration, types of pain, or severity.

ACUTE VERSUS CHRONIC PAIN

Acute pain typically occurs due to an identified event, and the pain usually resolves within days to weeks. Most of the time, acute pain is classified as nociceptive.[5] The IASP has defined chronic pain as pain that lasts beyond the normal healing time for the tissue.[8–10] The duration of chronic pain is indeterminate, and is typically more than 3 months. The etiology of chronic pain is not easily identifiable and sometimes has multiple causes. Chronic pain can be either nociceptive or neuropathic. It is also possible for patients with chronic pain to experience pain-free intervals.[8,11,12] Recent studies have shown that the determination of pain chronicity involved the ability of the complex limbic-cortical network helping to attenuate or intensify the emotional component of the nociceptive stimuli.[12] The most common causes of chronic pain are lower back pain, neck pain, and headaches. In the elderly, the most common cause of pain is degenerative joint disease. Other causes of chronic pain can be related to medical conditions such as cancer, vascular disease, or neuropathies.[6] Table 33.1 compares acute versus chronic pain.

TYPES OF PAIN BASED ON PATHOPHYSIOLOGY

Pain can be classified as nociceptive, neuropathic, or nociplastic.[13] Nociceptive pain, which may also be referred as physiologic pain, is triggered by stimulation of the primary afferent nociceptive fibers due to potential or actual tissue damage. It can be further subcategorized into somatic or visceral depending on the source of the stimulation of the sensory receptors. Somatic pain can be further subdivided into superficial and deep pain. Superficial somatic pain involves nociceptive input from skin, subcutaneous tissue, and mucous membranes. This superficial pain is well localized and is sharp, throbbing, or burning. Deep somatic pain involves input from deep tissue such as muscles, tendons, or bones. The quality of this pain is dull in nature and is not very well localized as compared to superficial somatic pain. Visceral pain is due to a disease process involving internal organs or their coverings. This pain involves sympathetic or parasympathetic input and signs and symptoms are related to the involvement of the nervous system. Parasympathetic input pain may be associated with nausea, vomiting, and diaphoresis, whereas sympathetic input pain involves the accompaniment of associated symptoms such as changes in blood pressure or heart rate.

Meanwhile, neuropathic pain can be generated either in the periphery, such as diabetic neuropathy, or centrally mediated (e.g., poststroke pain or spinal cord injury). According to the IASP, neuropathic pain may be defined as "[p]ain caused by a lesion or disease of the somatosensory nervous system."[1] It is associated with about 7% to 8% of adult pain and 25% of patients with diabetes. It may also occur in 35% of patients with human immunodeficiency virus (HIV) and is generally more difficult to treat or manage than other forms of chronic pain.[14] Other classic examples of neuropathic pain include herpes zoster, traumatic nerve injury, post-amputation pain, and trigeminal neuralgia. Generally, the site of nerve injury corresponds to the part of the body in which the person feels the pain. Patients often describe the pain as burning, tingling, or shooting down a part of the body and it can become very intense.

Nociplastic pain is a newer classification of pain that has been recently introduced by the IASP. Nociplastic pain is "[p]ain that arises from altered nociception despite no clear evidence of actual or threatened tissue damage causing the activation of peripheral nociceptors or evidence for disease or lesion of the somatosensory system causing the pain."[1] Examples of nociplastic pain are fibromyalgia, irritable bowel syndrome (IBS), and complex regional pain syndrome (CRPS) type I.[13]

Mixed types of pain exist, and a common example of both neuropathic and nociceptive pain can be observed in cancer-related pain. Cancer pain can be caused by the cancer directly growing on or pushing against nerves, soft tissue, or bone. It can also be a result of the cancer treatment side effects, such as vincristine-induced peripheral neuropathy.

THE PAIN PATHWAY

Pain is the consequence of the interaction between physiological and cognitive responses.[15,16] The physiological response is comprised of actions from the nervous and immune systems. To understand the pathology and therapies for pain, it is first necessary to appreciate the interactions between noxious and nonnoxious stimuli and the body's neural pathways, neurotransmitters, and neuropeptides. The pain pathway may be subdivided into four different segments: transduction, transmission, modulation, and perception.[17] *Transduction* is the conversion of mechanical, thermal, or chemical stimuli into electric charges within the neurons. In other words, this process converts noxious stimuli into electrical impulses so the signal can travel faster, further, and be conducted "freely" within neurons. When the electric signals travel and are conducted from one neuron to another, this process is called *transmission,* which allows the signal to propagate from the peripheral to central nervous system. During the transmission, *modulation* of these signals may take place at all levels of the nociceptive pathways via primary afferent neurons.[17] They follow different tracts by upregulation or downregulation of neurotransmitters. The *perception* of pain occurs when the nociceptive information is relayed to various cortical and subcortical regions in the brain, including the amygdala, hypothalamus, periaqueductal grey, basal ganglia, and regions of the cerebral cortex.[17]

Pain may also be observed without a noxious stimulus. This type of pain arises from injury of peripheral nerves or when there is interference to the normal pain process.[15] Because of nervous system adaptability, this type of pain can result in peripheral or central sensitization. Central sensitization occurs when the relay of pain signals is regulated at the spinal column which results in amplified transmission, also known as secondary hyperalgesia. Allodynia is described when there is a lowering of the pain threshold to a point where an innocuous stimulus produces a pain response.[18] Peripheral sensitization happens when the sensitivity of nociceptors to stimuli increases. An example of peripheral sensitization is when inflammatory messengers such as calcitonin gene-related peptide (CGRP) and substance P, which decrease pain threshold to produce a response, are present at the injury site. Signaling of pain can be affected at the supraspinal level through the descending pathway which originated from the brain to the spinal cord. This modulation on the descending pathway results in changing the perception to the stimulus. Because of this, there can be either increased or decreased sensitivity to pain.

ASSESSMENT OF PAIN

Pain is subjective, therefore, each assessment is specific for each individual patient.[19,20] Acute pain is generally easier and more reliably assessed. Chronic pain is more complex and requires deeper assessment. For example, baseline and serial evaluation of chronic pain should include assessment of function, cognitive function, and quality of life in addition to pain location, pain level and pain descriptors (e.g., throbbing, burning).[19] Many evidence-based tools exist to assess pain in specific situations. For example, the Wong-Baker FACES pain scale can be used in younger children or those who are nonverbal.[20]

STANDARDIZED TOOLS FOR MEASURING PAIN INTENSITY

The commonly used scales for measuring pain intensity are the verbal rating scale (VRS), numeric rating scale (NRS), visual analog scales (VAS), and the Wong-Baker FACES Scale.[19,21,22] These tools use self-reported pain scores to assess the severity of pain. For VRS, descriptive categories are provided so that a patient can select the descriptor that fits their pain such as "none" to "very severe." The NRS uses a verbal scale of 0 to 10 to quantify pain, with "0" being no pain and "10" being the worst pain imaginable. Visual analog scales use graphics to record scores. The VAS uses a 10 cm line that represents a numeric range from "no pain" to "worst pain" and the Wong-Baker FACES Scale uses faces to depict pain intensity (**Figure 33.1**). In either

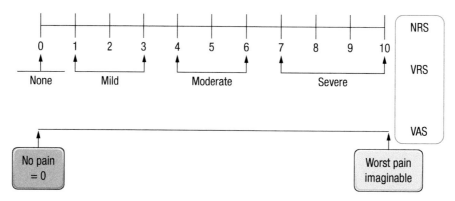

FIGURE 33.1 Visual analog scales for pain assessment.
NRS, numeric rating scale; VAS, visual analog scale; VRS, verbal rating scale.
Source: Reproduced with permission from Breivik H, Borchgrevink PC, Allen SM, et al. Assessment of pain. *Br J Anaesth.* 2008;101(1):17–24. doi:10.1093/bja/aen103; Garra G, Singer AJ, Taira BR, Chohan J, Cardoz H, Chisena E, Thode HC Jr. Validation of the Wong-Baker FACES Pain Rating Scale in pediatric emergency department patients. Acad Emerg Med. 2010 Jan;17(1):50-4. doi: 10.1111/j.1553-2712.2009.00620.x. Epub 2009 Dec 9. PMID: 20003121.

case, the patient can point to the value that represents their pain intensity.

STANDARDIZED TOOLS TO ASSESS NEUROPATHIC PAIN

In addition to the standardized tools used to assess general pain, there are tools specifically used for assessing neuropathic pain.[23-25] Screening questionnaires such as the Douleur Neuropathique (DN4) and PainDETECT are intended to be utilized in the diagnosis of neuropathic conditions by differentiating symptoms from other types of pain.

OTHER STANDARDIZED TOOLS

Function and quality of life are additional areas that can be assessed to evaluate pain. The Centers for Disease Control and Prevention (CDC) recommends assessment of these areas in people who suffer chronic pain using the Pain, Enjoyment of Life, General activity (PEG) tool for assessment of function.[26] It is a three-item scale that includes an NRS and asks how pain has interfered with enjoyment of life, as well as general activity.[27] Other functional assessments exist, but they lack validity compared to the previous tools mentioned.[28] Quality of life and daily activity with pain can be assessed as well. The Pain Disability Index is a tool for measuring the severity of interference with daily activities.[28]

MANAGING PAIN

Key concepts in pain management include identification of the underlying cause and determining whether a patient is opioid-naïve versus opioid-tolerant. Opioid-tolerant patients are defined by the U.S. Food and Drug Administration (FDA) as those receiving

treatment with opioids at the following doses or higher for at least 1 week: oral morphine 60 mg/day, transdermal fentanyl 25 mcg/hour, oral oxycodone 30 mg/day, oral hydromorphone 8 mg/day, oral oxymorphone 25 mg/day, or an equianalgesic dose of another opioid (**Box 33.1**).[29] The majority of the pain management is targeted toward opioid-naïve patients; however, there are guidelines to help with managing pain in patients who are opioid tolerant. Equianalgesic dosages of commonly used opioids are listed in **Table 33.2**.

ACUTE PAIN

Nonopioid analgesics are typically used as first-line therapy options for acute pain.[30] Comorbidities such as renal impairment, hepatic impairment, and heart disease guide therapy selection for pain management. For example, nonsteroidal anti-inflammatory drugs

---

BOX 33.1
OPIOID TOLERANCE AS DEFINED BY THE FEDERAL DRUG ADMINISTRATION

Opioid therapy of ≥1 week with any of the following medications:
- Oral hydrocodone, 60 mg/day
- Oral hydromorphone, 8 mg/day
- Oral morphine, 60 mg/day
- Oral oxycodone, 30 mg/day
- Oral oxymorphone, 25 mg/day
- Transdermal fentanyl, 25 mcg/hour

Source: Adopted from PL Detail-Document. Equianalgesic dosing of opioids for pain management. Pharmacist's Letter/Prescriber's Letter. August 2012.

TABLE 33.2 Equianalgesic Dosing of Opioids for Pain Management in Opioid-Tolerant Patients

Drug	Equianalgesic Dosing (in mg/dose)*	
	Parenteral	Oral
Morphine (parenteral, immediate-release oral)	10 mg	30 mg
Morphine (CR)	n/a	30 mg
Morphine (ER)	n/a	30 mg
Hydromorphone	1.5–2 mg	7.5–8 mg
Hydromorphone (CR)	n/a	7.5 mg
Oxycodone	n/a	20–30 mg
Oxycodone (CR)	n/a	20–30 mg
Oxymorphone	1 mg	10 mg
Oxymorphone (ER)	n/a	10 mg
Hydrocodone (with acetaminophen)	n/a	30–45 mg
Codeine	100–130 mg	200 mg
Codeine (CR)	n/a	200 mg
Methadone	Variable	Variable
Meperidine	75 mg	300 mg
Fentanyl**	0.1 mg	n/a

*Equianalgesic doses are approximate and provided only as a guideline. Dosing must be titrated to individual response. It is recommended to begin with a 50% lower dose than the equianalgesic dose when changing drugs and then titrate to a safe/effective response.

**All noninjectable fentanyl products are for opioid-tolerant patients only. Do not convert mcg for mcg among fentanyl products (i.e., patch, transmucosal lozenge, buccal tablet, buccal film, sublingual tablet, nasal spray).

CR, controlled-release; ER, extended-release; n/a, information not available.

Source: Adapted from PL Detail-Document. Equianalgesic dosing of opioids for pain management. Pharmacist's Letter/Prescriber's Letter. August 2012.

(NSAIDs) may not be appropriate for individuals with renal impairment, risk of gastrointestinal bleeding, or cardiovascular events.[30] Topical NSAIDs can be used for localized pain with decreased risks for the adverse effects that are seen with use of systemic NSAIDs.[31–33]

Opioids are often appropriate for management of severe acute pain.[30] When prescribed, they are used at the lowest effective dose and for the shortest duration possible. When indicated, the CDC recommends no more than a 7-day supply of opioids for acute pain. The CDC also suggests 3 days or less as sufficient for most acute pain management.[26,34] Extended-release opioid formulations are not appropriate for management of acute pain.

CHRONIC PAIN

When providing care for individuals suffering from chronic pain, it is important to establish the expectation that complete pain relief is unlikely to be achieved. Management of chronic pain should target improving function and quality of life. Clinicians and patients both need to understand that a 30% to 50% reduction in pain intensity is more likely to be achievable. Chronic pain care involves using different modalities of therapy that can target physical, cognitive, and emotional suffering to improve quality of life.[35]

Based on the CDC guidelines, opioids are typically not recommended as first-line therapy for chronic pain. The CDC recommends that nonpharmacologic approaches and nonopioids are the preferred agents to use first.[36] For neuropathic pain, antidepressants (e.g., serotonin–norepinephrine reuptake inhibitors [SNRIs] or tricyclic antidepressants [TCAs]) and gabapentinoids can be used. Topical lidocaine or capsaicin can be used for localized pain.[37]

A 2015 meta-analysis by Finnerup et al. assessed more than 200 studies of treatments for neuropathic pain. The number needed to treat (NNT) to achieve 50% pain intensity reduction was lowest for TCAs (NNT = 3.6). SNRIs were less effective (NNT = 6.4). Gabapentin and pregabalin were found to be have NNTs of 6.3 and 7.7, respectively.[38] Topical agents such as capsaicin were less effective, and lidocaine was not able to be evaluated because of low-quality evidence. The disadvantage of TCAs is that they are not as well tolerated as the other options. When deciding on a pharmacologic option for neuropathic pain, gabapentinoids, TCAs, and SNRIs should be first-line agents.[38]

Acetaminophen and NSAIDs are also widely used for both acute and chronic pain management. NSAIDs are classified as cyclooxygenase 2 (COX2)-selective (c2s) or nonselective (ns) and are discussed further below.[31]

Opioids can be appropriate for management of chronic pain with careful follow up and monitoring. It is always important to weigh the risk versus benefit of opioid use. Patients for whom opioid therapy is considered will need to provide informed consent regarding the risks and benefits of opioid therapy, as well as clear understanding of the expectations of the patient and clinician.[17]

Chronic pain is often a complex entity to treat. Interdisciplinary pain management programs have been shown to improve outcomes, be cost effective, and incorporate a patient-centered approach that includes pharmacologic and nonpharmacologic interventions.[32] Examples of nonpharmacologic therapies that appear to provide benefit for patients suffering from chronic pain include cognitive-behavioral therapy (CBT), physiotherapy, and peripheral nerve stimulation. There is some literature that suggests that acupuncture can be effective for many types of chronic pain, including migraine, osteoarthritis, and low-back pain. There is a lack of evidence supporting the use of chiropractic care or herbal treatments. Self-care for chronic pain includes activities which enhance function, improve mood, and decrease pain by targeting and influencing the emotional, cognitive, and behavioral responses to pain, such as mindfulness techniques.[39,40]

PHARMACOLOGY OF ANALGESIC AGENTS

NONOPIOID AGENTS

Acetaminophen

Analgesia should be initiated with the most-effective analgesic agent having the fewest side effects. Acetaminophen is considered a first-line analgesic for most patients due to its safety profile and tolerability. It is an antipyretic and pain reliever that lacks anti-inflammatory activity; it is thought to provide pain relief through central inhibition of the COX pathway and prostaglandin synthesis.[33,41] Acetaminophen is safe for use in patients with renal impairment and pregnancy, and it has few drug–drug interactions.[41] An important adverse effect known to be linked to acetaminophen is hepatotoxicity.[41] Consequently, the total oral acetaminophen dosage is typically limited to 4 gm/day in patients with normal renal and hepatic functions.[42,43]

Meanwhile, for the elderly with frailty and/or risk factors of hepatotoxicity, the maximum dose should be capped at 2 gm/day or 3 gm/day.[43,44] Acetaminophen should not be used with alcohol, which is known to induce CYP450 2E1 to further cause hepatic injury. Acetaminophen-induced hepatotoxicity occurs when the resulting metabolite, N-acetyl-p-benzoquinone imine (NAPQI) depletes hepatic glutathione which is required for conjugation of toxic metabolites. N-acetylcysteine (NAC) is an antidote to acetaminophen overdose that avoids toxicity by replacing and increasing glutathione and restoring conjugation to nontoxic metabolites (**Figure 33.2**).[45]

Nonsteroidal Anti-Inflammatory Drugs

NSAIDs inhibit prostaglandin synthesis by reversible or irreversible inhibition of COX.[30,33] There are two COX isoforms: COX-1 and COX-2. All NSAIDs carry well-documented risk of adverse gastrointestinal (GI), cardiovascular (CV), and renal effects, including GI bleeding, peptic ulcer, acute myocardial infarction (MI) and thrombotic events, and acute and chronic kidney injury.[46] However there are distinct differences between the different types of NSAIDs (COX2-selective [c2s] versus nonselective [ns]). Several recent clinical trials have compared efficacy and adverse event risks between c2s-NSAIDs and ns-NSAIDs. The PRECISION trial[47,48] compared a c2s agent (celecoxib) with two ns-NSAID (ibuprofen and naproxen); the CONCERN trial compared celecoxib to naproxen[49]; and the MEDAL trial[50] trial compared etoricoxib (c2s-NSAID) to diclofenac (ns-NSAID). All studied NSAIDs were equally effective analgesics for arthritis pain. CV adverse event rates were comparable for patients with or without preexisting CV disease in the PRECISION trial, lower in the celecoxib group versus the naproxen group in the CONCERN trial, and slightly lower for the subgroup of patients taking low-dose aspirin who were on etoricoxib versus diclofenac in the MEDAL trial. Co-administration of esomeprazole (a proton pump inhibitor [PPI]) was used in the PRECISION and CONCERN trials and recommended in the MEDAL trial. GI adverse events were assessed in all three, with significantly lower rates of GI bleeding, anemia associated with GI blood loss, and NSAID discontinuation due to GI adverse events in the c2s-NSAID—treated groups versus the ns-NSAID groups.[47–50] Of note, PPI use was found to be nonprotective for lower GI bleeding in all three trials. While not a primary endpoint, the PRECISION trial also found significantly fewer serious renal adverse events in the celecoxib group versus the ns-NSAID groups.[47] A study comparing NSAID combined with a PPI versus a histamine-2 receptor antagonist (H2RA) versus misoprostol also found to be more effective that H2RA or misoprostol in preventing GI adverse effects.[46]

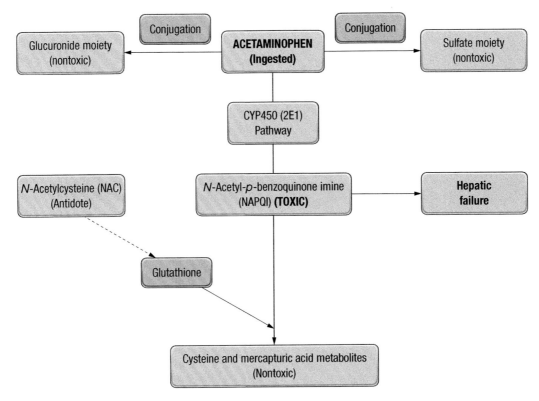

FIGURE 33.2 Acetaminophen metabolism and hepatotoxicity.

Source: Reproduced with permission from Athersuch TJ, Antoine DJ, Boobis AR, et al. Paracetamol metabolism, hepatotoxicity, biomarkers and therapeutic interventions: a perspective. *Toxicol Res.* 2018;7(3):347–357. doi:10.1039/C7TX00340D

COX-1 and COX-2 have different effects on renal function. COX-1 primarily controls hemodynamics and GFR; COX-2 primarily impacts sodium and water excretion. Blockade of these enzymes can therefore result in decreased renal blood flow and sodium and water retention.[51] Thus, NSAID use can cause or exacerbate hypertension and cause clinically significant edema. NSAIDs can also cause clinically significant renal dysfunction; however, the incidence is less than 1% of patients.[52] Risk factors that increase the probability of NSAID-induced renal impairment include age greater than 60 years, volume and/or sodium depletion, comorbid disease (diabetes, hypertensions, heart failure, hepatic, existing kidney disease), concomitant drug therapy (multiple NSAIDs, angiotensin-converting enzyme inhibitors, diuretics, oral steroids, warfarin), and current tobacco use.[52] The decision to use an NSAID, and which type, should be based upon individual patient's contraindications such as pregnancy (see Chapter 22) as well as risk factors for CV, GI, and renal adverse events

Key treatment recommendations based upon consensus guidelines and recent trials are summarized in **Figure 33.3**. Topical NSAID formulations provide an alternative to oral NSAIDs because of their low systemic absorption decreases the risk of systemic adverse events and drug–drug interactions. They have been studied extensively for use in treatment of osteoarthritis and can be considered for use in elderly patients and those with comorbid conditions in whom systemic NSAIDs should be avoided. Commonly used topical NSAIDs available in the United States include diclofenac sodium 1% gel and diclofenac sodium 1.5% solution.[53]

Serotonin–Norepinephrine Reuptake Inhibitors

Duloxetine and venlafaxine are the most commonly used antidepressants for the treatment of chronic and neuropathic pain.[54,55] SNRIs act primarily upon serotonergic and noradrenergic neurons, with minimal or no effect on cholinergic or histaminergic receptors. The proposed mechanism of action for SNRIs is that increased activity of noradrenergic and serotonergic neurons in the descending spinal pathway on the dorsal horn inhibits the activity of dorsal horn neurons, which suppresses excessive input from reaching the brain. The hypothesis is that the excess input reaching the brain is responsible for altered or heightened pain perception. Venlafaxine is predominantly a selective serotonin reuptake inhibitor (SSRI) at 75 mg/day; at higher doses such as 225 mg/day, it has more significant norepinephrine inhibition in addition to serotonin.[56,57] Both duloxetine and venlafaxine are good choices to treat patients with comorbid pain and depression. Dose titration for either duloxetine or venlafaxine should begin at the lowest dose with titration up every 7 days to an

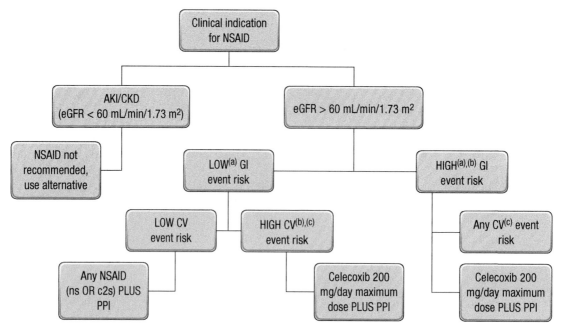

FIGURE 33.3 Algorithm for determining the use of NSAIDs in different patient groups.

(a)Both upper- and lower-GI risk must be assessed. PPIs do not prevent lower GI NSAID-induced adverse events. Celecoxib is associated with lower risk of both upper- and lower-GI tract adverse events than ns-NSAIDs.

(b)Risks and benefits of therapy should be weighed and alternative to NSAID considered.

(c)NSAIDs should generally be avoided in patients with known CV disease, current evidence supports low-dose celecoxib when benefit outweighs risk.

AKI, acute kidney injury; c2s, COX-2 selective; CKD, chronic kidney disease; CV, cardiovascular; eGFR, estimated glomerular filtration rate; GI, gastrointestinal; ns, nonselective; NSAID, nonsteroidal anti-inflammatory drug; PPI, proton pump inhibitor.

Sources: CDER statement: FDA approves labeling supplement for Celebrex (celecoxib). Food and Drug Administration. Published June 28, 2018. Accessed June 13, 2020. www.fda.gov/drugs/drug-safety-and-availability/cder-statement-fda-approves-labeling-supplement-celebrex-celecoxib; Chan FK, Ching JY, Tse YK, et al. Gastrointestinal safety of celecoxib versus naproxen in patients with cardiothrombotic disease and arthritis after upper gastrointestinal bleeding (CONCERN): An industry-independent, double-blind, double-dummy, randomised trial. Lancet. 2017;389(10087):2375–2382. doi:10.1016/S0140-6736(17)30981-9; Combe B, Swergold G, McLay J, et al. Cardiovascular safety and gastrointestinal tolerability of etoricoxib vs diclofenac in a randomized controlled clinical trial (the MEDAL study). Rheumatology (Oxford). 2009;48(4):425–432. doi:10.1093/rheumatology/kep005; Curiel RV, Katz JD. Mitigating the cardiovascular and renal effects of NSAIDs. Pain Med. 2013;14:S23–S28. doi:10.1111/pme.12275; Gwee KA, Goh V, Lima G, et al. Coprescribing proton-pump inhibitors with nonsteroidal anti-inflammatory drugs: Risks versus benefits. J Pain Res. 2018;11:361–374. doi:10.2147/JPR.S156938; Nissen SE, Yeomans ND, Solomon DH, et al. Cardiovascular safety of celecoxib, naproxen, or ibuprofen for arthritis. N Engl J Med. 2016;375(26):2519–2529. doi:10.1056/NEJMoa1611593.

effective dose that allows the patient to build tolerance to the potential adverse effects of the medication while improving symptoms of neuropathy. Because titration to an effective dose occurs over a period of weeks, it is important to review expected onset of action, titration, and expectations for symptom improvement. Duloxetine has been more extensively studied than venlafaxine for use in chronic pain, and thus has more specific dosing guidelines.[54–57] Table 33.3 lists the duloxetine and venlafaxine starting doses and dose ranges for common chronic pain conditions. Venlafaxine is approved for use in only patients aged 18 years and older.[57]

Adverse Effects

Both duloxetine and venlafaxine have a lower anticholinergic adverse-effect profile than TCAs; however, venlafaxine has a higher incidence of GI complaints (nausea/vomiting), sleep impairment, and sexual dysfunction than TCAs.[56,57] Duloxetine and venlafaxine are contraindicated with concurrent or recent (within 2 weeks) therapy with a monoamine oxidase inhibi-

TABLE 33.3 Starting Doses and Dose Ranges of Duloxetine and Venlafaxine for Common Chronic Pain Conditions

Drug	Starting Dose (mg/day)[a]	Maximum Dose (mg/day)
Duloxetine	30 mg[b]	60 mg
Venlafaxine (IR)[c]	25 mg	150 mg typical, 375 mg maximum
Venlafaxine (ER)[d]	37.5 mg	225 mg

(a)Titrate dose every 7 days to maximum dose as tolerated.

(b)Alternative titration: start 20 mg once daily; increase dose by 20 mg every week, up to 60 mg, as tolerated.

(c)Venlafaxine (IR): 25, 37.5, 50, 75 and 100 mg.

(d)Venlafaxine (ER): 37.5, 75, 150, and 225 mg.

ER, extended-release; IR, immediate-release.

Source: Adopted from Dhaliwal JS, Molla M. *Duloxetine.* StatPearls Publishing; 2020. https://www.ncbi.nlm.nih.gov/books/NBK549806; Singh D, Saadabadi A. *Venlafaxine.* StatPearls Publishing; 2020. https://www.ncbi.nlm.nih.gov/books/NBK535363.

BOX 33.2
COMMON AND SERIOUS ADVERSE EFFECTS OF DULOXETINE AND VENLAFAXINE

Duloxetine
Common Adverse Effects

Headache
Drowsiness
Fatigue
Insomnia
Dizziness
Tremor
Abdominal pain
Nausea
Xerostomia
Constipation
Decreased appetite
Diarrhea
Weight loss
Weakness
Diaphoresis
Libido changes
Erectile dysfunction

Serious Adverse Effects

Suicidality
Serotonin syndrome
Hepatotoxicity
Mania
Syncope
Syndrome of inappropriate antidiuretic hormone secretion
Hyponatremia
Acute angle glaucoma

Venlafaxine
Common Adverse Effects

Headache
Abnormal dreams
Blurred vision
Anxiety, tremor
Insomnia
Dizziness
Somnolence
Asthenia Nausea
Anorexia
Xerostomia
Constipation
Diarrhea, abdominal pain
Hypertension
Hypotension
Hypercholesterolemia
Impotence, decreased libido, and/or anorgasmia
Weight loss

Serious Adverse Effects

Suicidality
Serotonin syndrome
Hypomania/mania
Hyponatremia
Serotonin syndrome
Seizures
Acute angle glaucoma

Source: Adapted from Dhaliwal JS, Molla M. Duloxetine. [Updated June 19, 2020]. In: *StatPearls* [Internet]. StatPearls Publishing; 2020. https://www.ncbi.nlm.nih.gov/books/NBK549806; Singh D, Saadabadi A. Venlafaxine. [Updated November 3, 2020]. In: *StatPearls* [Internet]. StatPearls Publishing; 2020. https://www.ncbi.nlm.nih.gov/books/NBK535363

tor (MAOI) and in uncontrolled acute-angle glaucoma. Venlafaxine has an FDA black box warning regarding the risk of increased suicidality, depression exacerbation, hypomania/mania, acute-angle glaucoma, and seizures. Venlafaxine is also associated with abnormal bleeding, altered platelet function, anaphylactoid reactions, and potentially fatal skin conditions such as Stevens–Johnson syndrome, toxic epidermal necrolysis, and erythema multiforme. It can also cause deterioration of glaucoma angle closure and seizures. Both duloxetine and venlafaxine increase the risk of serotonin syndrome due to hyperstimulation of brainstem 5HT-1A receptors. Caution should be used in concomitant administration with other medications that inhibit serotonin reuptake.[56,57] Common and serious side effects of these SNRIs are outlined in **Box 33.2**.

Tricyclic Antidepressants

TCAs such as amitriptyline (the "prototypical" TCA), nortriptyline, and desipramine have been long used to treat chronic and neuropathic pain.[58] These medications are thought to exert analgesic effect by mechanisms similar to SNRIs and SSRIs. TCAs produce spinal and supraspinal analgesia by mechanisms independent of their effect on mood disorders through the inhibition of both norepinephrine and serotonin reuptake and muscarinic anticholinergic effects. The analgesic action of TCAs has not been fully described but is proposed to involve multiple mechanisms. Because TCAs provide more potent analgesia than SSRIs, it is thought that their noradrenergic mechanisms are more responsible for analgesia than the potentiation of serotonergic effects. TCAs also have moderately potent effects on sodium channel blockade and bind to *N*-methyl-ᴅ-aspartate (NMDA) receptors.[59]

Adverse Effects

Despite their well-documented efficacy use in various chronic pain conditions, TCAs are typically not first-line agents due to the adverse-effect profile. The muscarinic and histaminergic (H1) receptor antagonist effects of TCAs are primarily responsible for their common adverse effects (**Box 33.3**). The side effect of sedation may be used to some advantage to treat sleep disturbances that often occur in patients with chronic pain. TCAs are listed in the Beers Criteria as drugs to be used with caution in the geriatric population. TCAs are associated with several serious adverse effects including increased risk of QT prolongation and arrhythmias, ventricular fibrillation, and sudden death. They should be used with caution in patients with preexisting ischemic heart disease, and are *contraindicated* in those with a family history of prolonged QT syndrome or sudden cardiac death. TCAs are associated with increased risk of suicidality in patients aged 24 or younger. If prescribed in this population, close follow-up and assessment for suicidal ideation is essential.

Concomitant use of TCAs with MAOIs and SSRIs is contraindicated due to increased risk of serotonin syndrome. Of the TCAs, nortriptyline and desipramine are the least sedating and tend to have a better side-effect profile. TCAs should be started at low doses to help patients build tolerance to side effects, particularly sedation, with the dose titrated slowly over 6 to 8 weeks if the patient is tolerating the medications and reporting improvement in symptoms. A trial of maximum tolerated dose should be done for at least 2 weeks to see therapeutic benefit. Therapeutic benefit for chronic pain is typically seen at lower doses than those used for treatment of depression. If a patient is tolerating the medication but not seeing full benefit, consider continued dose optimization as benefits may vary based on patient metabolism.[58]

Gabapentinoids

Gabapentin and pregabalin inhibit calcium channels, much like the TCAs action upon sodium channels, to help stabilize nerve conduction and prevent pain signaling along the nerves.[60] These medications are gamma-aminobutyric acid (GABA) analogues and, therefore, reduce neuronal excitability. These medications have long been used for neuropathic pain and are typically well tolerated. The most common patient-reported side effect is sedation, which can be used as a benefit to help with sleep while patients become tolerant to that effect. When initiating the medication, it is important to monitor for sedation, edema, and central nervous system (CNS) disturbances. These drugs do

---

BOX 33.3
COMMON AND SERIOUS ADVERSE EFFECTS OF TRICYCLIC ANTIDEPRESSANTS

Common Adverse Effects

Constipation*
Dizziness*
Xerostomia*
Sedation
Blurred vision
Confusion
Urinary retention
Tachycardia
Orthostatic hypotension
Increased appetite
Weight gain
Transient elevation of liver enzymes

Serious Adverse Effects

Suicidality (more likely patients age 24 and under)
Prolonged QT interval
Cardiac arrhythmias, including ventricular fibrillation
Hepatitis/hepatotoxicity (rare)
Serotonin syndrome
Increased seizure activity in persons with preexisting epilepsy

*Most common side effects

Source: Adapted from Moraczewski J, Aedma KK. Tricyclic antidepressants. [Updated May 30, 2020]. In: *StatPearls* [Internet]. StatPearls Publishing; 2020. https://www.ncbi.nlm.nih.gov/books/NBK557791

---

not undergo hepatic metabolism; they are renally excreted (100%) so dosages should be reduced for renal impairment based on creatinine clearance (CrCl). For patients with history of opioid use disorder or illicit substance use, close monitoring and patient counseling should be provided on the potential for gabapentinoid abuse.[61,62] **Table 33.4** summarizes the classes of medications used for treatment of neuropathic pain.

OPIOID ANALGESIA AND SAFE OPIOID PRESCRIBING

Opioids have been the mainstay for both acute and chronic pain. Because of their inherent risks for dependence, misuse, and risk of serious adverse effects, including respiratory depression, overdose, and death, it is important to identify and assess patient risk before initiating opioid therapy.

TABLE 33.4 Agents Used for Neuropathic Pain

Medication	Approved Indication for Pain	Common Side Effects and Precautions
Tricyclic antidepressants (TCAs): amitriptyline, nortriptyline, desipramine	None	Anticholinergic adverse effects (e.g., blurred vision, confusion, urinary retention, constipation, somnolence); increased suicidality in patients aged 24 and younger; prolonged QT syndrome, cardiac arrhythmias, sudden cardiac death
Serotonin norepinephrine reuptake inhibitors (SNRIs): duloxetine, venlafaxine, milnacipran	Duloxetine: chronic musculoskeletal pain, fibromyalgia, diabetic peripheral neuropathy	Nausea is a common adverse effect; may increase blood pressure, bleeding risk; duloxetine is renally dose adjusted
Gabapentinoids: gabapentin, gabapentin enacarbil, pregabalin	Gabapentin/gabapentin enacarbil: postherpetic neuralgia Pregabalin: postherpetic neuralgia, fibromyalgia, diabetic peripheral neuropathy, neuropathic pain associated with spinal cord injury	Dizziness and drowsiness are common adverse effects; may cause peripheral edema; titrate slowly to an effective dose; dose adjustment in renal impairment; caution re: dependence/abuse potential

Source: Adapted from Gallagher HC, Gallagher RM, Butler M, et al. Venlafaxine for neuropathic pain in adults. *Cochrane Database Syst Rev.* 2015;(8):CD011091. doi:10.1002/14651858.CD011091.pub2; Hempenstall K, Nurmikko TJ, Johnson RW, et al. Analgesic therapy in postherpetic neuralgia: a quantitative systematic review. *PLoS Med.* 2005;2:e164. doi:10.1371/journal.pmed.0020164

Screening for Substance Use Disorder

Screening for substance use disorder can be done by evaluating individuals who are likely to be at increased risk for abuse, addiction, or opioid use disorder.[17] An assessment of multiple factors is required to accurately predict this type of risk. Risk factors include, but are not limited to, psychosocial history, genetics, and socioeconomic factors. Individuals who have a history of multiple occasions with substance use disorder are at increased risk for opioid misuse. Substance use disorders encompass illicit drugs, tobacco, and alcohol. There are many tools for the screening of opioid use disorder; however, there is no consensus as to which screening tool to use.[25,63] The Opioid Risk Tool (ORT) is commonly used for assessing risk for opioid use disorder; it takes approximately 1 minute to complete.[25]

Prescription Drug Monitoring Programs

In addition to clinician screening tools, aberrant controlled substance use may be identified by monitoring the state's Prescription Drug Monitoring Program (see chapter 9). The FDA created the Opioid Analgesic Risk Evaluation and Mitigation Strategy (REMS) program to ensure safe use of all opioids used on an outpatient basis. This program requires manufacturers to provide funding to develop continuing education (CE) courses based on the FDA's suggested guideline. Ongoing CE regarding opioid prescribing is required for physicians nationwide and is recommended for all opioid-prescribing healthcare clinicians.[64–66]

Naloxone Coprescribing

Expert opinion strongly supports the use of alternatives to opioid therapy when factors that increase risk for opioid-related harms are present. Risk factors that can increase risk for opioid-induced respiratory depression and overdose include concomitant therapy with sedating medications (e.g., benzodiazepines or other CNS depressants), increased age or comorbid disease states (e.g., untreated sleep apnea [central or obstructive], chronic obstructive pulmonary disease [COPD], renal impairment, hepatic impairment) and prior history of overdose, history of substance use disorder, and higher opioid dosages (>50 morphine mg equivalent [MME]/day).[26]

The 2016 CDC Guideline for Prescribing Opioids for Chronic Pain[26] includes recommendations for mitigating the risk of opioid therapy and assessing the need for naloxone coprescribing when opioid therapy must be initiated for patients at increased risk for respiratory depression or overdose. Naloxone is an opioid antagonist that can reverse severe respiratory depression. Studies have shown that educating patients' families about naloxone and training them on the appropriate use decreases opioid overdose deaths.[67,68] Resources for prescribing and naloxone in outpatient settings, including patient education materials, can be found on the Prescribe to Prevent website: https://prescribetoprevent.org.

OPIOID AGENTS

It is important to know the difference between opiates and opioids. Opiates include only morphine and codeine, which are found naturally in the opium poppy plant (*Papaver somniferum*).[69] Opioids are any molecule, including synthetic or partly synthetic molecules, that produce morphine like effects. The mechanism of opioid-induced analgesia is primarily through agonism at the mu-opioid receptor. Genetic differences of the opioid receptor mu-1

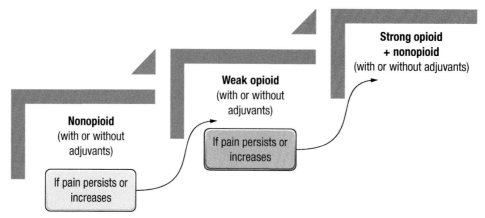

FIGURE 33.4 Analgesic ladder for treating cancer pain.

Source: Adapted with permission from World Health Organization. WHO's cancer pain ladder for adults. n.d. https://www.who.int/cancer/palliative/painladder/en

TABLE 33.5 Chemical Structural Classes of Opioids				
Phenanthrenes	**Diphenylheptanes**	**Phenylpiperidines**	**Benzomorphans**	**Miscellaneous**
Buprenorphine	Methadone	Fentanyl	Pentazocine	Tapentadol
Butorphanol		Meperidine		Tramadol
Codeine				
Morphine				
Hydrocodone				
Hydromorphone				
Levorphanol				
Nalbuphine				
Naloxone				
Naltrexone				
Oxycodone				
Oxymorphone				

Source: Adapted from Rang HP, Dale MM, Ritter JM, et al. Analgesic drugs. In: *Rang and Dale's pharmacology.* 7th ed. Elsevier; 2012:503–524.

(OPRM-1) gene create a variety of mu-receptor subtypes. The effect of these genetic differences results in a variety of responses in individuals, such as quick and slow metabolism. In general, patients who have quick metabolism of opioids, the effect and duration of action may be less. Patients who metabolize opioids slowly have a risk for accumulating the active metabolite, and the effect and duration of action may be greater.

Opioids are an effective treatment option in the management of nociceptive pain. The World Health Organization (WHO) stepladder approach to cancer pain management is appropriate for most nociceptive somatic and visceral pain (**Figure 33.4**).[70] If opioids are being used in opioid-naïve patients, initial doses should be conservative and then titrated based on the patient's response.

Opioid Structural Classes

Opioids are generally categorized by structural class or opioid receptor activity. There are five structural classes of opioids: phenanthrenes, diphenylheptanes, phenylpiperidines, benzomorphans, and miscellaneous (**Table 33.5**). The majority of opioids belong to the phenanthrene class. The ability to differentiate opioids based on structural class is important when selecting an agent for patients with hypersensitivities, or for opioid rotation for patients with opioid intolerances.[71] The most common reaction includes itching or rash due to the histamine release from cutaneous mast cells. True opioid allergies are rare, though cross-sensitivity across structural classes may occur. Because of the potential for a cross reaction when rotating to alternative opioids, the effects of opioids should be monitored closely.

Opioid Receptor Activity

The activity of opioids depends on their affinity for opiate receptors. There are three different subtypes: mu, delta, and kappa. *Mu* receptors are responsible for supraspinal analgesic effects and some of the adverse effects such as respiratory depression, euphoria, sedation, decreased gastrointestinal motility and constipation, and physical dependence. *Kappa* receptors contribute to analgesia at the spinal level and adverse effects including sedation, dysphoria, psychomimetic effects, respiratory depression, and dyspnea. *Delta* receptors found primarily

TABLE 33.6 Analgesic Effects at Opioid Receptors			
	Mu Receptors[a]	Kappa Receptors[b]	Delta Receptors[c]
Agonists			
Morphine	Agonist	Weak agonist	–
Codeine	Weak agonist	–	Weak agonist
Fentanyl	Agonist	–	–
Hydrocodone	Weak agonist	–	Weak agonist
Hydromorphone	Agonist	Weak agonist	Partial agonist
Levorphanol	Agonist	–	–
Meperidine	Agonist	–	Agonist
Methadone[d]	Agonist	–	–
Oxycodone	Agonist	Agonist	Agonist
Oxymorphone	Agonist	–	Possible antagonist
Tramadol[e]	Weak agonist	–	–
Mixed Agonist–Antagonist			
Buprenorphine	Partial agonist	Antagonist	–
Butorphanol	Partial antagonist	Antagonist	–
Nalbuphine	Antagonist or partial agonist	Agonist	–
Pentazocine	Weak antagonist	Agonist	–
Antagonists			
Naloxone	Antagonist	Antagonist	Weak antagonist
Naltrexone	Antagonist	Antagonist	Weak antagonist

[a]Mu 1: analgesia; mu 2: side effects (sedation, euphoria, respiratory depression, vomiting, constipation, urinary retention, physical dependence, pruritis).

[b]Analgesia, sedation, dyspnea, respiratory depression, psychomimetic and dysphoric effects, euphoria.

[c]Analgesia, spinal analgesia.

[d]Methadone also exhibits activity on *N*-methyl-D-aspartate (NMDA) and monoamine receptors.

[e]Tramadol is also a serotonin/norepinephrine reuptake-inhibitor (SNRI) and exhibits activity on numerous pain modulators, including NMDA.

Source: Adapted from Trescott AM, Datta S, Lee M, Hansen H. Opioid pharmacology. *Pain Physician.* 2008;*11*(2 suppl):S133–S153. https://www.painphysicianjournal.com/current/pdf?article=OTg3&journal=42; DrugBank Database. Accessed June 13, 2020. https://www.drugbank.ca.

in the brain and their effects are not well understood. They are responsible for weak analgesia at the spinal level, with effects of dysphoric and psychomimetic side effects.[72] Opioids are classified based upon their different types of receptor effects as agonists, partial agonist, mixed agonist-antagonist, and antagonist (**Table 33.6**).

Partial agonists and antagonists compete with agonists for opiate receptor sites.[72] Molecules that exhibit mixed agonist–antagonist activity may result in analgesia with less adverse effects. Efficacy and side-effect profile may also vary among agents because of receptor subtype differences.[73] Opioid choice should be based on pharmacokinetics, pharmacodynamics, adverse effects, possible drug interactions, patient's age, and patient's medical history (e.g., renal or hepatic impairment).

Adverse effects such as hallucinations, mood changes, sedation, nausea, vomiting, decreased GI motility, constipation, respiratory depression, dependence, and tolerance can be seen with all agents. Neurotoxicity can be observed in all opioids; however, it is more prevalent with morphine due to its active metabolites. Factors that may precipitate respiratory depression, sedation, and neurotoxicity include dehydration, renal impairment, hepatic impairment, advanced age, and drug–drug interactions. Tolerance to side effects generally develops over time, except for constipation.[72] Chronic opioid use can affect the hypothalamic–pituitary–gonadal axis, resulting in hypogonadism, loss of libido, infertility, depression, loss of muscle mass, and osteoporosis in both sexes; erectile dysfunction in men; and menstrual irregularities in women.[74] Opioids can be administered by a variety of methods, including oral, transmucosal, and parenteral (i.e., intravenous, intramuscular, or subcutaneous). The oral route is preferred for administration, if possible. Alternative routes of therapy may be necessary during episodes of acute severe pain or when the patient is unable to take oral medications. Alternative routes of administration include sublingual, transdermal, rectal, epidural, or intrathecal.

Opioid Agonists

Morphine

Morphine is generally considered the first-line opioid when managing moderate-to-severe pain.[72] Morphine has a wide variation of dosage forms (e.g., tablets, oral solution, intravenous, and suppositories) and routes of administration (e.g., oral, sublingual, rectal, intravenous, subcutaneous, and intramuscular), while also being cost effective. All opioids have variable bioavailability and are metabolized in the liver. Major metabolites of morphine include morphine-3-glucuronide (M3G) and morphine 6-glucuronide (M6G). Because morphine and its metabolites are renally cleared, these metabolites can accumulate leading to adverse effects such as neurotoxicity.[75] Opioid-induced neurotoxicity is dependent on both the dose and the duration of opioid therapy. It is essential to monitor for signs and symptoms of neurotoxicity when doses of opioids are rapidly escalated. These symptoms include hyperalgesia, allodynia, myoclonus, delirium, and seizures.

Hydromorphone

Hydromorphone has pharmacokinetic and pharmacodynamic properties similar to morphine, but it is five to seven times more potent and has a shorter duration of action. Hydromorphone can also be administered through the same routes of administration as morphine.[76] The active metabolite of hydromorphone is hydromorphone-3-glucuronide (H3G), which can accumulate in patients with renal impairment. Neuro-excitatory activity of H3G was observed in animal models (e.g., rats) however, it is not proven to exhibit neuroexcitation in humans.[77] Therefore, hydromorphone may be preferred over morphine in patients with renal impairment.[76]

Fentanyl

Fentanyl also has multiple dosage forms and routes of administration which include sublingual, transdermal, intravenous, and epidural.[76] For acute severe pain, intravenous (IV) fentanyl has a very short onset of action, as well as duration of action, and may be considered in patients who are morphine intolerant. Fentanyl is also considered safer to use in patients with renal impairment. Fentanyl patches can be considered for chronic pain management in patients who are not able to tolerate extended-release medications through the oral route. They should *never* be used in opioid-naïve patients or treating acute pain. The onset of action of transdermal fentanyl patches is approximately 12 to 18 hours after patch application, with a duration of action of approximately 72 hours. Transdermal fentanyl reaches its peak effect in approximately 36 hours after the patch is applied. Therefore, dose titration is difficult and must be approached carefully.

Meperidine

Meperidine was commonly used for pain management before safer alternatives were available. It has a shorter duration of action compared to morphine but has a similar pharmacokinetic profile.[76] Meperidine's active metabolite is normeperidine, which can accumulate in patients with renal impairment, increasing the risk for neurotoxicity, CNS hyperirritability, and seizures. Because of this risk, meperidine is no longer routinely used for acute or chronic pain management.

Oxycodone and Hydrocodone

Oxycodone and hydrocodone are potent oral opioid analgesics with similar analgesic and side-effect profiles, except for higher incidence of constipation among hydrocodone users. Both are available in immediate-release (IR) form in various dose combinations with either acetaminophen or ibuprofen.[76] The IR formulations of oxycodone and hydrocodone may be used for severe, acute pain and are preferred for patients with documented to morphine. In patients with renal impairment, combination formulation with acetaminophen is preferred over ibuprofen. Extended-release oxycodone and hydrocodone are reserved for chronic pain management.

Methadone

Methadone is a long-acting opioid commonly used for maintenance programs for patients who suffer from opioid use disorder. However, methadone also has benefits when used for pain management. Methadone exhibits agonist activity on the mu and delta receptors, as well as antagonist activity on NMDA receptors and inhibits reuptake of monoamines.[76] These properties may explain why methadone may be helpful for the management of neuropathic and nociceptive pain.

Methadone pharmacokinetics differ from morphine. It has a variable half-life (19–72 hours), higher bioavailability, and is metabolized primarily metabolized by the cytochrome P450 system in the liver.[78] Methadone is considered to be safe to use in patients with renal impairment, though urine pH does impact half-life.[79] Because of its variable half-life, it is difficult to titrate methadone to an effective dose. For this reason, as well as the risk of QT prolongation associated with methadone use, methadone should not be the first choice for a long-acting opioid. Additionally, clinicians who prescribe methadone must be familiar with its specific risk profile, provide informed consent, and closely monitor patients, including an electrocardiogram (EKG) before initiating therapy.[80]

Opioid Antagonists

Opioid antagonists such as naloxone and naltrexone compete with other molecules to bind to opioid receptors. Naloxone is commonly used to reverse the action of opioid agonists because it has a stronger affinity to the opioid receptors.[81] Before administering naloxone, a thorough assessment should be completed to rule out other causes of sedation or respiratory depression.

Possible adverse effects of naloxone include withdrawal, pain, acute respiratory distress syndrome, and pulmonary edema. Naloxone has minimal bioavailability when taken by the oral route.[76] Consequently, combination products that contain buprenorphine and naloxone are used to prevent misuse and abuse. By ingesting the combination product, naloxone has essentially no effect. However, if it is administered directly to the bloodstream, naloxone will bind to the opioid receptors which decreases buprenorphine effectiveness. Naltrexone is indicated for alcohol abuse. Low-dose naltrexone has limited evidence to support its use for pain management.[82] Although the mechanism is not clear, it is believed to have anti-inflammatory properties.

Atypical Opioids

Tapentadol is an opioid agonist with norepinephrine reuptake inhibition.[76] Tramadol is a weak opioid agonist with weak serotonin/norepinephrine reuptake inhibition. These additive effects are the proposed mechanisms for their effectiveness for neuropathic pain. Both tapentadol and tramadol lower seizure threshold and should be used cautiously in patients with increased risk for seizures.

Mixed Opioid Agonist–Antagonist

Buprenorphine is gaining popularity in chronic pain management due to its proposed agonist–antagonist opioid receptor activity and selectivity.[83] Buprenorphine is FDA indicated to treat pain and comes in six formulations: sublingual tablet, buccal film, transdermal patch, subcutaneous implant, and intravenous and intramuscular injection. It is important to note that buprenorphine is also available in a combination form (buprenorphine + naloxone) as both oral tablets and sublingual film,[76] which is used to treat opiate use disorder. The indications and prescribing requirements for buprenorphine for pain management versus buprenorphine (with or without naloxone) for opiate use disorder are outlined in **Table 33.7**.

Buprenorphine exhibits its analgesic effect through action on a multiple opioid receptors. It exerts partial agonist activity and high affinity for the mu-opioid receptor providing the analgesic effect. Buprenorphine is an agonist at the delta-receptor, providing analgesia and anxiolytic effects, and it is an antagonist at the kappa-receptor, limiting dysphoric effects. This combination results in pain relief and some anxiolytic effects while minimizing euphoria and therefore abuse potential compared to traditional opioids. This unique receptor selectivity is what has recently propelled buprenorphine into favor for the chronic management of pain. Additionally, buprenorphine has a slow dissociation rate from the mu-opioid receptors, improving pain relief and reducing withdraw effects if the medication is abruptly discontinued.[82]

Side effects to buprenorphine are similar to those of traditional opioids, including but not limited to respiratory depression, sedation, administration site reactions, headache, and GI upset.[82] The combined antagonist–agonist mechanism of buprenorphine results in a ceiling effect on the side effect of respiratory depression as compared to traditional opiates. As buprenorphine has a long half-life (approximately 11–37 hours) based on formulation. Extensive counseling should be provided to patients on expectations of pain relief and onset of action.

TABLE 33.7 Indications and Prescription of Buprenorphine for Pain Management Versus Opiate-Use Disorder

	Buprenorphine for Pain Management	Buprenorphine for Treatment of Opioid-Use Disorder
Authorized prescribers	MDs; NCs; PAs	MDs; NCs; PAs
DEA registration	Required (schedule II)	Required (schedule X)
Continuing education requirement	Varies by state and licensing board	MDs: subspecialty in addiction psychiatry/medicine or an 8-hour course in addiction medicine to qualify for waiver NCs and PAs: 24-hour course in addiction medicine to be eligible for waiver
Additional regulatory limits	None beyond state licensing and DEA registration	All: Maximum number of patients limited to 30 in first year after waiver approved; after first year, may apply for waiver to treat up to 275 patients concurrently NPs and PAs: states may apply lower patient limits (not <30) and additional practice setting, education, or reporting requirements

DEA, Drug Enforcement Agency; NC, nurse clinician; PA, physician assistant.

Source: Adapted from National Alliance of Advocates for Buprenorphine Treatment. 30–100 patient limit. Accessed June 13, 2020. http://www.naabt.org/30 _patient_limit.cfm; American Society of Addiction Medicine Staff. The Comprehensive Addiction Recovery Act—highlights for members. Published July 19, 2016. Accessed June 13, 2020. https://www.asam.org/Quality-Science/publications/magazine/read/article/2016/07/19/the-comprehensive-addiction-and-recovery -act---highlights-for-members.

Additionally, dose titrations should not occur sooner than every 3 to 4 days to prevent dose accumulation.

CONCLUSION

The approach to pain management begins with a determination of the underlying cause and categorization of pain as acute or chronic in nature. Understanding if the pain is the result of nociceptive, neuropathic, or mixed mechanisms will aid in choosing appropriate analgesic agents. While acute pain management is relatively straightforward and the need for analgesia is self-limiting, chronic pain management is complex and often requires an interprofessional approach including both pharmacologic and nonpharmacologic strategies.

CASE EXEMPLAR: Patient With Chronic Pain

MJ is a 31-year-old IT technician experiencing chronic L3–L5 low-back pain. He underwent a L4 microdiscectomy 10 months ago. According to MJ, the procedure has helped with his back pain only about "30%." He continues to have baseline 2 to 3/10 daily constant pain with exacerbations to 7 to 8/10. Initially these were limited to one to two times per month. Over the past 4 months these episodes have increased to three to four times per week. As a result, MJ has had to miss work three to four times per month. He expresses concern that he might "get fired." Due to his ongoing pain, which is causing functional impact and his concern with losing his job, MJ is requesting to start chronic opioid therapy.

Past Medical History
- L4 microdiscectomy 10 months prior
- Completed formal physical therapy sessions
- Participating in a home exercise program
- Cognitive behavioral therapy

Medications
- Acetaminophen, 1,000 mg q6–8h prn
- Hydrocodone and acetaminophen, 10/325 mg two tablets q4h for past 7 days

Discussion Questions

1. What are the key elements to consider before starting MJ on chronic opioid treatment?
2. What are the essential steps to complete prior to initiating chronic opioid therapy?
3. How much morphine extended-released (ER) should be prescribed to replace the dosing regimen of hydrocodone/acetaminophen that he is taking?

CASE EXEMPLAR: Patient With Shingles

LS is a 72-year-old woman who presents with pain on the skin of her upper back. She says this is in the location of her recent shingles episode that resolved about 3 to 4 months ago. Since then she has had persistent burning pain day and night that does not go away. She has found it difficult to sleep or be sociable with her friends and relatives. She has started to lose weight because the pain has interfered with her appetite. She has tried some creams and over-the-counter acetaminophen with no relief.

Past Medical History
- Osteoarthritis of the knees
- Systolic hypertension
- Glaucoma

Medications
- Acetaminophen, 500 mg one to two times daily
- Hydrochlorothiazide, 25 mg daily
- Latanoprost, 0.005% solution (1.5 mcg) in the affected eye(s) once daily in the evening

Physical Examination
- Height: 54 inches; weight: 122 lbs.; blood pressure: 152/78; pulse: 72; respiration rate: 16; temperature: 97.0 °F
- Well-developed, well-nourished female in no distress
- Lungs: clear
- Heart: regular rate and rhythm
- Skin: right posterior thorax with confluent scarring and hyperpigmentation in the T6 dermatomal distribution
- Psychiatric: flat affect, Beck depression index score 25 (moderate depression)

Discussion Questions

1. How would LS's pain syndrome be classified?
2. What medications might be effective in LS's treatment?
3. What special considerations are necessary in the selection of treatment for LS?

KEY TAKEAWAYS

- For many patients, an approach using combinations of drugs that target different mechanistic pathways may result in improved analgesia and fewer side effects because lower doses of each drug can be used.
- The duration of chronic pain is typically more than 3 months, is often multifactorial, and can be either nociceptive or neuropathic.
- Unlike nociceptive or neuropathic pain, nociplastic pain arises from altered nociception despite no clear evidence of actual or threatened tissue damage causing the activation of peripheral nociceptors or evidence for disease or lesion of the somatosensory system causing the pain.
- Key concepts in pain management include identification of the underlying cause and determination of whether a patient is opioid-naïve versus opioid-tolerant.
- Interdisciplinary pain management programs have been shown to improve outcomes and be cost effective for chronic pain, incorporating a patient-centered approach that includes pharmacologic and nonpharmacologic interventions, such as cognitive-behavioral therapy, physiotherapy, peripheral nerve stimulation, and acupuncture.
- Risk factors for opioid abuse include psychosocial history, genetics, socioeconomic factors, and a history of multiple occasions with substance use disorder (illicit drugs, tobacco, and alcohol).

REFERENCES

1. International Association for the Study of Pain. IASP terminology. Revised December 14, 2017. https://www.iasp-pain.org/Education/Content.aspx?ItemNumber=1698
2. Rosenquist RW, Vrooman BM. Chronic pain management. In: Butterworth IV JF, Mackey DC, Wasnick JD, eds. *Morgan & Mikhail's clinical anesthesiology.* 5th ed. The McGraw-Hill Companies; 2013:Chapter 47.
3. Elbinoune I, Amine B, Shyen S, et al. Chronic neck pain and anxiety-depression: Prevalence and associated risk factors. *Pan Afr Med J.* 2016;24:89. doi:10.11604/pamj.2016.24.89.8831.
4. Liu F, Fang T, Zhou F, et al. Association of Depression/Anxiety symptoms with neck pain: A systematic review and meta-analysis of literature in China. *Pain Res Manag.* 2018;2018:3259431. doi:10.1155/2018/3259431
5. Mackey S. The "continuum of pain" and the American Academy of Pain Medicine. *Pain Med.* 2015;16(3):413–415. doi:10.1111/pme.12695
6. Institute of Medicine. *Relieving pain in America: A blueprint for transforming prevention, care, education and research.* National Academies Press; 2011. doi:10.17226/13172
7. National pain strategy: A comprehensive population health-level strategy for pain. Interagency Pain Research Coordinating Committee. Accessed May 31, 2020. https://www.iprcc.nih.gov/sites/default/files/HHSNational_Pain_Strategy_508C.pdf
8. Treede RD, Rief W, Barke A, et al. Chronic pain as a symptom or a disease: The IASP Classification of Chronic Pain for the International Classification of Diseases (ICD-11). *Pain.* 2019;160(1):19–27. doi:10.1097/j.pain.0000000000001384
9. Dahlhamer J, Lucas J, Zelaya C, et al. Prevalence of chronic pain and high-impact chronic pain among adults—United States, 2016. *MMWR Morb Mortal Wkly Rep.* 2018;67:1001–1006. doi:10.15585/mmwr.mm6736a2
10. Treede RD. The International Association for the Study of Pain definition of pain: As valid in 2018 as in 1979, but in need of regularly updated footnotes. *Pain Rep.* 2018;3(2):e643. doi:10.1097/PR9.0000000000000643
11. Von Korff M, Scher AI, Helmick C, et al. United States national pain strategy for population research: concepts, definitions, and pilot data. *J Pain.* 2016;17(10):1068–1080. doi:10.1016/j.jpain.2016.06.009.
12. McCarberg B, Peppin J. Pain pathways and nervous system plasticity: Learning and memory in pain. *Pain Med.* 2019;20(12):2421–2437. doi:10.1093/pm/pnz017
13. Orhurhu VJ, Roberts JS, Cohen SP. *Ketamine in acute and chronic pain management.* StatPearls Publishing; 2020. https://www.ncbi.nlm.nih.gov/books/NBK539824
14. Murnion BP. Neuropathic pain: Current definition and review of drug treatment. *Aust Prescr.* 2018;41(3):60–63. doi:10.18773/austprescr.2018.022
15. Ringkamp M, Dougherty PM, Raja SN. Anatomy and physiology of the pain signaling process. In: Benzon HT, Raja SN, Liu SS, et al., eds. *Essentials of pain medicine.* 4th ed. Elsevier; 2018:3–10 https://www.clinicalkey.com/#!/browse/book/3-s2.0-C20140038373.
16. Yam MF, Loh YC, Tan CS, et al. General pathways of pain sensation and the major neurotransmitters involved in pain regulation. *Int J Mol Sci.* 2018;19(8):2164. doi:10.3390/ijms19082164
17. Herndon CM, Ray JB, Kominek CM. Pain management. In: DiPiro JT, Yee GC, Posey L, et al., eds. *Pharmacotherapy: A pathophysiologic approach.* 11th ed. McGraw-Hill; 2019:959–988.
18. Woolf CJ. Central sensitization: implications for the diagnosis and treatment of pain. *Pain.* 2011;152(3 suppl):S2–S15. doi:10.1016/j.pain.2010.09.030.
19. Breivik H, Borchgrevink PC, Allen SM, et al. Assessment of pain. *Br J Anaesth.* 2008;101(1):17–24. doi:10.1093/bja/aen103
20. Main CJ. Pain assessment in context: a state of the science review of the McGill pain questionnaire 40 years on. *Pain.* 2016;157(7):1387–1399. doi:10.1097/j.pain.0000000000000457
21. Lazaridou A, Elbaridi N, Edwards RR, Berde CB Pain assessment. In: Benzon HT, Raja SN, Liu SS, et al., eds. *Essentials of pain medicine.* 4th ed. Elsevier; 2018:39–46
22. Garra G, Singer AJ, Taira BR, et al. Validation of the Wong-Baker FACES Pain Rating Scale in pediatric emergency

department patients. *Acad Emerg Med.* 2010;17(1):50–54. doi:10.1111/j.1553-2712.2009.00620.x.

23. Attal N, Bouhassira D, Baron R. Diagnosis and assessment of neuropathic pain through questionnaires. *Lancet Neurol.* 2018;17(5):456–466. doi:10.1016/S1474 -4422(18)30071-1

24. Morgan KJ, Anghelescu DL. A review of adult and pediatric neuropathic pain assessment tools. *Clin J Pain.* 2017;33(9):844–852. doi:10.1097/AJP.0000000000000476

25. Assessment tools. Washington State Agency Medical Directors' Group website. Accessed April 10, 2020. http:// www.agencymeddirectors.wa.gov/AssessmentTools.asp

26. Dowell D, Haegerich TM, Chou R. CDC guideline for prescribing opioids for chronic pain—United States, 2016. *MMWR Recomm Rep.* 2016;65(1):1–49. doi:10.15585/ mmwr.rr6501e1.

27. Krebs EE, Lorenz KA, Bair MJ, et al. Development and initial validation of the PEG, a three-item scale assessing pain intensity and interference. *J Gen Intern Med.* 2009;24(6):733–738. doi:10.1007/s11606-009-0981-1

28. Turk DC, Fillingim RB, Ohrbach R, et al. Assessment of psychosocial and functional impact of chronic pain. *J Pain.* 2016;17(suppl 9):T21–T49. doi:10.1016/j.jpain.2016.02.006.

29. Food and Drug Administration. Extended-release (ER) and long-acting (LA) opioid analgesics Risk Evaluation and Mitigation Strategy (REMS). Updated June 2015. https:// www .fda.gov/downloads/drugs/drugsafety/postmarketdrug safetyinformationforpatientsandproviders/ucm311290.pdf.

30. Blondell RD, Azadfard M, Wisniewski AM. Pharmacologic therapy for acute pain. *Am Fam Physician.* 2013;87(1):766–772. https://www.aafp.org/afp/2013/0601/ p766.html

31. Ho KY, Gwee KA, Cheng YK, et al. Nonsteroidal anti-inflammatory drugs in chronic pain: implications of new data for clinical practice. *J Pain Res.* 2018;11:1937–1948. doi:10.2147/JPR.S168188

32. Danilov A, Danilov A, Barulin A, et al. Interdisciplinary approach to chronic pain management. *Postgrad Med.* 2020;1–5. doi:10.1080/00325481.2020.1757305

33. Candido KD, Perozo OJ, Knezevic NN. Pharmacology of acetaminophen, nonsteroidal antiinflammatory drugs, and steroid medications:Implications for anesthesia or unique associated risks. *Anesthesiol Clin.* 2017;35(2):e145–e162. doi:10.1016/j.anclin.2017.01.020

34. Mundkur ML, Franklin JM, Abdia Y, et al. Days' supply of initial opioid analgesic prescriptions and additional fills for acute pain conditions treated in the primary care setting—United States, 2014. *MMWR Morb Mortal Wkly Rep.* 2019;68(6):140–143. doi:10.15585/mmwr.mm6806a3.

35. Sturgeon JA. Psychological therapies for the management of chronic pain. *Psychol Res Behav Manag.* 2014;7:115–124. doi:10.2147/PRBM.S44762.

36. Centers for Disease Control and Prevention. Nonopioid treatments for chronic pain. Published April 27, 1016. https://www.cdc.gov/drugoverdose/pdf/nonopioid_treatments-a.pdf

37. Cohen SP, Mao J. Neuropathic pain: Mechanisms and their clinical implications. *BMJ.* 2014;348:f7656. doi:10.1136/bmj.f7656. Erratum in: *BMJ.* 2014;348:g2323.

38. Finnerup NB, Attal N, Haroutounian S, et al. Pharmacotherapy for neuropathic pain in adults: a systematic review and meta-analysis. *Lancet Neurol.* 2015;14(2):162–173. doi:10.1016/S1474-4422(14)70251-0

39. Zeidan F, Vago DR. Mindfulness meditation-based pain relief: a mechanistic account. *Ann N Y Acad Sci.* 2016;1373(1):114–127. doi:10.1111/nyas.13153

40. Kovačević I, Kogler VM, Turković TM, et al. Self-care of chronic musculoskeletal pain—experiences and attitudes of patients and health care providers. *BMC Musculoskelet Disord.* 2018;19(1):76. doi:10.1186/s12891-018-1997-7

41. Gerriets V, Anderson J, Nappe TM. Acetaminophen. [Updated August 11, 2020]. In: StatsPears [Internet].StatPearls Publishing; 2020. https://www.ncbi.nlm.nih.gov/ books/NBK482369

42. Fresenius Kabi USA. Prescribing information for acetaminophen injection. Updated October 2015. https://www.accessdata.fda.gov/drugsatfda_docs/label/2015/204767s000lbl.pdf

43. What dose of paracetamol for older people? *Drug Ther Bull.* 2018;56(6):69–72. doi:10.1136/dtb.2018.6.0636

44. Bacle A, Pronier C, Gilardi H, et al. Hepatotoxicity risk factors and acetaminophen dose adjustment, do prescribers give this issue adequate consideration? A French university hospital study. *Eur J Clin Pharmacol.* 2019;75(8):1143–1151. doi:10.1007/s00228-019-02674-5

45. Athersuch TJ, Antoine DJ, Boobis AR, et al. Paracetamol metabolism, hepatotoxicity, biomarkers and therapeutic interventions: A perspective. *Toxicol Res.* 2018;7(3):347–357. doi:10.1039/C7TX00340D.

46. Scarpignato C, Lanas A, Blandizzi C, et al. Safe prescribing of non-steroidal anti-inflammatory drugs in patients with osteoarthritis: An expert consensus addressing benefits as well as gastrointestinal and cardiovascular risks. *BMC Med.* 2015;*13*:55. doi:10.1186/s12916-015 -0285-8.

47. Reed GW, Nissen SE. NSAID choice: lessons from PRECISION. *Aging.* 2019;11(8):2181–2182. doi:10.18632/ aging.101930

48. Nissen SE, Yeomans ND, Solomon DH, et al. Cardiovascular safety of celecoxib, naproxen, or ibuprofen for arthritis. *N Engl J Med.*2016;*375*(26):2519–2529. doi:10.1056/ NEJMoa1611593

49. Chan FK, Ching JY, Tse YK, et al. Gastrointestinal safety of celecoxib versus naproxen in patients with cardiothrombotic disease and arthritis after upper gastrointestinal bleeding (CONCERN): an industry-independent, double-blind, double-dummy, randomised trial. *Lancet.* 2017;389(10087):2375–2382. doi:10.1016/S0140 -6736(17)30981-9

50. Combe B, Swergold G, McLay J, et al. Cardiovascular safety and gastrointestinal tolerability of etoricoxib *vs* diclofenac in a randomized controlled clinical trial (the MEDAL study). *Rheumatology (Oxford).* 2009;48(4): 425–432. doi:10.1093/rheumatology/kep005.

51. Harris R. Physiologic and pathophysiologic roles of cyclooxygenase-2 in the kidney. *Trans Am Clin Climatol Assoc.* 2013;124:139–151. https://www.ncbi.nlm.nih.gov/ pmc/articles/PMC3715909

52. Curiel RV, Katz JD. Mitigating the cardiovascular and renal effects of NSAIDs. *Pain Med.* 2013;14:S23–S28. doi:10.1111/pme.12275

53. Stanos SP. Osteoarthritis guidelines: a progressive role for topical nonsteroidal anti-inflammatory drugs. *J Multidisc Health Care*. 2013;6:133–137. doi:10.2147/JMDH.S35229.

54. Gallagher HC, Gallagher RM, Butler M, et al. Venlafaxine for neuropathic pain in adults. *Cochrane Database Syst Rev*. 2015;(8):CD011091. doi:10.1002/14651858.CD011091.pub2

55. Hempenstall K, Nurmikko TJ, Johnson RW, et al. Analgesic therapy in postherpetic neuralgia: A quantitative systematic review. *PLoS Med*. 2005;2:e164. doi:10.1371/journal.pmed.0020164

56. Dhaliwal JS, Sperling BC, Molla M. Duloxetine. [Updated June 19, 2020]. In: *StatPearls* [Internet]. StatPearls Publishing; 2020. https://www.ncbi.nlm.nih.gov/books/NBK549806

57. Singh D, Saadabadi A. *Venlafaxine*. [Updated November 3, 2020]. In: *StatPearls* [Internet]. StatPearls Publishing; 2020. https://www.ncbi.nlm.nih.gov/books/NBK535363

58. Moraczewski J, Aedma KK. Tricyclic antidepressants. [Updated May 30, 2020]. In: *StatPearls* [Internet]. StatPearls Publishing; 2020. https://www.ncbi.nlm.nih.gov/books/NBK557791

59. Belinskaia DA, Belinskaia MA, Barygin OI, et al. Psychotropic drugs for the management of chronic pain and itch. *Pharmaceuticals*. 2019;12(2):99. doi:10.3390/ph12020099

60. Patel R, Dickenson AH. (2016). Mechanisms of the gabapentinoids and α 2 δ-1 calcium channel subunit in neuropathic pain. *Pharmacol Res Perspect*. 2016;4(2):e00205. doi:10.1002/prp2.205

61. Evoy KE, Morrison MD, Saklad SR. Abuse and misuse of pregabalin and cabapentin. *Drugs*. 2017;77(4):403–426. doi:10.1007/s40265-017-0700-x

62. Buscaglia M, Brandes H, Cleary J. Special report: the abuse potential of gabapentin & pregabalin. *Pract Pain Manag*. 2019;19(4):50–53. https://www.practicalpainmanagement.com/treatments/pharmacological/non-opioids/special-report-abuse-potential-gabapentin-pregabalin

63. Kaye AD, Jones MR, Kaye AM, et al. Prescription opioid abuse in chronic pain: an updated review of opioid abuse predictors and strategies to curb opioid abuse: part 2. *Pain Physician*. 2017;20(2s):S111–S133. https://www.painphysicianjournal.com/current/pdf?article=ND-IwNA%3D%3D&journal=103

64. Woolf CJ. What is this thing called pain? *J Clin Invest*. 2010;120(11):3742–3744. doi:10.1172/JCI45178.

65. Federation of State Medical Boards. *Continuing medical education. Board-by-board overview*. Published November 20, 2019. http://www.fsmb.org/siteassets/advocacy/key-issues/continuing-medical-education-by-state.pdf

66. Jones MR, Viswanath O, Peck J, et al. A brief history of the opioid epidemic and strategies for pain medicine. *Pain Ther*. 2018;7(1):13–21. doi:10.1007/s40122-018-0097-6

67. McDonald R, Strang J. Are take-home naloxone programmes effective? Systematic review utilizing application of the Bradford Hill criteria. *Addiction*. 2016;111(7):1177–1187. doi:10.1111/add.13326

68. Adams JM. Increasing naloxone awareness and use: the role of health care practitioners. *JAMA*. 2018;319(20):2073–2074. doi:10.1001/jama.2018.4867

69. Mather LE. Trends in the pharmacology of opioids: implications for the pharmacology of pain. *Eur J Pain*. 2001;5(suppl A):49–57. doi:10.1053/eujp.2001.0280

70. Vargas-Schaffer G. Is the WHO analgesic ladder still valid? Twenty-four years of experience. *Can Fam Physician*. 2010;56(6):514–517. https://www.ncbi.nlm.nih.gov/pmc/articles/PMC2902929

71. Rang HP, Dale MM, Ritter JM, et al. Analgesic drugs. In: *Rang and Dale's pharmacology*. 7th ed. Elsevier; 2012:503–524.

72. Trescott AM, Datta S, Lee M, et al. Opioid pharmacology. *Pain Physician*. 2008;11:S133-53. https://www.painphysicianjournal.com/current/pdf?article=OTg3&journal=42

73. Pathan H, Williams J. Basic opioid pharmacology: an update. *Br J Pain*. 2012;6(1):11–16. doi:10.1177/2049463712438493

74. Colameco S, Coren JS. Opioid-induced endocrinopathy. *J Am Osteop Assoc*. 2009;109:20–25. https://jaoa.org/article.aspx?articleid=2093682

75. Matzo M, Dawson KA. Opioid-induced neurotoxicity. *Am J Nurs*. 2013;113(10):51–56. doi:10.1097/01.NAJ.0000435351.53534.83

76. Lexi-Drugs Online. Lexi-Comp; Accessed May 2019.

77. Wright AWE, Nocente ML, Smith MT. Hydromorphone-3-glucuronide: biochemical synthesis and preliminary pharmacological evaluation. *Life Sci*. 1998;63(5):401–411. doi:10.1016/S0024-3205(98)00288-4

78. Lugo RA, Satterfield KL, Kern SE. Pharmacokinetics of methadone. *J Pain Palliat Care Pharmacother*. 2005;19(4):13–24. doi:10.1080/J354v19n04_05

79. Nilsson M-I, Meresaar U, Änggård E. Clinical pharmacokinetics of methadone. *Acta Anaesthesiol Scand*. 1982;74:66–69.10.1111/j.1399-6576.1982.tb01850.x

80. Chou R, Cruciani RA, Fiellin DA, et al. Methadone safety: a clinical practice guideline from the American Pain Society and College on Problems of Drug Dependence, in collaboration with the Heart Rhythm Society. *J Pain*. 2014;15(4):321–337. doi:10.1016/j.jpain.2014.01.494

81. Schwartz JA, Koenigsberg MD. Naloxone-induced pulmonary edema. *Ann Emerg Med*. 1987;16:1294–1296. doi:10.1016/S0196-0644(87)80244-5

82. Younger J, Parkitny L, McLain D. The use of low-dose naltrexone (LDN) as a novel anti-inflammatory treatment for chronic pain. *Clin Rheumatol*. 2014;33(4):451–459. doi:10.1007/s10067-014-2517-2

83. Ehrlich A, Darcq E. Recommending buprenorphine for pain management. *Pain Manag*. 2019;9(1):13–16. doi:10.2217/pmt-2018-0069

Substance Use Disorder

James Anderson and Kathleen Nowak

- Describe the progression from substance use to substance abuse disorder.
- Outline the use of the *DSM-5* criteria in diagnostic decision-making related to substance use disorders.
- Define the agreement that must be made between the clinician and patient regarding the treatment goals in the pharmacologic management of alcoholism.
- Discuss the behavioral and pharmacologic interventions recommended for tobacco cessation including a review of the use of interventions using the five A's.
- Delineate the various components, including legal aspects, involved in managing the opioid addiction and treatment crisis.

INTRODUCTION

Substance use disorder (SUD) is a broad term that describes a functional and clinical impairment due to dependence on use of a substance, which may be a legal or illicit substance. In the United States, the most common substance use disorders include alcohol, tobacco, cannabis, opioid, stimulant, and hallucinogen use disorder. Over 19 million people in the United States are affected by SUD; the young adult population is disproportionately affected. Among those aged 18 to 25 years, 10% have been diagnosed with alcohol use disorder and 7.3% have SUD due to illicit drug use, compared with 5% and 2%, respectively, in adults aged 26 years and older.[1] Worldwide, tobacco use is responsible for nearly 6 million deaths annually.[2] In the United States, an estimated 37.8 million adults (15.5%) are current tobacco users, with a disproportionate prevalence among minority populations (nearly 32% of all American Indian/Alaskan Natives and 25% of mixed race individuals).[2]

Opioid use disorder (OUD) has become a significant public health concern in recent years and opioids account for more than 60% of all drug overdose deaths. The death rates associated with opioid overdose have increased 200% since 2000.[3] Moreover, the total economic burden related to prescription opioid misuse is estimated at $78.5 billion annually.[4] This includes the cost of healthcare, addiction treatment, lost productivity, and criminal justice involvement. In recognition of the magnitude of the opioid epidemic in the United States, the U.S. Department of Health and Human Services (DHHS) in 2015 developed a targeted initiative aimed at reducing opioid overdose and treating opioid dependence. The DHHS identified three priority areas to address the opioid crisis:

1. Prescriber education and training
2. Increasing community access to naloxone
3. Expanding access to medication-assisted treatment (MAT) for OUD.[5]

BACKGROUND

Substance use disorder is a complex brain disorder and mental illness that presents as a pattern of behavior involving compulsive use of a substance despite harmful physical, social, and/or psychological consequences.[6,7] SUD is generally considered a chronic, relapsing disorder that can be challenging to treat and manage for both the patient and clinician.

As a person progresses from substance use to substance abuse, and further to substance use disorder, there is a significant change in behavioral patterns and neurological imbalances. In particular, there is a recognized shift from impulsivity and positive reinforcement to compulsivity, as well as behavior driven by negative reinforcement. It is unclear what causes some individuals to progress to SUD and some to only use substances occasionally, but once a patient progresses to SUD, an addiction cycle develops. This cycle is comprised of three stages: (a) binge/intoxication, (b) withdrawal/negative affect, and (c) preoccupation/anticipation.[8]

The pathophysiology and neurobiology of SUD is still not completely understood, but chronic substance use is known to lead to long-lasting neuronal changes.[9] Each stage of addiction is associated with specific changes in neurocircuitry. In the binge/intoxication stage, activation of the mesolimbic dopamine system—or the reward system—leads to intoxication and repeated intake of the substance in escalating doses.[10] Many other neurotransmitters have recently been recognized as playing a major role in the drug-use reward system, including opioid peptides, gamma-aminobutyric acid (GABA), endocannabinoids, serotonin, glutamate, and acetylcholine.[8,10] Chronic substance use leads to development of tolerance, or an increased reward threshold.[11] When the substance is no longer available, a dramatic drop in dopamine, serotonin, and dysregulation of other neurotransmitters associated with the reward system results in the dysphoria seen in the withdrawal/negative affect stage.[11] Additional neuroadaptive changes in the brain, in response to repeated activation of the reward system, include dysregulation of the hypothalamus-pituitary-adrenal (HPA) axis and the brain stress system through increasing corticotropin releasing factor (CRF), norepinephrine, and dynorphin.[8,11] In acute withdrawal, this results in activated amygdala CRF and elevated levels of norepinephrine, as well as a reduction in neuropeptide Y levels.[11] This dysregulation of the brain stress and antistress systems is believed to be associated with the negative emotional state seen in withdrawal.[10]

The preoccupation/anticipation stage is proposed to be the crucial element driving relapses and has also been linked to the cravings described by substance users.[10] Activation of the prefrontal cortex during substance use and a glutamate-mediated response in various areas of the brain (e.g., nucleus accumbens, basolateral amygdala, ventral pallidum) is postulated to be associated with cravings, based largely on animal models and human brain imaging studies.[8,10] Human imaging studies have also revealed the likely mechanisms driving relapse: Executive function deficits and decreases in frontal cortex activity that mediates decision-making, inhibitory control, memory, and self-regulation.[10] Indeed, smaller gray matter volume in the frontal and prefrontal cortex was predictive of shorter time to relapse in one human imaging study in alcohol-dependent patients.[12]

DIAGNOSIS OF SUBSTANCE USE DISORDER

In August of 2015, the *American Journal of Psychiatry* published the *DSM-5* Criteria for "Substance Use Disorders: Recommendations and Rationale," which laid out the history of diagnostic criteria for addiction-related maladies. While many content experts have labored to settle on language related to addiction, it is important to note that there is not a diagnosis called "addiction." In an effort to develop consensus, the *DSM-5* Substance-Related Disorders Work Group discussed whether to retain the two main disorders, dependence and abuse—"whether substance use disorder criteria should be added or removed, and whether an appropriate substance use disorder severity indicator could be identified."[13] The new *DSM* version (*DSM-5*) combines the *DSM-IV* categories of substance abuse and substance dependence into a single disorder measured on a continuum from mild to severe. Each specific substance is addressed as a separate use disorder (e.g., alcohol use disorder, opioid use disorder); however, nearly all substances are diagnosed based on the same overarching criteria.[14] The *DSM-5* criteria offer clinicians a straightforward way to make diagnostic decisions related to the wide variety of substance use disorders. See **Box 34.1** for signs and symptoms consistent with substance use disorder.

TREATMENT OF SUBSTANCE USE DISORDER

ALCOHOL USE DISORDER

Prior to initiating pharmacotherapy, the clinician and patient should agree on treatment goals (e.g., reducing alcohol consumption, abstinence). This should also include a discussion about the patient's legal obligations, if any, and the risk of harming themselves and/or others with continued alcohol use.[15] It is also important to assess for other psychiatric conditions and use of other substances, including tobacco.[15] In recent years, the focus of treatment has shifted from achieving complete abstinence to recognizing harm-reduction outcomes, such as reducing heavy drinking days and increasing abstinent days. These consumption measures provided the basis for most of the evidence supporting pharmacotherapy. Very little data exists on health outcomes (e.g., quality of life, accidents or injury, mortality) associated with reduced consumption or complete abstinence. In addition to setting realistic goals, the American Psychiatric Association (APA) recommends the development of a person-centered comprehensive assessment (e.g., mental status examinations, physical examinations, laboratory testing) and treatment, including specific plans for addressing acute intoxication and both nonpharmacologic and pharmacologic interventions.[15]

Signs and Symptoms Consistent With Substance Use Disorder

1. Substance used in larger amounts or over longer periods than intended
2. Unsuccessful efforts to cut down or control substance use, despite the desire to do so
3. Considerable time spent in activities necessary to obtain and use substance or to recover from the effects of substance use
4. Craving or a strong desire to use the substance leading to onset of repeated substance use
5. Tolerance resulting in need for increased amounts of the substance to attain the desired effect, or diminished effect with continued use of the same amount of the substance
6. Withdrawal symptoms experienced, or the substance used to relieve or avoid withdrawal symptoms
7. Recurrent substance use resulting in failure to fulfill major role obligations at work, school, or home
8. Continued substance use despite having persistent or recurrent social or interpersonal problems
9. Social, occupational, or recreational activities discontinued or reduced as a result of substance use
10. Recurrent substance use in hazardous situations or environments
11. Continued use despite knowledge of having a persistent or recurrent physical or psychological problem that is likely to have been caused or exacerbated by the substance

Mild SUD is defined by two or three signs/symptoms of 11 listed.

Moderate SUD is defined by four to five signs/symptoms.

Severe SUD manifests as six or more.

Source: Adapted from American Psychiatric Association. *Diagnostic and Statistical Manual of Mental Disorders*. 5th ed. American Psychiatric Publishing; 2013. https://dsm.psychiatryonline.org/doi/book/10.1176/appi.books.9780890425596

Pharmacotherapy for Alcohol Use Disorder

According to the APA guidelines, pharmacotherapy should be offered to all patients with moderate-to-severe alcohol use disorder (AUD) in addition to nonpharmacologic treatments.[15] To date, three medications are approved by the U.S. Food and Drug Administration (FDA) to treat alcohol dependence: naltrexone, acamprosate, and disulfiram (**Table 34.1**). Many other medications have been investigated, including baclofen, buspirone, multiple antidepressants, topiramate, and gabapentin. Of these, only topiramate and gabapentin are noted as potential treatment options in the APA guidelines.[15] Naltrexone and acamprosate have the most evidence supporting their use and are the only "recommended" pharmacologic agents in the guidelines. Disulfiram, topiramate, and gabapentin are "suggested" as treatment options if the patient has a preference for one of these agents or has failed naltrexone or acamprosate.[15] Deciding on the specific treatment agent to use depends on many factors, including patient preference, treatment goals (e.g., abstinence, reduced consumption), comorbid medical or psychiatric conditions, other substance use, and potential adverse effects.

Acamprosate

Although acamprosate is FDA approved and recommended by APA guidelines, the evidence for its use in treating AUD is mixed. Some trials have demonstrated effectiveness at reducing drinking days, while others have found no significant difference when compared with placebo. The Agency for Healthcare and Research Quality (AHRQ) conducted a systematic review and meta-analysis in 2014 and revealed no significant difference in alcohol consumption outcomes between acamprosate and placebo for three trials completed in the United States. However, there was a 12% reduction in return to any drinking and an 11.2% reduction in number of drinking days compared with placebo among trials in other countries, primarily in Europe.[16] No significant difference was observed in return to heavy drinking or number of heavy drinking days for acamprosate compared with placebo.[16] The duration of treatment varied in the trials, with the majority between 12 and 24 weeks and a few with longer durations of 48 to 52 weeks. The 2018 APA guidelines recommend an individualized treatment plan with regard to treatment duration, taking into account disorder severity, relapse history, patient preference, clinical response, and patient tolerability.[15]

The mechanism of action of acamprosate is still not completely understood. It is thought that it may act by modulating glutamate or GABA, and its effects appear to be specific to alcohol use disorder based on animal studies.[17] It seems to have minimal effect on the CNS outside of the effect on alcohol dependence and exhibits no antidepressant, anticonvulsant, or anxiolytic activity.[17] The recommended dose is 666 mg (two 333 mg tablets) orally three times daily. It is generally recommended to begin treatment after a patient has achieved abstinence from alcohol and to continue treatment even during a relapse.[15,17] Acamprosate does not cause aversion to alcohol or any significant reaction if alcohol is ingested during treatment.

TABLE 34.1 Pharmacotherapy for Alcohol Use Disorder*

Drug	Dose	Mechanism of Action	
Naltrexone	Oral: 25–50 mg daily initially; titrate to 100 mg daily prn Long-acting injectable: 190–380 mg IM every 4 weeks, administered by a clinician	Reduces cravings; opioid receptor antagonist—highest affinity for mu receptors	Must achieve abstinence from alcohol before initiating treatment: 7–10 days for short-acting opioids, up to 2 weeks for long-acting opioids Oral naltrexone must be discontinued 48–72 hours prior to opioid/opiate therapy
Acamprosate	Oral: 666 mg tid	Unclear; modulating glutamate or GABA	Must achieve abstinence from alcohol before initiating treatment Contraindications: Known hypersensitivity or severe renal impairment (CrCl <30mL/min)
Disulfiram	Oral: 500 mg daily × 1 to 2 weeks, then 250 mg daily	Irreversibly inhibits aldehyde dehydrogenase	Contraindications: Use of metronidazole, paraldehyde, alcohol, or any alcohol-containing preparations; myocardial infarction, coronary artery disease, psychoses, hypersensitivity to disulfiram or other thiuram derivatives Adverse reactions: Flushing, tachycardia, nausea, vomiting, headaches, syncope, confusion, and blurred vision; can occur up to 14 days after discontinuing use

CrCl, creatinine clearance; IM, intramuscular; prn, as needed; tid, thrice daily.

*While not currently approved by the U.S. Food and Drug Administration for the treatment of alcohol use disorder, topiramate or gabapentin may be used in patients for which naltrexone or acamprosate has failed.

Acamprosate is contraindicated in patients with any known hypersensitivity to the agent and in patients with severe renal impairment (estimated creatinine clearance [CrCl] < 30 mL/min).[17] In patients with moderate renal impairment (CrCl 30–50 mL/min), a dose reduction is recommended.[17] Patients should also be monitored for and educated about the potential for depression and suicidal ideation, as this was observed in clinical trials, though infrequently (1.4%–2.4% of patients).[17] Other common side effects (>2%) reported in clinical trials included: diarrhea (16%), insomnia (7%), anxiety (6%), asthenia (6%), depression (5%), nausea (4%), pruritis (4%), dizziness (3%), flatulence (3%), anorexia (3%), pain (3%), and accidental injury (3%).[17]

Naltrexone

Studies evaluating the use of naltrexone in the treatment of AUD primarily in the United States have produced mixed results. The 2014 AHRQ meta-analysis found a 4% reduction in return to any drinking for any formulation of naltrexone compared with placebo; however, the injectable formulation did not meet statistical significance on its own.[16] Additionally, there was a 7% reduction in return to heavy drinking, and there was a trend toward greater effect sizes with the 50-mg daily oral dose compared with injectable naltrexone or the 100-mg daily dose.[16] However, there have been no head-to-head trials that compare the oral to the injectable formulation. Patients treated with naltrexone (any formulation) also had 4.6% fewer drinking days and 3.8% fewer heavy drinking days compared to those treated with placebo.[16] The majority of trials have evaluated short durations of treatment (12–17 weeks), with six trials using extended durations of 24

to 52 weeks. Again, the APA guidelines recommend an individualized approach to develop a plan for treatment duration, and do not provide specific guidance.[15]

Naltrexone is an opioid receptor antagonist with the highest affinity for mu opioid receptors. The mechanism in alcohol dependence is not entirely understood; however, based on preclinical data, it is believed to involve the endogenous opioid system.[18,19] Naltrexone is also thought to reduce cravings experienced by alcohol-dependent patients by an unknown mechanism.[20] Multiple dosing strategies for the oral formulation have been studied. The initial recommended dose is 50 mg daily, but this can be titrated to 100 mg daily if needed for efficacy.[15] The recommended dose for the long-acting injectable formulation is 380 mg intramuscularly (IM) every 4 weeks, administered by a clinician (not for patient self-injection).[19] Similarly to acamprosate, it is recommended that naltrexone be initiated when a patient has achieved abstinence from alcohol use; naltrexone is also not an aversive agent and does not cause a significant reaction if alcohol is ingested during treatment.[15,18,19] Patients must be abstinent from opioid use prior to starting naltrexone for at least 7 to 10 days for short-acting opioids and up to 2 weeks for long-acting opioids, such as buprenorphine or methadone.[18,19]

Naltrexone is contraindicated in patients receiving opioid analgesics or with current physiologic opioid dependence, since it can drastically reduce the effectiveness of analgesia due to opioid antagonism and precipitate opioid withdrawal.[18,19] It is also contraindicated in patients who are in acute opioid withdrawal and in patients who have not passed the naloxone challenge test or have a urine drug screen positive for opioids. Other contraindications include patients who have any history of hypersensitivity to naltrexone or to polylactide-co-glycolide or carboxymethylcellulose for the injectable formulation.[18,19] Patients should be educated on the effects of naltrexone on opioid use, the potential for precipitating opioid withdrawal, and the risk for opioid overdose if the patient resumes opioid use after stopping naltrexone due to reduced tolerance.

A naloxone challenge test can be used to determine the risk for precipitating opioid withdrawal in patients previously using opioids. It involves administering a dose of naloxone in a clinical setting and observing the patient for withdrawal symptoms. If no withdrawal symptoms occur, the patient will likely tolerate naltrexone; however, precipitated withdrawal has occurred in some patients despite passing a naloxone challenge test in a few case reports.[18,19] To prevent precipitated opioid withdrawal, it is recommended that patients stop use of opioids.[18,19] If reversal of naltrexone blockade and use of opioids is required for pain management in an emergent situation, it is recommended that the patient be closely monitored by anesthesia personnel since the dose of opioids required will likely be much higher than usual, putting the patient at increased risk for respiratory depression.[18,19] Clinicians should also be aware that naltrexone can cross-react with some immunoassays used for urine drug screens for opioids and may yield a false positive result.[18,19]

Naltrexone has been associated with hepatotoxicity, including acute hepatitis and asymptomatic transaminase elevations in clinical trials and postmarketing studies.[18,19] The APA guidelines recommend obtaining baseline liver chemistries prior to initiating naltrexone and completing further workup as needed.[15] Although there are no dose adjustments required in mild-to-moderate hepatic insufficiency (Child-Pugh Class A or B), it is recommended to avoid naltrexone in severe hepatic impairment (Child-Pugh Class C).[18,19] Increases in naltrexone AUC (area under the curve) of five-fold and ten-fold have been observed in patients with compensated (Child-Pugh Class A) and decompensated cirrhosis (Child-Pugh Class B or C).[18] Consider avoiding naltrexone in patients with any degree of hepatic impairment or closely monitor liver function tests during treatment. No dose adjustment is required when using naltrexone in patients with mild renal impairment (CrCl >50 mL/min); however, its use has not been evaluated in patients with moderate-to-severe renal impairment.[19] Given that naltrexone and its primary metabolite are primarily renally excreted, use caution in patients with moderate-to-severe renal impairment.[19] Caution should also be used when administering injectable naltrexone to patients with thrombocytopenia or coagulopathy, as with any intramuscular injection.[19] Depression and suicidal ideation have also been reported with naltrexone use. It is recommended to educate patients and caregivers to monitor for these symptoms.[18,19]

Common side effects (>2%) reported with naltrexone in clinical trials for use in alcohol use disorder include injection site reactions with the injectable formulation such as site tenderness, pain, induration, and swelling (50%). Other side effects may include headache (7%–18%), fatigue/malaise (4%–12%), insomnia (3%–12%), nausea (10%–11%), pharyngitis (11%), diarrhea (10%), abdominal pain (8%), anxiety (2%–8%), vomiting (3%–6%), arthralgia (5%), back pain (5%), dry mouth (4%), depression (4%), dizziness (4%), rash (4%), and anorexia (3%). In general, adverse effects appear to be more frequent in patients treated with the injectable formulation compared with oral tablets.[18,19]

The AHRQ meta-analysis found no significant difference between acamprosate and naltrexone for return to any drinking, heavy drinking, or number of drinking days.[16] The COMBINE trial, however, indicated that naltrexone may be superior to acamprosate in reducing the time to first heavy drinking and the percentage of abstinent days.[21] Given these mixed results, the APA guidelines recommend either naltrexone or acamprosate as first-line options and recommend using other patient-specific factors to decide between the two medications.[15] Factors to consider include dosing and administration with potential impact on adherence, cost, side effect profiles, patient comorbidities (e.g., renal or hepatic impairment), and the presence of cravings.

Disulfiram

The APA guidelines include disulfiram as a "suggested" treatment option, if the patient's treatment goal is to achieve abstinence and the patient understands the risks associated with alcohol consumption during treatment. Additionally, disulfiram is recommended if the patient was unable to tolerate acamprosate or naltrexone or otherwise did not have a sufficient response to acamprosate or naltrexone.[15] Disulfiram irreversibly inhibits aldehyde dehydrogenase, the enzyme responsible for breaking down acetaldehyde, which is an ethanol metabolite.[22] When a patient consumes alcohol within 12 to 24 hours of taking disulfiram, an accumulation of acetaldehyde occurs and can lead to a significant reaction, including flushing, tachycardia, nausea, vomiting, headaches, syncope, confusion, and blurred vision.[22] Severe reactions can include respiratory depression, arrhythmias, myocardial infarction (MI), acute congestive heart failure (CHF), convulsions, unconsciousness, and death.[22,23] Adverse reactions can occur with very small amounts of alcohol (e.g., cough syrups, mouthwashes, and even cooking) and for up to 14 days after discontinuing disulfiram use.[23] It should be noted that alcohol is present in many oral liquid formulations of commonly prescribed medications, including sertraline and ritonavir, and a review of the patients' current medication list for potential interactions is important prior to starting disulfiram. The fear of developing a disulfiram reaction acts as a deterrent to alcohol use.[15]

Indeed, adherence is very important for the effectiveness of disulfiram, and involving family members or roommates in treatment planning may be beneficial.[15] Disulfiram is not known to affect the neurobiology or influence cravings associated with alcohol dependence.

The AHRQ meta-analysis included four trials, all of which were completed in U.S. Department of Veteran Affairs (VA) medical centers. No significant difference was observed in return to any drinking compared with the placebo; however, there was a significant association between adherence and complete abstinence.[16] Only two trials reported the number of drinking days, one indicating no significant difference, while the other reported fewer drinking days with disulfiram 250 mg daily compared to disulfiram 1-mg dose or riboflavin alone (49% vs. 75.4% vs. 86.5%, respectively).[16,24]

The recommended dose of disulfiram is 500 mg once daily initially for 1 to 2 weeks, followed by maintenance dosing of 250 mg once daily.[22] APA guidelines state that there is no evidence regarding duration of treatment and recommend that duration be individualized based on patient preference, tolerability, severity of disorder and clinical response, and history of relapse.[15] Because of the potential severity of the disulfiram reaction, there is a Black-Boxox Warning stating that disulfiram should never be given to a patient without their full knowledge or when they are in a state of alcohol intoxication; physicians should instruct relatives accordingly.[22,23] It is important to educate the patient on the risks of alcohol consumption while using disulfiram and the various forms in which alcohol may inadvertently be ingested (e.g., cooking sauces, mouthwash, cough syrups). Disulfiram is contraindicated in patients who have recently received metronidazole, paraldehyde, alcohol, or any alcohol-containing preparations, and in patients with severe myocardial disease or coronary occlusion, psychoses, or hypersensitivity to disulfiram or other thiuram derivatives used in pesticides and rubber vulcanization.[22] Psychosis has been reported with concomitant use of metronidazole and isoniazid and may also be the result of unmasking an underlying condition. Consider testing for thiuram hypersensitivity if a patient has a history of rubber contact dermatitis.[22]

Since there is a possibility of accidental alcohol ingestion and disulfiram reaction, it is recommended to use extreme caution in patients who may be vulnerable to the effects of the reaction, including patients with diabetes, epilepsy, cerebral damage, chronic kidney disease or acute kidney injury, and hepatic impairment.[23] Hepatotoxicity, including hepatic failure, transplant, and death, have been reported with disulfiram use and may occur regardless of baseline liver function and even after months of treatment.[22,23] Patients should be educated about signs and symptoms of acute hepatitis and liver function tests monitored at baseline and regularly during treatment. Other adverse effects reported with disulfiram (frequency not defined) include hepati-

tis, optic neuritis, peripheral neuropathy, polyneuritis, rash, drowsiness, fatigue, impotence, headache, metallic or garliclike taste disturbance, and psychosis.[22,23]

Topiramate and Gabapentin
APA guidelines suggest topiramate and gabapentin as alternative treatment options for patients who prefer these agents or were unable to tolerate or did not achieve sufficient response to acamprosate and naltrexone.[15] Neither of these agents are approved by the FDA to treat alcohol use disorder. The APA provides no specific duration of treatment but recommends an individualized treatment plan.[15]

Topiramate has been associated with significant reductions in the number of heavy drinking days and any drinking days in many studies; however, some trials have not found a significant benefit.[15,16] Topiramate has also shown improvement in frequency of cravings and overall quality of life.[15] The doses used in trials ranged from 200 to 300 mg daily; however, gradual titration may result in fewer adverse effects.[15] Dose adjustment is required in renal impairment; reduce dose by 50% if CrCl is <70 mL/min.[25] Topiramate has been associated with serious adverse effects, including acute myopia and secondary angle-closure glaucoma, reduced sweating and hyperthermia, metabolic acidosis, nephrolithiasis, suicidality, cognitive dysfunction (e.g., memory difficulty, confusion, difficulty concentrating), behavioral disturbances, somnolence and fatigue, and hyperammonemia and encephalopathy.[25] Topiramate is also known to be teratogenic and can increase the risk for cleft lip and/or cleft palate.[25] It is recommended to use caution in the older adults as topiramate meets American Geriatrics Society (AGS) BEERS criteria.[26] Common side effects (>2%) reported with topiramate use include: abnormal serum bicarbonate (25%–67%), paresthesia (1%–51%), somnolence (6%–29%), dizziness (4%–25%), loss of appetite (10%–24%), weight loss (4%–21%), fatigue (6%–16%), nervousness (4%–16%), impaired psychomotor performance (2%–13%), fever (1%–12%), memory impairment (3%–12%), confusion (3%–11%), mood disorder (4%–11%), reduced concentration (2%–10%), and impaired cognition (2%–7%).[25]

In a randomized placebo-controlled trial by Mason et al., gabapentin treatment for 12 weeks was associated with significant improvements in rates of abstinence and no heavy drinking.[27] These effects appear to be dose related, with more patients achieving abstinence or no drinking days in the 1,800-mg/day group compared with the 900-mg/day group, divided into three doses with gradual dose titration to minimize adverse effects.[15,27] Benefits were also noted with regard to mood, insomnia, and cravings.[27] Dose adjustment of gabapentin is required in patients with renal impairment.[28] Serious adverse reactions reported with gabapentin include drug reaction with eosinophilia and systemic symptoms (DRESS), anaphylaxis and angioedema, suicidality, new and worsening of existing tumors, and central nervous system (CNS) depression and possible impairment.[28] Gabapentin also meets AGS BEERS criteria and should be used cautiously in older adults.[28] Common side effects reported with gabapentin use include: dizziness (28%), somnolence (21%), fatigue (3%–11%), viral disease (11%), peripheral edema (2%–8%), nystagmus (8%), nausea/vomiting (1%–3%), and ataxia (3%).[28]

Medications to Avoid

APA guidelines recommend against the use of antidepressants to treat AUD unless the patient also has a comorbid depression or anxiety disorder that would indicate use.[15] Antidepressants demonstrate minimal efficacy and have even been shown to worsen outcomes when used in patients without a comorbid psychiatric disorder.[15] Benzodiazepines are also not recommended for treatment of AUD unless the patient has a comorbid disorder for which a benzodiazepine would be indicated.[15] An exception is the treatment of acute alcohol withdrawal, where benzodiazepines are typically used. Chronic benzodiazepine use is not recommended without an identifiable indication, as there is no evidence supporting the use of benzodiazepines (or other sedative hypnotics) for primary treatment of AUD.[15] Additionally, use of benzodiazepines during alcohol intoxication increases the risk for respiratory depression and sedation.

TOBACCO USE DISORDER

The AHRQ 2008 guidelines for treating tobacco use and dependence and the U.S. Preventive Services Task Force (USPSTF) recommendation statement for behavioral and pharmacologic interventions recommend brief interventions at every office visit for known tobacco users.[29,30] These interventions should include the five A's:

- *Ask* about tobacco use.
- *Advise* the patient to quit.
- *Assess* willingness and readiness to quit.
- *Assist* in the quit attempt by providing prescriptions for medication or referring for counseling or other services as needed.
- *Arrange* for follow up to prevent relapse.[29,30]

If a patient is not willing to quit, the guidelines recommend using motivational interviewing strategies and plan to discuss tobacco use at the next visit.[29]

Intensive interventions have been shown to be more effective than the brief interventions described in the previous text.[29,30] If the patient has access to and expresses interest in intensive services, they should be offered to the patient. Intensive interventions generally involve more and more frequent counseling, including practical counseling (skills training, problem-solving) and social support.[29] This counseling is recommended to be used in addition to pharmacotherapy and may be delivered by any number of clinicians (e.g., physicians, nurses, pharmacists, trained tobacco cessation counselors, psychologists). There is also a national network that connects patients to local state tobacco quit-lines, 1-800-QUIT-NOW.[29] State quit-lines offer a variety of services, including individual counseling, information on cessation medications, assistance with cost of medications, and referrals to other resources. Individual, group, and telephonic counseling may be acceptable, should last longer than 10 minutes per session, and include at least four sessions.[29]

Pharmacotherapy for Tobacco Use Disorder

The AHRQ guidelines and USPSTF recommend that all patients attempting to quit smoking should be offered medication to assist the quit attempt, with the exception of those populations for which there is limited evidence (pregnant women, light smokers <10 cigarettes/day, smokeless tobacco users, and adolescents).[29,30] All of the FDA-approved medications used to treat tobacco dependence—nicotine patch, nicotine inhaler, nicotine nasal spray, nicotine gum, nicotine lozenge, bupropion SR, and varenicline—are considered first-line treatment options (**Table 34.2**).[29] There are two options which have been shown to be superior to the nicotine patch alone: varenicline 2 mg/day and the combination of a nicotine patch and nicotine gum, lozenge, inhaler, or nasal spray as needed.[29] Patient-specific factors such as comorbid medical and psychiatric conditions, potential side effects, and cost are likely to drive treatment choices. Other considerations include history of quit attempts and intensity of tobacco dependence. If a patient has had success with a specific medication during a prior quit attempt, then that medication may be considered for the next quit attempt as well. In highly nicotine-dependent patients, nicotine replacement therapy (NRT) has demonstrated efficacy, particularly combination NRT, and may be preferred over bupropion or varenicline.[29] In patients who are concerned about weight gain associated with tobacco cessation, bupropion and NRT may delay, but not prevent, weight gain.[29] Medications can be combined as well, and there is evidence to support combination NRT (nicotine patch + nicotine gum, lozenge, inhaler, or nasal spray) and NRT in combination with bupropion.[29] The combination of NRT with varenicline has been associated with increased rates of side effects and is not generally recommended.[29] The duration of treatment is generally recommended to be 6 to 12 weeks initially; however, longer durations of treatment (up to 6 months) may be beneficial in some patients to achieve long-term abstinence.[29] In fact, many patients continue occasional use of short-acting NRT, such as the lozenge or gum, long term.

Nicotine Replacement Therapy

NRT has been a mainstay of tobacco cessation treatment for many years. NRT is intended to be an

TABLE 34.2 Pharmacotherapy for Tobacco Use Disorder

Treatment	Dose	Side Effects
Nicotine gum	First cigarette within 30 minutes of waking: 4-mg First cigarette after 30 minutes of waking: 2-mg One piece q1–2h × 6 weeks; reduce to q2–4h × 3 weeks, then q4–8h (max: 24 pieces/day)	Common: Mouth soreness, hiccups, dyspepsia, jaw ache
Nicotine lozenges	First cigarette within 30 minutes of waking: 4 mg First cigarette after 30 minutes of waking: 2 mg One lozenge q1–2h × 6 weeks (min: 9 lozenges/d); reduce to q2–4h × 3 weeks, then q4–8h (max: 20 lozenges/day)	Common: Nausea, hiccups, dyspepsia, headache, cough
Nicotine patch	>10 cigarettes/day: 21-mg patch (step 1) × 6 weeks, then 14-mg patch (step 2) × 2 weeks, then 7-mg patch (step 3) × 2 weeks ≤10 cigarettes/day: 14-mg patch (step 2) × 6 weeks, then 7-mg patch (step 3) × 2 weeks	Common: Local skin irritation (50%), insomnia, vivid dreams
Nicotine inhaler	6–16 cartridges/d × 3–6 weeks (max: 16 cartridges/day) Best effect observed with continuous puffing for 20 minutes	Common: Local irritation of mouth or throat, cough, headache, rhinitis, dyspepsia, dysgeusia, hiccups, nausea
Nicotine nasal spray	1–2 doses (1 spray in each nostril)/hour; adjust dose prn (min: 8 doses/day; max: 5 doses/hour, 40 doses/day)	Common: Nasal irritation, nasal congestion, transient changes in sense of smell or taste, dyspepsia, rhinitis, throat irritation, cough
Bupropion SR	Initiate 1–2 weeks prior to quit date 150 mg daily × 3 days; increase to 150 mg bid	Common: Insomnia, rhinitis, dry mouth, dizziness, nausea, decreased concentration, anxiety, constipation, abnormal dreams, arthralgia/myalgia, rash, diarrhea, cough, anorexia, pruritis, taste perversion Serious: Seizures, suicidal ideation, neuropsychiatric effects, hypertension, anaphylaxis, Stevens-Johnson syndrome
Varenicline	Initiate 1 week prior to quit date 0.5 mg daily × days 1–3; 0.5 mg bid days 4–7; 1 mg bid thereafter	Common: Nausea, insomnia, headache, abnormal dreams, flatulence, constipation, dysgeusia, abdominal pain, fatigue, dry mouth, dyspepsia, vomiting, increased appetite. Serious: Neuropsychiatric effects, suicidal ideation, seizures, somnolence/loss of consciousness, cardiovascular adverse effects, angioedema anaphylaxis, Stevens-Johnson syndrome
Nortriptyline	Initiate 10–28 days prior to quit date 25 mg daily; titrate to 75–100 mg/day as tolerated	Common: Sedation, dry mouth, blurred vision, urinary retention, constipation, lightheadedness, tremor Serious: Suicidal ideation, CNS depression, orthostatic hypotension, SIADH, narrow angle glaucoma, serotonin syndrome, bone marrow suppression, bone fractures, arrhythmias
Clonidine	0.1 mg po bid or 0.1 mg/day td; titrate by 0.1 mg/day weekly prn	Common: Dry mouth, drowsiness, dizziness, sedation, constipation Serious: Bradycardia, CNS depression, hypotension

bid, twice daily; CNS, central nervous system; h, hour; max, maximum; min, minimum; prn, as needed; q, every; SIADH, syndrome of inappropriate antidiuretic hormone secretion; SR, sustained-release; td, transdermal.

alternative nicotine source to tobacco, thus reducing the dependence on tobacco products and the severity of withdrawal symptoms. There are five FDA-approved formulations of NRT: transdermal patch, gum, lozenge, nasal spray, and inhaler. Only the nasal spray and inhaler are available by prescription only, the other products are available over the counter (OTC), increasing access to treatment. Use of any NRT has been associated with an increase in the percentage of patients who achieve abstinence at 6 months (17% vs. 10% with placebo).[31] No significant difference has been found when comparing the different types of NRT. Use of combination NRT has been shown to result in a higher likelihood of achieving abstinence compared with use of a single NRT and is recommended as a first-line treatment strategy in the AHRQ guidelines.[29,31]

NRT is contraindicated only in patients with any history of hypersensitivity to nicotine or any component of the formulation.[32] As nicotine can increase blood pressure and heart rate, it should be avoided in patients with a recent MI (within 2 weeks), unstable angina, or serious arrhythmias.[29,32,33] Use caution and weigh the risks and benefits of NRT use versus continued smoking in patients with other cardiovascular disease. It is also recommended to use caution in patients with bronchospastic disease (for the inhaler), active peptic ulcer disease (PUD), hepatic or renal impairment, hyperthyroidism, pheochromocytoma, and insulin-dependent diabetes.[29,32,33] Patients should also be educated that continued smoking during NRT use can result in additive side effects due to higher-than-normal nicotine peak levels.[33] Nicotine nasal spray produces the highest peak levels compared with any of the other formulations and, as such, has a higher risk for dependence development.[33] For dosing and side effects associated with each dosage form, see Table 34.2.

Bupropion

Bupropion SR (sustained release) has been FDA-approved for use in smoking cessation since 1997 and has been shown to nearly double the likelihood of achieving abstinence at 6 months.[29,31] Data on the combination of bupropion with NRT are mixed, but there is evidence to support the combination, showing a modest increase in effect with the combination compared with bupropion alone.[29,31] Given bupropion's dual indication, it may be particularly beneficial in patients with comorbid depression. The mechanism of action in tobacco cessation is not completely understood, but is believed to be related to inhibition of norepinephrine and dopamine reuptake.[34] It is recommended to start bupropion SR 1 to 2 weeks prior to quitting smoking to allow for the drug to reach steady-state blood levels.[29,34] Dose titration is recommended to reduce the incidence of adverse effects; start with 150 mg once daily for 3 days, then increase to 150 mg twice daily, at least 8 hours apart.[29,34] Though no specific dosing is recommended, a dose reduction should be considered in patients with renal impairment and the maximum dose should not exceed 150 mg every other day in patients with moderate-to-severe hepatic impairment.[34] The duration of treatment should be 7 to 12 weeks initially, and some patients may benefit from up to 6 months of treatment.[29] If a patient has not yet quit smoking after 12 weeks of treatment, consider discontinuing bupropion SR.[34]

Bupropion can cause seizures and is contraindicated in patients with seizure disorders, eating disorders (e.g., anorexia and bulimia), and patients undergoing abrupt discontinuation of alcohol or sedative use (e.g., benzodiazepines, barbiturates, and antiepileptics).[34] Bupropion should be used cautiously in any patient who may have an increased risk for seizures, such as patients with severe head injuries, CNS tumors or infection, arteriovenous malformation, severe stroke, and concomitant use with other medications that lower the seizure threshold.[34] Due to the risk for development of suicidal thoughts associated with most antidepressants, there is a Black-Box Warning for risk of suicidality.[34] There is also a risk for developing other neuropsychiatric effects, including depression, agitation, psychosis, hallucinations, paranoia, and delusions.[34] Patients and caregivers should be educated about the risks for neuropsychiatric effects and advised to monitor for side effects. Bu-

propion can result in hypertension, particularly when used in combination with NRT, and should be used cautiously in patients with uncontrolled hypertension.[34] Bupropion is also contraindicated in patients with concomitant use of monoamine oxidase inhibitors (MAOIs) within 14 days and initiation in a patient who is receiving linezolid or methylene blue (both reversible MAOIs) due to increased risk for development of hypertension.[34] Additionally, severe hypersensitivity reactions such as anaphylaxis and Stevens-Johnson syndrome have been reported.[34]

Common (>2%) side effects reported with bupropion SR in clinical trials for tobacco cessation include: insomnia (31%–40%), rhinitis (12%), dry mouth (10%–11%), dizziness (8%–10%), nausea (9%), decreased concentration (9%), anxiety (8%), constipation (8%), abnormal dreams (5%), arthralgia (5%), myalgia (4%), rash (4%), diarrhea (4%), nervousness (4%), cough/pharyngitis (3%), anorexia (3%), pruritis (3%), taste perversion (3%), and abdominal pain (3%).[34]

Varenicline

Varenicline was approved by the FDA in 2006 for treatment of tobacco dependence. It may be the most effective at achieving abstinence at 6 months compared to other tobacco cessation aids based on a USPSTF 2015 evidence review, which showed that varenicline more than doubled abstinence rates at 6 months (28% vs. 12% with placebo).[29,31] Varenicline is a partial agonist at the alpha-4 beta-2 neuronal nicotinic acetylcholine receptors and, due to its high affinity for these receptors, also inhibits binding of exogenous nicotine, which is believed to disrupt the reinforcement and reward system.[35] It is recommended to start varenicline 1 week prior to quitting smoking, but the patient may also choose a quit date any time after day 7 of treatment and continue to work toward reducing tobacco use during varenicline treatment.[29,35] The dose should be titrated gradually to minimize adverse effects: 0.5 mg once daily for 3 days, then 0.5 mg twice daily for 4 days, then 1 mg twice daily.[35] Varenicline should be taken after a meal and with a full glass of water. For patients with severe renal impairment (CrCL <30 mL/min), the maximum dose should not exceed 0.5 mg twice daily.[35] No dose adjustment is necessary in hepatic impairment. If patients have successfully quit smoking during the first 12 weeks of treatment, consider extending treatment for an additional 12 weeks to further improve the chances of long-term abstinence.[35] If a patient experiences adverse effects on varenicline, consider a dose reduction to improve tolerance.

Varenicline is contraindicated in patients with a known hypersensitivity or skin reaction to varenicline.[35] Serious neuropsychiatric adverse events have been reported with varenicline in post-marketing reports. Reactions reported include depression, mania, psychosis, hallucinations, paranoia, delusions, homicidal ideation, aggression, agitation, anxiety, and suicidal ideation and attempts.[35] Patients and caregivers should be educated on the potential for these side effects and report any changes to the prescriber. Seizures have also been reported with varenicline use; use caution in patients with a history of seizures or who have other conditions or medications that may lower the seizure threshold.[35] Varenicline has also been reported to cause somnolence, dizziness, difficulty concentrating, and loss of consciousness.[35] Patients have reported increased intoxicating effects when combined with alcohol use as well as accidental injury and somnambulism (sleep-walking).[35] Patients with underlying cardiovascular disease may be at an increased risk for developing cardiovascular adverse effects, including nonfatal MI and nonfatal stroke.[35] Clinicians should carefully weigh the risks versus benefits of varenicline use versus continued tobacco use and the health benefits associated with tobacco cessation. Hypersensitivity reactions, angioedema, and serious skin reactions have been reported with varenicline use, including Stevens-Johnson syndrome and erythema multiforme.[35]

Common (>2%) side effects reported with varenicline in clinical trials include: nausea (16%–30%), insomnia (18%–19%), headache (15%–19%), abnormal dreams (9%–13%), flatulence (6%–9%), constipation (5%–8%), dysgeusia (5%–8%), abdominal pain (5%–7%), fatigue/malaise (4%–7%), upper respiratory tract disorder (5%–7%), dry mouth (4%–6%), dyspepsia (5%), vomiting (1%–5%), sleep disorder (2%–5%), increased appetite (3%–4%), somnolence (3%), and rash (1%–3%).[35]

Nortriptyline and Clonidine
Nortriptyline and clonidine are both recommended as second-line agents in the AHRQ guidelines; however they are not FDA-approved for tobacco cessation.[29] The USPSTF recommendations statement recommends only FDA-approved pharmacotherapy and does not address the use of either nortriptyline or clonidine.[30] As there is some evidence to support the use of these agents, they may be considered if first-line agents fail (alone or in combination) or if a patient has contraindications to first-line agents; however, prominent side effects may limit use.[29]

Nortriptyline is a tricyclic antidepressant. Its mechanism in treating tobacco dependence is not completely understood, but it is believed to be related to effects on norepinephrine and/or dopamine.[36] Nortriptyline is recommended to be started 10 to 28 days prior to the quit date to allow the drug to reach steady-state levels.[29] Doses should be titrated gradually to minimize adverse effects; initiate at 25 mg daily and titrate to 75 to 100 mg daily as tolerated.[29] The AHRQ guidelines recommend a duration of 12 weeks initially, which may be extended up to 6 months as needed.[29] There are no specific dosing recommendations in renal or hepatic impairment due to lack of data, but as nortriptyline is metabolized hepatically and eliminated renally, caution is advised.[37] Nortriptyline is contraindicated in patients with history

of hypersensitivity, those who are in the acute recovery phase of an MI, concomitant use with an MAOI within 14 days, or initiation in a patient taking linezolid or methylene blue.[37] There is also a Black-Box Warning for suicidal thinking, which can be precipitated with use of antidepressants.[37] Nortriptyline should be used with caution in the following conditions: decreased gastrointestinal motility, urinary retention/benign prostatic hyperplasia (BPH), xerostomia, cardiovascular disease, diabetes, seizure disorders, and bipolar disorder.[37] Patients should be monitored for and educated about potential serious side effects, including CNS depression, bone marrow suppression, bone fractures, orthostatic hypotension, syndrome of inappropriate antidiuretic hormone secretion (SIADH), narrow angle glaucoma, and serotonin syndrome (particularly when used in combination with other serotonergic agents).[37] Nortriptyline should not be abruptly discontinued due to the risk for a withdrawal syndrome.[37] Common side effects include sedation, dry mouth, blurred vision, urinary retention, lightheadedness, tremor, and constipation.[29]

Clonidine is used primarily as an antihypertensive; the mechanism of action in treating tobacco dependence is not well understood, but it is believed to lessen withdrawal symptoms.[38] The dosing of clonidine for tobacco cessation has not been standardized; doses ranging from 0.1 to 0.75 mg/day orally and 0.1 to 0.2 mg/day transdermally were used in clinical trials.[29] AHRQ guidelines recommend initiating at 0.1 mg orally twice daily or 0.1 mg/day transdermally, titrating by 0.1 mg/day weekly as needed.[29] Consider dose reduction in renal impairment; no dose adjustment is required in hepatic impairment.[39] Clonidine is contraindicated only in those who have a history of hypersensitivity, but caution should be used in patients with cardiovascular disease, cerebrovascular disease, and renal impairment.[39] Patients should be monitored for and educated about potential serious side effects, including bradycardia, CNS depression, and hypotension.[39] A gradual taper is required when discontinuing clonidine due to the risk for withdrawal syndrome with abrupt discontinuation.[39] Common side effects include dry mouth, drowsiness, dizziness, sedation, and constipation.[29]

Electronic Nicotine Delivery Systems
Electronic nicotine delivery systems (ENDS) or e-cigarettes have gained tremendous popularity in recent years, particularly among youth and adolescents. In 2018, more than 3.6 million middle and high school students had used ENDS within the past 30 days.[40] Among U.S. adults who use ENDS, the majority (58.8%) still smoke traditional cigarettes.[40] The USPSTF found insufficient evidence to recommend ENDS as a smoking cessation aid, though there is some data to support use of ENDS to increase the likelihood of long-term abstinence.[30,41] Indeed, many patients are utilizing e-cigarettes to replace regular cigarettes in an effort to improve their chances of quitting smoking, and more

patients are using this strategy compared with the FDA-approved tobacco cessation medications (35.3% of persons utilized ENDS during a recent quit attempt compared with 25.4% of persons who utilized the nicotine patch or gum).[42] However, ENDS are not currently recommended for tobacco cessation due to the lack of data on long-term health effects associated with chronic ENDS use and the need for more robust data indicating efficacy in smoking cessation.

OPIOID USE DISORDER

MAT, a term that originated in early 2000, is commonly used to describe the use of methadone, buprenorphine (with or without naloxone), and naltrexone to treat OUD. There is ongoing controversy about the use of this term, particularly related to the stigma that is often associated with OUD. The use of terms such as "replacement therapy" and "substitution therapy" may have implied and interpreted with other underlined meanings. Yet, current evidence indicates that methadone and buprenorphine do not simply replace heroin or other aberrant opioid use; their function is similar to traditional medication treatment of other chronic illnesses.[43,44]

Pharmacotherapy for Opioid Use Disorder

Evidence indicates that MAT is the gold standard for the treatment of OUD.[45] Although the effectiveness of methadone, buprenorphine, and IM naltrexone vary, all three medications have proven to be effective in treating OUD (**Table 34.3**).[45]

Methadone

Methadone has consistently demonstrated efficacy in the treatment of OUD, when compared to placebo or no treatment. According to a Cochrane meta-analysis, methadone results in longer stays in treatment for patients with OUD when compared to buprenorphine, and a rate equal to buprenorphine when reducing the use of illicit opioid agents.[46–49] Methadone is unique among the three MAT medications in that it is a full mu-opioid agonist. This binding, at adequate doses, can result in reduction of heroin or other aberrant opioid use by decreasing craving and withdrawal from other opioids.[50] While methadone is available in an injectable formulation, only the oral form has been used in opioid treatment programs. Methadone is slow to reach steady state, taking approximately 5 days (five half-lives). This is one of the features of methadone that dictates the need for knowledge and caution when prescribing. Compared to buprenorphine, it has no ceiling effect and is thought to carry a higher risk of overdose than buprenorphine because of its full-agonist action.

Methadone is fully absorbed via the gastrointestinal (GI) tract in approximately 30 minutes and reaches its daily peak between 2 and 4 hours. It may be prescribed for the treatment of pain like any other Drug Enforcement Administration (DEA) Schedule II controlled substance; however, it may not be prescribed by any clinician for use in treatment of OUD. This prohibition limits the use of methadone for treatment of OUD to federally approved opioid treatment programs only. The highly restricted nature of the use of methadone reflects the relatively high overdose risk. During the induction phase, where methadone dosing increases until the patient reaches a target dose, the risk of overdose may be very high; therefore, care must be taken in using a "low and slow" approach.[50] Induction protocols may vary, but all reflect the need for caution. A typical induction procedure would involve evaluating the patient using *DSM-5* criteria for OUD. Once a patient meets the criteria, methadone may be initiated at a maximum dose of 30 mg per day. Some patients may need to be inducted at a lower dose such as 10 to 20 mg, including those aged 60 and older, as well as those with concomitant use of sedating medication such as benzodiazepines, history of alcohol use disorder, other medications taken that may slow the metabolism of methadone, history of cardiac arrhythmias and bradycardia, known QTc prolongation, electrolyte abnormalities such as hypokalemia or hypomagnesemia, or compromised pulmonary function such as asthma and chronic obstructive pulmonary disease (COPD).

Qualified clinicians who are approved to prescribe methadone include nurse clinicians, physicians, physician assistants (PAs), and, in some settings, qualified pharmacists (PharmD). Clinicians would meet the patient at regular intervals (e.g., weekly), assess the patient, and titrate the dose in small increments until reaching the target dose. Typically, the "target dose" is a dose where the patient can stop using heroin or other opioid of abuse, does not feel sedated or overmedicated, and has little to no subjective or objective withdrawal symptoms.

In the early 2000s, researchers provided evidence that individuals may process and metabolize methadone at differing rates, related to methadone's racemic formulation (United States). Racemic methadone is a 50:50 mixture of R and S stereoisomers. The R isomer is thought to be the active component of the medication, both for prevention of withdrawal as well as analgesia. The relative activity of the R isomer is up to 50 times more active than the S isomer.[51] However, the R and S isomers can be metabolized at very different rates between individuals. Therefore, a relatively large dose of methadone in a patient who metabolized the R isomer at a fast rate may not be adequate for preventing withdrawal.[52,53] This sheds doubt on the use of serum levels to assess dose adequacy. Recommendations moved to using subjective, objective, and examination results to determine dose adequacy, rather than measuring the serum level of methadone. A 2016 study by Jiang et al.[54] also reached similar conclusions, noting the relative ineffectiveness of using serum levels to determine dose in most cases. While serum levels are thought not to be useful in assessing if someone's dose may be too high, there may be serum-level utility determining if a patient's dose may be too low.

TABLE 34.3 Pharmacotherapy for Opioid Use Disorder		
Drug	**Dose**	**Guidelines for Use and Side Effects**

Buprenorphine	SL tablet/film (combination product with naloxone preferred):
	  Induction: 2–4-mg initial dose, increase by 2–4-mg increments to clinical effect if no precipitated withdrawal after 60–90 minutes
	  Maintenance: 8–32 mg/day
	  Extended-release injection (used after induction and dose titration with SL formulation for at least 7 days):
	  300 mg SQ monthly for the first 2 months, then 100 mg SQ monthly
	  Dose may be titrated back to 300 mg monthly prn for clinical effect
	  Subdermal implant:
	  Insert four implants subdermally in the inner side of the upper arm
	  Remove after 6 months maximum, repeat on the other arm as desired
	  Discontinue use after one implant in each arm
		Patients must be opioid-free for 6–12 hours for short-acting opioid use or 24–72 hours for long-acting opioid use; begin induction after withdrawal symptoms appear.
		Common: Nausea/vomiting, dry mouth, diarrhea, constipation, fatigue, headache, dizziness, drowsiness
		Serious: CNS depression, respiratory depression, hepatotoxicity, angioedema/anaphylaxis, hypotension, QTc prolongation, infection (subdermal implant)

Methadone	Induction: 20–30-mg initial dose; if withdrawal symptoms not controlled after 2–4 hours, consider an additional 5–10-mg dose (maximum initial dose: 40 mg) Maintenance: Titrate cautiously to achieve suppression of withdrawal symptoms for 24 hours, reduced cravings, minimal sedation (usual dose: 80–120 mg/day)	Initiate therapy when there are no signs of intoxication or sedation and withdrawal symptoms are present. Common: Sedation, dizziness, lightheadedness, nausea/vomiting, constipation, diaphoresis, hypotension Serious: CNS depression, respiratory depression, hypotension, QTc prolongation, serotonin syndrome (in combination with other serotonergic agents)
Naltrexone	Oral: Initial dose: 25 mg; if no withdrawal symptoms, increase to 50 mg daily Alternative dosing schedules: 50 mg every weekday and 100-mg dose on Saturday; 100 mg every other day; 150 mg every 3 days Injection: 380 mg IM every 4 weeks by a clinician (not for self-injection)	Patients must be opioid free for 7–14 days prior to use; consider naloxone challenge (see text) or urine drug test Common: Syncope, headache, insomnia, anxiety, dizziness, abdominal pain/cramps, nausea/vomiting, diarrhea, decreased appetite, injection site reaction Severe: Acute opioid withdrawal, hepatotoxicity, eosinophilic pneumonia, suicidal ideation, severe injection site reactions, angioedema/anaphylaxis

CNS, central nervous system; IM, intramuscular; prn, as needed; SL, sublingual; SQ, subcutaneous.

Lexicomp. Buprenorphine. Lexi-Drugs. Wolters Kluwer Health, Inc. Accessed January 28, 2019. http://online.lexi.com; Lexicomp. Methadone. Lexi-Drugs. Wolters Kluwer Health, Inc. Accessed January 28, 2019. http://online.lexi.com; Lexicomp. Naltrexone. Lexi-Drugs. Wolters Kluwer Health, Inc. Accessed January 28, 2019. http://online.lexi.com; Pfizer. Nicotrol® Inhaler (nicotine inhalation system) [package insert]. revised 2008.

One unique potential adverse reaction to methadone is related to possible prolongation of QT interval on an electrocardiogram (ECG), resulting in increased risk of torsades de pointes (TdP), a fatal cardiac arrhythmia. While it is thought to be a rare reaction, evidence indicates that the risk is related to higher dose; other medications that may also lengthen the QT interval; family history of cardiac arrest, MI, or other cardiac diseases; and electrolyte balances. A QTc interval of more than 500 ms is thought to be significant and should prompt further workup, referral, and consideration of dose reduction. While protocols related to the QTc monitoring may vary, it is recommended that any clinician or agency ordering the dispensing of methadone for the treatment of OUD develop a protocol for assessing and monitoring cardiac risk related to the use of methadone.[50]

The use of methadone is recommended for pregnant patients with OUD. These recommendations have been made by an expert panel coordinated by the U.S. Substance Abuse and Mental Health Services Adminis-tration (SAMHSA), as well as the American College of Obstetricians and Gynecologists (ACOG).[55] Treating pregnant patients with OUD requires additional care in dose determination as well as supporting their efforts to sustain appropriate obstetric care. All pregnancies associated with OUD are considered high risk and require care from clinicians knowledgeable and experienced in working with this population. Other considerations include careful monitoring of the patient's dose effectiveness because there is increased metabolism during pregnancy. Methadone dose increase and/or division of the usual daily dose into two divided doses are options for consideration, particularly during the third trimester when methadone metabolism may become more rapid.[56]

Buprenorphine

Unlike methadone, buprenorphine is a partial agonist at mu-receptors. It binds tightly to CNS receptors and reduces the risk of overdose due to its blocking effect when other opioids are ingested together.[50] Studies have clearly

TABLE 34.4 Buprenorphine Formulations Approved for Opioid Use Disorder

Year Approved	Brand Name	Generic Ingredients	Notes
2002	N/A	Buprenorphine/naloxone sublingual tablets	Generic available in United States
	Subutex	Buprenorphine sublingual tablets	Brand discontinued in United States; generic tablet formulations still available
2010	Suboxone	Buprenorphine/naloxone sublingual films	Both brand and generic available in United States
2013	Zubsolv	Buprenorphine/naloxone sublingual tablets	Brand only
2014	Bunavail	Buprenorphine/naloxone buccal films	Brand only
2016	Probuphine	Buprenorphine intradermal implants	Brand only
2017	Sublocade	Buprenorphine extended-release subcutaneous injection	Brand only

demonstrated the effectiveness of buprenorphine and buprenorphine–naloxone for the treatment of OUD. While buprenorphine was originally approved for pain management, multiple formulations have emerged for the treatment of OUD and been approved per the SAMHSA Treatment Improvement Protocol 63 publication (**Table 34.4**).[50]

Oral (PO) buprenorphine is commonly combined with naloxone in order to reduce the risk of medication misuse or diversion. When taken orally, naloxone has little bioavailability; however, when injected intravenously, naloxone can rapidly induce precipitated withdrawal, therefore disincentivizing the misuse of the buprenorphine–naloxone combination. When starting a patient on buprenorphine, there is a risk of inducing opioid withdrawal if the patient is not in withdrawal. Patients who are taking short-acting opioids pre-induction need to stop the opioid medication for 6 to 12 hours to decrease the risk of precipitated withdrawal. Meanwhile patients taking long-acting opioids will need to stop taking the long-acting opioid for 24 to 72 hours before buprenorphine induction. Induction should not take place without significant opioid withdrawal.[50] The user-friendly Clinical Opiate Withdrawal Scale (COWS) is recommended when initiating oral buprenorphine induction, and it is recommended not to initiate induction until the patient scores 6 to 10 on the COWS.[57] A typical dosing of observed oral buprenorphine–naloxone induction should be started at 2 to 4 mg; dose may be repeated 2 to 4 hours later if the patient is still experiencing withdrawal, without signs of worsened withdrawal. Commonly the dose is increased up to 4-mg increments, with follow up in 3 to 4 days. Stable doses of buprenorphine are usually capped at 24 mg, although in some cases the dose may be increased to 32 mg/day. Similarly to methadone therapy, a "target dose" of buprenorphine is defined by cessation of heroin or other illicit opioid use, lack of sedation, and reduction/cessation of opioid withdrawal.

Naltrexone
Extended-release naltrexone is injected IM into the gluteal muscle. There is no restriction on nurse clinicians or PAs related to the ordering of naltrexone IM for OUD. Typically, injection is every 4 weeks by a clinician, with a usual dose of 380 mg. Naltrexone is an opioid antagonist, with the ability to displace opioids from receptors. Consequently, this medication is not appropriate for patients who currently have opioids in their system. Administering it to such patients can precipitate severe, acute withdrawal symptoms. Naltrexone is intended to decrease the risk of relapse in patients who have successfully tapered from an illicit or OUD-related opioid. Evidence also suggests that extended-release IM naltrexone is thought to be most effective when taken as part of a comprehensive management program, including counseling or other psychosocial components. Caution should be used in patients with active liver or renal disease or in patients who may attempt to take illicit opioid doses in amounts large enough to override the naltrexone blockade. Naltrexone is classified under pregnancy C category, noting its uncertain safety in pregnant patients.[58]

Expanding Access to Medication-Assisted Treatment
Expanding access to MAT for OUD is one of the key strategic priority areas identified for reducing opioid overdose and treating opioid dependence. One way to increase access is to expand the number of prescribers. For example, the role of nurse clinicians and PAs in the treatment of MAT is quickly expanded with increased opportunities for them to play key roles in the treatment of OUD. It was only in recent years that the American Society of Addiction Medicine (ASAM) recognized nurse clinicians and PAs as important members of this association.[59,60]

For decades, physicians have been the only group of prescribers that was allowed by law to prescribe MAT. In 2016, U.S. President Barack Obama signed the Comprehensive Addiction and Recovery Act (CARA) into law, which extended the prescribing privileges of buprenorphine to nurse clinicians and PAs. This law required a 24-hour training for nurse clinicians and PAs who prescribe buprenorphine for OUD; meanwhile, physicians were required to take an 8-hour training to receive a "Suboxone Waiver"[61] to prescribe medication for the same indication. This law also introduced the availability of what is known as an *X-Waiver* for nonphysician prescribers. In other words, this waiver would provide the nurse clinicians and PAs the privileges to prescribe MAT. In addition to the waivers, OTP (opioid treatment program) exemption may also be filed so other nonphysician prescribers may gain privileges to prescribe MAT.[62] It was put in place to allow nurse clinicians, PAs, and PharmDs to fully function in OTP settings. Unfortunately, this process is not well-known to many prescribers or regulators, posing a barrier for the full utilization. Various organizations, such as the American Academy of Physician Assistants (AAPA) in collaboration with the Society of PAs in Addiction Medicine (SPAAM), have offered a roadmap for navigation of the OTP exemption process.[63] The following steps are required for a federally approved OTP to obtain an exemption:

1. The OTP must be in a state that grants nurse clinicians/PAs Schedule 2 prescriptive authority.

2. The OTP must be in a state where there are no regulations prohibiting the practice of nurse clinicians/PAs in OTPs.
3. The OTP must have the support of the agency OTP medical director in seeking the exemption.
4. Every state has a SAMHSA-delegated State Opioid Treatment Authority (SOTA). The SOTA must be willing to approve a request for exemption from Guidelines for 42CFR Part 8. An initial contact with the SOTA should be set up to facilitate the approval process. The contact information for each state SOTA can be found at https://dpt2.samhsa.gov/regulations/smalist.aspx.
5. SAMHSA will consider the exemption request for approval.
6. Clinicians may not seek this exemption independent of their program sponsor, medical director, or State Opioid Treatment Authority.

SAMHSA provides a wide range of resources designed to help medical professionals administer MAT. See available resources on their website, www.samhsa.gov/homelessness-programs-resources/hpr-resources/useful-resources-medication-assisted-treatment.

CASE EXEMPLAR: Patient With Opioid Dependence

JJ is a 22-year-old college senior who attends a university on a football scholarship. He was injured early in the season, experiencing a medial collateral ligament (MCL) and anterior cruciate ligament (ACL) tear for which he underwent several surgeries. With each injury and subsequent surgery, hydrocodone was easy to acquire. He visits the clinician because he believes he is addicted to hydrocodone. He does not want to see the team medical staff or disclose to them anything about his feelings of dependence. He wants help.

Past Medical History
- MCL and ACL surgeries, 9 and 6 months previous
- Ambulatory with limp left side
- No known drug allergies
- No other surgeries or injuries

Medications
- Hydrocodone, 5/325 mg every 4 to 6 hours as needed for pain by prescription
- Street-obtained hydrocodone on a daily or every other day basis

Social History
- Drinks a six-pack of beer each weekend
- No tobacco use

- Uses food money and has shoplifted items to purchase street-obtained hydrocodone

Physical Examination
- Height: 76 inches; weight: 320 lbs.; blood pressure: 110/64; pulse: 90; respiration rate: 12; temperature: 98.2 °F
- Appears anxious, nervous, slight tremor in hands

Labs
- Liver function: Normal

Next Steps
- Plan medication-assisted treatment (MAT), refer for counseling

Discussion Questions

1. What criteria in the *Diagnostic and Statistical Manual of Mental Disorders (DSM-5)* does JJ meet to qualify him for intervention?
2. Which pharmacologic intervention should the clinician choose to manage JJ's addiction, and what is the rationale for this choice?
3. Which of the three medications commonly used to treat opioid addiction is a full mu-opioid agonist, and why would it be effective for JJ?

CASE EXEMPLAR: Patient With Tobacco Use Disorder

SS has been smoking one pack of cigarettes per day for more than 35 years and has tried unsuccessfully throughout the years to quit. She now suffers from emphysema, and her heart is affected by her lung condition. Her husband is adamant that she must quit smoking. He did so 1 year ago. She is at the clinic today seeking help to quit.

Past Medical History
- Diagnosed with chronic obstructive pulmonary disease (COPD) 5 years ago
- Hysterectomy 7 years ago
- Three children with no miscarriages
- No other surgeries or injuries
- No known drug allergies

Medications
- Levalbuterol, 45 mcg every 4 hours
- Furosemide, 40 mg once daily
- Digoxin, 140 mcg tablet once daily
- Lisinopril, 30 mg once daily

Social History
- Drinks wine with or after meals
- No illicit drug use

Physical Examination
- Height: 63 inches; weight: 88 lbs; blood pressure: 90/64; pulse: 90; respiration rate: 24; temperature: 98.2 °F
- Increased chest anteroposterior (AP) diameter
- Decreased breath sounds throughout all lobes
- Leans forward to aid in breathing, pursed lips

Labs and Imaging
- Arterial blood gas (ABG):
  - pH: 7.30
  - PO_2: 68
  - CO_2: 48
  - HCO_3: 30
- Hematocrit (Hct): 10
- Hemoglobin (Hgb): 31
- Red blood cells (RBC): 5.6
- Chest x-ray: Infiltrates throughout, lung and heart enlargement

Diagnosis
- Chronic COPD with possible cor pulmonale. Needs to stop smoking as soon as possible.

Discussion Questions

1. What initial interventional assessment should the clinician use with SS?
2. SS desires to quit smoking and assures the clinician that her desire is firm and that she does not see the support of her husband as negative. What intervention should the clinician choose for SS?
3. Describe additional potential interventions and follow-up.

KEY TAKEAWAYS

- SUD describes a functional and clinical impairment due to dependence on use of a substance, which may be a legal or illicit substance. In the United States, substance abuse disorders most often include alcohol, tobacco, cannabis, opioids, stimulants, and hallucinogens.
- OUD accounts for more than 60% of all drug overdose deaths, and rates associated with opioid overdose have increased 200% since 2000.
- DHHS identified three priority areas to address the opioid crisis: Prescriber education and training, increasing community access to naloxone, and expanding access to MAT for OUD.
- The binge cycle is comprised of three stages: Binge/intoxication, withdrawal/negative affect, and preoccupation/anticipation.
- The *DSM-5* combines the *DSM-IV* categories of substance abuse and substance dependence into a single disorder measured on a continuum from mild to severe. Each specific substance is addressed as a separate use disorder.
- In treating alcohol addiction, the APA recommends developing a person-centered comprehensive assessment (e.g., mental status examinations, physical exams, laboratory testing) and treatment (specific plans for addressing acute intoxication, nonpharmacologic and pharmacologic interventions).
- Pharmacotherapy should be offered to all patients with moderate-to-severe AUD in addition to nonpharmacologic treatments.
- Three medications are approved by the U.S. FDA to treat alcohol dependence: (1) naltrexone, (2) acamprosate, and (3) disulfiram. Each of these carries significant interactions.

Disulfiram requires patients to avoid alcohol entirely. If considered the drug of choice, naloxone must be used with caution in patients taking opiates for a concurrent diagnosis. A challenge test can determine the risk for precipitating opioid withdrawal in patients previously using opioids.

- The use of antidepressants is not recommended unless the patient also has a comorbid depression or anxiety disorder; benzodiazepines are also not recommended.
- For tobacco users, both behavioral and pharmacologic interventions are recommended. Intensive interventions involve more frequent counseling, including practical counseling (skills training, problem-solving) and social support.
- MAT—including the use of methadone, buprenorphine (with or without naloxone), and naltrexone—is considered the gold standard in the treatment of OUD. Expanding access to this treatment is key in reducing opioid overdose and treating opioid dependence.

REFERENCES

1. Substance Abuse and Mental Health Services Administration. *Key Substance Use and Mental Health Indicators in the United States: Results From the 2017 National Survey on Drug Use and Health (HHS Publication No. SMA 18-5068, NSDUH Series H-53).* Center for Behavioral Health Statistics and Quality, Substance Abuse and Mental Health Services Administration; 2018. https://www.samhsa.gov/data/sites/default/files/cbhsq-reports/NSDUHFFR2017/NSDUHFFR2017.pdf

2. Centers for Disease Control and Prevention. *Smoking & tobacco use: fast facts.* Accessed January 16, 2019. https://www.cdc.gov/tobacco/data_statistics/fact_sheets/fast_facts/index.htm

3. Rudd RA, Aleshire N, Zibbell JE, Gladden RM. Increases in drug and opioid overdose deaths – United States, 2000–2014. *Morb Mortal Wkly Rep.* 2016;64(5):1378–1382. https://www.cdc.gov/mmwr/preview/mmwrhtml/mm6450a3.htm

4. National Institute on Drug Abuse. Opioid overdose crisis. 2018. Accessed December 4, 2018. https://www.drugabuse.gov/drugs-abuse/opioids/opioid-overdose-crisis

5. U.S Department of Health and Human Services. HHS takes strong steps to address opioid-drug related overdose, death, and dependence. 2015. Accessed December 4, 2018. https://wayback.archive-it.org/3926/20170127185704/https://www.hhs.gov/about/news/2015/03/26/hhs-takes-strong-steps-to-address-opioid-drug-related-overdose-death-and-dependence.html

6. McLellan AT. Substance misuse and substance use disorders: Why do they matter in healthcare? *Trans Am Clin Climatol Assoc.* 2017;128:112–130. https://www.ncbi.nlm.nih.gov/pmc/articles/PMC5525418

7. Hesse M. What does addiction mean to me. *Mens Sana Monographs.* 2006;4(1):104–126. doi:10.4103/0973-1229.27609

8. Koob GF, Volkow ND. Neurocircuitry of addiction. *Neuropsychopharmacol.* 2010;35(1):217–238. doi:10.1038/npp.2009.110

9. Substance Abuse and Mental Health Services Administration; Office of the Surgeon General. The neurobiology of substance use, misuse, and addiction. In: Substance Abuse and Mental Health Services Administration; Office of the Surgeon General, eds. *Facing Addiction in America: The Surgeon General's Report on Alcohol, Drugs, and Health [Internet].* US Department of Health and Human Services; 2016. https://www.ncbi.nlm.nih.gov/books/NBK424849

10. Koob GF, Volkow ND. Neurobiology of addiction: a neurocircuitry analysis. *Lancet Psychiatr.* 2018;3:760–773. doi:10.1016/S2215-0366(16)00104-8

11. Koob GF, Simon EJ. The neurobiology of addiction: where we have been and where we are going. *J Drug Issues.* 2009;39(1):115–132. doi:10.1177/002204260903900110

12. Rando K, Hong KI, Bhagwagar Z, et al. Association of frontal and posterior cortical gray matter volume with time to alcohol relapse: a prospective study. *Am J Psychiatry.* 2011;168(2):183–192. doi:10.1176/appi.ajp.2010.10020233

13. Hasin DS, O'Brien CP, Auriacombe M, et al. *DSM-5 criteria for substance use disorders: recommendations and rationale. Am J Psychiatr.* 2013;170(8):834–851. doi:10.1176/appi.ajp.2013.12060782

14. American Psychiatric Association. *Substance related and addictive disorders.* Published 2013. https://www.psychiatry.org/file%20library/psychiatrists/practice/dsm/apa_dsm-5-substance-use-disorder.pdf

15. American Psychiatric Association. Practice guideline for the pharmacological treatment of patients with alcohol use disorder. *Am J Psychiatr.* 2018;175(1):86–90. doi:10.1176/appi.ajp.2017.1750101

16. Jonas DE, Amick HR, Feltner C, et al. Pharmacotherapy for adults with alcohol use disorders in outpatient settings: a systematic review and meta-analysis. *JAMA.* 2014;311(18):1889–1900. doi:10.1001/jama.2014.3628

17. Forest Pharmaceuticals, Inc. *Campral® (acamprosate calcium) delayed release tablets* [package insert]. Published August 2005. https://www.accessdata.fda.gov/drugsatfda_docs/label/2010/021431s013lbl.pdf

18. Duramed Pharmaceuticals, Inc. *Revia® (naltrexone hydrochloride tablets USP)* [package insert]. Published October 2013. https://www.accessdata.fda.gov/drugsatfda_docs/label/2013/018932s017lbl.pdf

19. Alkermes, Inc. *Vivitrol (naltrexone for extended-release injectable suspension)* [package insert]. revised 2018.

20. Anton RF. Naltrexone for the management of alcohol dependence. *N Engl J Med.* 2008;359(7):715–721. doi:10.1056/NEJMct0801733

21. Pettinati HM, Anton RF, Willenbring ML. The COMBINE Study-: An Overview of the Largest Pharmacotherapy Study to Date for Treating Alcohol Dependence. Psychiatry (Edgmont). 2006 Oct;3(10):36-9. PMID: 20877545; PMCID: PMC2945872.

22. TEVA Pharamceuticals USA, Inc. Disulfiram tablets USP [package insert]. Updated 2018.

23. IBM Micromedex. *Disulfiram*. Micromedex solutions. Truven Health Analytics, Inc. Accessed January 18, 2019. http://www.micromedexsolutions.com

24. Jonas DE, Amick HR, Feltner C, et al. *Pharmacotherapy for Adults with Alcohol-Use Disorders in Outpatient Settings*. Agency for Healthcare Research and Quality; May 2014. https://www.ncbi.nlm.nih.gov/books/NBK208590

25. Janssen Pharmaceuticals, Inc. *Topamax®* [package insert]. Updated October 2012. https://www.accessdata.fda.gov/drugsatfda_docs/label/2012/020844s041lbl.pdf

26. IBM Micromedex. *Topiramate*. Micromedex solutions. Truven Health Analytics, Inc. Accessed January 18, 2019. http://www.micromedexsolutions.com

27. Mason BJ, Quello S, Goodell V, et al. Gabapentin treatment for alcohol dependence: a randomized clinical trial. *JAMA Intern Med*. 2014;174(1):70–77. doi:10.1001/jamainternmed.2013.11950.

28. IBM Micromedex. *Gabapentin*. Micromedex solutions. Truven Health Analytics, Inc. Accessed January 18, 2019. http://www.micromedexsolutions.com

29. U.S. Department of Health and Human Services. *Treating tobacco use and dependence: 2008 update*. U.S. Department of Health and Human Services; 2008. https://www.ncbi.nlm.nih.gov/books/NBK63952

30. Siu AL, U.S. Preventive Services Task Force. Behavioral and pharmacotherapy interventions for tobacco smoking cessation in adults, including pregnant women: U.S. Preventive Services Task Force recommendation statement. *Ann Intern Med*. 2015;163(8):622–634. doi:10.7326/M15-2023

31. Patnode CD, Henderson JT, Thompson JH, et al. Behavioral counseling and pharmacotherapy interventions for tobacco cessation in adults, including pregnant women: a review of reviews for the U.S. Preventive Services Task Force. Agency for Healthcare Research and Quality; 2015. https://www.ncbi.nlm.nih.gov/books/NBK321744

32. Lexicomp. Nicotine. *Lexi-Drugs*. Wolters Kluwer Health, Inc. Accessed January 19, 2019. http://online.lexi.com

33. Pfizer. *Nicotrol® NS (nicotine nasal spray)* [package insert]. Revised 2010. https://www.accessdata.fda.gov/drugsatfda_docs/label/2010/020385s010lbl.pdf

34. GlaxoSmithKline. *Zyban® (bupropion hydrochloride) sustained-release tablets, for oral use* [package insert]. Updated July 2019. https://www.gsksource.com/pharma/content/dam/GlaxoSmithKline/US/en/Prescribing_Information/Zyban/pdf/ZYBAN-PI-MG.PDF

35. Pfizer. *Chantix® (varenicline) tablets, for oral use* [package insert]. Updated June 2018. https://www.accessdata.fda.gov/drugsatfda_docs/label/2010/020385s010lbl.pdf accessed date: 05/01/2019

36. Hughes JR, Stead LF, Lancaster T. Nortriptyline for smoking cessation: a review. *Nicotine Tob Res*. 2005;7(4): 491–499. doi:10.1080/14622200500185298

37. Lexicomp. Nortriptyline. *Lexi-Drugs*. Wolters Kluwer Health, Inc. Accessed January 19, 2019. http://online.lexi.com

38. Gourlay SG, Stead LF, Benowitz NL. Clonidine for smoking cessation. *Cochrane Database Syst Rev*. 2004;2004(3):CD000058. doi:10.1002/14651858.CD000058.pub2.

39. Lexicomp. Clonidine. *Lexi-Drugs*. Wolters Kluwer Health, Inc. Accessed January 19, 2019. http://online.lexi.com.

40. Centers for Disease Control and Prevention. *Smoking & tobacco use: About electronic cigarettes (e-cigarettes)*. Accessed January 21, 2019. https://www.cdc.gov/tobacco/basic_information/e-cigarettes/about-e-cigarettes.html

41. Hartmann-Boyce J, McRobbie H, Bullen C, et al. Electronic cigarettes for smoking cessation. *Cochrane Database Syst Rev*. 2016;(11):CD010216. doi:10.1002/14651858.CD010216.pub3

42. Caraballo RS, Shafer PR, Patel D, et al. Quit methods used by US adult cigarette smokers, 2014–2016. *Prev Chronic Dis*. 2017;14:160600. doi:10.5888/pcd14.160600

43. McLoone I. *Can we stop calling it "medication assisted treatment?"* Updated November 4, 2019. https://www.rehabs.com/pro-talk-articles/can-we-stop-calling-it-medication-assisted-treatment

44. Payte JT. The use of insulin in the treatment of diabetes: an analogy to methadone maintenance. *J Psychoactive Drugs*. 1991;23(2):109–110. doi:10.1080/02791072.1991.10472227

45. National Institute on Drug Abuse. *Effective treatments for opioid addiction*. Published November 1, 2016. https://www.drugabuse.gov/publications/effective-treatments-opioid-addiction/effective-treatments-opioid-addiction

46. Mattick RP, Breen C, Kimber J, et al. Buprenorphine maintenance versus placebo or methadone maintenance for opioid dependence. *Cochrane Database Syst Rev*. 2014 (2):CD002207. doi:10.1002/14651858.CD002207.pub4

47. Degenhardt L, Randall D, Hall W, et al. Mortality among clients of a state-wide opioid pharmacotherapy program over 20 years: risk factors and lives saved. *Drug Alcohol Depend*. 2009;105(1–2):9–15. doi:10.1016/j.drugalcdep.2009.05.021

48. Metzger DS, Woody GE, McLellan AT, et al. Human immunodeficiency virus seroconversion among intravenous drug users in- and out-of-treatment: an 18-month prospective follow-up. *J Acquir Immune Defic Syndr*. 1993;6(9):1049–1056. Pubmed PMID: 8340896.

49. Ball JC, Ross A. *The Effectiveness of Methadone Maintenance Treatment*. Springer Verlag; 1991.

50. Substance Abuse and Mental Health Services Administration. *TIP 63: medications for opioid use disorder*. 2018. Accessed December 1, 2018. https://store.samhsa.gov/system/files/sma18-5063fulldoc.pdf.

51. Eap CB, Buclin T, Baumann P. Interindividual variability of the clinical pharmacokinetics of methadone implications for the treatment of opioid dependence. *Clin Pharmacokinet*. 2002;41(14):1153–1193. doi:10.2165/00003088-200241140-00003

52. Leavitt SB, Shinderman M, Maxwell S, et al. When "enough" is not enough: new perspectives on optimal methadone dose. *Mt Sinai J Med*. 2000;67:404–411. Pubmed PMID: 11064491.

53. Maxwell S, Shinderman M. Optimizing response to methadone maintenance treatment: use of higher-dose methadone. *J Psychoactive Drugs*. 1999;31(2):95–102. doi:10.1080/02791072.1999.10471730

54. Jiang H, Hillhouse M, Du J, et al. Dose, plasma level, and treatment outcome among methadone patients in Shanghai, China. *Neurosci Bull.* 2016;32(6):538–544. doi:10.1007/s12264-016-0059-0

55. American College of Obstetricians and Gynecologists. *Opioid use and opioid use disorder in pregnancy.* Published August 2017. https://www.acog.org/Clinical-Guidance-and-Publications/Committee-Opinions/Committee-on-Obstetric-Practice/Opioid-Use-and-Opioid-Use-Disorder-in-Pregnancy

56. Drozdick J III, Berghella V, Hill M, et al. Methadone trough levels in pregnancy. *Am J Obstet Gynecol.* 2002;187(5):1184–1188. doi:10.1067/mob.2002.127132

57. Providers' Clincal Support Team for Medication Assisted Treatment. *Buprenorphine induction.* Updated November 27, 2013. https://pcssnow.org/wp-content/uploads/2014/02/PCSS-MATGuidanceBuprenorphineInduction.Casadonte.pdf

58. Substance Abuse and Mental Health Services Administration *Pocket guide for medication-assisted treatment of opioid use disorder.* Substance Abuse and Mental Health Services Administration; 2017.

59. Hurley B. Non-physicians and ASAM: Membership? ASAM Magazine. Published April 13, 2013. https://www.asam.org/Quality-Science/publications/magazine/read/article/2013/04/13/non-physicians-and-asam-membership-

60. American Society of Addiction Medicine. *ASAM associate membership.* Accessed December 3, 2018. https://www.asam.org/membership/the-associate-membership

61. American Society of Addiction Medicine. Treatment of opioid use disorder course. Accessed December 3, 2018. https://www.asam.org/education/live-online-cme/waiver-qualifying-training

62. Addiction Treatment Forum. *Opioid treatment program accreditation guidelines will not allow mid-levels; SAMHSA will work with states on exemptions.* Published April 21, 2015. http://atforum.com/2015/04/new-otp-accreditation-guidelines-will-not-allow-mid-levels

63. American Academy of Physician Assistants. *PA role in opioid treatment programs.* Published May, 2018. https://www.aapa.org/wp-content/uploads/2017/01/PA_Role_in_Opioid_Treatment_Programs.pdf

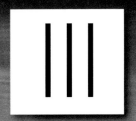

Health Promotion and Maintenance

Over-the-Counter Medications

Ashley Taylor, Janel Bailey Wheeler, and Kristi Isaac Rapp

INTRODUCTION

Over-the-counter (OTC) medications, or nonprescription medications, can be purchased by patients without a prescription from a clinician. OTC medications are often the first line of therapy for consumers treating a minor condition or symptom. According to the Consumer Healthcare Products Association, 81% of adults use nonprescription medications as a first response to minor ailments.[1] Eighty-six percent (86%) of consumers believe that the use of nonprescription medications helps lower their healthcare costs.[1] The accessibility and affordability of these products make them a critical component of the healthcare system.

There are more than 100,000 approved nonprescription products with over 400 active ingredients available in the United States.[2] These products must be both safe and effective for their intended use and have a wider margin of safety than prescription drugs. There are several conditions and symptoms that can be treated by nonprescription medications, including cough and cold, allergy, and pain. Natural products, dietary and nutritional supplements, and cosmetic agents are also available without a prescription. This chapter will discuss treatment options for conditions commonly managed with nonprescription medications.

OVER-THE-COUNTER MEDICATIONS FOR COUGH AND COLD

Cough is the most common symptom for which patients visit or consult their primary clinician.[3] Cough can be a valuable mechanism to clear secretions and foreign materials from airways.[4] A cough can be productive or nonproductive. Productive coughs may be valuable as they may expel secretions and mucus that may cause infections or inhibit ventilation if retained. Nonproductive coughs do not expel secretions and are often described as "dry or hacking coughs."

Selection of the appropriate OTC medication for the treatment of cough depends on the nature and etiology of the cough. Generally, nonproductive coughs are treated with antitussive medications that suppress cough; these medications should not be used to treat productive coughs. Expectorants work to thin mucus secretions and increase the amount of mucus expelled. **Table 35.1** lists U.S. Food and Drug Administration-(FDA) approved OTC cough medications, dosages, and formulations.

ANTITUSSIVES

Available OTC antitussives include codeine, dextromethorphan, diphenhydramine, and chlophedianol. Codeine, a centrally acting opioid that acts to suppress cough, is available without a prescription in many

TABLE 35.1 Over-the-Counter Antitussive and Expectorant Products Used for Treatment of Cough

Drug and Formulation	Dosage
Codeine (Oral solutions, liquids, suspensions, syrups in combination with other active ingredients)	>12 years: 10–20 mg q4–6h (max daily dose: 120 mg) 6–12 years: 5–10 mg every q4–6h (max daily dose: 60 mg) <6 years: Consult a clinician
Dextromethorphan HBr* (Oral capsules, liquids, lozenges, strips, suspensions, syrups)	>12 years: 10–20 mg q4h or 30 mg q6–8h (max daily dose: 120 mg); ER, 60 mg bid 6–12 years: 5–10 mg q4h or 15 mg q6–8h (max daily dose: 60 mg); ER, 60 mg bid 2–5: 2.5–5 mg q4h or 7.5 mg q4–8h (max daily dose: 30 mg); ER, 15 mg bid
Diphenhydramine citrate	>12 years: 38 mg q4h (max daily dose: 228 mg) 6–12 years: 19 mg q4h (max daily dose: 114 mg) <6 years: Consult a clinician
Diphenhydramine HCl (Oral capsules, liquids, elixir, strips, tablets, chewable tablets)	>12 years: 25 mg q4h (max daily dose: 150 mg) 6–12 years: 12.5 mg q4h (max daily dose: 75 mg) 2–5 years: Consult a clinician
Chlophedianol HCl (syrup)**	>12 years: 25 mg q6–8h (max daily dose: 100 mg) 6–12 years: 12.5 mg q6–8h (max daily dose: 50 mg) 2–5 years: 12.5 mg q6–8h (max daily dose: 50 mg)
Guaifenesin (Granules, ER tablets, IR tablets, liquid	>12 years: 200–400 mg q4h (max daily dose: 2,400 mg) 6–12 years: 100–200 mg q4h (max daily dose: 1,200 mg) 2–5 years: 50–100 mg q4h (max daily dose: 600 mg)

*Not for OTC use in children <4 years of age.

**Currently not available in the United States.

bid, twice daily; ER, extended release; h, hour; HBr, hydrobromic acid; HCl, hydrochloric acid; IR, immediate release; max, maximum; q, every.

Source: Data from U.S. Food and Drug Administration. Cold, cough, allergy, bronchodilator, and antiasthmatic drug products for over-the-counter human use. *CFR: Code of Federal Regulations*, Title 21, Part 341. Updated April 1, 2018. https://www.accessdata.fda.gov/scripts/cdrh/cfdocs/cfcfr/CFRSearch.cfm?CFRPart=341&-showFR=1; Lexicomp Online. *Diphenhydramine.*Wolters Kluwer Clinical Drug Information. Published 2019. http://webstore.lexi.com/ONLINE.

states as a Schedule V drug. These products must contain at least one non-codeine active ingredient and no more than 200 mg of codeine per 100 mL. The onset of action of codeine is 15 to 30 minutes with a duration of 4 to 6 hours. Common side effects of codeine at antitussive doses include sedation, constipation, dizziness, nausea, and vomiting.[5] The use of codeine may lead to respiratory depression and has the potential for abuse. Codeine is contraindicated in patients who have a hypersensitivity to codeine and should be used with caution in individuals with asthma, chronic obstructive pulmonary disease (COPD), and drug addictions.[5] The FDA recommends against the use of prescription codeine in children under 18 because the risk of misuse, abuse, overdose, and death outweigh the benefits in this population. The FDA is considering regulatory action for OTC codeine-containing products.[6]

Dextromethorphan is a nonopioid antitussive with a similar onset of action as codeine. It has a duration of action of 3 to 6 hours. Side effects associated with dextromethorphan include dizziness, drowsiness, gastrointestinal distress, nausea, vomiting, and stomach pain.[7] Patients with a known hypersensitivity to dextromethorphan should avoid its use. Dextromethorphan should not be used concomitantly with monoamine oxidase inhibitors (MAOI) or within 2 weeks of discontinuing

a MAOI.[8] At higher doses, dextromethorphan produces a euphoric effect; numerous cases of abuse have been reported. Clinicians should be aware of the abuse potential of this drug.[7]

Diphenhydramine is a first-generation antihistamine that acts centrally on the medulla to increase the cough threshold and suppress cough. Side effects include drowsiness, dizziness, excitement, insomnia, dry mucous membranes, and urinary retention.[9] Diphenhydramine is contraindicated in patients with a known hypersensitivity to diphenhydramine or other structurally similar antihistamines. It should be used with caution in persons with asthma, cardiovascular disease, increased intraocular pressure, angle-closure glaucoma, prostatic hyperplasia, bladder neck obstruction, genitourinary obstruction, and thyroid disorder. Diphenhydramine increases the central nervous system (CNS)–depressant effects of alcohol, sedatives, and tranquilizers.[9]

Chlophedianol is a centrally acting cough suppressant that has a slower onset of action and longer duration of action than codeine. It is available in combination with other cold and cough medications. Adverse effects of chlophedianol include excitement, hyperirritability, nightmares, and dry mouth. Drowsiness, hallucinations, nausea and vomiting, and vertigo may occur at larger doses.[8,10]

Camphor and menthol are topical antitussives available OTC. These products are most commonly available for the treatment of cough in lozenges, ointments, and steam inhalation liquids.[11]

EXPECTORANTS

Guaifenesin, the only FDA-approved expectorant, works by increasing hydration of the respiratory tract and promoting the removal of secretions by the natural clearance processes. Side effects of this medication include dizziness, drowsiness, headache, skin rash, nausea, vomiting, and stomach pain. There have been reports of nephrolithiasis with consumption in large doses. Guaifenesin is contraindicated in patients with a known hypersensitivity to guaifenesin.[12]

For the treatment of cold symptoms, decongestants and analgesics are often used to relieve symptoms of nasal congestion, sore throat, body aches, and/or fever. Decongestants and analgesics are discussed later in this chapter. Combination cough, cold, and allergy products are widely available for the treatment of colds.

HERBALS AND THE COMMON COLD

Natural products, including zinc and vitamin C, are available for use in treating the common cold.[13] Zinc at doses of greater than 75 mg/day have been found to reduce the average duration of a cold when taken within 24 hours of symptom onset. Healthy patients taking zinc are less likely to have symptoms beyond 7 days of treatment.[13] The role of vitamin C in the prevention and treatment of a cold is debatable. There is some evidence that suggests vitamin C in doses up to 2 g/day may shorten the duration and severity of symptoms. Studies suggest that there may be some benefit of vitamin C in patients exposed to severe exercise and/or cold environments.[13]

OVER-THE-COUNTER MEDICATIONS FOR ALLERGIC RHINITIS

Allergic rhinitis affects more than 14% of adults and 13% of children in the United States.[12] Symptoms include sneezing, rhinorrhea, nasal congestion, and itching.[14] Allergic rhinitis is considered mild when symptoms do not affect the quality of life of the patient; when symptoms affect patient quality of life, allergic rhinitis symptoms are classified as moderate to severe.[14]

The goals of treatment of allergic rhinitis are to prevent or reduce symptoms and improve patient functional status. Treatment is individualized to provide optimal symptom control. OTC options available to treat allergy symptoms include intranasal steroids, antihistamines, decongestants, and other agents.

INTRANASAL CORTICOSTEROIDS

Intranasal corticosteroids work to decrease inflammation in allergic rhinitis and are the preferred initial treatment of nasal symptoms associated with seasonal allergic rhinitis.[14] These products assist in reducing sneezing, rhinorrhea, itching, and congestion. OTC intranasal corticosteroids are listed in **Table 35.2**, along with dosages and brand names. Local side effects include epistaxis, pharyngitis, and nasal irritation. Patients should be monitored for systemic side effects, including adrenal suppression, impaired growth, infections, and ocular disease.[14]

ANTIHISTAMINES

Oral antihistamines are also utilized in the OTC treatment of allergic rhinitis.[14] They are helpful in reducing symptoms of itching, sneezing, and rhinorrhea; they have little effect on nasal congestion. Antihistamines

TABLE 35.2 Over-the-Counter Intranasal Corticosteroids

Drug	Dosage
Budesonide (Rhinocort® allergy relief)	≥12 years: Initial—two sprays in each nostril daily; once controlled, decrease to one spray in each nostril daily 6–11 years: One spray in each nostril daily; if uncontrolled, increase to two sprays in each nostril daily
Fluticasone propionate (Flonase® allergy relief)	≥12 years: One to two sprays in each nostril qd 4–11 years: One spray in each nostril <4 years: Do not use
Fluticasone furoate (Flonase® Sensimist)	≥12 years: One to two sprays in each nostril daily; do not use >6 months unless directed by a clinician 2–11 years: One spray in each nostril daily; do not use >2 months unless directed by a clinician
Triamcinolone	≥12 years: Initial—two sprays in each nostril qd; once controlled, decrease to one spray in each nostril daily 6–11 years: One spray in each nostril daily (max daily dose: two sprays in each nostril) 2–5 years: One spray in each nostril daily (max daily dose: one spray in each nostril)

max, maximum; qd, once daily.

Source: Data from Lexicomp Online. Wolters Kluwer Clinical Drug Information. Published 2018. http://webstore.lexi.com/ONLINE

work by blocking histamine binding at the histamine-1 receptor. Second-generation antihistamines are preferred over first-generation antihistamine agents because they cause less sedation and cognitive effects. Examples of available first and second-generation antihistamines can be found in **Table 35.3**.[14]

DECONGESTANTS

Oral and nasal decongestants effective in reducing nasal congestion are available OTC. These agents work by stimulating adrenergic alpha-1 receptors, thereby producing vasoconstriction. **Table 35.4** lists oral and nasal decongestants that are available without a prescription. Side effects of oral decongestants include tachycardia and increased blood pressure; these agents should be used with caution in patients with cardiovascular disease and uncontrolled blood pressure. Side effects of topical agents include burning, stinging, sneezing, and trauma from the tip of the device. Topical nasal decongestants should not be used more than 3 days to prevent rhinitis medicamentosa (rebound congestion).[8]

Combination products containing an antihistamine and decongestant are available for the treatment of allergy symptoms. If an OTC product contains a "D" after the name, it usually contains a decongestant.

OVER-THE-COUNTER MEDICATIONS FOR PAIN

Pain is a common symptom that many patients experience during their lifetimes. The intensity, duration, and location of pain are significant factors that may impact how to manage this undesirable sensory experience. For mild-to-moderate pain, many patients will initially try to alleviate symptoms by using OTC medications. More severe forms of pain typically warrant patients seeking out the advice of a clinician for stronger and longer acting analgesics.[15]

Pain symptoms may be acute or chronic. Acute pain presents briefly and quickly in response to musculoskeletal damage or injury. It may last for days up to months. Chronic pain presents with a gradual onset in response to a chronic process or prolonged tissue damage or injury. Chronic pain symptoms may persist for years after musculoskeletal damage/injury has occurred and may be burdensome and disabling for some patients.[14,16]

TABLE 35.3 Selected Over-the-Counter Antihistamines

Drugs	Dosage
First-Generation Oral Antihistamines	
Diphenhydramine	≥12 years: 25–50 mg q4–6h (max daily dose: 300 mg) 6–11 years: 12.5–25 mg q4–6h (max daily dose: 150 mg) 2–6 years: limited data available; 6.25 mg q4–6h (max daily dose: 37.5 mg)
Chlorpheniramine Brompheniramine	≥12 years: 4 mg q4–6h (max daily dose: 24 mg) 6–11 years: 2 mg q4–6h (max daily dose: 12 mg) 2–6 years: 1 mg q4–6h (max daily dose: 6 mg)
Second-Generation Oral Antihistamines	
Loratadine	≥12 years: 10 mg qd or 5 mg bid 6–11 years: 10 mg qd or 5 mg bid 2–5 years: 5 mg qd
Fexofenadine	≥12 years: 180 mg qd (max daily dose: 180 mg) or 60 mg bid (max daily dose: 120 mg) 6–11 years: Oral disintegrating tablets—30 mg q12h (max daily dose: 60 mg) 2–11 years: Suspension—30 mg q12h (max daily dose: 60 mg)
Cetirizine	≥6 years: 5–10 mg qd (max daily dose: 10 mg) 2–5 years: 2.5 mg daily; may increase to 2.5 mg bid or 5 mg daily (max daily dose: 5 mg) 12 months–1 year: 2.5 mg qd (max daily dose: 2.5 mg bid) 6–12 months: 2.5 mg qd
Levocetirizine	≥12 years: 5 mg qd (max daily dose: 5 mg) 6–11 years: 2.5 mg qd (max daily dose: 2.5 mg) 2–5 years: 1.25 mg daily (max daily dose: 1.25 mg)

bid, twice daily; h, hour; max, maximum; q, every; qd, once daily.

Source: Data from Lexicomp Online. Wolters Kluwer Clinical Drug Information. Published 2018. http://webstore.lexi.com/ONLINE

TABLE 35.4 Selected Over-the-Counter Nasal Decongestants

Oral Decongestants

Pseudoephedrine	≥12 years: 60 mg q4–6h (max daily dose: 240 mg) 6–11 years: 30 mg q4–6h (max daily dose: 120 mg) 2–5 years 15 mg q4–6h (max daily dose: 60 mg)
Phenylephrine	≥12 years: 10 mg q4h (max daily dose: 60 mg) 6–11 years: 5 mg q4h (max daily dose: 30 mg) <6 years: 2.5 mg q4h (max daily dose: 15 mg)

Topical Decongestants

Oxymetazoline	**0.05% solution:** ≥6 years: Two to three sprays in each nostril q10–12h; do not exceed two doses in 24 h; therapy should not exceed 3 days <6 years: Consult a clinician **0.025% solution:** <6 years: Two to three drops per spray in each nostril q10–12h; do not exceed two doses in 24 hours
Naphazoline	**0.05% aqueous solution:** ≥12 years: One to two drops/sprays in each nostril no more than q6h <12 years: Consult a clinician **0.025% aqueous solution:** 6–12 years: One to two drops/sprays in each nostril no more than q6h <6 years: Consult a clinician **0.05% water-based jelly:** 6–12 years: Place small amount in each nostril and inhale (with adult supervision) <6 years: Consult a clinician
Levmetamfetamine	≥12 years: Two inhalations in each nostril no more than q2h 6–11 years: One inhalation in each nostril no more than q2h <6 years: Consult a clinician

h, hour; max, maximum; q, every.

Source: Data from U.S. Food and Drug Administration. Cold, cough, allergy, bronchodilator, and antiasthmatic drug products for over-the-counter human use. *CFR: Code of Federal Regulations*, Title 21, Part 341. Updated April 1, 2018. https://www.accessdata.fda.gov/scripts/cdrh/cfdocs/cfcfr/CFRSearch.cfm?CFRPart=341&showFR=1; Lexicomp Online. Wolters Kluwer Clinical Drug Information. Published 2018.

Distinguishing the different types of pain that patients experience is extremely important in providing a recommendation for an appropriate treatment option. Clinicians can make recommendations on how to best manage pain if they are aware of the onset, duration, and intensity of the pain symptoms.

Analgesics may be used to reduce the intensity of pain symptoms. Several classes of analgesics are currently available OTC to treat mild-to-moderate pain. These products are indicated for the relief of acute pain for several conditions, including arthritis, gout, dysmenorrhea, fever, and headaches. Unlike acute pain symptoms, chronic and severe pain symptoms are not commonly treated with nonprescription medications. OTC medications available for the treatment of pain include nonsteroidal anti-inflammatories (NSAIDs), acetaminophen, and topical analgesics.[17,18] These agents are typically used for up to 10 days for pain relief.[16] See **Table 35.5** for characteristics of commonly used agents.

TABLE 35.5 Commonly Used Analgesics

Drug and Formulation	Dosage
Aspirin (Caplet, tablet, EC tablet)	≥12 years: 325–650 mg q4h (max daily dose: 4,000 mg)
Naproxen (Capsule, tablet)	≥12 years: 200 mg q8–12h (max daily dose: 600 mg)
Ibuprofen (Capsule, suspension, tablet, chewable tablet)	≥12 years: 400 mg q4–6h prn (max daily dose: 3,200 mg) ≥6 months–11 years: 10 mg/kg up to 400 mg (max daily dose: 240 mg)
Acetaminophen (Caplet, capsule, oral liquid, rectal suppository, oral suspension, tablet, chewable tablet, orally disintegrating tablet)	≥12 years: 650–1,000 mg q4–6h prn (max daily dose: 4,000 mg) <12 years: 10–15 mg/kg q4–6h prn (max daily dose: 75 mg/kg/day)

h, hour; max, maximum; prn, as needed; q, every.

Source: Data from Lexicomp Online. Wolters Kluwer Clinical Drug Information. Published 2018.

NONSTEROIDAL ANTI-INFLAMMATORY DRUGS

NSAIDs like aspirin, ibuprofen, and naproxen are first-line agents chosen by many patients to treat mild-to-moderate pain. All three medications work by inhibiting prostaglandin synthesis, which leads to a reduction in pain and inflammation. By inhibiting cyclooxygenase (COX) isoenzymes, COX-1 and COX-2, arachidonic acid binding is blocked. The results of this inhibition include analgesic, antipyretic, and anti-inflammatory pharmacologic effects. These agents have similar efficacy but vary in duration of action and onset. Common side effects associated with using NSAIDs are related to their effects on the gastrointestinal (GI) tract. Patients may complain of epigastric/abdominal pain, heartburn, or bloating. Aspirin is most likely to cause these reported effects. Aspirin may be used at low doses for its cardioprotective effects in addition to using the agent for analgesia. Combining low-dose aspirin with other NSAIDs significantly increases the risk for NSAID-induced GI events, including gastric ulcers, perforation, and bleeding.[17–20]

These analgesics may be available individually or in combination with other medications or analgesics to treat various pain symptoms. Other nonanalgesic active ingredients are combined with analgesics to augment their pharmacologic effects. Caffeine is routinely combined with analgesics to enhance their effects.[21]

Chronic NSAID use may decrease the effectiveness of antihypertensive medications, resulting in loss of blood pressure control. Over time, this may increase the risk of cardiovascular events. Use NSAIDs with caution in patients who have uncontrolled hypertension or cardiovascular disease. Combining NSAIDs with other antiplatelets or anticoagulants may increase bleeding risks. Systemic corticosteroids, which may be used for their anti-inflammatory properties, may also increase risk for GI bleeding in patients who are taking NSAIDs concurrently.[16]

ACETAMINOPHEN

Acetaminophen is a safe option to use in patients who have a history of hypertension or cardiovascular disease.[21] It should be used with caution in patients with a history of liver disease or patients who consume three or more alcoholic beverages daily. Inadvertent overdoses of this medication can occur in patients who use acetaminophen along with OTC combination products containing acetaminophen. It is extremely important that patients adhere to package labeling for acetaminophen regarding maximum daily dosage (see Table 35.5) and dosing frequency to avoid hepatotoxicity.[21]

TOPICAL AGENTS

Topical products may be utilized either alone for mild pain or in combination with systemic analgesics for moderate pain. While there are many combination products available for OTC use, the most common active ingredients will likely include menthol, capsaicin, methyl salicylate, or camphor.[15] These agents are useful for acute, localized pain and are usually applied up to four times daily. They should always be applied to intact skin. These agents may be commercially available individually or in combination with other topical products.

Both camphor and menthol are sensory irritants.[22] They produce a warming or cooling sensation on the skin once applied.[16] Camphor causes excitation in nerve endings, which induces a sensation of relief and masks the more severe sensation of pain. At high doses, it can cause GI distress and CNS toxicity, including seizures and headaches.[16] Menthol's activity when applied topically depends on the concentration of the formulation. It may have a local anesthetic effect or act as a sensory irritant. Menthol can also increase the absorption of other topical agents with which it may be administered.[16] Methyl salicylate increases blood flow to the skin by causing vasodilation. This is reported as a feeling of warmth on the skin by the patient. This agent also inhibits prostaglandin synthesis, which provides pain relief.

HERBALS AND NATURAL PRODUCTS

Herbal products are plant-based dietary substances that may be utilized by patients to treat and prevent a variety of conditions. These products are not approved by the FDA; they do not undergo safety and efficacy trials like nonprescription medications; therefore, patients should be aware that though these substances are plant-based supplements, safety and efficacy have not always been proven.[23] **Table 35.6** displays common herbal products, uses, and dosages. The products may have significant interactions with other prescription or nonprescription medications that the patients may be taking.[15] Patients should consult with healthcare professionals prior to using these agents.

NUTRITION AND SUPPLEMENTATION

VITAMINS AND MINERALS

Vitamins are found in foods consumed by individuals and may also be found in OTC supplements. They can be used to manage diseases due to deficiencies. There are two types of vitamins available: Lipid-soluble and

TABLE 35.6 Herbal Products: Uses and Dosages

Herbal Product	Indications and Dosages	Notes
Cranberry	Use: UTI prevention and treatment Dose: 300–400 mg bid or 8-oz juice tid (3)	Modest efficacy, good tolerability, no documented drug-drug interactions
Saw palmetto	Use: Symptom improvement in BPH Dose: 320 mg daily with extract	Increases bleeding risk with warfarin
Ginkgo	Use: Treat intermittent claudication, cognitive disorders Dose: 120–240 mg daily	Little evidence of efficacy; may cause mild GI upset, increased bleeding time
Garlic	Use: Lower blood pressure and cholesterol, prevention of common cold Dose: 300–1,000 mg extract daily	May cause malodorous scent with breath and body
Echinacea	Use: Decrease cold symptom duration and intensity Dose: 300 mg tid	Limited efficacy for treating infections
Ginseng	Use: Physical and cognitive performance enhancement Dose: 500–3,000 mg daily for root	May increase bleeding risk with other antiplatelets
Green tea	Use: Weight loss, cancer prevention Dose: Three to five cups brewed daily or 400 mg EGCG bid	May cause headaches and dizziness
Aloe	Use: Promote healing of wounds and burns Dose: Apply three to five times/day	—
St. John's wort	Use: Treatment of mild depression Dose: 900 mg daily in three doses of extract	May case mild GI symptoms; CYP3A4 inducer
Soy	Uses: Menopausal symptoms Dose: 40–120 mg daily isoflavones	—
Chamomile	Uses: GI spasms, sedative Dose: One cup tea qd–qid	—
Coenzyme Q-10	Uses: Cardiovascular disease, improve Parkinson's disease, reduce statin-associated side effects Dose: 300 mg daily	—
Glucosamine	Uses: Decrease osteoarthritis pain Dose: 1,500 mg daily	May be combined with chondroitin
Melatonin	Uses: Decrease jet lag symptoms, sleep aid Dose: 3–5 mg at bedtime	—
Fish oil	Uses: Hypertriglyceridemia Dose: 1,000–2,000 mg daily	May be labeled omega-3 fatty acids

bid, twice daily; BPH, benign prostatic hyperplasia; EGCG, epigallocatechin gallate; GI, gastrointestinal; qd, once daily; qid, four times daily; tid, thrice daily; UTI, urinary tract infection.

water-soluble. Fat-soluble vitamins include vitamins A, D, E, and K; all other vitamins are water-soluble.[24] **Table 35.7** lists common uses of selected OTC vitamins and minerals.

ENTERAL SUPPLEMENTS

Enteral nutrition refers to any method of feeding that uses the GI tract to deliver all or part of a person's caloric requirements.[25] Enteral nutrition products can be administered via feeding tube to provide nutrition to patients who are unable to ingest foods or liquids orally. These products are commonly used as nutritional supplements for persons who require additional nutritional sources to meet their caloric needs. They may also be used as a healthy and convenient alternative to skipping meals or consuming unhealthy foods.[26]

Enteral formulas are classified as polymeric, oligomeric, and modular.[24] Polymeric formulas are designed for individuals with normal digestion and are the most commonly used. These formulas usually contain carbohydrate, protein, and fat ranges consistent with the American diet and are generally safe when taken orally. Oligomeric formulas, also known as predigested

TABLE 35.7 Common Uses of Selected Over-the-Counter Vitamins and Minerals

Vitamins and Minerals	Common Uses
Vitamin A	Vision care, immune dysfunction
Vitamin B	B1 (thiamine): Beriberi, Wernicke's encephalopathy, muscle weakness B2 (riboflavin): Metabolism of fat, protein, and carbohydrates B3 (niacin): Pellagra, dyslipidemia B6 (pyridoxine): Peripheral neuropathy B12 (folate): Anemia, depression
Vitamin C	Enhance iron absorption, treat scurvy, decrease duration of symptoms for colds
Vitamin D	Enhance calcium absorption for bone health, rickets
Vitamin E	Peripheral neuropathy, retinopathy
Vitamin K	Blood clotting
Calcium	Osteoporosis, decreased bone mass
Chromium	Glucose metabolism
Fluoride	Prevent dental caries
Iodine	Thyroid supplement
Iron	Iron-deficiency anemia
Phosphorus	Bone maintenance
Zinc	Wound healing, skin integrity, immunocompetence

formulas, require minimal digestive capability. These formulas consist of less complex carbohydrates and an altered fat content to improve absorption. Oligomeric formulas are rarely consumed orally because of poor palatability and usually require medical supervision. Unlike polymeric and oligomeric formulas, modular formulas supply a single macronutrient. These products can be added to foods to increase the intake of the appropriate nutrients and/or calories.[26]

Enteral formulas are used by many individuals because they may be consumed right from their original container or reconstituted from a powder formula. Any unused formula should be reclosed, refrigerated, and used within 48 hours. After removing from the original container, the formula should be covered, refrigerated, and used within 24 hours. Formulas should be kept cool and never microwaved.[25] OTC specialty formulas are available for patients with specific disease states. These products should be used under medical supervision. **Table 35.8** lists commonly used enteral formulas along with nutritional content.

COSMETICS

According to the U.S. Federal Food, Drug, and Cosmetic Act, cosmetics are defined as articles intended to be rubbed, poured, sprinkled, sprayed on, introduced into, or otherwise applied to the human body for cleansing, beautifying, promoting attractiveness, or altering the appearance.[27] A multitude of products are included in this definition, including skin moisturizers, eye and facial makeup preparations, perfumes, lipsticks, shampoos, toothpastes, deodorants, and any material intended for use as a component of a cosmetic product.[28] For the purpose of this chapter, the products will be limited to products for the treatment of acne, dry skin, psoriasis, dandruff, alopecia, and warts.

OVER-THE-COUNTER MEDICATIONS FOR TREATMENT OF ACNE

Acne, a chronic, inflammatory condition that can cause pimples, lesions, papules, and cysts on various parts of the body, affects more than 50 million people in the United States.[29] Though it can affect most age groups, it is most common in adolescents and adults. Acne is caused by clogged hair follicles, bacteria, excess oil production, and complex inflammatory mechanisms. This condition may lead to permanent scarring, depression, poor self-image, and anxiety.[29]

Most OTC acne medications are topical treatments that help kill bacteria or reduce oil production. These products are available in a variety of formulations, including lotions, creams, and scrubs. Benzoyl peroxide, salicylic acid, and topical retinoids are nonprescription medications indicated in the treatment of acne.

Benzoyl Peroxide

Benzoyl peroxide has antibacterial, keratolytic, and comedolytic activity and is recommended as monotherapy for mild acne. It is available in strengths ranging from 2.5% to 10% and is used one to two times daily. Concentrations above 2.5% may not always result in improved efficacy and can increase the risk of adverse effects, including irritation.[27] It can also be used in combination therapy for more severe acne.

Salicylic Acid

Salicylic acid, a comedolytic agent for acne, is available for OTC use in concentrations of 0.5% to 2%. Like benzoyl peroxide, it is used one to two times a day.[27] Although mild, visible peeling may occur as a result of its action; depending on the vehicle used, skin reactions can range from cutaneous irritation to little or no reaction.[29]

TABLE 35.8 Nutritional Summary of Common Oral Enteral Products

Product*	Calories	Protein (g)	CHO (g)	Notes
Boost® Original**,***	240	10	41	Contains CalciLock® (builds and maintains strong bones) and PreBio™ (supports digestive health); available in compact (4-fl oz) size
Ensure® Original Shake**,***	220	9	32	Available in compact size (4 fl oz)
Ensure® Plus**,***	350	13	50	Therapeutic formulation available and used under medical supervision
Boost¯ High Protein**,***	240	15	33	Contains CalciLock® (builds and maintains strong bones)
Ensure® High Protein Shake**,***	160	16	19	Therapeutic formulation available and used under medical supervision
Ensure® Max Protein Nutrition Shake (11 fl oz)**,***	150	30	6	—
Ensure® Light Nutrition Shake**,***	70	12	2	Food supplement only; not to be used for weight reduction
Ensure™ Clear Nutrition Drink (10 fl oz)**,***	180	8	37	—
Jevity® 1.0 Cal**,***	250	10.4	36.5	Fiber-fortified therapeutic nutrition; use under medical supervision
Jevity® 1.2 Cal**,***	285	13.2	40.2	
Jevity® 1.5 Cal**,***	355	15.1	51.1	
Juven® (23-g packets)**,***	80	2.5	4.2	Use under medical supervision
Diabetes				
Boost® Glucose Control**,***	190	16	16	
Glucerna¯ Shake**,***	180	10	16	
Glucerna® Therapeutic Nutrition Shake**,***	220	10	26	
Glucerna® 1.0 Cal**,***	237	9.9	22.8	
Glucerna® 1.2 Cal**,***	285	14.2	27.1	
Glucerna® 1.5 Cal**,***	356	19.6	31.5	
Renal Disorders				
Suplena® with CARBSTEADY**,***	425	10.6	46.4	Use as an oral or feeding tube in patients with stage 3 or 4 CKD or nondialyzed patients without PEW; use under medical supervision
Nepro® with CARBSTEADY**,***	425	19.1	37.9	Use as an oral or feeding tube in patients on dialysis with stage 5 CKD; use under medical supervision
Renalcal®**,***	500	8.5	73	Calorie dense; use under medical supervision
Respiratory Disorders				
PULMOCARE® (1 L)**,***	1,500	62.6	105.7	Use under medical supervision

*Eight fluid ounces unless otherwise noted.
**Gluten-free.
***Kosher.

CHO, carbohydrate; CKD, chronic kidney disease; fl, fluid; L, liter; oz, ounce; PEW, protein energy wasting.

Source: Abbott Nutrition for Healthcare Professionals. *Adult products.* Accessed January 17, 2019. https://abbottnutrition.com/adult; Nestle Health Science. *Sitemap.* Accessed January 19, 2019. https://www.nestlehealthscience.us/info/sitemap

Topical Retinoids

Nonprescription topical retinoids are synthetic vitamin A also used to treat acne. Topical retinoids are effective due to their ability to normalize follicular hyperkeratosis and prevent formation of acne.[30] Adapalene 0.1% gel is the first FDA-approved, prescription-strength retinoid product available without a prescription.[31] It should be applied once at bedtime and therapeutic effects should be seen within 8 to 12 weeks. Common side effects include xeroderma, exfoliation of the skin, erythema, and burning or stinging of the skin.[32] In addition to the topical formulation, oral vitamin A and prescription products are also available.

OVER-THE-COUNTER MEDICATIONS FOR TREATMENT OF DRY SKIN, PSORIASIS, AND DANDRUFF

Dry skin, or xerosis, is caused by a decrease in the water content of the skin that leads to an abnormal loss of skin cells. Dry skin has a variety of causes including dry air; not drinking enough water; detergent use; dehydration; damage to skin; and long, hot showers. Symptoms include itching, roughness, scaling, loss of flexibility, and ichthyosis. The goals of treatment include restoring rehydration and function of the skin.[33]

Nonprescription medications are available to treat these conditions. Many of the treatment options may be used for more than one condition. Treatment of dry skin should include moisturizers, oils, and emollients that may be applied several times daily as needed.[33] Some products that may be applied topically include petrolatum, glycerin, lanolin, and ammonium lactate. They should be applied generously to the body shortly after baths or showers to lock in moisture. Emollients applied up to three times daily are optimal to keep the skin moisturized. Anti-itch medications, like topical corticosteroids, may also be used to minimize any discomfort associated with dry skin.[33]

Psoriasis is a chronic inflammatory disease caused by accelerated growth of skin cells that causes raised, red scales and patches to appear on the skin. Psoriasis can appear anywhere on the body, although it commonly affects the elbows, knees, and scalp. Symptoms of psoriasis include red patches on the skin with silvery scales; itching; burning; stinging; and dry, cracked skin. Psoriasis is not contagious.[34]

Topical medications are normally utilized as first-line treatment for mild episodes of psoriasis. The FDA recommends that mild cases (no more than a few isolated lesions, no larger than a quarter) of psoriasis be treated with nonprescription medications. For larger affected areas, the presence of joint pain, and involvement of the face, prescription medications are recommended. OTC options for the treatment of psoriasis include

salicylic acid, coal tar, anti-Malassezia products, and combination products.[34]

Dandruff is an inflammatory condition affecting the scalp. Due to the scalp scaling seen with dandruff, patients may be embarrassed by the condition since it carries a negative social stigma. Dandruff is the result of increased epidermal cellular turnover and keratinization. This process leads to flaking and pruritus. Treatment should focus on slowing the rate of epidermal cellular turnover, which will minimize itching and scaling. Agents used to treat dandruff include pyrithione zinc, coal tar, salicylic acid, selenium sulfide, and ketoconazole.[32] **Table 35.9** displays commonly used OTC medications for the treatment of these disorders.

OVER-THE-COUNTER MEDICATIONS FOR TREATMENT OF WARTS

Warts, a common skin disorder caused by human papillomaviruses, affect 7% to 10% of the population.[35] Common warts most often occur on the fingers, nails, and back of the hands and are usually skin-colored or brown and dome-shaped. Plantar warts occur in weight-bearing areas, like the soles of the feet, and grow flat and inward.[35]

Salicylic acid and cryotherapy are nonprescription products available for the treatment of warts. Salicylic acid concentrations of 5% to 40% are available in various formulations, including pads, strips, patches, disks, gels, and liquids. These products should not be used on moles, birthmarks, warts on the face, patients with diabetes, and patients with impaired circulation.[36] Cryotherapy works by freezing and destroying the wart tissue. A combination of dimethyl ether and propane are approved for OTC use for the treatment of both common and plantar warts. Improper use can cause damage to adjacent unaffected areas of the skin. A persistent wart can be treated only three times using these products. Complete removal of warts when using these products may take up to 4 to 12 weeks. If the wart is still present after 12 weeks of treatment, the patient should consult a clinician.[36]

This form of therapy should not be used on patients younger than 4 years of age, on those who are pregnant or breastfeeding, or on those who have diabetes or poor circulation.[36]

OVER-THE-COUNTER MEDICATIONS FOR THE TREATMENT OF ALOPECIA

Hair loss is a problem that affects up to 50% of the population.[33] Androgenetic alopecia, also known as male-pattern or female-pattern baldness, is a common cause of hair loss.[37] Minoxidil is the only FDA-approved agent indicated for the treatment of androgenic alopecia of the scalp. It works in several ways to cause a stimulation of hair growth. It causes vasodilation, which is increased cutaneous blood flow and stimulation of resting hair

TABLE 35.9 Commonly Used Cosmetics Products

Ingredient	Use	Formulation
Benzoyl peroxide	Acne	Cream: 10% Foam: 5.3%–9.8% Foaming cloths: 6% Gel and liquid: 2.5%–10% Lotion: 5%–10%
Hydrocortisone	Eczema, psoriasis, atopic dermatitis (mild-to-moderate), seborrheic dermatitis	Cream, ointment, and solution: 0.1%–2.5% Lotion: 0.1%–2%
Salicylic acid	Acne, hyperkeratotic skin conditions (including warts)	Gel: 2% Liquid: 2%–3% Solution: 16.7%–17% Pad: 0.5%–2%, 40%
Coal tar	Dandruff, seborrhea dermatitis, psoriasis	Foam and ointment: 2% Shampoo: 0.5%–10% Solution: 20%
Ketoconazole	Dandruff	Shampoo: 1%
Minoxidil	Alopecia	Foam: 5% Solution: 2%–5%
Pyrithione zinc	Dandruff, seborrhea dermatitis, hyperkeratotic skin conditions	Bar and shampoo: 2% Liquid (body wash): 0.5%
Salicylic acid (alone or in combination with coal tar or sulfur)	Dandruff, seborrhea dermatitis, psoriasis	Gel and shampoo: 2%–3%
Selenium sulfide	Dandruff, seborrheic dermatitis	Shampoo: 1%

Source: Data from Lexicomp Online. Wolters Kluwer Clinical Drug Information. Published 2018.

follicles.[38] It is recommended for use in men who have general thinning of hair at the vertex of the scalp and in women who have general thinning of hair in fronto-parietal areas.[39] Patients with heart disease should undergo a risk assessment prior to using minoxidil due to a potential risk of systemic absorption.[40] Minoxidil should not be used if the degree of hair loss is different than that shown on the product labeling; if no family history of hair loss is present or hair loss is sudden and/or patchy; if hair loss is associated with childbirth or the reason for hair loss is unknown; if the scalp is red, inflamed, infected, irritated, painful; or if other medicines are used on the scalp.[38] The product is also not intended for use in pediatric patients younger than 18 years of age.[39]

Patients should discontinue use and contact a clinician if they experience chest pain, rapid heartbeat, faintness, dizziness, or sudden unexplained weight gain after using minoxidil. The product should also be discontinued if swelling of the hands or feet occurs, scalp irritation or redness develops, unwanted facial hair growth occurs, or if hair regrowth is not seen in 4 to 6 months.[38] Common side effects include local erythema (6%), pruritus (6%), dryness, scaling/flaking, and local irritation or burning. Patients may experience hair discoloration with minoxidil use.[38]

FIRST-AID PRODUCTS

A variety of first-aid products are available OTC. These products may be recommended for the treatment of minor injuries, including minor burns, scrapes, wounds, and insect bites and stings. Antihistamines, analgesics, local anesthetics, antiseptics, and antibiotics are examples of products that may be useful in relieving pain, decreasing swelling and inflammation, disinfecting, and preventing infections.[41] Table 35.10 displays commonly used OTC first-aid products.

CONCLUSION

Patients may seek out nonprescription medications to treat and prevent a variety of medical conditions. Due to the large number of individual and combination products available for OTC use, clinicians must play an active role in helping patients choose the most appropriate therapy for their conditions. Clinicians should also help patients differentiate the various products available for use, be empowered to confidently recommend nonprescription medications, and instruct patients on how to safely utilize these products.

TABLE 35.10 Selected Over-the-Counter First-Aid Products

Active Ingredient	Use	Dosage
Bacitracin (alone or in combination with polymyxin B, neomycin, and/or pramoxine)	Prevention of infection in minor cuts, scrapes, or burns	Adult and pediatric: Apply qd–tid; do not use longer than 1 week unless recommended by a prescriber
Benzocaine	Management of pain and prevention of infection caused by minor skin irritations, burns, sunburn, and insect bites	Dermal irritation (adults and children >2 years): topical (external) spray 5% and 20% or ointment 5%—apply to affected area or use one spray qd–qid prn; in cases of bee stings, remove stinger before treatment Poison ivy/sumac: Topical (external) spray 5% (Ivy–Rid® only): Spray affected area until wet
Diphenhydramine (1%–2%)	Management of pain and itching associated with insect bites; sunburn; scrapes; minor cuts, skin irritations, and burns; rashes due to poison ivy, poison oak, and poison sumac	Apply to affected area qd–qid
Hydrocortisone (0.1%–2.5%)	Management of inflammation and itching associated with poison ivy, oak, sumac, insect bites, and minor skin irritation	Apply a thin film to affected area and rub gently
Hydrogen peroxide (1.5%–3%)	Antiseptic used to clean minor wounds or abrasions; mouthwash for minor dental irritations	Apply qd–tid or swish solution in mouth for 1 minute, then expectorate qd–qid
Iodine 2% solution	Antiseptic used to manage minor wounds	Apply to affected area prn; product may stain the skin; iodine tincture less preferred due to skin irritation
Isopropyl alcohol (70%)	Antiseptic used to prevent infections associated with minor burns or cuts/scrapes	Apply prn to clean intact skin
Lidocaine	Local anesthetic	Apply externally bid–qid

bid, twice daily; prn, as needed; qd, once daily; qid, four times daily; tid, thrice daily.
Source: Data from Lexicomp Online. Wolters Kluwer Clinical Drug Information. Published 2018.

CASE EXEMPLAR: Patient With Knee Pain Secondary to Osteoarthritis

MP is a 70-year-old female who presents to the clinician's office for a routine check-up. Her complaint at today's visit is the pain in her knees secondary to osteoarthritis for the last 3 days. She describes the pain as a 4 on a scale of 1 to 10. She has been using cold compresses on her knees every evening but has experienced little relief of her pain symptoms.

Past Medical History
- Gastroesophageal reflux disease
- Hypertension
- Osteoarthritis
- Seasonal allergies
- Atrial fibrillation
- No known drug allergies

Medications
- Cetirizine, 10 mg once daily
- Hydrochlorothiazide, 12.5 mg once daily
- Ranitidine, 75 mg once nightly
- Warfarin, 2.5 mg once daily (INR 2.7)
- Sotalol, 80 mg twice daily
- Multivitamin, once daily

Social History
- MP is a smoker, half a pack per day
- Reports rare consumption of alcohol

Physical Examination
- Review of symptoms unremarkable

Labs
- Within normal limits

Discussion Questions

1. Which health conditions may impact the over-the-counter (OTC) analgesic recommendation?
2. Which OTC analgesic is recommended for MP, and how should MP be counseled to take this medication?
3. MP has also requested a topical agent to rub on her knees. What OTC product is recommended?

CASE EXEMPLAR: Pediatric Patient With Nonproductive Cough

HM is a 6-year-old female who is brought to the clinic by her mother with complaints that HM's cough has gotten worse over the past 48 hours. It started with just an occasional cough and now the cough is keeping everyone awake at night.

Past Medical History
- No past history of surgeries or significant injuries
- Otitis media 1 year ago, treated successfully with antibiotics
- No known drug allergies
- Wore a helmet to correct cranial deformities at age 6 to 9 months

Medications
- Children's vitamins
- Acetaminophen for pain

Social History
- Outside in sun almost every day (pool in backyard)

Physical Examination
- Vital signs normal for age
- Afebrile
- Lungs: Clear with coughing; no wheezing

Next Steps
- Medication for cough and consider medication for allergies

Discussion Questions
1. What factors will the clinician consider when suggesting medications for HM?
2. What medication will the clinician choose to treat HM's cough?
3. When providing patient education to HM and her mother, what side effects associated with the recommended medication should the clinician highlight?

CLINICAL PEARLS

- Before recommending nonprescription medications, review current medications to ensure there are no potential drug–drug or drug–disease interactions.
- Counsel patients to pay attention to the active ingredients of OTC products and never take two medications with the same ingredients.
- Counsel patients about the importance of following product labeling to prevent unintentional medication overdoses or inappropriate use.
- Ensure that patients store nonprescription medications up and away from children to avoid inadvertent use.
- Advise patients to use proper measurement tools when administering nonprescription medications to children.
- Direct patients to discontinue nonprescription medication use if symptom resolution does not occur within the time frame listed on the package labeling.

KEY TAKEAWAYS

- OTC medications are often the first line of therapy for treating minor conditions or symptoms. Many adults use them as a first response, believing that use of nonprescription medications will help lower their healthcare costs.
- Nonproductive coughs are treated with antitussives such as codeine, dextromethorphan, diphenhydramine, and cloprednol. Guaifenesin, the only FDA-approved expectorant, works by increasing hydration of the respiratory tract and promoting the removal of secretions.
- Options available to treat allergy symptoms include intranasal steroids, antihistamines, decongestants, and other agents. Intranasal corticosteroids are the preferred initial treatment of nasal symptoms. Second-generation antihistamines are preferred because they cause less sedation and cognitive effects. Oral and nasal decongestants may pose a risk to hypertensive patients.

- OTC analgesics treat mild-to-moderate pain. Chronic and severe pain are not commonly treated with nonprescription medications. NSAIDs, aspirin, ibuprofen, and naproxen are first-line agents for moderate pain.
- Two types of vitamins are available: lipid-soluble (A, D, E, and K) and water-soluble (B and C). Fat-soluble can become toxic if taken in excess.
- Enteral formulas are classified as polymeric, oligomeric, and modular. Polymeric formulas are designed for individuals with normal digestion, oligomeric formulas require minimal digestive capability, and modular formulas supply a single macronutrient.
- Benzoyl peroxide, salicylic acid, and topical retinoids are nonprescription medications indicated in the treatment of acne.
- Topical medications are normally utilized as first-line treatment for mild episodes of psoriasis.

REFERENCES

1. Consumer Healthcare Products Association. *Statistics on OTC use.* Accessed January 17, 2019. https://www.chpa.org/about-consumer-healthcare/research-data/otc-use-statistics.
2. Sobotka J, Kochanowski BA. Self-care and nonprescription pharmacotherapy. In: Krinsky DL, Ferreri SP, Hemstreet BA, et al., eds. *Handbook of Nonprescription Drugs: An Interactive Approach to Self-Care.* 19th ed. American Pharmacists Association; 2018. doi:10.21019/9781582122656.ch1
3. U.S. Department of Health and Human Services, Center for Disease Control and Prevention, National Center for Health Statistics. *National ambulatory medical care survey.* Published 2015. https://www.cdc.gov/nchs/data/ahcd/namcs_summary/2015_namcs_web_tables.pdf
4. Irwin R. Introduction to the diagnosis and management of cough: ACCP evidence-based clinical practice guidelines. *Chest.* 2006;129:25S–27S. doi:10.1378/chest.129.1_suppl.25S
5. Lexicomp Online. *Codeine.* Wolters Kluwer Clinical Drug Information. Published 2018. http://webstore.lexi.com/ONLINE
6. U.S. Food and Drug Administration. FDA Drug Safety Communication: *FDA requires labeling changes for prescription opioid cough and cold medicines to limit their use to adults 18 years and older.* Published January 11, 2018. https://www.fda.gov/Drugs/Drugsafety/ucm590435.html
7. Lexicomp Online. *Dextromethorphan.*Wolters Kluwer Clinical Drug Information. Published 2018. http://webstore.lexi.com/ONLINE
8. U.S. Food and Drug Administration. Cold, cough, allergy, bronchodilator, and antiasthmatic drug products for over-the-counter human use. *CFR: Code of Federal Regulations*, Title 21, Part 341. Updated April 1, 2018. https://www.accessdata.fda.gov/scripts/cdrh/cfdocs/cfcfr/CFRSearch.cfm?CFRPart=341&showFR=1
9. Lexicomp Online. *Diphenhydramine.* Wolters Kluwer Clinical Drug Information. Published 2019. http://webstore.lexi.com/ONLINE
10. Lexicomp Online. *Chlophedianol.* Wolters Kluwer Clinical Drug Information. Published 2018. http://webstore.lexi.com/ONLINE
11. Tietze K. *Handbook of Nonprescription Drugs: An Interactive Approach to Self-Care.* 18th ed. American Pharmacists Association; 201.
12. Lexicomp Online. Guaifenesin.Wolters Kluwer Clinical Drug Information. Published 2018. http://webstore.lexi.com/ONLINE
13. Rondanelli M, Miccono A, Lamburghini S, et al. Self-care for common colds: The pivotal role of vitamin D, vitamin C, zinc and *Echinacea* in three main immune interactive clusters (physical barriers, innate and adaptive immunity) involved during an episode of common colds—Practical advice on dosages and on the time to take these nutrients/botanicals in order to prevent or treat common colds. *Evid Based Complement Alternat Med.* 2018;2018:1–36. doi:10.1155/2018/5813095
14. Dykewicz M, Wallace D, Baroody F, et al. Treatment of seasonal allergic rhinitis: an evidence-based focused 2017 guidelines update. *Ann Allergy Asthma Immunol.* 2017;119(6):489–511. doi:10.1016/j.anai.2017.08.012
15. Krinsky DL, Ferreri SP, Hemstreet BA, et al. *Handbook of Nonprescription Drugs: An Interactive Approach to Self-Care.*19th ed. American Pharmacists Association; 2018.
16. Pain. In: *Funk & Wagnalls New World Encyclopedia*; Funk & Wagnalls 2017:1. Accessed September 28, 2018. https://www.cc-pl.org/funk-wagnalls-new-world-encyclopedia
17. Shawn L. Essential oils. In: Hoffman RS, Howland M, Lewin NA, et al. eds. *Goldfrank's Toxicologic Emergencies.* 10th ed. McGraw-Hill; 2015. http://accesspharmacy.mhmedical.com/content.aspx?bookid=1163&sectionid=65094215
18. Lexi-Drugs Online. *Naproxen.* Wolters Kluwer Clinical Drug Information. Published 2019. Updated January 2, 2019. http://webstore.lexi.com/ONLINE
19. Lexi-Drugs Online. *Ibuprofen.* Wolters Kluwer Clinical Drug Information. Published 2019. Updated January 2, 2019. http://webstore.lexi.com/ONLINE
20. Lexi-Drugs Online. *Aspirin.* Wolters Kluwer Clinical Drug Information. Published 2019. Updated December 14, 2018. http://webstore.lexi.com/ONLINE
21. Lipton RB, Diener HC, Robbins MS, et al. Caffeine in the management of patients with headache. *J Headache Pain.* 2017;18(1):107. doi:10.1186/s10194-017-0806-2
22. Lexi-Drugs Online. *Acetaminophen.* Wolters Kluwer Clinical Drug Information. 2019. Updated January 2, 2019. http://webstore.lexi.com/ONLINE
23. Katzung BG, Kruidering-Hall M, Trevor AJ, eds. Dietary supplements & herbal medications. In: *Katzung & Trevor's*

Pharmacology: Examination & Board Review. 12th ed. McGraw-Hill; 2018. http://accesspharmacy.mhmedical.com/content.aspx?bookid=2465&sectionid=197947087

24. Fabian E, Bogner M, Kickinger A, et al. Intake of medication and vitamin status in the elderly. *Ann Nutr Metab*. 2011;58(2):118–125. doi:10.1159/000327351

25. Terrie E. *Medical food and meal replacement nutritional supplements*. Pharmacy Times Website. Published January 9, 2015. https:// www.pharmacytimes.com/publications/issue/2015/january2015/medical-food-and-meal-replacement-nutritional-supplements

26. Rollins C, Baker C. Functional and meal replacement folds. In: Krinsky DL, Ferreri SP, Hemstreet BA, et al., eds. *Handbook of Nonprescription Drugs: An Interactive Approach to Self-Care*. 19th ed. American Pharmacists Association; 2018.

27. U.S. Food & Drug Administration Website. *Cosmetics & U.S. Law*. Accessed November 30, 2018. https://www.fda.gov/cosmetics/guidanceregulation/lawsregulations/ucm2005209.htm#Intro

28. Abbott Nutrition for Healthcare Professionals. *Adult products*. Accessed January 17, 2019. https://abbottnutrition.com/adult

29. Zaenglein AL, Pathy AL, Schlosser BJ, et al. Guidelines of care for the management of acne vulgaris. *J Am Acad Dermatol*. 2016 May;74(5):945–73.e33. doi:10.1016/j.jaad.2015.12.037

30. Gollnick H, Cunliffe W, Berson D, et al. Management of acne: a report from a global alliance to improve outcomes in acne. *J Am Acad Dermatol*. 2003;49(1 suppl):S1–S37. doi:10.1067/mjd.2003.618

31. Galderma Laboratories. *Differin*. Accessed June 11, 2019. https://www.differin.com/healthcare-professional

32. Lexi-Drugs Online. *Adapalene*. Wolters Kluwer Clinical Drug Information. Published 2019. Updated June 7, 2019. http://webstore.lexi.com/ONLINE

33. Benner KW. Atopic dermatitis and dry skin. In: Krinsky DL, Ferreri SP, Hemstreet BA, et al., eds. *Handbook of Nonprescription Drugs: An Interactive Approach to Self-Care*. 19th ed. American Pharmacists Association; 2018.

34. Kim W, Jerome D, Yeung J. Diagnosis and management of psoriasis. *Can Fam Physician*. 2017;63:278–285. https://www.cfp.ca/content/63/4/278

35. Adkins DM. Warts. In: Krinsky DL, Ferreri SP, Hemstreet BA, et al., eds. *Handbook of Nonprescription Drugs: An Interactive Approach to Self-Care*. 19th ed. American Pharmacists Association; 2018.

36. Mansukhai RP, Volino L. Scaly dermatoses. In: Krinsky DL, Ferreri SP, Hemstreet BA, et al., eds. *Handbook of Nonprescription Drugs: An Interactive Approach to Self-Care*. 19th ed. American Pharmacists Association; 2018:chap 34. doi:10.21019/9781582122656.ch34

37. Mounsey A, Reed S. Diagnosing and treating hair loss. *Am Fam Physician*. 2009;80(4):356–362. https://www.aafp.org/afp/2009/0815/afp20090815p356.pdf

38. U.S. National Library of Medicine. *Androgenetic alopecia*. Accessed December 30, 2018. https://ghr.nlm.nih.gov/condition/androgenetic-alopecia#

39. Lexicomp Online, Lexi-Drugs Online. *Minoxidil*. Wolters Kluwer Clinical Drug Information. Published 2018. http://webstore.lexi.com/ONLINE

40. Lexicomp Online, AHFS essentials (Adult and Pediatric). *Minoxidil*. Wolters Kluwer Clinical Drug Information. Published 2018.

41. Bernard D. Minor burns, sunburn and wounds. In: Krinsky DL, Ferreri SP, Hemstreet BA, et al., eds. *Handbook of Nonprescription Drugs: An Interactive Approach to Self-Care*. 19th ed. American Pharmacists Association; 2018

Pharmacotherapy for Obesity

Seleda Williams and Dennis M. Styne

LEARNING OBJECTIVES

- Define obesity in adult and pediatric populations.
- Summarize the physiological control of weight and appetite.
- Complete a comparative list of hormones involved in weight gain and satiety.
- Categorize FDA approved pharmaceutical agents for weight control based on their physiologic targets.
- Summarize challenges specific to the therapeutic interventions for children, youth, and adults with obesity.
- Be able to discuss the indications, general dosing guidelines, contraindications, and side effects related to prescribing anti-obesity drugs.

INTRODUCTION

Three quarters of U.S. adults and 18.5% of U.S. children and adolescents are either overweight or obese.[1,2] This data is troubling because obesity is one of the major contributors to chronic disease in the United States today.[3] New obesity treatments, including medications, are being explored to complement lifestyle medicine approaches. Weight-loss drugs, also referred to as obesity and/or anti-obesity drugs, are used primarily in the treatment of overweight and obesity. These drugs should be used in conjunction with a reduced-calorie diet, a physical activity plan, and other lifestyle changes.

This chapter is composed of two sections: Part I, Adult Obesity, will discuss U.S. Food and Drug Administration (FDA)-approved weight-loss drugs used for the treatment of of adult overweight and obesity. Part II, Pediatric Obesity, will discuss challenges and recom- mendations for treating obese pediatric age groups with anti-obesity drugs.. It will also review anti-obesity drug pharmacology, safety, and efficacy, as well as key national guidelines on treatment of overweight and obesity. Part I of this chapter focuses on adult obesity, and Part II covers pediatric obesity.

PART I: ADULT OBESITY

DEFINITION AND PREVALENCE OF ADULT OBESITY

The U.S. Centers for Disease Control and Prevention (CDC) defines adult overweight as a body mass index (BMI) of 25.0 kg/m^2 to less than 30 kg/m^2 and obesity as a BMI of 30 kg/m^2 or higher.[4]

Data from the 2017 to 2018 U.S. National Health and Nutrition Examination Survey (NHANES) indicated that the age-adjusted prevalence of obesity in U.S. adults was 42.4%.[2] The situation is particularly dire for certain racial/ethnic groups, with the highest rate of obesity found in adult African American (AA) women, at a concerning rate of 56.9% compared to 39.8% for White females.[2] The prevalence of obesity among American Indian adults is reported at 36.9%.[5] The lowest rates are seen in non-Hispanic Asian adults at 17.4%.[2] Trends of obesity have shown that between 1980 and 2000, U.S. rates of obesity increased significantly for adult men and women[6] More recently, between 2005 and 2014, the prevalence of obesity increased significantly among women, but not for men.[6]

COMORBIDITIES ASSOCIATED WITH OVERWEIGHT AND OBESITY

Excess weight is associated with increased risk of coronary heart disease, ischemic stroke, hypertension, type 2 diabetes mellitus, metabolic syndrome, certain types of cancers, gallstones, osteoarthritis, benign prostatic hyperplasia, nonalcoholic fatty liver disease, and many other weight-related illnesses.[7] The estimated global cost of obesity has been as high as $2 trillion or 2.8% of gross domestic product (GDP).[7,8] In the United States alone, obesity cost was estimated up to $149.4 billion in 2014.[9]

ETIOLOGY OF OBESITY

It is clear from the evidence that the leading contributors to obesity are lifestyle related. Excluding metabolic and genetic abnormalities, environmental factors such as excessive intake of calories, inadequate physical activity, behavioral problems, and psychosocial stressors may all contribute to excessive weight gain.[10] Single gene defects and syndromes have been found to contribute to obesity but at a relatively lower rate compared to environmental and lifestyle factors.[10–12]

In general, research shows that obesity is a complex multifactorial disorder. For example, the history of slavery, racism, and inequalities in the United States has been found to contribute to the increased risk of overweight and obesity in the African American population.[13,14] Additionally, public health officials have noticed, among other factors, a correlation with rising obesity rates and the increased marketing and access to fast foods, larger portions, and decreased physical activity in the workplace.[15,16] However, this diet-centric theory still does not explain all the causes of obesity.[10] Biochemical studies have revealed other primary causes to include: melanocortin-4 receptor mutation, leptin deficiency, pro-opiomelanocortin (POMC) deficiency, and genetic syndromes such as Prader-Willi; Bardet-Biedl; and Cohen, Alström, and Froehlich. Neurological causes include brain injury, brain tumor, consequences of cranial irradiation, and hypothalamic obesity. Endocrine causes include hypothyroidism (in adult obesity), Cushing syndrome, growth hormone deficiency, and pseudohypoparathyroidism. Drug-induced causes include use of tricyclic antidepressants, oral contraceptives, antipsychotics, anticonvulsants, glucocorticoids, sulfonylureas, glitazones, and beta-blockers.[17] Psychological causes include depression associated with overeating and eating disorders, such as binge eating disorder. **Box 36.1** summarizes the primary and secondary causes of obesity.

In addition to medical and lifestyle treatment, underlying psychosocial causes of obesity in all Americans, including the built environment, socioeconomic status, incarceration rates, and education, are important additional factors to address the obesity epidemic in America today.

PHYSIOLOGIC PATHWAYS RELATED TO OBESITY

Scientific investigations have elucidated many of the gastrointestinal (GI), adipose and neuroendocrine pathways that affect hunger and satiety. This progress has also been occurring in parallel with drug research

---

BOX 36.1
PRIMARY AND SECONDARY CAUSES OF OBESITY

Primary Causes (Rare)
- Melanocortin-4 receptor mutation
- Leptin deficiency
- Pro-opiomelanocortin (POMC) deficiency
- Prader–Willi syndrome
- Bardet–Biedl syndrome
- Cohen, Alström, and Froehlich syndromes
- Other rare types of genetic conditions

Secondary Causes (Most Common)
- Environmental
- Endocrine: Hypothyroidism (adult obesity), Cushing syndrome, growth hormone deficiency, pseudohypoparathyroidism
- Psychological: Depression associated with overeating, binging, and eating disorders
- Neurologic: Brain injury, brain tumor, cranial irradiation, hypothalamic
- Drug-induced: Use of tricyclic antidepressants, oral contraceptives, antipsychotics, anticonvulsants, glucocorticoids, sulfonylureas, glitazones, and beta-blockers

---

on weight loss drugs and on how these biological pathways intersect with drug mechanisms of action. These satiety and hunger neuro-hormonal pathways are complex, and a detailed discussion is beyond the scope of this chapter. However, it is important to understand these pathways, in general terms, in the context of weight loss drug mechanisms of action.

Hunger and satiety are also associated with other organ systems such as vision, hearing, taste, and smell which trigger hunger or satiety signals to the GI, adipose, endocrine, and nervous systems. Animal and human research have identified key hormones in adipose tissue, as well as the stomach, intestines, pancreas, and liver, that interact with positive and negative feedback hormonal and neuronal pathways to the neuroendocrine systems in the pituitary, hypothalamus, and brainstem. For example, once food is ingested, distention of the GI tract is communicated to the brain. **Figure 36.1** illustrates the main physiological pathways and regulations of food intake.

SATIETY (ANORECTIC) HORMONES

Satiety is a state of inhibition over further eating that is regulated by various hormones that reduce appetite and

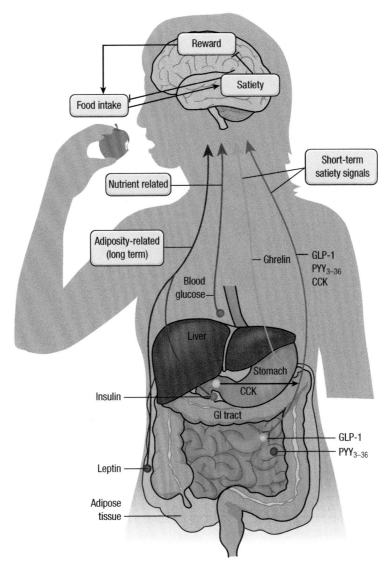

FIGURE 36.1 Hormonal and nutrient regulations of food intake.
CCK, cholecystokinin K, GI, gastrointestinal; GLP-1, glucagon-like peptide; PYY, peptide YY.

make one feel full. These hormones include peptide YY (PYY), secreted by the ileum and colon, and cholecystokinin K (CCK), secreted in the duodenum. There are also other gastric inhibitory hormones, such as gastric inhibitory polypeptide (GIP), secreted by K cells in the duodenum and jejunum, and glucagon-like peptide-1 (GLP-1), secreted by the L cells in the ileum. GIP and GLP-1 are primarily secreted in response to glucose and promote insulin secretion from the pancreas and satiety. Many of these signals are transmitted to the brain via the vagal afferent fibers that synapse in the nucleus tractus solitarius (NTS) in the hindbrain resulting in satiety. Another anorectic hormone that has been discovered to promote satiety is leptin, which is secreted from adipose tissue. It inhibits neuro peptide Y/agouti-related peptide (NPY/AgRP) neurons, which activate pro-opiomelanocortin/cocaine amphetamine-related transcript neuron (POMC/CART) secretion in the ar-

cuate nucleus of the hypothalamus. These pathways result in food reward, decreased food intake, and increased energy expenditure.[17,18] **Figure 36.2** illustrates the hormonal circuits regulating satiety.

HUNGER (OREXIGENIC HORMONE)

Hunger is initiated by complex central and peripheral orexigenic signals that promote feeding. Ghrelin is produced in the stomach and is considered the only known hunger-generating hormone to date.[7] Ghrelin also activates growth hormone secretion. It does this by activating the growth hormone receptor called growth hormone secretagogue receptor (GHS-R). It regulates feeding via the arcuate nucleus by activating GHS-R on the NPY/AgRP neurons in the arcuate nucleus. This increases expression of the NPY/AgRP neurons stimulating the release of gamma-aminobutyric acid (GABA) onto the

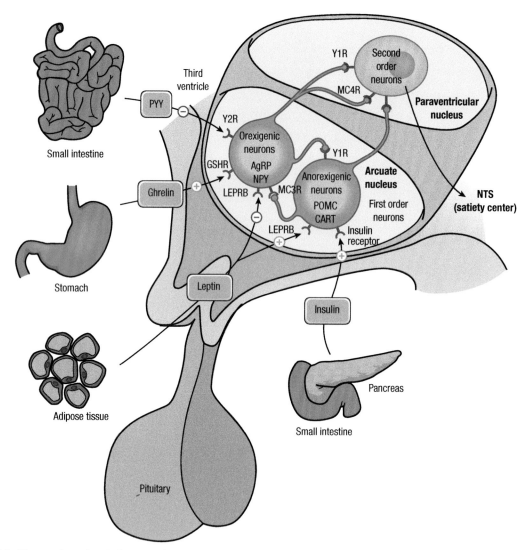

FIGURE 36.2 Hunger (orexigenic hormone). Hormonal circuits from the gut and fat that impact the sensations of hunger and satiety that are exerted via hypothalamic neuroendocrine pathways.

AgRP, agouti-related peptide; CART, cocaine- and amphetamine-regulated transcript; GSHR, growth hormone secretagogue receptor; LEPRB, leptin receptor; MC3R, melanocortin-3 receptor; MC4R, melanocortin-4 receptor; NPY, neuro peptide Y; NTS, nucleus tractus solitarius; POMC, pro-opiomelanocortin; PYY, peptide tyrosine–tyrosine; Y1R, NPY receptor 1 Y2R, NPY receptor 2.

Source: Adapted from Medical Biochemistry Page, LLC.

POMC neurons, reducing or suppressing the anorexic effects of the POMC neurons.[7] **Box 36.2** summarizes the key hormones and neurons in appetite control.

HISTORY OF PHARMACOTHERAPY FOR OBESITY

The treatment of overweight and obesity can be traced back to ancient history and includes descriptions in medical writings from ancient Egypt, Babylon, China, Greece, Rome, and Meso-America.[19,20] Early treatments recognized the value of a healthy lifestyle, but also included herbal preparations and tinctures. In the 16th century, tobacco was introduced in Europe; it contained nicotine, known to decrease appetite and increase energy expenditure, and was used as a treatment for obesity.[21] The advance of science led to the

isolation of "thyroid extract" in 1893, which was found to have weight-loss effects.[21] It later became apparent that inappropriate use of thyroid extracts could lead to hyperthyroidism and other sequalae.[22]

The 20th century led to the development of dinitrophenol (1934) and amphetamine (1937), which were found to have effects on body weight. However, these drugs came with significant side effects. For example, dinitrophenol can lead to cataracts and neuropathies, whereas amphetamine can lead to addiction and other cardiac and neurological side effects.[21,22]

Obesity drug treatments in the 19th and 20th centuries foreshadowed the future difficulties in finding safe and effective drug treatments for obesity. Over the past few decades, about 30 medicinal products have been approved internationally for treating obesity. However,

BOX 36.2
KEY HORMONES AND NEURONS IN APPETITE CONTROL

Orexigenic/Anabolic

- Ghrelin
- Arcuate nucleus: First-order NPY/AgRP neurons stimulated by ghrelin

Anorectic/Catabolic

- Leptin: Adipose tissue
- CCK: Secreted by the small intestine
- PYY: Secreted by the ileum and colon
- GLP-1: Cosecreted by L cells in the intestine; incretin effect—stimulates insulin
- POMC/CART neurons

CCK, cholecystokinin; POMC/CART: pro-opiomelanocortin/cocaine- and amphetamine-regulated transcript; GLP-1, glucagon-like peptide; NPY/AgRP, neuropeptide Y/agouti-related protein; PYY, peptide YY.

one study concludes that of 30 products reviewed, 25 of them have been withdrawn from the market because of concerns about serious side effects.[23,24] Furthermore, in 2012, James Rippe and Theodore Angelopoulos expressed dismay about the lack of drugs available to treat obesity in their 2012 book titled *Obesity: Prevention and Treatment.*[25]

At the same time in 2012, the combination drug phentermine hydrochloride/topiramate extended-release (ER; Qsymia®) and lorcaserin hydrochloride were approved by the FDA. However, in February 2020, the FDA requested the withdrawal of lorcaserin (Belviq® and Belviq XR®) from the market due to additional safety concerns (see further discussion on lorcaserin withdrawal in the "Long-Term Weight Loss Medications" section).

In October 2010, the FDA removed sibutramine (Meridia®) approved in 1997 from the market because of concerns about unnecessary cardiovascular risks to patients.[26]

In 2014, the FDA approved the combination drug naltrexone hydrochloride/bupropion along with liraglutide. However, these drugs have limited insurance coverage.[27]

CURRENT TREATMENT OF ADULT OBESITY

Nonpharmacologic Interventions

Lifestyle and behavioral interventions are the cornerstones of obesity prevention and treatment. These interventions include dietary and physical activity as well as stress reduction. According to the 2018 U.S. Preventive Services Task force (USPSTF), clinicians should offer "intensive, multicomponent behavioral interventions" to adults with a BMI of 30 kg/m^2 or greater.[28] These interventional programs can range from 3 to 12 months (or even longer) and have various components, including technology-based programs, counseling, and access to such specialists as registered dietitians, exercise physiologists, behavioral therapists, social workers, lifestyle coaches, and others.[28] The USPSTF systematic review found that at 12 to 18 months, intervention participants were more likely to lose 5% of their initial weight compared to control participants. Moreover, this review also found that interventions that combined pharmacotherapy with behavioral interventions reported greater weight loss and weight-loss maintenance compared to placebo. A decreased incidence of progression to type 2 diabetes was also observed in the combined treatment group. Additionally, the sustainability of these combined interventions may last up to 48 months compared to behavioral weight loss alone.[28,29]

In 2013 the American Heart Association (AHA), American College of Cardiology (ACC), and The Obesity Society (TOS) published the joint "Clinical Practice Guideline for the Management of Overweight and Obesity in Adults."[30] When released, orlistat was the only FDA-approved drug for weight loss, so pharmacologic options for the treatment of obesity were limited. In addition to lifestyle recommendations, the guideline recommended that adults with a BMI of greater than or equal to 40 kg/m^2 or patients with a BMI greater than or equal to 35 kg/m^2 plus two other cardiovascular risk factors such as diabetes or high blood pressure should be considered for bariatric surgery. But treatment guidelines did not recommend weight-loss surgery for patients with a BMI under 35 kg/m^2.[30] For the most current guidelines, please refer to the updated reports from the Endocrine Society and the American Association of Clinical Endocrinologists (AACE)/American College of Endocrinology (ACE).[17,31]

Pharmacologic Interventions

FDA-approved anti-obesity drugs are recommended for those individuals who have a BMI greater than or equal to 30 kg/m^2 and for individuals who have a BMI of greater than or equal to 27 kg/m^2 in the presence of one or more risk factors/comorbidities such as hypertension, diabetes, and dyslipidemia.[17] When clinicians are considering prescribing anti-obesity drugs, they should complete a medical and reproductive history, comprehensive weight history, surgical history, list of all medications, and physical examination, including anthropometric measurements such as BMI. Clinicians should also review all past attempts of weight loss, drugs used for weight loss, how long they were used, how many pounds were lost, and how long the weight loss was maintained.

There are two major categories of weight-loss drugs—those for *short-term* (**Table 36.1**) and *long-term* use (**Table 36.2**). Phentermine hydrochloride

TABLE 36.1 Weight-Loss Drugs Approved by the FDA for Short-Term Use (≤12 Weeks)

Drug	Action	Dose	Indications/Contraindications	Side Effects
Phentermine HCl (ADIPEX-P®, Lomaira™)[1-3]	Sympathomimetic amine, anorectic	Dosage may vary and should be individualized. ADIPEX-P®: 37.5-mg tablets and capsules Lomaira™: 8-mg tablets	Indications: BMI ≥30 kg/m² or ≥27 kg/m² in the presence of one or more risk factors/comorbidities such as hypertension, diabetes, and dyslipidemia. Contraindications: Cardiovascular disease, uncontrolled hypertension, hyperthyroidism, glaucoma, agitated states, history of drug abuse, pregnancy, breastfeeding, know hypersensitivity to sympathomimetic; do not use with MAOIs	Dry mouth, headache, constipation, difficulty sleeping, dizziness, feeling nervous or restless Caution: May increase blood pressure; may lead to dependence and tolerance; alcohol may result in adverse drug reaction

[1]FDA approved, controlled substances: DEA Schedule IV – phentermine, phentermine IR, and topiramate ER (Qsymia®); FDA approved, non-controlled drugs: Bupropion HCl/naltrexone HCl (Contrave®) and liraglutide (Saxenda®)

[2]Some brands have been discontinued (e.g., Ionamin®)

[3]Combination drugs with phentermine that included fenfluramine (Pondimin®) and dexfenfluramine (Redux®: commonly known as "fen-phen") were withdrawn from the market in 1997 due to risk of valvular heart disease. The association of phentermine alone with valvular heart disease cannot be ruled out; however, the drug is still FDA approved.

FDA, U.S. Food and Drug Administration; HCl, hydrochloride; MAOIs, monoamine oxidase inhibitors.

Source: KVK-Tech. *Lomaira full prescribing information.* 2016. https://www.lomaira.com/Prescribing_Information.pdf; Teval Select Brands. *ADIPEX-P highlights of prescribing information.* 2017. https://www.adipex.com/globalassets/adipex/adipex_pi.pdf

(phentermine) is the main prototype for short-term weight loss (i.e., <12 weeks) and has been on the market since 1959. Drugs approved for long-term use include orlistat, phentermine/topiramate, naltrexone hydrochloride/bupropion hydrochloride ER, and liraglutide. Except for orlistat, which is a gastrointestinal lipase inhibitor, most of the other FDA-approved anti-obesity drugs act primarily on the central nervous system, especially the hypothalamus and neuroendocrine axis, which regulate appetite and satiety. These drugs, usually in combination with a low-calorie diet, lead to an average 5% to 10% weight loss compared to placebo. This range can vary based on the type of weight-loss drug and length of therapy.[23,32–37]

A 2018 systematic review and meta-analysis found that centrally acting anti-obesity products were significantly more likely to cause at least a 5% reduction in baseline body weight than a placebo.[23] However, the review also determined that there were significant increases in the risks of several adverse events, including neurological, cardiovascular, and gastrointestinal side effects.[23] A previous review by Onakpoya et al.[24] identified 25 anti-obesity drugs withdrawn from U.S. and international markets between 1964 and 2009. Of the 25 withdrawn anti-obesity drug products included in the review, 92% were appetite-suppressants acting on monoamine neurotransmitters.[24] Therefore, prescribers should be aware of the history of drug withdrawals when prescribing appetite suppressants acting on monoamine neurotransmitters.

Prescribers of anti-obesity drugs should also be aware that several of these FDA-approved drugs are classified

as controlled substances. Schedule IV drugs include phentermine and phentermine/topiramate ER; they have been identified as weight-loss drugs that can lead to dependence. Orlistat and bupropion hydrochloride (HCl)/naltrexone HCl are not controlled substances.

It is beyond the scope of this chapter to discuss off-label use of drugs to treat obesity, such as metformin, topiramate alone, and antidepressants (e.g., fluoxetine and bupropion alone).

Short-Term Weight-Loss Medications

Phentermine Hydrochloride

Phentermine (ADIPEX®, Lomaira™) was approved in the United States in 1959 and is a sympathomimetic amine or noradrenergic agonist that is thought to suppress appetite in humans. It is considered to have lower abuse potential than amphetamines due to the insignificant release of dopamine when compared to amphetamines.[38,39] Phentermine in combination with topiramate is also FDA approved for long-term use.

Other drugs from this class include diethylpropion/amfepramone (Tenuate®, Tenuate Dospan®), phendimetrazine (Bontril®), and benzphetamine (Didrex®). Phendimetrazine and benzphetamine are rarely prescribed and commercial brands of these drugs tend to come and go off the market.[39,40] These sympathomimetic amines are classified by the U.S. Drug Enforcement Administration (DEA) as controlled substances due to their potentially addictive risks. Phentermine and diethylpropion are schedule IV controlled substances, whereas benzphetamine and phendimetrazine are

TABLE 36.2 Weight-Loss Drugs Approved by the FDA for Long-Term Use

Drug	Action	Dose	Indications/Contraindications	Side Effects
Orlistat (Xenical®, alli®)	Reversible inhibitor of gastrointestinal lipases	120-mg capsule (prescription strength) bid with each main meal or up to 1 hour after meal; also available as OTC (alli®; 60 mg)	Indications: BMI ≥30 kg/m² or ≥27 kg/m² in the presence of one or more risk factors/comorbidity (e.g., HTN, diabetes, dyslipidemia); may be used in children >12 years (under the care of a licensed pediatrician or pediatric endocrinologist) Contraindications: Pregnancy, GI malabsorption, cholestasis; may decrease cyclosporine exposure Delayed administration required in patients on levothyroxine and cyclosporine therapy	GI side effects, liver damage (rare); fat-soluble vitamin replacement necessary
Phentermine HCl / topiramate ER (Qsymia®)[a]	Sympathomimetic; anticonvulsant (GABA receptor modulation, carbonic anhydrase inhibition, glutamate antagonism)	3.75-mg phentermine IR/23-mg topiramate ER capsules 1 cap PO QAM x 2 wks, then 7.5 mg/46 mg PO QAM x 2 wks; increase dose every 2 weeks if needed to max dose of 15 mg/92 mg. Discontinue if weight loss is less than 5% in 12 weeks. Other dose combinations: 7.5 mg phentermine IR/46 mg topiramate ER 11.25 mg phentermine IR/69 mg topiramate ER 15 mg phentermine IR/92 mg topiramate ER	Indications: BMI ≥30 kg/m² or ≥27 kg/m² in the presence of ≥1 or risk factor/comorbidity (e.g., HTN, diabetes, dyslipidemia) Contraindications: Pregnancy	Parasthesia, dizziness, dysgeusia, insomnia, constipation, dry mouth Caution: Risk of fetal toxicity, suicidal behavior, tachycardia, acute myopia with angle closure, mood and sleep disorders, metabolic acidosis, cognitive impairment, increased creatinine
Naltrexone HCl/ bupropion (Contrave®)	Dopamine/ noradrenaline reuptake inhibitor; opioid receptor antagonist	8-mg naltrexone HCl/90-mg bupropion HCl 1 tab PO QAM x 1 wk, then 1 tab PO BID, then 2 tabs PO QAM and 1 tab PO QPM x 1 wk; max dose: 4 tabs/day.	Indications: BMI ≥30 kg/m² or ≥27 kg/m² in the presence of one or more risk factors/comorbidity (e.g., HTN, diabetes, dyslipidemia) Contraindications: Pregnancy, glaucoma, hyperthyroidism, and during or within 14 days of monamine oxidase inhibitors. Also known hypersensitivity or idiosyncrasy to sympathomimetic amines	Nausea, constipation, headache, vomiting, dizziness, insomnia, dry mouth, diarrhea Caution: Risk of suicidal behavior, increased blood pressure and heart rate, seizure, hepatotoxicity, angle-closure glaucoma
Liraglutide injection (Saxenda®)	GLP-1 receptor agonist (glucagon-like peptide-1-intestinal hormone)[b]	Saxenda@ (18 mg/3 mL): Starting at 0.6 mg SC per day x 1 wk, may increase 0.6 mg/day every week up to max of 3 mg/day. Victoza®: NOT for weight loss; used for type 2 DM	Indications: BMI ≥30 kg/m² or ≥27 kg/m² in the presence of one or more risk factors/comorbidity (e.g., HTN, diabetes, dyslipidemia) Contraindications: Multiple endocrine neoplasia syndrome; pregnancy	Nausea, hypoglycemia, diarrhea, constipation, vomiting, headache, decreased appetite, dizziness, increased lipase Caution: Risk of thyroid C-cell tumors in rodents, pancreatitis, gallbladder disease, renal impairment, increased heart rate

[a]United States Drug Enforcement Agency (DEA) controlled substances for obesity: Schedule IV—phentermine, Qsymia® (phentermine and topiramate ER); not-controlled agents for obesity—Orlistat (Xenical®); Contrave® (bupropion HCl/naltrexone HCl) and liraglutide (Saxenda®)

[b]Victoza® NOT for weight loss; used for type 2 diabetes mellitus.

DM, diabetes mellitus; ER, extended-release; FDA, U.S. Food and Drug Administration; GABA, gamma aminobutyric acid; GI, gastrointestinal; HCl, hydrochloride; HTN, hypertension; IR, immediate release; OTC, over the counter.

Sources: Data from Novo Norksisk Inc. Saxenda (liraglutide [rDNA origin] injection) [package insert]. https://www.accessdata.fda.gov/drugsatfda_docs/label/2014/206321Orig1s000lbl.pdf; Roche Laboratories. Xenical (orlistat) [package insert]. U.S. Food and Drug Administration website. https://www.accessdata.fda.gov/drugsatfda_docs/label/2012/020766s029lbl.pdf; Takeda Pharmaceuticals America, Inc. Contrave (naltrexone HCl and bupropion HCl) [package insert]. U.S. Food and Drug Administration website. https://www.accessdata.fda.gov/drugsatfda_docs/label/2014/200063s000lbl.pdf; Vivus, Inc. Qsymia (phentermine and topiramate extended-release) [package insert] U.S. Food and Drug Administration website. https://www.accessdata.fda.gov/drugsatfda_docs/label/2012/022580s000lbl.pdf

schedule II controlled substances.[7] A 2013 study examining U.S. national drug use estimated that from 1991 to 2011 phentermine was the most frequently prescribed weight-loss drug and sometimes used longer than the recommended 12-week treatment time.[41] In 2011, approximately 2.74 million patients used anti-obesity drugs, 2.43 million (close to 90%) of whom used phentermine.[41] Since then, newer drugs such as phentermine/topiramate, naltrexone/bupropion, and liraglutide have also been FDA approved and will most likely be utilized compared to phentermine products.

Dosage

Phentermine is approved for short-term use, up to 12 weeks' duration. It is available in capsules and tablets at a variety of dose strengths, depending on the brand name. ADIPEX-P is available in 37.5 mg, while Lomaira is available in low-dose tablets of 8 mg. Generics may be available in 15-mg and 30-mg forms. Dosages and frequency of administration vary; typically, patients will take 15 mg to 37.5 mg orally once a day in the morning on an empty stomach. Refer to prescribing information for further details.[42,43]

Side Effects, Contraindications, and Cautions

Common side effects include dry mouth, insomnia, constipation, headache, dizziness, palpitations, nervousness, tremor, and other sympathomimetic symptoms.[39,44,45] Phentermine can also increase blood pressure and must be used with caution in patients even with well-controlled hypertension. It should not be used in patients with poorly controlled hypertension and/or other cardiovascular disease. If phentermine is used in patients with well-controlled hypertension and no other cardiovascular disease, periodic blood-pressure monitoring should be done. Since obesity is associated with an increased risk for cardiovascular disease and other comorbidities, the clinician will find that phentermine is contraindicated for obese patients with poorly controlled hypertension and cardiovascular disease.[46–49] This contraindication is also applicable for the combination weight-loss drug phentermine/topiramate, thus limiting the clinician's choice of weight-loss drugs.

Efficacy

Even though phentermine has been on the U.S. market since 1959, there are relatively few long-term efficacy studies.[50–52] A 28-week randomized controlled trial comparing phentermine/topiramate (Qsymia) with its component drugs phentermine alone and topiramate alone, versus placebo, showed that subjects achieving a greater than or equal to 5% weight loss were 43.3% for 7.5-mg phentermine alone and 46.2% for 15-mg phentermine alone compared to 15.5% for placebo.[50] See **Figure 36.3** for mean percent weight loss over time (modified intention to treat [ITT]) versus placebo for phentermine, topiramate, and phentermine/topiramate.[50]

Long-Term Weight-Loss Medications

Orlistat

Orlistat (Xenical®) acts by inhibiting GI and pancreatic lipases. As a result, hydrolysis of triglycerides is blocked and fatty acid absorption by the intestine is reduced. When taking orlistat, it is estimated that about one-third of fatty acids consumed with food are not absorbed.[39,53] This can result in the inadequate absorption of fat-soluble vitamins, A, D, E and K, and requires vitamin supplementation.[39] Orlistat is generally well tolerated but has been associated with GI side effects, including flatulence and steatorrhea. It was approved by the FDA in 1999 and sold under various brand names such as Xenical and the over-the-counter (OTC) brand allī®.

Dosage

Orlistat is available commercially as an OTC preparation in 60-mg capsules. The prescription strength is available at 120-mg capsules. Both allī® and Xenical are usually taken three times a day with each main meal containing some fat (during or up to 1 hour after the meal). Orlistat can also interact with certain medications, including cyclosporine, levothyroxine, warfarin, amiodarone, antiepileptic drugs, and antiretroviral medications.[54] For patients on these therapies, orlistat doses should be taken at least 4 hours apart.

Orlistat is the only anti-obesity drug approved by the FDA to treat adolescent obesity for individuals older than 12 years of age.[55] However, the associated side effects of flatus and diarrhea often dissuade teenagers from continuing its use.

Side Effects, Contraindications, and Cautions

Other side effects of orlistat are oily spotting, fecal discharge and urgency, fatty/oily stool, increased defecation, and fecal incontinence. Rarely orlistat is associated with severe liver injury with hepatocellular necrosis or acute hepatic failure. Patients may also develop increased levels of urinary oxalate. It is important to monitor renal function in all patients and particularly those with renal insufficiency.[39,54]

Contraindications for orlistat include pregnancy, cholestasis, malabsorption, and known hypersensitivity to orlistat or any component of this product. It is not known if orlistat is present in human milk; thus, it is prudent to wait until nursing is completed before using orlistat.[54]

Efficacy

A 4-year, double-blind, randomized controlled prospective study of 3,305 participants (XENDOS Study) using orlistat versus placebo showed that 72.8% of patients taking orlistat plus lifestyle changes achieved weight loss greater than or equal to 5% after 1 year of treatment compared to 45.1% taking placebo ($P < 0.001$).[33] The mean weight loss after 4 years was significantly greater with orlistat versus placebo (5.8 kg vs. 3.0 kg with placebo; $P < 0.001$). Moreover, after 4 years of treatment, the

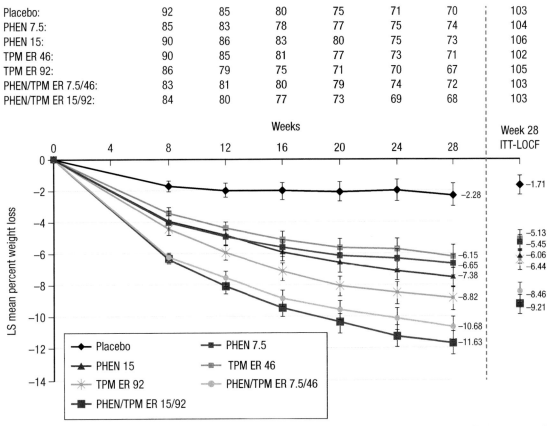

Placebo:	92	85	80	75	71	70	103
PHEN 7.5:	85	83	78	77	75	74	104
PHEN 15:	90	86	83	80	75	73	106
TPM ER 46:	90	85	81	77	73	71	102
TPM ER 92:	86	79	75	71	70	67	105
PHEN/TPM ER 7.5/46:	83	81	80	79	74	72	103
PHEN/TPM ER 15/92:	84	80	77	73	69	68	103

FIGURE 36.3 Phentermine/topiramate. Least squares mean percent weight loss over time (mITT) versus placebo for phentermine, topiramate, and phentermine/topiramate.

ITT-LOCF, intention to treat-last observation carried forward;PHEN 7.5, phentermine (immediate release - IR) 7.5 mg (alone); PHEN 15, phentermine (immediate release - IR) 15 mg (alone); TPM ER 46, topiramate ER 46 mg (alone); TPM ER 92, topiramate ER 92 mg (alone); PHEN/TPM ER 7.5/46, phentermine IR 7.5 mg / topiramate ER 46 mg (combination); PHEN/TPM ER 15/92, phentermine IR 15 mg / topiramate ER 92 mg (combination).

Source: Adapted from Aronne LJ, Wadden TA, Peterson C, et al. Evaluation of phentermine and topiramate versus phentermine/topiramate extended-release in obese adults. *Obesity.* 2013;21(11):2163–2171. doi:10.1002/oby.20584

cumulative incidence of diabetes was 9% with placebo and 6.2% with orlistat, corresponding to a risk reduction of 37.3% (*P* = 0.0032); see **Figure 36.4.**[35,53]

Lorcaserin (withdrawn from market in February 2020)

In February 2020, a FDA Drug and Safety Communication requested that the manufacturer of Belviq®/Belviq XR® withdraw them from the U.S. market due to safety concerns related to a clinical trial that showed an increased occurrence of cancer. The FDA has advised patients to stop taking lorcaserin and talk to their clinicians. In addition, the FDA has instructed healthcare professionals to stop prescribing and dispensing lorcaserin to patients. Per FDA recommendations, patients who are taking lorcaserin at the time of this announcement should be informed of the increased risks of cancer. Healthcare professionals were also advised to discuss alternative weight-loss medications or treatments.[56]

Lorcaserin, a selective 5-hydroxytryptamine 2C (5HT-2C) receptor agonist, has been found to target hypothalamic POMC neurons.[39,57] These neurons and their receptors regulate appetite and satiety.[18,58,59] It is still too early to determine why there is an increased risk of cancers with lorcaserin. When the FDA approved lorcaserin

for weight loss in 2012 they had required the manufacturer to do additional clinical safety testing, primarily to assess the risk of cardiovascular problems and look at other risks. This study found that several cancers occurred more frequently in the lorcaserin group compared to the control group, including pancreatic, colorectal, and lung.[56] As a result, the FDA recommended that the manufacturer withdraw lorcaserin from the market.

Liraglutide

Approved in the United States in 2014, liraglutide (Saxenda®) is a glucagon-like-peptide 1 (GLP-1) analogue, originally approved for the treatment of type 2 diabetes. It is an incretin hormone that is secreted after meals by the L-cells of the distal ileum, proximal colon, and the vagal nucleus of the solitary tract.[39] Incretins stimulate insulin secretion by the pancreas.[60] Liraglutide has a complex mechanism of action and acts through both peripheral and central receptor pathways. These affected pathways impact glucose homeostasis, food intake, and satiety.[38] Because of its incretin effects, liraglutide may be useful for obese individuals with insulin resistance or type 2 diabetes.

Dosage

Saxenda® comes as a solution for subcutaneous injection in the form of a prefilled, multidose pen that delivers doses of 0.6, 1.2, 2.4, or 3 mg (6 mg/mL, 3 mL pre-filled, single patient-use pen). It is administered as a subcutaneous injection with tiered dosing.[61] Another related brand, Victoza® (liraglutide subcutaneous injection 1.2 mg/1.8 mg), is used to treat type 2 diabetes and is not recommended for weight loss. Since Saxenda and Victoza have the same active ingredient (liraglutide), they should not be used together.[61]

Side Effects, Contraindications, and Cautions

The most frequent side effects associated with liraglutide are nausea, hypoglycemia, vomiting, diarrhea, constipation, headache, dyspepsia, fatigue, dizziness, abdominal pain, and increased lipase.[39,61] GI side effects are the leading causes for discontinuation of this medication.[62] There have been concerns about the increased risk of acute pancreatitis; however, long-term trials and meta-analyses suggest that pancreatitis does not seem to increase significantly.[39,62–64] Nevertheless, prescribers should be cautious when prescribing Saxenda and monitor their patients for pancreatitis because postmarketing reports of acute pancreatitis, including fatal and nonfatal hemorrhagic or necrotizing pancreatitis, have been observed with liraglutide. The manufacturer recommends discontinuing Saxenda if pancreatitis is confirmed and should not be restarted. Liraglutide may be associated with a slightly increased risk of cholelithiasis, most likely due to rapid weight loss.[65] There are additional cautions related to renal impairment, increase of heart rate, hypersensitivity reactions, thyroid C-Cell tumors, suicidal behavior, and ideation.[61]

Contraindications for liraglutide include pregnancy and personal history of medullary thyroid carcinoma or type 2 multiple endocrine neoplasia (MEN 2). There is no data on the presence of liraglutide in human milk, the effects on the breastfed infant, or effects on milk production;[61] thus, further research is needed in the area of lactation.

Efficacy

A review of five multicenter, randomized placebo-controlled trials examining the efficacy of liraglutide in conjunction with a prescribed diet and physical activity showed a 5% to 10% weight loss compared to placebo.[37] It was noted that liraglutide also improves glycemic control and is effective in obese patients with comorbidities (e.g., hypertension, dyslipidemia, type 2 diabetes, and obstructive sleep apnea).[37,39,66] Comparison data indicates that weight loss with liraglutide is greater than that seen with orlistat or lorcaserin, but slightly less than weight loss seen with phentermine/topiramate combination treatment.[37,65] A 2016 meta-analysis of 28 randomized clinical trials of 29,018 patients found that liraglutide was associated with a higher odds ratio of discontinuation due to adverse effects.[65]

Phentermine/topiramate (Qsymia®) is a combination weight-loss drug approved by the FDA in 2012. It has not yet been approved in Europe, mainly because of the lack of long-term data on the cardiovascular effects of phentermine and cognitive side effects of topiramate.[39] The AACE and ACE practice guidelines for obesity indicated that phentermine with topiramate ER, in combination with a lifestyle intervention, are effective in both weight loss and maintenance compared to lifestyle intervention alone.[31] This combination drug suppresses appetite by mechanisms that are still under investigation.[39,67] As previously discussed, phentermine is a sympathomimetic amine or noradrenergic agonist. Topiramate is a GABA agonist, glutamate antagonist, and carbonic anhydrase inhibitor. Topiramate has primarily been used in the treatment of various types of epilepsy, such as partial seizures.[67,68]

Dosage

Phentermine/topiramate is given in stepwise titrated doses starting at a low dose of ER formulation (3.75 mg/23 mg) daily in the morning for 14 days, followed by an increased dose of 7.5 mg/46 mg daily for 12 weeks. After the initial phase of dosing titration, if the weight reduction is less than 3%, the drug should either be discontinued, or its dose be further increased. Typically, the next dose titration would be at 11.25 mg/69 mg daily for the next 2 weeks, followed by 15 mg/92 mg daily for another 12 weeks, as tolerated. At this point, if the extent of weight loss is not equal to or greater than 5% from baseline, the drug should be discontinued.[39,52,68] If the increased doses are poorly tolerated, phentermine/topiramate should gradually be titrated down over the next 3 to 5 days, especially in patients with seizure disorders, as an abrupt discontinuation may precipitate a seizure.[68]

Side Effects, Contraindications, and Cautions

Common side effects of phentermine/topiramate include dizziness, paresthesia, insomnia, dry mouth, constipation and dysgeusia, anxiety, depression, suicidal ideation, sleep disorders, or cognitive impairment.[39,52,68] Other adverse side effects include fetal toxicity, acute angle-closure glaucoma, increased heart rate, and possible renal side effects such as metabolic acidosis and nephrolithiasis (secondary to carbonic anhydrase inhibition by topiramate). Thus, heart rate, electrolytes, and creatinine should be monitored periodically. For patients with impaired hepatic and/or renal function, dosing reduction is required. In these patient populations, phentermine/topiramate maximum dose should not exceed 7.5 mg/46 mg once daily.[52]

Phentermine/topiramate is contraindicated in glaucoma and hyperthyroidism. It is also contraindicated in patients taking monoamine oxidase inhibitors (MAOIs) due to severe drug–drug interactions.[31] Because of topi-

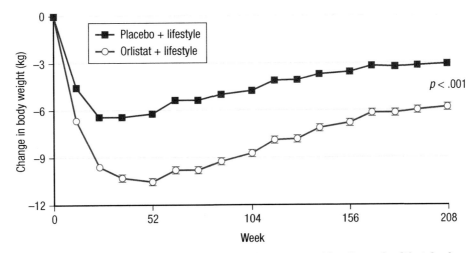

FIGURE 36.4 Orlistat. Weight loss (mean ± SEM) during 4 years of treatment with orlistat plus lifestyle changes or placebo plus lifestyle changes in obese patients (LOCF data).

<insert legend on new line>

LOCF, last observation carried forward.

Source: Adapted from Torgerson JS, Hauptman J, Boldrin MN, et al. XENical in the prevention of diabetes in obese subjects (XENDOS) study: randomized study of orlistat as an adjunct to lifestyle changes for the prevention of type 2 diabetes in obese patients. *Diabetes Care.* 2014;27(1):155–161. https://care .diabetesjournals.org/content/diacare/27/1/155.full.pdf

ramate's fetal toxicity, Qsymia is also contraindicated in pregnancy.[31,52,69,70] These active ingredients may be found in human milk and lead to serious adverse reactions in nursing infants;[52] thus, Qsymia should be avoided during breastfeeding.

Efficacy

One of the sentinel studies (the SEQUEL study) on phentermine/topiramate showed that the combination drug was associated with significant sustained weight loss by Garvey et al.[31] Similarly, another study demonstrated that combining phentermine with topiramate ER (7.5/46 and 15/92) results in greater weight loss than either drug when used as monotherapies (**Figure 36.4**).[50]

In a 2016 meta-analysis, data revealed phentermine/topiramate (Qsymia) combination had the highest odds of achieving at least a 5% to 10% weight loss, compared to all of the five FDA-approved agents at that time.[65] At 1-year follow-up, the significant excess weight loss compared to placebo for each formulation are: phentermine-topiramate, 8.8 kg reduction; liraglutide, 5.3 kg reduction; naltrexone-bupropion, 5 kg, reduction; lorcaserin, 3.2 kg, reduction; and orlistat, 2.6 kg, reduction.[65]

Naltrexone HCl/Bupropion Extended-Release

Naltrexone/bupropion ER (Contrave®) is a combination drug for weight loss, approved for long-term use by the FDA in 2014. Naltrexone is an opioid antagonist used in the treatment of drug and alcohol abuse. Bupropion is an aminoketone antidepressant and acts as a weak inhibitor of neuronal reuptake of dopamine and norepinephrine, which has been and is used to treat major depressive disorder, seasonal affective disorder, and to assist with smoking cessation.[71,72] These two drugs have complementary actions on the central

nervous system and act to reduce food intake via the anorexigenic pathway.[31,73] This formulation may work best in patients with eating disorders.

Dosage

Contrave®, the commercial brand sold in the United States, comes in 8-mg naltrexone HCl/90-mg bupropion HCl tablets. Dosing should be escalated over a 4-week period as tolerated.[73]

Side Effects, Contraindications, and Cautions

Frequent side effects of naltrexone HCl/bupropion ER include nausea, vomiting, constipation, dizziness, dry mouth, and headache.[36,71,74] Contrave® has a Black-Box Warning for suicidal thoughts and behaviors and has not been studied in pediatric patients.[73] It is contraindicated in patients with uncontrolled hypertension, seizure disorders, anorexia nervosa or bulimia, and those undergoing abrupt discontinuation of alcohol, benzodiazepines, barbiturates, and antiepileptic drugs. In addition, it should not be used in patients who are also taking other bupropion-containing medications, as well as those with chronic opioid use, those taking MAOIs, and those who are pregnant.[73]

Efficacy

The key historical research studies involved in the approval of Contrave® are the COR-I (Contrave Obesity Research I), COR II, COR-DIABETES, and COR-BMOD (COR in Adjunct to Intensive Behavioral MODification).[36,74–76] The COR-I study (phase 2 study) was a 2010 multicenter double-blind randomized control study of 1,742 enrolled overweight and uncomplicated obese patients, which included a diet plan and exercise, examining the efficacy and effects of naltrexone/bupropion

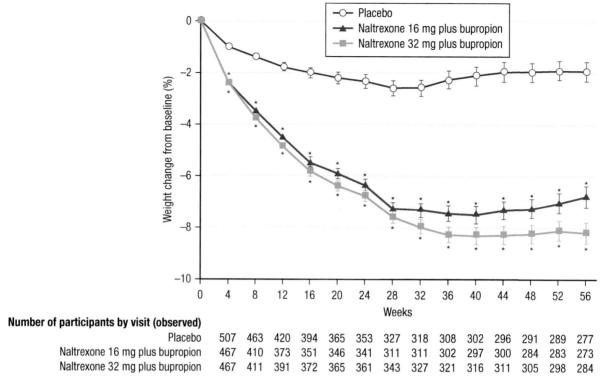

FIGURE 36.5 Naltrexone/bupropion. Change in bodyweight (naltrexone, 16 mg/bupropion, 360 mg and naltrexone, 32 mg/bupropion, 360 mg vs. placebo): Observed least squares mean (standard error) percentage from baseline bodyweight and number of participants at each visit during 56 weeks. * *p* < 0.0001 compared with placebo.

Source: Adapted from Greenway FL, Fujioka K, Plodkowski RA, et al. Effect of naltrexone plus bupropion on weight loss in overweight and obese adults (COR-I): a multicentre, randomised, double-blind, placebo-controlled, phase 3 trial. *Lancet.* 2010;376(9741):595–605. doi:10.1016/s0140-6736(10)60888-4.

sustained-release (SR) at 32 mg/360 mg and 16 mg/360 mg versus placebo over a 56-week period. Mean change in bodyweight was –1.3% in the placebo group, –6.1% in the naltrexone/bupropion SR 32 mg/360 mg group (*P* <0.0001 vs. placebo), and –5.0% in the naltrexone/bupropion SR 16 mg/360 mg group (*P* <0.0001 vs. placebo). In addition, 16% of participants assigned to placebo had a decrease in bodyweight of 5% or more compared with 48% of participants on naltrexone/bupropion SR 32 mg/360 mg (*n* = 226) (*P* <0.0001 vs. placebo) and 39% of participants on naltrexone/bupropion SR 16 mg/360 mg (*n* = 186; *P* <0.0001 vs. placebo); see **Figure 36.5**. This demonstrated that the naltrexone/bupropion SR combination therapy was generally well tolerated and associated with greater weight loss than placebo and showed a greater improvement in several cardiometabolic risk factors.[36]

The COR II study, a parallel phase 3 trial of naltrexone/bupropion SR, corroborated the COR I efficacy results showing a significantly greater weight loss in the treatment group versus placebo. For example, a 6.5% weight loss was observed in the treatment group versus 1.9% in the placebo group at week 28. Additionally, a weight loss of 6.4% was observed in the treatment group versus 1.2% in the placebo group at week 56 (*P* <0.001). Furthermore, both the COR-DIABETES AND COR-BMOD substantiated the COR-I and COR-II results of significantly more weight loss in the naltrex-

one/bupropion SR treated groups versus placebo.[75,76] In addition, the COR-DIABETES trial showed associated improvements in glycemic control and select cardiovascular risk factors.[75,76]

MEDICATIONS THAT CONTRIBUTE TO WEIGHT GAIN

Clinicians should be aware of drugs that may cause weight gain, including antidepressants (e.g., amitriptyline, mirtazapine, and paroxetine), antihyperglycemic agents (e.g., insulin, sulfonylureas, and thiazolidinediones), antihypertensives such as beta-blockers, atypical antipsychotic agents (e.g., clozapine, olanzapine, and risperidone), migraine medications, seizure control medications (e.g., carbamazepine, gabapentin, and valproate), hormonal contraceptives, and corticosteroids.[77] Where possible, alternative medications should be considered for individuals with overweight and obesity. For example, consider sodium-glucose-transporter-2 (SGLT2) inhibitors for weight-loss benefit in patients with diabetes instead of sulfonylureas.

CONCLUSION

Substantial progress has been made over the past century in the development of effective drugs to treat obesity and its comorbidities. Although multiple anti-obesity drug efficacy studies have shown only a modest amount of weight loss (usually ranging from 5%–10%), many of these studies have also confirmed that even this modest amount of weight loss in obese and overweight patients may result in improvements in glycemic control and reductions in cardiovascular risks.[23] When combined with lifestyle modification, appropriately selected anti-obesity drugs may lead to health benefits for overweight and obese patients. Treatment regimens should be individualized, taking into consideration social justice issues, environmental factors, and other socioeconomic issues surrounding the patient. Prescribers should also be aware of the various side effects and contraindications associated with anti-obesity drugs. More research is needed to further ascertain the safety and long-term efficacy of FDA-

CASE EXEMPLAR: Patient With Obesity and Unsuccessful Weight Loss

AM, a 45-year-old woman, is referred to you for management of her obesity. About 1 year ago she attempted to lose weight with lifestyle modification, including a low-calorie diet and physical activity plan over a 6-month period without successful weight loss. Her primary care clinician subsequently prescribed phentermine, 37.5 mg daily and she has been taking it for over three months. She has lost about 11 pounds since starting the phentermine. She states that she has been feeling well, except she has developed insomnia.

Past Medical History
- Obesity
- Depression
- Insulin resistance

Medications
- Phentermine, 37.5 mg daily
- Lisinopril, 20 mg daily
- Fluoxetine, 100 mg daily

Physical Examination
- Height: 67 inches; weight: 220 lbs.; BMI: 34.5; blood pressure: 148/94; pulse: 85
- Discoloration around neck consistent with acanthosis nigricans

Labs
- Hemoglobin A1C: 6.9%

Discussion Questions

1. In addition to a healthy diet and regular physical activity, what other treatment options may be considered for an obese patient with a BMI ≥ 30 kg/m²?
2. What anti-obesity drugs should not be used when an adult patient has uncontrolled hypertension?
3. What anti-obesity drugs are useful when an adult patient has insulin resistance? Type 2 diabetes?
4. What anti-obesity drugs are approved by the U.S. Food and Drug Administration to treat adult obesity?

KEY TAKEAWAYS

- The U.S. Centers for Disease Control and Prevention (CDC) defines adult overweight as a body mass index (BMI) of 25 kg/m² to less than 30 kg/m² and obesity as a BMI of 30 kg/m² or higher.
- Hunger is initiated by complex central and peripheral orexigenic signals that promote feeding; ghrelin is produced in the stomach and is considered the only known hunger–generating hormone.
- Lifestyle and behavioral interventions remain the cornerstones of obesity prevention and treatment, while interventions that combine pharmacotherapy with behavioral interventions are associated with greater weight loss and weight loss maintenance compared to placebo.

- FDA–approved anti-obesity drugs are recommended for those individuals who have a BMI greater than or equal to 30 kg/m² and for individuals who have a BMI of greater than or equal to 27 kg/m² in the presence of one or more risk factors/comorbidities such as hypertension, diabetes, and dyslipidemia.
- It is important to keep in mind that some FDA-approved weight loss drugs are classified as DEA controlled substances and may lead to dependence.
- Some antidepressants, antihyperglycemic agents, beta-blockers, antipsychotics, and anticonvulsants, as well as contraceptives and corticosteroids, may be associated with weight gain. Alternatives should be considered in patients trying to lose weight.

approved drugs for weight loss. Furthermore, there is a need for advocacy to ensure adequate coverage by public and private health plans. Until the efficacy and safety profiles of these drugs have been fully understood, they will most likely be underutilized.

PART II: PEDIATRIC OBESITY

Pediatric obesity is a growing public health problem worldwide affecting approximately 18.5% of U.S. children and adolescents.[2] Over the last decades, the prevalence of children with weight above the 95th percentile has increased fourfold.[78] According to the Endocrine Society, the etiology of child obesity has its basis in genetic susceptibilities influenced by a permissive environment starting *in utero* and extending through childhood and adolescence.[78] In general, obesity is present with various comorbidities and often leads to long-term health complications. Therefore, clinicians should screen patients regularly to detect and initiate appropriate treatment to prevent further complications. If not well managed, the psychological well-being of the individual and family may be significantly impacted. It is essential to provide mental health screening and counseling as indicated. In addition, genetic screening for rare syndromes should be provided when patients present with specific historical or physical features suggesting hereditary conditions. Generally, the prevention of pediatric obesity should be centered around healthy diet, activity, and environment and lifestyle modification. In addition to behavioral interventions, studies have shown modest success with pharmacotherapeutics; however, weight-loss medication use in childhood and adolescence is often restricted to clinical trials.[78] Recognizing the serious health effects of pediatric obesity, there is increasing interest in pharmacologic therapy under controlled circumstances as well as substantial research into bariatric surgery in older teenagers. This part of the chapter presents the current evidence on the use of weight-loss medications in the pediatric population.

DEFINITION OF PEDIATRIC OVERWEIGHT AND OBESITY

The definition of obesity in childhood differs from the various degrees of obesity considered in adults. Rather than a BMI of greater than or equal to 25 kg/m² indicating overweight and 30 through 40 kg/m² representing different degrees of obesity, overweight and obesity in childhood is defined by the percentile of BMI for age and sex (**Figure 36.6**). A BMI greater than or equal to 85th percentile but less than 95th percentile defines overweight, a BMI greater than or equal to 95th percentile defines obesity.[79]

New classifications of extreme obesity denote that children with BMI values more than 20% over the 95th percentile have class II obesity and a value more than 40% over the 95th percentile defines class III obesity.[80] The greatest increase in the prevalence of obesity is in these extreme categories.[81]

GENERAL CONSIDERATIONS OF TREATMENT FOR PEDIATRIC OBESITY

Lifestyle modification is the cornerstone of treatment of childhood obesity but shows modest effects in most studies; thus, prevention is of primary importance since the treatment of childhood obesity is difficult once developed. When evaluating the effects of weight-loss treatments, the outcomes monitored vary among studies. Since BMI will change with age, the *BMI standard deviation* for age is the best measure; however, publications often use BMI or weight as the outcome, which makes comparison between studies difficult. One of the reasons that 85% of the childhood population can be classified as obese is because the only U.S. weight charts that are valid in the present day are constructed with weight data collected decades ago before the obesity epidemic occurred.

Pediatric Weight-Loss Medications

The conservative approach to pharmacologic therapy as noted in the Endocrine Society guidelines arises from a concern over potential side effects of anorexic agents on the developing individuals' brain and neurotransmitters. Furthermore, there is extremely limited data on pharmacologic therapy for obesity in childhood and the data is often of low quality.[82] Due to the significant comorbidities of childhood and adolescent obesity, a careful focus upon the use of such agents in children and teenagers is warranted.[83]

At present, orlistat (Xenical or allī) is the only FDA-approved agent for use in children over 12 years of age. Drugs approved for adults with obesity often can be used only in younger individuals off-label. Additionally, drugs previously approved for other pediatric conditions could be repurposed for the off-label treatment of obesity. This is particularly true when there is inadequate testing in children but years of clinical experience supports the safety of off-label use for such medication. A prescriber wishing to use an agent off-label in pediatric patients should be cognizant of their state laws concerning off-label use.[83] Most legal actions brought for use of non-FDA–approved drugs occur in the setting of research studies and lack of informed consent. To date, there have not been lawsuits for the use of off-label drugs for the treatment of obesity. However, out of an abundance of caution, if any obesity drugs approved for adults are used in children, a statement placed in the medical record along the lines

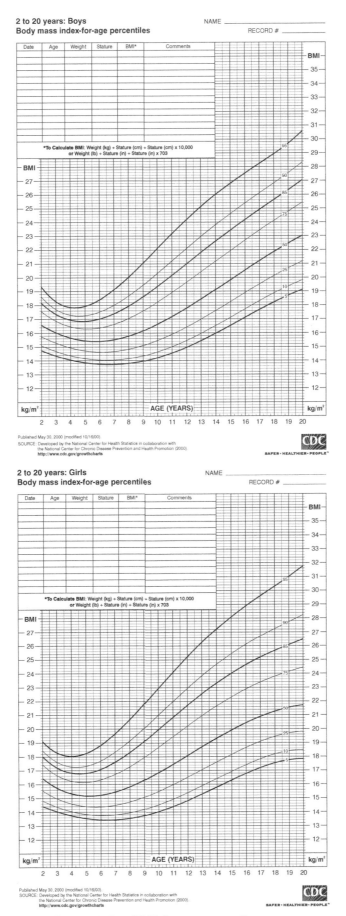

FIGURE 36.6 Boys (A) and girls (B) body mass index (BMI) for age percentiles.

Source: National Center for Health Statistics. Clinical growth charts. Updated October 16, 2000. https://www.cdc.gov/growthcharts/clinical_charts.htm

of informed consent would be appropriate to ensure that the parents understand the prescribers' rationales.

Orlistat

Orlistat inhibits GI and pancreatic lipases so that fats in the diet are not absorbed. This medication is approved for patients as young as 12 years of age in a dose of 120 mg PO tid with meals containing fat. It is generally considered safe and even ingestion by toddlers in large doses leads to only moderate GI distress.[84,85] The common side effects of flatus and diarrhea limit its clinical utility in all ages. Although fat-soluble vitamin deficiency may occur, liver abnormalities can develop in adults. The National Institute for Health and Care Excellence (NICE) in the United Kingdom suggests limiting the use of orlistat to children over 12 years of age with severe psychological or physiologic complications and in children younger than 12 only with exceptional complications.[86]

In clinical trials, there have been variable reported outcomes. A 6-month randomized controlled study of 120 mg of orlistat daily in 40 adolescents demonstrated no change in BMI.[87] However, a 1-year placebo controlled randomized trial of 539 adolescents taking 120 mg of orlistat demonstrated a decrease of BMI by 0.55 kg/m^2 compared to an increase by 0.31 kg/m^2 with placebo alone, and a decrease in fat mass measured by dual-energy x-ray absorptiometry (DEXA) and waist circumference in the orlistat group.[88]

More recently, a 10-week controlled single-blind study of 67 adolescents demonstrated reduced body weight, BMI, waist circumference, low-density lipoprotein (LDL) cholesterol, triglyceride and insulin levels, and decrease in caloric intake while on orlistat. In addition, flow-mediated dilation of the brachial artery increased significantly with orlistat with or without increased exercise.[89]

Phentermine

Phentermine is approved for teenagers over 16 years of age with a BMI greater than 27 kg/m^2 in the presence of at least one obesity-related comorbidity. A recent retrospective chart review that evaluated 25 patients with a mean age of 16.1 years treated with phentermine and lifestyle modification revealed better outcomes compared to 274 patients treated with only lifestyle modification.[90] Phentermine used over 6 months led to a 4.1% decrease in BMI. Heart rate and blood pressure were increased in phentermine-treated patients but there were no ill effects reported, although there is evidence in the literature of rare events of myocardial infarction with use of this agent in adults.[90] The dose for phentermine hydrochloride for those over 16 years is 15 to 37.5 mg orally every morning; this must be tapered off if discontinued.

Topiramate

Topiramate is another pharmacologic agent that has been evaluated for obesity management in pediatric patients. A randomized controlled double-blind placebo study demonstrated that topiramate combined with commercial meal-replacement products did not produce a significant decrease in weight compared to meal-replacement products alone.[91] Twenty-five percent of the patients taking topiramate experienced paresthesias and one with a preexisting history of depression became more depressed.[91] Additionally, topiramate is a teratogenic agent; therefore, contraception must be used for patients during the reproductive age. This therapy should not be discontinued abruptly as seizures may occur.

Lorcaserin

Although this agent has been approved for adult obesity, there are no pediatric studies involving lorcaserin to date. In February 2020, the FDA asked for voluntary recall of lorcaserin due to an association with increased incidence of cancer in those taking the medication.

Naltrexone/Bupropion Extended-Release

Naltrexone/bupropion ER is one of the options for treating obesity in the adult population; however, there is no current evidence supporting its indication for pediatric obesity, although bupropion does have some efficacy in the treatment of attention deficit/hyperactivity disorder (ADHD) and other pediatric behavior diagnoses.[92] The combination treatment carries a Black-Box Warning due to risk of suicidal ideation in young adults.

Liraglutide

Liraglutide, a glucagon-like peptide 1 agonist, has been found to improve glucose control in children with type 2 diabetes. Combined data from two studies of 32 subjects 8 to 19 years of age with extreme obesity demonstrated a 3.42% decrease in BMI compared to placebo. Despite the positive effects in weight loss, liraglutide was approved by the FDA for only type 2 diabetes, not as an anti-obesity drug for pediatric patients.[93] The dose for type 2 DM is 0.6 to 1.8 mg/day subcutaneously.

Metformin

Metformin is another anti-diabetic medication that has frequently been used as a weight-loss agent in pediatrics without FDA approval. A systematic review of 15 studies lasting over 6 months on the effects of metformin on weight in children demonstrated a possible beneficial effect on weight.[94] Another systematic review of 14 studies lasting 6 months demonstrated a 1.38 decrease in the BMI value compared to control or baseline.[95] These studies did not look at BMI standard deviations in most cases, which would be the most important indicator of effects on weight in growing children. The maximal dose is 2,000 mg/day. The patient starts with 500 mg with breakfast and if there is no ill effect such as abdominal distress 500 mg is added to dinner 5 days later. In another 5 days, 500 mg is added to breakfast, and finally 500 mg more is added to dinner.

Lisdexamfetamine

Lisdexamfetamine, a medication that is used to treat ADHD in children as young as 6 years of age, also showed weight loss in children taking the agent. There are no studies of this agent in obese children but those with ADHD have been shown to lose between 1 to 5 pounds depending upon age (6–18 years) and dosage according to the package insert[96] Lisdexamfetamine is associated with significant psychological changes, has caused severe cardiovascular disease, and cannot be used as a routine agent for weight loss in children.

Setmelanotide

Setmelanotide, an agonist of the melanocortin-4 receptor (MC4R), is one of the newest investigational anti-obesity drugs in children. It provides promising data in adults with MC4R pathway mutations, such as patients with POMC deficiency[97] and MC4R deficiency[98] It is also being tested in patients with leptin receptor (LepR) deficiency[99] Prader–Willi syndrome, Bardet–Biedl syndrome, and Alstrom syndrome[100] If approved, this medication will be a notable addition to the armamentarium of agents to treat the most seriously obese patients with monogenetic defects. In these cases, the agent is specifically tailored to the exact genetic defect compared to the other aforementioned agents, which were often developed for other uses and demonstrate anorexia as a side effect.

CONCLUSION

There is a need for more information on the use of pharmacologic agents in pediatrics. It must be emphasized that these agents should be used with caution. Prescribers should be familiar with their relative indications, benefits, side effects, and toxicities. The withdrawal of several agents approved for adults, that subsequently were linked to significant complications, emphasizes the caution necessary when considering pharmacologic therapy in children and adolescents.

Another consideration in pediatrics is how to determine the appropriate weight of a child for the calculation of dosages of any medication[101] The patient's actual body weight may not always be an appropriate dosing weight for patients with obesity. Currently, there is no agreement on this issue but considering the ideal body weight of the child for age as the weight to determine dosage is a reasonable approach.

CASE EXEMPLAR: Patient With Obesity and Fatigue

JG, a 16-year-old Hispanic male with a history of obesity, presents with increasing fatigue and sleepiness. His parents note that he has lost significant weight over the last several months and has been urinating several times each night. He complains of thirst, difficulty sleeping, and loud snoring.

Past Medical History
- Obesity

Family History
- Father: type 2 diabetes; myocardial infarction at 50 years of age

Physical Examination
- Body mass index (BMI): 61 kg/m² (>140% of the 95th percentile); blood pressure: 158/94; pulse: 120; respiration rate: 20
- Skin: Notable for brown-to-black, poorly defined, velvety hyperpigmentation in the neck and axilla (acanthosis nigricans)

Labs
- Serum sodium: 132 mEq/L
- Potassium: 3.9 mEq/L

- Carbon dioxide: 22 mEq/L
- Glucose: 350 mg/dL
- Alanine aminotransferase (ALT): 62 U/L (normal <25 for a boy)
- Triglycerides: 145 mg/dL (normal <130)
- Low-density lipoprotein (LDL): 140 mg/dL (normal <130)
- High-density lipoprotein (HDL): 30 mg/dL (normal >40)
- Non HDL cholesterol: 160 mg/dL (normal <145)
- Hemoglobin A1C: 12% (normal <5.5)
- Urinalysis: Large glucose but no ketones
- Serum C-peptide concentration: 5 ng/mL (normal = 0.5–2.0 ng/mL)
- Anti-islet cell: Negative
- Anti-insulin: Negative
- Anti-glutamic acid decarboxylase (GAD) antibodies: Negative

Discussion Questions

1. What is the most likely diagnosis for JG?
2. How should JG's obesity be classified?
3. What is the most appropriate management of JG's other conditions?

KEY TAKEAWAYS

- Pediatric obesity is a growing public health problem worldwide affecting approximately 18.5% of U.S. children and adolescents.
- Generally, the prevention of pediatric obesity should be centered around healthy diet, activity, environment, and lifestyle modification. Studies have shown modest success with pharmacotherapeutics.
- Overweight and obesity in childhood is defined by the percentile of BMI for age and sex.
- Lifestyle modification is the cornerstone of treatment of childhood obesity but shows modest effects in most studies. Prevention is of primary importance since the treatment of childhood obesity is difficult once developed.
- There is extremely limited data on pharmacologic therapy for obesity in childhood, and the data is often of low quality.
- At present, orlistat (Xenical or Allī) is the only FDA-approved agent for use in children over 12 years of age, while drugs approved for adults with obesity often can only be used in younger individuals off-label.

REFERENCES

1. National Center for Health Statistics. *Health, United States, 2017—Data Finder. Table 058: normal weight, overweight, and obesity among adults aged 20 and over, by selected characteristics: US, selected years 1988–1994 through 2013–2016.* https://www.cdc.gov/nchs/hus/contents2017.htm#Table_058

2. Hales CM, Carroll MD, Fryar CD, Ogden CL. Prevalence of obesity among adults and youth: United States, 2017–2018. *NCHS Data Brief.* 2020;(360):1–8. https://www.cdc.gov/nchs/data/databriefs/db360-h.pdf

3. National Center for Health Statistics. *Health, United States, 2016: with chartbook on long-term trends in health.* 2017. https://www.cdc.gov/nchs/data/hus/hus16.pdf.

4. Centers for Disease Control and Prevention. *Defining adult overweight and obesity.* https://www.cdc.gov/obesity/adult/defining.html

5. Subica AM, Agarwal N, Sullivan JG, Link BG. Obesity and associated health disparities among understudied multiracial, Pacific Islander, and American Indian adults. *Obesity.* 2017;25(12):2128–2136. doi:10.1002/oby.21954

6. Flegal KM, Kruszon-Moran D, Carroll MD, et al. Trends in obesity among adults in the United States, 2005 to 2014. *JAMA.* 2016;315(21):2284–2291. doi:10.1001/jama.2016.6458

7. Wadden TA, Bray GA. *Handbook of Obesity Treatment.* Guilford Publications; 2018.

8. Dobbs R, Sawers C, Thompson F, et al. *Overcoming Obesity: An Initial Economic Analysis.* McKinsey Global Institute; 2014. https://www.mckinsey.com/~/media/mckinsey/business%20functions/economic%20studies%20temp/our%20insights/how%20the%20world%20could%20better%20fight%20obesity/mgi_overcoming_obesity_full_report.ashx

9. Kim DD, Basu A. Estimating the medical care costs of obesity in the United States: systematic review, meta-analysis, and empirical analysis. *Value in Health.* 2016;19(5):602–613. doi:10.1016/j.jval.2016.02.008

10. Archer E, Lavie CJ, Hill JO. The contributions of 'diet','genes', and physical activity to the etiology of obesity: contrary evidence and consilience. *Prog Cardiovasc Dis.* 2018;61(2):89–102. doi:10.1016/j.pcad.2018.06.002

11. Reinehr T, Hinney A, de Sousa G, et al. Definable somatic disorders in overweight children and adolescents. *J Pediatr.* 2007;150(6):e618–e622. e615. doi:10.1016/j.jpeds.2007.01.0412

12. Speiser PW, Rudolf M, Anhalt H, et al. Childhood obesity. *J Clin Endocrinol Metab.* 2005;90(3):1871–1887. doi:10.1210/jc.2004-1389

13. Stepanikova I, Baker EH, Simoni ZR, et al. The role of perceived discrimination in obesity among African Americans. *Am J Prev Med.* 2017;52(suppl 1):S77–S85. doi:10.1016/j.amepre.2016.07.034

14. Mwendwa DT, Gholson G, Sims RC, et al. Coping with perceived racism: a significant factor in the development of obesity in African American women? *J Natl Med Assoc.* 2011;103(7):602–608. doi:10.1016/S0027-9684(15)30386-2

15. Brehm BJ, D'Alessio DA. *Environmental Factors Influencing Obesity.* Endotext; 2014. https://www.endotext.org.

16. Atkinson G, Fullick S, Grindey C, Maclaren D. Exercise, energy balance and the shift worker. *Sports Med.* 2008;38(8):671–685. doi:10.2165/00007256-200838080-00005

17. Apovian CM, Aronne LJ, Bessesen DH, et al. Pharmacological management of obesity: an Endocrine Society clinical practice guideline. *J Clin Endocrinol Metab.* 2015;100(2):342–362. doi:10.1210/jc.2014-3415

18. Morton GJ, Cummings DE, Baskin DG, et al. Central nervous system control of food intake and body weight. *Nature.* 2006;443(7109):289–295. doi:10.1038/nature05026

19. Haslam D. Weight management in obesity—past and present. *Int J Clin Pract.* 2016;70(3):206–217. doi:10.1111/ijcp.12771

20. Bray GA. *An Atlas of Obesity and Weight Control.* The Parthenon Publishing Group; 2003.

21. Bray GA. *A Guide to Obesity and the Metabolic Syndrome: Origins and Treatment.* CRC Press, Taylor and Francis Group; 2011.

22. Wadden TA, Stunkard AJ, eds. *Handbook of Obesity Treatment.* The Guilford Press; 2002.

23. Onakpoya IJ, Collins DRJ, Bobrovitz NJH, et al. Benefits and harms in pivotal trials of oral centrally acting antiobesity medicines: a systematic review and meta-analysis. *Obesity.* 2018;26(3):513–521. doi:10.1002/oby.22118

24. Onakpoya IJ, Heneghan CJ, Aronson JK. Post-marketing withdrawal of anti-obesity medicinal products because of adverse drug reactions: a systematic review. *BMC Med.* 2016;14(1):191. doi:10.1186/s12916-016-0735-y

25. Rippe JM, Angelopoulos TJ, eds. *Obesity: Prevention and Treatment.* CRC Press, Talor & Francis Group; 2012.

26. U.S. Food and Drug Administration. *FDA drug safety communication: FDA recommends against the continued use of Meridia (sibutramine).* Published October 8, 2010. https://www.fda.gov/drugs/drug-safety-and-availability/fda-drug-safety-communication-fda-recommends-against-continued-use-meridia-sibutramine

27. Gomez G, Stanford FC. US health policy and prescription drug coverage of FDA-approved medications for the treatment of obesity. *Int J Obesity.* 2017;42:495–500. doi:10.1038/ijo.2017.287

28. Curry SJ, Krist AH, Owens DK, et al. Behavioral weight loss interventions to prevent obesity-related morbidity and mortality in adults: US Preventive Services Task Force recommendation statement. *JAMA.* 2018;320(11):1163–1171. doi:10.1001/jama.2018.13022

29. LeBlanc ES, Patnode CD, Webber EM, et al. Behavioral and pharmacotherapy weight loss interventions to prevent obesity-related morbidity and mortality in adults: updated evidence report and systematic review for the US Preventive Services Task Force. *JAMA.* 2018;320(11):1172–1191. doi:10.1001/jama.2018.7777

30. Jensen MD, Ryan DH, Apovian CM, et al. 2013 AHA/ACC/TOS guideline for the management of overweight and obesity in adults: a report of the American College of Cardiology/American Heart Association Task Force on Practice Guidelines and The Obesity Society. *J Am Coll Cardiol.* 2014;63(25 Part B):2985–3023. doi:10.1016/j.jacc.2013.11.004

31. Garvey WT, Mechanick JI, Brett EM, et al. American Association of Clinical Endocrinologists and American College of Endocrinology comprehensive clinical practice guidelines for medical care of patients with obesity. *Endocrine Pract.* 2016;22(suppl 3):1–203. doi:10.4158/EP161365.GL

32. Kumar RB, Aronne LJ. Efficacy comparison of medications approved for chronic weight management. *Obesity.* 2015;23(suppl 1):S4–S7. doi:10.1002/oby.21093

33. Torgerson JS, Hauptman J, Boldrin MN, Sjöström L. XENical in the prevention of diabetes in obese subjects (XENDOS) study: a randomized study of orlistat as an adjunct to lifestyle changes for the prevention of type 2 diabetes in obese patients. *Diabetes Care.* 2004;27(1):155–161. doi:10.2337/diacare.27.1.155

34. Singh J, Kumar R. Phentermine-topiramate: first combination drug for obesity. *Int J Appl Basic Med Res.* 2015;5(2):157–158. doi:10.4103/2229-516X.157177

35. Fidler MC, Sanchez M, Raether B, et al. A one-year randomized trial of lorcaserin for weight loss in obese and overweight adults: the BLOSSOM trial. *J Clin Endocrinol Metab.* 2011;96(10):3067–3077. doi:10.1210/jc.2011-1256

36. Greenway FL, Fujioka K, Plodkowski RA, et al. Effect of naltrexone plus bupropion on weight loss in overweight and obese adults (COR-I): a multicentre, randomised, double-blind, placebo-controlled, phase 3 trial. *Lancet.* 2010;376(9741):595–605. doi:10.1016/s0140-6736(10)60888-4

37. Mehta A, Marso SP, Neeland IJ. Liraglutide for weight management: a critical review of the evidence. *Obes Sci Pract.* 2017;3(1):3–14. doi:10.1002/osp4.84

38. Srivastava G, Apovian CM. Current pharmacotherapy for obesity. *Nat Rev Endocrinol.* 2018;14(1):12–24. doi:10.1038/nrendo.2017.122

39. Pilitsi E, Farr OM, Polyzos SA, et al. Pharmacotherapy of obesity: available medications and drugs under investigation. *Metabolism.* 2019;92:170–192. doi:10.1016/j.metabol.2018.10.010

40. U.S. Food and Drug Administration. *Drugs@FDA: FDA approved drugs—adipex.* 2020. https://www.accessdata.fda.gov/scripts/cder/daf/index.cfm?event=overview.process&ApplNo=085128

41. Hampp C, Kang EM, Borders-Hemphill V. Use of prescription antiobesity drugs in the United States. *Pharmacotherapy.* 2013;33(12):1299–1307. doi:10.1002/phar.1342

42. Teval Select Brands. *ADIPEX-P highlights of prescribing information.* Updated March 2017. https://www.adipex.com/globalassets/adipex/adipex_pi.pdf

43. KVK-Tech. *Lomaira full prescribing information.* Published September 2016. https://www.lomaira.com/Prescribing_Information.pdf

44. Cercato C, Roizenblatt V, Leança C, et al. A randomized double-blind placebo-controlled study of the long-term efficacy and safety of diethylpropion in the treatment of obese subjects. *Int J Obes.* 2009;33(8):857–865. doi:10.1038/ijo.2009.124

45. Kang J, Park C-Y, Kang J, et al. Randomized controlled trial to investigate the effects of a newly developed formulation of phentermine diffuse-controlled release for obesity. *Diabetes Obes Metab.* 2010;12(10):876–882. doi:10.1111/j.1463-1326.2010.01242.x

46. Akil L, Ahmad HA. Relationships between obesity and cardiovascular diseases in four southern states and Colorado. *J Health Care Poor Underserved.* 2011;22(4 suppl):61–72. doi:10.1353/hpu.2011.0166

47. Kenchaiah S, Evans JC, Levy D, et al. Obesity and the risk of heart failure. *N Engl J Med.* 2002;347(5):305–313. doi:10.1056/NEJMoa020245

48. Manson JE, Colditz GA, Stampfer MJ, et al. A prospective study of obesity and risk of coronary heart disease in women. *N Engl J Med.* 1990;322(13):882–889. doi:10.1056/NEJM199003293221303

49. Must A, Spadano J, Coakley EH, et al. The disease burden associated with overweight and obesity. *JAMA.* 1999;282(16):1523–1529. doi:10.1001/jama.282.16.1523

50. Aronne LJ, Wadden TA, Peterson C, et al. Evaluation of phentermine and topiramate versus phentermine/topiramate extended-release in obese adults. *Obesity.* 2013;21(11):2163–2171. doi:10.1002/oby.20584

51. Cameron F, Whiteside G, McKeage K. Phentermine and topiramate extended release (Qsymia™). *Drugs.* 2012;72(15):2033–2042. doi:10.2165/11640860-000000000-00000

52. VIVUS Inc. *Qsymia, highlights of prescribing information.* Revised October 2020. https://qsymia.com/patient/include/media/pdf/prescribing-information.pdf

53. Heck AM, Yanovski JA, Calis KA. Orlistat, a new lipase inhibitor for the management of obesity. *Pharmacotherapy.* 2000;20(3):270–279. doi:10.1592/phco.20.4.270.34882

54. CHEPLAPHARM Arzneimittel GmbH. doi: 10.1592/phco.20.4.270.34882

55. Grandone A, Di Sessa A, Umano GR, et al. New treatment modalities for obesity. *Best Pract Res Clin En-*

docrinol Metab. 2018;32(4):535–549. doi:10.1016/j
.beem.2018.06.007

56. U.S. Food and Drug Administration. *FDA requests the withdrawal of the weight-loss drug Belviq, Bleviq XR (lorcaserin) from the market.* Published February 13, 2020. https://www.fda.gov/drugs/drug-safety-and-availability/fda-requests-withdrawal-weight-loss-drug-belviq-belviq-xr-lorcaserin-market

57. Thomsen WJ, Grottick AJ, Menzaghi F, et al. Lorcaserin, a novel selective human 5-Hydroxytryptamine$_{(2C)}$ agonist: in vitro and in vivo pharmacological characterization. *J Pharmacol Exp Ther.* 2008;325(2):577–587. doi:10.1124/jpet.107.133348

58. Miller LE. Lorcaserin for weight loss: insights into US Food and Drug Administration approval. *J Acad Nutr Diet.* 2013;113(1):25–30. doi:10.1016/j.jand.2012.08.028

59. Millington GW. The role of proopiomelanocortin (POMC) neurones in feeding behaviour. *Nutr Metab.* 2007;4(1):18. doi:10.1186/1743-7075-4-18

60. Rehfeld JF. The origin and understanding of the incretin concept. *Front Endocrinol.* 2018;9:387. doi:10.3389/fendo.2018.00387

61. Novo Nordisk. *Saxenda: prescribing information.* Revised March 2020. https://www.saxenda.com

62. Marso SP, Daniels GH, Brown-Frandsen K, et al. Liraglutide and cardiovascular outcomes in type 2 diabetes. *N Engl J Med.* 2016;375(4):311–322. doi:10.1056/NEJMoa1603827

63. Funch D, Gydesen H, Tornøe K, et al. A prospective, claims-based assessment of the risk of pancreatitis and pancreatic cancer with liraglutide compared to other antidiabetic drugs. *Diabetes Obes Metab.* 2014;16(3):273–275. doi:10.1111/dom.12230

64. Monami M, Nreu B, Scatena A, et al. Safety issues with glucagon-like peptide-1 receptor agonists (pancreatitis, pancreatic cancer and cholelithiasis): data from randomized controlled trials. *Diabetes, Obes Metab.* 2017;19(9):1233–1241. doi:10.1111/dom.12926

65. Khera R, Murad MH, Chandar AK, et al. Association of pharmacological treatments for obesity with weight loss and adverse events: a systematic review and meta-analysis. *JAMA.* 2016;315(22):2424–2434. doi:10.1001/jama.2016.7602

66. Wadden TA, Hollander P, Klein S, et al. Weight maintenance and additional weight loss with liraglutide after low-calorie-diet-induced weight loss: the SCALE Maintenance randomized study. *Int J Obesity.* 2013;37(11):1443–1451. doi:10.1038/ijo.2013.120. https://www.nature.com/articles/ijo2013120.pdf

67. Verrotti A, Scaparrotta A, Agostinelli S, et al. Topiramate-induced weight loss: a review. *Epilepsy Res.* 2011;95(3):189–199. doi:10.1016/j.eplepsyres.2011.05.014

68. Velazquez A, Apovian CM. Updates on obesity pharmacotherapy. *Ann N Y Acad Sci.* 2018;1411:106–119. doi:10.1111/nyas.13542

69. Patel DK, Stanford FC. Safety and tolerability of new-generation anti-obesity medications: a narrative review. *Postgrad Med.* 2018;130(2):173–182. doi:10.1080/00325481.2018.1435129

70. Vorsanger MH, Subramanyam P, Weintraub HS, et al. Cardiovascular effects of the new weight loss agents. *J Am*

Coll Cardiol. 2016;68(8):849–859. doi:10.1016/j.jacc.2016.06.007

71. Greig SL, Keating GM. Naltrexone ER/bupropion ER: a review in obesity management. *Drugs,* 2015;75(11):1269–1280. doi:10.1007/s40265-015-0427-5

72. Valeant Pharmaceuticals North America. *Wellbutrin XL: highlights of prescribing information.* Revised May 2017. https://www.accessdata.fda.gov/drugsatfda_docs/label/2017/021515s036lbl.pdf

73. Nalpropion Pharmaceuticals. *Contrave: highlights of prescribing information.* Revised August 2020. https://contrave.com/content/pdf/Contrave_PI.pdf

74. Apovian CM, Aronne L, Rubino D, et al. A randomized, phase 3 trial of naltrexone SR/bupropion SR on weight and obesity-related risk factors (COR-II). *Obesity.* 2013;21(5):935–943. doi:10.1002/oby.20309

75. Hollander P, Gupta AK, Plodkowski R, et al. Effects of naltrexone sustained-release/bupropion sustained-release combination therapy on body weight and glycemic parameters in overweight and obese patients with type 2 diabetes. *Diabetes Care.* 2013;36(12):4022–4029. doi:10.2337/dc13-0234

76. Wadden TA, Foreyt JP, Foster GD, et al. Weight loss with naltrexone SR/bupropion SR combination therapy as an adjunct to behavior modification: the COR-BMOD trial. *Obesity.* 2011;19(1):110–120. doi:10.1038/oby.2010.147

77. Malone M. Medications associated with weight gain. *Ann Pharmacother.* 2005;39(12):2046–2055. doi:10.1345/aph.1G3378.

78. Styne DM, Arslanian SA, Connor EL, et al. Pediatric obesity—assessment, treatment, and prevention: an Endocrine Society clinical practice guideline. *J Clin Endocrinol Metab.* 2017;102(3):709–757. doi:10.1210/jc.2016-25779

79. Centers for Disease Control and Prevention. *Defining childhood obesity.* Accessed November 1, 2020. https://www.cdc.gov/obesity/childhood/defining.htm80

80. Kelly AS, Barlow SE, Rao G, et al. Severe obesity in children and adolescents: identification, associated health risks, and treatment approaches: a scientific statement from the American Heart Association. *Circulation.* 2013;128(15):1689–1712. doi:10.1161/CIR.0b013e3182a5cfb81

81. Skinner AC, Ravanbakht SN, Skelton JA, et al. Prevalence of obesity and severe obesity in US children, 1999–2016. *Pediatrics.* 2018;141(3):e20173459. doi:10.1542/peds.2017-34582

82. Mead E, Atkinson G, Richter B, et al. Drug interventions for the treatment of obesity in children and adolescents. *Cochrane Database Syst Rev.* 2016;(11):CD012436. doi:10.1002/14651858.Cd0124383

83. Srivastava G, Fox CK, Kelly AS, et al. Clinical considerations regarding the use of obesity pharmacotherapy in adolescents with obesity. *Obesity.* 2019;27(2):190–204. doi:10.1002/oby.22384

84. O'Connor M. An orlistat "overdose" in a child. *Irish J Med Sci.* 2010;179(2):315. doi:10.1007/s11845-009-0429-85

85. Forrester MB. Pattern of orlistat exposures in children aged 5 years or less. *J Emer Med.* 2009;37(4):396–399. doi:10.1016/j.jemermed.2007.10.0586

86. National Clinical Guideline Centre. *Obesity: Identification, Assessment and Management of Overweight and*

Obesity in Children, Young People and Adults: Partial Update of CG43. National Institute for Health and Care Excellence (UK); 2014. https://www.ncbi.nlm.nih.gov/books/NBK2641687

87. Maahs D, de Serna DG, Kolotkin RL, et al. Randomized, double-blind, placebo-controlled trial of orlistat for weight loss in adolescents. *Endocr Pract.* 2006;12(1):18–28. doi:10.4158/EP.12.1.188

88. Chanoine J-P, Hampl S, Jensen C, et al. Effect of orlistat on weight and body composition in obese adolescents: a randomized controlled trial. *JAMA.* 2005;293(23):2873–2883. doi:10.1001/jama.293.23.28789

89. Yu CC, Li AM, Chan KO, et al. Orlistat improves endothelial function in obese adolescents: a randomised trial. *J Paediatr Child Health.* 2013;49(11):969–975. doi:10.1111/jpc.122590

90. Ryder JR, Kaizer A, Rudser KD, et al. Effect of phentermine on weight reduction in a pediatric weight management clinic. *Int J Obesity.* 2017;41(1):90–93. doi:10.1038/ijo.2016.1891

91. Fox CK., Kaizer AM, Rudser KD, et al. Meal replacements followed by topiramate for the treatment of adolescent severe obesity: a pilot randomized controlled trial. *Obesity.* 2016;24(12):2553–2561. doi:10.1002/oby.21692

92. Ng QX. A systematic review of the use of bupropion for attention-deficit/hyperactivity disorder in children and adolescents. *J Child Adolesc Psychopharmacol.* 2017;27(2):112–116. doi:10.1089/cap.2016.0193

93. Tamborlane WV, Barrientos-Pérez M, Fainberg U, et al. Liraglutide in children and adolescents with type 2 diabetes. *N Engl J Med.* 2019;381(7):637–646. doi:10.1056/NEJMoa19038294

94. Lentferink Y, Knibbe C, van der Vorst M. Efficacy of metformin treatment with respect to weight reduction in children and adults with obesity: a systematic review. *Drugs.* 2018;78(18):1887–1901. doi:10.1007/s40265-018-1025-95

95. McDonagh MS, Selph S, Ozpinar A, Foley C. Systematic review of the benefits and risks of metformin in treating obesity in children aged 18 years and younger. *JAMA Pediatr.* 2014;168(2):178–184. doi:10.1001/jamapediatrics.2013.42096

96. Shire US. Vyvanse: highlights for prescribing information. Revised January 2017. https://www.accessdata.fda.gov/drugsatfda_docs/label/2017/208510lbl.pdf

97. Kuhnen P, Clément K, Wiegand S, et al. Proopiomelanocortin deficiency treated with a melanocortin-4 receptor agonist. *N Engl J Med.* 2016;375(3):240–246. doi:10.1056/NEJMoa15126998

98. Collet T-H, Dubern B, Mokrosinski J, et al. Evaluation of a melanocortin-4 receptor (MC4R) agonist (Setmelanotide) in MC4R deficiency. *Mol Metab.* 2017;6(10):1321–1329. doi:10.1016/j.molmet.2017.06.015

99. Clément K, Biebermann H, Farooqi IS, et al. MC4R agonism promotes durable weight loss in patients with leptin receptor deficiency. *Nat Med.* 2018;24(5):551–555. doi:10.1038/s41591-018-0015-9

100. Srivastava G, Apovian C. Future pharmacotherapy for obesity: new anti-obesity drugs on the horizon. *Curr Obes Rep.* 2018;7(2):147–161. doi:10.1007/s13679-018-0300-4

101. Gade C, Christensen HR, Dalhoff KP, et al. Inconsistencies in dosage practice in children with overweight or obesity: a retrospective cohort study. *Pharmacol Res Perspect.* 2018;6(3):e00398. doi:10.1002/prp2.398

Index